Psychiatric and Mental Health Nursing

The craft of caring

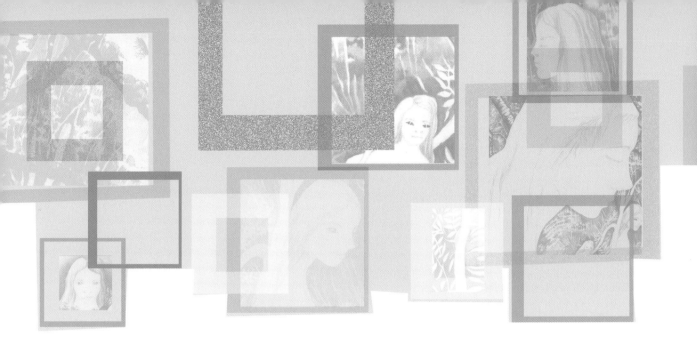

Psychiatric and Mental Health Nursing

The craft of caring

Edited by

Phil Barker PhD RN FRCN
Formerly Professor of Psychiatric
Nursing Practice, University of
Newcastle, UK
Visiting Professor at Trinity College
Dublin, Ireland
Director, Clan Unity (The International
Mental Health Recovery Agency)

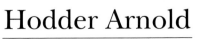

Hodder Arnold

A MEMBER OF THE HODDER HEADLINE GROUP

First published in Great Britain in 2003 by
Hodder Arnold, a member of the Hodder Headline Group,
338 Euston Road, London NW1 3BH

http://www.hoddereducation.com

Distributed in the United States of America by
Oxford University Press Inc.,
198 Madison Avenue, New York, NY10016
Oxford is a registered trademark of Oxford University Press

Whilst the advice and information in this book are believed to be true and
accurate at the date of going to press, neither the author[s] nor the publisher
can accept any legal responsibility or liability for any errors or omissions
that may be made. In particular (but without limiting the generality of the
preceding disclaimer) every effort has been made to check drug dosages;
however it is still possible that errors have been missed. Furthermore,
dosage schedules are constantly being revised and new side-effects
recognized. For these reasons the reader is strongly urged to consult the
drug companies' printed instructions before administering any of the drugs
recommended in this book.

British Library Cataloguing in Publication Data
A catalogue record for this book is available from the British Library

Library of Congress Cataloging-in-Publication Data
A catalog record for this book is available from the Library of Congress

ISBN-10: 0 340 81026 2
ISBN-13: 978 0 340 81026 2

4 5 6 7 8 9 10

Commissioning Editor: Georgina Bentliff
Development Editor: Heather Smith
Project Manager: Nora Naughton
Production Controller: Lindsay Smith
Cover Design: Amina Dudhia

Typeset in Berling 9.5/12pt by Fakenham Photosetting Limited, Fakenham, Norfolk
Printed and bound in Spain

What do you think about this book? Or any other Hodder Arnold title?
Please send your comments to www.hoddereducation.com

This book is dedicated to all people who have struggled to understand the messages contained within their experience of mental distress, and to all those – friends, family, professionals and fellow travellers – who have tried to help them on their recovery journey.

COMMENTARY ON THE COVER ILLUSTRATION

Phil Barker writes: The illustration used as the basis for the cover was painted by Ann Thomas, from Wallsend, New South Wales, Australia. Ann is a published book illustrator whom my wife, Poppy, and I met in the summer of 2001. She showed us some of her illustrations and we were so impressed that we asked her to contribute to the cover for this book. When she submitted the final illustration, Ann added the following commentary.

As a person who has schizophrenia, and who was once a successful book illustrator, I have a deeper understanding of mental illness than most artists. It is a true understanding that I have painted for the cover of this book.

I find that insight into the person behind the mental illness, and particularly that of a self-portrait that you see here, is not just of an illness, but also of a peculiar or particular type of person. Other patients commonly see each other as saints, angels or holy ones. In fact, the Bible promised the return of saints of old as poor Christians in days such as these. I am a sincere Christian who has feelings and perceptions of such manner, and we as people with illnesses truly have extra sensory perceptions of such things. Many of us have powers of prophecy that go far beyond the norm. I have self-prophecy powers that I have portrayed in this illustration, which are true and very real to my mind, my mentality, my life and my soul. Maybe some people can learn to see a little beyond an illness and see the fascination into these mysterious and fascinating lowly people.

With my love

Ann Thomas

Phil Barker adds: Ann reminds us all of the need to see beyond the 'patient' label to discover something of the person who lies within. As she notes, many people who have suffered the blight of mental illness have remarkable experiences, which often bewilder and confuse family, friends and professionals alike. Instead of dismissing these as 'merely part of the illness', we might exercise some genuine curiosity as to what they might say about the person. Through such curiosity we might learn something of lasting value about people, as opposed to 'patients'.

Contents

Contents

List of Contributors

Trevor Adams PhD MSc RMN RGN Cert Ed CPN Cert
Lecturer in Mental Health, European Institute of Health and Medical Sciences, University of Surrey, Guildford, UK

Phil Barker PhD RN FRCN
Visiting Professor, Trinity College Dublin, Ireland; Director, Clan Unity (The International Mental Health Recovery Agency)

Ian Beech BA (Hons) RMN RGN PGCE
Senior Lecturer in Mental Health Nursing, School of Care Sciences, University of Glamorgan, Pontypridd, Wales, UK

Judy Boxer RMN CQSW
Senior lecturer, School of Health and Social Care, Sheffield Hallam University, Sheffield, UK

Joy Bray MA RN Cert Ed ENB 650 RNT PGCE
Senior Lecturer, Homerton School of Health Studies, Homerton College, Cambridge, UK

Philip Burnard PhD RN
Vice Dean, School of Nursing Studies/ School of Nursing and Midwifery, University of Wales College of Medicine, Cardiff, UK

Andrew Cashin Dip App Science BHSC MN
The University of Technology, Sydney Faculty of Nursing, Midwifery and Health, Australia

Jon Chesterson RN RMHN Dip CPN DipAppSc BappSc FANZCMHN MRCNA
Mental Health Promotion Officer, Hunter Mental Health, NSW Australia; Project Officer (Credentialing), Australian and New Zealand College of Mental Health Nurses, Australia Conjoint Lecturer, University of Newcastle

Liam Clarke RN Dip Nurs Dip Ed Dip Theol Dip Med Ethics BA MSc PhD
Senior Lecturer in Mental Health, University of Brighton, Eastbourne, UK

David B Cooper RN FETC
Author, Editor and Consultant, Chulmleigh, Devon, UK

Seamus Cowman RPN RN RNT DipN London PGCEA MSc PhD FFNMRCSI
Professor and Head of Nursing, Royal College of Surgeons in Ireland, Dublin, Ireland

Susan Croom MSc BA (Hons) RN
Senior Lecturer and Research Fellow, Northumbria University and Newcastle, Northumbria and N. Tyneside Health Trust, UK

John Cutcliffe RMN RGN BSc (Hons) Nrsg PhD
Chair of Nursing, University of Northern British Columbia, Canada

Nancy Daniels MN APRN BC
Psychiatric Clinical Nurse Specialists, Alamo Mental Health Group, San Antonio, Texas, USA

Peter Dodds RMN
Senior Nurse, Oakburn Ward, Bradford, UK

Dianne Ellis RMN MSc
Affinity Healthcare and Northern Centre for Mental Health, UK

Mark Fenton RMN MA
Sociology and Community Mental Health (Essex), Research Nurse, Trial Search Co-ordinator, Cochrane Schizophrenia Group, Academic Unit of Psychiatry and Behavioural Sciences, School of Medicine, University of Leeds, Leeds, UK

Cheryl Forchuk RN PhD
Associate Professor, Nurse Scientist, University of Western Ontario, London Health Science Centre, Ontario, Canada

Elaine Fletcher RMN DipHE
Senior Nurse, St Nicholas Hospital, Gosforth, Newcastle upon Tyne, UK

Paul French RMN BA (Hons)
Senior Cognitive Therapist, Early Detection and Intervention Team, Psychology Services, Bolton Salford and Trafford Mental Health Partnership, Manchester, UK

Ruth Gallop RN MScN PhD
Professor and Associate Dean, Research, Faculty of Nursing, University of Toronto, Canada

Lyn Gardner
Lecturer in Mental Health Studies, University of Southampton, UK

Alec Grant BA (Hons) MA PhD RN Cert Res Meth PGCTLHE ENB 650 Cert
Principal Lecturer in Mental Health, InaM, University of Brighton, Eastbourne, East Sussex, UK

Amanda Haddock RMN RNMH
Acting Team Leader, Community Alternatives Practice Team, Waverley CMHC, Torbay, Devon Partnership Trust, UK

Michael John Hazelton RN BA MA PhD FANZC MHN
Professor of Mental Health Nursing, School of Nursing and Midwifery, The University of Newcastle, New South Wales, Australia.

Anne Helm BEd Diploma of Teaching LTCL
Consumer Advisor Healthcare Otago, Dunedin, New Zealand

Colin Holmes RN BA (Hons) Tcert MPhil PhD MRCNA
Professor of Nursing, (Mental Health) School of Nursing,
University of Western Sydney, New South Wales, Australia

Clare Hopkins MSc RMN
Crisis Assessment Team, St Nicholas Hospital, Newcastle;
Senior Lecturer in Mental Health Nursing, University of
Northumbria at Newcastle, UK

Elsabeth Jensen RN BA PhD (cand)
Research Co-ordinator, Lawson Health Research Institute,
London, Ontario, Canada

Mami Kayama PhD MNSc RN
Associate Professor, Department of Psychiatric Nursing,
Graduate School of Health Science and Nursing, University of
Tokyo, Japan

Janis Keen BA (Hons)
Senior Care Officer, St. Maur, Newton Abbot Community Care
Trust, South Devon, UK

Tom Keen RMN RNT MSc
Senior Lecturer, Mental Health Nursing, University of
Plymouth Institute of Health Studies, Exeter, UK

Richard Lakeman DipCpNsg DipHerb BN BA (Hons)
Clinical Nurse Consultant, Mobile Intensive Treatment team,
Townsville Intergrated Mental Health Service, Queensland,
Australia

Philip Luffman RMN ENB660 Diploma Group
Psychotherapy
UKCP Registered Adult Psychotherapy, Diploma Group
Psychotherapy, The Hazel Centre, Llandrindod Wells, Powys,
Wales, UK

Hugh McKenna PhD RMN RGN BSc(Hons) DipN(cond) Adv
Dip Ed RNT FFNRCSI
Professor and Head of School, Faculty of Life and Health
Science, University of Ulster, Jordanstown, County Antrim, UK

Mervyn Morris MA
Reader in Mental Health Faculty of Health and Community
Care, University of Central England, Birmingham, UK

Erina Morrison–Ngatai RCpN BHScN PgradCert MHN
Senior Lecturer, Mental Health Nursing, School of Health
Sciences, Massey University, Palmerston North,
New Zealand

Eimear Muir-Cochrane BSc(Hons) RN RMN Grad Dip Adult
Education MNS PhD
Senior Lecturer, Division of Health Sciences, School of
Nursing and Midwifery, University of South Australia,
Australia

Brendan Murphy MA RMN ENB 660 ENB 998
Department of Psychotherapy, Mill Hill Lane, Derby, UK

Anthony O'Brien RGN RPN BA MMPhil (Hons)
Senior Lecturer, Mental Health Nursing, School of
Nursing, University of Auckland Medical School, New
Zealand

Shaun Parsons CiPsychol PhD MSc BSc Registered
Nurse
Lecturer in Clinical Psychology and Chartered Forensic
Psychologist, University of Newcastle, Newcastle upon Tyne,
UK

Mark Philbin RPN DipN BSc (Hons) MA
School of Nursing, Dublin City University, Dublin, Ireland

Gary Platz
Consumer mental health consultant, Case Consulting Ltd.
New Zealand

William Reynolds PhD MPhil RMN RGN RNT
Reader in Nursing Turku Polytechnic, Salo, Finland

Gary Rolfe PhD MA BSc RMN
Reader in Practice Development, School of Health and Social
Care, University of Portsmouth, Portsmouth, UK

Denis Ryan RPN RGN CAC BSc (Hons)
Lecturer, Centre for Nursing Studies, Department of Life
Sciences, College of Science, University of Limerick, Limerick,
Ireland

Angela Simpson RMN BA MA
Lecturer in Mental Health, Department of Health Sciences,
University of York, York, UK

Mike Smith RMN BSc (Nurs) MA
Director of Nursing, Northern Birmingham Mental
Health Trust and Research Fellow University of Central
England, Centre for Community Mental Health, Birmingham,
UK

Shirley Smoyak RN PhD FAAN
Professor II, The Bloustein School of Planning and Public
Policy Rutgers, The State University of New Jersey, New
Jersey, USA

Elaine Stamina RN BA BAAN MSc PhD (C)
Clinical Leader Manager, St Michael's Hospital, Toronto, Canada

Chris Stevenson RMN BA(Hons) MSc (Dist) PhD
Reader in Nursing, University of Teesside, Newcastle upon Tyne, UK

Cynthia Stuhlmiller
Professor of Nursing (Mental Health) School of Nursing and Midwifery, Finders University of South Australia, Adelaide, Australia

Ann Thomas
Illustrator, Wallsend, NSW, Australia

Tracey Tully RN MSc PhD (cand)
Women's College Ambulatory Care Centre, Women Recovering from Abuse Programme, Toronto, Ontario, Canada

Kay Vaughn RN MS CS
Adjunct Faculty University of Colorado Health Sciences Center School of Medicine Department of Psychiatry and Regis University Department of Nursing, Colorado, USA

Paul Veitch RMN MSc
Senior Nurse, Newcastle, North Tyneside and Northumberland Mental Health NHS Trust, Newcastle upon Tyne; Senior Nurse, Homeless Service, Joseph Cowen Health Centre, Newcastle, UK

Cheryl Waters RN BSc (Hons) PhD
Senior Lecturer, Research Degrees Coordinator, Faculty of Nursing Midwifery and Health, University of Technology, Sydney, Australia

Martin Ward Mphil RMN DipNurs RNT Cert Ed NEBSS Dip
Director, MW Professional Development Limited and Independent Mental Health Nurse Consultant (Formerly, Director of Mental Health, The Royal College of Nursing), UK

Denise Webster RN PhD CS
Professor, University of Colorado Health Sciences Center, School of Nursing, Denver, Colorado, USA

Irene Whitehill BSc PhD
Independent User Trainer and Consultant (Mental Health), Section 36 Consultancy, Northumberland, UK

Jonathon Wigmore BSc RN Dip (Mental Health Nursing)
Investigation Manager, Office of the Health Service Commissioners, Millbank, London, UK

Gail Williams PhD RN
Associate Professor, Department of Family Nursing Care, The University of Texas Health Science Center, San Antonio School of Nursing, San Antonio, USA.

Peter Wilkin RMN MA
Primary Mental Health Service, Birch Hill Hospital, Rochdale, UK

Jerome Wright MSc REN RMN
Lecturer in Nursing, Department of Health Sciences, University of York, York, UK

The Cleansing has Begun

Chest deep in the Wainuiomata stream
Earth's energies combine with mine
Me the mighty super-conductor
Here to do God's will

Yes, the cleansing has begun

With Jehovah's name reverberating from the hills
Wainui's demons go screaming to the abyss
Ah Wainuiomata, New Jerusalem
River of life

The cleansing has begun

The cries of my disciples from the asylums of the world
Keep tearing at my soul
Hold on my followers, I'm coming

The cleansing has begun

Strapped to a sterile bed
Spiritual poison in my veins
Encrusting my heart, fogging my head
I'll keep fighting, my disciples

The cleansing has begun

Through days of haze
Hospital food
I keep sitting,
A god hunched
Looking for answers on the wall

Through days of haze
Hospital food
I see the answer

It's written in their eyes

I'm no god
Just a fool
Raped by heart and soul

The cleansing has begun

Then a power to be
Said you may go free
(I'll be tethered to him
With a chemical chain)
Oh try to get yourself a job

The cleansing has begun

Through days of haze
Timeless sleep
I lick my violated brain
Ah Wainuiomata
The cleansing has begun

Somehow I am much better now
I have taken that to be's advice
I'm searching the papers
Up dated my c.v.
Brought myself some shoes

Hey, wait a minute
You, out there
Do you have an opening
For a part time god
The cleansing has begun

Gary Platz

Gary Platz is a person who has the experience of mental illness. Since 1994 he has been a declared consumer of mental services in various consumer roles.

Currently he is a director of Case Consulting Ltd. involved in consultancy and education. He is also active in consumer networks in New Zealand.

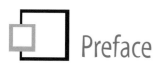 Preface

'Ultimately, man should not ask what the meaning of his life is, but rather must recognise that it is he who is asked. In a word, each man is questioned by life; and he can only answer to life by answering for his own life; to life he can only respond by being responsible'.[1]

Mental health care in the 21st century is a many-headed beast. Multidisciplinary teams, offer multi-dimensional care programmes that draw on multifarious theories and models. The options for practice multiply further as a multitude of professionals, paraprofessionals and consumer-advocates bring their own perspectives to bear on what, exactly, might be needed in the name of care and treatment. Everybody has a view on what needs to be done. Some employ complex meta-analyses, of equally complex scientific studies, to distil an evidence base for the best possible form of practice. Others advocate a more heart-felt form of analysis, employing personal experiences or the empathic appreciation of others' experiences or stories, which generate something more akin to human wisdom than a scientific body of knowledge. Increasingly, however, the appreciation of what anyone needs in the name of care has become a case of 'horses for courses' – those needs often being different, for different people, or even changing for the same person across time or life circumstances. Ironically, this recognition is dawning as much for those who claim to be social scientists as it is for the folk wisdom advocates.

There is a third group – those who claim to know (in an absolute sense) what mental health is and how it might be realized. This group seems almost as threatening as the experience of mental illness or disorder itself, which is synonymous with existential danger and disempowerment. Those possessed of such certainty about 'what needs to be done' in the name of care or treatment, risk obliging (or even forcing) others to conform to their stereotype of 'mental health', rather than helping people reach an understanding of what mental health means for them. I fear that those who believe that they know the answer to the many individual and social riddles associated with human experience, have not given full consideration to the questions involved.

When we ask 'What do people in mental distress need?', the answer is not at all clear. Or at least, it is not clear to me. After almost 35 years in the psychiatric and mental health field what does seem clear is that people need different things, at different times in their lives, in differing amounts, according to their differing needs, as persons. I emphasize that they are persons, for the common tactic of reducing them to patients, or clients, or consumers, or service users, is simply that – a tactic:

One way of dealing with the anxiety involved in confronting the question – 'how to respond to another person in distress?' This is a human question, as opposed to a social or scientific or psychological question. It also seems clear that, as such, this merits a human answer.

I never believed that producing yet another textbook of psychiatric and mental health nursing would be easy. In many fields of human enquiry – like biology, sociology or psychology – there is at least some consensus regarding what is known, and agreement about the evidence that supports these theoretical assumptions. This is not to say that the field is necessarily united, but the discourses are bound by at least some agreement as to its proper focus and the emergent knowledge base of the discipline. Most psychiatric and mental health nurses that I have met were in no doubt as to what nursing was all about and what it was worth in therapeutic terms. However, if asked to justify their views, based on undisputable evidence, many faltered and most could not even begin to frame a perspective of their chosen discipline in what might be called scientific terms.

I would have to count myself as just such a faltering voice, since I would find it difficult to *demonstrate* the value of psychiatric and mental health nursing. This is not to say that there is no demonstrable basis for the discipline; it simply means that much of what I believe is important about nursing has not been subjected to what might be called 'rigorous scrutiny'. Indeed, beyond counting the number of people who *believe* in the value of various aspects of nursing, and how nursing has affected their lives, I am not sure that any such demonstrations are possible. Nursing seems to occupy a similar territory as other human phenomena like belonging, love or friendship. We cannot begin to ask what they are worth without engaging in a discussion as to what these concepts *mean* to different people. Not surprisingly, we find that often they mean different things to different people although they all agree that this is what the concept *should* be called. Nursing is often so many things, and yet just one thing. When we try to unpack or dismantle the whole experience of nursing, we lose contact with the whole of the thing called 'nursing'. There is a story about the practice and receipt of nursing care, but I see no value in reducing it, metaphorically, to paragraphs, clauses or words. It is a story that can be told in many different ways, all of which are commentaries on the same experiential phenomena. Why not settle for such an uncertain answer to our question – what is nursing and what is it worth?

When I have asked people who claim to have benefited from nursing care, to tell me what really was important – what they really 'needed nurses for', as distinct from doctors, or social workers or psychologists – their answers frequently bordered on the mundane.[2] This encouraged me to believe that nursing was not so much a 'what' as a 'how'. In the words of the old song, 'it ain't what you do, it's the way that you do it'. Effective nursing – or at least what people who have experienced nursing say is effective – appears to involve particular ways of being with people, or doing often commonplace things, in an uncommon or extraordinary way. Most of the activities that nurses might describe as part of their core function, can – and often are – done by other people. What appears to be special about nursing is how nurses perform those activities, especially when they perform them for extended periods of time – as in supporting people in acute crisis – or across the illness-health continuum.

I have frequently compared psychiatric nursing with the work of a lifesaver or fire fighter. Anyone could save a person's life. People do so each and every day. However, to make lifesaving the focus of one's daily work, over a period of several years, transforms the activity from the commonplace to the extraordinary. Being a regular lifesaver or fire fighter requires dedication, skill and knowledge – if the lifesaver or fire fighter is not to end up consumed by the waters or flames within which she or he practices the discipline. Any discipline requires discipline, thus making it special, even when ordinary.

This is also true of the educational aspect of mental health nursing. Most people could help someone to deal with a situation by extending their personal knowledge – by learning something, about themselves, others or the world in general. However, to help people learn from painful or difficult experiences, some of whom may wish to avoid such learning, perhaps over an extended period of time, transforms the helper into an educator who is genuinely special.

These analogies sum up my appreciation of the thousand shades of grey that represent the psychiatric-mental health nursing continuum. In the course of their working lives, if not in the course of a working day, nurses shuttle back and forth across this shadowland. Or at least they appear to do so, as they shape-shift in response to the changing needs of the person, or family, or group. Effective nursing is framed more by the specific dimensions of the moment, than by any absolute, received wisdom, enshrined in journal papers or text-books.

Having said that, journal articles and chapters in text-books can help us to know what we already know better, or to point us in the direction of adding to our personal knowledge. There is no received wisdom, single perspective or unanimous agreement on what (exactly) psychiatric and mental health nurses do, and why this is important, despite what my own research has revealed. That said, there does exist a lot of agreement on these questions. Education is, arguably, more about questions than about answers. Knowledge is a moving target – no sooner do we think we have answered the question, than a whole new set of questions loom over the horizon. It was just such an acceptance of the inevitability of uncertainty that I brought with me when I began to put this book together. Now that the book is completed, I am even more acquainted with the diversity of the need for nursing and how nurses might respond to such needs. Being uncertain heralds the promise of new learning. This was true for me and I hope it will also be true for you, the reader.

I have brought together here some important voices from the mental health field. I hope they will help you become aware of some of the important questions about your practice, and perhaps also will help you feel that you are close to answering these questions better. I chose these authors for I believe that all of them are striving to answer the question *'How should I respond to another person in distress?'* Some appear more certain about what needs to be done than others, but I believe all of them are still developing their understanding of nursing. They are, therefore, growing expertise, rather than *experts*. In that respect they are like you and me. Some of us may appear to know more than others, but none of us is an expert – all of us are growing expertise. There is always more to learn.

Some of the authors are doing their learning as part of their routine working lives, in what are still called clinical settings. Some are educationalists and researchers, exploring such fundamental issues with their students, or with other professionals and people in care through various research projects. Others are involved in the development of grass roots level advocacy and support projects, exploring the need for human support at the critical *care face*.

Some of the authors have had direct experience of mental distress and have been cared for in a variety of ways; treated or abused by the psychiatric system. There are only two chapters written expressly from the user/consumer perspective, which develop the allusive understandings offered by *Gary Platz* in his introductory poem, and *Ann Thomas* in her cover illustration. However, many of the other chapters are informed by the dual experience of having been both 'patient' and 'professional', and the conflicts that often overshadow such a twinned experience. Increasingly, the boundaries between those who 'use' mental health services and those who deliver them are collapsing. Given the inherently human context of mental health problems, this can only be a good thing. 'If you prick us, do we not bleed?' as Shakespeare wisely noted. Mental health is the birthright of all women and men, and mental health problems – whether called madness or personality problems – know no national, social or cultural boundaries. Certainly, mental health professionals are not immune to their ravages. As humans we are all more alike than different.

However, the concept of mental health remains something of a bogey, if not an albatross around our necks. I mean no disrespect to my colleagues, my discipline, or the wider body of psychiatry when I acknowledge that, in general, psychiatry – and by implication, psychiatric nursing – has been largely unsuccessful in promoting the 'mental health' commonly held up as the *raison d'etre* of the field. Indeed, psychiatry has had a long association with abuse, marginalization and the wholesale diminishment of people. One of the important psychiatric tasks, as yet left undone, is to apologise to all those who suffered, needlessly, in the name of 'care and treatment'. In the same way that nations that oppressed people have felt a need to issue a 'backdated apology', I too believe that such an apology is needed if psychiatric nursing is ever to fully embrace the dream of 'mental health nursing'.[3]

Here I have offered some of my own views of psychiatric-mental health nursing. In this book, the reader will find some authors who appear to share some of my views about the nature of nursing and mental health and others who appear to hold radically different perspectives to my own. Such diversity is inherently healthy, reflecting the catholic nature of nursing knowledge and the state of flux that is the key characteristic of the inquiring mind.

I hope that the many and varied perspectives on psychiatric and mental health nursing offered here will stimulate the reader. I hope that the experience of reading these perspectives will help you to know better what you already know and, more importantly, become aware of the limitations of your existing knowledge. Doubt is the great Teacher. Through 'not knowing' we whet our appetites for more knowledge and a better understanding, all the while knowing that the task can never be completed.

I hope that you will enjoy the feast of accumulated knowledge and wisdom within these pages, but I sincerely hope that you will not be satisfied.

REFERENCES

1. Frankl V. Man's *Search for Meaning*. New York: Washington Square Press, 1963.
2. Barker PJ, Jackson S, Stevenson C. The need for psychiatric nursing: towards a multidimensional theory of nursing. *Nursing Inquiry* 1999; **6**: 104–112.
3. Barker PJ, Barker-Buchanan P. Apologising for our colonial past. *Open Mind* 2001; **112**: p10.

Phil Barker

Acknowledgements

I thank Aileen Parlane for giving me the original idea for this book and Georgina Bentliff and Heather Smith at Arnold for helping me bring the project to fruition.

I also thank Poppy Buchanan-Barker for collating the manuscript, and for keeping in almost daily contact with many of the authors, throughout the development of the book.

Thanks also is due to the University of Newcastle, which granted me a sabbatical to work on the book, and my colleagues in the Department of Psychiatry who kept the wheels turning in my absence.

Finally, I thank all the authors for writing for the book, and for their patience during the often-protracted editing period. Their collegiality is beyond measure.

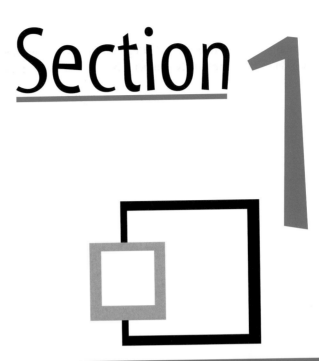

Section 1

The need for nursing

Preface to Section 1

Nursing is, or at least should be, a practical endeavour – focused on identifying what people need *now*, and exploring ways of meeting those needs. Before we begin to examine the various philosophies and processes, which support nursing care, it may be profitable to consider how nursing people with mental distress has changed down the ages and how the concept of care – and the need for nursing – is framed at the beginning of the 21st century.

This section begins with a brief consideration of what mental health *care* might mean, in human terms, and how nurses might approach the identification of the 'need for nursing'.

The discipline of nursing is a relatively recent phenomenon, although people have been 'cared for' or 'looked after' – in various ways – down the ages. Knowing where we have come from – the history of the *care and confinement* of people with mental distress – is important, if we are to ensure that developments represent progress rather than regress.

Understanding the value of nursing, and the *evidence* that signals an appreciation of its worth, is central to current developments in the field. However, the nature of evidence has become a vexed issue, often confused by ideology or political bias. A *careful* consideration of what evidence is and is not, will help the discipline clarify further its caring focus.

This leads us, naturally, to appraise contemporary developments within mental health nursing care. Debate has raged for at least a generation over whether nursing is an art or a science. Here, an alternative perspective – the concept of nursing as *craft* – is considered, and some thought is given to how we might *manage* the development of this craft in practice.

Finally, we turn full circle to connect again with the *people* who might need nursing and who, given their status, might help nurses clarify the proper focus of their craft. These contributions are framed positively, emphasizing how nurses might aid and abet the recovery process, helping people to reclaim ownership of lives blighted or overtaken by mental distress. The last two contributions in this section are, without doubt, the most important – reminding us of the *raison d'être* of nursing and the many dimensions of the craft of caring.

Chapter 1

PERSON-CENTRED CARE: THE NEED FOR DIVERSITY

Phil Barker

PEOPLE AND PROBLEMS

Case study 1.1: Mary

People have been noticing big changes in Mary over the past year – neighbours, friends and most of the all family. She gets up during the night, ransacking drawers and cupboards, searching for precious things she has lost, that she believes have been stolen. She says that, sometimes, she comes downstairs to find the living room full of strangers. Their presence does not appear to disturb her, but she does wonder who they are and what they are doing there. Her oldest son, Archie, who visits his mother regularly, has never seen these strangers but is reluctant to suggest that they might be a figment of her imagination. Mary, who is in her mid-70s, has been widowed for over a decade and recently had to have her pet dog put down. Her family doctor is worried about her and decides to refer her to the local mental health service for older people for further assessment.

Case study 1.2: Jake

Jake was a bright kid but seemed to have trouble making friends. Arguably the smartest in his family, his grades started to slip in his mid teens and he grew increasingly distant. Some nights his father would find him sitting naked in the garden, gazing at the stars. Last weekend he painted his whole bedroom black, when his family went to visit Jake's grandmother in hospital. His parents have separated twice before but always patched things up, for the sake of Jake and his two sisters. They argue a lot these days over Jake. His father thinks he is taking drugs but his mother says he is just a creative type. Sharon, his younger sister, is very close to Jake and he talks to her about some of the strange sensations he gets, like hands running over his body. Karen, the eldest, has a boyfriend who thinks Jake is 'seriously weird'. His teachers agree and he is referred to the school psychologist.

THE HUMAN DIMENSION

We begin this book with two short stories, since telling stories is the stock-in-trade of psychiatric and mental health nursing. As people present themselves to nurses they reveal something of their personal identities through their behaviour and a little more of whom they 'are' as people, through their contribution to the dialogue.

Of course, no one reveals *all* of themselves, for arguably, few of us know ourselves in any complete sense. However, this process of revelation is important not only for the nurses, who gain a degree of understanding of the person in their care, but also for the person, who may be able to add further insights into the nature of 'who' he or she 'is' and 'what' this might mean to others, as well as to themselves.

The nurses who encounter the two people who introduced this chapter would need to ask themselves some fundamental questions, such as: who exactly *is* Mary, and who *is* Jake? They need also to ask, what, exactly, is going on in their lives? However, only rarely do we get anything like a satisfactory answer. These are provocative questions since, by the nature of their human curiosity we are required to take a closer look at the person. Our apprehension about getting *too* close to people has bred the psychiatric tradition of viewing people through the lens of diagnosis and classification, where they become *objects of study* – like plants or animals – somehow set apart from us, their investigators. This is not an entirely foolhardy approach to understanding people, and some of the authors will later try to illustrate the value of choosing this approach to assessment. However, it seems clear that when viewed from a safe distance, or through the reverse telescope of diagnosis, which appears to *reduce* the complexity of the person, problems *seem* more distinct, tidy and intelligible. Things appear simpler from a distance. Viewing the person from a distance also often feels much safer. The closer we get, however, the less clear-cut and the more complex human problems become, and (invariably) the less comfortable we feel.

Through the psychiatric lens, Mary and Jake are classic examples of people at different stages of the development of different forms of 'serious mental illness'[a]. Traditionally, Mary's assessment would explore the possibility that she is depressed or developing a form of dementia. Jake might well just be a sensitive, creative type, but the psychologist will probably be looking for signs of substance abuse or the signs and symptoms of schizophrenia. While such an *examination* of the 'patient' might be useful – either in the short or longer term – it represents only one way of 'looking' at people in human distress. Even if we were able to state, categorically, based on rigorous clinical examination, backed up by laboratory tests, that Mary or Jake *had* a specific form of mental illness or psychiatric disorder, I would hope that nurses would still be primarily interested in knowing what the *experience* of dementia or schizophrenia was like for Mary and Jake.

The need for diversity

This is a book about *people* like Mary and Jake. Although there will be various references to clients, users, consumers, patients and survivors, I would hope that the reader would not lose sight of the human fact that all are *people*, first and foremost. The different contributing authors approach psychiatric and mental health nursing from different angles. However, all are interested in the people who become the focus of nursing care and attention. Their differing perspectives reflect the different philosophical and theoretical perspectives associated with psychiatric and mental health nursing in the 21st century. Although there is an emphasis on developing person-centred *care*, I recognize that such a focus rarely stands alone, and may even need the support or challenge of differing perspectives. Hopefully this book will show how these differing perspectives can be harmonized.

The various authors discuss how we might go about identifying what *exactly* might be going on in the lives of people like Mary and Jake, and how we – as a caring discipline – should respond.

- ❑ What is the *nature* of their present difficulties?
- ❑ How might we *support* Mary and Jake?
- ❑ How might our offer of help, whatever it entails, *fit in* with what other professionals might choose to do, or feel obliged to do?
- ❑ What will the *family* expect of us, as nurses?
- ❑ What will *Mary* and *Jake* expect of us?

The reality of human experience is that our *needs* are often subject to dramatic change. Sometimes we are like *this* and other times we are like *that*. The changeable nature of our experience – of ourselves, of others, and of the world in general – determines that what any person might *need* at any point in time, is also subject to change.

The different authors will adopt different approaches to working out an answer to the question: 'what does the person need *now?*' Some will begin, as I have done here, with part of someone's story, using this as a springboard for examining what might need to happen next. In a very real sense the author is trying to build a 'theory of the person' that might inform care. Others will begin from a formal theoretical perspective, using understandings about people *in general* to help us understand *this person* in particular. In my view, both approaches have different values but each, in the right context, is equally valid. Flexibility is one of the keys to opening the way to appropriate and, hopefully, enhanced human care. Hopefully the reader will come to appreciate, better, the need for flexibility of thought, as well as action, in the development of person-centred care.

---

[a] Although in common usage, the term 'serious mental illness' is objectionable for several reasons, not least for the implication that some forms of 'mental illness' are trivial, or 'not serious'.

Getting personal

A hallmark of professional practice is the establishment of a close, confiding relationship. We need to get close enough to the person emotionally to begin to appreciate the human nature of their difficulties. However, we need to avoid becoming so enmeshed in the person's experience, that we cannot distinguish our feelings from those of the person. This notion of the *boundary* between the nurse and the person in care is a thread that runs through most, if not all, of the chapters in this book.

Nursing is an interpersonal process, involving the establishment and development of complex relationships between nurses and the people in their care, their family and friends, as well as other health and social care disciplines. It also involves a complex of relationships between different aspects of the person who is the nurse.[1]

We should not forget that nurses too are people. They are women or men, who may be gay, straight or bisexual. They may have had multiple partners or may be celibate. They may be 'white' or 'black' or 'coloured', but on closer examination may be the product of a whole string of racial, ethnic and cultural influences. They may be the oldest or youngest members of a family, or have grown up in an orphanage. They may be the only child of a single parent, or the middle child of 13 siblings. They may be married, single, divorced, separated or widowed. They may be members of one of the traditional faiths – Christianity, Islam, Judaism, Hinduism or Buddhism; or belong to a little-known religious sect; or be an atheist, agnostic or 'fair-weather churchgoer'.

It goes without saying that nurses bring these dimensions of themselves to their relations with people in their care. On occasions, these personal aspects of the nurse may intrude into the professional aspects of the individual nurse. A key obligation of professional practice is to become aware of how such differing personal, social and cultural characteristics might influence our professional decision-making, and our relations with the person who is the patient or client.[2]

Nursing as a human service

Nursing is, first and foremost, a human service: offered by one group of human beings to another. The extent to which one group (nurses) really differs from the other (patients or clients) is debatable. However, within the power dynamic of care, where one person has a *duty* to care for the other, the relationship is often artificially distinguished. Before we begin to consider how psychiatric and mental health nurses might develop the knowledge and skills that might allow them to help Mary and Jake, I ask the reader two simple, yet important, questions:

1 If you were Archie, what would you want for your mother? Why would you want *this*, rather than anything else?

2 In the same vein, if you were Sharon, what would you want for your brother, Jake? And why would you want *this*, rather than anything else?

We should begin here – with these very *personal* questions – since your answers will say something about you, as a person, as distinct from you as a professional, whether you are a student or an experienced practitioner. Your answers will suggest some of the values, beliefs and prejudices – and perhaps even interpersonal problems – that have shaped you as a human being.

In most Western countries the first thing that might happen to Mary or Jake is that they might be admitted, perhaps against their will or wishes, to a psychiatric unit, or be obliged to receive a visit from a crisis team, or a member of a community mental health team. There, the problems Mary and Jake have been experiencing in their everyday lives will be examined by a whole string of professionals. Their problems will be subject to the highly unusual, and often frightening, spotlight of the psychiatric system. Putting them 'under the spotlight' may have been what you had in mind for your hypothetical 'mother' or 'brother', but I doubt it. I suspect that you were thinking of something a little less harsh, and certainly a lot less threatening.

For many years I have asked students and fellow professionals if they would be happy to admit one of their loved ones into the service with which they are associated. Few, if any, judged their services good enough for someone as valuable, in human terms, as their 'loved one'. Many of those whom I asked found the question challenging, some even suggesting that it was somehow 'unfair' or 'manipulative', tugging at the metaphorical heartstrings of these mental health professionals.

The question is in no way unfair or manipulative. Indeed, it represents a very useful place to begin our consideration of what we do, as nurses, and why we do this, as opposed to anything else. By putting ourselves, firmly, in the position of 'loved ones', we can begin to appreciate why Mary and Jake, Archie and Sharon and all the family and friends that make up their close social circle, often feel let down by the services we offer. Because they are inextricably linked to Mary and Jake, in all sorts of ways, their view of what their 'loved one' needs, may differ markedly from our objective, often distant, sometimes wrongheaded, view of the person's needs. By reminding ourselves that the person who is the 'patient' or 'client' is someone's *mother*, or *daughter*, *sister* or *brother*, *friend* or *lover*, we remind ourselves of the *human value* of the person. By focusing on the human being – the person – we remind ourselves of the potential weaknesses, or pitfalls, of what we might offer through a standardized professional service.

Various circumstances – such as inadequate funding, poor staffing, restrictive policies, or inter-professional disagreements – may militate against organizing and delivering the kind of care, which we consider appropriate or necessary. However, such circumstances should not influence our judgement as to what is really needed in the name of appropriate nursing care. When we view the need-for-nursing scenario[3] through the lens of our loved ones, all too often we can see the inappropriateness and deficiency of our nursing response writ large. It can offer a humbling, yet intensely revealing, perspective on the need for, and development of, individually focused care.

THE NATURE OF NURSING

Nursing is a social construct. People look after themselves, others, animals, the environment and all manner of 'things', in a range of ways, all of which might be called 'nursing'. The athlete who sustains some damage to a tendon or ligament is often said to be 'nursing an injury' – acting in such a way as to prevent the injury getting worse, and to promote healing. The seasoned drinker is often described as 'nursing a pint' – taking time over the consumption of the beer, trying to enjoy each mouthful in a vain effort to prolong the enjoyable experience. The nurseryman, responsible for planting and overseeing the growth and development of a new forest, 'nurses' his new shoots. The fragile new growth is sheltered from strong winds, and adequate drainage, irrigation and – most of all – *space* is made available, all of which are necessary if growth and development is to take place.[4]

In a social context, the most enduring example of nursing is the supportive care offered by parents, in most cultures especially by mothers, to their children. This form of care spans nations and cultures and is largely indistinguishable from that found in the animal kingdom. Parents, being responsible for their offspring, shape the immediate physical environment of their young, to ensure that the 'space' is safe *and* will provide adequate room for growth.

A few short weeks ago, the blackbirds in our garden built a nest under the eaves of the house, and now three small chicks are being fed frantically by their parents, who swoop dramatically over our heads, in a powerful display of territoriality and parenting. In only a few more weeks the chicks will be big enough to leave their shelter, to take their flight into adulthood and parenthood.

These birds remind us that the formal relations between parent and offspring involve a complex of interactions designed to foster the safety, sustenance and growth of the young. Ultimately, the point of these interactions is to foster their independence from the parent.

In the same vein, the ultimate *point* of nursing is to make it redundant. We care for one another in such a way that, following a reasonable degree of growth and development we hope we can relinquish the need for nursing. We need to care *enough* for people, so that – in time – they will not need our care, *at all*.

As health and social care is increasingly *organized*, and subject to the influences of economics and especially the political philosophy of the day, this fundamental appreciation of nursing can become lost in a morass of policies and protocols, legislation and language. In the final section, developments in mental health nursing in some very different countries around the world are examined briefly (Chapters 68–71). These illustrate some of the restrictions which delimit the expression of nursing, but also some of the possibilities for growth of the discipline, brought about by such social and political challenges.

Mental health and human development

The relationship between people in need of nursing, and those who care for them, is analogous to, but different from, that of the child–parent relationship. People who experience any one of the myriad threats to their personal or social identities, which are commonly called *mental illness*, or *mental health problems*, experience a human threat that renders them vulnerable. For some people this vulnerability – which waxes and wanes – may last for a considerable time. Such people – often called in health care jargon the 'enduringly mentally ill' – are not vulnerable every moment, of every day. However, such is the nature of their difficulties, or their circumstances, that this perceived vulnerability casts a shadow over their lives; and often limits their opportunities for further human growth and development. For others, their vulnerability is more sharply defined, and the perceived threats to their physical safety or emotional security are more marked. Often described as 'acutely' mentally ill, such a person's degree of vulnerability may also fluctuate. However, when it does present itself, this may represent a formidable challenge to the person, often suggesting the need for some intensive or sophisticated support, to address the emergent crisis.

Such physical, emotional and existential threats may, temporarily, disable or limit the person's capacity to operate, constructively, in the world. The greater the nature of the threat and concomitant vulnerability, the greater will be the person's perceived 'need for nursing'. In almost all societies, when a citizen's vulnerability or degree of concomitant incapacity is pronounced, provisions are made in law, to detain the person in a safe and supportive environment, until the threat has either abated or is, in some sense, 'under control'.

Such attitudes towards people who experience either

temporary or prolonged crises, involving their perceived 'mental health', reflect the moral scruples of society, especially in relation to its perceived need to care for those who appear unable to care, fully, for themselves. Once regarded as the hallmark of a civilized society, the development of organized forms of care (and treatment) for people viewed as being 'mentally ill' reflects the moral values commonly associated with parents and their off-spring. In much the same way as parents are (at least in principle) responsible for the safekeeping and physical, intellectual and emotional development of their children, so society adopts a similar role in relation to its members. Those who appear unable (or even unwilling) to care for themselves – or otherwise deal with their human prob-lems – receive the kind of support that might meet their needs, either now or in the future.

Given that so many people either reject, or are never able to access, the kind of support they believe they need to deal with their life difficulties, the view of a caring society sketched above may be false or idealistic. Given that readers of this book are interested in advancing *mental health* care, an idealistic stance might be the best place to begin. Through clarifying what, exactly, are the individual and collective needs of people deemed to be one state of mental illness or another, nurses might begin to develop *mental health* services that are genuinely worthy of the name. This might be very different from the mental *illness* services – often focused only on the amelioration of distress, or the management of crises – that commonly operate under the wholly inappropriate title of 'mental *health* services'.

The name is never the thing

Names – what we call people, and their various experi-ences, and the services that they receive – will play an important part in this book. Many of the everyday terms used already in this chapter – mental *illness*, mental *health, enduringly mentally ill, acutely mentally ill, patient, client* – are highly loaded terms. They mean different things to different people. Indeed, mental *illness* and mental *health* – two expressions that are fundamental to this book – possess no clear, accepted definition. However, they are used in everyday conversation *as if* their meaning is unambiguous.[5]

In a very real sense these linguistic confusions either do not matter, or may even be helpful. If we are unsure of what, exactly, these terms mean, we might be more care-ful in using them. Alternatively, if we believe that the meanings are obvious, we can simply get on with dealing with 'illness' and promoting 'health'. One of the key prin-ciples underlying the philosophy of this book is that nurses do *not* deal with illness, disease or disorder. Instead, nursing is a special kind of human response to the prob-lems of living that people experience when they are viewed as ill, disordered, diseased or dysfunctional. In that sense, nursing is focused on *human responses* to *human problems*.[6] Nursing may augment and complement the services provided by various other health and social care practitioners, but its unique focus is on providing a human response to some very special human problems.

Nurses are mainly involved in providing the kind of support that will help people to reduce the experience of distress, so that they might make decisions for themselves, act for themselves and live their lives as autonomously as possible, given their immediate circumstances. Given such a focus, quibbles over whether they are mentally ill or healthy will become redundant. Arguably, few people are fully healthy – if by that we mean 'whole'. Most people are, however, sufficiently healthy to be able to act for themselves and to influence, constructively, the direc-tion of their lives. Perhaps this focus, on how people live their lives and their capacity to transfer their constructive choices and decisions into a meaningful reality, should be the focus of nursing care plans. Nurses do not heal or otherwise cure people of their various ailments – physical or mental, emotional or spiritual. When nursing does suc-ceed in making a difference, however, the person is placed – as Nightingale famously remarked – in the right con-dition to be healed by Nature or by God.

The value of difference

In this book the reader will become acquainted with dif-ferent authors, from different countries and different philosophical, theoretical and practice backgrounds. This diversity will result in some cases, in different emphases being given within the chapters. These differing back-grounds influence our perception of what (exactly) are the human problems that people bring to the field of mental health care; what (exactly) might be the nursing response to such problems; and what (exactly) this might mean for the development of the discipline of nursing. I hope that the reader will view this diversity – as I have done – as a positive asset, reflecting the value of holding different, perhaps changeable, views of nurs-ing – *what it is, how it works* and what it might *mean* for health care. Given the complexity of 21st century mental health care, and the social and cultural worlds it inhabits, a single, monolithic, unchanging view of 'what needs to be done' seems as inappropriate as it does unlikely. I hope the reader will agree.

People first

What all the contributors to this book share is a concern for people. They may refer to the people who receive nursing as patients, clients, users or consumers, but these terms do not obscure their real interest – the person who lies behind the label of convenience. Over the past few years, debates have raged over what to call the people who use mental health services. In the UK the expression 'users' has become fashionable, although – given its older association with illicit drugs – the term is seen, by some, as problematic. In the USA and Australia, efforts to streamline health care along business lines led, indirectly, to the popularization of the term 'consumer'. However, the extent to which anyone who receives a mental health service has anything like the rights of the average 'consumer', is debatable, to say the least. The term 'client', well established in social work and counselling, has also enjoyed some popularity, arguably on the grounds that it acknowledges the independent status of the person using the service. The expression derives from the Latin *cliens*, which referred to a plebeian – a working class person of low birth – who was supported by a patrician – or nobleman. The *cliens* offered the patrician loyalty and service, in return for which he received support and security. To a great extent this reflects the power relationship between professionals and 'clients' in current mental health services, where much emphasis is given to compliance and the inherent wisdom of the professional. Although considered by many to be outmoded, the term 'patient' still has much to recommend it. Certainly people who receive mental health services often are required to exercise great patience as they await the outcomes of the deliberations of the nursing team, or as they wait, patiently, for nurses to recognize what are their true needs.

Our need to find ways of defining the people who receive mental health services has become something of a professional neurosis. It is not at all clear why we cannot simply call people who use nursing services, *people*! It seems likely that the collective names used to address *people* who receive psychiatric-mental health nursing will change, as fashions and legislation changes. Hopefully, the focus of nursing will remain unchanged, and we shall continue to focus on *people* and their human needs.

In responding to such human needs nurses will continue to develop a body of nursing knowledge that will acknowledge the wide range of complex factors, which define people and their needs. This will include consideration of:

❑ personal history;
❑ personal preferences, values and beliefs;
❑ social status;
❑ cultural background;
❑ family affiliations;
❑ community membership.

In the traditional world of health care – where the presumed 'illness' and its 'aetiology' were seen as all-important – this human dimension was often neglected.

We can become so focused on the person's illnesses or presumed disorder that we risk forgetting the human dimensions of people like Mary and Jake whom we discussed earlier. Some years ago, on a trip to New Zealand, I came across the Maori expression:

Ne aha te mea nunui ki te ao
Ne tangata Ne tangata Ne tangata.

Roughly translated this means:

What is the most important thing to the world?
It is the people, it is the people, it is the people.

The Maori culture recognizes that *who* people are, is very much a function of the family relations, culture and the heritage of the ancestors. This *people* focus offers a fitting frame for our consideration of what anyone might need by way of a nursing service.

❑ How might we help people to grow and develop, as human beings, so that they might become more aware of the *problems of living*, which they experience, which commonly are called mental illness or psychiatric disorder?
❑ How might we help people to address, deal with and perhaps recover from, or overcome, the *problems* and *difficulties* that distress them, or limit their ability to function effectively in the world?

PSYCHIATRIC AND MENTAL HEALTH NURSING

How nurses help people to live with, or overcome their distress, or develop themselves in such a way that they begin to overcome or recover from their difficulties, differs little from the nurturing approach to human development, practised by parents down the ages. Although the specifics of *what* nurses do, in the form of various interventions, or therapeutic approaches, may differ markedly, *why* they do this – the rationale, or underlying philosophy of nursing – is no different.

When people are in acute distress, and may be in some way a risk to themselves or others, the high drama of the situation often requires an equally dramatic nursing response. Such 'critical interventions', where the nurse might need to make the person and the environment safe and secure, often requires great skill and composure. This is akin to the work of the lifesaver who rescues someone from drowning, or the fire-fighter who needs to deliver a person from a burning building. The kind of care a person needs, when suicidal or acutely disturbed by the experience of hearing voices, for example, involves a kind of 'emotional rescue'. Here, the nurse provides the kind of supportive conditions that will reduce the experience of distress and prepare the way for a more detailed examination of what needs to be done next. When nurses respond to people's distress by helping to contain it, delimit it, or otherwise fix it, they might be seen as practising *psychiatric* nursing. Both the nurse and the person are locked in the present. The emphasis is on stemming the flow of distress, or keeping a watchful eye out for any signs of exacerbation of the original distress.

However, almost as soon as this 'crisis' has passed, and the person – or their circumstances – appear to have calmed down or quietened – the focus turns to something more constructive and *developmental*. Once the person has been dragged ashore and is judged to be 'safe' the emphasis switches to 'rehabilitation': what needs to happen now to help the person return to normal living. Where it is thought that the person may have played a part in their own crisis – whether by accidentally falling or intentionally jumping into the river – the focus turns to an examination of the person's motives, or understanding of the risks involved. This will involve, of necessity, a more careful, longer-term inquiry, which aims to ensure the person's safety and well-being *in the future*. This kind of developmental care involves much more active collaboration between the carer and the person being cared for. Often, it takes the form of an active alliance – where both work together to develop an understanding of the nature of the problem and what might be done – *now* – to begin to address or resolve it. Such a careful, paced, developmental approach to clarifying understanding of problems of living, and their possible solutions, might be called *mental health* nursing.[7]

Care – the precious gift

The term 'care' has lost some of its original currency in 21st century nursing. Many nurses in the late 20th century grew dissatisfied with the notion of *caring*, exploring instead the idea of nursing as a *therapeutic* activity – in particular a psychotherapeutic activity. It should go without saying that when nurses *care* effectively, what they do will be therapeutic – it will begin to provide the conditions under which the person can begin to be healed, as Nightingale said, by Nature or by God.[8] Psychotherapy originally meant the 'healing of the soul (or spirit)'. When nurses organize the kind of conditions that help to alleviate distress and begin the longer term process of recuperation, resolution or learning – helping the person to begin to feel the 'whole' of their experience – those activities might be considered to be therapeutic, engendering the potential for healing.

We might also value the term *care* since it emphasizes the caution, attention to detail and sensitivity that is necessary when handling something precious. The archaeologist who goes in search of some long lost treasure, may begin his work with strenuous and dramatic digging – excavating the site until there are signs that something of value might lie somewhere just below the surface. Then the powerful tools of excavation are exchanged for smaller tools, which are more focused and can be used more sensitively. Finally, when a 'find' begins to emerge, even these small tools are exchanged for brushes, which are used, even more *carefully*, to remove the layers of earth and dust that cover the treasure.

The archaeologist's *care*-ful approach to unearthing and finally revealing a possible find suggests a concern and respect for the treasure. The team may have unearthed a relic from a bygone age, or they may simply have uncovered another stone. Either way, their approach is characterized by *care, sensitivity* and *attention to detail*, for these 'finds' are priceless – whatever their market value.

If we can view a piece of pottery that was buried in the earth a thousand years ago as 'priceless', it should go without saying that a person, who is by definition unique, should be viewed, similarly, as invaluable. This respect for the person – irrespective of their age, class, nationality, creed or colour, where they are nursed or the presumed nature or origins of their presenting problems – lies at the heart of all the contributions in this book. I hope that readers will consider carefully what the different voices of the authors represented here have to say about nurses and nursing. I hope also that they will use the contributions made within this book to construct and develop further their own body of knowledge, which will inform their own practice.

REFERENCES

1. Peplau HE. *Interpersonal relations in nursing.* London: Macmillan, 1987.
2. Butterworth A, Faugier J, Burnard P (eds). *Clinical supervision and mentorship in nursing.* London: Nelson Thornes.
3. Barker P, Jackson S, Stevenson C. The need for psychiatric nursing. *Journal of Psychiatric and Mental Health Nursing* 1999; **6**(4) 273–82.
4. Barker P. *The philosophy and practice of psychiatric nursing.* Churchill Livingstone: Edinburgh, 1999.
5. Stevenson C. Living within and without psychiatric language games. In: Barker P, Stevenson C (eds). *The construction of power and authority in psychiatry.* Oxford: Butterworth-Heinemann, 2000.
6. The American Nurses Association. *Nursing: a social policy statement.* Kansas: American Nurses Association, 1980.
7. Barker P. The Tidal model: developing an empowering, person-centred approach to recovery within psychiatric and mental health nursing. *Journal of Psychiatric and Mental Health Nursing* 2001; **8**(3) 233–40.
8. Barker P. Reflections on caring as a virtue ethic within an evidence-based culture. *International Journal of Nursing Studies* 2000; **37**(4) 32–6.

Chapter 2

THE CARE AND CONFINEMENT OF THE MENTALLY ILL

Liam Clarke*

INTRODUCTION

In the beginning there was Bedlam: at first it was called the Priory of St Mary of Bethlehem (but later bowdlerized to Bethlem or Bedlam). In the 13th century it was the only lunatic enclosure in England. Stealing Elizabeth Shoenberg's phrase, Bedlam was the original 'castle of fantasy' but at a time when the fantasy could be realized for the price of an entrance fee. Freak shows were the order of the day and Bedlam was the classiest show in town, way above the level of circus side-show by virtue of its perceived philanthropy. Philanthropy aside, it was (at first) probably privately owned. Being small, (originally six patients) it was unlikely to tax the strength of its curious visitors.

Bedlam is important, not only as a starting point, but because much of psychiatry's reputation would come to rest on different perceptions of it and their reification over time. Superficially, we can see it as a place where the affluent paid to watch the 'antics' of confined, brutalized, terrified lunatics. The passage of time would canonize this image, perhaps as a contrasting backdrop against which the 'liberating' activities of Pinel in Paris or the Tukes in England could assume heroic form. Allderidge[1] notes that very little written about Bedlam derives from primary sources, resulting in easygoing assumptions about the nature of its provision and money-making proclivities. The brutality of chaining and whipping, which lasted until the 18th century is hardly denied but, as Allderidge shows, things are more complicated than has sometimes been portrayed. By 1677, for instance, Bethlem's rules stated that:

> None of the Officers or Servants shall at any time beat or abuse any of the Lunatics in the said hospital, neither shall offer any force unto them but upon absolute necessity for the better government of the said Lunatics.[2]

Force, in other words, while a real possibility, was not seen by the Bethlem authorities as ordinarily acceptable. Also, the existence of two wards for 'incurables' suggests that, for other patients, cure was not an unrealistic aspiration. In truth, the early asylums – built in the mid 18th century – were known for their weird and wondrous attempts to cure insanity. A Doctor Cox,[3] for instance, suspended patients from the ceiling in a contraption which rotated them 100 times a minute: unsurprisingly, many hastily reported a marked improvement in their condition. As Peter Ackroyd[4] observes, 'You have to be brave to be mad'.

*Liam Clarke has worked as a lecturer for Brighton University for twelve years and in that time has published widely on various matters pertaining to mental health and psychiatry. One of his particular interests has been the history of psychiatric nursing and its relationship to the management of hospitalized patients and especially their confinement and containment.

Liam Clarke is married with two grown-up children and is currently involved in developing ways of increasing psychiatric user participation in undergraduate nurse training programmes.

On paying to watch the lunatics, Allderidge says that the practice lasted hundreds of years, inferring that it had become custom and practice and not just a money earner: was there, perhaps, an element of almsgiving involved? In 1673, a new building, at Moorfields, took the place of the old Bethlem and while – like the later Victorian asylums – it had an outward appearance of grandness, it was anything but inside. Inmates continued to be put on display, this time along two galleries, one above the other. In addition, 'on each floor a corridor ran along a line of cells, with an iron gate in the middle to divide the males from the females'[4]. The practice of rigidly separating the sexes was to remain until the post-Thatcher closure of the mental hospitals.

Beyond Bedlam

After Bethlem, from the early 18th century other asylums sprang up usually on the basis of individual local initiative. These constitute the first wave of public asylums in England beginning in 1751 with St Luke's, London, under the guidance of William Battie whose 'Treatise on Madness' became influential. One of Battie's first actions was to ban asylum sightseers. St Luke's also broke with the past by accepting medical students. It seemed as if a new liberalism was about to dawn in English psychiatry. However, it was the invention of 'moral therapy' by a family of Quakers at York, which heralded a dramatic shift in how lunacy was conceived and managed. Following a suspicious death at the York asylum, heretofore an institution of good repute, the Tuke family opened their Retreat, also at York. Perhaps its most significant departure was to recognize that the community of carers and patients, together, could be a force for good. Rather than following established practices of trying to break the lunatic's will, by medicine fair or foul, the lunatic's will was gently coerced in the way that a kind parent would 'inculcate' goodness in a child. Their desire seems to have been to admonish, as well as praise, the behaviours of inmates so that they might re-capture their dignity and acquire self-control. In her history of the Retreat, Ann Digby[5] records that its liberalism was not new but that it was working on received ideas of ethical and rational justice coupled with the abandonment of physical restraints then becoming common. Yet the Retreat exerted little direct influence on contemporary asylum practices perhaps unsurprisingly given the uniqueness of its religious disposition. True, pockets of liberal treatment occurred throughout the early asylums and some of them showed commendable tolerance of their inmate's behaviour (see Porter,[6] Chapter 10). But they could never rid themselves fully of their custodial function, the sheer bricks and mortar density of their presence made liberalism extremely unlikely. For example, the outer walls of these asylums were fifteen feet high. Although this protected the inmates from the 'gaping at the lunatics' phenomenon which, despite Battie's efforts, had continued into the early 19th century, they were primarily intended to prevent escape. The windows in these hospitals were small and set high up in their inner walls, a deliberate invocation of claustrophobic menace. Smith[7] reminds us that the fine grounds were for walking in by fee-paying inmates only, and not for the pauper lunatics who had to take their exercise in airing yards. The frightening conduction of sounds, particularly at night, the poor diet, the bland hospital garb, the dead hand of routine, the bludgeoning of individuality and so on and on and on: all of this endured into the second wave of public asylums built by the Victorians.

Initial summary

To summarize, the history of professional psychiatry begins with the separation of the mentally ill into institutions. Bethlem was hardly a prototype but – within the story of confinement – it set a metaphorical standard which influenced how subsequent developments would be seen. For Roy Porter,[8] 'the epic of English madness opens in the late 18th Century' and with 'psychiatric institutionalization as the key to this history'. From its beginnings, confinement represents the basic conundrum of psychiatry – an excruciating conundrum for nurses – which is the problem of reconciling custody and care. At Bethlem, the natural impetus, for years, was to chain and punish. By the 16th century more enlightened minds prevailed and current opinion suggests that treatments as well as a measure of compassion were by this time becoming acceptable.[8,9] The unleashing of restraints at Hanwell (announced by John Connolly in September 1839),[10] although not an isolated act, represented a watershed mainly on account of the (large) size of Hanwell and Connolly's charismatic leadership. Leadership was needed, as attendants often required intense pressure to relinquish their attachment to chaining and other punitive measures.

By the mid 19th century, however, dissatisfaction with custodialism and coercion was coalescing into a social push for change. In 1845, change came in spades with the passage of 'arguably the most significant mental health legislation of the century'[7]. This required county magistrates to establish pauper lunatic asylums and with a remit that they reflect Connolly's principles of care.

Porter has argued that the 19th century asylums did not follow on the back of an earlier century of neglect and cruelty: the pauper lunatics certainly suffered inside their 17th and 18th century institutions but no more than they would have done had these institutions not existed. What the 19th century represented was an unprecedented public-spiritedness: 'Victorian England ... was, after all, a time of great men, of great vision, of great achievement'[11] and with a penchant for attacking problems with verve and tenacity. The Victorians did not invent compassion, nor (even) awareness of the plight of mad people. Despite the fact that the Victorian asylums lasted a mere century, theirs was an extraordinary optimism (and achievement) all the same.

MORAL STRICTURES

To what extent did moral therapy (at the Retreat) entail elements of moral *expectations*? And, did this constitute a more subtle form of restraint? Smith[7] observes that:

> Moral treatment comprised more than a gentle, considerate approach. There were also aspects which sought to alter inappropriate behaviour. By 1800, the conception was widely accepted that the doctor had to gain ascendancy over the madman, as a precursor to curative treatment.

This is important because even allegedly liberal psychiatric regimes can camouflage malevolent intentions. For example, therapeutic communities[12] have typically advocated principles of democratization, permissiveness, communalism and so on. However, these principles may cloak moral imperatives such that, if the workings of the community break down, more traditional forms of management will re-emerge to put matters right. Lindsay,[13] a resident in a therapeutic community, noted that whenever life became intolerable, conventional codes issued forth to redress imbalances and restore equilibrium. The implication is that, ultimately, therapeutic communities only work when they have – at least during crises – conventional moral codes to fall back on. A more complicated overlap between public and institutional moralities is where hospitals evince progressive features – such as unlocking doors, patients wearing their own clothes etc. – features which represent change and development at one level, but whose apparent liberalism is intended to make confinement more acceptable.

Michel Foucault[14] has much to say about confinement along these lines: he talks of the:

> invention of a site of constraint, where morality castigates by means of administrative enforcement ... institutions of morality are established in which an astonishing synthesis of moral obligation and civil law is effected.

Although Foucault hurled his edicts at the York Retreat and its works (for example the abolition of physical constraints, instigating a generally caring milieu), his injunctions just as easily castigate confinement generally. Foucault sees the Retreat as

> an asylum in which the free terror of madness is substituted with the stifling anguish of responsibility; fear no longer reigns outside the asylum gates, it now rages under the seals of conscience.

Rather than punish guilt, the asylum now organizes it, an illusion of therapy is created by a new age of rationality, which objectifies and distances the *experiences* of its inmates.

Insightful obeisance

Much of Foucault's work is premised on patients as unwilling or ignorant participants in their treatment when, actually, patients are often complicit in their treatment or even detention. For example, the first patients at the York Retreat were themselves Quakers and so probably did not experience their 'moral management' as irksome or unwarranted.

In addition, a libertarian agenda drives Foucault's writings and one suspects that his conclusions may not trustworthily reflect available evidence. Contrary to Foucault, Digby's account[5] of the York Retreat *is* consistent with the high praise that its humanitarianism has traditionally warranted. One measure of its openness, for example, was that less than 5% of inmates were restrained at any time and only if violent or suicidal. Most of its patients mixed freely with visitors; they dressed ordinarily, took tea with the governors and even, now and then, ventured outside the hospital walls.

However, Digby's version does support Foucault's assertions about moral control by listing the Retreat's implicit *threat* of restraint as well as its prevalent religious training and work regimes. The basic idea of Retreat was to allow people to regroup or recollect their senses and faculties. The Tuke Family believed in appealing to the unaffected faculties of its inmates, and were influenced, in this instance, by John Locke's assertion that insanity is a disturbance of *ideas*, not of the spirit, nor of the person. The problem with Foucault, however, is not his scepticism about the Retreat's achievements so much as the glib connections he makes between events, and the *wilfulness* he attaches to the medical colonization of thought and behaviour as he sees it. That a therapeutic community *might* elicit guilt from residents falling foul of its precepts is plausible enough; that this would preclude good therapeutic intentions as well sounds a bit one-sided. Also, was it necessarily wrong to implant guilt in the minds of 18th century pauper-lunatics if what was intended was an improvement in their moral probity? Such an admission might raise eyebrows today; but in an 18th century religious context?

Separation

A central theme of Foucault's is that in the 17th century a grand confinement of society's rejects and misfits took place, eventually culminating in the building of the Victorian asylums. However, as Roy Porter[8] points out, 17th century schemes of confinement were parochial in nature: much of the management of madness was in (often lucrative) private houses or in families (the latter classically evoked in Bronte's Jane Eyre) and it was not until the early 19th century that a widespread separation of the mad was attempted.

Separation means new rules – different rules – distancing the separated from everyday life, an implication of moral inferiority and societal threat. The conventional view is that the 'asylum separation' was a positive result of political altruism, as well as medicine's growing confidence in its ability to manage the insane. Commenting on this, Andrew Scull[15] stated:

> The very language that is used reflects the implicit assumptions which for many years marked most historians' treatment of the subject – a naïve Whiggish view of history as progress, and a failure to see key elements of the reform process as sociologically highly problematic.

Foucault's view of the pre-19th century world is that it is at ease with madness: in a sense, the village fool is indeed a fool 'but he's *our* fool': he possesses consensual worth because, as yet, no epistemology exists by which to debar him. Foucault postulates this so as to attack a psychiatric science, which he alleges objectifies patients, thus marginalizing them. He has a point, since the close of the 18th century sees the advent of philosophical and scientific rationalism with their offspring, sociology and psychology, when religious thought becomes superseded by humanist discourse. Psychiatry comes about because it invents a new concept of madness in which unreason is no longer considered virtuous. According to Foucault, the 'madman' – combined roughly of two parts noble savage and village buffoon – moves from a primitive, but socially viable status, to one of mental defective where, in the name of medical expertise, his social 'position' is severely thwarted.

According to Edward Shorter[16] this perspective is faulty. In the years before the asylums were built, people:

> were treated with a savage lack of feeling ... there was no golden era, no idyllic refuge from the values of capitalism. To maintain otherwise is a fantasy.

These are harsh words. However, in the sense of 'golden eras' they are true enough. That said, Foucault's point is not so much about how people treated one another – life was nasty, brutish and short for everyone – but that the mad were now confined on grounds of *disease*: the mad are now *conceptually* excluded by scientific advance.

THE PRINCIPAL ISSUE

An important issue is whether the asylums were a product of Victorian paternalism, or a result of increasing medical power, coupled with an impetus to protect society from the criminal and/or eugenic propensities of the mentally ill. The following view from Edward Shorter, gives a flavour of the discussion:[16]

> To an extent unimaginable for other areas of the history of medicine, zealot-researchers have seized the history of psychiatry to illustrate how their pet bugaboos – be they capitalism, patriarchy, or psychiatry itself – have converted protest into illness, licking into asylums those who otherwise would be challenging the established order.

And Andrew Scull noted:[15]

> The direction taken by lunacy reform in the nineteenth century is thus presented as at once inevitable and basically benign – both in intent and in consequences – and the whole process crudely reduced to a simplistic equation: humanitarianism \+ science \+ government inspection 5 the success of what David Roberts calls the great nineteenth-century movement for a more humane and intelligent treatment of the insane.

The issue is the extent to which elements from one or other (or both) of these strands holds true. Nietzche stated that, ultimately, all argument represents 'a desire of the heart' and this is certainly an arena where 'evidence' can lend itself to conflicting attitudes about the purposes of psychiatry. Possibly the interpretations of the anti-institutionalists, intent on revising status quo accounts, have been more inspired, more creative. That said, their central point was not without foundation. The 19th century reforms operated, not as a kind of noblesse oblige, an outpouring of Victorian benevolence, but from a desire to corral troublesome citizens.

Kathleen Jones,[17] while acknowledging the second class status of their patients, their use as cheap labour, as well as the recurring violence, smell and abuse of rights, nevertheless states that asylums were humane and intelligent. She believes that much that has been written about asylums is biased: 'we must', she says, 'get beyond prejudice, both old and new, assessing the asylum movement in the context of its own day'. What this means is that given the conditions of 19th century working class life, both in the workhouses and generally, asylum admission may well have been a blessing. For Jones, the removal of the mentally ill to rural hospital outposts protected them from 'the pestilence and open cesspools' of urban living. It may have helped. Eerily, Peter Ackroyd records[4] that Bethlem had a fresh water supply from an Artesian well which indeed provided a lifetime's freedom from cholera. But siting the asylums in rural areas was probably more to do with finance; the imperative to purchase building land in cheap non-urban settings.

So why did the Victorian asylums get built?

Certainly 'social control' cannot be discounted at a time of political concerns about public disorder. The asylums satisfied Victorian concerns about the plight of lunatics: their secondary purpose to make the streets safe cannot however have been far from their minds. Neither can the good or therapeutic intentions of interested parties be set aside as lightly as some have done. In Walton's view,[18] it may have been the promise of 'cure' that forced the development of asylum psychiatry. Undoubtedly, *some* anticipation of psychiatric cure existed, for at least some of the mental maladies. However, the new 'mad doctors' (as they were first called) needed a medical arena in which to work and, with the building of the public asylums they got it.

Scull's view is that asylums became appropriate places for the working classes to send relatives whose behaviour had rendered them unsuitable for family living, at a time when market economics was leading to a separation of home and workplace. So long as the insane needed to be looked after at home, they threatened the practicality of cottage industries. In support of his view, Scull[15] presents the *Lunacy Commissioners and Asylum Superintendents' Reports* for the 1890s that the asylums were populated by 'the impossible, the inconvenient and the inept'. Whereas the old madhouses had accommodated obvious cases of madness, the Victorian asylums housed a much broader clientele. Scull notes that in 1891 there were 15,853 institutionalized pauper lunatics in London but that this had increased to 26,293 by 1909. Since this sudden increase in hospital numbers could hardly reflect an increased incidence in mental illness the implication is that some form of 'social cleansing' was at play. The governing principle seems to be that whenever those in power restrict hapless, unproductive, people this probably represents

some coercive intent. If this interpretation is not to your liking, you can always subscribe to the more traditional view whose governing principle is that a Victorian faith prevailed, in which the mentally belligerent can be returned to normalcy through benevolence and the provision of programmes of mental hygiene. Walton[18] states that both views can cohere: there are examples of powerful magistrates and doctors incarcerating people so as to maintain social order but, equally, there are examples of relatives supplicating for such action to be taken, presumably in the 'best interests' of their relatives.

The nature of the beast

Although the 19th century asylums contained many that would today be diagnosed 'schizophrenic', the variation in cases was remarkable. Walton describes the case of 'Emma Blackburn, a 19-year-old, admitted to an asylum in 1871 after having been confined to Haslington workhouse for five months'. She was said to be suffering from 'political excitement' and the notes on her case are interesting:

> A fine healthy looking young woman, well nourished and of robust frame. Since admission has continued to shout and cry at intervals. Her countenance and eyes are much suffused. She does not occupy herself in any way and is occasionally quarrelsome. Frequently will not respond to questions put to her. Takes her food well but is restless at night.

Partly as a result of giving her morphine but also, I imagine, the sheer horror of her predicament, led to her deterioration and, after two years, she died. Such cases were hardly rare and although beliefs about women and madness varied across political and social dimensions (such as poverty), Elaine Showalter[19] states that:

> The prevailing view amongst Victorian psychiatrists was that … women were more vulnerable to insanity because the instability of their reproductive systems interfered with their sexual, emotional, and rational control.

Skultans[20] agrees saying that:

> women's reproductive role [was seen as] precluding her from intellectual activity which she engages in at the risk of insanity.

It is worth noting that emphasizing female anatomy and vulnerability increased, as women's demands for education – as well as their growing assertiveness about their historical social roles – was also increasing. It is also worth noting that the history of the confinement of women by a male oriented psychiatry is a neglected area of inquiry.

THE 1950s ONWARDS

From the 1950s, psychiatry painstakingly got its medical act together: concepts of pauper-lunatic were long gone and therapeutic zeal mushroomed. The eagerness to cure was practised along two different fronts. One of these was social in nature and was composed of two strands, namely therapeutic community 'proper' (typified by the work of Maxwell Jones at the Henderson Hospital) and a therapeutic community 'approach' reflected in less radical approaches concerning such things as unlocking doors and minimizing regimentation.[21]

A second front was the single-minded drive to unleash physical treatments that would halt mental illness once and for all. These two fronts could be complexly linked. For example, William Sargant – doyen of physical treatment methods – insisted that the advent of phenothiazine drugs sounded the death knell of the asylums since their administration allowed previously troublesome, withdrawn or disturbed patients to return to their families. Thus begins the mythical 'phenothiazine revolution', the supposed 'real' reason behind the unlocking of hospital doors and other liberal moves. In fact, the post-war period was more intricate than this with changing hospital practices coming about, for the most part, from changing attitudes towards mental illness and its causation. The sobering spectacle of soldiers going to war in (apparent) mental health and returning as psychological wrecks, suggested that mental illness could no longer be seen as, *necessarily*, a pathology of the nervous system. That mental illness could come about, or at least be mediated, by social events severely dented the role of asylums whose patients had traditionally been regarded as having the psychological status of inborn and irredeemable.

The shortfalls of benevolence

By the mid-20th century, the Victorian mental hospitals were becoming subject to criticism and review. David Clark,[22] medical superintendent at Fulbourn Hospital, split them into three groups:

❑ The first, influenced by therapeutic community principles, achieved a good level of care for their patients.
❑ A second, a much larger, group remained institutionalized but with a paternal/maternal approach and minimal punitiveness.

❑ The third group were 'the bins': large hospitals situated near cities, and operating at a low point of restrictive and punitive care.

Martin's 'Hospitals in Trouble'[23] chronicles the failures of this latter group as well as the abuses that they inflicted on patients. Writing in the 1950s, Johnson and Dodds reported[24] that:

> the attitudes of the hospital towards its patients is one of regarding them as unmitigated nuisances and undeserving malcontents (in Porter[6]).

The problem was partly the hospitals themselves. As Gittins[25] observes, 'class, gender and categorizing illness were literally built into the hospital infrastructure' (p. 5). Their architecture was closely linked to their function so that no matter how hard some enlightened staff might try to improve and encourage good care the institutions themselves affected the psychiatric practices, which occurred within them (see Scull,[15] Chapter 8). To this can be added the miseries of overcrowding and a demoralized nursing staff saddled with the thankless task of trying to contain ever-worsening situations while paying lip-service to notions of care and treatment. It says a lot about the human condition that, amidst sometimes fanatical regimentation, there exist innumerable stories of companionship between nurses and patients as well as, I suppose, the ultimate survival of most.

Confinement had always meant separating the sexes: eugenic fears of the mentally ill reproducing with abandon were always strong. At first sight, therefore, the abolition of separation in psychiatric wards (in favour of integration) always looked like progress. But it merely showed (again) how patients can be a means for the accomplishment of (ostensibly liberal) staff ends. Notwithstanding the serial humiliations of older people being placed in 'integrated' wards, this 1970s 'reform' went ahead anyway. It was well meant but, regrettably, the idea of asking patients what *they* might want was still some time off. The attitudes of these old people were rooted in an earlier (Edwardian) age and many were too polite, too circumspect to protest at the spectacle of their spouses being housed in mixed sex wards.

Into the community

If, over the years, the mental hospitals had weathered growing liberal condemnation, it was, at least, criticism that stemmed from professional and ethical concerns. By the 1970s, however, liberalism had become fair game for Thatcherite economics and the closure of expensive hospitals in favour of community care. The grossly precipitous implementation of community care, however, could only mean a shortfall of actual or efficient care; in fact, the 'plight' of the mentally ill under 'care in the community' became a sorry conclusion to a century that had started with such high hopes. Cataloguing community psychiatric grief is beyond the scope of this chapter, so I will focus on one or two aspects only.

Smith's outline[26] of assertive outreach shows how its initial intentions have quickly coalesced around primary concerns with medication and the professional difficulty of non-compliance. In Smith's view there has been:

> a re-emergence of old institutionally based ideas of biomedical illnesses requiring control, containment and, in particular pharmacological treatments – the very issues that led to 'learned helplessness' for so many people in asylums.

In effect, a therapeutic bureaucracy ensnares patients, so that their continued monitoring by professionals – their continued membership of the community – becomes contingent on complying with medication.

Hemming *et al.*,[27] concerned that the restrictive functions of assertive outreach might take hold in the public imagination, tried to provide a definitive (warmer) account of it but which, in its detail, matches Smith's foreboding. Hemming *et al.* describe a world where patients are a problem *per se*. They typically fail to comply with their treatments and are in need of *clinical* supervision, especially in relation to risk assessment. Associating the mentally ill with concepts of risk is part of a process of fixing them within a neighbourhood in such a way as to sustain the policing role of community psychiatric nurses.[28] Just as Bethlem had insisted that those of its inmates going begging in London's streets wear a tin badge fixed to their arm, so is this echoed in the maintenance of 'at-risk registers' of patients in the community, patients who may need to be quickly identified and treated either in their own abode or through re-confinement.

The Italian experience?

Beginning in the 1960s, a radical psychiatric movement called Psychiatrica Democratica (led by Franco Basaglia) forced the Italian government to formally legislate mental hospitals out of existence in 1978. The hospitals would be replaced by community services and reflected a marked reduction (or abolition) of medical influence. Influenced by the British therapeutic community movement, the Italian reformers were a more politicized group, Italian psychiatrists being less likely to deny the political and economic implications of their trade and its potential for institutional abuse. The impression created (in Britain) was that something truly radical had occurred in Italy and with much talk of its possible relocation to British hospitals.

The question quickly turned on what *had* occurred and how widespread the change was. Significantly, Professor Kathleen Jones re-emerged[29] to insist that the 'Italian Experience', as it had come to be known, was not all it seemed to be. The debate which followed revived much of the rhetoric and discourse of the past concerning the moral worth of psychiatry as a medical speciality. Professor Jones visited various centres in Italy and her reports contradicted those which had praised the Italian changes as revolutionary and widespread.[30] In fact, stated Jones,[29] the successful closure of mental hospitals had only happened at Trieste, with other centres only partially implementing community programmes because hindered by ongoing lack of resources. In some ways, Jones's account sobered up what had become accepted at face value whereas what actually was happening in Italy was more piecemeal and problematic. But Jones's account was more than this. Stung by the criticism that she favoured mental hospitals, but, more so, dismayed that the Italians exulted at the idea of hospital closure Professor Jones went on to reiterate her lifelong contention that 'what matters is the quality of care, not where they are housed'.[29] This, of course, misses the point because it *does* matter where psychiatry is practised: the architectural environment of psychiatric patients does encourage deterioration and stereotypical behaviour.

Trieste was the natural home of Italian reform and Jones praised it as a fascinating experiment in human relationships. She describes a carnival atmosphere combined with a refreshing rejection of professionalism with everybody on first name terms and everyday life replicated as far as possible. However, the problem, she believed, was that, by and large, the Trieste experiment was not replicated elsewhere other than in a watered down or half-hearted fashion. Also, some categories of patients, for example those with dementia, were excluded. Referring to an 'Italian Experience' was, says Jones, a major misnomer. This is a fair point but is a common mistake which Jones herself also makes when she refers to Britain's 'open door movement of the 1950s'.[29] The opening of doors was, as I have shown,[31] fairly patchy and hardly constituted a 'movement'.

In the long run, the ideas that propelled Italian radicalism are what matter because, in principle, the central criticism of psychiatry is its possession of unacknowledged political intent. The role of psychiatric dissidence is to critique psychiatry's rationale as much as the vagaries and mishaps of its actual practice. This is why criticism is viewed as intolerable by the psychiatric establishment. So Professor Jones ends her commentary on Trieste with references to 'frolic radicalism' as well as its appeal 'to the non-rational side of the human mind'. There is a stern warning that the Italians are not above confusing politics with the dispensation of psychiatry, added to which is the admonition that 'in a country with a Catholic heritage, symbols and dogma still have a considerable power'. The implication being, I suppose, that a dogma-free Britain – still less encumbered by symbols – is hardly the place for non-rational versions of psychiatry. Granted, British practitioners would hardly align themselves with political parties or even claim that their work was directly political. Yet few would deny that mental illnesses are managed within conventional (and typically under-examined) agreements of what constitutes the norms of mental health; norms that closely match what counts as acceptable social behaviour by the majority.

Psychiatric practices probably do not travel well – as current British difficulties with ethnic minority patients demonstrates – and what works in Trieste might not go down well in Tunbridge Wells. Nevertheless, *Psychiatrica Democratica* reminded us that psychiatry is still perceived in some quarters as a malevolent force, particularly when it ignores the political and economic dimensions of mental distress.

ACCOMMODATING LOSS

As we try to accommodate losing our mental hospitals, combinations of legal restrictions and concerns with 'non-compliance' echo older desires to confine 'the mad' whether for their own or society's good. The Victorians believed that their lunacy mansions were a solution; we came to dislike their *form* while continuing to respect their function. But these hospitals were the visible reminder of *our* repressive impulses and so we needed to devise less obtrusive ways to manage insanity, to devise systems with the power to treat when required and even if objected to by patients. Such objections, in any event, are transformed by psychiatrists to a symptomology, which can be over-ruled. To attribute legitimacy to such objections is seen as immoral and heartless; heartless, that is, not to treat the symptoms even when this requires preliminary confinement. Such confinement will henceforth rest more on community processed restrictions, such as at risk registers, assertive outreach programmes and compulsory treatments. As psychiatry becomes ever more medicalized and dependant on biotechnology, its self-assuredness may become less susceptible to incursions from non-medical thinking. To be fair, psychiatric radicals more often than not arise within psychiatry's own ranks but almost always as a reaction to psychiatry's capacity for, and inclination towards, reductionist thinking and benevolent coercion respectively.

And yet the insistence (and optimism) of psychiatric nurses on working therapeutically with patients is undiminished. This insistence is not misguided, nor is it cynical. It is an aspiration, which finds expression in a million and one encounters between nurses and patients. Regrettably, personal expressions of humanity have had to contend with a collective commitment which errs on the side of confinement if, in many cases, this is seen as a prerequisite to providing care. Even if, as has been argued,[28] a policing role is endemic to psychiatric nursing, it is the *regrettable and objectionable* necessity of that role, which should govern its expression. In psychiatry, confining people has become a daily activity so lacking in moral wakefulness as to be almost banal: the effect of a psychiatric diagnosis is to collapse any ethical doubts which might attend removing people's rights. Yet we know, from disparities in the diagnoses and confinement of ethnic minority groups, that psychiatric diagnosis is hardly a scientific activity. Perhaps confinement is a necessary prerequisite to caring and treating recalcitrant patients? If so, is it not wise, therefore, to keep the Trieste flag flying, to continue to be wary of a profession which, although largely benign in its intentions, confirms the marginalization of people nevertheless and which historically has made the denial of human freedoms a highly respectable activity.

REFERENCES

1. Allderidge P. Bedlam: fact or fantasy. In: Bynum WF, Porter R, Shepherd M (eds). *The anatomy of madness: essays in the history of psychiatry*, Vol. II. London: Tavistock Publications, 1985: 17–33.
2. Minutes of the court of governors of Bridewell and Bethlem. March 30th, 1677.
3. Cox JM. *Practical observations on insanity in which some suggestions are offered towards an improved mode of treating diseases of the mind to which are subjoined Remarks on medical jurisprudence as connected with diseased intellect*, 2nd edn. London: Baldwin and Murray, 1896.
4. Ackroyd P. *London: the biography*. London: Chatto and Windus, 2000.
5. Digby A. Moral treatment at the Retreat 1796–1846. In: Bynum WF, Porter R, Shepherd M (eds). *The anatomy of madness: essays in the history of Psychiatry*, Vol II. London: Tavistock Publications, 1985: 52–72.
6. Porter R. *The Faber book of madness*. Porter R (ed.) London: Faber & Faber, 1991.
7. Smith LD. *Cure comfort and safe custody*. London: Leicester University Press, 1999.
8. Porter R. *Mind-forg'd manacles*. Harmondsworth: Penguin Books, 1990.
9. Andrews J, Briggs A, Porter R. *The history of Bethlem*. London: Routledge, 1997.
10. Jones WL. *Ministering to minds diseased: a history of*

psychiatric treatment. London: William Heinemann Medical Books, 1983.

11. Winchester S. *The surgeon of Crowthorne: a tale of murder, madness and the Oxford English Dictionary*. London: Penguin Books, 1999.

12. Jones M. *The therapeutic community: a new treatment method in psychiatry*. New York: Basic Books, 1953.

13. Lindsay M. A critical view of the validity of the therapeutic community. *Nursing Times: Occasional Papers* 1982; **78**: 105–7.

14. Foucault M. *Madness and civilisation: a history of insanity in an age of reason* (Trans. R Howard). London: Tavistock Publications, 1967.

15. Scull A. *The most solitary of afflictions: madness and society in Britain, 1790–1990*. London: Yale University Press, 1993.

16. Shorter E. *A history of psychiatry: from the era of the asylum to the Age of prozac*. Chichester: John Wiley, 1997.

17. Jones K. The culture of the mental hospital. In: Berrios GE, Freeman H (eds). *150 years of British psychiatry 1841–1991*. London: Gaskell, 1991: 17–28.

18. Walton JK. Casting out and bringing back in Victorian England: pauper lunatics, 1840–70. In: Bynum WF, Porter R, Shepherd M (eds). *The anatomy of madness: essays in the history of psychiatry*, Vol II. London: Tavistock, 1985: 132–46.

19. Showalter E. *The female malady: women, madness and English culture, 1830–1980*. London: Virago Press, 1987.

20. Skultans V. *English madness: ideas on insanity 1580–1890*. London: Routledge and Kegan Paul, 1979.

21. Clark D. *Administrative therapy*. London: Tavistock, 1964.

22. Clark D (personal communication).

23. Martin JP. *Hospitals in trouble*. Oxford: Blackwell Science, 1984.

24. Johnson D, Dodds N. *The plea for the silent*. London: Christopher Johnston, 1957.

25. Gittins D. *Madness in its place: narratives of Severalls hospital, 1913–1997*. London: Routledge, 1998.

26. Smith M. Assertive outreach: a step backwards. *Nursing Times* 1999; **95**: 6–7.

27. Hemming M, Morgan S, O'Halloran P. Assertive outreach: implications for the development of the model in the United Kingdom. *Journal of Mental Health* 1999; **8**: 141–7.

28. Morrall P. *Mental health nursing and social control*. London: Whurr, 1998.

29. Jones K, Poletti A. The Italian experience reconsidered. *British Journal of Psychiatry* 1986; **148**: 144–50.

30. Rotelli F. Changing psychiatric services in Italy. In: Ramon S, Giannichedda MG (eds). *Psychiatry in transition: the British and Italian experiences*. London: Pluto Press, 1991.

31. Clarke L. The opening of doors in British mental hospitals in the 1950s. *History of Psychiatry* 1993; **iv**: 527–51.

Chapter 3

EVIDENCE-BASED PRACTICE IN MENTAL HEALTH CARE

Hugh McKenna*

INTRODUCTION

You meet some friends who you have not seen for some time. They are not health professionals and over a coffee they ask you what is 'new' in the field of mental health nursing. You mention that evidence-based practice is currently a popular phenomenon. When they ask you what this means you say that it involves providing people with care and treatment that is based on the most up to date knowledge. They look puzzled and ask: 'is this not something that nurses have *always* done?'

A member of your family is receiving psychiatric care and the treatment regime being used is out of date and possibly dangerous. Furthermore, the nurses have received no clinical updating or professional development in years and they do not appear to keep up to date through reading nursing journals. You also find out that your family member's treatment is quite different from that offered to patients with similar problems allocated to another team in the same region.

It is worrying that these scenarios reflect reality in many parts of the mental health nursing world. Someone somewhere today is receiving care or treatment that is out of date or that is not underpinned by sound evidence. If they perceive themselves as the patients' advocates, mental health nurses should be very concerned about this. People coming into care have clear legal and moral rights. One such right is to be cared for and treated in the best possible way within available resources. If the above scenarios are true reflections of reality, even in a small number of cases, then these nurses and these services are undermining the laws and moral codes at the foundations of the nursing profession.

Whether you go into McDonald's for a hamburger, or to Starbucks for a coffee, or drink Coca Cola, or have a Bushmills malt, you have a clear expectation before purchasing. You expect that the product will be of consistent quality. Similarly, you expect consistency regardless of whether you buy these products in Edinburgh, or Dunedin, in Belfast or Baltimore. But if you are admitted for psychiatric care the service may be different depending on who 'serves you' or where you are undergoing care. While one should not compare patients with commercial products, it could be argued that psychiatric care is also about providing a service and how we serve and what we serve should be underpinned by good evidence.

WHAT IS EVIDENCE IN PSYCHIATRIC-MENTAL HEALTH NURSING?

There are many definitions of evidence-based practice. Here are just some of them:

*Dr McKenna is Professor and Head of School of Nursing at the University of Ulster. He has 16 years experience in general and psychiatric nursing. He has over 100 publications, many of which relate to mental health care. He is married with two children and lives in Jordanstown, Northern Ireland.

- ❑ An approach to decision making in which the clinician uses the best evidence available.[1]
- ❑ Conscientious and judicious use of current best evidence in making decisions about the care of individual patients.[2]
- ❑ An approach to health care that promotes the collection, interpretation and integration of valid, important and applicable patient-reported, clinician-observed and research-derived evidence.[3]

There are various types and grades of evidence. The types relate to the robustness of the source of the evidence. The grades relate to how well you can trust a specific type of evidence. Many authors who write about evidence-based practice identify a hierarchy of evidence.[1,4] This hierarchy is illustrated in Table 3.1.

TABLE 3.1 Levels of evidence

■ **Level I**	meta-analysis of multiple randomized controlled trials (RCTs)
■ **Level II**	experimental studies (at least one)
■ **Level III**	well-designed, quasi-experimental studies
■ **Level IV**	well-designed non-experimental studies (comparative, correlational, descriptive, case studies)
■ **Level V**	case reports, clinical examples

Strength of evidence

You will notice that this hierarchy of evidence is influenced by a particular philosophy of science (see Table 3.2). Level I evidence is perceived clearly to be the best possible evidence. It has its basis in the positivist tradition of quantitative research designs.[5] The same goes for Level II and Level III. While Level IV could incorporate some qualitative designs, what are really being referred to are large quantitative surveys. Interestingly Level V is probably the most important level for psychiatric-mental health nursing yet it comes bottom of the hierarchy.

TABLE 3.2 Strength of evidence

A	Level I evidence or consistent findings across Levels II, III or IV
B	Consistent findings from Levels II, III, or IV
C	Evidence of Levels II, III, or IV; findings inconsistent
D	Little or no evidence or Level V only
E	Panel consensus; opinion of experts

In the foreword to the textbook *Mental Health Nursing: An Evidence-Based Approach*, Goldberg asserts that 'well conducted meta analyses are probably the best that we can present and are certainly preferable to the rules of thumb of eminent practitioners however distinguished they may be'.[6]

This above hierarchy is useful but it has inherent problems that are not always addressed.[7] For instance, evidence databases can be incomplete; publication biases affect what is available in the literature and the emphasis on randomized control trials (RCTs) skews information because it is relevant only to patient populations included in the trials and may not match the people who nurses see in daily practice. Therefore, while the hierarchy of evidence has some strengths, it has several weaknesses. It might be more useful for psychiatric-mental health nurses if turned upside down (see Table 3.3).

TABLE 3.3 How nurses might evaluate evidence

■	**Level I**	Nurses' experiences
■	**Level II**	Patient preferences and narrative accounts
■	**Level III**	Opinion and views of experts
■	**Level IV**	The results of qualitative studies and quality improvement/audit activities
■	**Level V**	The results of quantitative research

But how do you decide whether a patient's narrative account should come above or below the experience of nurses? It depends on circumstances and for some situations the preference of patients would be paramount but for others evidence at a different level would be better. Similarly, a qualitative researcher would have difficulty constructing a hierarchy of evidence. How would you decide whether to place grounded theory above feminist methodology, phenomenology or ethnography? Hierarchies seem to belong to the world of positivism, where scientists have always pursued the goal of classification and categorization.

What is clear from many of the articles and books written about evidence-based practice in health care is that word of mouth or observations are not regarded as good evidence.[4] This is not the case in all professions. In the legal profession such evidence is highly valued and includes circumstantial evidence (indirect evidence affording a certain presumption) and the testimony of witnesses. Here word of mouth or observed behaviour is accepted and is sufficient to put a person in jail or in some countries to be executed. In contrast, such sources are denigrated in most textbooks and articles about evidence-based practice in nursing.

Evidence is also a victim of time. What was evidence last year may not be evidence this year. Perhaps at one time there was evidence that prefrontal lobotomies or insulin coma therapy were perceived as good ways of controlling some psychiatric symptomatology. In the last century continuously spinning patients in specially constructed chairs or harnesses was thought to cure certain psychiatric illnesses. Today, such interventions would be perceived as barbaric. I have no doubt that in fifty years time, therapies currently used as best evidence will be disparaged. It is always dangerous to crystal ball gaze, but I suspect electroconvulsive therapy (ECT) will be one of these, as will the use of major tranquillizers.

To bring this section to a close, it can be stated that what *is* and *is not* evidence is fluid and relies as much on timing and choice as it does on methodology. The rule of thumb should be that it is not the best possible evidence that is required, it is the best available at a particular time for a specific patient in a specific situation. This means that in some situations the patient's preference will be the best evidence while in others it may be the results of an RCT. In other words different kinds of evidence have different uses in different contexts.

After reading this you might be forgiven for thinking that everything is evidence in one form or another. To some extent this is true but evidence-based practice does undermine ritualistic, routine and traditional behaviours and ungrounded opinions as a basis for nursing intervention. Indeed, it highlights the importance of consensus among recognized experts, confirmed experiences and patient accounts as well as research findings and quality improvement data.

How do practitioners access 'best' evidence?

The search for evidence normally begins with a question. For instance, a nurse working with older people with dementia may ask if reminiscence therapy is effective in caring for her patients. To seek an answer to this question they may simply ask one of their colleagues who has used this therapy effectively (or seen it used effectively) in other settings. Alternatively, the nurse may have to search for the answer to her question elsewhere, and this takes time and effort. If the nurse is lucky enough to have access to the Internet she may be able to peruse databases such as the Centre for Reviews and Dissemination or Cochrane Collaboration Centre (see Appendix 3.1). She may also access publications such as *Evidence-based Nursing* or *Evidence-based Mental Health*, which provides evidence in bite size user-friendly synopses. If she still cannot find any evidence it does not mean that it does not exist. She may decide to browse through hundreds of journal articles or textbooks looking for relevant information. To do this she needs time and a well-stocked library near her place of work or home.

The *British Medical Journal* publishes a compendium of the best available evidence for effective health care. The fifth issue of this compendium (June 2001 available on CD-ROM) had the following entries: Alzheimer's disease, bulimia nervosa, depressive disorders, generalized anxiety disorder, obsessive compulsive disorder, post traumatic stress disorder, and schizophrenia. However, the philosophy underpinning these entries tends towards the positivist hierarchy of evidence alluded to earlier. Nonetheless, the nurse may find her answer there: it indicates that there was insufficient evidence on the effects of reminiscence therapy[8] and music therapy on people with dementia. She also notes that there is evidence that reality orientation improves cognitive function and behaviour compared with no treatment.[9]

Increasingly, publications on evidence-based practice are taking into account sources other than RCTs. For instance, *Evidence-based Mental Health* has changed considerably since it was first published in 1998. Most of the papers at that time were based on the results of RCTs and other quantitative studies. However, in 2000 it began to include evidence that emanated from qualitative studies and from quality improvement activities. In the November 2000 issue the results of a qualitative study on the experiences of seclusion were published as were the results of a quality improvement project that showed the benefits of physician feedback plus telephone care management, on people with depression.

Do nurses always use best evidence?

It seems logical that if we possess knowledge about the best way to practise we should use it to improve patient care. Although it might appear heretical, this is not the case. Evidence may be a necessary but it is not a sufficient condition to change practice. There may be many reasons why practising psychiatric-mental health nurses do not use evidence, even though they possess it.[10] There may be issues relating to cost, for to be clinically effective does not necessarily mean we will be cost effective. It could be morally reprehensible to use a costly intervention on one individual patient when for the same cost we could care for or treat many individuals. Our conscience or religion could also be reasons for not using best evidence. While electroconvulsive therapy may be effective for acute depression,[9] some nurses may decide to ignore this evidence and choose not to participate in this treatment. Patients too may decide that they do not wish to be treated in a specific way even though the proposed intervention is founded on the best available evidence.

In essence, psychiatric-mental health nurses, at their best, must be knowledgeable about the various sources of evidence available to them and they must participate with the patient and others in making the best decision for a specific problem in a specific context. This requires a high level of competency and not one that comes easy to novices. Like all skills it must be learned through practice and study.

Is evidence-based practice a managerial and educational straitjacket for practitioners?

Evidence-based medicine has been criticized as leading to a 'cookbook' kind of medicine where individual practitioner judgement is downgraded and the doctor has to adhere slavishly to the dictates of distant researchers who have provided an evidence-based guideline.[2] To veer from the guideline could be interpreted as ignoring the best available information on which to base an intervention. It is not beyond the bounds of possibility that patients and their families could sue a doctor who has ignored clinical guidelines. Could a patient instigate litigation against a psychiatric nurse because the nurse based an intervention on her experience rather than on a research based guideline emanating from a university department? If this were commonplace then positive risk-taking and innovation would be severely curtailed to the detriment of the nursing profession. In this regard the evidence would be a straitjacket and would stifle practice.

Sackett used the phrase 'judicial use of evidence'.[2] This suggests that the professional judgement of the practising nurse based on confirmed experience could lead to best evidence not being used. Like most professional people, nurses have always had to take such decisions. However, nursing as a discipline can often be guilty of 'paralysis through analysis' where academic arguments pervaded the journals on whether models are theories or conceptual frameworks or whether standards are guidelines or criteria. Nonetheless, regardless of what the books and articles dictated, practising nurses had to make decisions on how useful was the model or theory when they were assessing patients and how useful was the prescribed standard when they were assessing quality of care. This must also be the case with evidence-based practice. While I have spent half of this chapter delving into what is and what is not evidence, hard pressed practising nurses must get on with caring for and with patients in the most effective way possible. As a principle, the judicial use of evidence ensures that the nurse is not detracted from patient care by a slavish adherence to research-based guidelines.

How can psychiatric-mental health nurses use evidence in a meaningful way?

It has already been stressed that psychiatric-mental health nurses must be aware of new evidence. To be in this position they must keep abreast of the latest developments and thinking in mental health care, but this is just the first step. They also have to weigh the evidence and be convinced that it will work in the setting or situation confronting them. Once this has been agreed with colleagues, patients and/or their families, the most difficult part of using evidence emerges. The use of new evidence requires change, which can be difficult and threatening: in most cases it also requires extra resources.

Take the example of a psychiatric-mental health nurse who works with children and adolescents. She reads relevant journals on a regular basis, scans appropriate research databases on the Internet, attends relevant conferences and discusses innovations with her multidisciplinary colleagues. She comes across an article showing that cognitive behaviour therapy relieves the symptoms of depression in adolescents.[11] She discusses with her colleagues whether this would be effective with a specific group of young people currently in her care. There is consensus that it could be beneficial and so she discusses its use with the young people and their families. Even when agreement has been reached the therapy cannot begin. Those using it will have to be trained and the means of evaluating its effectiveness will have to be agreed. It is also possible that this change in practice could bring initial unease for the adolescent or for professional colleagues who favour another therapeutic approach. This example shows that seeking, sifting, using and evaluating new evidence is not a straightforward task. While one can see how some nurses would feel more comfortable with routine and ritual, psychiatric-mental health nursing has to grow and develop and the pursuit of appropriate best evidence is a moral responsibility for any professional nurse worthy of that title.

What are the barriers to using best evidence in mental health care?

According to the Oxford English Dictionary a barrier 'is an obstacle that bars progress and success and prevents communication'.[12] A range of barriers to research application is slowing down the progress and effectiveness of psychiatric-mental health nursing.

A 1997 Australian study identified the entrenched attitudes of practising psychiatric-psychiatric-mental health nurses as being the single most significant barrier to their use of research findings.[13] Ignoring evidence and basing practice on tradition has immense benefits for some practitioners: they don't have to question why or how they practise; they feel comfortable with routines, which were often learned from an authority figure and such routines have universality because everybody appears to do it that way. Routines are often a mechanism for keeping control in a busy clinical area where there were unpredictable and ever changing conditions and where staff are forever altering in numbers and qualifications. Encouraging evidence-based practice in such a setting is not seen as a priority.

A positive correlation has been found between the adoption of evidence into practice and nurses' reading of journals.[14] In a US study it was found that practising psychiatric-psychiatric-mental health nurses did not read research.[15] It appeared that since they did not develop the habit of reading these type of articles during training, it followed that because of increased responsibilities and pressures, they were unlikely to start once qualified. Tisdale argues that this is a major barrier to applying evidence in practice.

However, the notion that if clinical nurses read and uncover evidence they will begin to use it and change their practice accordingly does not take into account what is in reality a complex change process. Nurses are no different from other people and evidence is not seen as an adequate reason for changing their behaviour. There are many research papers on the dangers of fatty foods and smoking but many people ignore this evidence.

In one study, most of the respondents saw lack of management commitment as the greatest barrier to research utilization.[14] This was supported by results from an Australian study which showed that senior mental health managers do not perceive research as a core element in the provision of nursing services.[13] It is a truism that in a setting with competing demands no one is really going to believe that research is truly important unless the boss makes it important.[16]

According to findings from a UK study, managerial perceptions can act as an important barrier to evidence-based practice.[17] It was found that rigorous and systematic research activities are still considered by UK managers to be inappropriate and incompatible with good nursing and a direct threat to the very essence of nursing.

It is well documented that senior clinical nurses were often products of a system that fostered unconditional obedience and an unquestioning disposition towards their role. Traditionally, students who asked too many questions were often perceived as troublemakers and ended up being sent to the so-called 'back wards' – traditional practice wanted obedience, not enquiry. This has implications for the search for and use of best evidence. For instance, in the UK it was found that patient interventions often reflect what the practitioner remembers from their formal training rather than on current best knowledge.[18]

Psychiatric-mental health nurses must question practice continually and take chances with new knowledge and this must be perceived as a legitimate use of their time. Evidence-based decision-making must be incorporated into the organization's culture rather than being superimposed upon it.

Most psychiatric-mental health nursing courses today have modules on evidence-based practice and these place emphases on students being able to search for evidence, critique it and analyse its possible effects. These are laudable objectives. However, being evidence aware and being able to critique the commoner methods used to obtain evidence is fine but the students may still not be motivated to base their practice on such evidence, or to encourage others to do so. In other words the skills required to find and assess best evidence are being taught in splendid isolation from the skills required to use it in practice.

Educators must ensure that this generation and the next generation of psychiatric-mental health nurses are advanced practitioners – who use sound and relevant evidence to inform their practice. Educational programmes on the **4As** should be the norm: these are being able to *appreciate*, to *access*, to *appraise* and *apply* best evidence.

In 1997 I used an adapted form of Funk's Barriers to Research Utilization Tool to collect data from 71 psychiatric-psychiatric-mental health nurses who work in Ireland.[19] Demographic details indicated that 37% were community-based, 33% worked in long-term settings and 26% in acute care settings. Forty-two per cent were senior nurse managers, 32% were charge nurses/ward sisters and 26% were staff nurses. While 49% were currently enrolled on education programmes, only two of the 71 respondents held a bachelor's degree and one had a master's degree.

The average number of barriers identified per respondent was 17. Part of the study entailed them being asked to identify the top three barriers. These were:

1 Insufficient time on the job to implement new ideas.

2 Other staff are not supportive.

3 The nurse does not see the value of research in practice.

I compared clinical nurses' responses with those of managers and noted some key differences. Although both groups perceived time as a barrier, practitioners tended to see lack of management commitment to be a major barrier. In contrast, nurse managers identified a major barrier to be the unwillingness of the nurse to change and try out new ideas. These results reflect the findings of other studies in the USA[15] and Australia.[13]

CONCLUSION

No reasonable person would deny that people who have mental health problems should be cared for and treated using interventions that are based on the best available evidence. While the ability to produce evidence is restricted to a small number of individuals in most professions, the knowledge of how to search for it, assess it, disseminate it and apply it in practice must be a major part of the mind set for every psychiatric-mental health nurse. The mere existence of evidence cannot alter the care of patients; it has to be used.

A note of caution though: psychiatric-mental health nurses should not apply evidence in an unquestioning manner. The thoughtless or inappropriate use of evidence may do a great deal of harm and may become just as much a ritual as the habitual acceptance of traditional routines.

Psychiatric-mental health nurses are still individually accountable to the public for the delivery of high quality care and for seeking ways to improve that care through evidence-based practice. Therefore, to look favourably on the use of evidence is to look favourably on quality of patient care. This means the willingness to accept that our favourite views and practices may be wrong. Alvin Toffler wrote, 'The illiterate of the 21st century will not be those who cannot read and write, but those who cannot learn, unlearn, and relearn'.[20]

REFERENCES

1. Muir Gray JA. *Evidence-based healthcare: how to make health policy and management decisions.* New York: Churchill Livingstone, 1997.
2. Sackett DL, Richardson WS, Rosenberg W, Haynes RB. *Evidence-based medicine: how to practice and teach EBM.* New York: Churchill Livingstone, 1997.
3. McKibbon KA, Walker CJ. Beyond ACP Journal Club: how to harness Medline for therapy problems [Editorial]. *Annals of Internal Medicine (ACP Journal Club Supplement 1)* 1994; **121**: A10.
4. Newell R, Gournay K (eds). *Mental health nursing: an evidence-based approach.* Edinburgh: Churchill Livingstone, 2000.
5. McKenna HP. *Models and theories of nursing.* London: Routledge, 1997.
6. Goldberg D, Foreword. In: Newell R, Gournay K. *Mental health nursing: an evidence-based approach.* Edinburgh: Churchill Livingstone, 2000.
7. Ridsdale L (ed.) *Evidence-based practice in primary care.* Edinburgh: Churchill Livingstone, 1998.
8. Spector A, Orrell M. *Reminiscence therapy for dementia.* Cochrane Library Issue 3, Oxford, 2000.
9. *Clinical evidence: a compendium of the best available evidence for effective healthcare.* London: British Medical Journal Publications, 2001.
10. McKenna HP, Cutliffe J, McKenna P. Evidence-based practice: demolishing some myths. *Nursing Standard* 2000; **14**(16): 39–42.
11. Harrington R, Whittaker J, Shoebridge P, Campbell F. Systematic review of efficacy of cognitive behaviour therapies in childhood and adolescent depressive disorder. *British Medical Journal* 1998; **316**: 1559–63.
12. OED. *The Oxford English dictionary.* Oxford: OUP, 1986.
13. Deans C, Lea D, Geyer R. Nursing research 'down under'. *Journal of Psycho-social Nursing* 1997; **35**(2): 25–31.
14. Funk SG, Champagne MT, Wiese RA, Tornquist EM. Barriers: the barriers to research utilisation scale. *Applied Nursing Research* 1991; **4**: 39–45.
15. Tisdale NE, Williams-Bernard CL, Moore PA. Attitudes, activities and involvement in nursing research among psychiatric-psychiatric-mental health nurses in a public sector facility. *Issues in Mental Health Nursing* 1997; **18**: 365–75.
16. Funk SG, Tornquist EM, Champagne MT. Barriers and facilitators of research utilisation. *Nursing Clinics of North America* 1995; **30**(3): 395–407.
17. Hicks C. The dilemma of incorporating research into clinical practice. *British Journal of Nursing* 1997; **6** (9): 511–15.
18. Hynes BR, Sackett DL, Grey JMA, Cook DJ, Guyatt GH. Transferring evidence from research into practice: 1. *Evidence-based Medicine* 1996; **1**(7): 196–7.
19. McKenna HP. *Barriers to using evidence in mental health nursing.* Unpublished report. University of Ulster, 1997.
20. Toffler A. *Future shock.* New York: Random House Publications, 1970.

APPENDIX 3.1

Useful websites

1 www.shef.ac.uk/~scharr/ir/netting/menu.html
Netting the Evidence Resource Guide from the University of Sheffield.

2 www.nelh.nhs.uk
National Electronic Library for Health

3 www.nlm.nih.gov/nichsr/nichsr.html
National Information Centre on Health

4 www.york.ac.uk/inst/crd/welcome.htm
NHS Centre for Reviews and Dissemination at the University of York

5 www.shef.ac.uk/~nhcon/
Nursing and Healthcare Resources on the Internet

6 www.omni.ac.uk
The UK's Gateway to high quality health information

7 www.jr2.ox.ac.uk/bandolier
Evidence-based Journal (Bandolier)

8 http://hiru.mcmaster.ca/acpjc/default.htm
ACP Journal Club (Canada)

9 www.ahcpr.gov/
Agency for Healthcare Research and Development

10 www.nurseresearcher.com
Canadian Nurse Researcher Database

11 www.public-health.org.uk/casp/
Critical Appraisal Skills Programme (CASP)

12 www.evidence.org/homepage.htm
Clinical Evidence Journal Homepage

13 www.cma.ca/cpgs/index.asp
Clinical Practice Guidelines Info-base

14 www.update-software.com/clibhome/clib.htm
Cochrane Library

15 http://nhscrd.york.ac.uk/
NHS Centre for Reviews Databases

16 www.fons.org
Foundation of Nursing Studies Homepage

17 http://hebw.uwcm.ac.uk
Health Evidence Bulletins (Wales)

18 www.windsor.igs.net/~nhodgins/literature_searches.html
Online literature search workshop

19 www.healthatoz.com/
Health A to Z resource guide

20 www.n-i.nhs.uk/crest/index.htm
CREST Guidelines (N.I.)

21 www.doh.gov.uk/ntrd/chain/chain.htm
CHAIN Contacts, Help, Advice and Information Network

22 www.man.ac.uk/rcn
RCN R&D Co-ordinating Centre

23 www.nice.org.uk/pics/new_uk.ipg
NICE Homepage

24 www.healthgate.co.uk
Health Gate UK Homepage (Healthcare Databases)

25 www.guideline.gov/STATIC/whatsnew.guide/asp
National Guideline Clearing House (Index of Guidelines)

26 www.shef.ac.uk/uni/projects/facts/
FACTS Framework for Appropriate Care Throughout Sheffield

27 http://libsun1.jr2.ox.ac.uk/prise/
PRISE Primary Care Sharing the Evidence

Chapter 4

THE CRAFT OF PSYCHIATRIC–MENTAL HEALTH NURSING PRACTICE

Peter Wilkin*

> You have made fair hands, you and your crafts! You have crafted fair!
>
> William Shakespeare, Coriolanus, Scene VI

INTRODUCTION

It is your first day on the ward. You are suddenly approached by a middle-aged man who, seconds ago, was a complete stranger to you. His face is fixed, creased with overwhelming concern. He addresses you, although his eyes do not, with the words: 'I did but taste a little honey with the end of the rod that was in mine hand, and, lo, I must die'[a]. Slowly, his gaze rises until it meets your own. His eyes project his pain, his hopelessness and his guilt. What do you say? What do you do? How can you engage him as he begins to turn away from you, already tried and convicted by the internal demons that persecute him? How do you craft your nursing response to this man who is hell-bent on scripting his own crucifixion?

The answer, of course, is that there is no right answer – although a thousand 'experts', if pressed, would undoubtedly offer a thousand possible responses: some remarkably similar, yet all slightly different. Such hypothetical dilemmas, neatly constructed within the black-and-white of the scholarly text, can only ever lift the curtain on any psychiatric episode. If such an incident were to unfold before your eyes as a psychiatric-mental health nurse it would be loaded with unique possibilities too numerous to imagine. This leads us to ask, 'how can any nurse hope to master (sic) a craft when the materials that make up each psychiatric situation are never the same?'

Psychiatric-mental health nursing is primarily 'being' and 'becoming' with people who are suffering (either directly or indirectly as carers) the effects of mental dis-ease and distress. It does not – should not – involve working out people's problems and finding solutions for them. To do so would be to invalidate the person's experiences, robbing him of his right to navigate his own recovery.[1] For much of the time, psychiatric-mental health nursing is about 'not knowing' and tolerating the anxiety that this emptiness generates within us. It can be compared to what Keats[2] described as 'negative capability': an ability to tolerate 'uncertainties, mysteries, doubts, without any irritable reaching after fact and reason'. Your willingness to 'be'

*Peter Wilkin is the Primary Mental Health Service Leader in Rochdale and Clinical Supervision Module Leader at Manchester Metropolitan University. His professional priorities are the welfare and development of his colleagues and the personal growth of psychiatric service users. His therapeutic approach is conversational, combining pragmatism with unconditional regard.

[a] In the bible Jonathan uttered this as a response to his father, Saul's, proclamation of death upon the person who had incurred God's wrath upon his army. (Following investigation, this turned out to be Jonathan himself, who had unwittingly broken the fast that his father had imposed.) It seemed to be an incredibly harsh sentence (which was, indeed, eventually revoked) passed out of bitterness for a very minor misdemeanour. *1 Samuel, XIV, verse 43*.

(to stay with), rather than 'do' (or flee) during such situations transmits a valuable message to the other. You are saying, non-verbally: 'I have the time, the patience and the commitment to journey with you through your distress; I am genuinely interested in you'. The psychiatric-mental health nurse must function from within a developmental stage that never ends: she must become good enough to forge therapeutic alliances with most of the people, most of the time, and to tolerate and learn from those inevitable occasions when she does not.

With this vital premise constantly in mind, our brief passage together through this chapter becomes a journey of purpose. We shall gather together the raw materials that enable us, as psychiatric-mental health nurses, to practice our craft as life-long learners and eternal students, being taught by those who always know better than us – our patients.[3]

CRAFTING OUR PRACTICE

Rather than explaining psychiatric-mental health nursing as an art or a science, Barker[4] offers us a more relationship-based interpretation which echo's Peplau's[5] philosophy of interpersonal relations. Truly collaborative caring, he believes, is based on an implied 'contractual relationship' between the psychiatric-mental health nurse and the person being nursed. It is a 'craft of caring' that focuses upon the human development of people in mental distress. Choosing to accept psychiatric-mental health nursing as a craft may imply that we must reject either scientific or artistic contributions towards the creation of our product (whatever that might be). That is not so. The psychiatric-mental health nurse 'needs to speak, however hesitantly, two different and yet related languages: the language of science and the language of art'[6] to form a feelings language – 'a language of the heart'.[7]

Any occupation that is predominantly relationship-based must rely heavily on the social sciences to explore the human factors that might inform future practice (e.g. how do some people respond to a particular approach in a given situation?). Similarly, breaking down a particular therapeutic approach into structured stages of application helps the psychiatric-mental health nurse adopt this technology and achieve a level of competency in its application. The same can be said of art, whereby the nurse's artistic interventions figure prominently within the caring relationship. In the broadest sense, many psychiatric-mental health nurses have integrated the 'arts' into their practice as alternative pathways towards personal growth and emotional healing (painting, music, dance, drama, storytelling). And if we were to break down psychiatric-mental health nursing into its component parts, we would surely acknowledge the art of conversation, as we ' "spontaneously" choose words, expressions and gestures that express ... forms of feeling'.[8]

Yet the application of science and technical skills, blended together with the creativity of conversational brush strokes, does not constitute the whole of our craft. Technical knowledge, or skill, must always be wrapped with ethical knowledge to deliver a response that fits each individual. The guiding principles that form our belief systems will always need to be modified to fit the unique circumstances that we, as psychiatric-mental health nurses, encounter. This process of application is even more complex when one realises that every nursing intervention can be influenced by the history, tradition, race, culture, gender and faith of both the nurse and the other, who is the 'patient'. These are the incalculable 'ifs' that govern all our actions. Who will tell us, for example, that prudence may be the best nursing response, at any given moment: where prudence may be a word, a gesture, a procedure – or even a retreat? Scientific theory and technical artistry may inform practice, but cannot deliver it. Only we, as psychiatric-mental health nurse practitioners, are capable of deciding 'where to go' in any given psychiatric situation. And it is only having reached a particular therapeutic destination (which always is unique) that we can say, in retrospect, how we came to be there.

The craft of caring involves a person-centred agenda that sits surrounded by a consideration of the 'whole'. The psychiatric-mental health nurse needs to view the psychiatric situation with maximum depth of field, whilst focusing sharply on the eyes of the other. It is a craft that relies heavily upon a pragmatic approach to caring akin to Bergson's 'le bon sens'[b]. Rather than searching for explanations, a pragmatist tries to identify how best to cope with and respond to a particular set of circumstances.[9] Yet such pragmatism nestles safely beneath warming blankets of training, experience and a desire to do no harm. It is no 'bootstrap theory', but rather is a moving vehicle from which to see the situation from many different perspectives.

Every psychiatric moment begins for the nurse as she tries to make some sense of a situation. It is a naïve and

---

[b] *Le Bon Sens* was a term used by the French Philosopher, Henri Bergson, to describe a form of 'common sense'. Contrary to scientific dogma, 'Le Bon Sens' advocates a combination of tactfulness, morality and human relationship as the primary guiding principles towards human relating. It is cited in: Gadamer H-G. *Truth and method*, 2nd edn. London: Sheed and Ward, 1989, p. 26. Unfortunately, the original paper is only available in French. Bergson H. *Écrits et paroles*. Paris: Presses Universitaires de France, 1957: 84–94.

muted picture that she sees; a hastily drawn sketch that can only gain colour and form through the other – the experiences of the person who is 'patient'. A genuine understanding of the other can only dawn through him and his view of the world. We must pay attention to the other and create conversations that are inspired through him. He is always the leader and the instigator of 'the glory of discovery'.[10] He alone holds the key to the craft-work cupboard. Unless the nurse consults him and looks at life from his viewing gallery, she will fashion an object that is precious only to herself. The craft of caring is always dependent upon the other, whose own personal growth becomes a catalyst for the incidental development of the nurse.

Creating conditions for growth and development

The concept of emotional or spiritual growth is ambiguous and difficult to measure. Unlike the fruit on the tree, the human being shows no external signs of psychological ripening. Yet the ethereal nature of personal growth is quantifiable beyond all reasonable doubt merely through verbal confirmation. People tell us, through their stories, of the growth taking place within them. If we listen 'actively'[c] we will hear those words that signify human growth and change. Such statements usually demonstrate greater understandings, clearer pictures, changed perspectives and a more positive sense of self. The craft of psychiatric-mental health nursing involves modifying the climate of the caring relationship to bring about 'the necessary conditions for the promotion of growth and development'.[11]

A person once described to me her grief. It was 'paralysing' and made her feel 'dead inside'. When we finally parted company, she was feeling 'released' and 'able to get on with living'. This common theme of disablement surfaces in various guises, irrespective of the mental trauma. It is the part of the problem that enervates and pervades one's being as drizzling grey rain, lethal black ice or demoralizing mirages.

When these disabling emotions begin to subside, the person becomes able to channel her intent and energies outwards once more. The rutted winter months of distress begin to melt away and new shoots of purpose slowly begin to surface. This healing process – this period of growth by way of understanding and discovery of more fruitful ways of living – is all part and parcel of the nurse–other alliance. The opportunity to

grow through and with the other is just as much an option for the psychiatric-mental health nurse as her partner. What a privilege to practise a craft that enables us to set sail each working day on a voyage of 'becoming with'.

Becoming with the other: a journey of togetherness

'Becoming with' means picking up the tempo of the other and joining with by joining in. It is a tune called and conducted by the other. The role of the psychiatric-mental health nurse is to identify the melody and harmonize accordingly. Sometimes, this is a conscious process, where the nurse pays attention to the messages being broadcast by the other. Guided by her feelings, she works out her best responses to the emotional pain and distress of the other.

From my own lived experiences as a psychiatric-mental health nurse, I find myself firstly enveloped by certain feelings during this process. These feelings, generated by the other, become my guiding light through a formulatory process that involves a conversation within myself. I begin to ask myself, if I were this 'other', I mean *really* were this particular other, what would I be feeling or believing now? Walsh[12] calls this process of understanding 'shared humanity': a 'being-in-the-world-with-patients' that 'makes the ordinary extraordinarily effective in helping patients'. Gradually, I begin to check out just how close I am to understanding with the other. I begin to put together a hypothesis that I can tentatively share: 'So, I'm not too sure, yet, but I wonder if . . . ?' A furrowed brow, a considered sigh and a moment's hesitation all signify that I have further to travel before I can bathe in the warm glow of that shared understanding. Often, the response from the other is silent and deafening: the sudden eye contact that speaks louder than any words: 'Oh! You've touched my heart'; the rocking motion that says: 'You're getting close, too close right now – back off!'; the body that suddenly switches to a different frequency with inaudible voices that do not speak to me, is the body that transmits a signal telling me I have been tuned out.

At other times the psychiatric-mental health nurse will become oblivious to her own otherness. She will have crossed the threshold of conscious separation and joined the other person in all but body. She will see no colour on the walls, no curtains at the windows, no features on the face of the other. She has temporarily ceased to be aware of her own existence and plunged

---

[c] 'Active Listening' was coined by Gerard Egan, and describes the total presence of the listener. As well as attending to the verbal content, active listening includes non-verbal behaviour, hearing the words in the context of the person's whole life situation and, finally, the 'spin' that the speaker puts on her story. Egan G. *The skilled helper: a problem-management approach to helping*, 6th edn. USA: Brooks/Cole, 1998.

into the wholeness of togetherness. In Buber's[13] terms, this has become an *I–Thou* moment: a potential space of exclusivity where man (sic) steps 'out of the glowing darkness of chaos, into the cool light of creation'. As the psychiatric nurse plies her craft, it is always *with* the other.

Those magic I–Thou moments are inevitably swathed in blissful ignorance – and can only be acknowledged by reflective after-light. I can recall my own such experiences of subliminal togetherness, best described, perhaps, as spiritual confluence, devoid of any doing – pure becoming. Such therapeutic closeness, to my mind, is artless metaphor untempered by and defiant of theoretical reduction. It is beautiful knowing that cannot be explained but can be completely understood through experience. As Keats[14] so elegantly wrote, 'Beauty is truth, truth beauty – that is all ye know on earth and all ye need to know'.

Collaborative healing

Somewhere within this I–Thou alliance exists the spiritual dimension of healing: a collaboration of the two 'others' that defies and always will defy any analysis. Indeed, the merest attempt to explain separates us from this process like the sudden roar of the outboard motor kills the joy of the tranquil loch. The only theoretical device capable of carrying the spiritual component of nursing is metaphor, which is born out of experience. When I grope and feel my way towards such experiences, which lie within my own nursing practice, I can recall heart-melting moments of spiritual togetherness. Hobson,[15] in his own inimitable style, offers his own interpretation for those sublime, spiritual moments between two people in therapy: 'aloneness-togetherness' … 'an imaginative activity which discloses the possibility of creating a kind of loving that lies within and between persons'.

Collaborative caring is the journey of two fellow (sic) travellers 'into the flow of life'.[16] Only when people step into the life-stream together are they able to make sense of what it is to feel hard pebbles under their feet, or the cool rush of noisy water against their skin. Making sense of things reduces fear and introduces new possibilities, new options, and new ways of being. The road ahead is cleared of debris and despondency gives way to hope. Without hope, there can be no wind change and, indeed, no 'X' on 'the treasure map of the territory of care'.[17] When the chains of emotional distress prove just too heavy, it is the psychiatric-mental health nurse who offers the 'tender leaves of hope' by showing a genuine belief in the other.

To offer hope, the psychiatric-mental health nurse must trust and believe in the other without reservation.

Perhaps this is her most challenging responsibility? Or perhaps not? Benner[18] suggests that 'Nurses establish a healing relationship and create a healing climate by mobilizing hope in themselves … and the patient'. Having faith in our selves constitutes the very first step, as we journey through the rivers of distress with the other. Each subsequent step is taken in tandem with that other person until the banks of the river are within reach. The psychiatric-mental health nurse becomes an emotional lifeguard, on hand to prevent the other from drowning. Should the other stumble and fall from his stepping stone, the likeliest consequence is that, despite becoming emotionally drenched, he will scramble back onto the stone himself.[19] The most that we will have to do is offer a handhold, together with a message of support: 'Come on – I know you can do it'.

Emotional life saving,[20] however, is a final response that we rarely have to resort to. Most of the time we sit with the other and admire his resilience and commitment to survival. By far the greatest amount of time is spent being and responding, keeping apace as he chooses which stepping stone to try next. As we approach the riverbank, we can drop back a step, enabling the other to reach dry land first. Through our relationship with the other, we are able to nurture a positive concept within him and reinforce his potential to become.[21] Depending on the depth and rapidity of the water flow, emotional river crossing can be a harrowing experience. If we are to engage in healing relationships, we must be willing to accept that we, too, are as susceptible to being emotionally wounded as any other is. If the psychiatric-mental health nurse is feeling emotionally fragile, irrespective of the reasons why, she needs to put herself first and tend to her own wounds. This may mean seeking extra supervision and support from her colleagues, engaging in some form of personal therapy or even taking time out for a while. It is perfectly acceptable for nurses to ask for help. Collectively, psychiatric-mental health nurses need to acknowledge the demanding nature of their role and be available for each other at all times.

As you read this text, my words may draw you into a shared understanding of the craft of psychiatric nursing. Conversely, they may sail past your heart like passing ships in the night. They may reflect pictures of psychiatric nursing that mimic images of your own. Or they may not. Look on these words as waves within the psychiatric ocean. Sail on them or sail past them. Like reading a book, the craft of psychiatric nursing involves constant searching for meaning with the other. It is a voyage of perpetual discovery. Do not become disheartened or disabled if you struggle to grasp the reasoning and supposition within this chapter. More importantly, each and every time you engage with the other you are living and learning your craft.

GEORGE'S STORY

Case study 4.1

Let us return to the beginning of this chapter, to the hospital ward where I first met George, tried and sentenced by his own internal judge and jury. Our paths first crossed in the dramatic fashion I described in the opening paragraph. Detained under a section of the Mental Health Act, he had been medically diagnosed and prescribed a hefty regime of psychoactive drugs to treat his mental illness. George had not worked for several years, although he had held an officer's commission in the Salvation Army until his recurrent mental ill health had caused him to take early retirement. A very knowledgeable man, with a degree in theology, much of his conversation was related to his religious beliefs.

Being heavily sedated, he would sleep for long periods during the day. During his wakeful moments he would sit with glassy eyes and spittled mouth, slowly and self-consciously raising both his cup and saucer to his lips, as his noticeable tremor caused the tea to flow over the brim. Little by little, George disclosed his persecutory beliefs to me. He believed that he had contributed significantly to the demise of Christianity and that he, alone, was responsible for the recent closure of a nearby church. God had spoken to him many months ago, telling him that it was his mission to boost the congregation and save the church. Alas, he had failed to do so.

Conversation with George was, sometimes, very one-sided. He would leave our conversational frequency and engage in dialogue with God. He would eventually join me once more and share with me what God had said to him. I would listen with the utmost respect and, at times, revel in the gift of his extensive biblical awareness. On such occasions, George and I would lose ourselves together as we wandered through the wilderness of his torment.

Six weeks after my privileged meeting with him, George began to emerge from the desolation of his psychosis. By now, I had come to know his wife and, during an evening visit on the ward, the three of us sat together drinking tea. We were making the final preparations for George's weekend leave, in preparation for being discharged home. I remember his wife suddenly turning to me and placing her hand on my arm. Sincerity shone in her eyes as she expressed her gratitude to me for 'being so nice to George and helping him get through everything'. I decided to ask George what it was that had helped him to survive and transcend his emotional ordeal. He responded by saying that he thought his medication had played a vital role in his recovery. His wife agreed and added that she had prayed continually for God to look after George and 'heal him'. George nodded his support and reflected for a moment. 'Yes', he smiled, 'Yet when I first came into hospital I thought He'd abandoned me'.

Soon afterwards, George did, indeed, return home. For a week or so, I missed his presence: the intrigue and exclusivity of his divine experiences; the privilege of having an open door that led into his life; and, latterly, the conversations that decorated the borders of his road to recovery. Several months later I received a letter from George. It was a lovely surprise, particularly as it confirmed that he was feeling 'completely regenerated'. Towards the end of his letter, George made reference to a student nurse, Laura, who was on placement during his stay with us. 'Please tell her just how much I appreciated her kindness. I'm not sure if I saw her as a daughter figure, but she treated me as I imagine she would her own father. She seemed so genuine in her desire to do whatever I needed her to do in order to speed my recovery. She encouraged me to the breakfast table when eating had ceased to be a priority and she made the ward bathroom my own personal space in her attempts to rekindle my interest in myself'.

Finally, George turned to our relationship, as he wrote, 'At one stage, I thought I had entered hell. It was the most frightening experience of my life. I felt tormented and terrified. I just could not understand why you had followed me there, but you had. You were with me, Peter, and that's just where I needed you to be. Rather than trying to convince me that I was hallucinating (which would have been completely pointless, others tried and failed miserably) you chose simply to stay with me. And more than once. For that, I will be eternally and everlastingly grateful. I was in the lion's den – you dared to be there with me'.

George's letter is confirmation enough that I helped to sustain him during those awful psychotic episodes. It also bears witness to the most memorable psychiatric nursing interventions during his almost unbearable moments of madness: Laura's kindness and loving interventions and my willingness to be with him. The craft of our caring was cast in collaboration with George. Nothing was done for him, rather, he was engaged with: encouraged and spiritually (and, on occasions, physically) held through his emotional trauma. There were times when he was so troubled he did not know how he could be helped. There were no therapeutic skills to be employed, nor any clever words to interpret or console. During such times, the craft of psychiatric nursing practice is simply to be with in readiness to become with.

Both student nurse Laura and myself exercised our craft with George sensitively and productively. The craftwork that took place always involved George. On admission, he was trapped in and bedevilled by his psychotic experiences. With George's permission, we joined with him as often as possible as privileged wayfarers as he wandered through difficult terrain: two, sometimes three, sets of footprints all heading in the same direction. Time passed by and George reached a stage of development where he no longer needed our company. He would craft his own life once more from outside the hospital ward. The finished product of mental healthfulness was of the utmost value to George. The fact that he was able to enjoy the fruits of our labours together strongly suggests that I practised my craft well enough. Yet I know that, at times, I failed to respond as perhaps I should have. I failed to listen carefully, said the wrong thing; acted in my own interests rather than his; or acted out of impatience and anxiety, instead of waiting and being. Such second-class craftings are to be expected. They will always happen, even to the most experienced psychiatric nurse practitioner. When they do, they become golden opportunities for us to learn from and grow. The craft of psychiatric nursing can only ever be practised, never mastered (sic).

EMPOWERMENT

Relationship as a gift

Over recent years, psychiatric nurses have introduced the word empowerment into their vocabulary.[22] In one respect it is a misnomer and detracts from the real craft of care. It implies that the psychiatric-mental health nurse must carry with her an agenda that includes 'giving' or 'handing over' chunks of power to psychiatric service patients. As power is an abstract construct, that is of course impossible.[23] A person can only ever feel to *have* power or *be* powerful. The science within the craft of caring is purely an awareness of, and belief in this. That willingness to be with the other leads both players to the edge of the water – only one step away from a significant shift of feeling from powerless to powered.

If the psychiatric-mental health nurse is to play any part in empowering the patient, (other than by cheerful accident) she, herself, must feel empowered. Through the process of being with the other, the nurse is able to learn how to become in order to give her best response. If the patient has a need to be empowered, it is he who will have shown the nurse what she needs to do. She will offer her response from this position of empowerment and, if the patient is ready, he will step into the pool – always slightly ahead in terms of knowing himself better than the nurse knows him.

Once the other feels sufficiently supported and sustained to wade into the waters, there dawns the realization of the potential self. The psychiatric-mental health nurse has cultivated the conditions of growth by 'sus-

taining the other as a subject of action rather than attempting to negate' (him).[24] She has fostered the patient and (under his expert direction) utilized his potential to be and become. Whilst power is, indeed, at play here, the nurse learns how to become a 'channel for the perspective of the other',[25] releasing him and enabling him to use his freedom productively.

Frequently, psychiatric-mental health nursing care is delivered through surveillance: either overtly under the watchful eye of the nursing sentinel or more covertly (and possibly more intrusively) through clinic appointments and home visits. Fox[26] describes this as the 'vigil of care', which he sees as 'the continual subjection of care's clients and increasingly, all aspects of the environment in which they live to the vigilant scrutiny of carers'. When nursing practice is driven by vigilance, a heavy shadow is cast, which intimidates the other and blocks out sunrays of hope. It involves a nurse–patient relationship driven by a model of care based on sameness and repetition. The feelings of power predominantly belong to the nurse, as she uses her badge of office to impose the controlling structure of the organization onto every patient. It is a relationship constructed on the foundations of power and knowledge that shape the interventions of the psychiatric-mental health nurse. According to Cixous,[27] it is a relationship that springs from within the masculine realm of what she terms the 'proper': a relationship that seeks to possess, to profit, to pleasure and to measure success in terms of 'return'. By contrast, Cixous offers the feminine relationship-as-gift, where she 'with open hands, gives herself – pleasure, happiness, increased value, enhanced self image' without ever trying 'to recover her expenses'.[28] Even within the most panoptical institutional setting, there is room for the individual to grow by way of his relationship with others.[29]

Each and every time care is gift-wrapped with kindness and consideration, a climate of possibility has been created between nurse and other. The other has been liberated enough to make choices rather than following the prescriptive route markers of a depersonalizing system. He has become 'deterritorialized': his quarantine has been lifted and new 'lines of flight'[d] drawn to wherever he chooses. 'You are suffering from schizophrenia', 'You need to take this medication', and 'You need to stay in hospital for a while' may constitute professional recommendations delivered in the patient's 'best interests'. Yet they are really no more than paternalistic impositions and, as such, are loaded with control. There is no negotiation, no shared understandings and, often, no

---

[d] In their seminal text '*A thousand plateaus*', Deleuze and Guattari use the expression 'deterritorialization' to describe the process of breaking free from a restrictive or oppressive discourse (such as the disempowering consequences of a regime of psychiatry based upon subjugation). Deterritorialization is achieved by creating a new 'line of flight' – an escape route – towards becoming what Deleuze and Guattari term a 'nomad': free to travel 'beyond' and discover new, more liberating ways of being. Deleuze G, Guattari F. *A thousand plateaus*. London: Athlone Press, 1988.

room for manoeuvre. They are interventions, which carry the agendas and prejudices of the psychiatric provider and, as such, they negate the experiences of the other. The person who is patient remains unrecognized in his distress and, as such, is unable to live it and survive it.

At every given opportunity, the craft of psychiatric-mental health nursing embraces the act of offering what rightly belongs to the other. In order to survive an experience, a person must experience that experience as it is for him (and not as someone says it is for him). The craft of caring involves a decolonizing of the other by enabling him to reclaim his own territory. If the psychiatric nurse is to play any part in this returning home, it is merely to 'gently guide the tiller'[30] in response to the navigational prompts of the other. Each response needs to be blessed by 'a universal common sense'[31] that is always applied to the difference of the other. It is the way she says things that takes precedence over her need to influence outcomes. Her 'words (must) take their meanings from other words rather than by virtue of their representative character'.[32] Otherwise, genuine conversations will either degenerate into sterile inquiry or become distorted and meaningless for the other. The only acceptable nursing agenda 'is to keep the conversation going'[33] and the door open to brand new ways of being.

CONCLUSION

Like any other craftsperson, the psychiatric-mental health nurse fashions a product to please a customer. As nurses, we have come to call our product 'care'. Unless we engage with those customers by asking questions and actively listening to their responses, our craftwork will become an artefact of our own design. It will be of no value to our customer. As Barker and Whitehill so poignantly declare, 'If we are to develop a craft of care in psychiatric nursing, then we need to know what the experience of mental ill health *means* (author's italics) to the person who is "in" that experience'.[34] The craft of our caring, then, must always follow a pattern fashioned by our customer – the person in need of our care.

As each new working day begins, we enter our workshop with the other knowing only that the material to be crafted will be familiar, but always will be different from that which we have previously encountered. We will be faced with interesting and challenging situations that materialize through the togetherness of the nurse–patient relationship. Because the psychiatric-mental health nurse can never be sure what her craft-

mate will bring, she will always need to improvise. Although she will, by necessity, have her tool bag to hand full of interventions, she must first engage the other as the primary director of his care. This may take time and patience and involve lengthy periods of rejection and not-knowing for the psychiatric-mental health nurse. Accepting this and showing a genuine willingness to wait and still be available is a crucial component of our craft. It is only when the other person feels secure enough within the caring relationship that the conditions can sustain that person's growth and recovery.

Psychiatric-mental health nursing is an occupation that carries a salary, enabling us to pay our mortgages and feed our families. We are employed by an organization to practice our craft. Yet, without a steady stream of customers, we would be redundant. I find it sobering that our world is constructed in such a way that we, as psychiatric-mental health nurses, rely upon the psychological suffering of others to pay our wages. It would be crass, therefore, to say that we choose to nurse by way of a 'calling' and nothing more: there is *always* something more in it for the psychiatric-mental health nurse. Yet, as far as the 'other' goes, we really should expect nothing from him, only 'the common wages'[e] that all relationships are capable of yielding.

While this comprehensive textbook will, hopefully, become your constant companion throughout at least the formative years of your career in psychiatry, you can only ever learn your craft with the other. Paradoxically, the emotionally disabled person who turns to you for succour will become your most reliable guide and teacher. Follow his lead and resist any desire to forcibly re-describe his experiences – for those experiences are his only proof that he exists.

REFERENCES

1. Chamberlin J. The medical model and harm. In: Barker P, Campbell P, Davidson B (eds). *From the ashes of experience: reflections on madness, survival and growth.* London: Whurr Publishers, 1999: 171.
2. Keats J. Letter to George and Thomas Keats, 21 December, 1817. In: Barnard J (ed.) *John Keats: the complete poems*, 3rd edn. London: Penguin Books, 1988.
3. Peplau H. *Interpersonal relations in nursing.* Basingstoke: Macmillan Press, 1988: 84.
4. Barker P, Whitehill I. The craft of care: towards collaborative caring in psychiatric nursing. In: Tilley S (ed.) *The mental health nurse: views of practice and education.* Oxford: Blackwell Sciences, 1997: 15–27.

---

[e] A line from Dylan Thomas's aptly named poem, '*In my craft or sullen art*', which refers to the spontaneous and esoteric rewards that relationships yield: solidarity, rapport and, perhaps most importantly, an acceptance of individual limitations. *The Dylan Thomas omnibus.* London: Phoenix Giants, 1995.

5. Peplau, H. *Interpersonal relations in nursing.* Basingstoke: Macmillan Press, 1988.

6. Hobson RF. *Forms of feeling: the heart of psychotherapy.* London: Tavistock Publications, 1985: xiii.

7. Hobson RF. *Forms of feeling: the heart of psychotherapy.* London: Tavistock Publications, 1985: 15.

8. Hobson RF. *Forms of feeling: the heart of psychotherapy.* London: Tavistock Publications, 1985: 93–4.

9. Menand L. An introduction to pragmatism. In: Menand L (ed.) *Pragmatism: a reader.* New York: Vintage Books, 1997: xi–xxxiv.

10. Barker P, Kerr B. *The process of psychotherapy: a journey of discovery* Oxford: Butterworth-Heinemann, 2001: 135.

11. Barker P, Whitehill I. The craft of care: towards collaborative caring in psychiatric nursing. In: Tilley S (ed.) *The mental health nurse: views of practice and education.* Oxford: Blackwell Sciences, 1997: 20.

12. Walsh, K. Shared humanity and the psychiatric nurse–patient encounter. *Australian and New Zealand Journal of Mental Health Nursing* 1999; **8**: 7.

13. Buber, M. *I and Thou.* Edinburgh: T. & T. Clark, 1958: 41.

14. Keats J. (1820) Ode on a Grecian urn. In: Barnard J (ed.) *John Keats: the complete poems,* 3rd edn. London: Penguin Books, 1988.

15. Hobson RF. *Forms of feeling: the heart of psychotherapy.* London: Tavistock Publications, 1985: 279–80.

16. Barker P. *The philosophy and practice of psychiatric nursing.* Edinburgh: Churchill Livingstone, 1999: 127.

17. Barker P. *The philosophy and practice of psychiatric nursing.* Edinburgh: Churchill Livingstone, 1999: 119.

18. Benner P. *From novice to expert: excellence and power in clinical nursing practice.* California: Addison-Wesley, 1984: 213.

19. Watkins P. *Mental health nursing: the art of compassionate care.* Oxford: Butterworth-Heinemann, 2001: 57.

20. Barker P. The Tidal Model: the development of personal caring within the chaos paradigm 8 pages, *The Tidal Model,* Internet, 25th May 2001, available: http://members.nbci.com/_XMCM/drphilbarker/Phil_Barker~2/Tidal_paper.html

21. Graham IW. Seeking a clarification of meaning: a phenomenological interpretation of the craft of mental health nursing. *Journal of Psychiatric and Mental Health Nursing* 2001; 8(4): 335–45.

22. Barker P, Stevenson C, Leamy M. The philosophy of empowerment. *Mental Health Nursing* 2000; **20**(9): 8–12.

23. Watkins P. *Mental health nursing: the art of compassionate care.* Oxford: Butterworth-Heinemann, 2001: 78.

24. Crossley N. *Intersubjectivity: the fabric of social becoming.* London: Sage, 1996: 147.

25. Crossley N. *Intersubjectivity: the fabric of social becoming.* London: Sage, 1996: 147.

26. Fox NJ. *Beyond health: postmodernism and embodiment.* London: Free Association Books, 1999: 81.

27. Cixous H. Sorties: out and out: attacks/ways out/forays. In: Cixous H, Clément C (eds). *The newly born woman.* London: Tarris, 1996: 87.

28. Cixous H. Sorties: out and out: attacks/ways out/forays. In: Cixous H, Clément C (eds). *The newly born woman.* London: Tarris, 1996: 87.

29. Wilkin PE. From medicalization to hybridization: a postcolonial discourse for psychiatric nurses. *Journal of Psychiatric and Mental Health Nursing* 2001; 8(2): 115–20.

30. Barker P, Kerr B. *The process of psychotherapy: a journey of discovery.* Oxford: Butterworth-Heinemann, 2001: 156.

31. Gadamer H-G. *Truth and method,* 2nd edn. London: Sheed and Ward, 1989: 17.

32. Rorty R. *Philosophy and the mirror of nature.* Oxford: Blackwell Publishers, 1980: 368.

33. Rorty R. *Philosophy and the mirror of nature.* Oxford: Blackwell Publishers, 1980: 377.

34. Barker P, Whitehill, I. The craft of care: towards collaborative caring in psychiatric nursing. In: Tilley S (ed.) *The mental health nurse: views of practice and education.* Oxford: Blackwell Sciences, 1997: 21.

Chapter 5

MANAGING DEVELOPMENTS IN THE CRAFT OF CARING

Angela Simpson*

INTRODUCTION

The therapeutic focus of psychiatric-psychiatric-mental health nursing appears to have become lost and devalued within chaotic clinical settings characterized by rapid change and managed care. Indeed, *managing* care has become a dominant nursing preoccupation. As a consequence, we need to consider how nurses might restabilize the clinical environment so that they might focus once again on the therapeutic practice of their craft. Nurses need to adopt a style of open and flexible management so that a new learning environment may be developed. This, in turn, might best be supported through the application of transformational (*feminine*) leadership, which fosters creativity and is empowering in nature.

Transformational leadership has already been linked to the development of advanced nursing practice.[1] A supportive and empowering form of clinical leadership, as opposed to traditional management, might reawaken nurses' natural curiosity in the therapeutic potential of nursing itself and foster growth and maturity in nursing. Where these conditions are in place it may be possible to facilitate new approaches to practice that are both creative and investigative in nature. These might right-

fully focus on evaluating the discrete practice of psychiatric-mental health nursing, asking what *exactly* is the contribution of nursing to the overall mental health programme?

NURSING AS A MATURING FORCE

Peplau originally envisaged nursing as a maturing force.[2] In developing the theory of interpersonal relationships she identified concepts and principles that 'underlie interpersonal relationships and transform nursing situations into learning experiences'. This led her to advocate her belief in the therapeutic potential of nursing in its own right. Peplau foresaw nurses advancing practice to the point of being able to contribute to caring, not just for the individual, but *for* and *with* the wider community. This vision of nursing as a healing force in the wider community was ambitious and, in its purest form, has yet to be fully realized.

Developing the practice of psychiatric-mental health nursing to this point perhaps hinges on facilitating the growth and role maturity of nursing. This raises several interesting questions:

*Angela Simpson RMN, BA, MA, is Lecturer in Mental Health Nursing at the University of York. Her interests include Mental Health Service User and Carer Collaboration and Nursing Practice Development. She maintains a fervent interest in developing nursing practice *in* practice having led an acute psychiatric inpatient nursing team to accreditation as a Nursing Development Unit.

❑ How might nurses develop such role maturity?

❑ What are the organizational conditions that support growth in the practice of psychiatric-mental health nursing?

❑ How might nurses nurture the potential for growth in each other?

These lead to the wider question:

❑ How might psychiatric-mental health nurses investigate and evaluate the impact of therapeutic nursing?

These issues are discussed here in the context of managing developments in the craft of caring. First of all, however, I shall consider how, traditionally, nurses have managed each other.

Managing to nurse

Nursing has a well-documented history dating back to the turn of the 20th century. At this time, men strictly controlled the position of women in society. This was also the case within nursing, led by the male dominated medical profession, which managed hospitals and was the powerful decision-maker. Nurses with management responsibilities at this time were from the upper classes. It is perhaps due to this factor that autocratic management became the accepted norm. Rawdon[3] observes that the class divisions present within nursing contributed to a climate of subservience and noted that nursing was influenced as much by its own class divisions as it was by the sexist attitudes present at that time. These combined influences contributed to Rawdon's view that nursing became a rigid profession with its ultimate control firmly in the grip of the predominantly male medical staff.

Nursing still retains some aspects of this early subservience to and dependence upon medicine. These are best observed within the routines of task orientated practice, where nurses engage in clinical roles without questioning their purpose or timeliness.[4] Today, it would appear that nursing is still attempting to free itself from its past. Although nurses are predominantly female, beyond first line (clinical) management, nursing continues to be disproportionately managed by men.

Although management styles within nursing have remained fairly static, over the years the environment within which nurses work, has changed greatly. The modernization of health services in the UK, driven by a desire for high quality, cost efficient health care, necessitated a reorganization of clinical services. Consequently, nurses face a new and challenging organizational culture that appears highly competitive and is constantly changing. Traditional management styles – involving hierarchy, underpinned by bureaucracy – are inappropriate within such a climate. Their inherent inflexibility results in work environments that are slow to adapt and change. However, abandoning the tradition of autocratic management represents a huge cultural shift for nursing and has many implications.

Few would argue against the need for nursing to adopt a more responsive and creative management style. This is essential at all levels in nursing but especially at the clinical interface, between service user and service provider, where important impressions of care are generated. Here, observations of the person's experience of the service can be collected and used to improve the quality of care provided. Receiving and acting on 'customer-led feedback' requires a genuine commitment to listening and responding to the views of those using the service. This kind of power shift requires the nurse to acknowledge the expertise of people in care, as they judge the therapeutic value of the service they receive. Initially, nurses might feel threatened by devolving this judgement process. However, by developing a conjoint therapeutic and management model, the voice of the person in care is heard and, subsequently, empowered. Although the maturing, self-confident nurse might rightfully take pride in facilitating such an empowering approach to care, she might also be staring into the eyes of her most potent fear – her professional undoing. Psychiatric-mental health nursing can only benefit from further investigation of this fear. It will reveal how health care workers in general, often stifle the distress, or silence the voices, of people in mental health care. However, such an enquiry requires a highly supportive nursing management style; one that respects both the experience of the nurse as well as her need to grow and develop.

Managing nurses and developing the practice and discipline of nursing are closely related concepts. These involve parallel journeys with common aims and values and are best undertaken within a climate of safety, and in a spirit of mutuality, respect and common understanding.

The advancement of the practice of nursing hinges on nurses' belief in their potential. Embracing this belief is a constructive starting point, but it can be jeopardized by the failure of nurses to define adequately what it is that they do.[5] Without such 'self' identity psychiatric-mental health nursing risks remaining an insecure occupational group expected to soak up the administrative burden of managed care. This common feature of current clinical practice often results in a blizzard of paperwork that further limits the nurse's capacity to engage the person who is patient. However, it is possible to streamline procedures or employ administrative staff, thereby allowing nurses more time to engage, clinically, with those in their care.[6] Although simplifying administrative procedures would considerably ease the administrative burden on nurses, there is concern that nursing has developed an unhealthy obsession with managing care. Indeed some nurses might now view this as the most important focus of their work. Where this is the case the ward or team may find it increasingly difficult to accept new ideas that fall outside of their current practice.

GROWING NURSING – LEARNING TO LEARN

If psychiatric-psychiatric-mental health nursing is to develop, its success is likely to hinge upon the ability of nurses at all levels (but especially first-line nurse managers) to *redefine* the ward atmosphere or team culture. Such redefinition would see a significant shift in atmosphere towards recognizing the clinical area as a responsive learning environment in which mutual growth through, shared partnerships at all levels, becomes a real possibility. Nurses can help develop an environment in which it might become possible for people in care to learn something of real value about themselves.

The Maori language incorporates a word that means both teaching and learning, indicating that perhaps the process of developing knowledge is *simultaneous* and might not be taught or learned in the 'educational' sense. This kind of learning takes place *within* the person. The nurse is responsible for facilitating the opportunity for this self-knowledge to be realized within an environment that supports the person's individual experience. In this new climate it would be expected that nurses would challenge traditional modes of practice, launch investigations into their role and functions, and explore the full potential of accepting patients as 'experts'. The clinical environment thus becomes a two-way street, where nurses and patients can learn from one another.

However, the therapeutic efforts of the ward or clinical team need to be harmonized with supportive and encouraging clinical management. Just as people in care are enabled to explore and face their individual problems, so nurses must take a similar 'journey,' exploring the human challenges of everyday practice. Such 'journeying' involves looking at nursing through new eyes, getting out of the groove of routine practice and looking far beyond this. Such active 'doing' involves the nurse in being attentive and mindful to the core task of being with another person throughout their individual experience of distress and sharing the discomfort and rewards that such close proximity brings. Within the earthiness of such nurse–patient encounters, the healing seeds of nursing are planted and the nurse's real learning begins.

Some nurses might assume that this kind of learning might be achieved through reading or attending a short course. However, the real lessons in nursing practice can only be learned through the 'active doing' of nursing *in practice*. Such an approach might release nurses' natural curiosity and so might then be more inclined to undertake informal experiments in nursing and its outcomes. Knowledge can be drawn from books and courses but the supportive learning atmosphere of the ward or team alone will help *transform* knowledge into a new clinical practice reality.

Senge[7] stated that:

real learning gets to the heart of what it means to be human. Through learning we re-create ourselves. Through learning we become able to do something we never were able to do. Through learning we re-perceive the world and our relationship to it. Through learning we extend our capacity to create, to be part of the generative process of life.

This illustrates how learning cannot be divorced from practice. The 'active doing' of putting new knowledge into practice (and observing its consequences) lets us *know* and *understand* nursing. However, this process depends on managerial support. Effective clinical management helps create the freedom in which nurses can experiment, choose their own direction and evaluate progress. Such conditions nurture and develop the practice of nursing, facilitating a growth-promoting climate for nurses and patients alike.

Zen wisdom acknowledges that 'the tighter you squeeze the less you have!' This illustrates how nursing has the potential to flourish, if it can release itself from the constraining grip of autocratic management, administration and routine practice. Nursing needs to locate itself at the centre of developing practice. Psychiatric-mental health nursing is limited, more, by the way nurses think about their craft, than by any other factor.

DISTINGUISHING MANAGEMENT FROM LEADERSHIP

Nursing management was defined by Yura *et al.*:[8]

The use of delegated authority within a formal organization to organize, direct or control responsible subordinates.

This illustrates the distinguishing characteristics of managers, who are *appointed* to, and occupy, formal positions of organizational authority, and use legitimatized power to *command*, *reward* or *punish* the workforce. Contrast this with leaders, who *emerge* from the workforce and attract followers, often with little power with which to influence the actions of colleagues. Leaders are those who can communicate and resonate with their followers.[9] Unlike management, leadership does not sit comfortably in a world of hard and fast rules. If it did however, those rules would doubtless be softer and slower by comparison.

Kouzes and Posner[10] noted that the root of the two words, manager and leader, distinguished them. 'Manage' originated in the word meaning 'hand'. *Managing* then, is about *handling* or organizing things while maintaining order. 'Leadership', by contrast, refers to 'going or travelling'. The metaphor of the leadership journey is described in Nelson Mandela's *Long Walk to Freedom*:[11]

> ... a leader is like a shepherd. He stays behind the flock, letting the nimble go ahead – whereupon the others follow not realizing that all along they were being directed from behind.

The notion of 'leading from behind' is interesting. While those who follow might perceive the leader to be at the front – leaders themselves are to be found within the pack steering and guiding those around them. In doing this, leaders are involved closely in the primary roles and functions of core tasks. Perhaps because of this they are viewed as having legitimate expertise. They lead by example and are expert *role models*. Leaders are acutely aware of the delicate relationship of *influence* over *authority*, recognizing that meaningful change cannot be forced, and will happen only at its own speed.

The leader pays close attention to the movement of the workforce on the journey towards its agreed goal – encouraging novel or creative approaches to traversing this new territory. Where leaders differ most from managers is in their intense interest in the journey itself (as opposed to possessing an overwhelming desire to achieve the goal for its own sake). Leaders recognize that by the time the goal is achieved it is already past its 'sell-by date' and the next goal has already emerged. Change is the only constant. Leaders understand what motivates people, and are concerned with finding out how to support and promote that forward movement. They know that this is highly valuable for a maturing workforce. Hence, leadership is a broader and more interpersonal concept than management, and hinges upon personal relationships.

Over the years theorists have tried to identify the distinguishing characteristics of leaders, recognizing that the leadership styles of men and women vary significantly.

LEADING LADIES: THE GENDER AGENDA

Rosener,[12] recognized that men and women offer very different descriptions of leadership. Men frequently describe using *power* and *authority*. Typically, men viewed management performance in terms of transactions, utilizing the traditional skills of command and control. Women's descriptions of leaders differed, and included getting other people to support the task, and express concern for achieving broader organizational goals. Conflict avoidance was recognized in women's desire to find *win–win* solutions, now very popular in business circles. Also, women who described themselves as *feminine* or *gender neutral* reported higher levels of 'followership' among women workers, than those who describe themselves in masculine terms. Women adopting a feminine style of leadership are viewed as *transformational*. They adopt:

❑ an interactive participative style of leading;
❑ fostering participation and involvement;
❑ validating others;
❑ delegating authority; and
❑ sharing in the decision-making process.

While women were found to have a natural orientation toward transformational leadership, men can also use similar leadership skills. The term 'feminine' leadership illustrates the softer focus of this approach and distinguishes it from more traditional power base management.

The feminine approach to leadership has a softer, more creative focus. This is highly desirable within organizations that face persistent change.[13] However, such skills are often not regarded highly within traditional organizations with a dominant masculine (or *macho* culture), resulting in the commonly held belief that only by adopting typically masculine traits can one be perceived as competent. Although nursing has been slow to embrace the potential of feminine leadership, many businesswomen have adopted this with great success. Anita Roddick, founder of the Body Shop, based her business around feminine principles,[14] defining these as:

> principles of caring, making intuitive decisions, not getting hung up on hierarchy, having a sense of work as being part of your life – not separate from it and putting your labour where your love is!

Adopting a feminine or transformational approach to leadership might be the creative release necessary to advance the craft of psychiatric caring. Pearson[15] suggested that nurses must 'confront' the ever-present, dominant masculine ideology that underpins modern health care. However, it is questionable if 'confronting' anything or anyone fits with this softer focus. The best way forward is for nurses to adopt feminine approaches to team leadership, explicitly aiming to creatively explore the therapeutic nature of nursing – through active/constructive 'doing'. Developing nursing practice hinges on constructive action not confrontation.

Transformational leadership: the art of empowering employees

Transformational (feminine) leadership values interpersonal communication, mutuality and affiliation. The transformational leader:

❏ Gets to know staff, taking an active interest in them and their development.
❏ Seeks to empower the workforce delegating tasks and giving praise.
❏ Seeks to promote excellence beyond mere tasks.
❏ Encourages employees to become ideas-orientated and solution-focused.

Bass and Avolio[16] identify transformational leaders as those who can:

❏ Stimulate interest among followers to view work from a fresh perspective.
❏ Generate an awareness of a vision, towards which the team is headed.
❏ Develop followers to higher levels of ability and potential.
❏ Motivate followers to look beyond their own interests, towards those that will benefit the group.

Transformational (feminine) leaders go far beyond mere task attainment. Work is a developmental opportunity, within which the leader and followers are motivated to produce higher levels of performance. Transformational leadership facilitates a culture in which others might become empowering leaders themselves.[1]

Transformational leadership is not, however, a magical quality possessed by a few.[10] It is an observable set of core behaviours that can be learned and developed. Nurse leaders in nursing development units appear (naturally) to adopt transformational styles of leadership in practice.[17]

Seven lessons in leadership guide the process of transformational leadership.[18]

Lesson 1: Leaders don't wait

Leadership is an adventure requiring a pioneering spirit.[18] In nursing this begins with a shift in attitude. Capturing this pioneering spirit involves swapping the cynicism or despair that frequently inhabits clinical environments, for the belief that things have the potential to be better. Changing attitudes does not involve additional resources – it is free! Success hinges rather on the leader's ability to view the world differently – to 'let go' of the constraining attitudes and beliefs present in everyday practice. How easy (or difficult) this will be, depends on the team and its motivation to 'let go'. An Indonesian story illustrates this beautifully.

Hunters setting traps for monkeys, cut holes in coconuts that are just the right size for a monkey to put his hand through. The hunter then secures the coconut to the bottom of the tree, places a banana inside and hides in wait. The monkey sees the banana and places his hand through the hole to take hold of it. The hole however is crafted so the monkey can pass his open hand through it, but when he clenches his fist round the banana, he cannot withdraw his hand. The solution is simple. To free himself, all the monkey has to do is to release hold of the banana. Most monkeys however, do not let go. And so, they are trapped!

Many nurses are clutching a (metaphorical) banana, in the shape of some aspect of practice that does not work for them, their clientele or both. They find it hard to engage in the creative, 'break-through thinking', needed to advance practice.

Break through thinking is often subtle and grounded in the everyday practice of nursing, rather than located in some complex organizational reconfiguration, or the latest Government guidelines. The word 'innovation' often conjures up the notion of far-reaching change. This need not be the case. Indeed, truly creative approaches to nursing practice might be 'blinding' only in their relative simplicity. Meaningful change is often small scale and subtle but, nevertheless, makes a significant contribution towards improving care and developing practice.

Leading a new venture, within a turbulent organizational climate, is often seen as overwhelmingly difficult. We often believe that positive change can only occur within stable conditions. However, much of the stress involved in change is a function of our human need to control or resist change. A more constructive view is to accept the pace of change. Instead of resisting, we should take an active interest in change. Learn to roll with it rather than against it. Nurse leaders who are serious about launching a voyage of discovery recognize that textbook conditions never apply in practice. They don't wait for favourable organizational conditions – but get on with it, in a spirit of optimism, accepting that the journey will involve as much fair weather as foul. Tom Peters[19] observed that 'if you sense calm, it's only because you are in the eye of the hurricane!'

Lesson 2: Character counts

Personal qualities, like courage, conviction, honesty, being forward looking and inspiring, are all powerful leadership attributes.[18] These result in the leader being viewed as a credible source of information, who are viewed as 'standing for something', tapping into a value system. Their work assumes a moral, rather than simply professional focus. As decisions become based around a belief or value system there is added stability through predictability (even within chaotic conditions) because decisions hold true to certain fundamental values. Leaders are closely in touch with their own personal values but more importantly, involve others in developing a set of shared team beliefs. This fosters a philosophical approach to practice. Burns viewed transformational leadership as taking the team to a higher moral level:[20]

> at the highest stage of moral development persons are guided by near universal ethical principles of justice such as equality of human rights and respect for individual dignity.

This is consistent with the principles that guide psychiatric-mental health nursing.

Lesson 3: Leaders have their heads in the clouds and their feet on the ground

Leaders are credible. They work from within the pack and have a strong sense of personal direction, which others feel inspired to follow. They do this by creating an uplifting picture of the future and inviting others to join the journey.[18]

Psychiatric-mental health nursing needs to consider where it is *now* and where it wants to *go*. Currently, nursing appears constrained, perhaps with good reason. Inadequate resources play a significant part in demoralizing nurses. However by succumbing to these factors, nursing might allow its very spirit to become imprisoned, in a self-imposed claustrophobia, within which nursing loses its will to determine its own future. In such cases, the oppressor is more clearly within than without. Breaking free of such constraints involves developing the belief that nursing has its own value – it's own unique potential. The old adage 'for those who believe, no proof is necessary; and for those who don't believe, no proof is possible' seems appropriate. Richard Bach was correct when he observed 'Sooner or later those who win are those that believe that they can.'

Lesson 4: Shared values

People have a tendency to drift when they become unsure or confused about what they should be doing. Stabilizing the team involves articulating shared values that are also consistent with organizational aims. Where this constancy exists there are benefits for both employees and the organization: strong feelings of personal effectiveness, and reduced levels of job stress and tension.[10,18] Transformational leadership is 'values' leadership.[21]

Identifying and sharing core values within the nursing team is only a useful exercise if the core principles are 'alive' at ward level or within the team. Reducing this task to a dry philosophy statement pinned to the office wall isn't enough. Significant meaning can be derived from this invisible code through the development of a practice philosophy clearly articulated within core beliefs. These beliefs become a touchstone and facilitate team maturity when used, for example within clinical supervision – where critical incidents are explored in relation to core team values. Nurses are then able to assess how close they are in the clinical context to the values they aspire to practice. If each team member is likened to members of an orchestra, then the role of the ward manager is similar to that of the conductor. To what extent is each member playing 'in tune', with the articulated values of the whole team.

Lesson 5: You can't do it alone

There is no leadership without a team. The collective efforts of the whole have greater value than any one individual. Leaders seek the active involvement of those around them to achieve mutually agreed goals. Competition between group members is counterproductive. Instead the collective will of all involved.[18] Nurse leaders often go beyond their own locality for personal inspiration. Developing this 'outsight' involves establishing contact with other leading clinicians, or well established nurse academics. The Internet often makes such contact easy to accomplish. You might link your team, for example, with a similar one in another continent, exchanging experiences of different approaches to care, stimulating further debate and interest among your colleagues.

Lesson 6: The legacy you leave is the life you lead

People are moved by deeds. It is actions that count – talking is never enough.[18] Effective leaders *walk the talk* – performing the deeds consistent with the shared values of the team. In leading nursing, involvement and participation are the keys to success. In a work environment that is constantly changing, leaders bring stability through behavioural predictability. Leaders do what they say they will do.

Lesson 7: Leadership is everyone's business

The idea that leaders are born not made is a myth. Leadership is not a magical quality possessed by a lucky few – is an observable set of practices that can be learned.[10,18]

> those who are most successful at bringing out the best in others are the people who set achievable goals that stretch both themselves and the people involved in achieving them.[18]

Leaders hold a fundamental belief in their ability to develop the talents of others. Leadership is:

> the process that ordinary people use when they are bringing forth the best in themselves and in others.

Nursing has a long humanistic tradition. The conditions that support the potential for growth for people in care are also the conditions that support the growth and developing maturity of nursing. In Peplau's original words[2] nursing is 'a maturing force'. Just as people in care need trust to be placed in them, so that they may examine their circumstances and choose future directions, so nurses also need trust to be extended to them, so that they might experiment with creative approaches to developing practice. Transformational leadership is the best way of restabilizing the clinical environment, so that nurses might be released to take constructive action in the development of their discipline. This might result in nurses enjoying more open and creative thinking, and lead to significant advances in the craft of psychiatric caring.

IN SEARCH OF TRANSFORMATIONAL NURSING

To develop nursing further careful analysis of the re-emerging centrality of the nurse–patient relationship is unavoidable. Through such an investigation, psychiatric-mental health nursing might finally define its own core purpose and refine the value of its own unique therapeutic potential.

This is best facilitated through the application of a conceptual framework or model of nursing practice. The need to investigate the potential of nursing through the introduction of models of nursing practice has not always been well supported by nurses.[22] It is likely that the failure of nursing to clarify its unique functions has contributed to a subculture, within which nursing is easily marginalized.

A new model of mental health care holds great practical utility in the further development and clarification of psychiatric-mental health nursing. The *Tidal Model*[23] develops the focus of interpersonal relationships pioneered by Peplau[2] and is constructed specifically to allow nurses to re-establish purposeful, active, working relationships with people in care. The model is based around four core assumptions:

1 The interactive and developmental nature of the nurse–patient relationship.

2 The centrality of the person as an 'expert' in terms of his/her unique potential to understand and derive meaning from the experience of illness.

3 The nurse and patient are involved in a relationship of mutual influence, opening the door to the potential for growth.

4 The everyday nature of nursing practice is harmonized with the problems of everyday living experienced by the person in care.

The Tidal Model[23] is underpinned by the values of mutuality, respect, empowerment and growth. As such, it sits comfortably with the transformational (feminine) learning culture proposed here. With all of these elements in place it is possible to foresee a new form of 'investigative' nursing, which values its traditional origins (interpersonal relationships), based on the creative advancement of the nurse–patient relationship (through active participation), and which seeks continuously to identify, clarify and evaluate emerging developments in practice.

New adventures in nursing

In comparison with other occupational groups nursing is still in its relative infancy. As nursing matures, psychiatric-mental health nurses must become more involved in generating nursing knowledge. The potential of developing the processes of care *for* nursing practice *in* practice, is 'the' single most exciting aspect of the Tidal Model.[23]

The development of nursing knowledge raises questions about the kind of research needed to support it. Currently, the wider trend is towards traditional 'scientific' or quantitative approaches to researching specific treatments or interventions.[24] Such investigations form the research 'evidence' base for specific treatments or interventions. However these offer only limited ways of understanding human behaviour. Scientific experiments are undertaken under controlled conditions, to predict specific outcomes. However, human experience is complicated and compounded by its ever-changing nature, rendering pure scientific examination problematic to say the least. Alternatively, qualitative investigation is likely to reveal more of the 'experience' of living *with* a particular condition, or *in* a particular set of circumstances, and is especially relevant to nursing. However, such enquiry is often considered 'soft science'. Nevertheless this kind of knowledge is more likely to advance the craft of psychiatric caring than the narrow reductionist approaches used to support the meta-analyses within, for example, the Cochrane studies.

Nursing must question the validity of randomized control trials to describe the impact of nursing practice. Superimposing scientific research (relevant to medicine) on the nursing domain, which is more akin to a craft, is at best inappropriate. The way forward for psychiatric-psychiatric-mental health nursing involves developing practice *within* a practice context – for example, through action research. This might allow practice settings to develop the three core elements of advanced nursing practice (*practice, research* and *teaching*) within a practice setting.

The current health care agenda seeks to align nursing with medicine and other occupational groups. While medicine is concerned with cure, nursing is concerned with understanding the impact of illness on a person's everyday experience of living. While health service managers are concerned with controlling resources, nurse leaders are concerned with motivating employees towards higher performance, releasing creativity and facilitating innovation. And while scientific approaches to research are concerned with reducing knowledge to a number of predictable outcomes, nursing might rightfully seek to expand knowledge, to seek further insights into the human problems of living. Nurses and nursing should not shy away from such challenges. The solution rests in active doing.

Back to the future

The focus of nursing's long humanistic tradition has become lost within clinical environments characterized by rapid change and managed care. The absence of a focus on therapeutic caring clinically does not mean that the focus of interpersonal relationships is inadequate or somehow redundant. People experiencing psychiatric distress will continue to need to further their understanding of such experiences. The core focus of psychiatric-mental health nursing is to support and facilitate such enquiry with particular emphasis on how the experience of mental ill health affects the ability of the person to live everyday life.

The future of psychiatric-mental health nursing practice is dependent on the development of clinical learning environments within which nurses are led, rather than pushed or pulled, towards a greater understanding of what is, or is not, quality care.[25] This is a 'real life agenda', where the potential of individual nurses, and their teams, is explored creatively, within an atmosphere of support and respect. Advancing psychiatric-mental health nursing will continue to be a feat of inclusion over isolation, care over control, moral responsibility over professionalism and simple human magic over clever science.

REFERENCES

1. Manley K. A conceptual framework for advanced practice. In: Rolfe G, Fulbrook P (eds). *Advanced nursing practice*. Oxford: Butterworth-Heinemann, 1998.
2. Peplau H. *Interpersonal relations in nursing*. London: Macmillan: GP Putnam, 1988.
3. Rawdon R. *Managing nursing* London: Baillère Tindall, 1984.
4. Walsh M, Ford P. *Nursing ritual research and rational actions*. Oxford: Butterworth-Heinemann, 1989.
5. Barker PJ. *The philosophy and practice of psychiatric-mental health nursing*. London: Churchill-Livingstone, 1999.
6. Hurst K, Wistow G, Higgins R. Managing and leading psychiatric-mental health nursing. *Nursing Management* 2000; **7**(1): 8–12.
7. Senge PM. *The fifth discipline: the art and practice of the learning organisation*. New York: Doubleday, 1994.
8. Yura H, Ozimek D, Walsh MB. *Nursing leadership: theory and process*. New York: Appleton Century Crofts, 1981.
9. Adair J. *Effective leadership*. London: Pan, 1988.
10. Kouzes JM, Posner BZ. *The leadership challenge: how to keep getting extraordinary things done inside organisations*. San Francisco: Jossey-Bass, 1995.
11. Mandela N. *Long walk to freedom*. London: Abacus, 1994.
12. Rosener JB. Ways women lead. *Harvard Business Review* 1990; **Nov–Dec**: 119–25.
13. Aburdene P, Naisbitt J. *Megatrends for women: women are changing the world*. London: Random House, 1994.
14. Helgesen S. *The female advantage: women's ways of leadership*. New York: Doubleday, 1990.
15. Pearson A, McMahon R. *Nursing as therapy*. London: Chapman and Hall, 1991.
16. Bass BM, Avolio BJ. *Improving organisational effectiveness through transformational leadership*. London: Sage, 1994.
17. Bowles A, Bowles NB. A comparative study of leadership development in nursing development units and conventional clinical settings. *Journal of Nursing Management* 2000; **8**: 69–76.
18. Kouzes JM, Posner BZ. Seven lessons for leading the voyage of the future. In: Hesselbein F, Goldsmith M, Beckard R (eds). *The leader of the future*. San Francisco: Jossey Bass, 1996.
19. Peters T. *The Tom Peters Seminar: crazy times call for crazy organisations*. London: Macmillan, 1994.
20. Burns JM. *Leadership*. New York: Harper and Row, 1978.
21. Fairholm GW. Values leadership: a values philosophy model. *International Journal of Value Based Management* 1995; **8**: 65–77.

22. McKenna H. The effects of nursing models on quality of care. *Nursing Times* 1993; **89**: 43–6.

23. Barker P. The Tidal Model: developing an empowering, person-centred approach to recovery within psychiatric and mental health nursing. *Journal of Psychiatric and Psychiatric-Mental Health Nursing* 2001; 8: 233–40.

24. Chalmers I, Altman DG. *Systematic reviews.* London: BMJ Publishing Group, 1995.

25. Barker P. Advanced practice in mental health nursing: developing the core. In: Rolfe G, Fulbrook P (eds). *Advanced Nursing Practice.* Oxford: Butterworth-Heinemann, 1998.

Chapter 6

THE CONCEPT OF RECOVERY

Irene Whitehill*

SURVIVING THE SYSTEM

To put the concept of 'recovery' and the role of the mental health nurse into context I consider it helpful to take a brief look at my own psychiatric career.

I have used psychiatric services for over twenty years. I experienced my first hypomanic episode in 1981 while writing up my doctoral thesis. I heard voices and thought I was the Virgin Mary. I was hospitalized for three months during which time I was given the label of 'manic depressive (bipolar disorder)' and prescribed lithium carbonate. This was the first of fifteen psychotic events in twenty years, which led to hospitalization.

My reaction to that first episode changed the whole direction of my life. I determined that I wanted to gain more information about mental health issues and become involved with people who had gone through similar experiences. I joined a local MIND group (the National Association for Mental Health in the UK) and soon became a representative at Regional and National levels. At the same time I became a founder member of MindLink, MIND's consumer network. This involvement with fellow service users formed the bedrock upon which 'My Journey to Recovery' was founded. Following a career in Further Education, I retrained in Health Promotion before moving into the voluntary sector in

1988. For the past thirteen years I have worked in Advocacy and User Involvement, setting up my own consultancy, Section 36, in 1993.

Between 1981 and 1998 I experienced one psychotic episode each year. The early episodes were extremely traumatic and reflected my initial 'spiritual crisis'. I believed I was Emily Pankhurst and Wayne Sleep and was sectioned on four occasions. In March 1999 I experienced my worst event and was hospitalized for three months. I had both physical and psychiatric symptoms. The consultant thought that as well as my usual psychosis that I could be suffering from a viral infection. I recall that I first brought my Emily Pankhurst persona to life at a striking miner's rally in Yorkshire, when I leapt on to a table and tried to rally the miners' revolutionary fervour. On another occasion I danced down the street, in full Wayne Sleep ballet mode, despite having no dancing ability to speak of. On reflection, these personas, which my psychiatrists perceived as 'delusional states', reflected aspects of my personality, which had lain buried for years. My great compassion for my fellow woman and man, had found its voice in Emily Pankhurst, and my great need to free myself from the past, found its shape in Wayne Sleep's inimitable ballet dancing.

I view my periods of hospitalization as a form of 'containment' rather than a therapeutic process. Service

---

*Dr Irene Whitehill was writing up her doctoral thesis in biology when first diagnosed with manic depression and has endured a further fifteen episodes during the past twenty years. She became a lecturer, but later retrained in health promotion and set up advocate and user/carer involvement projects in the voluntary sector. Since 1993 she has worked as a User Trainer and Consultant offering training and research skills to a wide variety of agencies across the Northern Region of England.

users are just expected to sit in the lounge, watch television, sit in the smoking room, play pool or go to occupational therapy. When I am in hospital I focus on *surviving* the experience. I just try to live by the rules and keep my head together. In my own way I try to adopt the Buddhist concept of just 'being'.

On leaving hospital my self-esteem and self-confidence are always severely undermined. Although I may well be pining for the sanctity of my own home, the most difficult task is to start rebuilding my life once I have been discharged. This was particularly difficult following the severe episode I experienced in March 1999. I felt extremely vulnerable, shell-shocked, emotionally wounded and lacking in energy. I cried myself to sleep most nights throughout the first six months after discharge. I was grieving for all the major losses in my life – the cot death of my younger brother at two months; the incarceration of my mother into a large psychiatric hospital for ten years; broken family ties; the death of both my parents; the emigration of my brother; my hysterectomy; being without a partner; failed relationships; having to give up my consultancy – Section 36; the trauma of fifteen psychotic episodes. It took three months before I felt physically and emotionally resilient enough to attend a creative writing course for women and six months before I was able to start work again, in a voluntary capacity.

Thankfully, I have not experienced a psychotic event for over three years. Most days my mood is stable and I feel extremely positive about life. However, twice a year I go into a depressive phase which lasts for three weeks. Fortunately, my self-management skills enable me to survive these phases, safe in the knowledge that I will come out the other end. Emotionally, I often feel extremely vulnerable but these periods do not last forever and I am learning to deal with my emotions more effectively.

I agreed to contribute to this chapter because I believe that mental health nurses have a key role in working with service users to help them on their 'journey to recovery'. I base these observations on my various roles as service user, project manager and user consultant.

Meanings of 'recovery'

Before considering the impact that nurses can have upon the recovery of service users we need to define exactly what we mean by the term. The Chambers 20th Century Dictionary's[1] definition of 'recover' is – 'to cure'.

In the context of mental health 'recovery' is generally not accepted as being synonymous with 'cure'. From her work with service users Repper observed that:

> Recovery does not mean that all suffering has disappeared, or that all symptoms have been removed, or that functioning has been completely restored.[2]

Pat Deegan, a clinical psychologist with a late childhood diagnosis of schizophrenia recognized that 'recovery' is not a 'cure' but sees no reason for despair.

> Being in recovery means I know I have certain limitations and things I can't do. But rather than letting these limitations be an occasion for despair and giving up, I have learned that in knowing what I can't do, I also open up the possibilities of all I can do.[3]

In contrast, Dan Fischer and Laurie Ahern,[4] from the National Empowerment Centre, in the USA, have developed an empowerment model for 'recovery', believing that people can fully 'recover' from even the most severe forms of mental illness. However, they accept that people need time to heal emotionally:

I do not feel totally 'cured' of manic depression. The major highs seem to be in abeyance but I still experience minor mood swings a few times a year. The emotional pain bubbles up to the surface when I am least expecting it. Most days, however, I feel a sense of 'well-being'. I have developed a greater insight into my condition and learnt how to self manage my highs and lows more effectively. I now recognize the importance of being able to have more control over my emotions. I have been teaching myself to resign them to the 'left luggage', so to speak, until I feel able to deal with them. These behavioural changes cannot be achieved overnight. Recovery is not so much an event, as a process. For many people, including myself, this may well be a lifelong quest.

Acceptance is a key factor in the recovery process. Again, Pat Deegan notes that:

> ... an ever-deepening acceptance of our limitations. But now, rather than being an occasion for despair, we find our personal limitations are the ground from which spring our own unique possibilities. This is the paradox of recovery ... that in accepting what we cannot do or be we begin to discover what we can be and what we can do ... recovery is a process. It is a way of life. It is an attitude and a way of approaching the day's challenges.[5]

After a great deal of soul searching, I have been able to accept that although my journey to recovery may last a life time, it is possible for me to value myself and get back into the driving seat of my life. I have come to accept that:

- ❏ I really do have infinite self-worth.
- ❏ I can confront my own vulnerability without feeling inadequate.
- ❏ I am worthy of love and friendship.

❏ I need to be able to ask for support from both pro-fessionals and friends, without feeling embarrassed or inadequate.

❏ I need to acknowledge that I can be as much of a friend as my friends have been to me.

❏ I am not a failure because I had to give up my busi-ness and am now working in a voluntary capacity and living on disability benefits.

❏ I subjected myself to too much stress and turned into a 'workaholic'. Too much of my 'persona' was tied up in my work.

❏ I have a great deal of expertise and practical skills that will enable me to put something back into the community and enjoy a good life.

Following my period of hospitalization three years ago I thought that I was 'stuck' and would never be able to get my life back together, let alone move forward. However, I have learnt to develop my self-management skills. By adopting the concept of 'Being Your Own Scientist' I have found that it is possible to become more aware of my moods and how to manage them.[6] More recently, I attended a self-management training course organized by the Manic Depression Fellowship (2001) which con-solidated a great many of the issues I had discussed with my colleague, Professor Phil Barker.

However, despite the improvement in self-manage-ment skills the pace of my life was too fast and I still found it impossible to balance work, socializing, and time for myself. I found it very difficult to relax. I was labelled a 'workaholic' but no-one was offering me any solutions. Finally, after eighteen years in the system, I was referred to a psychotherapist. At first I was very sceptical, but as the weeks went by I realized what a luxury it was to meet with someone on a regular basis, who listened to me without being judgemental. We have worked together for the past three years. During that time we have focused upon the following themes which I have tried to integrate into my daily life:

❏ **Balancing** – getting the balance right between work, socializing and time alone.
❏ **Pacing** – learning to live my life at the pace that suits me.
❏ **Boundary setting** – letting things or people into my life that are acceptable to me.

Trust soon developed and we have developed a good working partnership. Therapy is not an easy option. I have had to work in the gaps between the sessions and sometimes it has been extremely painful. However, three years down the line I know that it has been a life-changing process.

The path to recovery also relies upon positivity. Over the years I have read a great many books on positive thinking, self-help and personal development. I have not always found my reading very profitable. It is one thing to read a book but another to put any suggested behav-ioural changes into practice. However, one book, which I have found particularly helpful is *You Can Heal Your Life* by Louise Hay.[7] She believes that developing a posi-tive attitude to daily life can overcome any dis-ease. I was very fortunate to participate in a one-day training course which promoted her thinking. On the day I developed my own set of 'positive affirmations' a copy of which I have tacked to the wall in my office and refer to them every day:

Irene's affirmations

■ You are a unique and independent woman. You choose not to compare yourself with other people.
■ You are in 'control' of your life and approve of yourself.
■ You are capable of handling everything you choose to do and stay well at the same time.
■ You let go of other people's business and look after yourself.
■ You enclose yourself in a protective bubble and feel peaceful.

The psychotherapy sessions and training in positive thinking have helped me to redefine who I am. It's as if I have reinvented myself. There has been a distinct change in my 'self'. Simon Champ, a prominent Australian mental health activist, also views recovery as a lifelong process which requires important changes in 'self':

> I have come to see that you do not simply patch up the self you were before developing schizophrenia, but that you have to actually recreate a concept of who you are that integrates the experience of schizophrenia. Real recovery is far from a simple matter of accepting diagnosis and learning facts about the illness and medication. Instead, it is a deep searching and questioning, a journey through unfamiliar feelings, to embrace new concepts and a wider view of self. It is not an event but a process. For many, I believe it is a lifelong journey.[8]

These changes have been painful at times but have brought with them great periods of personal growth. Anthony has written :

> Recovery is described as a deeply personal, unique process of changing one's attitudes, values, feelings, goals, skills, and/or roles. It is a way of living a satisfying, hopeful and contributing life, even with limitations caused by the illness. Recovery involves the development of new meaning and purpose in one's life as one grows beyond the catastrophic effects of mental illness.[9]

I try to live 'one day at a time'. Most days I experience a sense of well-being and feel good about myself. I am learning to live my life at a pace that suits me and to appreciate the simpler things – such as my morning walk to the local shops; watching cloud formations from the bus window; walking along the beach; the arrival of the first daffodils; rediscovering a favourite piece of music; trying out a new recipe. I have different priorities. I work hard to ensure that my voluntary work does not envelop me completely! I need time for my hobbies, seeing friends and time for myself. Most days I feel in a state of equilibrium, safe in the knowledge that if I did experience a mood swing I could deal with it myself or, if necessary, seek out the appropriate professional support.

AIDING THE RECOVERY PROCESS

I consider myself extremely fortunate as a great many *things* and *people* have come into my life over the past twenty years, which have aided my journey to recovery:

❑ **Resilience** – My father brought me up to fight my own battles and be able to deal with whatever life threw at me. As I was growing up I often felt that he was being too harsh. However, my struggle with manic depression throughout the past twenty years has shown me how right he was, to work at promoting my resilience.

❑ **Spirituality** – I have always believed that a higher power had a hand in every part of my life. Throughout my childhood, teenage years and early adulthood I accepted that the higher power was the living God. However, in my forties, I discovered Buddhism, which proved to be far more helpful than Christianity in promoting my recovery process. The concept of 'being present in the moment' has helped me not just survive but grow through my periods of hospitalization.

❑ **Stability** – I have lived in the same former mining village for thirteen years, putting down roots.

❑ **People** – I live in a small community. People are very friendly but respect my privacy. I enjoy a good rapport with people serving in shops, plus a sense of belonging.

❑ **Home** – My home is away from the main road, is quiet with a garden and looks out onto trees. I have access to a local park and feel safe and secure in my own space. Certain practical things help – preparing the evening meal, the ritual of setting the table, listening to the radio, watching television or a video, reading books/magazines which have nothing to do with mental health, and getting enough sleep.

❑ **Self-medication** – This is a daily ritual. I check daily to ensure that I do not run out of tablets and always carry a pill-box with me when out for the day.

❑ **Relaxation** – Although I enjoy seeing my friends I do crave a certain amount of solitude. I am learning to relax. I can now allow myself to watch a video knowing that there's a pile of dishes in the sink! I am trying to banish guilt and perfectionism and to challenge hopelessness in a positive way.

❑ **Pampering myself** – Everyone needs to find ways of pampering themselves. The highlight of my month is a 'full-body aromatherapy massage' and an 'Indian head massage'. I have an oil burner in every room and use oils in the bath. I just adore having a leisurely bath by candlelight and lounging around afterwards in my towelling robe. I also enjoy having a leisurely breakfast and sitting in the garden reading the local newspaper.

❑ **Self-presentation** – Pampering myself and engaging in some voluntary work helped to increase my self-confidence. I began to take more notice of my appearance. I sorted out my wardrobe. I now wear make-up more often and dress-up for meetings and nights out with my girlfriends.

❑ **Neighbour** – I am very friendly with a neighbour upstairs, who has looked after my cats and cut my grass when I was in hospital. Often we meet to catch up on gossip.

❑ **Friends** – I have a good network of friends locally, few of whom work in mental health. Friends in different parts of country and abroad keep in touch by telephone and e-mail. I support them just as much as they support me. They tend to ask me if I have any problems related to mental health.

❑ **Colleagues** – I enjoy long-standing collaboration with colleagues, which is very supportive. They do not set any deadlines for me rejoining our various projects, understanding that I needed a time for recuperation.

❑ **Voluntary work** – This boosts my self-esteem and self-confidence and encourages me to develop my skills and expertise.

❑ **Professional support** – My care is managed under the Care Programme Approach (CPA). My progress has been so good that now I only meet with the team once every six months. However, I do have a direct line to my psychiatrist and community psychiatric nurse (CPN) should a serious mood change occur between appointments.

❑ **Advocate** – My advocate is a social worker, which is useful when dealing with system. She is a personal friend and has supported me through several hospital admissions. She usually attends the CPA meetings, which occur early after discharge.

❑ **Community psychiatric nurse** – My CPN visits me on a regular basis. I value both her ordinariness and professionalism.[10] She relates to me very much as a 'person' and not a 'label'. She has helped me with a variety of issues such as choosing the colour scheme for my lounge, drafting up a list of triggers for manic and depressive episodes and helping me to claim disability benefits.

- ❑ **Psychotherapist** – My referral to the psychotherapist was a life-changing event. It has not always been easy integrating 'balancing', 'pacing' and 'boundary setting' into my daily life. However, I reflect on my behaviour each day and aim to do better the next.
- ❑ **Home-care worker** – She helps me with the housework and provides a friendly face twice a week. At first I felt awkward about accepting such a service in my mid-forties. However, I soon realized that she would be able to help me keep on track more effectively and help me slide back into my life after a period in hospital.
- ❑ **Information** – As I work in the system it has been relatively easy for me to gather information about my condition, medication, available services and how to complain. Socially, I have a habit of picking up leaflets, reading notice boards and getting myself on arts and music mailing lists. I may not be able to afford to go to everything I used to, but I can have interesting conversations with friends who have been to a particular play etc!

BLOCKING THE RECOVERY PROCESS

There is always a downside. Some things and people have conspired to block my recovery process.

- ❑ **Friends** – Friends can be overprotective. They don't believe that I should be moving on in a particular direction. I have felt hindered sometimes because they do not approve of me 'getting back into the driving seat'.
- ❑ **Relatives** – My brother fails to understand why I work in mental health and believes that it would be far better for my health if I worked in a flower shop, for example. While I appreciate his concern I will not let my diagnosis limit my lifestyle. I do not wish to feel as if the 'sword of Damocles' was hovering over my head. If I cannot take risks, even experience failure, I may as well be institutionalized.
- ❑ **Stigma** – I have frequently experienced the stigma and prejudice associated with mental illness. On meeting people for the first time I have had to gauge when and how much to disclose. I baulk against this because I am not ashamed of who I am. However, when you are in the early stages of recovery it can be very painful to be faced with rejection because of your health status. Quite often people have spoken to me as the 'label' and not the 'person'. My own sister-in-law thinks that anyone labelled with a mental illness should be 'carted off to the funny farm'. Many service users only have professionals or fellow service users as friends because they are frightened of being stigmatized if they 'come out'. They find it very difficult to socialize outside of user groups. I am fortunate in that once I have recuperated I have enough confidence to join an evening class, for example, and make friends outside of mental health.
- ❑ **Benefits trap** – Service users need to have good budgeting skills to exist on benefits for long periods. It is very difficult to make that leap from living on benefits back into employment. Many service users do not feel able to take the risk in case they cannot get back onto benefits should they need to.
- ❑ **Impatience** – On occasions I do get extremely frustrated when I think of the possibilities of me ever getting back to paid work. However, I recognize that I need to practice the art of patience and live each day to the full rather than hankering after something I may never achieve.

MENTAL HEALTH NURSES AND RECOVERY

Mental health nurses are the key personnel working with service users on the ward and in the community. They have an essential role in supporting service users in their journey to recovery. The list below illustrates the critical aspects of the relationship between the mental health nurse and the service user from admission to discharge:

- ❑ **Service users as 'people' not 'labels'** – Many mental health nurses are prejudiced towards people in their care. There is a tendency for mental health nurses to relate to the diagnosis and not the person, especially when the service user has been admitted on several occasions (the 'revolving door' patient). Quite often mental health nurses have limited expectations of people in their care because they know very little about their lives outside of hospital. Some mental health nurses are frightened of giving up their power by relating to service users on an equal level, while others have been trapped in the office doing paperwork for so long that they have forgotten how to relate to service users as ordinary people.
- ❑ **'Caring with' not 'caring for'** – The mental health nurse forms a partnership with the service user to support them through the recovery process.[10,11] The trustworthy nurse acts as an ally and brings to the relationship both ordinariness and professionalism. The attitudes, beliefs and expressed needs of the service user should be accepted at every stage, and the user knows that the advice of the nurse may not necessarily be accepted.

- **On admission** – A mental health nurse needs to be present on admission to make the process less threatening and to add a sense of continuity when the service user moves onto the ward.

- **Assessment** – A mental health nurse needs to carry out the initial assessment with the service user. The assessment should be carried out in such a way that service users feel comfortable about expressing their views. All experiences should be accepted as 'true' and not dismissed as 'hallucinations' and added to notes without discussion. What does the service user feel caused their admission and what do they feel they need to address these problems?

- **Aids/blocks to 'recovery'** – A mental health nurse needs to work with service users to identify things/people, which might aid or block recovery.

- **Skills assessment** – A mental health nurse needs to work with the service users to identify skills that are required to promote recovery. Service users may not feel able to identify skills or join in any self-management/recovery groups. There is a right time for everything and the service user must be allowed to dictate the pace of their own recovery.

- **Facilitating self-management/recovery groups** – Specifically trained mental health nurses facilitate a selection of groups informed by the skills assessments carried out with service users. Contents could include: assertiveness; decision-making; building self-esteem and self-confidence; self-presentation; self-management skills; dealing with psychosis; living with voices; mental health promotion; self-medication; complementary therapies, etc.

- **Nurse training** – All mental health nurses need to undergo training in 'positive images' and 'user involvement' facilitated by an 'independent user consultant' or representatives from a local 'user group'. Specific preparation in one-to-one, and group work is necessary, so that nurses might be more effective in working with individual service users and facilitating self-management/recovery groups.

- **Acting as a 'link'** – The mental health nurse needs to act as a link with other professionals involved in the individual's package of care. Acts as user's voice within multidisciplinary team meetings. If acceptable, makes links with carers/friends/advocate to ensure that they are kept informed of individual's progress and to ascertain what role they will play when service user is discharged. If appropriate, introduces service user to the on-site Welfare Rights Officer.

- **Promoting social inclusion** – The mental health nurse needs to make links and collect information about appropriate agencies (housing, benefits agency, employment, job clubs, skills centre, self-help groups, social groups, women's groups, play groups, adult education classes) operating within the hospital's catch-ment area. Prior to discharge, the mental health nurse should work with the service user to consider their needs once they have moved back into the community. The nurse then contacts the agencies to ensure that they do indeed meet the needs of the service user. A CPN is appointed who can support the service user once they have moved back into community. The mental health nurse informs the CPN about the service users progress on their path to 'recovery' and feeds back the information she has gleaned from the agencies which she/he has contacted.

- **Discharge** – Prior to discharge, the service user meets with the CPN to discuss her/his expressed needs and how the CPN can support them now that they are moving back into the community.

MAIN CHALLENGES FOR MENTAL HEALTH NURSES

Three main challenges face mental health nurses in the 21st century:

1 A paradigm shift is needed, from 'containment' to 'therapeutic experience'. Mental health nurses need to break out of the mechanistic routine, which restricts their dialogue with service users. This ranges from giving orders – 'come down to the dining routine it's time for meds'; 'It's Tuesday, put clean sheets on your bed' – to relating with service users as people.

Nurses often base themselves in the office doing paperwork and only come out at specific times, to take out the drugs trolley, serve the meals, or periodically observe different service users. The people who spend most time talking with service users are nursing assistants and domestic staff. In the twenty years I have been using services, I have found the quality of nursing to be based more upon the intrinsic personal qualities of particular nurses – compassion, empathy, active listening ordinariness – rather than specific nurse training.

2 Mental health nurses must be prepared to undergo specific training which would enable them to 'care with' not 'care for' service users. Phil Barker and his colleagues[12] have developed a model of mental health care that puts the person at the heart of the 'caring' process, and which focuses on the possibility of recovery, for everyone.

3 Having taken the leap from containment to therapeutic experience it would be counterproductive if an attempt was not made to promote 'social inclusion' when service users move

back into the community. Mental health nurses will need specialist training so that they might form a bridge between service users and community services.

Above all, mental health nurses must be the bearer of hope and believe in the 'recovery' of service users no matter what particular path they have had to follow.

REFERENCES

1. MacDonald AM (ed.) *Chambers 20th Century Dictionary*. London: Chambers Harrap Ltd. 1978.

2. Repper J. Adjusting the focus of mental health nursing: incorporating service users' experiences of recovery. *Journal of Mental Health* 2000; **9** (6): 575–87.

3. Deegan PE. Recovering our sense of value after being labelled mentally ill. *Journal of Psycho-social Nursing* 1993; **31**: 7–11.

4. Fisher D, Ahern L. People can recover from mental illness. *National Empowerment Center*. Newsletter Article at the/website, 1999. http://www.power2u.org

5. Deegan PE. The independent living movement and people with psychiatric disabilities: taking back the control of our own lives. *Psycho-social Rehabilitation Journal* 1992; **15**: 3–19.

6. Barker P. Personal communication, 1993.

7. Hay L. *You can heal your life*. London: Eden Grove Editions, 1988.

8. Champ S. A most precious thread. In: Barker P, Campbell P, Davidson B (eds). *The ashes of experience: reflections on madness, survival and growth*. London: Whurr Publishers, 1999: 113–26.

9. Anthony WA. Recovery from mental illness: the guiding vision of the mental health service system in the 1990s. *Innovations and Research* 1993; **2**: 17–24.

10. Barker P, Jackson S, Stevenson C. What are psychiatric nurses needed for? Developing a theory of essential nursing practice. *Journal of Mental Health and Psychiatric Nursing* 1999; **6**: 273–82.

11. Barker P, Whitehill I. The craft of care: towards collaborative caring in psychiatric nursing. In: Tilley S (ed.) *The mental health nurse: views of practice and education*. Oxford: Blackwell Science, 1999.

12. Barker P. The Tidal Model: developing an empowering, person-centred approach to recovery within psychiatric and mental health nursing. *Journal of Psychiatric and Psychiatric-Mental Health Nursing* 2001; **8**: 233–40.

Chapter 7

RECOVERY AND RECLAMATION: A PILGRIMAGE IN UNDERSTANDING WHO AND WHAT WE ARE

Anne Helm*

THE UNIVERSALITY OF THE TASK

Recovery is rapidly becoming the 'in' word of psychiatric practice. As a long-time user of the mental health system I find the word ambiguous in its resonance. The importance of understanding that 'nothing ever stays the same' is, I believe, a given. We who are service users can rebuild our lives, defined by us in terms of quality. More so, you (the reader) and I (the service user) are, from birth to death, in a constant process of 'recovery'. The complexity of early relationships provides in itself much for some of us to recover from. Add to that the difficult adolescent voyage towards self-identity and the uncertainty of adult life and it could be asked of anyone reading this chapter, has she/he recovered? Recovery is not a destination, but the journeying task of making sense of life itself, and I ask the reader to accept the universality of the task. We are all in recovery. There are no *patients* to seek recovery for, no *nurses* to map the waterways and guide the boats on the voyage. We are all fellow wayfarers, who can share experiences and insights from our own lives, thereby facilitating each other's progress.

Humanness, in the 21st century, means we are constantly called to make sense out of our experience and incorporate it into our lives. For those of us with the experience of mental illness, making sense and giving value to that experience can be likened to doing a jigsaw puzzle with no picture to work from. In doing the task, we often discover several different puzzles have been placed within the same box. For me, some of my puzzle pieces may always be missing. The challenge to understand who and what I am is constant. However, I do get more of an integrated sense of self as I get older and wellness accompanies that. My quest for wellness was amidst horrific practices that are thankfully outmoded and relegated to psychiatric nursing history. My journey has therefore been mostly an internal one and my contributions to this chapter will reflect that.

MY BACKGROUND OF MOVING FROM SURVIVAL TO RECOVERY

I had my first experience of psychosis at the age of nineteen. My struggle for sanity and understanding through it took place in the context of nursing in the late 1960s onwards in New Zealand. This was a time when lock-ups, seclusion cells, sleep therapy, and the threat of

---

*Anne Helm is a musician and consumer advocate in Dunedin, New Zealand.

electroconvulsive therapy (ECT) as a means of control, were common. This was a time when wards of the forgotten were housed, fed, watered and medicated and sometimes strapped to their beds. The nursing staff came from the surrounding countryside by night and day and drove back along the long, sealed driveways to their lives on the outside. They brought their gossipy news of their socialized lives to share with each other, excluding us from their conversations as if we were inanimate objects. We, the crazed, were removed from the community and placed in institutions with sadly ironic names like 'Cherry Farm' and 'Sunnyside'. There was no flow-through traffic from the wider community and many of us – abandoned by families who were unable to deal with the shame or cope with the insanity of their kin – were placed daily in front of television to work out where we were in time and place, with no human reference points.

The reflections I have about it now are of a period when body and thoughts were dulled by heavy anti-psychotic medications. Disinterest was the all-pervading, emanating characteristic of the trained nursing staff, as heavy roll-lock keys swung and jangled at the jailers' sides. My last long-term hospitalization was in 1979. In one way it 'worked' – I had gained a slight but smouldering sense of self that would never allow my being to be placed in an institution again, and I never did.

I developed a theory about who was helpful and who didn't give a damn. Almost without exception the more stripes on the shoulder and medals that swung from the breast the less caring and humanly interactive the staff became. The first time I was bathed after the barbarity of seclusion a young, dark-haired endorsed nurse (one step above a nurse aid) gently washed my hair, touching my scalp with delicate massaging fingers. The simple experience of that act of caring was immensely powerful, as human touch had been so long denied me. I lay in the bathtub and as I looked up at her I felt I was in the presence of a different kind of human being all together. She was an angel, and goodness was in existence in my world.

THE SIMPLICITY OF THE SOLUTION

I have read much about the principles of the recovery focus in mental health. Words like partnership, acceptance, empathy, respect, building on strengths, hope, and compassion are to be found there. The task of rebuilding my life feels for me like a much more solo-navigated journey, as much of it had to be done out of isolation – away from what *was* my life. I do know though, that the stars that shone upon my craft came in the form of simple acts of human kindness from people such as the nurse I have just mentioned. Write as many words about recovery as you wish, one word fits all. It is of course *love*. This is the essential healer. Poets, musicians and spiritual leaders tell, and retell us. What counts *was* love, *is* love and *will always be* love.

Coming through a period of psychiatric institutionalization, where the act of loving in caring practices was the exception, made me hold onto those drops of nourishment, which helped restore my own sense of dignity and enabled me to begin the journey of reclamation. In spite of the anguish of my struggle I know from rubbing shoulders with certain gentle humble people of this world, that healing is possible and life can be fully and joyously lived amidst the crisis events of our lives, and in spite of diagnosis.

HEALING RELATIONSHIPS

The importance of realness in relationships

I was held by a long time committal in that hospital, and so began to look for quality relationships within its walls. I sought out the nurse aids, gardeners and cooks for real conversations about their lives and they listened with interest to the fragments of what I could tell them about mine. Practical down-to-earth people with their own struggles and openness in sharing helped give me a frame of reference to reflect my own life against. This place was a wasteland of the rejected where the institution existed to support the needs of the staff who ran it. Meaningful caring was not part of the ethos. The less trained were different. Simple acts of human kindness – like kitchen staff putting boiled water aside for me at morning tea time so I did not have to drink the mass-served, luke-warm, highly sweetened milky tea – became a sign of my own individual worth.

One or two special events stick in the memory and had a profound effect. The following is one of them.

I was very sensitive to sound of any kind. Unable to deal with the noise of socialization I had been constantly returned to a barren, bed-less seclusion cell. I had broken this pattern to progress to a locked, but more pleasant room, with a bed and a cabinet. One evening in a talent quest I had found my voice to sing and stunned the hall into silence. I carried my little green vase, given to me as the winner, back to the villa and placed it on the cabinet. Medicated and locked in for the night I thought how strange it was that this little vase was all I amounted to at that time. In the morning I awoke to an abundance of velvet red roses in bloom beside me. One of the aids, an older man who I had often dragged out of his reticence into conversation, had gone home and cut them for me from his much-loved garden. I learnt much from that quiet, retired seaman. He is prominent in the league of the gentle, humble angels to whom I owe pure, deep gratitude.

Many of the unqualified aid staff were splendid people. It was the aids that took me during their lunchtime to the swimming pool so I could use the pool alone, diving deep like a porpoise, swimming underwater to find my sense of aliveness and weightless freedom. And it was the aids who would unlock my room, and the day room, at dawn before shift change, so my fingers could find their way over a piano again.

Authentic relationships and commonalities

Nowadays we have fewer stories of long institutional lives unlived, and yet within the community-care model, patronizing attitudes of mental health professionals who 'know' and the recipients of their 'help', who 'doesn't know', still prevail.

Much is now written about the 'therapeutic relationship' in nursing practice. However, I still have to ask 'what the hell is that?' I have used the Psychiatric District Nurse system here in New Zealand and the best relationship I have had is with a nurse who battled with her own family alienation issues because of her sexual orientation. This nurse and I had parallel issues about stigmatization and our relationship, as a result, was gritty and real. Whether any of us function or do not function depends on our self-concepts as we live among the wider community, and that is universal. Effective relationships are, as Mary Auslander, the American consumer advocate says, about 'looking for the commonalities amongst us rather than the differences we discern from diagnosis.'[a]

The most therapeutic happenings in my journey have been with people who share of their own lives.

Seeing us as other

If the nurse sees us as 'other' – observing behaviours as symptoms of the illness – barriers are erected to relating, and to understanding what is going on for us. Some behaviour is hard to see beyond, yet I do believe that whatever is presented, a process of searching lies within it. Here is a challenging example.

A young woman in manic scattered psychosis has been placed in a barren seclusion cell. Naked except for an ill tying gown, she has a rough blanket for sleeping on, and a plastic bucket for her toileting. The practice of the day meant she had been given initial sedation of paraldehyde, which left her struggling like a wounded animal to even pick up her body from the cold lino floor. Heavy brown brogue shoes of fat-calved charge nurses periodi-cally pushed food in plastic bowls towards her. No-one spoke, no-one told her where she was, and the only touch given to her was the prizing open of the jaw to pour the thick brown anti-psychotic syrup down the throat. She was left for days. In psychosis she did not experience 'delusion' as clinicians had said. In fact her psychosis had much beauty and a sense of connectedness to the world. Awareness of the emotions of the human condition had been sharply intense. She had witnessed in many faces extremities of despair, anguish and human angst, being contrasted with the sheer joy and lightness of the simple act of smiling and giving of affection. Her world had sparkled. In that cell, all perceptions of her universe were boxed in and removed. Drugs took over. Any interaction with her now was as a jailer to a beast. New thoughts formed as she tried to make sense of her incarceration and where she was. Perhaps she really had lost the plot and had gone mad. She thought in her madness she must surely have killed a child, something dearly loved and innocent. Only an act such as that could warrant the disdain with which she was treated. She pleaded with her inner god that it had not been so and with the blanket wrapped around her, rocked and crooned for days, struggling to find a section of her mind that would assure her she had committed no crime. She lay there for weeks.

One day she changed things in her world. She held the only material available in her hands and painted the walls of the cell, fingers and palms exploring the texture and flowing designs. In the timelessness of day into night into day again, and left without human interaction, she had found a minute speck of something of herself and within herself. This act of doing and creating was the beginning of piecing herself together again. She had been in the cell for weeks and had discovered something very basic. To 'do' is to be human. Who would ever understand this behaviour, this regressed faeces smearer?

I do. I was that young woman. We are the experts of our own experience.

CONSUMER DEFINED RECOVERY

Definition of self

Recovery is a self-defined process. To me recovery means just getting on with life. 'Getting over it' as my kids would say. It means incorporating the experience into the fullness of all my living. How can someone 'get over' mental illness when the severity and complexity of reasons for diagnosed conditions are so variable? Does it mean the successful suicide has failed to get over it? How do I write of recovery and believe I am well down

---

[a] Mary Auslander, quoted by Tregoweth J, *Awhi Tautoko Aroha. Celebrating recovery-focused mental health workers.* Wellington New Zealand, Mental Health Commission, 2001: 23.

that path, when I still have 'a diagnosis' and an occasional visit to the psychiatrist, and am at present on maintenance medication? Once again I state that recovery is not a place to get to but a process. The starting point of this process is a belief in one's own value.

To some of the people I work with, recovery is seen as a negative term associated with an illness being 'cured'. The medical model looks to return the patient to the not-ill state. But people have mental illness as an experience, not an objective reality. It is woven into the fabric of who and what they are. Sometimes recovery is expressed as 'learning to live with it'. This feels similarly disempowering to me. My 'it' is part of me and always has been. I am more than the sum of my genetics and have tried to avoid subscribing to the brain-disease/chemical-imbalance medical focus, to describe my reality. I would have remained in an institution without the healing power of bare feet upon wet grass if I had believed these constructs were all I amounted to.

Recovering what?

Recovery indicates gaining something that was lost, but the depth of the journey is much richer than that. I would say it was finding something of my explicit uniqueness and wonder as a human being, along the way. It is a voyage towards integration of the self. Who am I and what am I? are questions we all ask ourselves from time to time. Those of us with mental illness are probably called upon to ask the question more often. The challenge of my journey has been whether I will weave the experiences of 'illness', my psychotic state, into an integrated sense of self, or regard the 'illness' as being part of an 'otherness'. This is the challenge, and as long as nursing practice focuses on the 'otherness' our self-perception and fragmentation is affected. If recovery is 'a state of mind' as has been said, making sense of who I am, as experienced through my mind, can be difficult.

Actualizing wellness

The recovery journey then comes from an internal desire for wellness. It should have no clinical definition, as it is the service user who must define what the outward display of that means for herself/himself. On one level there may be functional abilities to recover – such as the ability to concentrate to read and keep the hand steady enough to write, to converse without the slurring of the heavy medicated tongue and fogginess of the mind. Oftentimes, medicated sedation and their side-effects are the greatest hindrance to this basic reclamation. As we move into clearer functioning we wish to claim the functions of the wider community, like the right to drive

a car, work, make love, and have children. Then there are the more external things to realize and recover. Our illness will always put us on the back foot economically. Returning to education, establishing a home base, restoring old friendships and building new ones, and finding our place again within our families of origin, can be an overwhelming challenge. For some of us the returning to our families of origin can never be part of our wellness plans, as our madness was born out of them.

The internal journey lies at the core of all this reclamation. Courage, self-responsibility, realizing we are more than our illness, feeling good about ourselves and finding peace in the integration process, are just some of the elements that we have to find for the work required.

Integrating into community

Other people are essential to confirming our wellness. Our sense of who we are is often fragmented. Some of us have lost our work place and therefore have no definition by our jobs. If abandoned by family and friends we have no human context from which to glean a sense of the self, and no reflectors or interactions that will tell us we are OK people. As we bridge back into our local communities we meet hesitation and uncertainty in the eyes of people who know you have a mental illness. Fear of the unknown and therefore the 'dark' nature of mental illness is a reality, and our group's coverage in media does nothing to allay such fears. In such an environment working out our self-identity as other than *the mentally ill* takes much weaving, discarding many threads and choosing others. The choice will be affected by the affirmations of people around us.

CARING NURSING PRACTICE

My wellness came as a result of many simultaneous processes at work. I have spoken at length about the internal processes, and hope this sharing is helpful. There are obvious attitudes and behaviours that are not helpful to the rebuilding work we have to do. I came through a period of 'care' that exemplified many of them. Among these were: belittlement, lack of human respect and the loss of human dignity; lack of validation of the 'patient's' experience and our accompanying emotions; seeing us only as a set of behavioural deviants. And then there was the distant expert who seldom entered into conversations with the patients but knew what was 'best' for us and kept institutions functional for staff by his decisions. (Historically the 'experts' were always male.) Even now as a service user I meet health professionals who, with superior attitude, know more about my 'illness' than I do myself, and who can jettison my sense of wellness and of place.

The fine-tuning required to strike an empowering attitude of care is a delicate thing. 'Do-gooders' with a sense of helping the unfortunate, while nobly motivated, can be a pain in the proverbial arse. By its nature this model means that the professional occupies a state of the 'more' to the 'less than' in what is, undeniably, a patronizing relationship.

What really helps is the acknowledgement of our own resourcefulness and innate talents and capabilities. What is needed for such real relationships to happen is a certain humility. I return to my opening paragraph about the universal nature of making sense out of life or 'recovery' if you like. Sharing what *you* know and what *I* know needs to ebb and flow between us. The reward for relatedness is that we learn from each other.

CONTINUAL RECOVERY AND ANGELS ON THE JOURNEY

I have thought a lot about this word *recovery* and how it resounds within me. Part of my early story involved recovery from addictive substances. This proclivity did nothing for my already ignited disposition towards mania. Contextually that part of my life was real journeying both in the mind and on foot! I was dealing with the death of my mother, the loss of my family home, and a broken late-adolescent marriage and the subsequent removal of my first child. Trying to nullify the pain by self-medication and seeking psychedelic experiences seemed a good way to go. On reflection I can see a young woman trying to work out where she was going and who she was in the midst of all this.

The continuing search for identity

Our baby was born amidst young relationship dysfunction and I entered a period of deep grieving for my mother, made complex by my own sense of maternal inadequacy and anxiety. I had postnatal depression they said, and when my anxieties became manifest as the crying voice of my own baby I was 'crazy again'. Baby and mother were separated and hospitalizations followed. There was no family that could extend support. I had lost contact with my university friends and lived in a depressive flat above an early morning drinkers' pub overlooking the city gas works. Motherhood was a foreign experience to me. I remember lacing up my white roller skating boots I had from childhood and skating around the wooden floor of the old disused 1920s ballroom at the back of the flat in an attempt to hold onto something of the person I was and had known. Now there was a small helpless little baby girl dependent on me and on me alone. I was overwhelmed by the intensity of the responsibility. The baby's father was only a teenager himself, but he was a young man going places. He worked long hours and I befuddled my way through days of confusion and displacement in the grime of my surroundings. The music enthusiast, classical singer, and student once so enthusiastic with life and living had gone. I battled with my task of caring for my child until one day, knowing I was not mother enough, and fearing the snapping of my own sanity, I locked the baby's door, filled a bath, and slit my wrists after overdosing on as much as I could find. Providence – in the form of the pub sandwich-maker needing to use an unblocked toilet – meant I survived that act, an act I had chosen with such clear certainty. In a strange sense another angel had been put my way.

The ebb and flow of the journey

I see the journey towards wellness as an upward spiral motion. Sometimes the bottom of the spiral touches the base line of where we have been before, but it is often moving in an ebb and flow motion.

The climb back to finding life worth living again was a very long haul. I was encouraged to play the piano again. I had a very special doctor, another humble angel, who would bring in the music of his favourite arias for me to learn and place them beside my bed. When it came to group activities he would just say 'Anne will not be involved, she will be at the piano again.' I began to experience the joy of singing again and slowly over a period of time regained a sense of centre from which to rebuild. My baby was placed elsewhere and my husband took off up north in an exciting career move. The feeling surrounding my baby's removal and its subsequent effects are part of the weave of my life. The day she was taken, I gave my bridal veil to a young kid in the street for a dress-up and started self-medicating the pain of accumulated loss.

Drugs and hitching on the side of the road where the traffic was heaviest became my way of life. Drifting among the care-free days of the 1970s, thinking I was doing the hippie thing and living amidst the glorious drop-out people, eating home-made bread and dropping acid until life was like a series of psychoses, was both wonderful and frightening. Intuitively I knew I was on a road to burnout and possible death. I gradually sought a new group of people with hippie values and a life code of no drugs.

I was well on the road to recovering my sobriety when the universe provided that ultimate sanity tester. I fell deeply in love with a poet. The beauty of the universe sparkled sublime as I entered my mania. Weeks of road travel, singing with the planets and taking no food but the air I breathed, placed me in a detox unit. I was after all an 'addict in recovery' but there is no detoxification process for love. I was taken 'crazy' to one of the most notoriously feared institutions in New Zealand, incarcerated and certified. Much of the experience of this narrative occurred in this dreaded place. This was an irony. I had recovered from drugs only to be smitten by the most powerful drug of the gods themselves. What was I to recover from now?

In conclusion: a return to the simplicity of the solution

No singular action or interaction within the institution's walls could have been the pivotal catalyst for recovery. Days and nights came and went, as did the seasons. I needed someone to validate my human worth. It came in the form of a music tape sent into the hospital. A musician friend had composed a series of songs for me, and in Cat Stevens-like cleverness sang of our friendship and his caring. I sat hour upon hour playing and replaying it on the small tape recorder in the corner of the day room in the geriatric villa. I was so removed from the outside world and yet now so connected to it. There was a refrain at the end of one song: 'and if a friend can say that he loves you, that's all there is to be said'. It kept floating through my mind. My family had given up on me, the friends of my Faith had visited once but, embarrassed by the asylum nature of the place and unable to

relate to it – or me – had never come back. My uniquely poetic and special boyfriend of that time had bowed to the pressures of his family who were against our marrying because of my diagnosis, and he left the area. I had sat for months amidst the long-term abandoned geriatric senile/mentally 'ill', embarrassed by mass bathing practices, and spoon-feeding, and by my own menstruation. I was 28 years old and the idea that I was OK could not be realized without outside intervention. That tape gave me life. My dear musician friend died young but he holds the special ranking of humble angel closest to my heart. His songs were the turning point in recovery. 'Love' after all, is all there is to be said.

Final salutations

Sometimes on reflection one can point to significant events that changed the journey. My struggle to make sense of my life and who I am has and is happening internally and with the kindness of others.

I urge health professionals to find an openness of heart that can offer meaningful, simple acts of caring kindness. Those of us who walk this journey from illness to recovery will confirm the status of humble, gentle angel upon you. May many of you be found in the humane practices of your profession, and in sharing with us may God speed you on your own journeying.

Section 2

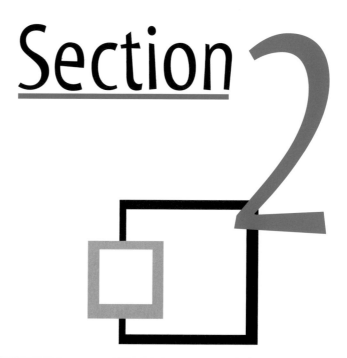

Assessment in practice

Preface to Section 2

The heart of nursing practice lies in asking questions – exploring the experience of the person in care, trying to identify what needs to be done, and how. Indeed, assessment represents the bookends of care. The developing story of the person's journey through the caring experience, is tightly wedged between the initial, exploratory assessment and the final assessment for discharge. However, assessment pops up on almost every page of the story of care, as nurses try to gauge what effect their caring intervention is having on the person or the family.

The Section opens with a general consideration of the importance of assessment, locating it as the key building block in the development of nursing care.

The following two chapters explore the kinds of methods, which are at the nurse's disposal for gaining different kinds of picture of people and their problems of living, and look in detail at the interview, which is by far the most commonly used assessment medium.

In recent years nursing has begun to emphasize the importance of engaging the person in care in the assessment process. Collaborative assessment provides openings to a wide range of caring interventions, which offer challenges to nursing practice but also hold the promise of more mutually satisfying nurse–patient relationships.

Few problems of living do not involve the family in one way or another. The assessment of people and their problems within the context of their family groups is rarely easy, but offers the promise of a more rounded picture of the person in the often chaotic, but intensely natural habitat of the real world.

Finally, we return to one of the commonest foci of nursing assessment – the private world of the person in care. What kind of feelings, thoughts and beliefs are relevant to the present problems of living and how do we go about gaining access to these important secrets of personal experience?

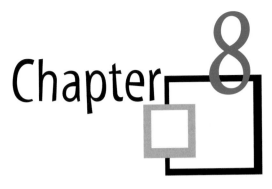

Chapter 8

ASSESSMENT – THE FOUNDATION OF PRACTICE

Phil Barker

THE NATURE OF ASSESSMENT

Although vitally important, assessment can be a very ordinary activity. People assess one thing or another, day after day, night after night. What are the chances of our soccer team winning the next round of the FA Cup, or of our daughter qualifying for the next round of the chess tournament? What are the chances that the accused person will be set free or receive a punitive sentence? These questions all involve a consideration of 'probabilities' – how can we read the mind of Fortune? Will it work for us, or against us?

The answer to such questions – or at least the educated guess – lies in an assessment of various factors, set against a sea of possibilities. Is assessment no more than an educated guess? I doubt it. Assessment may be informed by scientific principles but, by definition, it is more of an art form than a scientific endeavour. When we assess people in mental distress, we are interested to know, what is going on within them, and what might they do next? In this sense, the assessment process is, at best, a matter of highly qualified judgement. This reminds us that assessment in nursing involves more than trying to predict the future on the basis of present knowledge. It also involves clarifying our understanding of what is happening *now*.

In mental health care, most people's lives are upset or out of kilter. Many people are bewildered and bemused by their experiences. One of the commonest questions asked by people in mental distress – down the ages – is, 'what is happening to me?' We – the helpers – can never know, exactly, what is happening to the person, far less what it might mean. So, a key aspect of our assessment becomes focused on caring *with* the person, exploring and considering all the available information or experiential evidence, which might help the person come to understand, better, what is *happening* – and what it might *mean* on a personal level. Increasingly, we live in an 'evidence-based' mental health culture. We should not lose sight of the fact that the most prized evidence of all lies in the person's *experience* of mental distress and its associated meanings.

A judgement for all seasons

I began drafting this chapter in the middle of a hard Scots winter. In keeping with the British obsession with the weather, my neighbours have become, overnight, amateur meteorologists. At bus stops or in supermarket queues they discuss at length the prevailing weather conditions, and make all sorts of predictions about the likelihood of further snow or the chance of a thaw. By the time I finish this chapter, my neighbours will be on the look out for signs of 'good weather', as they begin to think about the summer vacation. Of course what constitutes 'good' or 'bad' weather is different for different people. For the young person who hopes to go tobogganing, the chance of snow will be a 'good' sign. For the more frail members of my village this is 'bad', carrying the threat of slippery pavements or being trapped indoors. Similarly, strong sunlight is welcomed by some as the chance to bronze their bodies and top of their store of vitamin D. For the very fair-skinned among us it means lashing on the sun block or retiring to the shade. Everyone judges the elements according to their present store of knowledge and personal wisdom. This knowledge 'frames' their construction of the weather. It could hardly be otherwise.

Each day, people everywhere assess the weather, each one judging the role it might play in the fabric of their lives. Of course they do not talk about assessment, yet, this is exactly what they are doing. It is just one part of the set of routines we use to make sense of our lives and our selves. Much of what nurses do with the people in their care also involves assessment although they do not necessarily talk about it as such. In mental health care, most of what we do involves asking questions.

This weather analogy is particularly relevant to mental health care. Like the various atmospheric events that we call 'the weather', people are complex and often highly unpredictable. Even the highly qualified meteorologists, who front our television weather programmes, often 'get it wrong', and predict sun when rain prevails. This does not mean that the science, which underpins their forecasts is invalid, merely that it is sorely limited to make sense of such complex phenomena. The same is true of people. Although we have pursued the dream of developing a 'scientific' approach to assessment in mental health, this is a pointless search. Making sense of people – understanding the significance of events in their past, in the light of the present – is remarkably complicated. Any judgement of what may or may not happen in the future can be no more than guesswork.

Assessment is linked strongly to evaluation, which also involves making judgements. How we judge the value of a work of art differs little from the process of evaluating our children's performance at school. In each case, having collected some information about the situation, we are then in a position to comment upon what we have observed. We can make judgements – is the painting worth the asking price? Is our daughter making progress with her studies? Each example shares an important feature, which is the hallmark of all assessments. They are rarely done for their own sake, but are undertaken with a view to some future action.

THE VALUE OF ASSESSMENT

My weather assessment helps me to decide whether I should take an umbrella or sunglasses. My assessment of the painting helps me decide whether or not I can afford

to spend money, or help judge the wisdom of borrowing. In health care, some assessments are done for statistical purposes: such as the clinical audits of services. However, even such an audit may suggest the need to change the nature or organization of the service. When we consider nursing assessment we realize that its aims are largely the same as those already quoted. In a small number of cases we collect information to help study the service offered. However, in the majority of cases assessment is undertaken with a view to understanding better what is 'going on' in the person's life, so that we might plan, and then evaluate, a specific pattern of nursing care.

Assessment lies at the core of the nurse's function. Nurses cannot offer valid and reliable forms of nursing care without valid and effective assessment. People often present with a wide range of problems of living, many requiring highly individual forms of attention. Consequently, the notion of 'scientific assessment' may be an inappropriate concept.

Assessment can identify the characteristics that different people have in common (*nomothetic*). It also plays an important role in telling us how one person differs from another: what makes the person unique (*idiographic*). The emphasis given to theory building, and the use of nursing models, in recent years illustrates how nursing is becoming more methodical and systematic. One consequence of these developments is that we are beginning to develop a common language of assessment, where different nurses describe and attempt to measure the phenomena associated with mental distress.

Most English dictionaries offer a fairly restrictive definition of 'assessment'. Traditionally, this referred to taxation, where an assessor fixes the value of something. More recently we have come to understand the term as having something to do with estimating the character of something or someone. This seems more relevant to psychiatric and mental health nursing. We are interested in estimating the people in our care in terms of who they are and what they might become, in the immediate future. People are, quite literally, priceless and this meaning emphasizes the inherent worth of a person.[1] This idiographic view contrasts with traditional medical diagnosis, which seeks to identify the nature of the pathology of the patient: looking for what was wrong with the person. Although people may appear to be having similar experiences when they are in mental distress, their experience is unique – framed by the unique context of the person's life history. One of the great challenges of nursing assessment is to make sense of this unique phenomenon. As Hilda Peplau noted, the key focus of any assessment – observation – is transformed by interpretation into a meaningful explanation.[2]

In search of the whole person

Over the past two decades in the UK, and over almost four decades in the USA, nurses have begun to move away from the strict use of a medical–diagnostic model, in favour of an assessment of the worth of the individual. The voice of the nursing process movement[3] urged all nurses to show concern for the person behind the patient label, reminding us to look for 'worth' amid what might seem like insurmountable problems. Today, there is a grave risk that nursing might drift back into a reductionist approach to care delivery, using medical diagnosis as the primary determinant for the design of care.[4–6] Private health care insurance companies in the USA will not authorize care and treatment unless the person is accorded a medical psychiatric diagnosis. Some advanced nursing practitioners are now authorized to make a psychiatric diagnosis. To some extent this reinforces the view that the diagnosis is central to the planning and delivery of 'care', rather than merely an economic necessity.

After almost 35 years in psychiatric and mental health nursing, I remain in agreement with Hilda Peplau's view that although diagnosis represents a useful way of talking about groups of people, with similar problems of living, it is largely irrelevant to the consideration of what any individual might need, now, in the name of nursing care. We can answer that question only by exploring the widest possible personal context, which will allow us to gain some insight into what is meaningful for this particular person, as opposed to what might be considered 'appropriate' for a group of 'patients'.[7]

Peplau noted that nurses increasingly had made the claim that:

> consideration of (the patients) their needs and interests as persons having dignity and worth, are primary values inherent in the design and execution of nursing services. These values should be implicit in a nursing approach for the care of patients having a diagnosis of schizophrenia. In keeping with these claims, it would behove nurses to give up the notion of a disease, such as schizophrenia, and to think exclusively of patients as persons.[8]

She spoke for many nurses who recognized that psychiatric nursing was concerned, first and foremost, to address the person's *human response* to problems involving his relationship to himself or others.[9] We might distinguish this approach from the work of doctors, who assess: 'the atypical, socially unacceptable behaviours which are called symptoms, and view them as indicators of disease.'[10]

It seems axiomatic that if nursing assessment involves valuing anything, it is the evaluation of the person's *human responses* to general or specific mental health problems. When nurses ask the simplest of questions – 'how are you doing?' – by implication they are asking:

> what is your human response, now, to whatever is happening to and for you now, in the context of what has been happening to and for you recently?

FORMAL AND INFORMAL ASSESSMENT

In a formal assessment the structure is apparent: using checklists, questionnaires and rating scales, and an organized interview plan. In an informal assessment the information is collected by less structured means and might appear quite haphazard.

Although formal and informal methods appear to have much in common this similarity is often only superficial. An interview can be formal or informal. In both cases the person is asked questions and the replies noted. However, in a formal interview questions will be prepared out carefully in advance. The informal interview lacks this structure. The nurse merely asks the questions she considers important at that time in the way she thinks appropriate. Although both kinds of assessment are in common use, we should be aware that any formal system has important advantages over less structured ways of looking at people-in-care. The rules, guidelines and specific procedures that are established in a formal system may help us to assess all the people in our care in more or less the same way. As a result, our own prejudices and idiosyncrasies are reduced. The outcome of the assessment should be much the same, whoever does it. The same cannot be said of more informal methods. Here our biases, opinions and other 'value judgements' influence the conduct of the assessment. Such factors can have a big influence on the kind of information collected.

The key assessment questions

A nursing assessment calls for information about the nature and scale of the person's problem.

❑ What is the person's problem?
❑ To what extent does it distress the person?
❑ To what extent does it interfere, in what way, with everyday living?
❑ To what extent is the person able to exercise any kind of control over the problem?[11]

In some situations the choice between formal and informal methods is determined by the person-in-care. Where the person is talkative, intelligent and anxious to communicate, the nurse may gain most of her information from open-ended conversations. Where the person is less articulate or communicative, more focused behavioural assessment of how the person 'appears' might be the best place to begin. This might be followed by use of standardized rating scales, rather than casual interviewing, and will be more formal as a result.

The focus of assessment

Mental distress and its consequences are expressed on a range of *levels of living*.[12] These become the focus of the assessment. Here we gain an appreciation of 'what is happening' for the person and what resources the person has that might begin to resolve the problem.

Levels of living

Everyone functions on several levels of human experience, at one and the same time.

❑ We function at a *physiological* level (or self). Although we are not sensitive to this level of living our biochemical existence is vital, literally, to the stability of our lives. This molecular or biochemical level of functioning is clearly the most basic level of our lives, but supports the function or expression of the other levels of living.

❑ At the next level lies our *biological* self. Here, our various organs work constantly to maintain the outward appearance of 'life', supported by our complex muscular and skeletal system, of which we have only the crudest awareness. Usually, we are only aware of this level of experience when we experience pain on exertion.

❑ At a third level lies our *behavioural* self. This is the level which attracts most attention in mental health care. At this level the person *thinks*, *feels* and *acts*. How we think and what we feel has a major effect on how we behave. By the same token, only a small proportion of our behaviour is not a function of thought and emotion. Consequently, the nursing assessment usually pays a lot of attention to *how* these three are interconnected.

❑ At the fourth level lies our *social* self. This is characterized by our relationships with the many people who make up our world. Some are close to us, such as family and friends. Others are simply the rest of 'humanity'.

❑ At the last level lies what might be called our *spiritual* self. Here we live in the world of our hopes, dreams and – perhaps most of all – our beliefs. Here we experience views of ourselves, and of the world around us. Often our experiences at this level are obscure, symbolic or vaguely defined. The very nature of our spiritual self might suggest that it is

impossible to define. Many of the more unusual experiences associated with mental distress are located at this level of living: loss of identity, waking-dream states, and many of the powerful realization and sensations that, sadly, are often dismissed as 'symptoms' of psychosis.

The real challenge of any assessment is to decide which of these levels of living, should be the assessment focus and, in reading the results, to relate this 'focused' assessment to the person's functioning on any or all of the other levels of living.

The life story

All people are storytellers. Some tell more exciting or interesting stories than others, but everyone expresses their 'lived experience' through story. The key aim of any nursing assessment is to get a *whole* sense of what is happening for the person, and what might need to be done to address this. Although it is often practical to focus on one or more of the levels of living – how the person *feels*, what the person *thinks* etc. – the person's experience is always *whole*. Feelings are a part of thinking, which is related to beliefs, which are expressed through behaviour, which is expressed through biological functioning, which ultimately is dependent on deep physiology. Although we cannot gain direct access to this 'whole lived experience' we can view it indirectly – through the person's story.

People know who they are and they become more knowledgeable about themselves, their lives and their problems, by talking about themselves. In Hilda Peplau's insightful words: 'people make themselves up as they talk'.[13] This illustrates the storytelling nature of people. Three hundred years ago, Enlightenment philosophers, like David Hume and John Locke, tried to account for our human identity solely in terms of psychological states or events. Regrettably, much the same tradition continues today, with over-simplistic neuroscientific or cognitive explanations of 'how people work'. These accounts fail to take account of the background to human identity: the stories that people are *born into*, and *become part of*, through the telling of their own story.

The life narrative

Just as history is not a simple catalogue of events, or a long list of characters, so the story of a person's life involves more than the events which the person experiences. The philosopher MacIntyre suggested that:

It is through hearing stories about wicked stepmothers, lost children, good but misguided kings, wolves that suckle twin boys, youngest sons who receive no inheritance but must make their own way in the world, and eldest sons who waste their inheritance on riotous living and go into exile to live with swine, that children learn or mislearn what a child and a parent is, what the case of characters may be in the drama into which they have been born and what the ways of the world are.[14]

Although such background stories vary from one country and culture to another, the power of story is universal. For this reason it is vital that the nursing assessment tries to get some sense of the background stories that frame the developing script of the story of the person, here and now.[15]

When nurses begin an assessment they are obliged to ask, 'who is this person?' This is a very different question from, 'what is wrong with this patient?' In so doing, they cannot divorce the person (and their story) from all the stories that helped the person become who (s)he is. As MacIntyre said, if we deprive children of stories we may 'leave them unscripted, anxious stutterers, in their actions as in their words'.

This philosophy carries a profound message. If we are to understand the people who are in our care, we need to listen to the stories of their lives. I am the story that I tell about myself – or that sometimes is told about me. This is also, obviously, true for the people in my care. In MacIntyre's words:

I am the subject of a history that is my own and no-one else's, that has its own peculiar meaning. When someone complains – as do some of those who commit suicide – that his or her life is meaningless, he or she often and perhaps characteristically complaining that the narrative of their life has become unintelligible to them, that it lacks any point, any movement toward a climax or telos.[16]

MacIntyre's use of the Greek word telos signifies how life is in constant flow towards some endpoint, whether we are aware of it or not. Viktor Frankl would have argued that the person whose life has lost its meaning, has simply lost his or her awareness of the presence of meaning.[17] One of the aims of assessment is to help people describe, explore and come to appreciate more where they are on their life path and what they think all of this might mean for them. In this sense, the assessment heralds the possibility that the intimate, constructive relationship between the nurse and the person-in-care will lead to the re-authoring of the person's own story, which they will eventually name recovery.

THE TERRORISM OF NORMALITY

If this seems an optimistic view of the potential of assessment, then it may be a necessary one. The Western view of madness is inherently pessimistic, predicated on the assumption that something 'abnormal' is going on within the person. This assumes, of course, that there is such a thing as 'normality'. Although there are various statistical ways to define 'normality' these all collapse when we begin to consider the individual. People who are exceptionally intelligent, or creative, or strong or tall, are all abnormal. In a more trivial, but equally important, sense 25 years ago it was unusual (ergo abnormal) for women to wear trousers to work. Now, this is part of the everyday dress code of many women. If it has not become normal, it has at least become commonplace.

However, we do not try to treat, fix or otherwise contain tall, creative, intelligent or strong people – or women who wear trousers – because we assume that their attributes are valuable – to them, us or society at large. Madness in its various manifestations is often seen as a social problem not because it is abnormal, but because it has no social value. However, some of the experiences that are associated with, 'serious' forms of madness – like hearing voices, or seeing visions, or descending to the depths of despair – have been used by people down the ages as the basis for creative experiments in art, literature and even the sciences.[18] The critical issue appears to be how do people respond to the experience of mental distress. If they can use this constructively as part of the development of their life story, it may be distressing, but is still of value. If people cannot make sense of, or otherwise learn from, the experience, then it is deemed to be worthless. Not surprisingly, people want to get rid of things that are worthless and which cause them discomfort or even emotional pain.

It is important to recognize that the person defines what is normal or abnormal – given the context of their own life story, and all the important stories that adjoin it. There is no 'gold standard' for normal/abnormal behaviour or experience. Indeed, social definitions of normality have been changing down the centuries and, in my own lifetime, have changed dramatically, often from year to year. Sexual preference and drug use are two examples of behaviour patterns, which once were deemed illegal, immoral or symptomatic of some psychological disturbance, but are now accepted as examples of personal choice or orientation. Homosexuality was classed as a 'mental illness' until fairly recently. However, it is clear now that heterosexuality is not so much normal as commonplace. We might remember this when we are tempted to judge the relative normality of any pattern of behaviour or reported experience.

What makes a problem?

Our interest in assessment lies mainly with the study of the person-in-care's behaviour: what he says, does, thinks, feels, etc. However, although it may be a relatively straightforward exercise to identify and measure such patterns of behaviour, it is more difficult to answer the question 'What does it all mean?' Once we have assessed a pattern of behaviour, how do we go about judging whether it is normal or abnormal? How do we determine whether or not any pattern of behaviour is a problem? Arriving at such a decision is rarely easy, since normal behaviour can vary from one person to the next, from one culture to another, and can be influenced by different laws even within the same country.

Our behaviour is, however, associated most with the culture within which we live. Most of our behaviour is learned: human beings appear to be poorly supplied with instincts, unlike our animal and insect relations. Even infants of only a few weeks old have already begun to learn how to respond to their environment: their behaviour is not preprogrammed before birth. We have no instincts or other biological endowments that help us to tie shoelaces, cook food, order a beer, comb our hair, catch a bus or open a window for fresh air. All these mundane behaviours are acquired through learning and are all part of the culture to which we belong. Were we to move to a different culture like an underdeveloped country or a hospital ward such behaviour might be redundant or might even be discouraged. Those features of our behaviour that are at present normal might become 'abnormal', deviant or at the very least unusual.

When we come to consider the behaviour of people in the psychiatric setting there is a common assumption that their behaviour is *either* normal or abnormal. It might make our task a lot easier were this absolute situation in fact the case. Reality is never quite so black and white. Normal behaviour appears to be defined by cultures. Even within a culture, discrete subcultures may determine different patterns of behaviour. In the UK newsagents magazine stands carry many magazines, aimed at younger men, which feature scantily clad or naked women on the covers. Within Western culture the appreciation of undressed women is seen as 'normal' male behaviour. Young men who might disparage the publication of such pictures – for intellectual, religious or moral reasons – will likely be scorned by the majority for what will be seen as their soppy, effeminate, 'un-masculine' stance.

Which of these attitudes is right? It seems clear that each is 'right' given the subcultural context. However, one is statistically 'normal' – occurring among most young men; the other statistically 'abnormal', occurring within a minority group. Divergence can occur, within social groupings, cultures, subcultures and even the sexes.

There are few, if any, universal norms as far as behaviour is concerned. One might assume that murder, incest and child abuse would be viewed as unacceptable by all societies and cultures. Sociologists would argue that this is not the case. Many cultures, admittedly some of them 'uncivilized' by Western standards, will tolerate, even encourage, such practices under certain conditions. We should not forget that even manifestly exceptional behaviour such as the experience of hallucinations is relatively common in some cultures. Romme and Escher's Dutch research into the prevalence of 'hearing voices' – what psychiatry calls an auditory hallucination, illustrated that sizeable proportions of 'non-patient' groups, reported hearing voices. Such findings question some of our established beliefs about the nature of 'madness', many of which are culture-bound by the Western tradition.[19]

The work of Romme and Escher is merely the latest chapter in the demythologizing of madness. In a study in the early 1960s Lee noted that one third of a random sample of Zulu women had reported visual and auditory hallucinations, involving 'angels, babies and little short hairy men'.[20] In the same study he found that more than half of the women engaged in 'screaming behaviour', often yelping for hours, days, even weeks. Either of these reported behaviours would be viewed as grossly abnormal in the West. Yet few of these women showed any other signs of mental disorder. Within their own culture their hallucinations and screaming were legitimate. More recently, African psychiatrists have reported that persecutory delusions are more frequent in African, Jamaican and Caribbean subjects than in any other groups. They explain this finding by attributing the delusions to beliefs in witchcraft and voodoo, common to their cultures.[21] This has been reported for over 30 years by other researchers,[22] who suggest that the beliefs (which we call delusions) held by West Indians diagnosed as psychotic, are the same as those held by 'normal' West Indians. The only difference between the two groups appears to be the abnormal reaction (or behaviour) of the so-called 'psychotics' to these beliefs.

THE SEARCH FOR AN EDUCATED GUESS

Here I have tried to emphasize the ordinariness of assessment. It is different only in quality from assessing how much seed will be needed to cover the bare patches on the lawn, or how we might undertake a trip around the world. Anyone can make a wild guess as to what these exercises might involve. There is no substitute, however, for the 'educated guess' made by the keen gardener or the regular traveller. Such calculations, by a genuinely interested party, are based upon knowledge and experience. In Chapters 9 and 10 I shall discuss some of the specific approaches to assessment. However, knowing how is never a substitute for knowing *why*.

Mark Twain famously said, 'give a man a hammer and he will treat everything as if it is a nail.' Knowing *how* to complete a checklist, fill out a rating scale or conduct an interview is a valuable skill. However, it is only valuable if we have first established *why* such a 'tool' is appropriate for the job in hand. The hammer used by the silversmith is quite different – in form and function – from the hammer used by the blacksmith. We can do a lot of damage by using the tools of assessment inappropriately. The silversmith and the blacksmith engage in similar behaviours – *hammering*. The crucial differences are:

❑ *how* they use the hammer (sensitivity);
❑ the *nature* of the hammer itself (tool); and
❑ the *selection* of one tool or another (rationale).

Asking people questions can seem like a fairly innocuous activity. We assume that even if it does not deliver anything of value, at least will not harm the person. This is one of the myths of psychiatric practice. The inappropriate administration of anything – from distant 'observation' to close-up, in-depth interviews – can do great damage to the vulnerable person on the receiving end. Our motto should be 'seek first to understand'.

❑ To begin to understand the person in care we must first understand fully what are our options – how might we explore and examine the situation with the person, their *experience* of what is happening.
❑ Then, we must understand why we have chosen one approach over another. (Why have they chosen to use this tool, in this particular way?) In a very real sense, nurses must understand themselves – their feelings about those in their care, and the motives underlying their attitude towards them. But most of all, nurses need to understand how little they really know about the people in their care.

A well-planned and carefully executed assessment may help the nurse learn something of value, about the person and their experience. In so doing, this will rid the nurse of some of the ignorance that often bars the way to the delivery of personally appropriate care in mental health. If the nurse is fortunate, a well-planned assessment might pave the way for the re-authoring of the person's own life story.

REFERENCES

1. Barker P. Assessment in psychiatric and mental health nursing: in search of the whole person. Cheltenham: Stanley Thornes, 1997.
2. O'Toole AN, Welt SR (eds). *Hildegard E. Peplau. Selected works. Interpersonal theory in nursing.* Basingstoke: Macmillan, 1984.
3. Ashworth P, Castledine G, McFarlane IK. The process in practice. *Nursing Times* 1978 (Suppl. 30 November).
4. Baguely I. Evaluation of the Tameside Nursing Development Unit for psycho-social interventions. In: Brooker C, White E (eds). *Community psychiatric nursing: a research perspective*, vol. 3. London: Chapman and Hall, 1995.
5. Gournay K. What to do with nursing models. *Journal of Psychiatric and Mental Health Nursing* 1995; **2**(5): 325–7.
6. McMinn B. Diagnostic classification systems and nursing diagnosis of collaborative problems. *Australian and New Zealand Journal of Mental Health Nursing* 1995; **28**(4): 124–31.
7. American Nurses Association. *Nursing: a social policy statement.* Kansas City, MO: American Nurses Association, 1980.
8. Peplau HF. Another look at schizophrenia from a nursing standpoint. In: Anderson CA (ed.) *Psychiatric Nursing 1974–94: A Report on the State of the Art.* St Louis, MO: Mosby Year Book, 1995.
9. O'Toole A, Loomis M. Classifying human responses in psychiatric and mental health nursing. In: Reynolds W, Cormack D (eds). *Psychiatric and mental health nursing: theory and practice.* London: Chapman and Hall, 1990.
10. Peplau HF, 1995, *op. cit.*
11. Barker P. The tidal model: the lived-experience in person-centred mental health nursing care. *Nursing Philosophy* 2001; **2**(3): 213–23.
12. Barker P, 1997, *op. cit.*
13. Peplau HE, personal communication.
14. MacIntyre A. The story-telling animal. In: Bowie L, Michaels MW, Solomon RC (eds). *Twenty questions: an introduction to philosophy.* London: Harcourt Brace Jovanovich, 1988.
15. Barker P, Kerr B. *The process of psychotherapy: the journey of discovery.* Butterworth-Heinemann: Oxford, 2000.
16. MacIntyre A, 1988, *op. cit.*
17. Frankl V. *Man's search for meaning.* London: Hodder and Stoughton, 1964.
18. Barker P. *The philosophy and practice of psychiatric nursing.* Edinburgh: Churchill Livingston, 1999.
19. Romme M, Escher S. The new approach: a Dutch experiment. In: Romme M, Escher S (eds). *Accepting voices.* London: MIND Publications, 1993.
20. Lee SM. *Stress and adaptation.* Leicester: Leicester University Press, 1961.
21. Ndtei DM, Vadher A. Frequency and clinical significance of delusions across cultures. *Acta Psychiatrica Scandinavica* 1984; **70**: 73–6.
22. Kiev A. Beliefs and delusions of West Indian immigrants to London. *British Journal of Psychiatry* 1963; **109**: 356–63.

Chapter 9

ASSESSMENT METHODS

Phil Barker

INTRODUCTION

In principle, assessment is simple. It merely involves collecting information, with a view to making a judgement about something. However, although this may be the case with *things*, people belong to a different order. In human affairs assessment is never simple. One person judging another is invariably fraught with all manner of complications. In mental health care, assessment is usually (hopefully) conducted so that a decision may be reached about what 'needs to be done' *next*.

How we go about collecting the information that generates the assessment *per se* is the **method**. When nurses try to establish a format of assessment that is *reliable*, irrespective of who undertakes assessment, and which will provide *valid* information about the actual people and their problems of living, the **methodology** they will use will – in one way or another – be scientific.[1]

1 Information about people can be collected in two ways. We can ask the person to *report* his situation. This might involve simply answering questions, or completing some kind of a record of his or her experience. Either way, we need to be confident that the person is *willing* (motivated) and *able* (competent) to provide such subjective reports. We also need to be assured that the person has no reason for wishing to mislead us. If we are not confident that the information we shall glean from the person is accurate, such a self-report may be worthless.

2 The alternative is to invite other people to make observations on the person Family members might use their proximity to the person to report on her or him from close range. Where the person is in care, members of the care and treatment team can provide differing kinds of 'observation', from their various vantage points in relation to the person in care. However, in both cases such observations are bedeviled with practical and ethical problems.

In every case, the aim of assessment is simple, yet complex. We aim to answer the question:

> What is really going on here, and how will this help us work out what we need to do, by way of a caring response?

Information channels

The methods discussed in this chapter involve *subjective* or *objective* reports. Wherever possible, information should he obtained *direct* from the person, either in the form of some kind of 'self report' or via observation. The ideal form of assessment is *collaborative* – see Chapter 11 – where the person in care and the professional explore the problem together, marrying their differing perspectives in a new construction of the problem of living.

'Second-hand' observations, obtained from fellow professionals, family or friends come a very poor second in this respect. We should be aware, however, that in some cases the person may be unwilling or unable to provide the information needed, requiring the nurse to fall back on the reports provided by others.

The comments and observations of other people may be important for the simple reason that they involve information known only to them, corroborating or contradicting the story offered by the person. This is particularly important where the person is in care. Junior staff members often have more contact with the person than senior staff. The person may also behave differently with staff they assume to be of a more junior status, perceiving them to be less threatening by dint of their inexperience or lack of authority. Often, people confide in junior staff because they feel closer to them than to more senior staff or other specialist therapists. Paradoxically, therefore, less-experienced staff may be a more useful source of information, or access point for assessing the person in care.

The views of 'significant others' – family, or friends who know the person well – are also invaluable in helping to develop the 'bigger picture'. Even if their perspective appears to contradict the story offered by the person her or himself, ultimately this can be useful – if only in illustrating how different parties have different views on the problem or its inherent nature.

Collecting information from the person or his 'significant others' usually involves some *informal* method of assessment. Highly structured (*formal*) assessments invariably make people uncomfortable and may prejudice the chance of gaining accurate information. By contrast, information supplied by staff will likely be more formal, involving the use of some standardized method of observation or recording. The specific *aim* of the assessment, and the particular people involved, will determine which form of information *channel* is selected.

❑ If we need to know how the person *thinks* or *feels*, or if we need to identify the person's values or beliefs, we need to **ask the person** (see Chapter 13).
❑ If we need to know what *other people* think, or feel, or believe about the person, we need to **ask those other people** (see Chapter 12).
❑ If we need to know how the person behaves under certain conditions, either we ask the person to observe or reflect on her/his own behaviour, or we ask someone else to observe the person. (These two options may provide completely different reports.)

PSYCHO-SOCIAL ASSESSMENT

Given the complexity of the human being who is the person, it is important to assess the person across a wide range of dimensions. The primary focus of nursing assessment is, however, on what might be called the psycho-social plane. For at least the past decade, nurses have been developing conceptual frameworks to aid the assessment of psycho-social care.[2]

Nurses might he expected, for example, to: participate in the collection of body fluids and their analysis; undertake routine physical assessments; or support physicians undertaking more complex diagnostic assessments such as computerized axial tomography (CAT) or positron emission tomography (PET) scans. These biomedical assessment activities are often a critical part of the diagnostic process for some people, and may represent a valuable contribution to determining appropriate medical intervention. However, although important, these assessment functions do not represent the 'proper focus' of nursing. Nurses focus upon, address and subsequently become involved in the person's *interaction* with her/his environment, which includes other people, groups, organizations and aspects of the expressed culture, which lie within that environment. Given this focus psychiatric and mental health nursing assessment methods emphasize this psycho-social world.

The term *psycho-social* includes consideration of a wide range of personal and interpersonal factors. These include *psychological* and *biological phenomena*:

❑ functional (behavioural) performance;
❑ self-efficacy.

and *ecological factors*, including:

❑ relationships within the family;
❑ relationships with the wider social environment;
❑ interpersonal communication;
❑ social resources.

THE MAJOR METHODS OF ASSESSMENT

There are four main methods of assessment, each of which has a different function, and produces a different kind of *data* – or information – from the others. What passes for assessment in most clinical settings, often involves a complex mix of these different approaches.[3]

1. Interviewing

In an interview the nurse questions the person about feelings, thoughts, beliefs or specific views of the person's behaviour. These questions may relate to life in general or may be specific to particular problems of living or aspects of care and treatment. An interview can simply involve 'sitting down and chatting with the person'. In other contexts the interview may involve asking the person to answer 'Yes' or 'No' to a series of questions. These represent the extremes of highly *unstructured* and *structured* formats. Somewhere between the two lies the *semi-structured interview*.

In the semi-structured interview the person is asked a range of *exploratory* questions on various topics. The answers usually generate additional questions, which need to be answered before moving on to the next topic. By contrast, wholly unstructured 'chatting' may be too rambling to lead to any useful conclusions. The rambling nature of the inquiry might even make the person uneasy, feeling that the conversation isn't going anywhere. At the other extreme the highly structured 'quizzing' of the person may seem impersonal and officious.

Where the nurse uses a fixed interview schedule, there is very little room for manoeuvre, as all the interactions are determined by the questions on the paper.

The semi-structured format is a common preference in virtually all situations. The conversation is orderly, without being regimented. There is room to break off at tangents, as appropriate, without losing one's place. This allows the conversation to flow, affording both nurse and person some security.

The success or failure of any interview is dependent on the nurse's behaviour. Sources of error in the use of interviews are most often associated with the nurse's relationship with the person, and less often with the person her or himself.

The relationship

The success of the interview depends largely on the nature of the relationship established between the nurse and the person-in-care. The interview should always be undertaken in a relatively quiet and relaxed setting. This need not be a formal interview room, but privacy and comfort are essential. The nurse should open with general questions, aiming to achieve rapport and put the person at ease. The purpose of the interview should be stated at the outset, in language that is appropriate to the intellectual and emotional status of the person.

Nurse: 'I am really pleased to meet with you, to talk about what is happening for you and how we can begin to work out what you need right now. I've got a few questions that I would like to ask, but please stop me at any point if you want to ask something. I would like this to be more of a conversation than an interview. How do you feel about that?'

Motivation

Some people will feel threatened by the prospect of the interview. They may feel inclined to deny, minimize or exaggerate their problems of living. Consequently, it is important to encourage the person to complete the interview fully and accurately. Often, this can best be achieved by linking the interview to the care planning process that follows.

Nurse: 'What we talk about here will help us work out what kind of care you need right now and maybe also over the days ahead. So I'd like you to take your time with this. We can come back to any things that you are not sure of later, if you like. OK?'

The nurse's attitudes

Before beginning the interview, the nurse should consider, carefully, her attitudes towards the person and the problems of living that are likely to emerge. If the interviewer feels uncomfortable, or negatively predisposed towards the person, this may prevent the person getting fully involved in the interview. Where the person's problems generate some attitudinal conflict for the nurse, this should be addressed in clinical supervision (see Chapter 64).

Recording

Most interviews require that some record be made of the person's responses. Ideally, this should be done during the interview, the person's words being clarified and amended before committing to paper. Recording the interview after it has been conducted is fraught with difficulties, not least problems with remembering what exactly was said, and the risk of interpreting the person's responses.

The role of the interviewee

The interview can have a profound effect on the information supplied by the person and can also affect his or her feelings during the interview. The time of day can be crucial, especially where the person is affected by time-related variations in mood. On completion of the interview, the person should always be offered an opportunity to discuss the interview – in whole or in part – with the nurse.

Advantages of the interview

The interview has several advantages:

❑ Interviews are popular because of their inherent simplicity. Many nurses can 'converse' with the person with little or no training. Of course, they might converse a lot better if they were properly trained. The interview may be most appropriate where the person is unable to use any kind of self-assessment. This is especially the case where the person has literacy problems, or is able to speak the common language but finds it difficult to express this in writing. This may be the case where the person belongs to an ethnic minority population.

- ❏ The interview also allows the nurse to check the person's understanding of a particular question. If the person appears hesitant or puzzled she can rephrase the question, or amplify it in some way, to help the person answer. This is not possible where the person is left to fill in a questionnaire or rating scale unaided.
- ❏ The interview also allows the person to provide as much detail as he thinks is necessary. The semi-structured format allows the person to develop a theme, which seems on reflection, important. This is rarely possible by any other means. Of course this is only possible if the nurse has the ability to recognize that something significant has been said and can encourage the person to pursue this, so amplifying the response.
- ❏ Finally, the interview usually allows the nurse to design the rest of the assessment. Interviews are often the first port of call in the assessment process. The preliminary interview gives us the clues regarding what might be important aspects of the person and/or the person's life, which might be explored further through other interviews or other forms of assessment.

Disadvantages of the interview

Among the disadvantages of the interview are the following:

- ❏ Interviewing can be time-consuming. In a difficult (or badly handled) interview, a lot of time may be spent for little reward. A successful interview may be equally costly: a lot of time is spent preparing the ground, asking general questions, probing the details and recording the person's replies. This does not take account of time lost pursuing 'red herrings'.
- ❏ Secondly, the interview is dependent on the expertise of the interviewer. Many nurses are obliged to assess the people in their care, often with little or no training. Where the person is very confused or otherwise distressed we must challenge the wisdom of this policy, not to mention the ethics. Where the person is not manifestly distressed, but is anxious to resolve his problems, this may also tax the expertise of the nurse. Highly intelligent and articulate people can be as demanding as those who are less intellectually gifted or educationally enabled. In either case the nurse interviewer needs a lot of skill to cope with the person's difficulties or expectations. One way to resolve this problem is to allow junior staff to develop their interviewing skills gradually, beginning with the highly structured 'quiz', which usually

greets the person on admission to the service, working gradually towards a more semi-structured format.

- ❏ The nurse may have a negative effect upon the person. Some people become anxious during interviews, especially when they are uncertain about the aims of the interview or find it difficult to supply the answers. They may also be anxious about how their replies are being interpreted. It is clear that similar anxieties may be present when a person is asked to fill in a form. However, interview anxiety seems to stem from being looked at, when the person may feel that she or he is being scrutinized or put under the spotlight. The interpersonal nature of the interview may cause problems for some people.

2. Diaries and personal records

A more formal way of collecting information involves asking the person to reflect on her or his experience. This may be undertaken in a variety of ways, all of which involve recording details of behaviour, feelings or thoughts as they occur, during the course of everyday activity. A *log* or a *diary* will provide details of the experiences the person had, as they were engaged in different activities, with different people. The diary may be completed once a day, such as in the evening. Or the person may complete the log or diary, as events occur, or at prescribed points in the day – lunchtime, at the end of the afternoon, before retiring. There are no rules as to what constitutes a log or a diary. Ideally, the person should choose her or his own format and also should choose how to complete it. That said, the nurse needs to let the person know what kind of information would help the team, but beyond that the form of the log or diary needs have no boundaries – and may include drawings, poems, pictures of other accumulated 'scraps' of information, which communicate something of the person's lived experiences.

Advantages of the log or diary

The main advantage of the diary is simplicity. It can also be seen as cost-effective, since it can reveal a wealth of information for minimal staff time. This information can be 'qualitative' – focused on stories, notes or other reflections on experience; or 'quantitative' – recording discrete information regarding how *often* or for how *long* the person engaged in a particular form of behaviour (such as hand-washing or social interaction). Where the person is already a diary keeper, these notes may be seen as a simple extension of routine 'self-study'. Where the person is less confident about committing experiences to paper, it may be necessary to tailor the recording format to suit the person, perhaps even helping the person design the kind of recording format which would be most appropriate. For example, if a person described a feeling of anxiety that came and went throughout the day, it might be helpful to monitor this. If the anxiety appeared to prevent her or him from doing things, the nurse might suggest recording:

❏ any activity that was disrupted;
❏ when the anxiety began and ended; and
❏ how severe was the feeling of anxiety.

Such information not only provides more details about the presenting problem, but can be used to evaluate progress at a later date.

It is also apparent that, when used appropriately, the self-study nature of the log or diary can have an inbuilt therapeutic effect, and may reduce the scale of a problem even before treatment even begins. In many cases, the use of the diary or log becomes an integral part of the subsequent therapy.[4]

Disadvantages

There are several disadvantages associated with this approach:

❏ Although diary formats require little investment of nursing time to complete, they can be costly in terms of analysis, especially where the person commits a lot of information to paper.
❏ If the nurse asks the person to study only one area of life experience, this may prejudice the person's observations, resulting in a failure to be open to the wider context of the problem.
❏ If the person is advised to record every instance of a particular problem – like hearing voices or becoming anxious – the person may increase awareness of the problem, appearing to enlarge the scale of the problem.
❏ The nature of going 'looking for' instances of particular problems may also heighten the person's emotional awareness, potentially adding to the person's present 'emotional burden'.
❏ Alternatively, if the person is asked to make notes on the number of times he avoided a drinking binge or lost his or her temper, the person may record less of these than expected, for the simple reason that the person is aware of their 'undesirable' nature.
❏ Because they are so simple – even commonplace – the person may forget to complete them. If this is the only information being collected then the assessment of the person can be delayed considerably. This is a good reason for tailoring such diaries to suit the person, rather than issuing standardized formats that have no personal connotations.

3. Questionnaires and rating scales

Questionnaires and rating scales are designed to gain *specific* measures of a problem area (although this general rule can he broken). These methods are usually developed from research projects, or are designed to augment scientific research (see Chapter 18). Various drafts of the measuring device are tried out on a sample population, and revisions or modifications are made depending on its success. When the research is complete, the questionnaire or rating scale should provide a reliable and valid measure of a specific problem for the minimum of effort.

A vast assortment of such methods has been developed to assess various psychiatric phenomena: e.g. depression, dependency, disorientation or 'social competence'. Each problem is a construct rather than a reality. Each problem comprises various behavioural, emotional or cognitive 'problems'. The questionnaire or rating scale provides only a global, or general, estimate of its severity.

Questionnaires

If the nurse wishes to assess only one aspect of the person's functioning, a questionnaire might help her do this *for* little effort. Many questionnaires require only Yes/No answers, which can then be scored giving a total score for a particular construct – like assertiveness. This allows a judgment to be made as to 'how assertive' the person is, compared to available group norms. Such questionnaires can be completed by the person alone, or as the basis for a structured interview.

Although such forms of questionnaire are simple, the responses (information) provided are equally simple.

Rating scales

The rating scale may also specify a problem area. However, here the person is asked to rate the *severity* of a problem or to rate his *performance*; or to indicate the extent to which he *agrees* or *disagrees* with certain statements (see Chapter 18). In principle, the rating scale may assess any area of human functioning. Particular patterns of *behaviour* may be assessed – e.g. 'How often do you brush your teeth': 'Never' (1) through to 'More than twice a day' (5). Alternatively the scale may focus on measures of *belief*: 'Success in life depends on luck' – 'I agree strongly (1) through to 'I disagree strongly' (5).

Although there is considerable variation in such scales, all rating scales end in a numerical score. This score will reflect the extent to which some emotion is *felt*, some behaviour is *performed*, some thought is *experienced* or some belief is *held*.

The Likert scale

Many rating scales are described as 'Likert' scales after the originator of this scaling method. Likert found that the best results were achieved by five categories of response.[5] Rating scales invariably measure a problem using a scale that extends from:

- ❑ 0 = 'Not present' or 'Not at all' or 'Never' to
- ❑ 5 'Extreme' or 'All the time' or 'Maximum'.

In principle, the Likert scale can be used to measure any phenomenon, and might also be used to measure 'change':

- ❑ 0 'No change' to
- ❑ 5 'Significant improvement'.

Advantages of the questionnaire or rating scale

There are three main advantages related to the use of standardized questionnaires or rating scales:

- ❑ Such standardized formats generate a quantifiable 'measure' of a problem for the minimum investment of time. Whereas we might spend 20 minutes interviewing the person about 'how they feel', the rating scale may require only a few minutes' explanation and a further few minutes' completion, and might generate a more manageable body of information about the person's feelings.
- ❑ Since the same facets of the problem are assessed in different people some comparison can be made between one person and another. Published questionnaires and rating scales include 'norms', reflecting the range of scores obtained from the study of different populations – e.g. hospitalized patients or 'normal subjects'. It is possible therefore, to compare the person's score with the available norms. It is possible to say that (for example) 'this person is very dependent, depressed, lonely, anxious'. Such judgements are not opinion but are made in the light of available knowledge regarding how people (in general) function.
- ❑ Such standardized methods often break problems into various component parts. This may help both team members and the person-in-care to appreciate what the problem involves. A scale measuring depression (for example) might cover aspects of the person's motivation, mood, libido, appetite, etc. An anxiety scale might measure a range of anxiety-related factors: feeling tense, panic attacks, sweating, urge to pass urine, etc. These analyses are not simply whimsical exercises. The various items on the scale or questionnaire have been arrived at through careful study and experimentation. They refer to the phenomena experienced or exhibited by *most* people who are described as suffering from anxiety, depression, etc. These methods are the psycho-social equivalent of the measuring tape, thermometer and the sphygmomanometer.

Disadvantages

There are at least three disadvantages to the use of such standardized methods.

- ❑ The rigid and highly structured nature of questionnaires and ratings scales prevents the nurse from exercising the flexibility and responsiveness to the person found in direct interviewing. The person may gain the impression that she or he is being 'processed', and that we are only interested in parts of them and their problems, rather than in them as 'whole people'.
- ❑ Many people find it difficult to express themselves using a structured format. Where the questionnaire demands a 'Yes/No' response, the person may want to answer 'Sometimes' or 'Just in the morning'. The scale, however, may make no concession to these varieties of experience. Where ratings are involved the person, again, may feel compromised if asked to choose between 'agree' or 'disagree' categories. The person may say that sometimes this rating applies but at other times another rating is more accurate. This may frustrate or even infuriate the nurse, who might think that the person is simply being difficult. Such a difficulty, however, may only illustrate the uncertainty of his experience.
- ❑ Finally, it is apparent that some people-in-care are unhappy with the written format, even when this is completed by the nurse. The demands of the exercise may unnerve them completely, adding to their distress. For this reason it may be necessary to be selective where questionnaires or rating scales are involved.

4. Direct observation

This approach involves, potentially, the most rigorous and methodical of all assessment methods. However, by virtue of the rigour required, it is the least practised of all the methods discussed here. However, just because direct observation is difficult should not discourage us from considering its potential value.

Direct observation may be carried out in a variety of ways:

- ❑ by the person himself ('self-monitoring');
- ❑ by members of the staff team;
- ❑ or, less frequently, by members of the person's family.

Although the principles behind self-monitoring and direct observation are similar, they are discussed here separately to aid clarity.

Self-monitoring

Self-monitoring is an extension of the diary/log format discussed above. However, here the self-assessment is made more formal. The person is helped to identify specific targets for self-observation, which are defined clearly and unambiguously, so that some kind of *measure* can be taken across time. The person may self-monitor any aspect of his experience, but in practice specific *behaviours*, discrete *thoughts* and clearly defined *feelings* may be appropriate targets.

Following the initial assessment the nurse discusses with the person the specific problems of living or aspects of problems that might be the most appropriate targets for self-monitoring. A decision is made regarding the kind of measure that might be appropriate. Usually this involves an estimate of *frequency* (how often the person engages in a pattern of behaviour, or has a particular experience) – or *duration* – how long the behaviour or experience lasts.

In self-monitoring *frequency* the person might record each time s/he:

- had a panic attack;
- drank alcohol;
- felt angry;
- spoke to a stranger;
- completed a task.

The only requirement is that each incident should be broadly similar in size or severity to the others. Before beginning, it may be appropriate to ensure that the person can distinguish (for example) between 'anger' and 'jealousy' or even 'annoyance'. The simplest way to ensure this is to ask the person to say what s/he might *do* or *say* when angry, jealous, annoyed, etc.

If the intention of the assessment is to help the person clarify the nature of his problems, it might be appropriate to distinguish (for example) between 'feeling angry' and 'losing my temper'. In some instances the definition can be quite specific:

- 'drinking alcohol' can be defined in terms of *units* of alcohol consumed, rather than glasses of beer or gin and tonic;
- 'speaking to a stranger' might be defined in terms of the sort of interaction that might be involved, and could also include some 'exclusion criteria', such as 'saying hello to a passer-by'.

The best targets for a frequency count are those actions that have a clear beginning and end. The person might record each time s/he:

- drinks one unit of alcohol;
- introduces himself to a stranger;
- swears at his wife;
- slaps his son;
- smokes a cigarette;
- thinks 'I'm a failure';
- eats a sweet biscuit;
- refuses to do someone a favour;
- hears the voice of his dead mother.

These events have fairly clear-cut beginnings and endings. Some may be more independent than others. However, the person could distinguish each occurrence, ending up with measure of at least one facet of his 'drinking', 'bad temper', 'greed', 'unassertiveness' or 'hallucinatory experience'.

For other patterns of behaviour it may be more helpful to measure how long the person spends engaged in the action. This is indicated where the action may be short-lived (shouting for a few seconds) but on others it may last much longer (e.g. a violent argument lasting 20 minutes). Instead of counting the number of times the person loses his temper, washes his hands, checks the doors and windows or has a conversation with a workmate, s/he is asked to note roughly how long s/he spent engaged in the activity.

In a few cases a slightly different kind of time measure may be appropriate. Where the person is particularly slow at doing something, such as 'summoning up the courage to say "Hello" to someone' or making decisions, s/he might measure how long s/he takes to complete these actions. The person might record how long s/he takes to:

- get up in the morning;
- get dressed;
- answer a question;
- select a particular brand of peaches;
- sit down to dinner;
- answer the telephone.

These examples were all problems for one person, who described these problems-of-living variously as:

- 'I can't be bothered getting up';
- 'I can't decide what to wear';
- 'I can't think of anything to say';
- 'I can't make up my mind';
- 'I'm too busy, I'll be with you in a minute';
- 'I'm frightened who might be on the line'.

Using a traditional psychiatric approach, these problems might be described variously as:

- apathy;
- indecisiveness;
- insecurity;

❑ obsessionality;
❑ anxiety.

Given the nurse's focus on the psycho-social domain of life, all these problems have a common denominator: the person took a long time to complete any of these actions.

Self-monitoring is rarely easy. The person is required to 'watch' her/himself virtually all day long. If s/he has too many things to monitor, the activity may simply overwhelm the person. If the assessment requires the person to make detailed notes, this may interfere with everyday life and s/he may give up. Appropriate assessment targets and a simple observational method are of crucial importance. The person could be given a tally counter so that s/he could clock up every instance of a 'worrying thought' or each time s/he thought people were laughing at me', without anyone noticing. Other ideas for frequency measures might involve placing ticks on the:

❑ inside back page of a diary;
❑ top of a newspaper;
❑ back of his hand with a felt-tipped pen;
❑ corner of a desk blotter.

These 'ticks' could be tallied up at the end of the day or week, whichever is appropriate. Alternatively the person might carry a plastic container of tiny cachous. Each time s/he felt 'gripped by panic' s/he might suck one of the cachous. If s/he counted the number of sweets in the box each morning and night, by subtraction, s/he could record the frequency of panic attacks each day.

Measuring time is more complex. However, with the advent of the microchip almost everyone is now sporting a stop-watch within their wristwatch. Providing that one remembers to set and stop it, highly accurate timings are possible. These may be transferred to the top of the newspaper, back of the hand, etc. Such self-monitoring is unlikely to be noticed, since many people fiddle continuously with watches.

Just because a simple measurement system is selected, however, offers no guarantee that the person will continue with the self-monitoring. Unless s/he already is an avid 'self-watcher' – such as a diarist – s/he is likely to tire of the chore. Consequently it is necessary to provide regular boosts of encouragement or offers of alternative ways of collecting the information. Otherwise the exercise may simply become another problem on top of many.

Being creative?

Some nurses think that their 'patients' would not be capable of such apparently complex forms of self-observation. Although the methods outlined above may appear complicated, depending on the context, they may be simplicity itself. The issue here is not so much the method as the degree of collaboration with the person-in-care.

People can be empowered by the process of self-monitoring. Almost 20 years ago, I published a book, which included several examples of self-monitoring, in many cases involving people with highly complex and disabling mental health problems.[6] The key to the success of those methods was the ingenuity of the nurses involved and the degree of empowering collaboration with the people concerned. Nothing has changed down the years. Nurses can use the principles of self-monitoring in a limitless range of possible ways. The more creative and personalized is the ultimate recording format, the more the person in care will identify with it, and the more likely that s/he will use this as part of the self-assessment process.

Staff monitoring

In traditional psychiatric practice, much of the assessment information is based on staff observations – how the person:

❑ *presented* at interview;
❑ *behaved* during the course of a period of in-patient assessment;
❑ *behaved* during a family meeting or in a group.

These observations are focused on what is visible or audible to professionals. Regrettably, professionals rarely keep objective records of behaviour, or fastidious notes on presentation, preferring instead to make judgements on the significance (perceived or actual) of what they have witnessed.

Consider the case of Henry, resident in an intensive-treatment facility.

Case study 9.1

It is 9.00 am. Henry leaves the breakfast table and goes to his room. On the way he taps the wall and skirting board, every few paces. He remains in his room for the next hour, pacing back and forth. Every so often he stops and rushes over to the window, which he opens and closes repeatedly for several minutes. His pacing is accompanied by rhythmic waving of his arms, which he raises aloft and by making what appears to be the 'sign of the cross' on his chest and head. He talks aloud to himself, although it is difficult to make out what he is saying. Occasionally he shouts a word aloud. Again the word is unclear and may not even be English. Every few minutes he stops, kneels down and puts his head in his hands and sways backwards and forwards.

What sense can the staff team make of this behaviour?

- ❑ Is this some kind of psychotic manifestation?
- ❑ Is he engaged in some strange obsessional ritual?
- ❑ Is he praying?
- ❑ Given that he knows that we are watching him (albeit from a distance or intermittently) is he 'putting on an act' for our benefit?

It seems obvious that trying to answer these questions without Henry's assistance (however limited) will prove fairly fruitless. We risk ending up with a highly prejudiced and potentially wild set of assumptions concerning the 'reality' of Henry's experience.

By law, nurses are required to make notes on the presentation of the people in their care (see Chapter 54). These records should be as objective and free of unnecessary interpretation as possible. Irrespective of the situation – inpatient ward, rehabilitation unit, group therapy session, outpatient clinic appointment, family meeting – the nurse should record only observable facts: what she *saw* and *heard*. This objective information can be supplemented with a range of information, which can be drawn from other sources:

- ❑ From the person in care her/himself.
- ❑ From family members and friends (where appropriate).
- ❑ From other therapists or team members.

All assessment is focused on answering the question: *what is really going on here?* These people will provide their own perspective on what they believed was *really* going on, if only from their own perspective.

In Henry's case, the nurse has several options available. S/he might:

- ❑ Visit Henry in his room and ask him, directly, what is happening for him when he 'appears to be crossing himself' or 'shouts aloud'.
- ❑ Arrange to meet with Henry and share with him her/his observations of how he appears to be behaving. Then s/he might ask Henry if he would like to comment on the nurse's observations.
- ❑ Ask family members and friends if they have ever noticed Henry doing anything like this, and ask if he has ever said anything about this.
- ❑ Ask other members of the team – medical staff, therapists etc. – if Henry has ever said anything that might help clarify the meaning or significance of these patterns of behaviour.

In each and every case the search is on for 'evidence'. Although there is a great emphasis on the importance of evidence for health care (see Chapter 3) in routine psychiatric practice there is often a surfeit of opinion, judgement and conjecture. In asking different people for their differing perspectives on 'what is going on here', the ultimate aim is to partial out the wheat from the chaff – the solid, reliable information from that which might well be only opinion or conjecture. This is rarely easy, which may be why so many nursing reports are replete with banal commentary on what the nurse *believed* was really going on.

The focus of assessment

Assessment invariably involves dipping into a complex bag of tools in search of the one tool (or combination of tools) that will unlock our understanding of the person's problems – or shared understanding with person of what is 'really going on, and what might be done in response to this'. Assessment rarely involves only one function. We might assess people:

- ❑ To find out *who they are* – as in the life profile;
- ❑ To describe and measure specific 'problems of living' – as in the problem-oriented interview; or
- ❑ To describe their assets and personal and social resources – as in the strengths assessment.

We might also try to assess the *scale* of these problems or *assets*; here assessment becomes an evaluative tool, judging whether problems (or assets) appear to be diminishing, increasing or remaining at the same level.

Common to all these areas is the hope that through assessment we might grow to understand the *meaning* or *human significance* of the person's problems. Historically, psychiatry has tended to view the patient's *presentation* or behaviour, as merely *symptomatic* of some greater distress, or something below the surface of life. Increasingly, we view many psychiatric 'problems of living' as a function of some biochemical anomaly or genetic influence. However, given that nurses are involved in helping people to identify, describe and ultimately deal with or live with problems in their everyday experience, there is a virtue in focusing on what is *happening* in a practical sense, rather than what we believe might be *causing* whatever is happening. It is for this reason that psychosocial assessment has been emphasized here. Since the person's behaviour – how they act or the stories they relate – is the stimulus for the generation of our theories about one form of mental 'illness' or psychiatric 'disorder', the behaviour of the person, and the stories told through interviews etc., should be the main focus in the assessment process.

ASSESSMENT STAGES

We have discussed four ways of describing the person. Through interviewing we build a picture of how s/he functions on various levels of experience and how s/he and others *perceive* that functioning. This is the most specific form of assessment. However, invariably, it is just the starting point for a complex series of stages of assessment.

1   An unstructured interview will elicit a vast amount of information about the person, his interactions with others, his beliefs, ambitions and hopes and dreams. Most of this information will be non-specific and general and characterized by its fuzzy outline. A structured interview will begin the process of defining the person and her/his situation more clearly. Interest in the person's stream-of-consciousness may begin to wane, as we start to narrow our focus – looking for more specific answers to increasingly more focused questions. Naturally, the person's freedom to talk begins, also, to be curtailed. By the end of the structured interview we should have identified the areas of the person and her/his life that need to be addressed, to develop appropriate care.

2   We may now wish to describe these significant aspects in more quantifiable terms, perhaps beginning by asking the person to summarize aspects of his life, his behaviour or his beliefs (his thoughts) through rating scales or questionnaires. These may produce a quantifiable measure of some specific construct – e.g. anxiety, social interaction, independence, depression. These will reflect either how the person sees her/himself or how s/he is perceived by others. These are only indirect measures. They are based upon the person's *perception* of her/himself. At a stage slightly beyond this lies the perception of the person held by others, e.g. staff, family or friends.

3   At the next stage, we could narrow the focus further by assessing the discrete patterns of behaviour that have been highlighted through the more indirect forms of assessment. By studying what the person *does*, and *where*, *when* and *with whom*, s/he engages in such behaviour, we can begin to quantify in greater detail the nature of the person and her/his problems, that we see before us. Staff or family members might (for example) record how often, or for how long, s/he engages in certain patterns of behaviour, under different circumstances. This would bring us closer to understanding 'what is really going on'.

4   This is finally achieved when the person can study her/himself closely under a range of conditions. Using logs, diaries, self-ratings, or and any one of a number of creative, yet simple self-monitoring techniques, the person can begin to describe what is really happening for and to her/him, in different life settings.

These methods may represent a form of 'personal science' wherein the person might study himself in much the same way as a naturalist might study a butterfly or bird. The person-in-care has an advantage over the naturalist, as s/he can assess thoughts and feelings as well as her/his patterns of behaviour.

CONCLUSION

When we talk about assessment, we should think of a toolkit. Each tool has a different function, but taken together all the tools are intended to illuminate our shared understanding of the person and her/his problems. If our intention is to reveal something of the mystery that is the individual person, we need to acknowledge that this is unlikely to be a simple affair. The person *lives* on a variety of levels of experience – emotional, cognitive, behavioural, interpersonal, social and spiritual. This should make us aware that a range of methods might be necessary to do justice to the assessment of such human complexity.

Although much emphasis is given, today, to the need for valid and reliable assessment instruments, we should not forget that, given the complexity of people, we need also to be *creative* in developing assessment methods. Wherever possible, we should work *with* people, in the exploration, examination and evaluation of their experiences – whether personal, interpersonal or social. Through such collaboration we may use general principles, to inform the development of personally appropriate forms of assessment.

REFERENCES

1. Barker P. *Assessment in psychiatric and mental health nursing: in search of the whole person.* Cheltenham: Stanley Thornes, 1997.
2. Evans ME. Using a model to structure psycho-social nursing research. *Journal of Psycho-social Nursing and Allied Mental Health Services* 1993; **30**(8): 27–32.
3. Barker P *op. cit.* For examples of standardized assessment tools in routine practice, see Appendix.
4. Barker P, Kerr B. *The process of psychotherapy: the journey of discovery.* Oxford: Butterworth Heinemann, 2000.
5. Likert RA. A technique for measurement of attitudes. *Archives of Psychology* 1932; **140**, 140–55.
6. Barker P, Fraser D (eds). *The nurse as therapist: a behavioural model.* London: Croom Helm, 1985.

Chapter 10

INTERVIEWING AS CRAFT

Phil Barker

INTRODUCTION

The interview is the simplest way to learn about the person-in-care but can also be the most complex. The interview in a psychiatric context differs little from the job interview. Both involve an imbalance of power and may involve 'open' as well as 'hidden' agendas. Only the questions and format will differ. The common aim is to build up a picture of the person through conversation – albeit a fairly one-sided one.

Interviews usually involve a face-to-face meeting between two people. Interviews may be conducted over the telephone but this is usually reserved for special situations. The meeting is focused on finding out something. The pattern of interaction between interviewer and respondent are highly specialized. We need no special qualification or training to be an interviewee. People undergo interviews almost everyday – when seeking employment, asking for advice from their boss or a friend, applying for unemployment benefit or a bank loan. By contrast, the interviewer needs special training to handle the potential complexity of the interview situation.

The need for focus

Inadequate assessment will result in inadequate care. The person's problems need to be seen as a whole, which requires the nurse to avoid assuming too much, trying instead to view problems against the 'backdrop' of the person's whole lived experience. However, we can never find out everything about a person, or even about a specific problem. Neither should we want to. The interview needs to be thorough, but we should avoid examining areas of the person's experience that are either irrelevant or unnecessary for our needs.

Critics of traditional psychiatric interviewing estimated that three-quarters of the material covered could be omitted without any appreciable loss, since it played little or no part in the plan of treatment.[1] Such interviewing is not only inefficient but raises an ethical issue: what right have we to subject aspects of the person-in-care's life to needless enquiry? Interviews need to be planned carefully. By engaging in idle chatter we may end up exploring aspects of the person's life that are of little or no relevance to care or treatment. We also risk addressing areas that are of crucial significance. The golden rule is:

> Find out everything you need to know and no more.

Idle curiosity has no place in a professional interview.

THE RELATIONSHIP

Interviewer characteristics

If the goal of interviewing is to shine a light upon the person and her/his problems the nurse needs to collect as much *relevant* information as possible by the shortest possible route. Consider first what the interviewer needs to *avoid* doing.

Someone who is abrupt, rude or officious is unlikely to be popular, far less effective as an interviewer. Similarly, if the nurse is cold or indifferent this will not generate the trust needed to allow talk about delicate or highly personal material. In many situations people will make statements that may appear shocking – admissions concerning:

❑ suicidal intent;
❑ sexual practices;
❑ past misdeeds which have inspired guilt; or
❑ material considered bizarre or delusional.

These may be disturbing, especially to the novice interviewer. Any expression of surprise, astonishment, reproach or even stunned silence, will stifle any further admissions or self-examination.

Any interviewer should appear warm, friendly and accepting. These are especially important in the psychiatric field. Your intention should be to help the person think that: 'Here is someone I can talk to'; 'Here is someone who understands me; and who is not sitting in judgement over me'. Interviewer characteristics such as empathy, warmth and genuineness can help promote self-disclosure and self-examination.[2]

The questions, and how they are asked, are of equal importance. The nurse should set a number of targets, aiming for accuracy, objectivity and organization – these will help her record important information, reflecting a minimum of bias. At the same time she should display signs of warmth, empathy, genuineness and unconditional positive regard, to encourage the person or the family to tell their stories.

The need for accuracy

It is not enough to obtain information. This should be accurate and should be reliably recorded for future reference. Some nurses have tried to resolve this problem by writing down everything the person-in-care says in a verbatim transcript. Although this is rarely used in practice it emphasizes some important principles.

First of all, inaccuracies can creep in even when interviews are written up as soon as they have taken place. Even if we set aside time to record the interview as soon as it has taken place, we are bound to get some of this 'reporting' wrong. This may have something to do with the sheer demand of having to record so much information in a short period of time. An alternative is to summarize the interview. However, when we condense the interview we may isolate and report upon certain items that are relatively unimportant; and we neglect others that are crucial. Clearly, some kind of compromise is needed, as far as writing up the interview is concerned.

Some nurses tape-record interviews, using this as a memory aid when writing up their notes. However, this may be too time-consuming. Perhaps the simplest procedure is to decide in advance upon the focus of the interview. This might function as headings, to which we can append brief notes during the interview. These can then he extended into longhand (if necessary) as soon as possible after the interview. We must accept that we are likely to make mistakes in reporting our conversations. The reporting process that we finally adopt should attempt to reduce the risk of mistakes.

The idea of a verbatim transcript is interesting. We write down *word for word* what was said. We do not report what we *thought* the person meant, only what was said. In the early stages of any assessment there is a great advantage in describing the events of the interview. Our aim in writing a report is to have something to reflect upon, something to remind us of what took place, so that we can give more thought to what was said. When we are in the heat of the interview – trying to listen attentively, making brief notes, thinking of the next question – it may be difficult to digest what has been said. For this reason we need a verbatim account of what the person actually did say. We can then study these notes, recollecting how certain comments were made, and come to some conclusion about what it all means for the care planning process.[3]

The other advantage of the verbatim account is that we can discuss with other members of the care team what the person said. Instead of saying: 'I interviewed John today and felt that he was very depressed; almost suicidal', we can tell our colleagues that 'I interviewed John today and these were the sort of comments he was making'.

It is all too easy to stray from what was said by adding layer upon layer of unnecessary professional judgement.

BELIEFS, VALUES AND ATTITUDES

Interviewers need to be non-judgemental. Often, the person's life-philosophy, values and attitudes towards her/himself and others, may conflict with those of the nurse. It is important to avoid appearing narrowminded, especially where the person is describing material that might be viewed as bizarre, irrational or unorthodox. It is important to accept the person's value system, even where it conflicts with that of the nurse. We are not being asked to agree or disagree. We are not being asked to join his life, far less to live it. We are simply being asked to acknowledge who and what the person *is*.

Nurses should keep their own selves out of the relationship. This raises the criticism that the so-called 'collaborative relationship' is somewhat one-sided. This seems only appropriate, since it is not the nurse who is in need of care. Consequently, the focus is very much upon the person. The nurse can act as an important model during psychotherapeutic treatment, where she might disclose feelings or thoughts of her own, to help the person identify with her. However, there is little room for such disclosure within the assessment stage. Discussion of the nurse's views, experiences or problems may serve only as distractions.

The need for patience

Few interviews are without difficulties. The person may appear uncooperative, uncommunicative or inarticulate. Such characteristics often result in a lengthy, and possibly frustrating, interview.

Some people are unwilling to talk about any aspect of their problem. They may have been over the same ground repeatedly with other members of the health care team. The person needs an explanation of why *this* interview is important and *different*. The person also needs time to find out about the interviewer, and time to change their attitude towards the interview process.

Others may find it difficult to answer questions, the material they wish to discuss being too distressing. Or they may find it difficult to find the 'right words'. Again, patience is essential. In other cases the person may appear to be skirting around the subject, going off at tangents, taking a long time to answer a question or avoiding answering at all. This may be an indication of difficulty. Again the person needs time, not criticism – whether overt or veiled. Avoid showing signs of impatience.

One way of dealing with the time constraints of an interview is to ask the person to 'keep time'. Not only might this 'empower' the person, but will allow the nurse to give the person full attention. By asking: 'How much time do we have left?' or 'How are we doing for time?' the nurse offers the person a degree of control over the process of the interview.

Resolving conflicts

Few nurses like everyone that they meet in the course of their work. Some people exasperate us, others bring past actions, or possess personalities, attitudes or values which we find repugnant. However, we do not need to like or approve of people, to be able to offer them help. In pursuing the ideals of the craft of caring we should take care not to:

❏ argue with the person;
❏ belittle the person;
❏ blame the person for her/his failings.

In general, we need to avoid being moralistic. Many people-in-care have had more than their fair share of conflict already. What they *have been*, or what they *are* may be in conflict with what they would *hope to become*. Mental health professionals should avoid adding to that conflict.

The collaborative relationship

Interviews frequently pose significant problems for the person in care. The interview is an unnatural form of conversation. This is especially true for most people who enter the psychiatric system. At least nurses have a chance to become more 'natural' through practice. The unusual nature of the interview may promote considerable anxiety. The person may be unaware of why he is being interviewed; or may simply feel uncomfortable when questioned closely about the private corners of his life. This is only natural. Most of us feel uneasy when under such 'direct fire'. The nurse should be sensitive to this, even when the anxiety is not obvious.

Many people disguise their discomfort, displaying their uneasiness indirectly through hesitant answers, short replies, or apparent 'striving to please' – always answering 'Yes', or agreeing with everything the nurse says. Appropriate questioning may reduce this. The interview should always begin by addressing non-threatening material; simple questions about the person where s/he lives, etc. These should be phrased to allow very short answers. Avoid asking for opinions or 'self-analysis' in the early stages, as it is too demanding. If the interview has progressed beyond this stage and the person again becomes anxious, postpone questions that appear upsetting. If the person becomes manifestly distressed it may even be appropriate to return to more mundane topics, allowing the person to regain composure. The interview can return to the 'threatening' material gradually, allowing the person to regain confidence through active participation.

It may be appropriate to ask the person directly if s/he is ready to return to a particular line of questioning:

❏ 'We spoke earlier about ... do you feel ready to return to that? If you don't want to discuss it just now, just say so.'

Giving the person a chance to influence the direction of the interview is crucial. This fosters a sense of partnership and reduces feelings of being manipulated by the interviewer. This partnership should begin early. The nurse's first responsibility is to tell the person what is the plan for the interview, what is the rationale for this process and what will be the person's role in the whole proceeding.

The simplest question is most often the one that might get to the very nub of the issue by the shortest possible route. It also offers the person the greatest room for manoeuvre.

❑ 'What have you brought along with you today?' or
❑ 'What brings you here?' or
❑ 'So . . . how would you like to use this time?'

Such questions hold no obvious 'hidden agenda' but represent the simplest forms of enquiry. The last question is perhaps the most sensitive, and offers the person an opportunity to control the proceedings. This kind of question may well help build the kind of confiding relationship that the nurse most desires.

Another important question, which should be asked at the outset is:

❑ 'Do you want to ask anything before we begin?'

This may be the best guard against anxiety, since it removes much of the threat of the unknown.

The person may well be unenthusiastic about being interviewed. This is often true when people are first admitted into care. The person may already have seen a long line of such interviewers and may be irritated by the prospect of another. The nurse should acknowledge that such irritation or annoyance is natural and appropriate. The nurse should acknowledge how the person might be feeling. Indeed, it is useful to emphasize exactly how *this* interview will be different and also how important the person is to the development of the interview. Indeed, the nurse should spell out clearly how the person will be helping the nurse, through the telling of the story. The person should be placed firmly in the driving seat.

Traditionally, psychiatric professionals employ the concept of *resistance* to explain difficulties in the interview process. However, instead of blaming the person for her/his poor cooperation, there may be value in trying to see the interview from the person's angle, so that we might prevent such resistance developing.

Some people may be unhappy about being grilled or cross-examined. This seems only reasonable. Why need the interview be so unpleasant? It must be something to do with the line of questioning or the way that questions are being asked. We should not assume that the person does not want to answer our questions. The interview should be designed to encourage participation. Even where people are not resistant they may not be overly enthusiastic. Again this may be a reflection of the interview format. Are we rushing through a routine checklist, ticking off answers, looking as if we have done this a hundred times before, and have a lot more pressing work ahead of us? If this is so, the person may feel that this is not very important, and may be disinclined to 'work' at the interview. There is great value in trying to make each interview a stimulating prospect, for the person and interviewer alike. Even if this is the hundredth interview this month, we should try to tailor the interview to suit the person: making it something personal and special. The focus of the interview is the person's life. How can it *not* be special?

OVERVIEW OF THE INTERVIEW

Phrasing the question

Questions are the central feature of the interview. The first priority is to avoid confusing the person who may already be confused or at a loss.

Be specific

The first priority in phrasing a question is to avoid ambiguity. Avoid questions that may have more than one meaning. Focus the question so that it will draw information on one aspect of the person's functioning or experience. If you do not get the answer you expected, you may not have asked the question you meant to ask.

Keep it short

Brevity is also important. Avoid asking long rambling questions. Avoid making general observations about the person or his situation, including a question hidden somewhere within this statement.

Don't ask
'You were saying earlier that you feel pretty tense all the time . . . that must be pretty awful. I can see that you are tense right now. You're sitting all sort of hunched up . . . is that what you mean? Like you said a moment ago, I mean . . . is that how you feel . . . all tense, anxious, nervy, like you said. Is it?'

Do ask
'You said a moment ago that you often felt tense.' (Pause)
'Tell me more about that.' (Await reply)
'When you feel tense . . . what does that mean for you?' (Await reply)
'So . . . how do you feel right now?' (Await reply)
'You are sitting sort of hunched up. Is that how you usually are when you feel tense?' (Await reply).

If the question is not specific it is more difficult to answer and may increase the person's anxiety. The same is true of the string of questions. Ask one question at a time, unless you have very good reasons for acting otherwise.

Sharpen the time focus

The question should also specify the time clearly, where appropriate. 'How do you feel *now*?' or 'How have you been feeling over the past *two or three days*?'

Where the time-scale is necessarily vague, you might ask: 'Can you tell me what sort of *things* you were able to do *when you felt you were well*?' or 'How did you *feel* when you were well?' following up the reply by asking 'And how *long ago* was that?' Be aware that many people who are highly distressed feel that they have 'always' been like this. Help them sharpen the time focus.

Open and closed questions

There are two kinds of question: those that elicit a *short* reply and those that require fuller answers.

❑ 'Are you still feeling depressed?'
❑ 'Your husband left you. Do you think that made you depressed?'
❑ 'Do you hear voices a lot?'

All these **closed** questions can be answered 'yes', 'no' or 'don't know'.

❑ 'How are you feeling today?'
❑ 'How did you react to your husband leaving you?'
❑ 'You say that someone is talking to you, in your head. Tell me more about that.'
❑ 'Can you give me an idea of how you are feeling right now.'

All these **open** questions provide the person with an opportunity to talk at length, should s/he choose to do so.

Closed questions may be appropriate in the initial stages of the interview, as they put fewer demands on the person-in-care. In this sense they are also appropriate when the person is very distressed or withdrawn. Open questions will, however, provide more information about what it is like to be the person, providing more information about the person's experience.

The value of reflection

When the person says something that appears interesting or significant, the nurse may choose to develop this theme, or gain more information. The simplest and least intrusive way to do this is to *reflect* – or bounce back – the reply.

Person: 'I get so confused sometimes I just don't know whether I'm coming or going'.
Nurse: 'Coming or going?'
Person: 'That's right. I mean … I just don't seem to be able to cope with things. I feel so useless all the time'.
Nurse: 'I see … you feel useless? Tell me more about that'.

Emphasis should be given to certain words to show that you are phrasing a question, and not simply repeating what the person has said. However, reflection needs to be used with discretion. If the nurse repeatedly reflects the person's answers s/he might think that s/he was answering the questions badly, or that the nurse was poking fun.

Reflection can be taken a stage further by using the person's actual phrasing to frame another question:

❑ 'You say that you don't know whether you are coming or going. Can you tell me what you mean by that?'

The key feature of reflection is that the nurse provides the minimum of guidance, interrupting the flow of the conversation no more than is necessary. This allows for more efficient interviewing. More importantly, it provides the person with an opportunity to talk as much as possible, without losing the necessary structure.

Threatening questions

Some questions will be disturbing to the person. Avoiding such questions is not a solution. Instead, questions about sensitive or distressing subjects should be carefully framed to reduce their impact. It is not possible to list all such perceived threats since these vary from one person to another. However, even in today's liberated society detailed questioning about sex is often perceived as a threat. The same is true of domestic violence and sometimes psychotic states.

Don't ask
❑ 'How often do you and your partner have sex?'
❑ 'Do you ever hit the kids?'
❑ 'How long have you been having these auditory hallucinations?'

Do ask
❑ 'You talked about you and your partner … is there any aspect of your relationship with which you are not entirely happy?'
❑ 'What happens when you lose your temper at home?'
❑ 'What can you tell me about the voices?'

If the person feels threatened by direct questioning s/he may simply deny the existence of any problem. By taking a more oblique line of questioning the 'glare' of the searchlight is reduced. Such indirect questioning may make it easier for the person to admit to problems of which s/he is ashamed.

The need for a framework

An interview needs a structure, which can be rigid or flexible depending on the demands of the situation. Structure most commonly refers to the order and nature of the questions asked. For example, a typical interview might begin with very open-ended questions:

❑ 'Would you like to tell me what's bothering you at present?'

Gradually, more specific queries can be introduced:

❑ 'How often has this happened?'

Eventually, the person's perception of the problem can be narrowed down to finer detail:

❑ 'How severe is this at present, on a scale of 1 to 10?'

These stages – beginning, middle and end – show how the interview begins with very broad concerns and gradually sharpens the focus on one or two problems. The first interview might be devoted entirely to drawing up a list of the person's problems. Subsequent interviews might take individual problems as topics, devoting the time to trying to understand each one better, through closer analysis.

A flexible framework, where the line of questioning is developed within the interview itself, is usually reserved for the expert interviewer. Most of us need a simple framework of questions to provide some security, so that we don't get lost for words. Our aim is to have a conversation with the person, so we want to talk as normally as possible. A general outline of the questions we want to ask and the areas we want to explore, may help us – and the person – feel more comfortable.[4]

Troubleshooting

Interviews rarely turn out the way we plan. It is important to prepare for problems.

Failure to respond

The person may find it difficult to give the information asked for, especially at the first interview. How far should you press him? Should you press him at all? If the person fails to answer to your satisfaction perhaps the question was badly phrased. Try presenting the question from a different angle.

❑ **Poor question**: 'When there is conflict within the family, what kind of coping strategies do you employ under such conditions?' (No answer try again)
❑ **Alternative**: 'Well, let me put it this way ... when there's an "atmosphere" at home, how do you deal with that?'

Difficult to answer

The person may answer, but may be unsatisfied with the reply. Offer some words of encouragement, helping the person to find the words needed to express her/himself. Beware, however, of putting words into the person's mouth. Instead, try to help shape up the answer through discreet feedback.

Nurse:	'So how did you feel when that happened?'
Person:	'Oh, I don't know. Just lost ... sort of... eh ... I – oh, I don't know'.
Nurse:	'Uh-huh, you felt "lost": lost in what way?'
Person:	'Lost, yes. Didn't know what to do ... what to say'.
Nurse:	'Lost for words?'
Person:	'Yes ... lost for words. Didn't know what to say to her. Felt powerless. No, that's not right. Can't seem to think straight'.
Nurse:	'You were lost for words. You didn't *know* what to say to her – or you felt that you *couldn't* tell her how you felt?'
Person:	'Well, maybe that's true. I knew how I felt, but I just couldn't face her. Yeah, I guess I couldn't *bring myself* to tell her how I felt'.

Dealing with refusal

Sometimes the person may not answer at all – which is an answer of sorts: 'I am not willing (or ready/able) to answer'. What should we do?

❑ Rephrase the question?
❑ Try to nudge the person gently?
❑ Or simply respect the person's wishes, leaving this issue for another time, or another place?

The last solution is probably best, although there are always occasions when it might be appropriate to try the others. If we choose to 'postpone' a question, however, we should let the person know why we have done so.

❑ 'You don't seem to be too happy with that question'. (Pause)
❑ 'Maybe it was the way I put it. Or maybe you don't feel ready to discuss that with me just yet?' (Pause)

- 'Maybe we could come back to it some other time, when you think you're ready. OK?' (Pause)
- 'We were talking a moment ago about . . .' (Move on to the next topic).

Going off at tangents

Rarely do we get all the answers to our question in a single interview. Ideally, one question leads to another and may span several interviews. In practice, however, one question usually produces a number of answers, some aspects of which are relevant, others less so. The nurse must decide whether or not to follow up such 'tangents' or to stick to the core question. If you decide to deal only with *some* of the person's replies make it clear that you are doing this.

Nurse: 'You were talking yesterday about going shopping in town'.

Person: 'Oh, I don't know. I get terribly tense in the crowds. Then there's my Henry, I should have rung him. He doesn't really manage well on his own. I worry about him ever so much ... and I promised to take Johnny – he's just 11 ... to the game on Saturday. I keep letting him down. He can hardly look at me. It's all so pointless'.

Nurse: 'Uh-huh. I see. Your family obviously mean a lot to you. That's why you worry about them. Maybe we need to spend some time just talking about that. Do you want to talk about that *now*, or do you want to carry on discussing the shopping trip you planned?'

The nurse had a decision to make here: either to respond to the person's 'need' to discuss her worries about the family or to stick to the agenda of the interview. By turning the decision over to the person, the nurse empowered the person's decision-making. No agenda is ever fixed. The interview may follow any course that is deemed appropriate. It is important to gauge the flow of the conversation carefully.

The interview setting

The interview is a 'formal' conversation, the outcome of which is crucial to the person. Interviews need not, however, be structured in a formal manner. Sometimes it may be appropriate to interview the person in her/his bedroom on the ward; the sitting room at home; a consulting room off the ward; or an interview room at a clinic. It may be just as practical, however, to interview the person in the hospital grounds or while walking the dog in the park. The important consideration is:

Will we have privacy, peace and quiet?

The person is unlikely to discuss personal problems within earshot of other people and may become distracted if there are repeated interruptions. In some cases walking in the park may feel more private and distraction-free than a consulting room, where people may be heard talking through the wall.

The setting is also important for putting the person at ease. A distressed person may feel more comfortable chatting over a cup of coffee in the corner of the hospital cafeteria or when walking in the fresh air. The restrictions of a small interview room may enhance the person's anxiety and may make communication more difficult. However, in some cases it is appropriate to pick an awkward setting. If the person has identified a situation that appears to trigger a problem it may be appropriate to conduct the interview there. We might take someone with social anxiety out into the street. If the person was suffering from a grief reaction, we might take her/him to a setting that evoked special memories of the loved one. The setting selected would serve as a trigger for certain emotions, thoughts and memories, which might be less evident in a more formal interview setting.

The power of ordinary communication

Some people do not like being interviewed. This may stem from bad experiences in other interview situations at the hands of the over-efficient, or the cold and probing interviewer. In addition to being warm, empathic, genuine and non-judgemental, it is also important to talk to the person in language s/he understands. The person may be baffled by professional language, by jargon, vocabulary or grammatical structures that are beyond her/his capabilities. In addition to easing tensions, the use of a common language – especially where the person speaks in some dialect – may help establish rapport.

Nurse: 'You're looking pretty down today, Derek. Is there something troubling you?'

Derek: 'Oh, I'm just proper ... scunnered, like. Been like this for weeks'.

Nurse: 'You feel *scunnered* (emphasis). What ... with everything?'

Derek: 'Yeah, just sick of everything. But especially myself'.

Nurse: 'Tell me more about that'.

By picking up on the person-in-care's use of the expression 'scunnered' meaning sick or tired of – the nurse develops rapport. The person may think, 'this person is someone I can *really* talk to'. The nurse need not actually know the exact meaning of the key words picked up and reflected back. By using Derek's language the nurse encourages him to amplify the point he is making. The more he is encouraged to express himself, the more information he gives and the more the nurse can build up a picture of 'what it is like to be this person'.

The power of respect

In the same context it is worth picking up the use of more technical terms – like 'depressed', 'anxious', 'alienated', 'paranoid', 'hostile'. These have very special meanings in professional language, but have become part of the vernacular. However, we should not assume that because such expressions are in everyday use their meaning remains the same. Where the person uses such technical expressions we need to ask her/him to clarify their meaning.

In a related vein, it is important to avoid translating the person's words into our own convenient shorthand:

Nurse: 'Tell me more about how you feel'.
Jane: 'Oh, blue'.
Nurse: 'You mean that you're depressed'.
Jane: (Sighs) 'I guess so'.

Here, the nurse missed an opportunity to engage with Jane by using the words she used to describe her experience. If she had intended to say she was depressed, she would have chosen that word. This is not mere semantics. Using the person's language is respectful. We acknowledge that the person knows her/his experience better than anyone. Indeed, only the person has access to that experience. The value we place upon those words denotes the value we accord to the person.

In some situations it may be appropriate to encourage the person to talk about the problem without even naming it. Where the problem is a source of embarrassment, or the person does not feel prepared to trust the nurse, talking about the problem in the abstract may be a solution.

Nurse: 'I get the feeling that you are not ready to talk about this situation yet. I understand ... in fact ... there is no need to tell me about this ... whatever it is. Not until you are ready to. What about if we just called it X? Maybe you could tell me how X is a problem for you?'

Alternatively, the nurse could ask:

❏ 'How does X make you feel?' or
❏ 'How long has X been a problem for you?' or
❏ 'When did X first become a problem for you?'

Providing that this arrangement is acceptable to the person the nurse can explore the problem fully without ever asking the person to define 'X' specifically. Where the person is discussing some taboo (like a sexual abuse scenario) or an experience that is normally considered implausible (like being possessed by demons), s/he might feel empowered by the opportunity to disguise the issue in this manner.[5]

THE PRESENTATION OF THE INTERVIEW

Preparation

The nurse should always aim to know:

❏ the aim of the interview;
❏ how best to conduct it; and
❏ how much time is available.

The aims of the interview vary enormously from one interview to another. Some preparation is necessary to ensure that you cover all the points you wish to cover. A general outline is helpful for the following reasons.

❏ It acts as a guide to the line of questioning, guarding against being unduly sidetracked.
❏ It helps foster a logical, sensitive line of questioning, beginning with non-threatening material building up gradually to more sensitive material.
❏ It guards against duplication of lines of questioning.
❏ It guards against taxing the person's concentration (e.g. by being unduly long), and guards against time-wasting (e.g. by spending too much time on general issues) before reaching the key questions.

The nurse should plan to conclude the interview at least 10 minutes before necessary, thus allowing the person time to regain composure or to ask any further general questions.

The plan

In considering the various ways of phrasing questions, it is helpful to distinguish between *higher*, and *lower* order questions.[6]

Lower-order questions

There are four main kinds of lower-order question.

1 The first involves the *recall of information*. The person might be asked:
   ■ 'Have you ever felt this bad *before*?' – to which he can answer 'Yes' or 'No'. Alternatively, he might be asked to recall *more* information:
   ■ 'When did you *last* feel this bad?'

2 The second kind involves *rephrasing* or rewording certain concepts or ideas:
   ■ 'Can you tell me, in your own words, what you mean by "helpless"?'

3 In the third class the person is asked to *compare* or *contrast* situations or experiences:
   - 'In which *situations* do you normally feel worst?'
   - 'Can you tell me, then, *where* you would feel OK?'

4 The last class invites the person-in-care to present *alternatives* to what they have done in the past:
   - 'How could you handle that differently?'
   - 'Given what we have just discussed, how would you tackle that situation in the future?'

Higher-order questions

This class of questions involves more complex replies, inviting the person to *analyse a situation*, giving some indication of why s/he believed that something happened. These motives or causes cannot, of course, be drawn simply from memory; the answer needs to be more 'creative' and is therefore more difficult.

- 'Why do you think your wife stopped talking to you?' or
- 'How do you think you came to be depressed?'

This class also contains questions that invite the person to make *predictions* or to discuss *complex ideas*:

- 'What would happen if you did that?' or
- 'What would be so bad about that?'

Ideally, the plan of the interview should begin with lower-order questions, which require the person-in-care to dip into memories or require simple problem-solving answers. As the interview progresses, or as the person becomes more comfortable, more complex questions, relying on complex reasoning, may be introduced.

Seating

Classically, interviewers sit behind a desk, with the interviewee facing. Such a job interview arrangement is clearly inappropriate given the inherent messages about power and control that are communicated. Where two people face each other *directly*, it may appear confrontational. Where a desk is used it may appear to represent a shield (suggesting that the interviewer wishes to remain at a distance) or barrier (placing the interviewee at a disadvantage).

The height and design of chairs are also important. If the interviewer sits on a higher chair, this may appear to confer an advantage. If the person is given a stiff, high-backed chair, while the nurse sits in an easy chair, again there may appear to be an advantage; the nurse in the easy chair appearing more relaxed and comfortable. Ideally, both should sit on the same kind of chair, at roughly 60 degrees to one another. This allows easy eye contact and orientation, as found in most normal social interactions.[7] Where matching chairs are not available the nurse should offer the person first choice. Where the nurse visits the person at home s/he should ask where the person would like the nurse to sit.

The seats should be close together, registering the privacy and intimacy of the conversation. If they are far apart, this may be interpreted as a gulf that is difficult to bridge. As with other aspects of the interview, check with the person that such arrangements are acceptable before beginning.

Opening

The nurse should begin by advising the person of the aims of the interview, asking if s/he has any queries or objections.

- 'Hello Mr Jackson. My name is Jacqueline and I am responsible for your care while you are here. I am aware that this all might seem strange to you and that you are still trying to get your bearings, but I would like to spend a little time with you, getting to know you a bit better'. (Pause)
  'I'd like to talk with you about what led up to you coming in to hospital'. (Pause)
  'That will help me get an idea about what kind of care you might need while you are here. At the same time, if you have any questions for me, I hope that you will feel OK about asking me. Is that OK with you?'

The nurse makes it clear who she is and what she wants to do. She also tries to acknowledge how the person might be feeling, trying to make the interview as non-threatening as possible. She pauses briefly throughout her introduction, giving him time to speak, or to allow her words to register. This kind of opening may reduce the person's natural anxiety. The emphasis upon collaboration – '*talk with you*' – may also enhance the person's self-esteem.

The interview core

The structure of the interview should emphasize the beginning and end of each section with summaries where appropriate.

Example

1 'To begin, I'd like you to tell me a bit about yourself.' This general question may be followed immediately by a series of specific queries: e.g. 'Do you live on your own? Who does your shopping for you? Where did you work before you retired?'

2 'Good. Maybe we could talk a bit about how you

came into hospital? Now you said that you lived alone ...' Having recapped on some of the points covered in (1) above the nurse might move on to more open-ended questions: 'When did you first feel that you needed help? Who did you discuss these problems with? How did you feel about being on your own?'

3 'That's fine. I have found that very helpful. Perhaps we might discuss some of the problems you have mentioned in more detail? Are you ready for that just now?' If the person agrees, further questions of a 'who', 'where', 'when', 'what' and 'how' variety might be asked: 'Where did that first happen? Were you on your own at the time? What would be so bad about that? In what way is that a problem for you?'

4 'From what you have said a number of things appear to be a problem just now. These voices appear to be distressing you a lot. Is that the case?' The information collected can now be summarized briefly. At the same time the nurse can check that her interpretation of the 'facts' is correct.

Promoting responses

The nurse's key role as interviewer is to encourage the person to tell the story that will help in the development of appropriate care. In addition to the actual questioning, the non-verbal dimension of the interview also is important.

The 'good' interviewer expresses her/his skills most often through non-verbal behaviour. Or rather, the person is likely to perceive the nurse positively or negatively on the basis of how the nurse stands, sits, uses gestures and looks at the person. The following is a very 'rough guide' to the importance of body language in interviewing.

Spatial behaviour

Sitting close to the person, suggests intimacy and being on an equal footing. This also suggests the absence of status. If you wish to 'control' the other person, you try to look down at him or sit behind a desk. Sitting side-by-side will likely communicate your liking for the person, or at least acceptance, and may give reassurance.

Posture

Try to appear relaxed and comfortable, communicating self-confidence. At times, a change of posture will enhance the conversation – leaning forward if the person is discussing confidential material or is distressed, or settling back in the chair if the person appears to want to talk at some length. These postural changes communicate confidentiality or a willingness to listen. In general sitting turned slightly towards the person – leaning slightly in her/his direction – is most helpful in facilitating conversation.

Facial expression

Our faces provide a regular commentary on our speech, as we flash our eyebrows, smile, frown or grimace. Try to follow the person's conversation by displaying appropriate facial expression. However, this should always be controlled, otherwise it may look theatrical and insincere. Partner the person, showing that you appreciate the meaning or significance of what is being said.

Eye contact

Usually, we look at other people in order to pick up non-verbal cues. However, gaze has another function: it adds emphasis to our speech and can be used to 'reply' to the other person. Although the amount of eye contact varies from one situation to another, rarely do we ever gaze constantly at others, except when madly in love or enraged with anger. Normal gaze patterns involve looking and quickly looking away. If we give more than around 70% of gaze-contact time we may appear confrontational (although this varies greatly across cultures and subcultures). Alternatively, we may look embarrassed, ashamed or suspicious if we do not give sufficient eye-contact for the given situation.

CONCLUSION

Conversation allows us to gain insights into the unique world of the person-in-care, focusing the person behind the patient label, studying his experience of 'being-in-his-world'. The basic interview format needs to be adapted to suit factors such as age, sex, cultural background, values, beliefs and presentation. These adaptations influence the structure of the interview, what we do and say, how long it lasts, where it takes place and how we record the outcome.

The interview has no single purpose apart from eliciting information. Instead, it may be used for a multiplicity of purposes, from learning about the patient as a person, to evaluating how things are changing in relation to specific aspects of everyday living. Throughout this range of conversations some basic principles remain constant. The interview should be seen as a *two-way* process and the person should be given every encouragement to collaborate, being informed regularly of the progress of the interview, and wherever possible informed *in advance* of 'what is coming next'.

The person should be encouraged to play a part in controlling the interview, for example, being asked to decide when s/he is ready to discuss certain topics. Or being asked to 'keep time'. The interviewer must be unbiased, isolating any preconceptions or prejudices that might influence the conversation that will develop. The person's value system should be accepted, although this need not mean that it is given active approval. The person's perception of his world and himself is used as the vantage point from which the assessment will develop. The interviewer tries to see the world through the person's eyes, at least for the time being.

The assessment interview should be a highly sophisticated interaction and often can be therapeutic. If handled properly the person may discover things of which s/he was unaware. Sometimes, however, these revelations can be traumatic and the person may require support afterwards.

In general, a 'good interview' will ultimately benefit the person. Even a difficult or distressing interview will yield some fruit. However, the nurse should never use her status to manipulate the person. Collaboration is essential for the development of purposeful care.

REFERENCES

1. Peterson DR. *The clinical study of social behaviour.* New York: Appleton Century Crofts, 1968.
2. Truax CB, Carkhuff RR. Towards effective counselling and psychotherapy training and practice. Chicago, IL: Aldine Press, 1967. [For detailed discussion.]
3. Barker P, Buchanan-Barker P. *The tidal model.* London: Brunner Routledge 2003.
4. Romme M, Escher S. *Accepting voices.* London: Macmillan/Mind, 1993. [For an example of the use of a specific structure to elicit information about hearing voices.]
5. Barker P. *Assessment in psychiatric and mental health nursing: in search of the whole person.* Cheltenham: Stanley Thornes, 1997.
6. Hewit FS. Communication skills: questions and listening. *Nursing Times* 1981; **25 June**: 21–6. [Format quoted in the text is adapted from this work.]
7. Argyle M. *Bodily communication.* London: Methuen, 1975. [For a detailed review.]

Chapter 11

DEVELOPING COLLABORATIVE ASSESSMENT

Tom Keen* and Janis Keen**

INTRODUCTION

Psychiatric assessment, or diagnosis, is essentially an attempt to attribute a person's suffering to an underlying illness, and thereby identify appropriate treatment. Insofar as psychiatric nurses assist psychiatry, nursing assessment may be understood as a part of this diagnostic process.[1] Assessment is conducted by observation, interviewing (the patient and significant others) and measuring (using tests, questionnaires etc.). Objectivity, benevolent neutrality, professional knowledge and expertise are assumed. The psychiatric nurse is a scientist, armed with knowledge of psychiatric classification and psychopathology; psychological processes; and an understanding of potential pathogenic stressors. At the end of the process, a comprehensive assessment should be reducible to concise care plans, consisting of a few briefly specified goals, and accompanying plans as to how they will be attained – what the patient will do, and how psychiatric treatment and nursing care will help. The virtues of this approach may be summarized as professional unity, objectivity and, paradoxically, simplicity. People generally understand how to be a patient in relation to illnesses, doctors and nurses. If they accept both this status, and a medical perspective on their lives, then their com-

pliance with the service enables unambiguous treatment prescription and goal selection. Proponents of psychiatrically subordinate nursing emphasize the empirical evidence-based strength of close allegiance to well-researched medical practice.[2] However, if formal psychiatric approaches are applied too rigidly, the service risks inducing excessive dependence, negativistic hostility, or passive aggressive behaviour because various routine assessment procedures, clinical cultural styles or staff attitudes may be perceived as personally invalidating, patronizing or even oppressive and threatening.[3–6]

However, it is possible to construe psychiatric-mental health nursing otherwise – as primarily concerned not with the identification and treatment of disease, but with understanding and helping people to overcome *their* real-life problems, fulfil *their* needs and achieve desirable, realistic *personal* goals. These may be socioeconomic, spiritual, intellectual, psycho-social or physiological in nature. From this perspective, assessment becomes not an objective task at all, but rather a more open-ended and uncertain process in which the nurse attempts to gain insight into the person's own subjective experiences and aspirations.[7]

Recent UK policy documents and professional reviews[8–12] have repeatedly emphasized the importance

*Tom Keen lectures in mental health at the University of Plymouth. He previously worked as a nurse, therapist or manager in various situations, including acute admission wards, adolescent psychotherapy, therapeutic community and community mental health centres. Previous teaching experience includes sharing responsibility for staff development in Torbay Mental Health Unit, England.
**Janis Keen has been a senior staff member of a therapeutic-community based rehabilitation hostel in Newton Abbot, Devon for 15 years. She has a special interest in personal exploration and development using structured programmes of groupwork.

of nursing becoming more collaborative. 'Collaboration' is used in two senses. It can relate to the goal of enhanced inter-professional communication, and refer to cross-agency communication, co-ordinated action, or to multidisciplinary teamwork.[13] However, 'collaboration' also refers to the promotion of users' views, choices and responsibility in care and treatment programmes. This chapter discusses 'collaborative assessment' in this latter sense of increasing users' autonomy by not merely involving them in decision-making, but working fully in partnership to formulate care. Patients should not be relatively passive recipients of care, but full participants in the process.[7,14] This shift in policy reflects the evolution of professional language that has seen the term 'patient' transformed into 'client' before being reconstructed as 'user'. It is a moot point, however, whether the changes in terminology have been accompanied by equivalently profound developments in clinical attitudes and behaviour.[15,16]

HOW COLLABORATIVE IS COLLABORATIVE?

The concept of collaboration is not as straightforward as may be assumed. When used to denote a working relationship with patients, little operational distinction is made between 'collaboration', 'involvement', 'consultation', 'participation', 'alliance' and 'partnership'. It may be thought of as simply an expression of politeness or courtesy to patients, so that they feel respectfully involved and decently treated.[17] It may function as a euphemism for paying lip-service to patient-involvement.[18] This may be achieved by having a tick-box on an assessment form labelled something like 'Level of patient consultation: (if appropriate)' or asking patients to sign their care-plans. Such half-hearted attempts at collaboration may arise from a belief that therapeutic partnership may be at best an unrealistic ideal, or at worst clinically abusive, for people considered seriously mentally disordered. Gamble and Brennan suggest that seriously mentally ill users can at least be involved in their assessment by having an opportunity to discuss the results of formal tests before care plans are drawn up. These authors go on to suggest that 'using and choosing appropriate assessments is the foundation on which successful collaborative intervention is built'.[19] Other authors describe 'the semi-structured interview' as the basis for collaborative care and emphasize the importance of establishing rapport and having patients' feel involved in their care.[20] Cognitive-behavioural therapists generally refer to Beck's concept of a collaborative relationship, but differ as to the relative significance attached to its development during assessment. Some emphasize 'working from the patient's perspective' and explicitly advocate allowing time and working flexibly,[21]

while others describe the early use of formal batteries of tests.[22] Some practitioners are clearly prepared to meet their clients halfway in formulating treatment, although the strictures imposed by modern 'managed care' often place unrealistic pressures on staff to complete assessments rapidly, and provide excessively brief emollient treatment.[23]

However, collaboration in its fullest sense implies a fundamentally different relationship between nurses and patients than commonly found in the tightly managed and basically medical culture of most modern psychiatric services.[12] It may also require fundamental shifts in the relationships of 'services' to 'patients', along the lines often indicated by radical critics and service-users' movements[16,24,25] and require staff to defend more patient, flexible, client-centred assessment practices against organizational demands for a brisker clinical tempo.[23] Nurses are certainly challenged to find ways of achieving genuine collaboration within a service geared more explicitly to coercive social control[26,27] and may argue that a more authoritative approach is essential for effective risk management. Morgan[28] however insists that service users should be deeply involved in both assessing and planning how to manage any risks they pose to themselves or others. Collaborative risk assessment is not only ethically sound, it is also less disempowering, and more effective than making actuarially informed guesses from a position of detached professional isolation.[29]

There has been little authoritative exploration or clarification of the preferred nature and extent of collaboration. Perkins and Repper[18,30] insist that it is not sufficient simply to take account of patients' views. Rather the 'patients' themselves must be fully involved and their views and choices should be central to the whole process of care. Too often patients' views are subordinated or ignored completely while care and treatment are reduced to whatever results from the impact of competing professional ideologies upon the supposedly collaborative multidisciplinary team.

> Most mental health strategy documents pay lip-service to the importance of responding to users' views and wishes – to giving users choice. If this is to be more than empty rhetoric then it is vital that as providers we accept the wishes of people with mental health problems wherever possible, even if they are at odds with our own opinions. We cannot expect clients to trust us unless we can demonstrate that we trust them by responding to and acceding to their views. We may explain our reservations about their opinions, but ultimately the choice is theirs.
>
> Clearly there are times when the law requires that we override the client's judgement, but there are many other ways in which we deny the individual's right to choose.

In particular we fail to make them aware of the range of options available; fail to help them pursue their chosen course of action when it differs from what we think best; and make one form of help or support contingent upon another.

(Perkins and Repper, 1996)

Stuart and Laraia[31] define collaboration somewhat circularly as 'The shared planning, decision-making, problem-solving, goal-setting and assumption of responsibilities by people who work together co-operatively and with open communication.' They mention three key ingredients:

❑ Active and assertive contributions from each person;
❑ Receptivity and respect for each person's contribution;
❑ Negotiations that build on the contributions of each person to form a new way of conceptualizing the problem.

A collaborative assessment process enables both parties to engage with each other in a mutual process of discovery. The nurse should discover the person's abilities, needs and aspirations as clearly as they can be discerned so that the service as a whole is enabled to respond helpfully. Meanwhile, the patient should be assisted to explore the culture, methods and concepts enshrined within the service, discover how that could help, and also how best to engage with the service.

ASSESSMENT AS EXPERIENTIAL RESEARCH

The process of assessment can be understood as a form of research – a single-case study where the experimenter is in close and constant interaction with the subject (person) of enquiry. 'New paradigm' research models such as 'collaborative inquiry' and 'experiential research methodology'[32] provide conceptual and operational frameworks that translate readily to the assessment process. The assessor understands that the clinical environment, process of assessment and the nurse himself are part of the interactive reality being assessed, not phenomena that exist in isolation from the person as object of study.[33,34] The problems, needs or goals being assessed are not assumed to be aspects of categories predefined by the psychiatric service, whether conceptualized as disease process, behavioural deficits or excesses, inappropriate cognitions, unconscious conflicts or emotional tensions. The issues may be initially defined within the patient's frames of reference, and elaborated dialectically with those held by the assessing nurse.

Traditional assessment is based on an underlying, often unconscious paradigm (amounting to a psychiatric and nursing schema) in which the assessor has ownership of interpretation, meanings, attributions, categories and hypotheses. Conceptual frameworks and clinical decision-making come within the ambits of professional knowledge (e.g. symptomatology), belief systems (e.g. diagnostic categories) and organizational imperatives (e.g. risk assessment formats). This ownership has consequences in terms of the power balance within a supposedly caring relationship. Not only the kind of knowledge, but the justification for knowing it, the methods of acquiring it, the right to and means of challenging or disputing any of those things are all within the control of the professional services.[35] Apart from the obstacles this situation poses to the development of trust and a therapeutic relationship, there are issues about the authenticity, validity and reliability of the information collected by such means. Such knowledge is at best narrow and exclusive, at worst artificial, sterile and inapplicable to everyday realities. Collaborative, relatively loosely structured assessment may produce much richer information, which is closer to the reality of the person being assessed.[36,37]

Collaborative assessment should concentrate on the meanings of experiences and behaviours within their social context, which can include the clinical situation and the assessment dyad itself, as well as the family and wider socio-economic environments. Thus, collaborative modes of assessment address people's reality, and privilege 'objective difficulty' aetiological explanations over 'personal defectiveness', or disease model, attributions (see Smail).[38] The emphasis should be upon sharing and interaction, in which both parties discuss the meanings attributed to specific behaviours and experiences, rather than their becoming clues to the allocation of diagnoses. The assessor accords especial priority and significance to the patient's own terminology and interpretations, so that subjective data become the central focus of the assessment inquiry.[39] This perspective displaces and relegates the supposedly more real objective material. In doing so collaborative assessment up-ends conventional hierarchies of evidence, and privileges single-case study as the 'gold standard' for psychiatric-mental health nursing over the highly structured objective RCT – the gold standard of the medico-psychiatric paradigm. Hypotheses and formulations emerging from collaborative assessment are not intended or likely to readily generalize to whole diagnostic classes of people. The collaborative analysis should conform to inductive rather than deductive processing. That is, theories, explanations, hypotheses are searched for *within*, and allowed to emerge *from*, the information uncovered, rather than the assessor using the data revealed to confirm pre-existing hypotheses (e.g. diagnoses, schema-modes or behavioural deficits). This enables unexpected or unaware concerns to be discovered. Creative solutions can be explored more confidently.[39] Beck's term 'collaborative empiricism' implies a similar inquisitive fascination with the shared discovery of meanings to help create therapeutic alliances:

> A young man dressed in an oddly anachronistic and colourful fashion approached a senior nurse who entered his ward and struck up a conversation. Although the two had never met before, the young man stood very close to the nurse and stared straight into her eyes as he carefully enunciated 'Hello, who are you? I hope you don't mind my talking to you. The staff say that I'm too nosy and that I put people off by my eye contact.'
>
> Nurse: 'Well, you are standing very closely – does that help your nose to make sense of me?'
>
> Patient: 'I've got to go to pottery soon. I enjoy pottery, but I'm much more interested in archaeology. Would you like to see my pots?'
>
> Nurse: 'Are they ancient pots or modern ones?'
>
> Patient: 'They're modern of course, but they might become ancient, if they live longer than me. How old are you?'
>
> Nurse: 'Forty-five. You know, to me all these things about you seem connected.'
>
> Patient: 'Well they're all part of me, aren't they, and I'm connected?'
>
> Nurse: 'Yes, I suppose so. Archaeology is all about finding out about what once happened and has become hidden; staring closely at people might help you know what thinking is happening but is hidden; and pottery is about finding out what might be hidden within some clay, that you could make happen in the figure. How much do you like to find out about what might be hidden, and maybe how to effect what happens?'

The terminology and concepts used in assessment summaries should be uniquely tailored to the individual because it has emerged from their experience and has employed their own language and experience as both enzyme and substrate. The use of 'ordinary, poetic and picturesque language' is also emphasized in accounts of therapeutic change as a process of re-writing one's life story, rather than being a participant in the medical elimination of problems. Such a process necessarily begins at the very beginning – the assessment. White and Epston noted: 'A therapy situated within the context of a narrative mode of thought would privilege the person's lived experience ... and encourage a sense of authorship and re-authorship of one's life and relationships'.[40]

By taking seriously the sense-making constructs that patients use, collaborative assessment challenges the potential falsification or narrowing of real-life experience. Such phenomenological constriction is a possible outcome of confining assessment to pre-determined structural formats, questionnaires etc.[39] In traditional modes of assessment, self-reportage is restricted to replies to questions previously determined by professionals. Without full collaboration, patients' realities are explored using only the system of knowledge and tools possessed and authenticated by the assessing professional service. It is like a walk through a landscape by two people – the person who lives there, and a visiting expert on one or more (but probably not all) of various admittedly relevant subjects. These may include botany, zoology, geology, meteorology, history, painting, photography, poetry etc., but will exclude intimate local knowledge. The conversation during the walk is controlled by the expert who chooses the various subjects that will be discussed during the walk and poses questions to the subordinated local whose home terrain is under investigation.

Nurses trained to be the dominant figure during assessment may fear being 'suckered' – duped by tall stories spun by mischievous, confused or deluded patients. After all, although it is important for people to feel believed or see that their relative is treated respectfully, it may feel equally important not to find that the key-worker is a fool. Would we be in danger of discrediting professionalism, and appearing credulous idiots, to establish our assessments on such a respectful, believing attitude? Although we may find ourselves apparently accepting fantastic rubbish, how much worse might it be, from a user's perspective, to reject the truth as madness? Effective collaborative assessment is not in a sense simple detective work, where the professional strives to uncover absolute truth. It is often more important to help the person clarify their personal story or narrative. Life needs to make sense if people are to confidently take control of their personal affairs again. A recovery focus may require that eventually people confront and accept the truth of their situation, but in the early stages of rescue, probing for literal truth may be less important than other therapeutic aims, such as:

❑ containing and clarifying underlying emotions;
❑ exploring meanings through metaphorical elements of personal storytelling;
❑ devising plot-lines or narrative threads that may suggest desirable future possibilities.

ASSESSING NEEDS, PROBLEMS OR SOLUTIONS

Nearing the end of a formal initial assessment after admission to a rehabilitation hostel, a young man of limited intelligence suffering from schizophrenia was asked a specified question about future employment:

Nurse:	"What work would you like to do when you leave here?"
Resident:	"I'm going to be a racing driver."
Nurse:	"Oh really? What attracts you about being a racing driver?"
Resident:	"I want to be like David Coulthard."
Nurse:	"So what do you admire about him?"
Resident:	"He's got lots of money, and he's always with beautiful women."
Nurse:	"Yes, that's true! What other things do you like about him?"
Resident:	"He's really confident and sure of himself – you have to be to go that fast."
Nurse:	"So how confident are you? Are you confident enough to become a racing driver?"
Resident:	"Not now."
Nurse:	"Did you used to be more confident then?"
Resident:	"Yes, but I lost it."
Nurse:	"How did that happen?"
Resident:	"When I was on a training scheme. They used to laugh at me a lot and make me do things I didn't want to."
Nurse:	"So would it help if we tried to get your confidence back while you're living here?"

Bradshaw[41] addresses the question of how *needs* are defined, and whose definition is given priority. He distinguishes four categories of need: *normative need*, which is professionally defined; *felt need*, which is the subjective dissatisfactions experienced by individuals; *expressed need*, which refers to the explicit demands made of the service by clients; and *comparative need* which is the prioritized, permitted needs identified during assessments. A needs-based collaborative assessment in effect requires the nurse to suspend his preoccupation with professional formulations of need and hold in abeyance the tendency to make judgements based on clinical categories, diagnoses and psychopathological aetiologies. The next step is to enable users to contact, explore and express felt-needs, and arrive at a formulation which expresses in positive terms what life would be (and is) when each need is met. Then the partnership studies the desirability, achievability, and ecological impact (on others, and other aspects of the person himself) of each identified aspiration. This process takes time, and certainly cannot be completed in an hour on the day of admission – it is an ongoing process.

Perkins and Repper[18,30] advocate such alliances, and point out that 'needs-led' assessment may be little different from 'problem-based' assessment unless professionals pay attention to their own attitudes and beliefs, the mystifying effects of clinical language,[42] and the partnership forged with users. 'Needs-led assessment' does not necessarily constitute a real shift from 'problem-based' assessments while professional definitions of problems and service-led priorities hold sway. As one influential report on overcoming engagement difficulties with mistrustful patients states 'Specialist mental health staff must be needs-led in their approach and allow the users' priorities to set the agenda'.[11]

> Arabella was a young woman diagnosed as having a borderline personality disorder. She cut her arms and breasts daily, and frequently burned her hands with cigarettes. The staff's clinical priorities were that she stopped this mutilating behaviour and concentrate on helping them to find some suitable supported accommodation. Arabella thought that she needed to spend much more time with her pony, Jasper. She felt sure she could get back her work as a stable-girl, and would happily sleep in the stable loft for accommodation. It took six months sojourn in an admission ward to convince her key-worker and consultant psychiatrist that she did not self-harm when with her beloved Jasper.

Recently, solution-focused and narrative forms of conversational, client-centred therapy have claimed considerable success.[40,43–45] Hoyt[23] summarizes some significant differences between such approaches and conventional psychiatric attitudes:

Possibility versus certainty

Fascinated curiosity and the identification of possibilities typify collaborative approaches, whereas formal assessment is predicated on discovery of fact or based on an assumption that there is a truth to be uncovered – the problem, disease diagnosis, or unmet need. The often intensely audited economic strictures imposed on modern clinical services create pressures not only to discover the truth (what it is that's wrong) quickly, but to do something effective about it just as quickly. If certainty cannot be achieved, then humans tend to devise temporary formulations or hypotheses as working models (heuristics) to explain the phenomena under investigation. These heuristics often become reified and frozen into professional quasi-scientific certainties (e.g. see Dorothy Rowe[46,47] on 'self-esteem' or Pilgrim[48] on 'personality disorders'). Collaborative assessment practice should insist that such hypotheses are explained and discussed with the user, and abandoned or reformulated if unacceptable. These seemingly innocent heuristic devices, which in truth may be no more than metaphorical constructs, easily assert their grip on professional thinking, and nurses can become convinced of their reality and applicability.

Egalitarian versus expert

Nurses (and other clinicians) should not allow their possession of clinical knowledge, technical skills and therapeutic attitudes to delude them into believing they have life-changing expertise. Having some insights into human conditions does not bestow absolute authority of wisdom about *The Human Condition*, and certainly doesn't imply intuitive comprehension of the condition of the individual human being assessed. Patients are potentially disempowered by such professional hubris, and prefer the sense of partnership they derive from feeling understood and equal.[49] Treatment is more likely to be effective when the patient shares ownership of the plan with the professionals.[50,51] This is best achieved by a collaborative conversation between equals. Professionals use terms like 'consultation' to describe situations where one partner begins by being apparently more competent. Collaboration is a different process.

Competency versus pathology

Collaborative assessment is characterized by the nurse being solution-focused (see De Shazer[43,44]) and strengths-based.[30] The primary interest is to establish what the patient wants and what skills and abilities they have or need to achieve their goals. Even when faced with very deranged, disturbed or distressed behaviour, a collaborative assessor will retain a respectful belief that the person has disguised, hidden or temporarily misplaced competence, and seek to elicit it. Mills[52] recognizes that collaboration can be scary for both professional and patient, but stresses the importance of 'the person with psychosis working alongside the professional … Both parties have a role to play in the development of new understandings and coping methods'. On the other hand, Morgan[53] discusses strengths-based assessment and emphasizes how much 'fun' can be had for client and practitioner. Conventional assessment procedures tend explicitly or subliminally to explore aspects of pathology (defect, deficit or weakness) even when couched in the recommended rhetoric of 'needs' rather than 'problems'.[16,30]

Systemic versus unilateral thinking

By focusing on the patient's experiences and constructs, a nurse undertaking a collaborative assessment would be led to embrace wider perspectives than narrowly focused individual pathology. This systemic gaze could involve exploring the reverberating interactions occurring in someone's family[54,55] or getting to grips with the reality of someone's social and economic stressors.[56] Working with problems embedded in family belief systems and communication matrices requires a fundamental shift in how nurses construe interpersonal aetiology. In order to sensibly understand the repetitive patterns of interaction within families, it helps to distinguish between *linear* and *circular* causality. A circular, reciprocal view of problem formation and maintenance stresses how the action of each person influences the other, whose behaviour in turn influences them. This is fundamentally different from linear explanations, which presuppose that one person's behaviour simply determines how another thinks, feels or acts: as though one person *makes* another do something, who then forcibly influences a third, in a sort of inter-psychic pecking-order.[55] A second, even wider systemic perspective requires nurses to take account of the openness and vulnerability of individuals and families to political, economic and cultural influences on behaviour, thought and feeling. Sadness, anxiety, anger and obsessive weirdness may have roots in threatening, absurd or alienating world events and situations, just as much as in defective neuro-signalling processes.[56] However wide or variously targeted the systemic gaze is, it takes full account of the 'fundamental attribution error' in not overestimating individual dispositional causes of difficulties (which an illness-focus may very easily entail) or underestimating situational, environmental factors.[57] This includes of course the impact on the patient of the clinical environment, of which the personality, attitudes and behaviour of the nurse-assessor and the internal relationships between him and the rest of the clinical team are significant components.[58]

USER COLLABORATION AND INTEGRATION WITH POLICY

Increased collaboration is just one of several themes in recent mental health policy. Indeed, Rogers and Pilgrim[15] argue that user collaboration is a policy that may already have climaxed, and is destined to be relegated against other policies, such as public safety. Currently, user collaboration is augmented, balanced, contradicted or undermined by other policy themes:

- ❑ Strengthening the social control function of psychiatric services, and developing more effective means of compelling people to accept either treatment or behaviour-management.[59,60]
- ❑ Basing treatment and care on effective methods that have been reliably demonstrated or 'evidenced-based practice'.[9,61]
- ❑ Establishing more effective communication between

professional disciplines and integrating practice within multi-professional care planning using a synthesis of clinical models, usually under the aegis of psychiatric conventions.[62–64]

❑ Using more formal assessment tools to improve evaluation of effectiveness and enhance communication between agencies and disciplines.[12] See also Refs 19 and 65.

These policies sometimes synergize effectively. For instance, Integrated Care Pathways[66] unify two objectives: enhancing professional integration and formal assessment methods. They may also appear to be in conflict or tension, as when users who otherwise agree their needs have been properly assessed, do not feel that their strengths and abilities were taken into account.[16] Nurses also frequently experience dilemmas when prioritizing clinical policies.[30] The clinical virtue of enabling a person to plan their own care is often weighed uncertainly against a managerial risk-avoidance imperative, e.g. when working with personality disordered people, or people with paranoid feelings that may lead to withdrawal, violence or self-harm. Similarly, there is often a tension between wishing to enhance autonomy or develop a trusting relationship by preserving confidentiality, instead of feeling obliged under Care Programme Approach provisions to share intimate revelations with other professionals.[67]

Increased use of formal assessment tools may conflict with the goal of full collaboration, if not with the step of enhanced user participation. Psychiatric nursing has prioritized concise, cogent and communicable formulations of patients' needs and risks[12] and emphasized the use of structured interview processes, rigorous observation schedules and formal assessment tools.[19] These emphases are sometimes softened by employing concepts like 'holism' to differentiate nursing assessment from medical examination[68] or referring to 'the semi-structured interview' as a means of involving patients.[20] However, the assumptions remain that clinical models will be employed for conceptual definition, that difficulties will be allocated by nurses to professionally defined categories of need, and that nurses will lead and structure the interview, employing formal tests when they consider it appropriate.

The variety of tools used within a service reflects the range of treatment models on offer. Each model of care or treatment develops its own assessment measures, designed to determine problems or needs as defined within the particular treatment paradigm, whether biomedical, cognitive-behavioural or nursing models are favoured. These models are not simply the treatment preferences of otherwise open-minded professional helpers. They also reflect the professionals' ideas about human nature, and specifically the nature and causes of human distress or disturbance.[69] The person undergoing assessment may well entertain quite different notions about human nature and his specific personality, needs or preferences. While the professional continues to view the person through the lens of her particular clinical world-view, then sapiential authority has been unilaterally imposed upon an already unbalanced power relationship. The professional has both statutory and structural authority and therefore potential power over the patient. The imposition of sapiential authority, via pre-determined and un-negotiated models of pathology and allied assessment measures, completes the patient's invalidation and may lead to either oppositional conflict or excessively compliant dependence. Speedy[70] claims that in the absence of an already established alliance, nurses' use of psychiatric concepts and language invalidates the users' experiences and renders them powerless. It certainly jeopardizes the attainment of a collaborative working partnership,[42] even though nurses may attempt to involve patients in negotiations about treatment decisions.[71]

Although some use of formal tools may be a necessary response to clinical or managerial imperatives,[12] a richer picture, or a thicker narrative may be obtained by synthesizing such methods with a collaborative, conversational approach. Embedding formal assessment tools within the matrix of a previously established, genuinely collaborative relationship is likely to enhance the clarity, accuracy and relevance of the results gleaned from assessment tools.[65] Patients are likely to feel more co-operative, more attentive and less anxious or mistrustful of the assessment procedure once they have been involved in determining and agreeing their use.[3,21,72]

People entering mental health services as patients, clients or customers often express a wish for less formal, more empathic processes of exploration of their difficulties and discovery of solutions.[73,74] They would like to be involved, but commonly feel excluded from the whole assessment process, despite evidence that when there is collaboration, or at least participation, quality of care improves, and satisfaction with the service increases.[10,16,64] People needing nursing care experience such complex, subtle difficulties and conflicting or unrealistic aspirations that more informal, exploratory and responsive processes are necessary to enable shared understanding of their struggles to develop within an essentially conversational relationship.[75,76]

Full collaboration requires that not only formal assessment measures but also formal professional thinking are understood and engaged with willingly by the patient. This can only happen if the *model* from which a tool derives, and whose concepts and categories it has been designed to measure or classify, has also been discussed, however minimally, and accepted, however uncertainly.

A person whose mental health is being assessed may be experiencing potentially disabling cognitive difficulties or emotional distress. In traditional assessments, if a model of treatment or care is to be discussed, the onus is on the professional to not only present concepts clearly and accessibly, but also relate them to the individual's experiences.[5] Collaborative assessment would relegate the proposal of a tool and the explanation of underlying theory (if it should happen at all) to some point after the user's perspective has been fully explored. Collaboration begins with the professional nurse attempting to set aside personal or professional prejudice; suspend clinical or philosophical certainties; and reach out to experimentally embrace or contain the patient's current way of experiencing the world, however deranged that may seem. Then *negotiation* can truly begin, rather than the *imposition*, however subtly managed, of the professional, clinical perspective. 'Imposition tends to generate opposition.'[23]

Marsha Linehan[77] explores this stance of empathic acceptance in relation to working with people diagnosed as borderline-personality-disordered. She refers to such deep validation as a 'core strategy': 'The essence of validation is this: The therapist communicates to the patient that her responses make sense and are understandable within her current life context or situation. (The nurse) takes the patients responses seriously and does not discount or trivialize them.' The initial adoption of a professional 'one-down' respectful stance may give the therapeutic alliance a working chance especially when there is a high degree of defensive sensitivity. However, collaboration is not thence best achieved by the worker simply switching conventional roles with the 'good patient' and transforming into a compliant pussycat. The energy needed to transfigure a cosily collusive relationship into a dynamically effective working partnership may well derive from the dialectical tensions that result from the juxtaposition and sustained interaction of opposing points of view. When both perspectives are recognized and validated at the same time, resolution can occur with the emergence of a third possibility that may resemble a compromise, or be some apparently entirely unrelated possibility. Dialectical collaboration involves the partnership's uncovering and exploring the impact of contradictory demands made by the person's own competing or conflicted self-states or schema modes (such as being a supportive father as well as a freaky fantasy figure); irreconcilable socio-cultural or environmental stresses (such as the practical demands of modern urban existence and an earth-empathic ecological commitment); and interpersonal relationships – including not only within families and other social groups, but also those between patients, nurses and other members of the multidisciplinary team.[77]

Johnstone[4] describes some of the difficulties, such as defensiveness, mistrust and breakdown of communication, created by 'the contrast between service users' desire for a psycho-social understanding of their difficulties and the primarily medical model of the professionals'. However, nurses who adapt and incorporate deep collaborative processes into their assessment practice may find that their nursing relationships move from polite formalism, grateful subordination, negativistic opposition, stagnation or helpless dependency to productive dialectic. The happy virtue of full collaboration may often not be achieved in practice. Many people are perhaps initially far too damaged to participate much in their own care. That is however no reason not to keep full collaboration in mind as the gold-standard of decent psychiatric-mental health nursing care, and to constantly strive to move nursing practice from imposed formulations and coercion through compliance, consultation, negotiation, participation, to collaboration and finally, professional redundancy.

REFERENCES

1. Ritter S. *Bethlem Royal and Maudsley Hospital manual of clinical psychiatric nursing principles and procedures*. London: HarperCollins, 1989.
2. Newell R, Gournay K. Introduction. In: Newell R, Gournay K (eds). *Psychiatric-mental health nursing: an evidence-based approach*. Edinburgh: Churchill Livingstone, 2000: 1–7.
3. Barham P, Hayward R. The lives of 'users'. In: Heller T, Reynolds J, Gomm R, Muston R, Pattison S (eds). *Mental health matters*. Basingstoke: Macmillan Press and Open University, 1996.
4. Lindow V. Survivor-controlled alternatives to psychiatric services. In: Newnes C, Holmes G, Dunn C (eds). *This is madness: a critical look at psychiatry and the future of mental health services*. Ross-on-Wye: PCCS Books, 1999.
5. Johnstone L. *Users and abusers of psychiatry*, 2nd edn. London: Routledge, 2000.
6. Faulkner A. *Strategies for living*. London: Mental Health Foundation, 2000.
7. Barker P. *Assessment in psychiatric and psychiatric-mental health nursing*. Cheltenham: Stanley Thornes, 1997.
8. Psychiatric-Mental Health Nursing Review Team. *Working in partnership: a collaborative approach to care (The Butterworth Report)*. London: Department of Health, 1994.
9. Department of Health. *Modernising mental health services: safe, sound and supportive*. London: HMSO, 1999.
10. Department of Health. *National service framework*

for mental health: modern standards and service models. London: HMSO, 1999.

11. Sainsbury Centre for Mental Health. *Keys to engagement: review of care for people with severe mental illness who are hard to engage with services.* London: Sainsbury Centre for Mental Health, 1998.

12. Standing Nursing and Midwifery Advisory Committee. *Addressing acute concerns.* London: Department of Health, 1999.

13. Watkins M, Hervey N, Carson J, Ritter S (eds). *Collaborative community mental health care.* London: Arnold, 1996.

14. Barker P, Whitehill I. The craft of care: towards collaborative caring in psychiatric nursing. In: Tilley S (ed.) *The psychiatric-mental health nurse: views of practice and education.* Oxford: Blackwell, 1998: 15–27.

15. Rogers A, Pilgrim D. *Mental health policy in Britain,* 2nd edn. Basingstoke: Macmillan Press, 2001.

16. Rose D. *Users' voices.* London: Sainsbury Centre for Mental Health, 2001.

17. Sugden J. The process by which nursing intervention is facilitated. In: Sugden J. with Bessant A, Eastland M, Field R (eds). *A handbook for psychiatric nurses.* London: Harper and Row, 1986.

18. Perkins R, Repper J. *Working alongside people with long-term mental health problems.* London: Chapman and Hall, 1996.

19. Gamble C, Brennan G. Assessment: A rationale and glossary of tools. In: Gamble C, Brennan G. *Working with serious mental illness: a manual for clinical practice.* London: Baillière Tindall, 2000.

20. Fox J, Conroy, P. Assessing clients' needs: the semi-structured interview. In: Gamble C, Brennan G. *Working with serious mental illness: a manual for clinical practice.* London: Baillière Tindall, 2000.

21. Fowler D, Garety P, Kuipers E. *Cognitive behaviour therapy for psychosis.* Chichester: Wiley, 1995.

22. Kingdon DG, Turkington D. *Cognitive-behavioural therapy of schizophrenia.* Hove: Psychology Press, 1994.

23. Hoyt MF. *Some stories are better than others: doing what works in brief therapy and managed care.* Philadelphia: Brunner-Mazel, 2000.

24. Lucas J. Multi-disciplinary care in the community for clients with mental health problems: guidelines for the future. In: Watkins M, Hervey N, Carson J, Ritter S (eds). *Collaborative community mental health care.* London: Arnold, 1996.

25. Newnes C, Holmes G. The future of mental health services. In: Newnes C, Holmes G, Dunn C (eds). *This is madness: a critical look at psychiatry and the future of mental health services.* Ross-on-Wye: PCCS Books, 1999.

26. Howell V, Norman I. Steering a steady course in an era of compulsory treatment: Taking psychiatric-mental health nursing into the millennium. *Journal of Mental Health* 2000; **9**: 605–16.

27. Morrall P. *Psychiatric-mental health nursing and Social Control.* London: Whurr Publications, 1998.

28. Morgan S. *Clinical risk management: a clinical tool and practitioner manual.* London: Sainsbury Centre for Mental Health, 2000.

29. O'Rourke M, Bird L. *Risk management in mental health: a practical guide to individual care and community safety.* London: Mental Health Foundation, 2001.

30. Perkins R, Repper J. *Dilemmas in community mental health practice: choice or control?* Oxford: Radcliffe Medical Press, 1998.

31. Stuart GW, Laraia MT. *Stuart and Sundeen's principles and practice of psychiatric nursing,* 6th edn. St Louis, Missouri: Mosby, 1998.

32. Reason P, Rowan J (eds). *Human inquiry: a sourcebook of new paradigm research.* Chichester: John Wiley, 1981.

33. Rowan J, Reason P. On making sense. In: Reason P, Rowan J (eds). *Human inquiry: a sourcebook of new paradigm research.* Chichester: John Wiley, 1981: 113–37.

34. Rowan J. Research ethics. *International Journal of Psychotherapy* 2000; **5**: 103–11.

35. White M. Deconstruction and therapy. In: Gilligan S, Price R (eds). *Therapeutic conversations.* New York: W.W. Norton, 1993.

36. O'Hanlon WH. Possibility therapy: from iatrogenic injury to iatrogenic healing. In: Gilligan S, Price R (eds). *Therapeutic conversations.* New York: W.W. Norton, 1993.

37. May-Stewart V-D. Working single mothers and stress: A collaborative inquiry. *Dissertation Abstracts International: Humanities and Social Sciences* 2000; **60** (7-A): 2708.

38. Smail D. *The origins of unhappiness: A new understanding of personal distress.* London: Constable, 1993.

39. Coolican H. *Research methods and statistics in psychology.* London: Hodder and Stoughton, 1994.

40. White M, Epston D. *Narrative means to therapeutic ends.* New York: W.W. Norton, 1990.

41. Bradshaw J. The conceptualisation and measurement of need: a social policy perspective. In: Popay J, Williams G (eds). *Researching the people's health.* London: Routledge, 1994.

42. Johnstone L. 'I hear what you're saying': how to avoid jargon in therapy. *Changes* 1997; **15**(4): 264–70.

43. De Shazer S. *Keys to solution in brief therapy.* New York: Norton, 1985.

44. De Shazer S. *Clues: investigating solutions in brief therapy.* New York: Norton, 1988.

45. Gilligan S, Price R (eds). *Therapeutic conversations.* New York: W.W. Norton, 1993.

46. Rowe D. *Guide to life.* London: Harper Collins, 1995.

47. Rowe D. Self-esteem – buy now while stocks last. *OpenMind* 2001; **110** (July/Aug): 7.

48. Pilgrim D. Disordered personalities and disordered concepts. *Journal of Mental Health* 2001; **10**(3): 253–65.

49. Burns D, Auerbach A. Therapeutic empathy in cognitive-behavioural therapy: does it really make a difference? In: Salkovskis PM (ed.) *Frontiers of cognitive therapy*. New York: Guilford Press, 1996.

50. Ryle A. *Cognitive-analytic therapy: active participation in change*. Chichester: John Wiley, 1990.

51. McGinn LK, Young JE. Schema-focused therapy. In: Salkovskis PM (ed.) *Frontiers of cognitive therapy*. New York: Guilford Press, 1999: 182–207.

52. Mills J. Dealing with voices and strange thoughts. In: Gamble C, Brennan G (eds). *Working with serious mental illness: a manual for clinical practice*. London: Baillière Tindall, 2000.

53. Morgan S. *Community mental health: practical approaches to long-term problems*. London: Chapman and Hall, 1993.

54. Proctor H, Pieczora R. A family oriented community mental health centre. In: Carpenter J, Treacher A. *Using family therapy in the 90's*. Oxford: Blackwell, 1993.

55. Dallos R, Draper R. *An introduction to family therapy: systemic theory and practice*. Milton Keynes: Open University Press, 2000.

56. Smail D. *How to survive without psychotherapy*. London: Constable, 1996.

57. Ross L, Amabile T, Steinmetz J. Social roles, social control and biases in social perception. *Journal of Personality and Social Psychology* 1977; **35**: 485–94.

58. Goodwin I, Holmes G, Newnes C, Waltho D. A qualitative analysis of the views of in-patient mental health service users. *Journal of Mental Health* 1999; 8(1): 43–54.

59. Department of Health. *Review of the Mental Health Act 1983: Report of the Expert Committee. (The Richardson Report)*. London: Stationery Office, 1999.

60. Department of Health. *Reforming the Mental Health Act*. London: Stationery Office, 2000.

61. Department of Health. *Treatment choice in psychological therapies and counselling: evidence-based clinical practice guideline*. London: DoH, 2001.

62. National Health Service Executive and Social Service Inspectorate. *Effective care co-ordination in mental health services: modernising the care programme approach*. London: Department of Health, 1999.

63. Department of Health. *Building bridges: a guide to arrangements for inter-agency working for the care and protection of severely mentally ill people*. London: HMSO, 1995.

64. Ramon S. Contextualising innovation: macro and micro issues. In: Ramon S (ed.) *A stakeholders' approach to innovation in mental health services*. Brighton: Pavilion Publishing, 2000.

65. Tunmore R. Practitioner assessment skills. In: Thompson T, Mathias P (eds). *Lyttle's mental health and disorder*, 3rd edn. Edinburgh: Baillière Tindall, 2000.

66. Jones A. Modernised mental health services: the role of care pathways. *Journal of Nursing Management* 1999; **7**(6): 331–8.

67. Liese BS, Franz RA. Treating substance use disorders with cognitive therapy. In: Salkovskis PM (ed.) *Frontiers of cognitive therapy*. New York: Guilford Press, 1996: 470–508.

68. Maphosa W, Slade M, Thornicroft G. Principles of assessment. In: Newell R, Gournay K. *Psychiatric-mental health nursing: an evidence-based approach*. Edinburgh: Churchill Livingstone, 2000.

69. Messer SB, Winokur M. Ways of knowing and visions of reality. In: Arkowitz H, Messer SB (eds). *Psychoanalytic therapy and behaviour therapy: is integration possible?* New York: Plenum Press, 1984.

70. Speedy S. The therapeutic alliance. In: Clinton M, Nelson S. Advanced practice in psychiatric-mental health nursing. Oxford: Blackwell Science, 1999.

71. Castillo H, Allen L, Coxhead N. The hurtfulness of diagnosis: user research about personality disorder. *Mental Health Practice* 2001; **4**: 16–19.

72. Tarrier N. Management and modification of residual positive psychotic symptoms. In: Birchwood M, Tarrier N (eds). *Psychological management of schizophrenia*. Chichester: John Wiley, 1994.

73. Beeforth M, Conlon E, Grayley R. *Have we got views for you: user evaluation of case management*. London: Sainsbury Centre for Mental Health, 1994.

74. Sainsbury Centre for Mental Health. *Pulling together*. London: Sainsbury Centre for Mental Health, 1997.

75. Hulme P. Collaborative conversation. In: Newnes C, Holmes G, Dunn C (eds). *This is madness: a critical look at psychiatry and the future of mental health services*. Ross-on-Wye: PCCS Books, 1999: 165–78.

76. Watkins P. *Psychiatric-mental health nursing: the art of compassionate care*. Oxford: Butterworth-Heinemann, 2001.

77. Linehan MM. *Cognitive-behavioral treatment of borderline personality disorder*. New York: Guilford Press, 1993.

Chapter 12

THE CONTEXT OF ASSESSMENT – FAMILIES

Chris Stevenson*

Jack feels Jill is greedy
because Jill feels Jack is mean
Jill feels Jack is mean
because Jack feels Jill is greedy[1]

INDIVIDUAL OR SYSTEM OR BOTH?

During the 20th century, psychiatry has been predicated on linear cause and effect explanations. It has been pre-occupied with the idea that some pathology (biological, psychological or social) leads to mental distress. Until fairly recently, psychiatric-mental health nursing has been based in similar assumptions. General system theory (GST), articulated by von Bertanlanffy during the 1940s,[2] offered a different way to account for phenomena that did not seem to lend themselves to traditional ideas of cause and effect. A systemic approach to understanding the world seemed to:

> ... provide a unifying theoretical framework for both the natural and social sciences, which needed to employ concepts such as organisation, wholeness and dynamic interaction, none of which lent itself easily to the methods of analysis employed by the pure sciences.[3]

According to GST, we can identify a system, the system's environment or suprasystem, and the system's components or subsystems. From this position, linear cause and effect are not helpful in understanding the system as a whole. For example, it is too simplistic to think that someone becomes depressed due to a social loss. In GST, causality is seen as a circular process. It has no beginning or end. GST is often illustrated with reference to a thermostat. The thermostat is a mechanism that monitors the ambient temperature (for example of a room). If the temperature drops to below a certain point, the thermostat responds by switching on the heating system. If the temperature rises, the thermostat responds by switching off the heating. Thus, it operates on both positive and negative feedback to produce a steady state (homoeostasis).

In applying GST to families and family therapy, a child's temper tantrum may be seen by the family as the cause of their distress. However, the temper tantrum may be a response to mother's ideas about strictness, which are a response to father's more easy-going attitude. The stricter mother becomes, the more temper tantrums erupt. The more temper tantrums erupt, the more easy-going father becomes, the more strict mother becomes etc. Symptoms are seen by family therapists to have a positive or negative feedback function in maintaining the balance or stability (homoeostasis), of the system, just as the thermostat uses positive and negative feedback in order to maintain the required temperature.

*Chris Stevenson is Reader in Nursing at Teeside University, England. Her doctoral research focused on family work and she has been a Community Psychiatric Nurse, Manager and Family Therapist, and presently retains an active engagement in clinical practice, working with families.

With such circular causality, the 'here and now' becomes much more the focus. Problem behaviour is actively maintained in the present. Although the balance achieved by the family may not be satisfactory, in terms of personal development of those concerned, it may be perceived (consciously or unconsciously) by family members, as preferable to the family break up which imbalance could trigger. For example, the temper tantrums may be a way of side-tracking the parents from their own marital disagreements, which might ultimately end in separation and divorce. Yet, the tantrums are not a pleasant experience for the child or other family members.

As the symptoms are embedded in social life, some family therapists, notably Jay Haley, refused to meet with 'incomplete' families. However, as Gorrell-Barnes notes,[4] different forms of family organization are increasing, and no clear boundaries exist to decide on what constitutes the 'family unit'. This has led some family therapists to be less attached to the idea of assessing 'whole' families. While there are differences in family therapy schools, there are some unifying ideas. It is worthwhile clarifying where commonalties lie as the suggestions for assessing families that follow are based in these common assumptions rather than being related to specific approaches.

Most family therapy approaches set the 'pathological' individual in a system of inter-related players. For example, Laing and Esterson state:[5]

> ... we are interested in what might be called the family nexus, that multiplicity of persons drawn from the kinship group, and from others who, though not linked by kinship ties, are regarded as members of the family. The relationships of persons in a nexus are characterised by enduring and intensive face-to-face reciprocal influence on each other's experience and behaviour.

Most family approaches have shared the view that problems and their solutions should be explored in relation to the patterns of information exchange that occurs between family members. For example, Gregory Bateson explored paradoxical communication within double bind communications.[6] Bateson noted that all communication has two levels, a report level, which is the content, or information that is being conveyed, and a command level, or meta communicative level. This level is concerned with conveying a message *about* the information. The two levels may be matching or clashing.

For example, the psychiatric-mental health nurse who tells the patient that it is no bother to find some clean towels, whilst looking exasperated at being disturbed while writing a care plan, is simultaneously presenting conflicting messages. The report level is usually based in words, while the command level is usually non-verbal. Take this example from family life. A mother goes shopping in the sales and buys her teenage daughter two T-shirts, one blue and one red. The girl is delighted with them and rushes upstairs to try them on. She comes down stairs to show her mother, wearing the red T-shirt. Her mother looks and says, 'Oh, so you didn't like the blue one'. The innocuous words (content) are accompanied by a higher-level communication of criticism. The girl is trapped in a no-win situation. She cannot wear two garments at once and so no matter what she chooses can always be accused. Bateson did not think that isolated incidents of this kind could cause schizophrenia (as popular fallacy has often argued), but he did believe that sustained paradoxical communication would lead to breakdown.

By now it should be clear that family therapists share an interest in the relationships and communication between family members. Therefore, it is of paramount importance to explore these within a family meeting. In the rest of this chapter, action and verbal approaches to helping the family offer their understandings are presented which are equally applicable to the work of psychiatric-mental health nurses.

EXPLORING THE FAMILY

Genograms – enhanced family trees

One way of breaking the ice with a family is to collaboratively draw their family tree. It is usually especially useful if there is someone in the family who is especially nervous, and with families where children are involved. One family member may be elected to be the 'scribe' to increase the level of involvement. A family tree, which has been completed earlier can be used to re-join with the family, for example, to assess whether there have been any changes in family life following involvement in family meetings.

Family therapists call a family tree a *genogram*. Within family work it tends to chart who's who, but also can be the site for additional information, for example about occupation, significant family events, etc. Never assume that events that are talked about are not significant – record them anyway. The genogram is often used to begin to build up a picture of closeness in the family, for example, is the mother in the family close or distant to her own mother/her husband's mother.

A common set of symbols is used to map a genogram (see Fig. 12.1). Sometimes, with families, it is easier to use colours. A large flip chart can be useful, as family organization is not always simple! In Figure 12.2, the Dinsdale family are represented.

Genogram symbols

☐	Male	☐₁₉₇₅○	Marriage and year
○	Female	☐₁₉₉₄○	Divorce and year
⊠	Death	☐₁₉₈₂○	Separation and year
▣	Index patient	☐₁₉₉₁○	Not married, year started
●	Spontaneous abortion		living together
○	Induced abortion	☐₁₉₈₆○	Solid or dashed line indicates
△	Pregnancy	○○	individuals living together
○△○	Dizygotic twins	⋀⋀⋀	Conflictual relationship
○△○	Monozygotic twins	-------	Distant relationship
☐	Adopted	═══	Close relationship
66 ☐ John	Year of birth Name	═══	Overly close relationship
⊠ 78	Age at death	⟶	Dominant relationship
'66–'96 ⊠ CA	Year of birth and death Cause of death	☐⋀⋀○	Marital discord
⊡	Carriers of sec-linked or recessive genes	☐ ○	Unmarried partners

FIGURE 12.1 Genogram symbols

You might like to write a short paragraph about your impressions of the family, gained through 'reading' their genogram. Think about the family structure and what questions it may be interesting to ask around that.

Sculpting

With this technique, the relationships between family members are recreated *in space*, through the formation of a physical tableau. This symbolizes the emotional position of each member of the family in relation to others. The therapist may ask the family to 'try out something a bit different', emphasizing that it will involve them all. If the therapist is enthusiastic enough it will help to overcome the family's initial reluctance. The therapist chooses one family member to act as the sculptor. The rest of the family are the 'clay' that the sculptor has to mould. The rationale for who is chosen as the sculptor is variable.

For example, the identified patient may be selec-

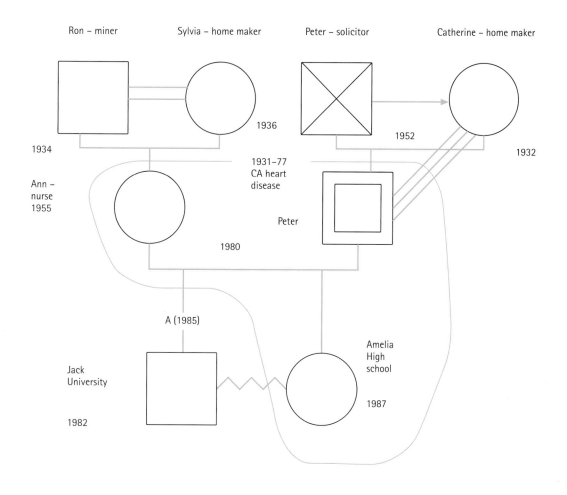

FIGURE 12.2 Family genogram

ted because s/he is already responding to perceived issues in family life; or a family member who seems less connected to the family may be offered the role as a way of making her/him more included. Once the sculptor is selected, the therapist asks the rest of the family to stand up and to move into whatever position the sculptor asks them to (Fig. 12.3). Once the sculptor starts to move the family members around, the therapist moves into an observing role. The therapist may ask the sculptor questions about what is happening.

For example, whether the family member has moved close enough to another family member; what each position is meant to represent. The family members who are being positioned may be asked questions also, for example, how they are feeling at that precise moment in terms of their physical position. In this scenario people often use emotion-laden words like 'being put down'; 'pushed out' etc. These spatial descriptions are often reflections of the emotional positions that family members occupy in relation to each other. It is not difficult for the family to make connections between relationships, communication and the family issues.

When the sculpting is complete, the therapist may ask the sculptor to find a place for her/himself. As well as representing the future, the sculptor may be asked to position family members in relation to how things were in the past, for example, when grandma died; to how things would change in a particular future; to how different degrees of closeness (indicated by interpersonal space) can have ripple effects in other family relationships.

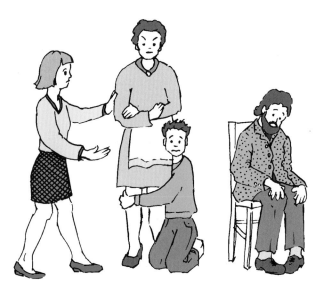

FIGURE 12.3 Sculpted family. Reproduced from Walrond-Skinner[3] with kind permission from Routledge

ASKING INTERESTING QUESTIONS

Ann Rambo and her colleagues suggest that the best therapists are those who have a natural curiosity.[7] But being curious is an attribute that can be translated into the ability to ask questions. Most staff with training in psychiatric-mental health nursing can make a distinction between open and closed questioning. Both of these types are useful in working with people, as techniques for opening up or closing down conversation. However, there are many questions of a different order that are used in working with families. These are described as circular questions. Circular questioning is a system of questioning developed by the (early) Milan group that helped them to test hypotheses generated by the team from referral information.[8] Linking questions to hypotheses can create a purposeful and coherent interviewing pattern that reveals new information and people's different perceptions of the problem. How this information is discussed becomes the basis for ongoing work.

Circular questions are based on triads, i.e. where people are asked to comment on the thoughts, behaviour and relationships of other family members. For example, the therapist might ask the mother in a family:

❑ 'Since your father-in-law came to live with you, has the relationship between your daughter and son been better or worse?'

Circular questions can be grouped for convenience into six rough categories which have some overlap: specific interactive sequence questions; before and after questions; attempts to solve problems; classification/ranking questions; mind-reading questions; and hypothetical questions. Each of these is discussed below.

1 *Specific interactive sequence questions* involve more than one person. For example:
   ■ 'When Ann (mother) is depressed what do father and daughter do?'
   ■ 'When father is angry with son, what does mother do?'

2 *Before and after questions* – changes that indicate a change in behaviour before and after a specific event. For example:
   ■ **Sister**: 'Helen and Joanne are very close to each other'.
   ■ **Therapist**: 'Did they get close to each other before or after your mum died?'

3 *Attempts to solve problems questions* – ask what worked, who helped. For example:
   ■ 'When Jane last became depressed, what was helpful?'

4   *Classification/ranking questions* – putting people, events and explanations in hierarchies according to specific criteria. For example:
■ 'Who in the family is most upset?'
■ 'Between A, B and C, who do you think is closest to D?'
■ 'Of the explanations given by mother, which one do you think dad agrees with most?'

5   *Mind-reading questions* – can give information on closeness in the family and reveal differences of opinion between people over important issues. For example:
■ **Therapist**: 'If your sister were alive today, what do you think she would say?'
■ **Mother**: 'She would say it had to happen.'
■ **Therapist**: 'In a moment I'm going to ask your brother whether he agrees or disagrees with your sister's view. What do you think he will say?'

6   *Hypothetical questions* – about (past/current/future) situations, ideas or explanations. For example:
■ **Therapist**: 'Let's suppose that you got a job and would be able to afford to rent a place of your own, which of your parents would be most upset when you moved out?'

You may have noticed that some questions combine well together. The last example combines a hypothetical and ranking question.

As well as circular questions, there are other important kinds of questions in working with families: future oriented questions; comparison questions; observer perspective; gender questions; relative influence questions.

1   *Future oriented questions* – the most famous of these is the miracle question:
■ 'If a miracle were to happen tonight while you were asleep and tomorrow you awoke to find this problem was no longer a part of your life, what would be different? How would you know that this miracle had taken place? How would other people be able to tell without you telling them? How would you act to try and maintain the new situation?'

2   *Comparison questions*. For example:
■ 'Is your parents' relationship better or worse lately?'
■ 'Have you felt more like a daughter or more like a wife this week?'
■ 'Was that always the case, or was it once different?'

3   *Observer perspective*. For example:

■ 'What do you imagine he feels when he gets into this situation?'
■ 'How do you think your GP sees the problem?'
■ 'When your father gets into an argument with your sister, what does your mother usually do?'

4   *Gender questions*. For example:
■ 'Do you believe that men should be sad/afraid/in need of approval?'
■ 'Do you believe that women should feel angry/be assertive/competitive/entitled to put themselves first?' (Asked of both genders).

Gender questions can be used to explore intergenerational beliefs about men's and women's roles:
■ 'Did either of your parents have a hard time meeting their parents' expectations about femininity/masculinity?'
■ 'If your father/mother disapproved of the manner in which you are a man/woman, how would you know that?'

Gender questions can combine well with some other kinds of question, for example, in future oriented questions:
■ 'If you have a son/daughter, would you like him/her to feel differently about his masculinity/femininity?'
■ 'Would your parents approve if you raised your children with different ideas about being a man/woman in the world?'

5   *Relative influence questions*. These questions invite two different descriptions of family members' association with the problem. The first is a question about the influence the problem has in their lives (directed to all family members). For example:
■ 'When Tom is hearing voices, how does the family find itself operating differently?' (This is passive influence).

The second is a description of the influence of family members in the life of the problem (active influence). For example:
■ 'When Tom is hearing voices, what do the family members do to try to make the voices go away or be less of a nuisance for Tom?'

So far, approaches to questioning as part of assessment have been set out. It remains unclear how far such questioning has in and of itself a *therapeutic* function. To end the chapter, I will outline an approach to care in which questioning and therapy are merged together. This theme will be revisited and expanded in Chapter 23.

EXTERNALIZING THE PROBLEM

Externalizing the problem is an approach used by Michael White[9] with people who feel entangled with some problem, which is making a mess of their lives. For example, families often offer accounts which are a 'problem-saturated description of family life'.[9] White presents the case of Nick, who was a six-year-old boy with a long history of soiling. Nick was making a 'play mate' of the poo. 'He would streak it down walls, smear it in drawers, roll it in balls and flick it behind cupboards and wardrobes, and had even taken to plastering it under the kitchen table'.[9] Externalizing the problem has several potential benefits:

❑ It encourages people to objectify and sometimes personify the problems they are experiencing.
❑ It is useful when the problem is thought to be inherent to the person and is seen as very fixed.
❑ It offers a new story that can free people from the fixed and dominant story they have about a problem.

I have broken the approach into three phases. Although my version is less sophisticated than White's own, I have found it useful in practice and I offer real practice world illustrations:

1 **Ask relative influence questions.**
   ■ 'What influence is the problem having on your life?' For example: 'When you wake up in the morning and feel sad, what can you not do that you would like to be able to do?'
   ■ 'What influence are you having on the "life" of the problem?' 'What do you *do* to try and make the problem go away or get less?' 'When you begin to feel anxious, how do you try to get on top of the feelings?' Sometimes the strategies people use to rid themselves of the problem actually become the problem, e.g. where a person constantly tries to 'cheer up' someone describing her/himself as depressed.

2 **Gain a definition of the problem to be externalized.**
   ■ Take the person's definition (whether specific or general) as sacrosanct. e.g. 'He has tantrums when . . .'; 'I have low self-esteem'; 'We have a communication problem'.
   ■ The definition of the problem may change over time as people struggle to describe their experience, as they move from the general to the specific. For example, sometimes people say 'I have schizophrenia'. However, over time they may say, 'I have the experience of hearing a voice which torments me by telling me that I am a pervert.'
   ■ When people use professional descriptions of their problems (e.g. 'I am depressed'; 'Jim is

schizophrenic'), try to find a less expert and more popular definition. For example, Jason's family had been told by a doctor that he was schizophrenic. This was revealed by asking for an observer perspective: 'How did the doctor at out-patients see the problem?'

■ Once, when working in a family team, which included a consultant psychiatrist who was not attached to diagnosis as a helpful means of understanding people's distress, the family asked him what the diagnosis meant. He replied: 'Personally, I don't find it useful to describe someone's reality disagreement as schizophrenia. There is a lot of negativity attached to that name. I prefer to find a way to describe what has been happening for you all and beginning to think about how we can address some of the issues.'

■ Through this process, we find a description of the problem that is mutually acceptable, and that is not located in the person. Extending the example above, Jason believed that his difficulties would resolve if he found work. His parents were concerned because he would spend all night moving from room to room, smoking and 'muttering' to himself and thought this behaviour needed some form of moderation. This difference was 'exposed' through asking circular questions, e.g. 'Jason if I asked your dad what he thinks the problem is, what would he say?' 'Mum, if I asked Jason what the problem is, what would he say?' However, despite these differences in perspective, all the family members were concerned that Jason would lead an unfulfilled life, by which they meant that he would not be able to develop financial and social independence.

■ If necessary, use characters/personifications, etc. Many staff members do this naturally, for example, they might ask a patient: 'How are the voices today?' However, here is a more conscious use of personification that has been helpful. Jane was constantly taunted by skeletons in her head. It was possible to describe these as events from the past or 'skeletons in the cupboard'. The skeletons in the cupboard had somehow escaped and needed to be re-confined.

3 **Find unique outcomes.**
   ■ There will always be an instance of the problem not being there, or being dealt with better than at another time. This is an example of a 'comparison question'. Sometimes, the questioner needs to be persistent. In Jane's case

the skeletons could not come out of the cupboard when she was reading the Bible.

- Start with current unique outcomes that are present as you meet with the person – e.g. respond to the person who says, 'I am always afraid of speaking about the problem', with, 'You are here speaking with me today'.
- If you cannot find a unique outcome in the present go to the past. For example, sometimes a patient will say, 'I'm too depressed to be able to think'. In this case, you might say (comparison question), 'When you were getting married, how did you conquer your nervousness?' Or, 'I understand that you worked as a bus driver. How did you manage to keep up being pleasant and cheerful even when you were having a hard day?'
- Future unique outcomes involve the person's plans to escape the problem. Ask 'What can you do to salvage your life?' Or the 'miracle question', followed by, 'What will you do to help the miracle to occur?' In this, and previous searches for unique outcomes, you are making a pre-supposition that something is possible. This is means of giving hope. For example, in running a group, ask people to say which animal they most identify with and why. One man once said he was unable to offer anything. He was too 'flat'. I then asked him to imagine that I had an animal encyclopaedia on my knee that I was flicking through. He would stop me when I reached the page where 'his' animal was. He immediately said, 'Deer'. It breaks the pattern of being immersed in the problem.

Why does externalizing the problem work? When people identify unique outcomes, of necessity, they change their relationship to the problem. They recognize they can resist the problem. It has become external to them. They refuse to submit to the problem and its effects. The problem becomes less effective.

CONCLUSION

When nurses begin to think about working with families, the prospect can be very daunting. This chapter has suggested some simple approaches to questioning which can aid the nurse and family in exploring relationships and communication patterns. I have often been impressed by the tolerance of families when I have been groping to find the next question in interviews. I have often been worried that my questioning might in some way 'make things worse'. With the benefit of practice experience, I am assured that this is rarely the case. I end, therefore, by encouraging nurses to 'have a go' with the questions presented her. Admit to the families you meet that you are new to a family approach and do not be afraid to take a prompt sheet with you. Families are very forgiving.

REFERENCES

1. Laing RD. *Knots*. New York: Pantheon Books, 1970: 51.
2. von Bertalanffy L. *General systems theory*. Harmondsworth: Penguin, 1968.
3. Walrond-Skinner S. *Family therapy: the treatment of natural systems*. London: Routledge and Kegan Paul, 1976: 12.
4. Gorrell-Barnes G. *Working with families*. London: Macmillan, 1984.
5. Laing RD, Esterson A. *Sanity, madness and the family*. Harmondsworth: Penguin, 1964: 21.
6. Bateson G, Jackson D, Haley J, Weakland J. Toward a theory of schizophrenia. In: Jackson D (ed.) *Human communication I*. LA: Science and Behaviour Books, 1968.
7. Rambo A, Heath A, Chenail RJ. *Practising therapy: exercises for growing therapists*. New York: Norton, 1993.
8. Pallazzoli MS, Boscolo L, Cecchin G, Prata G. Hypothesising – circularity – neutrality: three guidelines for the conductor of the session. *Family Process* 1980; **19**: 3–12.
9. White M. The externalising of the problem and the re-authoring of lives and relationships. *Dulwich Centre Newsletter*, Summer, 1998/89 reprinted in M. White *Selected Papers*. Adelaide: Dulwich Centre Publications, 1989: 5–8.

Chapter 13

THE ASSESSMENT OF FEELINGS, THOUGHTS AND BELIEFS

Mark Philbin*

INTRODUCTION

For mental health nurses, assessment represents an attempt to 'get to know' people-in-care[a]. Of course, there is a limit on the extent to which any person can know another. Human beings are complex, constantly changing and always capable of surprises. Furthermore, people are always selective in what they notice about others and so nurses' knowledge of people-in-care can only ever be partial. Nonetheless, it is important that nurses make a serious effort to comprehend and appreciate the people that they are trying to help. Such effort is necessary for a number of reasons.

First, nurses have a better chance of helping people when they know those people as individuals and have a sense of what they are experiencing.

Second, nurses' attempts to gain such understanding can help people-in-care to develop a different, perhaps more useful, understanding of their own situation. When nurses ask questions about particular experiences or issues, they may encourage people-in-care to examine and reflect upon what is happening within their lives. This might in itself help people to develop a clearer perspective on their situation, work out why certain experi-

ences have occurred or notice something else about themselves that is significant.

Third, in trying to understand, nurses can signal that they have a genuine interest in, and respect for, people-in-care. If people-in-care detect this signal, they may develop positive perceptions of the personal qualities of nurses and of the potential value of a relationship that can be had with them. Some research from the field of psychotherapy has suggested that these kinds of positive perceptions are associated with positive outcomes.[1]

So, given the potential benefits that are associated with getting to know people-in-care and trying to understand their experiences, the question arises as to how this might be achieved. This question is difficult to answer comprehensively but it seems reasonable to suggest that an effort to get to know and understand people should partly involve an assessment of how they *feel*, what they *think* and what they *believe*. In this chapter, then, the focus is on how and why mental health nurses can assess each of these matters as well as the inter-relationship between them. Given that the person in care is the real 'expert' on their thoughts, feelings and beliefs, the chapter adopts a clinically focused, rather than theoretically driven, approach.

---

*Mark is a lecturer in Dublin City University. He leads a newly developed postgraduate educational programme for community mental health nurses and is currently co-ordinating a project that involves the development of a solution-focused approach in nursing practice.

---

[a] This term, along with people, will be used in preference to patients, clients, service users or consumers.

INQUIRING INTO FEELINGS

A *feeling* can be a physical sensation, an emotion or a combination of the two. There is a range of ways that nurses can approach the assessment of feelings. These are addressed in turn.

Talking with people that identify feelings as a problem

Often, people-in-care are very aware of how they feel and consider 'feeling bad' as a major aspect, perhaps the most important aspect, of their problems. This can often be a useful starting point for an 'assessment interview' as an examination of the following excerpt from an interaction illustrates (where P is a person-in-care and N is a nurse):

Person: 'I've been feeling really down for the past month'.
Nurse: 'What's it like when you feel down?'
Person: 'It's like a dark cloud has descended on me. I'm gloomy and I don't feel like doing anything. Everything is such an effort'.
Nurse: 'What else do you notice about yourself when this dark cloud descends? ... '

Here, the person-in-care defined his problem in terms of how he feels and the nurse has encouraged him to elaborate in more specific detail on what this feeling involves. If this were continued, the nurse would gain a clearer sense of what 'feeling down' meant for this person and might also display her commitment to understanding this. To pursue this line of inquiry further, the nurse might have encouraged the person to talk about the following kinds of things:

❏ A specific example of a *time* when he was feeling 'most down' – what he was *doing*, the nature of the *situation*, the involvement of *other people*, what he was *thinking*, what *happened afterwards*, a *rating* of how bad the feeling was.
❏ The course of the problem – the timing of the initial onset, when he has felt better, when he has felt worse, factors that seem to be associated with feeling better or worse.
❏ The implications of the negative state of feeling – for his level of activity, for his relationships with other people, for his view of the future, for his enactment of social roles and responsibilities.
❏ The events in his life – what changes have occurred in his life circumstances, the relevance of such changes to how negatively he feels, things that are happening in his life that are somehow problematic.

As well as contributing to a clearer picture of people's experience of their problems, conversation about these kinds of issues can help nurses to begin to understand why people are feeling so bad. For example, it might become apparent that there is a connection between a person's negative feelings and certain kinds of situation such as an argument with relatives. On recognizing such a connection, a nurse has an indication of one issue that she might usefully focus upon in trying to help this person. Furthermore, this kind of connection might usefully be made by a person-in-care. For example, some stressful life event might have occurred before the onset of a problematic feeling but may not have been identified as significant. Through discussion with the nurse as part of an assessment, a person may come to view this event as relevant and therefore have been assisted in his or her efforts to try to understand why the problematic feeling is being experienced. If people-in-care are helped to view their problems as explicable in this way, this in itself can be helpful. Sometimes, people appear to have a need to understand the reasons for their problems as a basis for believing that such problems can be resolved. This need for *reasons* (and meaning) has been particularly emphasized in the work of Victor Frankl,[2] a seminal figure in the development of existential psychotherapy.

Searching for feelings

To summarize the discussion so far, some helpful consequences can emerge from enabling people to talk in detail about feelings that they identify as problematic. However, there are other scenarios in which mental health nurses assess feelings. One of these scenarios involves nurses in a quest for feelings that they assume to be significant even when this significance may not be immediately evident to people-in-care. This kind of situation is conveyed in the following excerpt from an initial interview between a community mental health nurse and a woman whose baby had died four weeks before:

Nurse: 'How have you been since your baby died?'
Person: (Smiling) 'Fantastic. I'm doing really well. My doctor referred me here because he knows that I've had psychiatric problems in the past but there was no need. I've been flying. My family are really pleased with me because they feared the worst, they thought I wouldn't be able to cope but I'm fine. Things are going really great, I have that feeling you have when you're on holiday'.
Nurse: 'What happens to holiday feelings after a holiday?' (Pause)
Person: 'They disappear when you have to face reality'. (Starting to cry) 'I've got a really long way to go, haven't I?'

In this situation, the nurse made an assumption about the feelings that are appropriately associated with the experience of grief. One reason for this assumption was a familiarity with the bereavement literature and the idea of a 'grieving process,' developed by people like Colin Murray Parkes.[3] While the idea of a grieving process that is universally appropriate has been challenged, the nurse was concerned by the person-in-care's assertion that she 'felt great'. To spell this out more clearly, the nurse quickly suspected that this assertion was a sign of 'denial' and that there was a need to help this person to express feelings that were associated with the reality of her loss. In a gentle way, the nurse successfully prompted such emotional expression and, from that point onwards, was able to discuss with the person the circumstances of her bereavement and the experiences that were involved.

This interaction represents an example of how nurses can search for people's feelings as part of an assessment. There are, of course, other ways.

Nurses often *observe* the behaviour of people-in-care and make *inferences* about whether they are feeling angry, sad, happy, anxious, contented and so on. These observations and inferences can be a basis for useful dialogue with people-in-care and can highlight, for example, inconsistencies between how they appear and how they feel 'inside'. Some people feel anxious and assume that their anxiety is highly visible to others. Indeed, this assumption can in itself be a source of greater anxiety. A nurse might observe a person, in this situation, and suggest that they appear a good deal calmer than they actually feel. Discussion of this observation might encourage the person to evaluate and even challenge the original assumption that others can see how he or she feels. Furthermore, observations of, and inferences about, feelings might help nurses to recognize sequences or patterns in people's behaviours and modes of relating to others. For example, a nurse might notice that an apparent feeling of agitation recurrently precedes a particular kind of behaviour such as violence towards another person. This recognition could then inform an early intervention to diffuse the impetus towards such behaviour.

Other methods of assessing feelings

Some people-in-care find it difficult to put their feelings into words. Observational approaches to assessment can take on an additional importance in such circumstances. However, there are some other methods of assessing feelings that can also be appropriate. Creative activities like art, drama, storytelling and writing can give some people-in-care an opportunity to express feelings that have been difficult to verbalize. Indeed, one of the benefits of these approaches is that they often enhance people's ability to articulate what they are feeling.

Questionnaires can also be helpful in this respect. There are a number of self-report questionnaires that are designed to assess things like anxiety, agoraphobia and depression. A number of these have been reviewed by Phil Barker.[4] Although these questionnaires are often used for diagnostic purposes, many of the individual items relate to statements about feelings. After people have completed such questionnaires, it can be useful for nurses to read each item that has been rated because they might discover information that has not arisen in the course of their discussions with people-in-care.

Only negative feelings?

When people discuss a particular way of feeling, they often re-experience that feeling in talking about it. This could be a positive thing because a person might, for example, have experienced traumatic events like sexual abuse and have been denied a proper opportunity to express how he or she feels. In this kind of a situation, a person might meet a nurse, as part of an initial assessment, and use the opportunity to re-experience and discharge feelings that he or she has 'contained' for a long period of time. This kind of emotional discharge is often called 'catharsis'. Although the value of catharsis is under-researched, some people-in-care talk about the relief that they feel as a consequence of 'getting things off their chest'. The possibility that people can gain such relief is another reason that nurses should focus on people's negative feelings, and encourage their expression, as part of an assessment. However, there is a question of whether mental health nurses should only focus on people's negative feelings, rather than any other kind, during an assessment. The concept of catharsis is relevant to a consideration of this question.

Barry Duncan and his colleagues are a group of solution-focused therapists who have emphasized an important principle of relating to people – that an issue is often amplified when it is focused upon.[5] This can be illustrated by reference back to the idea of catharsis. A nurse could make an inquiry about a person's childhood and, in response, be told that it was an unhappy one. On making this reply, a person might also begin to look a little upset. The nurse might notice this and ask what is upsetting about the memory of childhood. In response, the person might become still more upset and tearfully recount memories of parental neglect or abuse. With each question the nurse asks, the conversation might focus in more detail on the person's unhappy memories and, in so doing, amplify the feelings that are associated with those memories in the present moment. As has been mentioned, the person might gain some relief from this and the nurse might gain some understanding. However, what this example suggests is that if nurses continuously attend to people's negative feelings then they might encourage people-in-care to do the same. In other words, if nurses only inquire into what is wrong with the way people are feeling this might prompt people to feel worse on an ongoing basis and may therefore be unhelpful.

In the light of this danger that nurses can *over-assess* negative feelings, they also need to pay attention to positive feelings. Nurses need to inquire into the detail of such feelings and the circumstances in which they occur. Such inquiry might serve to amplify people's experience of 'feeling better' and expand their awareness of their own ability to do things that are associated with feeling good. Furthermore, this kind of inquiry can help nurses to develop a broader understanding of people-in-care. This broader understanding involves an awareness of people's strengths, abilities and successes as well as their problems, traumas and setbacks.

ASSESSING THOUGHTS

Thoughts consist of the words that people say to themselves in their own minds (what some cognitive-behaviour therapists call 'self-talk') and the images that pass through their minds. One reason that mental health nurses should assess what people think is that people's problems are often, in part, problems of thinking. If mental health nurses want to understand such problems then they need to give careful attention to what people are thinking and how this relates to how people are feeling.

Thinking problems

Sometimes, people-in-care identify their thoughts as the principal feature of a problem. For example, a person might describe a nagging thought about the possibility of some kind of awful event occurring, which cannot be defused by recognition that such an event is unlikely. On the other hand, many people may not be so clear about the role of thoughts in their problems and may be preoccupied by their feelings or some other kind of issue. In both these scenarios, nurses should inquire into the specific details of thoughts that are involved in experiences that are problematic. This is because thoughts are an important element in any experience and so a full picture of any problem that a person experiences has to include the thoughts that were, or are, involved. In addition, knowledge of what people are thinking at a given moment is often the key to making their feelings or behaviours intelligible. For example, it might become apparent as part of a discussion of a person's panic attacks that these experiences involve feeling a particu-

lar sensation (like a pain in the chest), interpreting that sensation as a symptom of an impending heart attack and then feeling increasingly panic-stricken. The person's panic becomes understandable when it is clear that he or she thinks that death is imminent from a heart attack that is signalled by chest pain. Furthermore, it might become apparent that the person has a systematic tendency to interpret bodily sensations (that are associated with anxiety) as a sign of serious illness and, still more widely, that he or she has a habit of expecting the worst possible things to happen.

So, problematic experiences can be particularly associated with negative thoughts that occur in given patterns. This insight has been particularly emphasized in the cognitive-behaviour therapy literature. One highly influential figure within that literature is Aaron Beck who detailed the various kinds of thoughts that are associated with particular emotional problems and who gave a number of examples of the patterned ways in which people can negatively interpret themselves, their experiences and their futures.[6] One question that arises for nurses from all of this is how these negative thoughts can be identified.

Identifying negative thoughts

Of course, the simplest way to find out about negative thoughts is to ask people about them. Often, this involves focusing on a particular situation where a person experienced a problem and asking for details of what specifically he or she was thinking at the time. This is illustrated in the following example of an interaction:

Person: 'I get these pains in my stomach and I get convinced that I have cancer.

Nurse: 'Tell me about the most recent time that you had these pains and this conviction'.

Person: 'Just this morning, after breakfast, I was sat in this chair and feeling really uncomfortable in my stomach. I started to think that I was sure it was stomach cancer'.

Nurse: 'What exactly was passing through your mind, when you were thinking about this?'

Person: 'I was thinking about dying'.

Nurse: 'Dying?'

Person: 'Yes, I imagined myself on my deathbed and I could see my family stood around me looking upset. Then I thought to myself that it's only a matter of time before this will be happening'.

Nurse: 'How much did you believe that thought?'

Person: 'Oh, I believed it'.

Nurse: 'Out of 100, how strongly would you rate this belief at the time that you were thinking it'.

Person: 'I'd say maybe 98%'.

By focusing on a particular situation in which pains were being experienced, the nurse was able to gain an impression of some of the actual thoughts that were associated with having cancer. However, it is not always as straightforward as this because people can sometimes have considerable difficulty in specifying these kinds of thoughts. Instead, people may have a tendency to talk in a generalized way in terms of what they were thinking about rather than what they were actually thinking. This can be because of difficulties to do with recall and the way that memories of an experience can quickly fade. Alternatively, people may find such memories distressing and may be reluctant to 're-visit' a disturbing thought. Or they might be concerned about what nurses might think of them if they were to acknowledge certain kinds of thoughts, especially ones that might be thought bizarre.

David Clark, a cognitive-behaviour therapist, has identified each of these potential difficulties in the recall of specific thoughts and has suggested some ways of helping people to overcome them.[7] These include the use of role-play or imagery to re-live a particular experience and therefore gain more immediate access to the thoughts that were involved. Alternatively, there are times when it seems apparent that a person's emotional state has suddenly changed and that, for example, he or she has become noticeably more anxious. On these occasions, it can be helpful to notice this emotional change and inquire into what the person is thinking at that moment.

Nurses could certainly use either of these approaches as part of an assessment. Furthermore, nurses can suggest assignments in which people are asked to monitor their emotional state and to identify thoughts that are associated with negative feelings. These kinds of assignments, and their use by nurses, have been discussed by Phil Barker.[4] One approach involves people-in-care keeping a written record on a form that is divided into three columns:

❑ In the first column, a person describes the details of a situation in which negative feelings were experienced;
❑ In the second, the person identifies those negative feelings and rates their severity;
❑ And in the third column, the person specifies the thoughts that passed through his or her mind and rates the extent to which these thoughts were believed.

Through these different methods, people can be assisted to notice and specify their negative thoughts. Something that nurses need to consider is the helpfulness of such assistance as part of an assessment.

The value of noticing thoughts

When a person is asked to notice negative thoughts that are associated with particular negative feelings, this can be helpful in at least two ways. First, the person may find it helpful to establish that there is a link between their thoughts and feelings. People can sometimes be bewildered by the way that they are feeling and they often view their problems as more explicable when they recognize the ways in which their thoughts shape their feelings. Second, nurses can devise ways to help people once they are aware of the particular thoughts, and patterns of thoughts, that are associated with particular difficulties. If, for example, nurses discover that a person is pre-occupied by the possibility of a terrible event that, objectively, is unlikely to happen then it might follow that this person could be helped by encouraging him to pay realistic attention to the probabilities of that event.

Although these positive consequences can stem from helping people to notice their negative thoughts and their relationship to negative feelings, it does not follow that this is the only kind of attention to thoughts that nurses should promote. It has already been observed that nurses can be overly pre-occupied with negative feelings and this can be said about negative thoughts for the same reasons. In addition, some people can become quite demoralized by the idea that their thoughts are a 'problem' because they view thinking as an automatic thing that cannot be consciously controlled or changed. Partly for these reasons, it is often valuable for nurses to encourage people to attend to thoughts that are not part of their problems but that instead are a part of 'exceptions' to problems.

For example, it can be useful to ask people to identify what they were thinking on an occasion when they were coping most effectively. Such a request encourages people to focus on their experiences of success and can promote a belief in the possibility of further success. Another potentially useful inquiry that nurses can make about thoughts concerns what people *would be* thinking if their problems had disappeared. This can be helpful as part of a discussion of how people would like their lives to be different and might encourage them to selectively attend to signs that a preferred scenario is developing or that it has already developed in some sense. These kinds of inquiries, and their empowering possibilities, are explored in more detail in the chapters on solution-focused therapy (see Chapter 23).

ASSESSING BELIEFS

Beliefs are the things that people accept as true and incorporate implicit assumptions that people make as well as what they explicitly and consciously profess to believe. Nurses have often been taught to respect people's beliefs but the implications of this idea have not always been fully explored. One such implication is that mental health nurses need to identify which beliefs should be respected.

Respecting beliefs

Nurses have always made routine inquiries about people's religious beliefs. These inquiries are focused on some details of a person's religion like the particular practices and outlooks that are involved and the extent to which the person observes them. One purpose of these inquiries is to provide information that will enable nurses to manifest respect for people's religious beliefs. And manifesting this kind of respect involves recognition that such beliefs are potentially important for a range of reasons. As Frankl[2] observed, people's religious beliefs can be a basis for the meanings that they find in adversity and therefore help them to endure such adversity. Nurses, then, recognize that religious beliefs can be a factor in people's ability to cope and respect for such beliefs is one way that nurses support people's ways of coping.

Hence, as part of an assessment, nurses often inquire about people's religious beliefs because these can be a positive factor in people's ability to 'get by' in life. However, there are many other kinds of beliefs that are relevant to how people cope and so nurses have to be broad in their understandings of beliefs that they should respect. For example, people have beliefs about themselves in relation to:

❑ how able they are to succeed;
❑ how much control they have over their lives;
❑ how attractive they are to others, how loveable or valuable they are.

The importance of such beliefs has been recognized in the field of psychology where they are expressed in concepts like self-efficacy, locus of control, body image and self-esteem. Sometimes, the positive implications of these kinds of beliefs are clearly expressed by people-in-care as the following interaction illustrates:

Nurse: 'You've told me that, over the years, you have had a lot of torment from voices in your head and have had to deal with some really weird and disturbing things. Yet you've had very little contact with psychiatric services'.

Person: 'Yes, that's right. It's eighteen years since I was in a psychiatric hospital. I don't really like having contact with doctors and nurses. I try to stay away from them. I don't need them. I can get by in life – I look after my flat, I pay my bills, I have a boyfriend, I don't hassle anybody and nobody really hassles me. I don't want to depend on psychiatrists and the drugs that they give me'.

As this conversation progressed further, it became increasingly clear that this person valued her own independence and believed in herself as a person that could 'stand on her own two feet'. This belief seemed justified in the sense that she was able to attend to the everyday aspects of living even though, from the nurse's perspective, she was experiencing psychosis for much of the time. Importantly, this ability to cope appeared to be founded on her belief that she could do so.

In this situation, then, the nurse was able to identify beliefs that 'worked' for a person-in-care. However, this person's beliefs involved a rejection of the nurse's conventional way of working that involved administering and monitoring medication as well as visiting people, on her caseload, on a frequent basis. Yet the nurse developed an approach to this person that showed respect for her beliefs. She kept a certain distance, signalled her availability and provided help with certain practical matters, like repairs to her council flat, when the person asked for it. Of course, the nurse could be criticized for failing to assert the value of medication to this person because of evidence that people with her diagnosis benefit from such medication. Yet there is also some evidence that people tend to benefit from care and treatment that accommodates their beliefs.

For example, Priebe and Gruyters undertook a small randomized controlled trial of day hospital treatment for people with a diagnosis of schizophrenia.[8] They found that positive outcomes were more associated with tailoring treatment to people's wishes than with the provision of a standardized service. In other words, people made greater progress when they received help that was consistent with their beliefs about the kind of help that they needed.

Although this study was small and its results should be viewed with a degree of caution, it does highlight the possibility that a service that reflects a respect for people's beliefs may also be effective in meeting their needs. Hence, mental health nurses need to assess people's beliefs and understand their positive implications as a basis for such a service. However, beliefs can also have problematic implications and this also needs to be a focus for assessment by mental health nurses.

Problematic beliefs

There are times when people hold beliefs that are manifestly false but this in itself is not very significant. What is significant is a situation in which a false belief has problematic consequences such as emotional distress or harmful behaviour. For example, a person might be terrified because of a false belief that his neighbours want to kill him. This belief might pre-occupy him to the extent that he has is monitoring the behaviour of his neighbours and tending to interpret their actions as indicative of their murderous intentions even though, objectively, they are just going about their daily business. In this kind of situation, people's beliefs are clearly a prominent part of their difficulties. Perhaps less obviously, people hold beliefs that are not blatantly untrue but are somewhat unrealistic. For example, a person might believe that decent parents never lose their temper or get impatient with their children. If this belief is strongly held, the person might be very self-critical for shouting at her children on a particular occasion and might therefore feel guilty about falling below her standard of parental behaviour. Beck[6] observed a range of ways in which these kinds of unrealistic beliefs shape patterns of negative thinking that give rise to negative emotions.

Hence, people's beliefs are often an important aspect of the problems that they experience. Both nurses and people-in-care therefore need to identify the beliefs that are associated with a problem in order to understand it. Furthermore, by identifying such beliefs, a basis can be created for challenging and changing them.

Exploring beliefs

So, nurses and people-in-care often need to identify problematic beliefs as well as those that should be respected. Furthermore, such beliefs need to be explored in terms of their consequences, the extent to which they are firmly held and perhaps also their relationship to the person's wider biography. This can be relatively straightforward when the focus is on beliefs that the person consciously espouses. However, many important beliefs are implicit assumptions that people rarely or never reflect upon. In assessing these kinds of beliefs, it will probably be insufficient for a nurse to simply ask, for example, 'what are your beliefs about yourself?' Instead, a nurse can often detect themes in a person's actions or in his or her accounts of various issues. One such theme might be perfectionism and this can reflect the person's belief that he or she always has to get things right and must never fail. Of course, such themes can also often be identified by people-in-care themselves once they have the opportunity to reflect upon their own situation and upon the questions posed by nurses.

CONCLUSION

Assessment is a process in which mental health nurses, and people-in-care, are active participants. The idea that assessment is something that nurses do *on* or *to* people-in-care should therefore be discarded. Instead, the assessment of what people feel, think and believe should be approached with a view to the benefits that can be gained by both nurses and people-in-care from processes of *inquiry* and *discovery*. These processes are ongoing and are not confined to any 'stage' in a person's nursing care. Assessment is an ongoing endeavour and the information generated can only ever be provisional as people change and new things are discovered. Indeed, the very notion of assessment should be a developing one and subject to continuing refinement and alteration.

REFERENCES

1. Metcalf L, Thomas FN, Duncan BL, Miller SD, Hubble MA. What works in solution-focused brief therapy: A qualitative analysis of client and therapist perceptions. In: Miller SD, Hubble MA, Duncan BL (eds). *Handbook of solution-focused therapy.* San Francisco: Jossey-Bass, 1996: 335–49.
2. Frankl V. *The will to meaning.* London: Souvenir Press, 1971.
3. Parkes CM. *Bereavement: studies of grief in adult life,* 3rd edn. London: Routledge, 1996.
4. Barker PJ. *Assessment in psychiatric and mental health nursing: in search of the whole person.* Cheltenham: Stanley Thornes, 1997.
5. Duncan B, Hubble M, Miller S. *Psychotherapy with 'impossible' cases: the efficient treatment of therapy veterans.* New York: Norton, 1997.
6. Beck AT. *Cognitive therapy and the emotional disorders.* Harmondsworth: Penguin, 1989.
7. Clark DM. Anxiety states: panic and generalized anxiety. In: Hawton K, Salkovskis PM, Kirk J, Clark DM (eds). *Cognitive behaviour therapy for psychiatric problems.* Oxford: Oxford University Press, 1989: 52–96.
8. Priebe S, Gruyters T. A pilot trial of treatment changes according to schizophrenic patients' wishes. *Journal of Nervous and Mental Disease* 1999; **187**: 441–3.

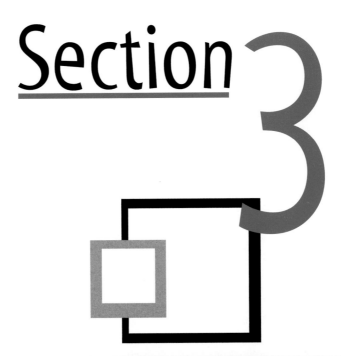

Section 3

The structure of care

Preface to Section 3

For the past 25 years the nursing process has provided the basis for defining the structure of care. However, as care moves to the wider, less controlled, context of the community, new ways of viewing people and their problems will prove necessary. The formal, rational, highly structured basis of the nursing process is close to redundancy if not already obsolete. As new care contexts emerge demands are placed on nurses to develop more flexible ways of organizing information about people in care and to develop more extensive plans for the caring process.

Nurses are confronted with such a wealth of information about the person in care that, often, this can prove overwhelming. This section begins with a consideration of the history and current development of classification systems in psychiatry and how they offer a means towards clarifying the emerging picture of people and their problems of living.

Nursing diagnosis was proposed as an adjunct to medi- cal diagnostic systems, aiming to broaden the approach to classifying the human problems that form the foci of care and treatment. Nursing diagnosis is not, however, without its problems, both methodological and practical and some of these are addressed here, as we ask 'what is the most appropriate way to frame problems of living, from a nursing perspective?'

Increasingly, individual patients are not the focus of the care plan, but are rather the most important members of a complex social unit, to which nurses need to relate in an effort to shape the offer of support that help ameliorate current problems and speed the development of more integrated personal and interpersonal experiences. In the final chapter in this section we address the complexities of working collaboratively with families, who represent the traditional social support group of the person in care. How might the families aid and abet the care planning process and how do nurses enlist family members as part of the therapeutic medium of care?

Chapter 14

CLASSIFICATION AND NURSING

Shaun Parsons*

In this chapter the process of psychiatric classification will be explored. Classification is placed in a historical context allowing the relevance of psychiatric classification to nursing to be explored.

WHAT IS CLASSIFICATION?

Classification is the process of naming objects in our daily lives and organizing them within larger groups, for example, a Rolls Royce (name of object) is a type of car (larger grouping). We name and group all kinds of objects and events, from ourselves to the objects around us. Such naming is a classification process. We accept this process as a central part of the human condition. Why? The main reason is one of convenience. By classifying objects we immediately remove the need to describe them in detail when trying to convey our meaning to others. For example, imagine that instead of simply being able to say we were going to get a taxi home it was necessary to describe the concept of a 'taxi' in detail. How would we convey this in conversation? Perhaps we would have to say something like 'I'm going to get the motor driven metal box on four wheels which is steered by someone whom I will have to pay for my journey'. This is extremely complicated and cumbersome. No-one would dream of doing this in everyday life. Although a

simplistic and fairly crude example, this shows that by using a standard classification system, we can employ a term that immediately conveys a meaning to others who share our language and culture. Surprisingly, this very useful process was only formally extended into the natural sciences in the 17th century when botanists began to name plants and to group them into similar types. This approach then spread from botany to the other physical sciences with perhaps the best example being in chemistry where the elements are named, ranked and grouped together by their physical properties in the periodic table.

In the 19th century the emergent discipline of scientific medicine embraced this process wholeheartedly and a classification of diseases, into groups depending upon their signs, symptoms and course, was undertaken. This form of classification – where diseases are grouped together by their properties (i.e. signs and symptoms), rather than by their causes – is known as a *descriptive classification system*. As knowledge of physical illnesses and their underlying causes increased, illnesses were increasingly grouped by their causes – a system known as an *aetiological classification*. For example, illnesses such as chickenpox were originally classified only by their symptoms but later, after the discovery of viruses, they were also classified by their causative virus. The advantages of such classification were the same as the advantages of

*Shaun Parsons is a Lecturer in Clinical Psychology at the University of Newcastle and he practises as a Forensic Psychologist in the NHS. His research interests include the monitoring and treatment of sex offenders in community and prison settings and the interaction between the police and people with mental health problems.

classifying objects in our day to day life. The meaning and concept of a complex disorder could be communicated in a few words instead of several hundred.

In physical medicine this process was initially controversial with considerable debates occurring around the cause of disease, for example the causes of cholera. However, as the causes of illness became clearer the process became more accepted, and less controversial, until in physical medicine today we have an almost entirely aetiological classification system. However, the same is not the case in psychiatry were there have been considerable debates not just about the causes of disorder but even their very existence.

Psychiatric classification – from ancient times to the current day

The earliest records of mental disorder are ancient and date back to 3000 BC when the Egyptian Prince Ptah-hotep was described as having symptoms which are now clearly recognizable as Alzheimer's disease. Later, in the second millennium BC, the ancient Greeks described melancholia and hysteria in terms we would understand today. By the late 19th century the newly emergent disciplines of psychiatry and psychology were describing and classifying disorders that would evolve into the current concepts of schizophrenia and depression. For example, Charcot described, in considerable detail, the symptoms associated with hysteria and in 1896 Kraepelin used descriptive methods to produce the first modern classification system when he hypothesized that a group of patients with the same symptoms and course of illness, had the same underlying disease. Kraepelin produced a textbook of psychiatry in which he named disorders based upon his descriptions of symptoms. The table of contents of Kraepelin's book became the foundation of modern psychiatric classification.

Early in the 20th century the American Medico-Psychological Association and the National Committee for Mental Hygiene developed a list of 22 psychiatric diseases for use in the United States. These classifications evolved over the middle of the 20th century into the *Diagnostic and Statistical Manual* version I (DSM I) in 1952.[1] The *World Health Organization* had also assumed responsibility for the *International Classification of Diseases* and produced a less comprehensive classification in the section on mental disorders in *ICD*-6. In 1980 the American Psychiatric Association produced DSM III, which was an attempt to produce an evidence based scientific classification system. In this sense scientific means that DSM III,[2] and its successors DSM III-R and DSM IV, were meant to define disorders that could be identified by objective criteria and then tested using experimental techniques. To this end the Authors of DSM III and its successors have relied heavily upon research evidence when writing and revising the diagnostic criteria of psychiatric disorders.

The DSM system has been criticized from a number of different standpoints. The DSM system's acceptance of psychiatric disorders as discrete diagnostic entities, which are real in the same way as physical disease, has been criticized at a fundamental level. Some researchers arguing from a social constructionist and post-modern perspective have argued that psychiatric disorders are illusionary and have been constructed by mental health professionals, and particularly psychiatrists, to further professional power and to service the needs of society. An English psychologist, Mary Boyle, argued in 1990 that psychiatric classifications are flawed at a fundamental level and that they have not been constructed using scientific techniques.[3] She argued that in psychiatry the observable symptoms of mental illness are fitted into constructs, which have been previously determined by committees. She contended that this was the opposite of the scientific method, as employed in the natural sciences, where the *observable* phenomena define the classifications they are accorded. For example, an element's position on the periodic table of elements is defined by its atomic weight. Boyle, and others holding similar views, suggested that psychiatric diagnoses are damaging as they reduce people to a diagnostic label rather than an individual with specific needs and an independent life. Those arguing in support of psychiatric classification (for example Frances *et al.*[4]), have asserted that DSM IV was intended to be experimental and pragmatic, and should be considered a work in progress under continuous revision. Consequently, the disorders listed were intended to be hypotheses, which could be used for clinical work, and as a framework for further research, which pursues an aetiological classification such as exists in physical medicine.

A further criticism of the DSM system is that the number of psychiatric diagnoses classified under DSM has grown considerably over the half century since DSM II was written. In DSM II there were 85 disorders, this grew to 265 in DSM III and 297 in DSM IV. There are three possible reasons for this change:

1 The researchers who devised DSM have become increasingly adept at recognizing various types of psychiatric disorder and at naming them.

2 Variations of existing disorders may have been categorized as new psychiatric disorders.

3 There may, indeed, have been a genuine increase in the number of new disorders recognized.

There is no clear agreement amongst researchers as to which of these explanations is correct. It seems likely that the correct answer is almost certainly a combination of all of these factors. It is possible that genuinely 'new' disorders have been discovered, using modern investigation techniques, coupled with the huge volume of research being carried out in psychiatry. It is also possible that over-zealous researchers have used ever more finely tuned diagnostic criteria to split disorders into two or three new disorders, when in fact they would have been better left as one. This last argument is often made in criticism of the personality Disorders in DSM IV where a number of researchers (for example Livesly[5]), argued that the evidence for the 10 personality disorders defined in DSM IV is ambiguous, and that the fact that the personality disorders are rarely diagnosed *apart from each other*, suggests that they would be better classified in a different way.

A final problem of the DSM, and indeed all psychiatric classification and psychological measurement, is the dilemma of when to decide whether a disorder is present or not. Again the situation in psychiatry is different from physical medicine. In physical medicine the presence or absence of an illness can often be confirmed by physiological examination based upon presenting symptoms. Indeed, when physical disorders have not had a clear aetiological basis and a clear diagnostic test, there has often been an attempt to move them into psychiatry. The recent controversy over the diagnosis of myalgic encephalomyelitis or ME is a good example. In psychiatry there has, historically, been no such certainty of the presence of a disorder, and psychiatric symptoms have tended to occupy a spectrum or continuum. For example feelings of low mood can be anything from a slight sadness up to thoughts of complete hopelessness, worthlessness and despair. The current psychiatric systems tend to provide a cut off point when a diagnosis is present or not, and these are known as categorical systems. However, these cut-offs can appear arbitrary. Within categorical systems it is necessary to define normal and abnormal and imply that there is a clear boundary between the two. However, this position is problematic. Firstly the definition of normal and abnormal is often subjective and dependent upon the wider definitions of normal behaviour within society. In psychiatry this definition is rarely without controversy. Even symptoms, which may appear by their very nature to be 'abnormal', can be disputed. For example, Romme and Escher[6] have argued that hearing voices, one of the defining symptoms of psychosis, is in fact a fairly common phenomenon and can exist on a continuum extending from being a positive experience for some people, whilst distressing for others. In such circumstances, providing a clear distinction between abnormal and normal, when the very constructs being judged are disputed, can appear to be an arbitrary process.

The alternative to this approach is to adopt a *dimensional system* where, rather than employ a 'cut off' point, the degree to which a symptom is present and affecting the individual's daily functioning is described. The problem of such systems is that they negate one of the main functions of classification: that of deciding whether a disorder is present or not. Dimensional systems also do not allow epidemiological and statistical data to be easily gathered. This may not seem to be a significant problem but such data are an essential part of planning health provision. However, despite the problems of classification and diagnosis there has been an attempt to create nursing's own classification system.

NURSING DIAGNOSIS

There has been an attempt to introduce a classification system to nursing which is based upon the concept of Nursing Diagnosis. In 1973 the foundations of what was to become the North American Nursing Diagnosis Association (NANDA) were laid when the first taskforce to name and classify nursing diagnoses was founded. The work of the taskforce was to identify problems that nurses defined which could be seen as separate to medical diagnoses and to then name and classify them. The taskforce continued throughout the 1970s and worked with other groups such as the nurse theorist group in identifying, refining and promoting the use of nursing diagnoses. In 1982 NANDA was created to unify and co-ordinate the work of the various groups working on nursing diagnosis and in 1986 a classification system called Taxonomy 1 was created, which attempted to classify nursing diagnoses. The American Nurses Association then attempted to gain the acceptance and credibility of a major classification system by trying, unsuccessfully, to have the World Health Organization include nursing diagnoses as a chapter in the International Classification of Diseases (ICD) system. If this attempt had been successful then NANDA's classification would have been included in the tenth version of ICD, ICD-10, published in 1992.[7] If ICD-10 had included NANDA's classification then it would have rapidly spread and been adopted across the world. However, the absence of the classification has ensured that nursing diagnosis as a concept has spread more slowly and in a less comprehensive way than it might have done.

Nursing diagnosis has become a popular, and some might argue, dominant method for nurses' description of patients' problems in North America. More recently it has spread to some European countries such as Sweden, Germany and France,[8] but it has not become popular or used to any great extent in the UK or Southern Europe.

What is nursing diagnosis?

Nursing diagnosis is, like all classifications, a naming or labelling of a phenomenon or group of phenomenon for the purpose of improving communication and reducing the need for long descriptions. The International Classification for Nursing Practice (ICNP) defines nursing diagnosis as terms for nursing factors which are recorded as diagnoses or problems and which indicates a reason for nursing care, International Nursing review 1994, cited in Hogston.[8] Nursing diagnosis can exist alongside a medical diagnosis to which it is usually related. Nursing diagnosis is an attempt to acknowledge that the problems people face through ill health are separate from the physiological fact of the illness. This situation is true even in physical illness. For example, for a person in the terminal stages of lung cancer the physical facts of the disease, and its progression, can be tightly defined using objective criteria, such as the extent of the tumour as seen in an X-ray and the histology of a biopsy taken from the tumour. The nursing problems are less concerned with these issues and are more concerned with the physical and psychological problems faced by an individual. For example, the nurse may be primarily concerned with the fear and anxiety that impending death may be bringing an individual.

Nursing diagnosis can therefore be seen as something of a paradox in that there is an attempt to highlight the differences between medical and nursing concerns but, by using diagnoses and classification, nursing diagnosis appears to be adopting a medical or at least pseudo-medical approach. The reasons for adopting nursing diagnosis are often presented as a need to have a common language of nursing problems that can be understood by all nurses. It can also be seen as an attempt for nursing to develop a language which is similar to medicine, and which can therefore raise the professional status of nursing. The need for nursing to have its own classification system and indeed the relevance of classification to nursing will now be discussed.

CLASSIFICATION AND NURSING

It has been argued that classification is a convenience, a way in which simple labels or names can be used to convey the meaning of complex concepts. In medicine perhaps the most important aspect of a classification is the usefulness of the description in identifying *caseness*, meaning whether a disorder is present or not, and predicating the treatment course. Although it has been argued by some that psychiatric classifications are not real but rather artificial constructions (for example

Boyle[3]), there has been increasing evidence, and a growing consensus in neuroscience over the 1990s that at least the major disorders are real entities with solid pathology underpinning them. However, we can to a large extent sidestep this debate when we examine the usefulness of classification systems to nursing, and particularly to psychiatric nursing. As discussed above even in physical medicine knowing a medical diagnosis often tells us little about the individual's problems. Congestive cardiac failure may lead us to surmise that the individual will be short of breath, have pitting oedema and poor mobility, but it tells us little about the concerns of the person with congestive cardiac failure.

❑ How does the individual feel about their lack of mobility?
❑ Who is looking after the dog at home?
❑ What is the most comfortable position they have found in dealing with dyspnoea over weeks of long nights awake at home as the illness developed?

These, other similar questions, often concern the nurse, in addition to the medically driven concerns such as administering drugs and oxygen. The same is true in psychiatry, perhaps even to a greater extent. A diagnosis of depression tells us that an individual may have a low mood, early morning wakening and difficulty in completing daily tasks. However, it tells us nothing about what the individual thinks about in their low mood or how they cope with their early morning wakening. In other words the diagnosis gives only a broad idea of the individual's problems but tells us nothing about the person themselves and what those problems and experiences mean to them. Again the psychiatric nurse may acknowledge the diagnosis, administer the medication prescribed and assist with the administration of electroconvulsive therapy. However, the nursing tasks, which matter most to the person experiencing depression, are likely to involve far simpler and, dare we say, more human concerns. The role of the nurse is often simply *being with* the person, talking to them, helping them help themselves stay safe and get through daily life. None of this diminishes the role of classification but emphasizes its irrelevance to most daily nursing activity. Nurses are concerned with people's day to day problems, their pain, their anxiety and worries. It is here that the proper focus of nursing lies.

As we have seen nursing diagnosis acknowledges this argument but then uses the language of classification to produce nursing diagnoses. This process may be useful if it allows nurses to explain complex concepts in simpler terms and aids communication and nursing care. However, there is a risk that in attempting to generate nursing diagnoses a person's problems are compartmentalized, reduced and standardized, to the detriment of their nursing care. The proponents of nursing diagnosis need to show that by adopting such a system, nursing care will be enhanced and an individualized approach to the person maintained.

SUMMARY

Classification or naming is simply an extension of an ordinary human process which we undertake every day of our lives. In medicine it has considerable benefits in being able to identify similar cases with similar underlying pathology. It is also essential in planning health care provision and services and in determining future needs. However, it has also been argued here that for most nurses classification is an irrelevance, even in physical medicine, as nurses are concerned with day to day problems and human concerns and not with diagnoses. This is by no means a rejection of the validity and importance of medical and psychiatric diagnoses, or their importance in medical practice. Rather, this is an acknowledgement that the proper focus of nursing lies with the individual, their human concerns and their perception of their problems, rather than directly with the disease or disorder they are experiencing.

REFERENCES

1. American Psychiatric Association. *Diagnostic and statistical manual of mental disorders*, 1st edn. Washington DC: APA, 1952.
2. American Psychiatric Association. *Diagnostic and statistical manual of mental disorders – revised*, 3rd edn. Washington DC: APA, 1987.
3. Boyle M. *Schizophrenia a scientific delusion*. London: Routledge, 1990.
4. Frances A, Mack AH, First MB *et al*. A forum for bioethics and philosophy of medicine. DSM-IV meets philosophy. Foundations of the new nosology. *Journal of Medicine and Philosophy* 1994; **19**: 204–97.
5. Livesley J. Past achievements and future directions. In: Livesley WJ (ed.) *The DSM-IV personality disorders*. New York: Guilford, 1995: 497–506.
6. Romme M, Escher S (eds). *Accepting voices*. London: MIND, 1993.
7. WHO. *The ICD-10 classification of mental and behavioural disorders*. Geneva: World Health Organization, 1993.
8. Hogston J. Nursing diagnosis and classification systems: a position paper. *Journal of Advanced Nursing* 1997; **26**(3): 496–501.

Chapter 15

THE VALUE OF NURSING DIAGNOSIS

Dianne Ellis*

INTRODUCTION

Imagine for a moment that someone has entered into your life and made a judgement about some aspect of it – be it your thoughts, appearance or behaviour. If this were to happen how might you feel? Perhaps you will feel relieved that at last someone has acknowledged, explained or named an issue that has been troubling you for some time. Alternatively you might be very anxious because in some way you feel different from other people, not whole or not perfect. You might be angry or even furious at his or her impertinence. You may simply disagree and want to discuss it further. Whatever your reaction it will be unique because it will be your own and you are entitled to experience and express the emotions stirred within you.

As a psychiatric-mental health nurse you will frequently be invited into the lives of other people in order to help them. This chapter focuses on how and why you would make a nursing diagnosis, bearing in mind the possible feelings that can emerge during this process? Both the value and the disadvantages of this process are given an appraisal with discussion about how you can respond to the individual's experiences and opinions? First of all we shall examine what diagnosis is and is not. This focuses on the practical purpose and process of nursing diagnosis. Then we shall discuss some of the different ways that knowledge can be 'ordered' before using for diagnosis. Finally we shall consider the potential negative impact that diagnosis can have upon people and discusses the benefits of collaborative working.

DIAGNOSING DIAGNOSIS

Given that nursing should be delivered in a manner that is professionally, legally and morally appropriate, a systematic approach to nursing is invariably seen as helpful. Assessment and diagnosis are components of the nursing process which aims to provide such order and direction to nursing practice by helping nurses to arrive at decisions, predict the outcomes and evaluate the consequences of care.[1] There are five stages to the nursing process, which provide a methodical approach to nursing:

1 Assessment.
2 Diagnosis or problem identification.
3 Planning.
4 Implementation.
5 Evaluation.

*Dianne Ellis has worked within Adult Mental Health Services as an RMN since 1985 with much of her experience as a community nurse. She completed an MSc in Mental Health and Psychiatric Nursing at Newcastle University where her research dissertation focused upon collaborative care, examining how nurses interacted with people receiving care.

The term 'nursing diagnosis' is often used synonymously with the term 'problem identification' to refer to the second stage of the Nursing Process. Despite differences of opinion within nursing literature[2] about the two terms, both provide a statement about the person's needs following an assessment.

Diagnosis is commonly associated with medicine, where a doctor determines the nature of a person's illness and treatment plan. Nursing diagnosis has been greatly influenced by the medical diagnostic system whereby the nurse forms a hypothesis in relation to the person's problem and its cause following assessment. This enables the nurse to decide what else needs to be known, or understood, for a diagnosis to be made. This process has, however, a much broader application than health care. For example, both mechanics and teachers use diagnosis as 'a step in any decision making process'.[3] The term diagnosis comes from the Greek word 'diagignoskein' meaning to discern – 'perceive clearly with the mind or the senses. Make out by thought or by gazing or listening'.[4] Such a basic definition needs further qualification, however. Given some of the curious assumptions that often lie behind the concept of diagnosis, it is important to note what nursing diagnosis **is not** before exploring what it might be.

❑ Nursing diagnosis should not be:
- An *essential* requirement of nursing but rather should be one method of approaching nursing.
- *Restricted* to one method, since there are numerous approaches to the diagnostic process.
- *The end-product* of care, but an element in the process of care.
- *A static statement*, because any nursing diagnosis made will continue to evolve in response to new information and the individual's changing needs.[5]
❑ Nursing diagnosis should be:
- A *statement* about the person's health problem.
- Based upon information gained from *assessment*.
- Based upon a problem that *requires nursing care*.
- *Validated* by the person.[6]

Assessment is a continuous process and, like a kaleidoscope, the diagnostic picture can change at every turn. To maintain a well-informed understanding of the person's needs it is essential to listen and take on board what that person has to say.[7] Being too focused upon a 'diagnosis' can prevent a nurse from actually hearing this important voice.

The information made known during the assessment is compared against a diagnostic framework so that a decision – in the form of a statement – can be made about the nature of those needs. It should:

❑ be a short and clear statement of the health problem;
❑ offer a concise description of the diagnosis;
❑ include the factors that support this diagnosis; and
❑ include the factors that are causing, influencing or maintaining it.

As such, diagnosis refers to:

1   A *process* by which nurses
2   *determine knowledge* from
3   *a classification system*.

CLASSIFYING CLASSIFICATION

Classification can be described as a process, which refers to the cataloguing of information. It is one means of dealing with an otherwise overwhelming amount of data, by ordering it into categories (with shared characteristics) so that it can be easily retrieved when needed.[8] This process is also referred to as Codification or Taxonomy. There is a vast and diverse body of information available in relation to mental health, which is growing continually. As a result various systems for processing such information have been created. Classification in health care has a multitude of functions for example:

❑ to order phenomena to enable communication among professionals;

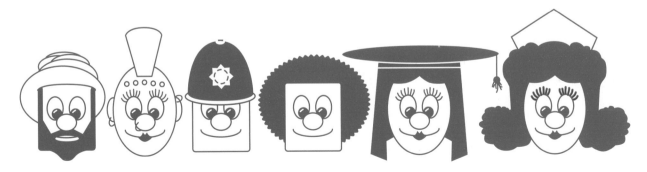

FIGURE 15.1 Classifying people. Would you classify these people by Gender? Hats? Culture? Beliefs? Occupation? Age? Hobbies? Size? Position?

❏ to categorize information from research;
❏ to facilitate literature reviews;
❏ to develop theory;[9]
❏ to develop diagnostic systems.

Figure 15.1 depicts six individuals each with unique characteristics. How would you go about the process of classifying these people?

It is clear that many characteristics are involved and so the task of classifying is problematic. Given the uniqueness and complexity of human nature, classification in health care is intricate unlike say, the traditional classification systems of mathematics.[10]

Standardized classification systems are those taxonomies of knowledge, which are intended for universal application. As an example, for the past four decades the Diagnostic Statistical Manual for mental disorders (DSM) published by the American Psychiatrist Association and the International Classification System (ICD) developed by the World Health Organization,[11] have been used by psychiatrists to diagnose mental illness. The two systems share a unified theoretical belief that mental illness is the result of behavioural, psychological or biological dysfunction.[12]

From the perspective of medicine, which underpins this diagnosis, postpartum depression is used to describe a pathological reaction, a symptom, syndrome, disorder or illness. For Samantha (Case study 15.1), this had a major impact upon her self-concept, marital relationship and future care. Because postpartum depression heralds a bipolar disorder requiring immediate medical treat-

---

Case study 15.1: Samantha has a case of 'the blues'

The 'blue' feelings experienced by Samantha following the birth of her daughter became progressively worse. Feeling very distressed she sought help from her general practitioner and was referred to a Consultant Psychiatrist. An assessment was subsequently completed and the reported symptoms and observed signs were compared against the DSM classification system. After ruling out physical illness the psychiatrist reached the following conclusions:

■ Changes from a previous level of functioning were noted.
■ Distress, social impairment and occupational impairment, all were noted.
■ Symptoms of depression weight loss, insomnia, and feelings of guilt and fatigue were evident.
■ This appeared to be a singular episode.
■ The onset was between 2 weeks and 12 months after delivery. (Postpartum).
■ A global assessment of Samantha showed a functioning level of 60 (moderate symptoms of disturbance).
■ Using these data, the psychiatrist made the following diagnosis, using the DSMIV – *(296.22f) single episode, Postpartum Major Depressive Disorder with moderate symptoms.*

---

ment[13] the diagnosis became the focus of further assessments and treatment plans. She was prescribed antidepressant medication and was referred to a day hospital

---

TABLE 15.1 A nursing diagnosis based on an assessment of Samantha's needs using Roy's Adaptation Model

Nursing diagnosis	Supporting data	Outcome criteria	Short-term goal
Nutrition less than body requirements	Unable to take a balanced diet. Has lost weight since birth of daughter outside of normal range for build	Samantha will resume her usual appetite She will gain weight to that appropriate for her height and build	Complete a teaching programme about maintaining a healthy diet Complete a nutritional assessment Weigh weekly
Inadequate pattern of activity and rest	Reports poor sleep pattern and worrying thoughts	Samantha will resume her usual sleep pattern	Education programme about relaxation Involve in daily activities
Ineffective pattern of aloneness and relating. Avoids friends and work because of how she feels.	Samantha does not want to return to work, or to spend time with friends	Resume usual relationships with family and friends Initiate social activities	Attend one activity session per day Discuss two other ways of dealing with the need to withdraw socially

for a comprehensive nursing assessment and medication/symptom monitoring.

The nursing team used the Roy Adaptation Model (1964), which is an example of a theoretical framework for nursing practice with its own classification system, in their assessment of Samantha (Table 15.1). With regard to diagnosis it offers a 'Typology of Commonly Recurring Adaptation Problems' and a 'Typology of Indicators of Positive Adaptation.'[14] The model itself cannot be discussed here, but its typology can be used to demonstrate a further diagnostic process. Assessment is guided by the underpinning theory and compared with the typology. A diagnostic statement can then be made to inform care planning.

It has been argued that nursing should have its own standardized classification system to provide a precise, universally recognized language for nurses.[15] The *International Nursing Review* (1994) reported that this system would describe specifically what nurses do (**nursing interventions**) in response to differing patient conditions (**nursing diagnosis**) with what effect (**nursing outcomes**). In the 1970s the *Nursing Diagnosis Movement* was initiated in the USA and in 1973 the first *Nursing Diagnosis Conference* took place, aiming to develop a classification system for nursing.[16] Such standardized systems either relate specifically to one theoretical viewpoint (for example the medical model discussed above) or employ a more flexible umbrella system, which can work alongside various theoretical positions. The *North American Nursing Diagnostic Association* (NANDA) developed a system in 1973 based upon Human Response Patterns to Diseases or Conditions.[17,18] This is an amalgamated system aiming to ensure that nurses pinpoint the areas that they treat and can then therefore measure the achievement of outcomes successfully. When this system was reviewed in 1992 there were over 100 diagnoses available – all described as based on research and, following audit, shown to be valid and reliable.

NANDA define diagnosis as:

> a clinical judgement about individual, family or community responses to actual and potential health problems/life processes, which provides the basis for the selection of nursing interventions and outcomes for which the nurse is accountable.[19]

Samantha subsequently encountered the standardized NANDA taxonomy (Table 15.2). Because of the success of cognitive-behavioural approaches[20] in the treatment of depression, a referral was made for her to see a psychologist. During this assessment period the psychologist learned that not only was George (Samantha's husband), unsupportive, but that he was also emotionally and physically violent towards her. (Research shows that people involved, long-term, in family violence, have higher levels of depression and self-contempt. It is estimated that 15–25% of women suffer violence during pregnancy.)[21] Due to the psychologist's diagnosis of family violence, her psychotherapy became orientated towards them as a couple, with George's behaviour the

TABLE 15.2 An example of NANDA nursing diagnosis based upon a dysfunctional family model·

NANDA nursing diagnosis – ineffective individual coping
NANDA definition – related to helplessness and feelings of low mood
Supporting data – depression, social anxiety, poor sleep/diet and weepy
Expected outcome – to have definite plans in order to change her current situation

Short-term goal	Intervention	Rationale
Samantha will state that violence has decreased by (date)	Continual assessment of violence and abuse Emphasize need and strategies for safety Discuss emergency and crisis services and contact numbers	Validates seriousness of situation and maximize safety
Samantha will be free from self-harm	Continually monitor self-harm potential Identify other options and contacts	Due to potential towards self-harm
Samantha will make decisions about her future by (date)	Encourage Samantha to examine situation and alternatives Reinforce the use of problem-solving skills	When in a dependent situation people find decision-making difficult
Samantha will have made two behavioural changes by (date)	Explore ways to make changes Assist in decision-making regarding her future	Directs assessment towards positive areas and can improve self-esteem
Samantha will identify resources and supporters that are important by (date)	Assist by discussion and activities	Identification of support and active support from nurse will help coping

TABLE 15.3 An example of collaborative nursing diagnosis

Person's diagnosis	Person's goals	Nursing plan	Rationale
I have difficulty sleeping	I will get some sleep each night	Education about relaxation Teach techniques to use Encourage activity Discuss Samantha's anxieties weekly	Sleep is easier when the body and mind are relaxed
I have little energy - not eating	I will gain energy and feel less tired	Education about high energy foods Prescription for high energy drinks Keep a check of weight	With no appetite small high energy foods will help
I am afraid about the future because of work and my daughter	I will feel supported with this problem	Listen to me when I'm scared Help me to think of solutions Help me get sick pay until things are sorted Reduce my day hospital attendance because child care is hard to manage	Practical help and support
I don't know what to do about George Can George change?	I will know what to do about George	Listen to my feelings about the psychology appointments Help me to make sense of what is happening	Needs support to deal with what she is learning about her relationship

focus. Samantha was introduced to a community psychiatric-mental health nurse for additional support. At this point in her life Samantha was assessed and diagnosed in terms of 'adaptive and maladaptive behaviour in response to life events'. Samantha and her family were viewed as a 'dysfunctional family'.

Although Samantha found her medication and therapy very helpful, she found the nursing emphasis upon her diagnosis and treatment frustrating. Day care was a burden because of having to make child care arrangements. This was ironic given that Samantha's main anxieties were:

❑ returning to work and leaving her baby at home; and
❑ finding someone who she could trust to look after her baby.

When the psychology appointments began with George she had been relieved, but soon Samantha felt 'pushed out, as her needs were not being met'. This illustrates how assessment and diagnosis direct care, rather than contribute to it. Consequently, important issues may be missed.

The Tidal Model[22] recognizes, through researching the views of people who use mental health services, that nursing needs to strike a balance between the 'ordinary' and the 'professional' nurse.[23] Nursing should deal with the 'person's description of their own immediate needs'. Care should gradually extend outward into the wider world of the person's experience.[24] It is important, therefore, to ensure that people like Samantha are involved within the diagnostic process. Collaborative working ensures that both nurse and individual influence the decision-making process. Here, if you like, the lens or theoretical viewpoint, is that of the individual.

It could be argued that Samantha's own diagnosis represented in Table 15.3 is merely 'problem identification', since it does not use a classification system. This highlights the debate mentioned briefly earlier. Here, however, we risk 'throwing the baby out with the bath water'. Samantha has been more than able to express her anxieties and to identify the areas with which she needs help. For some people this is not easy. Nurses need to be flexible in their response to individuals. It would be possible, however, to use the NANDA classification alongside Samantha's description of her needs. For example:

❑ Diagnosis – Sleep pattern disturbed.
❑ Description – 'I have difficulty sleeping.'

Although professional knowledge is frequently linked with words such as *fact, certainty, reality* and *truth*, this has been the subject of philosophical debate for centuries.[25] The theory of knowledge, or epistemology, constitutes myriad opinions about how we understand or know what is true (or untrue) about our world and ourselves.[26] Much of the knowledge or beliefs about mental health is subject to a similar debate, with differing views of people's experiences of mental distress. Such differences of opinion can be more noticeable between different health care disciplines. However, all diagnoses incorporate theoretical frameworks based upon philosophical and ethical assumptions.[27] Such frameworks encompass the systems of classification through which our lives (and problems of living) are examined (and hopefully understood).

This situation is analogous to the work of a microbiologist. The laboratory slide represents the *problem* being examined, the microscope the diagnostic tool and the lens the *theoretical viewpoint*. We cannot forget, however, that the microbiologist brings individual characteristics, attitudes, other forms of knowledge and experience, all of which can influence the *interpretation* of what is seen through the lens of the microscope.

Samantha's brief experience of the psychiatric system illustrates the diversity of nursing assessment and diagnostic systems available. Each one corresponds to a particular set of theoretical assumptions about psychiatric-mental health nursing. The nurse's difficulty is to decide which one to use. How does a nurse determine which body of knowledge to apply to a particular set of circumstances? In most areas of medicine the theory upon which supports medical diagnosis is common to practitioner and patient. However, when those judgements are about thoughts, feelings and actions, conflict between the practitioner and patient can occur. In particular, diagnoses, applied to human relationships, have the potential to cause harm to the individual.[28] An important consideration therefore when using any diagnostic system is to consider how the diagnosis will affect, both positively and negatively, the individual receiving care.

UNRAVELLING THE DIAGNOSTIC KNOT

One finger in the throat and one in the
Rectum makes a good diagnostician.
Sir William Osler (1849–1919)

Diagnoses are very similar to knots in that they can both be useful and annoying. Children often harass their parents with laces riddled with knots and yet rock climbers would be on dicey ground (or mountains) without them. Likewise, a diagnosis can steady a person who is dealing with mental distress but it can also create obstacles on the path of recovery. For many people with mental health problems, being given a diagnosis can have a negative impact upon their lives. The degree of this negative impact is often underestimated and yet these experiences can be used to inform the wise application of nursing diagnosis so that nursing might help people to feel safe and secure but not bound and gagged.

❏ People who disagree with a diagnosis that has been made about them can feel misunderstood and alone.[29] When such disagreement is vocalized often individuals are labelled as being difficult, anti-social, non-compliant or as having no insight. This can then affect the way in which other people behave towards them.[30]

❏ Nursing diagnosis can lead to the stereotyping of a person. Describing the depersonalization, disempowerment and isolation that he experienced as a result of being given a diagnosis, Coleman stated: 'Two years ago I gave up being a schizophrenic and decided to be Ron Coleman'.[31]

❏ Once a person has received a diagnosis, often, all aspects of their lives then become subject to assessment. This can create a situation where an individual is fearful of discussing the nature of their experiences, and so important information is withheld.[32]

❏ Often very practical problems in relation to housing or finance for example can emerge due to a diagnosis.

❏ In 1986 a cross-national study revealed significant differences between American and British psychiatrists' diagnoses when using the DSM. Anthropological research has also revealed cultural differences in relation to perceptions of mental illness. It is essential to keep individual and cultural difference in mind when making a diagnosis.[33]

❏ Not all nursing theories are compatible with the diagnostic process. Those with a focus upon problem/needs (such as Orem's Self-Care Model, which categorizes the activities of daily, living), fall neatly into a diagnostic process. However models such as that developed by Rosemarie Rizzo Parse (Human Becoming Theory) state that nurse–client interactions are not limited by prescriptions.[34]

❏ Not all nurses are orientated towards problem-solving approaches and the controlling of human behaviour. Indeed, some nurses are orientated towards accepting, understanding and being with the person. The issues of judging another person can cause tension for the nurse with such ideals.[35]

❏ Diagnosis can encourage a focus upon problems constructing a negative view of mental health with pessimistic treatment goals. For example schizophrenia can be viewed as a chronic condition with a poor outcome. It could be argued that by focusing upon illness, other aspects of the person (including strengths) are missed.[36]

The level of control that a theory has and the rigour with which it is applied are significant issues in relation to the individual receiving care. If diagnosis is acknowledged as being, the exercise of power of one person over another, then the potential to dominate an already vulnerable person becomes more apparent. It is a nursing responsibility to have this awareness and to avoid the unhelpful effects of the diagnostic process by respecting the individual's opinions and feelings.

CONCLUSION

We take a handful of sand from the endless
Landscape of awareness around us and call
That handful of sand the world.[37]

Robert Pirsig described how the knife of classification could separate the sand into categories of colour, size or

TABLE 15.4 A sense of balance

The nurse is the expert	'Balance'	The patient is the expert
Always use	Use when appropriate and helpful	Never use
There is **one** standardized classification system, which informs practitioners about mental health	There is no one universal truth about mental health and so nurses should be flexible, creative and responsive to the varying needs	Each person is unique and so Information about mental health should never be ordered/classified
Diagnosis is central to and drives the care planning process	Diagnosis is a narrative device to help make sense of what is happening	Diagnosis serves no positive purpose. It rules out all possibilities towards understanding the person's problems
Diagnosis identifies the cause and treatment of the person's problem	By formulating and naming person's problems that person can benefit from the order brought into a chaotic life but if presented as the absolute truth can cover up reasons	Giving the person a label is stigmatizing and it disempowers people

texture, and how this process could go on and on because ultimately each grain is unique in some sense. This analogy demonstrates how the process of classification has the potential to be both creative and destructive.

Some nursing diagnoses can help aid understanding, providing a concise account of a person's health needs and the beginnings of approach to offering a nursing response. Following assessment, a succinct statement defines the nursing purpose guiding the interventions and determining the outcomes. The diagnostic process aims to 'improve accuracy in relation to the classification of disease states'.[38] Several typologies can be used to complement a theoretical viewpoint and the diagnostic process can support the production of well-organized care plans. So, nursing diagnosis may benefit nurses, managers and auditors. But what about the people receiving care? The individual may benefit from a well-informed and designed care plan but, as noted, the diagnostic process can also be stigmatizing.

Nursing diagnosis can affect a person's self-concept, liberty and life. The divide between the individual and the nurse can widen when it should be being bridged. Being labelled as 'a one of 57 varieties' can create distance.[39]

Despite its implementation in America at some point during the 1970s nursing diagnosis has not been fully integrated into nursing practice in other countries.[40] Concerns have been raised regarding cultural influences, and not being able to provide accuracy from a list of options and difficulties measuring multi-professional outcomes.[41]

Table 15.4 observes the 'black and white' thinking that can exist in relation to nursing diagnosis. The two viewpoints are extreme and, to be successful, nurses might opt for a more 'balanced approach'.

Open-mindedness and creativity are essential ingredients to ensure that nursing assessment and diagnosis are to be framed by the individual.[42] With sufficient thought and skill, people who receive psychiatric-mental health nursing needn't be reduced to labels, which describe them as 'dysfunctional'. The road to recovery can be difficult enough without generating more obstacles.

REFERENCES

1. Stuart GW. Implementing the nursing process: standards of care. In: Stuart GW, Laraia MT (eds). *Principles and practice of psychiatric nursing.* Missouri: Mosby, 1998: 177–93.
2. Hammers JPH, Huijer Abu-Sad H, Halfens RJG. Diagnostic process and decision making in nursing: a literature review. *Journal of Professional Nursing* 1994; **10**: 154–63.
3. *The Collins English Dictionary.* London: HarperCollins, 1998.
4. *The Oxford English Dictionary.* Oxford: Oxford University Press, 1996.
5. Barker PJ. Arrested development. *Mental Health Care* 1999; **21**: 393.
6. Barker PJ. *The Tidal Model: theory and practice.* Unpublished. Newcastle: University of Newcastle 2000.
7. Rambo A, Heath A, Chenail. *Practising therapy: exercises for growing therapists.* New York: Norton, 1993.
8. Crowe M. Constructing normality: a discourse analysis of the DSM-IV. *Journal of Psychiatric and Psychiatric-Mental Health Nursing* 2000; **7**: 69–77.
9. Vincent KG, Coler MS. A unified nursing diagnostic model. *Image Journal of Nursing Scholarship* 1990; **22**: 93–5.

10. Hogston R. Nursing diagnosis and classification systems: a position paper. *Journal of Advanced Nursing* 1997; **26**: 496–500.

11. Sartorius N. *The ICD-10 Classification of Mental and Behavioural Disorders: Clinical descriptions and diagnostic guidelines*. Geneva: World Health Organization,1992.

12. Trubowitz J. Mental health: theories and therapies. In: Varcarolis E (ed.) *Foundations of psychiatric psychiatric-mental health nursing*. New York: Saunders, 1998: 29–64.

13. Stuart GW. Emotional responses and mood disorders. In: Stuart GW, Laraia MT (ed.) *Principles and practice of psychiatric nursing*. Missouri: Mosby, 1998: 348–82.

14. George JB (ed.) *Nursing theories: the base for professional nursing practice*, 4th edn. USA: Appleton and Lange, 1995: 251–79.

15. Mills C, Howie A, Mone F. Nursing diagnosis: use and potential in critical care. *Developments in Practice* 1997; **2**: 11–16.

16. Griffiths P. An investigation into the description of patient's problems by nurses using two different needs-based nursing models. *Journal of Advanced Nursing* 1998; **28**: 969–77.

17. Taptich B, Iyer P, Bernocchi-Losey D. *Nursing diagnosis and care planning*. Philadelphia: Saunders, 1989.

18. Farland GKM. *Nursing diagnosis and interventions*. St Louis: Mosby, 1993.

19. Carpentio LJ. In: Griffiths P. An investigation into the description of patients' problems by nurses using two different needs based nursing models. *Journal of Advanced Nursing* 1998; **28**: 969–77.

20. Varcarolis EM. Depressive disorders. In: Varcarolis EM. *Foundations of psychiatric psychiatric-mental health nursing*, 3rd edn. Pennsylvania: Saunders, 1998: 552–88.

21. Smith-Dijulio K. Families in crisis: family violence. In: Varcarolis EM. *Foundations of psychiatric psychiatric-mental health nursing*, 3rd edn. Pennsylvania: Saunders, 1998: 387–416.

22. Barker P. The Tidal Model: developing an empowering, person-centred approach to recovery within psychiatric and mental health nursing. *Journal of Psychiatric and Mental Health Nursing* 2001; **8**: 233–40.

23. Jackson S, Stephenson C. What do people need psychiatric and psychiatric-mental health nursing for? *Journal of Advanced Nursing* 2000; **31**: 378–88.

24. Barker PJ. Mental health: it's time to turn the tide. *Nursing Times* 1998; **94**: 70–72.

25. Harrison-Barbet A. *Mastering philosophy*. London: Macmillan, 1990.

26. Morris T. *Philosophy for dummies*. USA: IDG Books Worldwide, 1999.

27. Bracken P, Thomas P. Post modern diagnosis. *Post psychiatry: Openmind* 2000; **106**: 19.

28. Mitchell GJ. Nursing diagnosis: an ethical analysis. *Image: Journal of Nursing Scholarship* 1991; **23**: 99–103.

29. Crawford P, Nolan PW, Brown B. Linguistic entrapment: medico-nursing biographies as fictions. *Journal of Advanced Nursing* 1995; **22**: 1141–8.

30. Tilley S, Pollock L. Discourses on empowerment. *Journal of Psychiatric and Psychiatric-Mental Health Nursing* 1999; **6**: 53–60.

31. Coleman R. *Is the writing on the asylum wall? power to partnership*. Gwynedd: Handsell, 1995.

32. Reed A. Economies with 'the truth': professional's narratives about lying and deception in mental health practice. *Journal of Psychiatric and Psychiatric-Mental Health Nursing* 1996, **3**: 249–59.

33. Trubowitz J. Mental health: theories and therapies. In: Varcarolis E (ed.) *Foundations of psychiatric psychiatric-mental health nursing*. New York: Saunders, 1998: 29–64.

34. Hickman JS, Rizzo Parse R. In: George JB (ed.) *Nursing theories: the base for professional nursing practice*, 4th edn. USA: Appleton and Lange, 1995: 335–54.

35. Mitchell GJ. Mitchell GJ. Nursing diagnosis: an ethical analysis. *Image: Journal of Nursing Scholarship* 1991; **23**: 99–103.

36. Morgan S. *Helping relationships in mental health*. London: Chapman and Hall, 1996.

37. Pirsig RM. *Zen and the art of motorcycle maintenance*. London: Corgi, 1986.

38. Bennett M. Nursing diagnosis: in the beginning. *Australian Journal of Advanced Nursing* 1986; **4**: 43–6.

39. Barker P. *The philosophy and practice of psychiatric nursing*. London: Churchill Livingstone, 1999.

40. Mason G, Webb C. Nursing diagnosis: a review of the literature. *Journal of Advanced Nursing* 1993; **2**: 67–74.

41. Chambers S. Nursing diagnosis in learning disability nursing. *Journal of Advanced Nursing* 1998; **7**: 1177–81.

42. Watkins P. *Psychiatric-mental health nursing: the art of compassionate care*. Oxford: Butterworth Heinemann, 2001.

Chapter 16

COLLABORATING WITH PATIENTS AND FAMILIES IN THE DEVELOPMENT OF CARE

Tom Keen* and Mandy Haddock**

INTRODUCTION

UK mental health policy has for many years aspired to increase professional collaboration with users and their carers,[1,2] culminating in the establishment of statutory consultation under the provisions of the 2001 NHS Reform Bill.[3] There is consistent evidence that mutually respectful collaborative alliances between professionals and patients are of central importance in determining the outcome of any therapeutic strategy, regardless of specific treatment modality.[4–7] Service users, however, report disappointing levels of involvement in their own personal care and treatment, as well as in the planning and development of services.[8] Similarly, families and carers of service users with serious mental disorders have often felt excluded from decision-making, care and treatment processes[9] and historically many families, especially relatives of people diagnosed as schizophrenic, have felt blamed by professionals for the plight of their diagnosed relatives.[10]

Traditional assumptions about sickness and medical treatment derive from notions about the doctor as expert, nurses as kindly healers and the patient as needing to accept treatment and care as prescribed by doc-

tors and administered by nurses. These concepts dictate service structure; define appropriate relationships between sufferers and professionals; and are generally subsumed within terms like *the medical model* and *the sick role*. Even in the relatively uncontroversial fields of general medicine and physical illness, this unbalanced relationship of medical authority and patient dependency has long been subjected to critical analysis. It seems important for optimal recovery that medical and surgical patients feel as much as possible in *control* of their care and treatment.[11] People increasingly recognize that, whilst disease may be attributable to a single pathogenic cause, the impact that superficially simple illnesses have on individual and family life is complicated by many factors. Moreover, peoples' susceptibilities and responses to disease pathogens are exacerbated in subtle and complex ways: personal choice, lifestyles, values and beliefs; sociocultural differences; environmental and economic stressors.[12]

If these truths apply to relatively straightforward medical conditions like tuberculosis, where underlying organic causes are clearly identified, how much more true must it be of complex and uncertain disorders like psychiatric diagnoses which are mostly descriptively

*Tom Keen lectures in mental health at the University of Plymouth. He previously worked as a nurse, therapist or manager in various situations including acute admission wards, adolescent psychotherapy, therapeutic community and community mental health centres. Previous teaching experience includes sharing responsibility for staff development in Torbay Mental Health Unit.

**Mandy Haddock is a senior member and leader of a crisis intervention and resolution team based in Torquay, South Devon. She previously worked as a staff nurse on Torbay Mental Health Unit's acute admission centre, having begun her career as a learning disabilities nurse.

formulated? It may be sensible when suffering from an uncontroversial medical ailment to forgo collaborative equality and adopt the sick role – trusting, in one's weakness, the professionals' unclouded judgement and greater wisdom, expertise and psychological fitness (albeit at the risk of iatrogenic regressive dependency and compromised recovery). But psychiatric diagnoses are rarely aetiologically simple, frequently controversial, and often the subject of conflicting therapeutic approaches.[13] The majority of mental health clients have very complex needs, which should entail the abandonment of professionally imposed, rigid formulations of care, treatment and cure or rehabilitation.[14] Unilaterally imposed professional formulations are acceptable where there is both severe incapacity and a clearly delineated, uncontroversial illness. In psychiatry and psychiatric-mental health nursing, however, multi-faceted conceptualizations of disease like Zubin and Spring's 'stress-vulnerability diathesis'[15] and Ciompi's 'psycho-socio-biological' models of schizophrenia[16] clearly reveal the aetiological complexity of mental distress, even when there is strong evidence of genetic and organic causation. The resulting heterogeneous client groups are unlikely to benefit greatly from the mere attribution of a specific diagnosis and attached treatment protocols, even if the award of an identifying diagnosis provides initial relief for both sufferers and staff. Diagnosis provides clear treatment structure and direction, but such clarity may be gained by over-simplification of the patient and family system's complex dynamics, and by discounting individuals' unique characters, temperamental strengths, aspirations and resources. Some recent research strongly suggests that mental health patients most highly value opportunities to discuss and make sense of their symptoms, rather than passively receiving structured services and medication.[17] As Perkins and Repper assert,[18] mental health service users generally prefer 'alliance, not compliance'. Full collaboration with patients and families is based on the establishment of partnerships, or therapeutic alliances,[19] not dependence on professionals, however benign or well meaning their presentations of themselves and their service.

COMPONENTS OF COLLABORATION

Hoyt describes three factors considered essential components of effective collaboration:[20]

1 **Alliance**: being able to sublimate one's own professional concerns within a genuine partnership; being prepared to work *with* the other person's goals, formulations, preferences etc., not labouring *on* their symptoms or social deficits; nor aiming

interventions *at* their illness (the aggressive metaphor suggests one source of the potential resistance that can be induced by subliminally authoritarian clinical styles). A meta-analytic survey of 24 separate studies identified three characteristics of effective therapeutic alliances:[21]
   - The client believes in the relevance of the shared problem formulation and the effectiveness of suggested treatment options.
   - The client and professional agree on both the necessary and likely short and medium term expectations of care.
   - An affective component; a warm relationship based upon a professional ability to appear caring, sensitive and sympathetic.

2 **Evocation of resourcefulness**: being mindful that the person (however much apparently disabled by events or symptoms) has acquired abilities, intelligence, experience, skills and positive attributes. Nurses should attempt to mobilize and maximize these residual abilities, rather than risk colluding with patients' disowning their worth. To simply fulfil people's regressive needs for dependency may satisfy nurses' needs for approval, respect etc. but may not be in service users' best long-term interests. From a nursing point of view, this factor suggests it is unhelpful to inculcate in users a sense of passivity – being subjected to treatment and control – rather than an expectation of active participation. We should establish clinical cultures wherein people feel they are *working* with staff on their problems, rather than being treated, trained and restrained.

3 **Achievable therapeutic goals**: Ideally *we* (the professionals) should be in search of *their* (the users') solutions. Psychiatrically defined clinical outcomes may be appropriate for drug trials, but often bear little relevance to the demands of ordinary life. For many people, complete loss of symptoms or absolute cessation of problem behaviour may be impracticable. The *solution-focused* approach to problem-solving[22] represents one practical example of effective collaborative goal-setting. Each goal should be something that matters to the individual, not simply to the treatment team. Goals should be small enough to achieve, and stated in clear, operational terms, so that the person will know when they have achieved their intention. Each goal should be checked against other aspects of the person's private life or social ecology, lest an apparently desirable gain in one area of personal functioning cause a corresponding breakdown in some other significant relationship.

Recently developed frameworks for psychiatric-mental health nursing such as the 'Tidal Model' [23] and aspects of the Sainsbury Centre's 'Acute Solutions' project[24] incorporate elements of all the above three factors. The 'Tidal Model' advocates an essentially curious and un-dogmatic stance towards people's problems that privileges the user's own account of distress; personal meanings derived from their subjective experiences; and preferred solutions to their difficulties over 'off-the-shelf' psychiatric formulations. It also presupposes that people's situations are fluidly dynamic, and that problem-status changes frequently – often several times in the course of a day, especially when enjoying or enduring active, collaborative care. This means that rigid or stagnant 'care plans' that conventionally remain unchanged for weeks or months are little use. The nurse–patient partnership should collaboratively review and rewrite care plans as often as understanding of the person's difficulties and potential solutions changes. Such apparently professionally subordinate approaches could be construed as irresponsible collusion or cowardly failure to promote clinical insights and professional expertise. However it rarely helps to dismiss the validity of people's actions or beliefs (e.g. suicidal behaviour redefined as a cry for help; or discounting the experiential evidence for delusional thought). Psychological distress and disorder may involve misinterpretation of events and situations, but the phenomena themselves are not usually wrongly recalled.[25]

Case study 16.1

Joan was diagnosed as suffering from a schizo-affective disorder and deemed by her psychiatrist and the ward staff to be deluded, as she insisted that she was being poisoned by the medication she was being compelled to take. Joan distrusted ECT because she believed that the anaesthetic and muscle-relaxant were also poison. One nurse thought Joan's claims made sense, and that she may be suffering from unsettling side-effects. The staff discounted the idea of using a tool like LUNSERS as they deemed Joan too disturbed to answer the questions properly. The dissenting nurse thought that Joan's agitated, anxious restlessness may well be a form of akathesia and despite her colleagues' scorn, requested a visit from the pharmacist. He confirmed that Joan was suffering from her medication and recommended a more suitable prescription.

Case study 16.2

Mrs Chidgey was a middle-aged lady from a superficially jolly and supportive farming family who regularly if infrequently broke down and was well-known to staff as a relapsing paranoid schizophrenic. One of the symptoms of her illness was her belief – identified by staff as a recurrent delusion – that her husband and daughter (aged 19) slept together whenever Mrs Chidgey was away. This lady's illness had for many years been only partly effectively treated by neuroleptic medication of various kinds, until the family moved and came under the clinical responsibility of a clinical team that advocated family-based approaches to all clinical referrals. After a few sessions of therapy, it transpired that members of the family often shared the parents' large bed when either spouse was alone, and especially when mum was in hospital and the family felt distressed. To the rest of the family, it had never been a secret, nor even an issue, but had never previously been clinically broached.

Collaboration is an integral part of a *therapeutic alliance*. Zetzel[26] coined this term, analogous with nursing's more customary *therapeutic relationship*, five years after Carl Rogers' classic account of *client-centred therapy*[27] gave the humanistic creed its clearest clinical formulation: that empathic understanding, genuineness (congruence) and acceptance (warmth or unconditional positive regard) are not only essential components of caring, but also sufficient conditions of care and treatment for people to begin to recover or change.[28]

Rogers' connection between *acceptance* and *change* is echoed by recent strategies for working with seriously personality disordered people. Marsha Linehan identifies 'acceptance versus change' as one of the key paradoxical tensions or *dialectics* that professional staff need to maintain in their work with damaged personalities.[29] Linehan uses the term 'validation' to refer to the professional's deeply held conviction that a patient's pathological, self-damaging or aggressively sabotaging behaviour should be responded to by understanding it as making sense from within the person's current situation, emotional status and belief system. Last century, the psychologist George Kelly insisted that humans are essentially personal scientists, who attempt to create hypotheses or constructs that make sense of their experience, and behave accordingly.[30] Following Kelly's insights, systemic family therapy teams have long embraced the idea that people's apparently pathological behaviours could be interpreted as 'attempted solutions' to underlying psychological, interpersonal or socio-economic problems.[31]

Case study 16.3

Mrs Smith was referred to the Day Hospital diagnosed as suffering from an obsessional-compulsive disorder. In the words of her psychiatrist, she 'exhibited trichotillomania'. Mrs Smith spent hours each day trying to achieve absolute symmetry by plucking single hairs from two almost perfectly circular bald patches she had created above her forehead. Despite his wife's obvious distress, Mr Smith would leave home each day for work, and Mrs Smith's mother would usually come around to help her daughter settle her anxiety by measuring the diameter of the bald patches. Sympathetic and curious nurses at the Day Hospital soon learnt that Mrs Smith had felt lonely and unloved for many years; was terrified of going out alone; and felt unable to discuss her feelings with her rather taciturn husband. Her hair-pulling, far from worrying or annoying her husband seemed to have gained some pity, perhaps confirming his sense of masculine superiority and role of provider. It also led to a rare agreement between Mr Smith and his mother-in-law, and re-established a strong supportive bond between daughter and mother.

NOT ALL IN THE MIND

Despite the common-sense validity of Zubin and Spring's 'stress-vulnerability' formulation,[15] psychiatric custom and practice tends to locate the source of difficulties primarily within the patient's disease – people suffer because they are ill and therefore vulnerable. However, a genuinely collaborative account of problem-development and resolution would focus attention at least equally on the other side of the equation – the objective stress that people suffer. (This approach is increasingly established in family work, especially for those families that include individuals diagnosed as schizophrenic. Aspects of the diagnosed person's behaviour comprise potent stressors for close kin, whilst other family members are reciprocally construed as potentially stressing their vulnerable relative by excessive criticism, hostility or emotional over-involvement.)

In attempting to accurately attribute the causes of illness behaviour, traditional psychiatric formulations may overstate personal, individual, internally located factors (such as genetic defect, constitutional weakness, personality type or organic pathology) and underestimate the significance of situational, objective, externally located causes (such as social deprivation, economic difficulty, interpersonal abuse or cultural alienation). Collaborative nursing can help to correct this imbalance by not discounting a person's own perceptions and understanding of their circumstances and by deeply validating their struggles to cope with life's very real pressures and stresses. Professionals can resist imposing their own clinical priorities and problem-definitions, but instead work with clients to identify and prioritize their own, often more mundane, needs and aspirations. By practical collaboration and liaison

with other professionals and agencies, nurses can help people with important practicalities like benefits, accommodation difficulties, neighbourhood disputes etc. Furthermore, there is evidence that nurses who are empowered to directly perform helpful tasks themselves by working with their patients on such jobs as simple DIY, decorating, shopping could achieve stronger therapeutic alliances by embedding the relationship in more immediately productive soil than the potentially sterile clay of clinical and administrative procedures alone.[32]

The psychologist David Smail employs this kind of argument to substantiate a rigorous critique of specific models of psychotherapy. Smail[33,34] claims that people need effective, practical assistance to deal with the very real difficulties they encounter in life. Whenever psychotherapeutic care seems effective, it is because individuals indirectly obtain three important resources:

❏ *Comfort*,
❏ *Clarification* and
❏ *Encouragement*.

'**Comfort**' refers to the therapist offering support and personal validation – aspects of what Hoyt[20] refers to as 'alliance'; Linehan[29] believes vital to effective helping; and Rogers calls 'unconditional positive regard' and warmth – two of the 'necessary and sufficient conditions for change'.[28] In nursing terms, a collaborative relationship requires the nurse to care *about* as well as *for* the person. This is not always easy to maintain, and certainly cannot be achieved simply by reciting a nursing creed of moral imperatives to be kind at all times. It requires the nurse to confront his or her own emotional needs, and clarify reactions and responses to patients and clinical interaction through deep personal reflection and supervision.

'**Clarification**' refers to some explanation of how the person's problems originated and developed. Such explanatory theories of psychopathology or life-difficulties exist but differ in every school of psychotherapy, regardless of effectiveness. People need a story about their life that makes sense, and especially a narrative thread that could suggest a pathway out of their current difficulties. Some highly collaborative forms of therapy for psychosis based on narrative exploration and reconstruction exploit this insight,[20,35,36] which lends itself readily to conversational application by mental health nurses.

'**Encouragement**' refers to the ongoing support, confrontation, guidance and reinforcement that needs to accompany an individual's attempts to dare to be different or attempt another way of behaving, either specifically or in general, once problem-maintenance factors and potential solutions have become clearer. Equally, encouragement may be needed to help people tolerate or cope with socio-economic circumstances that remain stubbornly immune to practical efforts to improve them. Recently, assertive outreach schemes have devised increasingly creative and flexible means of practical encouragement, unashamedly offering rewards to help people work on towards goals (like medication compliance or obtaining employment) that may be proving difficult or when the struggle becomes temporarily more painful (as when a relationship deteriorates, symptoms flare-up or side-effects feel crippling) (see Table 16.1).[37]

TABLE 16.1 Elements of collaborative conversation

Rogers' 'Necessary and sufficient conditions for change'[a]	Smail's 'Components of psychotherapy'[b]	Hulme's 'Aims of collaborative conversation'[c]
Unconditional positive regard and warmth	**Comfort (or solidarity)**	**Reflection (not drowning)**
'A non-possessive caring acceptance of the client, irrespective of how offensive the person's behaviour might be. Unconditional positive regard helps to create a climate that encourages trust.' 'Conditional regard implies enforced control and compliance dictated by someone else.' 'Non-possessive warmth springs from an attitude of friendliness, is liberating and non-demanding.'[d]	'The comfort to be derived from sharing your deepest fears and most shameful secrets with a 'valued other' who listens patiently is one of the most potently therapeutic experiences to be had.' 'Comfort does not cure anything. The provision of therapeutic comfort is not unlike administering short-acting tranquillizers – it works, is addictive, but it will have to be withdrawn sooner or later.'[b]	'When we are drowning in our experiences we are unable to separate ourselves from them. They govern us completely.' 'Reflection is the capacity to separate consciousness from its contents. We can step back, inspect and think about our experiences. We become capable of changing our relationship with them and altering their meanings for us.'[c]
Genuineness (congruence)	**Clarification**	**Relativism (not dogmatism)**
'The degree to which we are freely and deeply ourselves and are able to relate to people in a sincere and undefensive manner.' 'Genuineness encourages client self-disclosure, while appropriate therapist disclosure enhances genuineness.'[d] 'Genuineness entails meaning what you say and do. It does not necessarily entail revealing all that you think. Paul Halmos wrote about being 'a vessel of honesty floating on a sea of concern'.[e]	'The point of establishing how you got to be the way you are is to disabuse yourself of mistaken explanations, not the least of which is that you are responsible for it.' 'People are often mystified about the causes of their suffering, and an important aspect of their coming to understand what they can and cannot do about their predicament is to be demystified'.[b]	'Dogmatism is to beliefs what drowning is to experiences.' 'In the absence of doubt there is little incentive to change one's mind about anything: we do not hesitate to put our beliefs into immediate action when the situation seems to demand it.' 'The antidote to dogmatism is relativism … We acknowledge that we have no monopoly on the truth, that we understand and experience the world at best imperfectly from a particular viewpoint or perspective.'[c]
Empathy	**Encouragement**	**Relatedness (not disowning)**
'The ability to step into the inner world of another person and out again.' 'Empathy is trying to understand another's thoughts, feelings, behaviours and personal meanings from their own internal reference frame.' 'For empathy we have to respond in such a way that the other person feels understood, or that understanding is being striven for.' 'Empathy is a transient thing. We can lose it very quickly.' Literally it means 'getting alongside'.[d]	'Nothing will ever change the need for human solidarity, whatever form it comes in.' 'The courage needed for a tiny powerless organism to take a chance on the nature of its reality must be colossal, and can only be acquired through a process of encouragement, in which loving recognition of the uniqueness of the baby's perspective is central to the nurture and instruction offered.'[b]	'When we disown aspects of our experience they do not necessarily cease to influence what we feel, think and do. We disown experiences that would otherwise engulf us. We disown conclusions that conflict with cherished beliefs.' 'Relatedness is the capacity to consciously acknowledge and relate to what we are experiencing. Without the capacity to own and reflect we remain helpless victims of our own inner life.'[c]

[a]Rogers C. *On becoming a person: A therapist's view of psychotherapy*. London: Constable, 1967.
[b]Smail D. *How to survive without psychotherapy*. London: Constable, 1996.
[c]Hulme P. 'Collaborative conversation'. In: Newnes C, Holmes G, Dunn C (eds). *This is madness*. Ross-on-Wye: PCCS Books, 1999.
[d]Stewart W. *An A–Z of counselling theory and practice*, 2nd edn. Cheltenham: Stanley Thornes, 1997.
[e]Halmos P. *The faith of the counsellors*. London: Constable, 1978.

COLLABORATIVE CONVERSATIONS: BEING USEFUL WHEN PEOPLE WANT TO TALK

Peter Hulme[38] has outlined a useful framework for developing collaboration within a normalizing conversational approach to psychiatric-mental health nursing. Hulme criticizes the potentially oppressive rigidity of many conventional psychiatric formulations and expands Smail's notions about the importance of 'clarification', 'solidarity' and 'encouragement'. Both mental health professionals and distressed people in need of care often become too psychologically inflexible and rigid. Psychiatric beliefs, behaviours and attitudes are sometimes just as obstinate and unhelpful as so-called delusions, compulsions or depressions. Hulme uses the phrase 'collaborative conversation' to describe the context in which fixed beliefs, habits and feelings on both sides can begin to be dissolved away and replaced with more expansive possibilities. There are three elements of such *collaborative conversations*:

❏ Reflection, Not Drowning;
❏ Relativism, Not Dogmatism;
❏ Relatedness, Not Disowning.

Reflection, Not Drowning

Rather than experience themselves 'drowning' in overwhelming difficulties, people need to be able to separate themselves temporarily from their lives; to separate their consciousness from chaotic experience and learn to *reflect* upon their situation. Collaborative conversation aims to help people feel a sense of rescue, so that the absolute (and usually apparently awful) nature of truth and reality can be considered more calmly and other possible meanings and perspectives explored. Distressed people can be aided to achieve this by experiencing the reflective calm of their potential rescuer. Sometimes, especially when faced with chaotic acting-out or threatened violence, it may be necessary for professional nurses to 'act-as-if' and non-verbally feign such confident detachment, while verbally acknowledging the apparently extreme mess that their dependent partner is experiencing.

Relativism, Not Dogmatism

Secondly, it is helpful if both nurse and patient can cease to rely upon deeply engrained certainties or 'dogmatism' and challenge their own beliefs or assumptions about themselves and their world. Nurses can help people generate alternative explanations and even point out unusual beliefs that might initially uncomfortably challenge previously unshakeable world-views. Paradoxically, the emerging possibility of doubt can be a step towards greater autonomy, freeing people from the usually unhelpful rigidity that has previously characterized their personalities. The development of such doubt and the consequent *relativism* helps dissolve unhelpful beliefs in the same way as reflection helps us to cope with difficult experiences.

Relatedness, Not Disowning

Thirdly, people often blame others for their difficulties long after any original damage may have been done to them. They deny any destructive, defective or negative attitudes on their own part; or simply refuse to face-up to consequences, connections or causes. People need help to discern and accept the connections, patterns or relationships between external events and their internal feelings and thoughts. They also need to learn how their subsequent behaviours are interpreted or construed by others and how these constructs then determine reciprocal behavioural responses that may in turn generate further hurt and misunderstanding, or elicit other negative emotional reactions. This *relatedness* is the undermining challenge to 'disowning', and brings denied problems or solutions back into focus, and thence into possible reconstruction and resolution (see Table 16.1).

BETTER THAN COLD WAR: THERAPEUTIC COMMUNITIES AS COLLABORATIVE ENVIRONMENTS

A common emphasis in psychiatric nursing is to identify and locate problems *inside* people, rather than within relationships (*between* people) or between people and real life (*around* people). This emphasis can create obstacles to progress and personal growth, if that includes coming to terms with *relatedness* and the reciprocal effects of emotion, thinking and behaviour within relationships. Shared clinical environments, whether residential units or day-centres, can usefully provide opportunities for socially reinforced learning provided that people are allowed some scope for expressing their difficulties and supported in receiving feedback from others about their behaviour. Patients can be helped to collaborate with each other's efforts to gain personal control and work towards recovery, rather than simply accept treatment passively from the professionals. This is after all what goes on informally and often surreptitiously within the subcultures of dormitory and smoking room. Nurses sometimes feel excluded from this community, and mistrust it, or feel unable to incorporate its potential benefits into the formal matrix of care.[39]

Outside of conventional psychiatric service organization, with its emphasis on one-to-one nurse–patient or psychotherapeutic relationships, perhaps the best example of shared collaborative responsibility is found within the various *therapeutic community* models of treatment.[40] This model of recovery-based mental health care grew from the military hospitals caring for soldiers damaged by the stress of the Second World War. Hierarchies of patients and professionals were abandoned and replaced by a communal, democratic model of organization, planning, decision-making and problem-solving. In most models of therapeutic community practice, staff as far as possible abandon their clinical authority (although they do not entirely abdicate it, but rather hold it in abeyance) until forceful prescriptive interventions are essential to prevent serious harm. Staff and patients alike are expected to both support and confront people with observations and interpretations of ordinary, everyday acted-out behaviour, so that social, interpersonal and intra-psychic learning is maximized and opportunities to avoid the implications of dysfunctional or damaging personal traits all but disappear. Responsibility for all aspects of day-to-day functioning are shared, and the community becomes in effect a socio-psychological clinical laboratory for clarification of problems and a testing-ground for more constructive behaviour.[41] This model of care thrived during the 1960s and 1970s, but shrank considerably during the 1980s and 1990s, as the political climate in the U.K. and overseas swung from co-operative communal, social or municipal models of progress to embrace more competitive, individualistic ideals. The use of so-called 'community meetings' on some clinical units represents a vestigial survival of therapeutic community practice. Unfortunately modern management procedures, confused treatment ideologies and rigid clinical hierarchies often mean that these meetings are shorn of their full democratic status. Instead of being a forum for dynamic problem-solving and collective decision-making, the community meeting's purpose often seems more a symbolic means of enforcing staff authority than an exercise in therapeutic liberalism. It has become a mechanism for staff announcements; ordering meals and complaining about food; and apportioning blame or punishment for overnight acting-out. Recently however, the drive to develop effective methods of helping people with severely disordered personalities has brought therapeutic community philosophy and practices back into political favour. The same principles could reinvigorate community-based acute and rehabilitation units.[42]

THE SICK SELF AND OTHERS: COLLABORATING WITH FAMILIES

When working with families collaboration becomes even more problematic, multi-dimensional and full of

potential pit-falls. Even when working individually, in an ecological sense nurses are usually and often unawarely working with the front-end of at least one family – a complex human system of friends and relatives. Families of people needing psychiatric services are rarely harmonious collectives. Behind each individual referral, there is usually a long history of grief and worry; emotional and social difficulties; pain and disappointment or conflict and recriminations. How can nurses collaborate with every part of an internally conflicted system?

Case study 16.4

An on-call nurse in a community mental helath centre received a demanding phone call from an angry father 'You'd better get round here now and sort my daughter out – she's gone mental'. The nurse was refused permissed to talk to the daughter herself. After their GP was contacted and made a referral, the family were offered a day-time appointment but instead turned up at the CMHC that evening when only the Crisis Team remained on duty. The daughter, a 17-year-old schoolgirl, seemed distraught, and collapsed when told that the family should keep the appointment they had been offered. A nurse from the Team took the girl, Lisa, away and spoke to her alone for over an hour, while a colleague interviewed her parents.

Lisa was a bright highly achieving A-level student, but confessed to being 'totally at the end' and unable to stay at home 'It's doing my head in'. She'd been thinking about suicide, and yesterday had cut her arms superficially and packed a case to leave home – thus prompting the phone call to the CMHC from her father. Lisa described an atmosphere of constant hostility between her father and mother, with father bearing the brunt of mother's frequent violent rages, supposedly to stop her beating her own daughter. She was unable to identify a just reason for this rage, except that mum had had a 'terrible childhood – full of sexual abuse and that'. Dad had begged her never to leave home, as 'that would kill your mother' and he himself would be broken hearted. Lisa felt that she had to stay at home to prevent real harm coming to either parent, but at the same time dreaded staying for her own psychological and physical health.

Functional analyses of family systems suggest that effective communication is one of the most important components of healthy families.[43, 44] Other key functions include affective responsiveness; emotional involvement; problem-solving; behaviour control; and allocation of roles and responsibilities.[43] Families that manage their own problems and seem to require little outside help demonstrate clear, direct communication patterns. When members of healthy families need to express their feelings, or achieve a particular task, they generally seem to understand what role they and others have in the situation, and speak directly to involved relatives in a lucid, unambiguous manner.[44,45] After years of traumatic stress, families with difficulties often manifest the opposite characteristics – they have fragile, permeable or impenetrable personal boundaries; show limited abilities to deal responsively with each other's emotions, and can tolerate only a restricted range or intensity of feelings. Fractured, unclear or indirect communications characterize their interactions. People make faulty assumptions about the meaning of other's behaviour. They impute thoughts, feelings or motives that mismatch each other's beliefs about themselves, and then react to each other on the basis of these erroneous assumptions, thus establishing self-fulfilling spirals of distorted attitudes and interactions which over time become deeply engrained. The 'bow-tie' method of graphically depicting communication circularities is a simple heuristic devise that can sometimes dramatically clarify apparently bafflingly complex family interactions [46] (see Figure 16.1). Nurses can help families to consider each other's thoughts and behaviour differently, and identify new possibilities for tolerance, shared feelings or problem-solving, by helping them to clarify vague or mismanaged communications between individuals.

Nurse:	'So Lisa, when you see Mum being so wild with Dad, what do you think, or how do you feel?'
Lisa:	'I feel angry with her, frightened for him, and I feel so stuck, I want to die.'
Nurse:	'and what do you actually do then, when you feel all that?'
Lisa:	'I usually go to my room, and cry.'
Nurse:	'How does Lisa's withdrawl and tears affect you, Mrs Jones?'
Mrs Jones:	'I feel guilty, of course I do, but it seems unfair as well – I get even angrier with John.'
Nurse:	'And what do you do when you feel guilty?'
Mrs Jones:	'I try to talk with Lisa about my frustration and tell her I'm sorry, but I always end up going off at her again.'
Nurse:	'What's that like, Lisa?'
Lisa:	'I'm sure she wants me dead, or different, but I can only be me.'
Nurse:	'Mr Jones – do you think that your wife wants Lisa dead or different?'
Mr Jones:	'I know she doesn't, but it must seem that way to Lisa.'
Nurse:	'A diagram of how this works out between you might make it clearer to me. Would you mind if we sketched it on paper? So, Lisa how does mum's nagging affect you again?'
Lisa:	'I think she hates me, and I want to get away – but I worry about dad.' ... See Figure 16.1 ...
Nurse:	'That's really very sad. How can you help each other with this fear that Mr Jones is no good, and Lisa could become like her?'

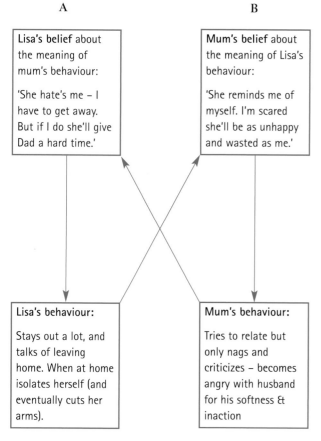

FIGURE 16.1: A's belief about B governs A's behaviour, which justifies B's belief about A, which governs B's behaviour, which justifies A's belief, which ...

On giants' shoulders – paying one's clinical dues

Recently family management-based Thorn courses and PSI training schemes have become popular with clinicians, managers and nursing educators. These programmes emphasize medication compliance strategies; educating people about relevant psychiatric diagnoses; enhancing people's preferred coping methods; teaching and applying problem-solving techniques; and altering family communication patterns. However, many collaborative strategies for working with families predate these developments. Although some family therapists have since been accused of unhelpfully detached authoritarianism,[47] many early pioneers stressed the necessity of making good relationships not only with the family as a whole, but also with each individual member. Salvador Minuchin described the processes of 'joining' and 'accommodation' that professionals need to negotiate successfully when engaging with families.[48] 'Joining' a family involves accepting its unique organization and blending with its cultural style. Nurses should adjust their own self-presentation (or 'accommodate') to achieve effective joining. Maintaining a formal, stereotyped, professional image is less important than gaining the families trust and being allowed to experience their pain, pleasure and possibilities at first hand. Nurses should consciously allow spontaneous, natural imitation of communication (or 'mimesis') to help facilitate accommodation, and follow (or 'track') family conversational threads and themes, rather than stick doggedly to pre-set questioning or interview formats. Minuchin also felt it essential to maintain 'balance' within the therapeutic system, so that whenever he supported one member over a particular issue, he would seek an early opportunity to ally with other members who might have felt their point of view disregarded. Nurses can adapt such techniques within their unique professional matrix to therapeutically transform the kind of social, conversational or more formal, organizational role-bound interactions that many have with patients and their relatives.

Jay Haley outlined a structure for conducting first and subsequent meetings with families.[49] He emphasized the importance of beginning the session with a 'social phase' during which the professional can make contact and engage with each member in turn by being genuinely interested in positive aspects of their life and personality, separate from any discussion of the family's problems. This phase is followed by a 'problem' stage in which each family member is invited to contribute their perspective on the family's difficulties and his or her preferred outcomes. Nurses need to be respectful of each person's contributions, and firm enough to conduct the session by facilitating other family members' listening while each person speaks. During the third 'interaction' stage the family is encouraged to talk together to share observations on a specific issue; understand each other's perspectives or behaviour; and start to identify shared viewpoints or resolutions. Nurses need to be ready to intervene during this stage to maintain balance, prevent 'scape-goating' or other damaging interactions and ensure that family members continue to listen to their relatives. During the final 'goal-setting' stage, nurse and family collaborate to identify, clarify and plan behavioural tasks and contracts involving all relevant family members in constructive change or support. Haley's framework offers nurses a structure to make more productive use of family meetings in both residential and sessional environments.

Collaborative conflict

Even with very careful attention to joint engagement, professionals can develop distorted perceptions of family processes, determined not only by their clinical orienta-

tion, therapeutic belief system and working practices but also by their own personality development and family experiences. Any unexplored or disowned aspects of self; personality rigidity; or prejudicial narrowness in professional education or cultural background may predispose a clinician to non-collaborative practice of one kind or another. Similarly, defensive interpersonal behaviours may stimulate emotional reactions in either nurses or clients; and unmet emotional needs may result in parataxic or projective distortion of working relationships. Regular personal supervision and staff sensitivity or support meetings are necessary if nurses are to avoid being disabled by unresolved needs or negativity.

Just as families (and individuals) are often internally riven with conflict, so also the history of working clinically with families demonstrates considerable theoretical and methodological dispute. Some forms of family therapy have been accused of 'blaming' families for the plight of a sick member,[10] whilst family management practitioners have been indicted for unnecessarily pathologizing vulnerable members and hypocritically deceiving relatives.[50] The diagnosis of schizophrenia has been an especial focus of disagreement.[51] As mentioned above, a useful concept deriving from early family therapy theory involves construing all family members' apparently pathological or unhelpful behaviours as 'attempted solutions' to perceived or underlying problems. The strangeness of a young schizophrenic may be interpreted as the result of efforts to escape the stifling conformity of a rigidly judgemental family culture[52] or simply but stubbornly create a different culture more suited to the individual's emerging personality.[53] Violent tantrums, bizarre behaviour, withdrawal or suicidal acts may all serve the purpose of detouring conflict – focusing attention and concern onto an apparently disturbed individual and away from unexpressed or unresolved conflict between other family members.[46] Equally, a family's displays of strongly judgemental criticism or hostility may reveal evidence of ambivalent grief or frustrated weariness, developed after years of ineffectual care and concern for a sick relative. Their well-meaning efforts may have been reacted to by resentment or rejection. They may have failed to dissuade an unwell relative from reckless deviance, unhappily odd preoccupations or dangerously careless behaviours. The family may desperately want to persuade the unwell member to conform to social or behavioural codes they sincerely believe to be better for their relative's welfare.[54]

All kinds of interpretation can fit the complex dynamics of a family in crisis. They are not mutually exclusive or contradictory.[55] However, it is precisely this kind of difference in perspectives that has resulted in recrimination between clinicians from different schools of professional family work. *Family therapy* theories construe families as complex organic systems. Diagnosed pathology in an individual may be understood as the result of chronic pressure or conflict within the whole family system revealing itself by breakdown of the most vulnerable family member. *Family management* theories view the situation from the other end, and assume *a priori* the existence of disease in one individual. The unwell family member's relatives experience chronic stress, anxiety, frustration or grief. This in turn induces weariness, compassion fatigue or unhelpful responses such as excessive criticism, hostility or emotional over-involvement.[56] Bennun[57] provides a brief exploration of issues around these dichotomous approaches. In both cases, however, therapeutic progress is made by helping the family to change some aspect of its structure or function; either because the family itself is seen as the primary unit of pathology; or because it has become less than optimally beneficial for all its members and ineffectively supportive as a caring network.[55] Whatever psycho-pathological perspective a clinical team works from, nurses should work to ensure that families experience a user-friendly service. Nurses can establish more informal, responsive relationships with both patients and relatives and avoid the arrogant dogmatism and technical excesses that have bedevilled various schools of family work.[47] Nurses can use their relationships with both diagnosed individual and family relatives to work towards helping family members collaborate more with each other. Alternatively, there is a risk that nurses who remain unmindful of or insensitive to significant family dynamics may develop relationships with either diagnosed patients or family carers that mimic the debilitating effects of high expressed emotion. They may themselves become hostile critics; over-involved and emotionally invasive,[58] or ally with one part of the family against another.[59]

REFERENCES

1. Department of Health. *Modernising mental health services: safe, sound, supportive*. London: Department of Health, 1999.
2. Standing Nursing and Midwifery Advisory Committee. *Addressing acute concerns*. London: Department of Health, 1999.
3. Department of Health. *National Health Service Reform and Health Care Professions Bill*. London: The Stationery Office, 2001.
4. British Psychological Society Division of Clinical Psychology. *Recent advances in understanding mental illness and psychotic experiences*. London: British Psychological Society, 2000.
5. Department of Health. *Treatment choice in psychological therapies and counselling: evidence based clinical practice guideline*. London: Department of Health, 2001.
6. Frank AF, Gunderson JG. The role of the therapeutic alliance in the treatment of schizophrenia: Relationship to course and outcome. *Archives of General Psychiatry* 1990; **47**: 228–36.
7. Roth A, Fonagy P. *What works for whom?* New York: Guilford Press, 1996.
8. Rose D. *Users' voices*. London: Sainsbury Centre for Mental Health, 2001.
9. Corry P. *Care before compulsion: charter for consensual treatment*. London: Mental Health Alliance, 2001.
10. Kuipers L, Leff J, Lam D. *Family work for schizophrenia*. London: Royal College of Psychiatrists/Gaskell, 1992.
11. Sarafino EP. *Health psychology: biopsycho-social interactions*, 2nd edn. New York: John Wiley, 1994.
12. Widgery D. *Some lives*. London: Simon and Schuster, 1993.
13. Coppock V, Hopton J. *Critical perspectives on mental health*. London: Routledge, 2000.
14. Keene J. *Clients with complex needs*. Oxford: Blackwell Science, 2001.
15. Zubin J, Spring B. Vulnerability – a new view of schizophrenia. *Journal of Abnormal Psychology* 1977; **86**: 103–26.
16. Ciompi L. Affect logic: an integrative model of the psyche and its relations to schizophrenia. *British Journal of Psychiatry* 1994; **164** (suppl. 23): 51–7.
17. Faulkner A. *Strategies for living*. London: Mental Health Foundation, 2000.
18. Perkins R, Repper J. *Dilemmas in community mental health practice: choice or control?* Oxford: Radcliffe Medical Press, 1998.
19. Watkins P. *Psychiatric-mental health nursing: the art of compassionate care*. Oxford: Butterworth-Heinemann, 2001.
20. Hoyt MF. *Some stories are better than others: doing what works in brief therapy and managed care*. Philadelphia: Brunner-Mazel, 2000.
21. Horvath AO, Symonds BD. Relation between working alliance and outcome in psychotherapy. *Journal of Consulting and Clinical Psychology* 1993; **38**: 139–49.
22. De Shazer S. *Clues: investigating solutions in brief therapy*. New York: Norton, 1988.
23. Barker P. The Tidal Model: developing an empowering, person-centred approach to recovery within psychiatric and psychiatric-mental health nursing. *Journal of Psychiatric and Psychiatric-Mental Health Nursing* 2001; **8**: 233–40.
24. Warner L. *Acute inpatient care*. London: Sainsbury Centre for Mental Health, 2001.
25. Chadwick P. *Schizophrenia: the positive perspective*. London: Routledge, 1997.
26. Zetzel ER. Current concepts of transference. *International Journal of Psychoanalysis* 1956; **37**: 369–76.

27. Rogers C. *Client-centred therapy*. Cambridge, MA: Riverside Press, 1951.

28. Rogers C. *On becoming a person: a therapist's view of psychotherapy*. London: Constable, 1967.

29. Linehan MM. *Cognitive-behavioral treatment of borderline personality*. New York: Guilford Press, 1993.

30. Kelly G. *A theory of personality: the psychology of personal constructs*. New York: Norton, 1963.

31. Watzlawick P, Weakland L, Fisch R. *Change: principles of problem formation and problem resolution*. New York: Norton, 1974.

32. Perkins R, Repper J. *Working alongside people with long-term mental health problems*. Cheltenham: Stanley Thornes, 1997.

33. Smail D. *The origins of unhappiness: a new understanding of personal distress*. London: Constable, 1993.

34. Smail D. *How to survive without psychotherapy*. London: Constable, 1996.

35. White M, Epston D. *Narrative means to therapeutic ends*. New York: W.W. Norton, 1990.

36. Gilligan S, Price R (eds). *Therapeutic conversations*. New York: W.W. Norton, 1993.

37. Sainsbury Centre for Mental Health. *Keys to engagement: review of care for people with severe mental illness who are hard to engage with services*. London: Sainsbury Centre for Mental Health, 1998.

38. Hulme P. 'Collaborative conversation'. In: Newnes C, Holmes G, Dunn C (eds). *This is madness*. Ross-on-Wye: PCCS Books, 1999.

39. Griffiths P, Pringle P. *Cassell Monograph No. 1: Psycho-social practice within a residential setting*. London: Karnac, 1997.

40. Kennard D. *Introduction to Therapeutic Communities*. London: Jessica Kingsley, 1999.

41. Hinshelwood RD. *Thinking about institutions*. London: Jessica Kingsley, 2001.

42. Barnes T. The legacy of therapeutic community practice in modern community mental health services. *Therapeutic Communities* 2000; **21**, 165–74.

43. Epstein NB, Bishop D, Ryan C, Miller D, Keitner G. The McMaster Model view of healthy family functioning. In: Walsh F (ed.) *Normal family processes*. New York: Guilford Press, 1993: 138–60.

44. Cleese J, Skynner R. *Families and how to survive them*. London: Methuen, 1983.

45. Beavers R. *Successful families*. New York: Norton, 1990.

46. Dallos R. *Family belief systems, therapy and change*, 2nd edn. Milton Keynes: Open University Press, 1994.

47. Treacher A, Carpenter J. User-friendly family therapy. In: Carpenter J, Treacher A. *Using family therapy in the nineties*. Oxford: Blackwell, 1993.

48. Minuchin S. *Families and family therapy*. London: Tavistock, 1974.

49. Haley J. *Problem-solving therapy*. San Francisco: Josey-Bass, 1987.

50. Johnstone L. Family management in 'schizophrenia': Its assumptions and contradictions. *Journal of Mental Health* 1993; **2**: 255–69.

51. Keen T. Schizophrenia: orthodoxy and heresies. *Journal of Psychiatric and Psychiatric-Mental Health Nursing* 1999; **6**: 415–24.

52. Laing RD, Esterson A. Sanity, madness and the family. London: Tavistock, 1964.

53. Stevens A, Price J. *Evolutionary psychiatry: a new beginning*, 2nd edn. London: Routledge, 2000.

54. Atkinson J, Coia DA. *Families coping with schizophrenia*. Chichester: Wiley, 1995.

55. Burbach F. Family-based interventions in psychosis – an overview of, and comparison between, family therapy and family management approaches. *Journal of Mental Health* 1996; **5**: 111–34.

56. Leff J, Vaughan C. *Expressed emotion in families*. New York: Guilford Press, 1985.

57. Bennun I. Family management and psychiatric rehabilitation. In: Carpenter J, Treacher A (eds). *Using family therapy in the nineties*. Oxford: Blackwell, 1993.

58. Gamble C. Using a low expressed emotion approach to develop positive therapeutic alliances. In: Gamble C, Brennan G (eds). *Working with serious mental illness: a manual for clinical practice*. London: Baillière Tindall, 2000: 115–23.

59. Goldstein JM, Caton C. The effects of the community environment on psychiatric patients. *Psychological Medicine* 1983; **13**, 193–9.

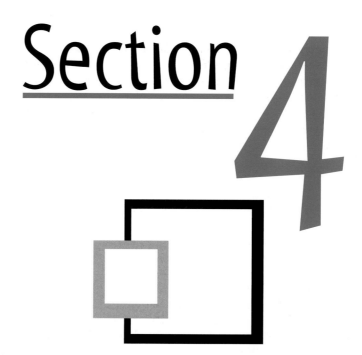

Section 4

Some models of therapeutic practice

Preface to Section 4

A wide range of theories of human nature, conduct and development informs nursing practice. Traditionally, nurses have borrowed from psychology and sociology to provide a frame of reference for the individual patient, in the context of the family and the wider community. However, the key challenge has been to identify a practical mechanism for engaging productively with the individual or the group.

Over the past 50 years a wide range of models has been developed, which serve as templates for the development of ways of relating to people in care and their families and friends. Nursing practice is invariably an intimate relationship, often located in the most ordinary of social surroundings. For this reason we begin our examination of models of therapeutic practice with a consideration of the therapeutic one-to-one relationship, and the development of empathy. If nurses are to get close to the people in their care they need to understand *how* this might be achieved, and they need also to know how to make the person aware that they appreciate the story, which is unfolding.

Most nursing practice is predicated on storytelling, either as an individual encounter or in a small social group. Working with children and adolescents provides special challenges, which illustrate that working with adults, individually or in groups, is different yet often remarkably similar. The next three chapters emphasize the psychodynamic basis of the relationship between nurses and individuals or groups, of whatever age. Nurses need to be aware that the relationship is always mutual and that much of its power is dormant or invisible.

The next three chapters illustrate three broad models of therapeutic practice, which provide different practical ways of shaping the one-to-one or group relationships already described.

The section ends with a consideration of loss, which is both a specific problem of human living, and also a facet of the wider experience of illness, disability and handicap that frames many other problems of living.

Chapter 17

DEVELOPING THERAPEUTIC ONE-TO-ONE RELATIONSHIPS

Bill Reynolds*

INTRODUCTION

The therapeutic nurse–patient relationship is not a nebulous, kind-hearted, well-intentioned relationship. The purpose of the nurse–patient relationship also differs from the purpose of the doctor–nurse relationship and social relationships with friends and chums. The nurse, more than the physician must relate positively to the reaction of patients to illness, including the psychological and social changes that illness force upon the patient. The nurse spends more time with the patient than does the physician, and therefore has more opportunity not only to observe but also to talk with and come to know the patient. Thus the nurse has an opportunity to help the patient become aware of, and make sense of, reactions to illness, particularly in terms of long-term personal consequences.

All nurse–patient contacts provide opportunities to implement the purpose of nursing: to come to know patients as human beings in difficulty, and to help the patients to stretch their capabilities in order to achieve more favourable health outcomes. For the patient, illness can be a source of new learning that can be applied in subsequent life situations. In order to provide this kind of meaningful relationship, the nurse must be a sensitive observer and have a range of theories within which to interpret and extend observations, and on which to base the interpersonal actions of the nurse.

In this chapter the concept of the one-to-one therapeutic relationship in nursing is introduced. Operational definitions of a therapeutic relationship are examined and the aims or purposes of the therapeutic relationship are discussed. It is argued that the therapeutic relationship is the crux of clinical nursing. Practical examples (cases) of the therapeutic relationship in action are provided and evidence supporting the importance of one-to-one relationships to health care outcomes is reviewed.

OPERATIONAL DEFINITIONS OF THE THERAPEUTIC RELATIONSHIP

Therapeutic relationships are the cornerstone of nursing practice with people who are experiencing threats to their health, including, but not restricted to, those people with mental illness. The concept of the therapeutic nurse–patient relationship evolved from the work of Hildagard Peplau in the 1950s.[1] Peplau introduced an interpersonal relations paradigm for the study and practice of nursing that was grounded in the clinical experiences of herself and her graduate students.[2] The

*Bill Reynolds is Reader in Nursing at Turku Polytechnic, Salo, Finland

paradigm held that nurse and patient participate in and contribute to the relationship and, further, that the relationship itself could be therapeutic. Theorists' studying the focus of psychiatric nursing[3] have also acknowledged the importance of the input of the patient in a two-way relationship. They stated that:

> The proper focus of psychiatric nursing is located in the careful (i.e. methodological) examination of the whole lived experience of people in care. This examination demands an active, collaborative relationship between nurse and patient. . . .

The idea that the one-to-one nurse–patient relationship has the potential to influence positive health outcomes for patients, (i.e. is a form of treatment), has been stated in the nursing literature for several decades. Reynolds cites Kalkman, who (in the 1960s) referred to the nurse–patient relationship as relationship therapy.[4] The following description illustrates that view:

> relationship therapy refers to a prolonged relationship between a nurse-therapist and a patient, during which the patient can feel accepted as a person of worth, feels free to express himself/herself without fear of rejection or censure, and enables him/her to learn more satisfactory and productive patterns of behaviour.

The view that the therapeutic nurse–patient relationship should be used to establish an interpersonal climate for nursing assessment and ultimately enable patients to learn more satisfactory and productive patterns of behaviour has prevailed until the present time. For example, it has been suggested that using therapeutic communication, the nurse can begin to assess the individual in crisis[5] and, it has been shown how a non-defensive relationship with nurses relieved embarrassment and anxiety in incontinent patients.[6] This is an important finding since it has been pointed out in the literature that severe anxiety can result in impaired problem-solving ability.[7]

In a similar vein Peplau informs us that anything that is not talked about, merely acted out, is less likely to be understood and addressed by the nurse or the patient.[8] Her theory of interpersonal relations provides an explanation for why people do the things that they do in respect of concepts such as anxiety, negative self-views, and hallucinations. However, the opportunity to assist patients to struggle toward full development of their potential for productive living is dependent upon nurses' ability to understand and apply such concepts within the context of a therapeutic nurse–patient relationship. Evidence supporting the efficacy of the nurse–patient relationship in clinical nursing is considered later in this chapter.

The aims or purposes of the therapeutic relationship

The therapeutic nurse–patient relationship is an important goal for working with individuals in most situations. In spite of the fact that psychiatric or mental health nurses have used Peplau's theory most frequently, the literature shows that it transcends all clinical nursing specialities. This is particularly true of the therapeutic relationship since a great deal of clinical nursing is based on the interpersonal process and relationship that develops between nurse and patient. This point was emphasized recently by an Australian nurse academic[9] who stated that:

> regardless of the apparently different clinical knowledge and skills required to function effectively in different clinical specialities, there is one reliable constant across all nursing settings, and that is the nurse–patient relationship.

Irrespective of the context of the therapeutic relationship, it has the same aims or purposes.[10] These include:

1　Initiating supportive interpersonal communication in order to understand the perceptions and needs of the other person.

2　Empowering the other person to learn, or cope more effectively with their environment.

3　The reduction or resolution of the problems of another person.

The achievement of these aims requires nursing strategies that orientates the patient to the purpose of the relationship, and aids the patient to resolve obstacles that stand in the way of full development and health. Obstacles are primarily of two kinds: (i) disturbances in thought, feeling, and action, which might be called pathological use of one's potential; and (ii) lacks and gaps in the development of intellectual and interpersonal competencies that are essential for healthy social interaction and positive health.[11] The nursing strategies needed to address such matters will facilitate the therapeutic nurse–patient relationship from beginning to end and requires that the nurse attends to the interpersonal processes that occur between nurse and client.

PHASES OF THE THERAPEUTIC RELATIONSHIP

The work of theorists, referred to in this chapter, identifies the nurse–patient relationship as the crux of nursing.[12–14] The early studies of the therapeutic relationship revealed that it evolves through identifiable overlapping phases. The phases include orientation, working, and resolution. The relationship form developed by Forchuk and others.[15] provides an overview of the nurse and patient behaviours at each phase (see Appendix 17.1).

Orientation phase

The initial phase of the relationship is the orientation phase where the nurse and patient comes to know each other as persons and the patient begins to trust the nurse. This phase is sometimes referred to as the strangers phase because the nurse and the patient are strangers to each other. The time in orientation phase can vary from a few minutes of an initial meeting to weeks or months of regular contact. During this phase the nurse is often confronted with interferences or blocks that hinder progression to the working phase of the relationship.

Common interferences are that the patient is unaware of the purpose of the relationship and has not learned to trust the nurse. Patients' confusion about the purpose of the nurse–patient relationship is illustrated by the following patient statements to my students during their clinical work: 'what do you want to talk about nurse?' and, 'I'm not very interesting nurse.' This indicates that the role expectations of the patient are unclear. What goes on between nurses and patients seems to be related to the expectations that each hold of the sick role and nurse role. At the beginning of a new relationship the patient needs to be provided with an explanation for one-to-one contacts. Since the role of the nurse is more diverse and unlike the role of other professionals (who may only provide formal counselling or psychotherapy), patients are often unclear why nurses are talking to them. Since the eventual outcome of the nurse–patient relationship is unknown during orientation phase, it is sufficient to provide a simple explanation that does not produce unrealistic expectations that might not be met. For example:

❑ 'I would like you to talk a bit about yourself as a person. This will help me to understand your needs as you see them and to understand what I can do as a nurse to help you.'

The dialogue arising from providing simple explanations provides the nurse and the patient with an opportunity to assess the 'boundaries' of the relationship, i.e. the purpose and limitations of the relationship.[16] It is also worth remembering that at this stage the patient needs time to learn that the nurse can be trusted. This can be particularly problematic when patients have extensive experience as an inpatient since it has revealed that the number and length of hospitalization is significantly related to movement through orientation phase.[17] During orientation phase the patient is closely watching the nurse. Trust will be established if nurses carry out their stated intentions over a period of time.

Sometimes patients will test out nurses in order to see whether stressors such as hostility and avoidance forces nurses to reject them. The following account (Figure 17.1) from one of my student's diaries describes testing out behaviour.

> ### Case study 17.1
>
> I invited my patient to meet with me for half an hour each day at 10a.m. in a semi-private part of the ward. The explanation that I gave was that it was his time to talk about what was important to him. He agreed to talk but on the first day he didn't turn up. My supervisor told me to stay in the arranged meeting place for the arranged time. On the second day he didn't turn up, but staff noticed that he was checking to see whether I was there. Between scheduled one-to-one meetings I approached him and said: 'I'm sorry that you were unable to come and talk to me today but I will be there each day in case there is anything important to you that you would like to discuss.' Eventually he came, but at first, he rarely stayed for the entire half hour. I always told him that I would stay just in case he felt the need to return. Eventually he always turned up on time and talked for the scheduled period of time. I felt that he now trusted me and understood the purpose of our relationship.

This case study is a good example of how being consistent can help your patient to trust you. Acceptance of the patient's difficulties and the physical presence of the nurse, within identified time limits demonstrates that the nurse is consistent and will deliver what has been promised.

Working phase

The second phase of the relationship, the working phase, is subdivided into identification and exploitation subphases. In the identification subphase the patient begins to identify problems to be worked on within the relationship. The nature of the problems identified can be as diverse as the scope of nursing practice. Examples include loneliness, anxiety, and unresolved relationship difficulties. The exploitation subphase occurs as the patient makes use of the services of the nurse to work through identified problems. The nurse does not usually 'solve' the patient's problems, but rather gives the patient an opportunity to explore options and possibilities within the context of the relationship with the nurse. The following clinical data from nurse–patient verbal interaction illustrates some of the clinical work that needs to be done during the working phase.

Case study 17.2

Patient: 'I felt confused, uncertain what to do when my daughter left home. I try to keep the peace, but the thing is, her father doesn't realize how upset she is by his interference.'

Nurse: 'Sounds as if you were really upset at that time; what did you feel?'

This is an example of a nurse working with her patient during the identification subphase of the relationship. It is a good example of an investigative response that does not challenge the relief behaviour or symptoms of the patient. It resulted in the patient confirming that she felt anxious. For example:

Patient: 'I avoided confronting him because I knew that would make things worse for me. I felt "in a million pieces," didn't know where to turn, felt anxious I suppose.'

Since the patient confirmed that she was anxious the nurse was able to move to exploitation subphase by asking:

Nurse: 'What were you doing to avoid being anxious?'

Essentially, the clinical work of the nurse during the working phase of the nurse–patient relationship should be investigative. Nurses should assist patients to investigate their experience of threats to their health and to meet needs in a manner that reflects their preferences. Nurses should always view patients as autonomous and free persons. The language of the nurse is intended to provide prompters that stimulate the work that the patient needs to do for his/her own therapeutic benefit. Patients often use vague generalizations rather than description, for example 'I had a lousy day in town today.' Unless this statement is investigated neither the nurse nor the patient will learn anything. The nurse should say something like, 'I have 20 minutes, talk about that experience.' If the patient does not begin, the nurse could say, 'What happened at that time?' Only by listening and hearing a full description from the patient, can the nurse understand the meaning of the patient's experience.

Resolution phase

The resolution phase of the relationship is the final phase that is sometimes referred to as the termination phase. Resolution is usually a gradual weaning off process where dependence is relinquished and the patient resumes independence. Ideally resolution should be done by mutual agreement when the patient has demonstrated a greater level of functioning. In practice it more often occurs with patients in an unplanned manner. This can be a problem since it has been reported that abrupt termination of nurse–patient relationships due to a change in staff, resulted in patients returning to orientation phase after completing this phase.[18] As a consequence nurses should anticipate and prepare the patient for resolution at a very early stage.

Assuming that resolution can be planned, there is no single criterion sufficient to demonstrate readiness to terminate a relationship. However, the following criteria are useful indicators.

1 An improved sense of autonomy, i.e. ability to 'stand on your own feet'.

2 A reduced need to be defensive.

3 The ability to use new-found insights to adaptively alter day-to-day functioning.

The resolution phase of the relationship can be viewed as a separation of what was unique to the nurse and the patient, and temporarily shared in a one-to-one relationship. It replicates some of the feelings of disconnectedness that follow bereavement. Termination of a relationship can engender feelings of discomfort, pain and anger. The difficulties confronting the nurse may be similar to those confronting the patient. Nurses, too, need to overcome an unwillingness to separate and to give up exalted roles the patient has assigned to them. Although the therapeutic relationship ends with an expanded appreciation of the stories and convictions that motivate the patient, it can also end on the same conflictional note on which it began, with expressions of ambivalence and a recounting of successes and failures. The nurse may have to endorse sadness, the patient's disappointment in them and their own disappointment in themselves.

The following case study highlights some of the problems that emerge during resolution phase of the therapeutic relationship. This example has been selected

---

Case study 17.3

A young student nurse who was providing a daily counselling service to a young male adult, scheduled a final counselling session on the final day of his clinical placement. Previously his patient had regularly turned up for appointments, and on the surface, appeared to be enjoying interaction with his nurse.

The patient failed to appear for his final counselling session and the student spent a frustrating hour waiting for him in the appointed place. He felt confused and angry.

Later, on seeking an explanation from his patient, the student was told: 'You are leaving to get on with better things, while I am stuck in this dump.' This response indicates regression on the patient's part that, he has returned to a more dependent state. It also reveals that the relationship has reverted back to orientation phase.

The student had failed to prepare the patient for termination, in fact it had never been spoken about. Following consultation with his supervisor the student identified his failure to prepare his patient for termination and immediately scheduled a further meeting with his patient to discuss termination.

> During that session the patient was assisted to identify ways of coping with termination. The remainder of the day was spent introducing the patient to other patients and a new nurse therapist. The friendship relationships and the new nurse–patient relationship would act as interpersonal support networks when the student left the clinical area.

from the author's work while supervising nursing students' clinical work in the USA.

In conclusion, the nurse must be alert to the surfacing of any behaviour during resolution phase of a relationship that indicates that the relationship has moved back to an earlier phase. Behaviours to be concerned about include regression, repression, anger, denial and sadness. The nurse may respond by repeatedly observing that the client is not addressing the issue of impending separation, and may move to explore this avoidance. The patient who reverts to a previously abandoned life pattern with the message, 'I can't make it without you', demonstrates regression. When the patients are regressing they give no evidence of an emotional response.

The following therapeutic interventions offer a humanistic approach to the resolution phase of a relationship.

1 Identify the circumstances under which the relationship may be terminated.

2 Assist the patient to discover new interests, such as hobbies, friendship relationships and personal achievement.

3 Encourage transference of dependence to other support systems, such as spouse, relative, employer, neighbour, friend or new therapist, for emotional support.

4 As the patient's independence from you grows, allow time and space for interaction with significant people in his/her life.

5 As the time for termination nears, increasingly focus on future orientated material.

6 Assist the patient to work through feelings associated with the resolution phase.

The course of termination is influenced by the work that precedes it. The more that patient and nurse discuss their successes and failure, their gratitudes and disappointments, the more that the patient will have benefited from the therapeutic relationship.

THE CLINICAL SIGNIFICANCE OF THE THERAPEUTIC NURSE–PATIENT RELATIONSHIP

A considerable amount of evidence exists in the literature to support the view that the therapeutic nurse–patient relationship is a significant variable in health care and that it can enable people to cope more effectively with threats to their health. The evidence varies from the theoretical to research evidence accumulated from different types of research designs. The cumulative evidence is encouraging and some of it is reviewed in the next section of this chapter.

Some of the evidence relating to the clinical significance of the nurse–patient relationship has been elicited from the recipients of health care, the patients themselves. A review of the literature reveals that patients are in a position to advise professionals about how to offer a therapeutic relationship. A paper reporting the findings from two qualitative studies conducted on opposite sides of the Atlantic[19] showed that the type of relationship that psychiatric patients wanted from their nurses in Canada and Scotland is similar. This indicates that the concept of the therapeutic relationship, that has its origins in the USA, can cross some national boundaries. Since cultural sensitivity can facilitate open, non-defensive relationships, that is an important finding. In both studies patients identified the relationship with the nurse as important to their overall recovery. Listening, availability and a friendly approach were identified as critical in the nurse–patient interaction in the Canadian study. Participants wanted to see that action was taken on issues that were identified.

In the Scottish study, similar themes were identified. Patients wanted nurses to listen, be sensitive to feelings, seek clarification of confused messages, help them to 'anchor' accounts of problems in the personal time and setting of the problem, help them to focus on solutions to problems, and to sound warm and genuine. Canadian patients valued help to see things more clearly, Scottish patients valued nurses' attempts to help them gain more detail about the emotional experience. The clinical significance of these data is indicated by the consensus in the literature[20] that the consumer of health care is an important, active collaborator in treatment and outcome goals.

Patients' perceptions of the nurse–patient relationship have been a focus for studies in various types of clinical contexts. For example, the findings of a pilot study into nursing observation from the perspective of the patient, showed that the experience was predominately negative for the majority of patients. A key variable in positive experience was a therapeutic relationship with the observing nurse and the provision of information about the observation process.[21] In a different type of clinical environment,[22] chemotherapy patients and their families placed a high value on a warm reciprocated personal relationship with a nurse. They claimed that it could create a supportive atmosphere in what might otherwise be a threatening environment for patients. Data from these studies indicate that the nurse–patient relationship can help to humanize care.

Several other studies show that there is now widespread belief in the therapeutic relationship as a means of generating favourable outcomes for patients. In a Hong Kong study[23] ten registered nurses were interviewed on their perceptions of caring behaviours in their clinical settings. Findings showed that respondents valued the importance of interpersonal relationships in providing holistic care. In a Japanese study[24] experienced psychiatric public health nurses revealed that they used an empowering relationship with families, neighbours, educators and employers in order to enable their patients' healthy living in the community. Finally, a German study[25] used clinical vignettes and observed that nurses used their relationship with psychotic patients to understand psychotic functional behaviour and that this enabled patients to return to the non-psychotic world.

The efficacy of the nurse–patient relationship is further supported by a Canadian study that revealed that overlapping hospital and community services enabled the therapeutic nurse–patient relationship to be maintained after discharge from hospital. Findings revealed improved quality of life for discharged patients, reduced re-admissions, and a saving to the taxpayers in Western Ontario of $500,000 in the initial year.[26] Subsequently, a major randomized controlled study in Western Ontario has revealed that the continuation of the therapeutic nurse–patient relationship in the community for a short period after discharge has reduced re-admission rates by 50%.[26]

The Canadian study is currently being replicated in the Highland Region of Scotland. The intervention is viewed as a solution to the very high relapse/re-admission rates to acute psychiatric wards in that region due to the inability of many individuals to adjust to community living. The supportive relationship with hospital staff is generally lost during discharge. It has been reported[27] that it can take several weeks to form a new working relationship with community staff, thus individuals are often left with minimal support at a time when they need to mediate the stress of the adjustment to community living. Discharge programmes that involve bridging therapeutic relationships from hospital to community build on the work of Forchuk in Canada and Reynolds in Scotland. The conclusions drawn from this work are that quality of interpersonal relations has a large bearing on quality of life[28] and that supportive interpersonal relationships will promote less need for expensive interventions in mental health, such as hospitalization.

CONCLUSION

The literature indicates that psychiatry is focusing on a biomedical approach to mental health. The work of the psychiatrist incorporates ongoing brain research and pharmaceutical research, and utilizes sophisticated equipment for forms of laboratory measurement, and the study of within-body phenomena of psychiatric patients. It would therefore seem urgent that mental health nurses develop their area of interest, the human responses of psychiatric patients. Examples of human responses observed by nurses, during their relationships with psychiatric patients, include anxiety, self-esteem problems, loneliness, grief and hallucinations. Mental health nurses need to study such problems, make themselves experts in a humanistic alternative approach to such problems of psychiatric patients and to speak out on the prevention of such problems. Such human responses, of patients, can only be studied effectively in a therapeutic (investigative) relationship that enables a person to investigate life experiences.[30]

Since research is now starting to provide evidence of the clinical significance of the nurse–patient relationship, any factors that place a constraint on nurses' ability and opportunity to offer such a relationship is a concern. Like all other helping professions, nursing exists to help people, and the nurse who offers a therapeutic relationship will be more able to help people than nurses who are unable to offer an interpersonal experience that is therapeutic.

REFERENCES

1. Forchuk C, Reynolds W. Guest editorial – Interpersonal theory in nursing practice: The Peplau Legacy. *Journal of Psychiatric and Mental Health Nursing* 1998; **5**(3): 165–6.

2. Peplau H. *Interpersonal relations in nursing.* London: Macmillan Education, 1988.

3. Barker P, Reynolds W. The proper focus of psychiatric nursing: a critique of Watson's caring ideology. *Journal of Psycho-social Nursing* 1994; **22**(5): 17–23.

4. Reynolds W. *The measurement and development of empathy in nursing.* Aldershot: Ashgate Publishing, 2000.

5. Smith D. Flight to Los Angeles: crisis at 30,000 feet. *Journal of Psycho-social Nursing* 2000; **38**(10): 38–45.

6. Shaw C, Williams K. Patients' views of a new nurse-led continence service. *Journal of Clinical Nursing* 2000; **9**(4): 574–82.

7. Barry F. *Psycho-social nursing: care of physically ill patients and their families.* Baltimore, MD: Lippincott, 1996.

8. Peplau H. Interpersonal relations model: theoretical constructs, principles and general applications. In: Reynolds W, Cormack D (eds). *Psychiatric and mental health nursing: theory and practice.* London: Chapman and Hall, 1990.

9. Martin T. Something special: forensic psychiatric

nursing. *Journal of Psychiatric and Mental Health Nursing* 2001; **8**(1): 25–32.

10. Forchuk C, Reynolds W. Clients' reflections on relationships with nurses: comparisons from Canada and Scotland. *Journal of Psychiatric and Mental Health Nursing* 2001; **8**(1): 45–51.

11. Reynolds W. Peplau's theory in practice. *Nursing Science Quarterly* 1997; **10**(4): 168–70.

12. Peplau H. Interpersonal techniques: the crux of psychiatric nursing. *American Journal of Nursing* 1962; **62**: 50–54.

13. Forchuk C, Hildegard E. *Peplau: interpersonal nursing theory*. London: Sage Publications, 1993.

14. Reynolds W, Scott A, Austin W. Nursing, empathy and perception of the moral. *Journal of Advanced Nursing* 2000; **32**(1): 235–42.

15. Forchuk C, Brown B. Establishing a nurse–client relationship. *Journal of Psycho-social Nursing* 1989; **27**(2): 30–34.

16. Lego S. *Psychiatric nursing: a comprehensive reference*. Baltimore, MD: Lippincott, 1996.

17. Forchuk C. The orientation phase: how long does it take? *Perspectives in Psychiatric Care* 1992; **28**(4): 7–10.

18. Ibid.

19. Ibid.

20. The Scottish Office. *Designed to care: renewing the National Health Service in Scotland*. London: The Stationary Office, 1997.

21. Jones J, Lowe T, Ward M. Inpatients' experiences of nursing observation on an acute psychiatric unit: a pilot study. *Journal of Mental Health Care and Learning Disabilities* 2000; **4**(4): 125–9.

22. Walker A, Wilkes L, White K. How do patients perceive support from nurses? *Professional Nurse* 2000; **16**(2): 902–4.

23. Yam B, Rossiter J. Caring in nursing: perceptions of Hong Kong nurses. *Journal of Clinical Nursing* 2000; **9**(2): 293–302.

24. Kayama M, Zerwekh J, Thornton K, Murashima S. Japanese expert public health nurses empower clients with schizophrenia living in the community. *Journal of Psycho-social Nursing* 2001; **39**(2): 40–47.

25. Teising M. 'Sister, I am going crazy, help me': psychodynamic-orientated care in psychotic patients in inpatient treatment. *Journal of Psychiatric and Mental Health Nursing* 2000; **7**(5): 449–54.

26. Forchuk C, Jewell J, Schofield R, Sircelj M, Valledor T. From hospital to community: bridging therapeutic relationships. *Journal of Psychiatric and Mental Health Nursing* 1998; **5**(3): 197–202.

27. Contact Bill Reynolds for further details of the Scottish Transitional Discharge Study, at University of Stirling, Department of Nursing and Midwifery, Highland Campus, Inverness, Old Perth Rd, IV2 3FG (e-mail: WJR2@stir.ac.uk)

28. Peplau H. Quality of life: an interpersonal perspective. *Nursing Science Quarterly* 1994; **7**(1): 10–15.

29. Peplau H. Investigative counselling. In: O'Toole A, Rouslin S (eds). *Hildegard E Peplau: selected works*, Chapter 16. London: Macmillan, 1994.

APPENDIX 17.1 Phases of the Therapeutic Relationship

	Non Therapeutic Relationships		Therapeutic Relationships		
	Mutual withdrawal	Grappling	Orientation Start	Working phase Identification	Resolution phase Exploitation / Resolution
Client:	Forgets appointments/planned times Cannot remember who nurse/service provider is Unaware if nurse/service provider is available Content kept superficial Actively avoids nurse/service provider	Frequent changes of topics and approach Increasing frustration Sense of lack of connection Begins to dread meetings	Seeks assistance Conveys educative needs Asks questions Tests parameters Shares preconceptions and expectations of nurse due to past experience	Identifies problems Aware of time Responds to help Identifies with nurse Recognizes nurse as a person Explores feelings Fluctuates dependence, independence and interdependence in therapeutic relationship with nurse Increases focal attention Changes appearance (for better or worse) Understands purpose of meeting Maintains continuity between sessions (process and content) Testing manoeuvres decrease	**Exploitation:** Makes full use of services Identifies new goals Attempts to attain new goals Rapid shifts in behaviour: dependent–independent Exploitative behaviour Realistic exploitation Self-directing Develops skills in interpersonal relationships and problem solving Displays changes in manner of communication (more open, flexible) **Resolution:** Abandons old needs Aspires to new goals Becomes independent of helping person Applies new problem solving skills Maintains changes in style of communication and interaction Positive changes in view of self Integrates illness Exhibits ability to stand alone
Service provider:	No time for client meetings Client meetings very short if they occur at all Focus on instrumental tasks Decision that client is a typical of usual relationship Avoids client contact	Frequent changes of the rapeutic approach Sense of lack of connection Increasing frustration Length of meetings vary Place of meetings vary	Respond to emergency Give parameters of meetings Explain roles Observes and listens Help client identify problem Help client plan use of community resources and services Reduce anxiety and tension Practice non-directive listening Focus client's energies Clarify preconceptions and expectations of nurse	Maintain separate identity Unconditional acceptance Help express needs, feelings Assess and adjust to needs Provide information Provide experiences that diminish feelings of helplessness Do not allow anxiety to overwhelm client Help client to focus on cues Help client to develop responses to cues Therapeutic use of language	**Exploitation:** Continue assessment Meet needs as they emerge Understand reason for shifts in behaviour Initiate rehabilitative plans Reduce anxiety Identify positive factors Help plan for total needs Facilitate forward movement of personality Deal with therapeutic impasse **Resolution:** Sustain relationship as long as patient feels necessary Promote family interaction Assist with goal setting Teach preventive measures Utilize community agencies Teach self-care Terminate nurse–client relationship

Copyright revised Cheryl Forchuk 2000

Note: Phases are overlapping

Please mark on the following scale where the check marks are concentrated within the above table. Check lists are designed to assist in the evaluation phase.

Mutual withdrawal	Grappling	Orientation	Identification	Exploitation	Resolution

Chapter 18

DEVELOPING EMPATHY

Bill Reynolds*

INTRODUCTION

Empathy is known to be crucial to all forms of helping relationships. While there is a considerable debate about whether empathy is a personality dimension, an experienced emotion, or an observable skill, empathy needs to involve the patient's actual awareness of the helper's communication in order that patients know whether they are being understood. Accurate empathy is a form of interaction, involving communication of the helper's attitudes and communication of the helper's understanding of the patient's world. It is an essential component of the therapeutic, one-to-one nurse–patient relationship discussed in Chapter 17, since, without empathy, there is no basis for helping.

In this chapter, the historical and theoretical background to empathy will be discussed. Different definitions of empathy will be considered and a construct of empathy that is relevant to clinical nursing will be described. Clients' views of their relationships with nurses and other research evidence will be presented to illustrate that empathy is crucial to the goals of clinical nursing.

EMPATHY: HISTORICAL AND THEORETICAL BACKGROUND

Essentially the concept of empathy originated from the German word *'Einfühlung'* as used by Lipps,[1] which liter-

ally means feeling within. This contribution led to empathy being viewed for many years as a perceptual rather than a communicating skill. For several decades references to empathy as a trait or human quality indicate that a necessary condition of empathy is that the observer understands in some sense the affective state of the other person. The tendency to conceptualize empathy as a kind of attitude or way of perceiving, which therapists assume, and not to something that they say or do, is illustrated by the following quote from the early 1960s.[2]

> In order to help, one has to know the patient emotionally. One cannot grasp subtle and complicated feelings of people, except by this emotional knowing the experiencing of another's feeling that is meant by the term empathy. It is a very special mode of perceiving.

The work of many individuals in the helping and health care disciplines, over several decades, has helped us to recognize that empathy has many more components than was originally recognized. This work has clarified the meaning of empathy and helped professionals to know when they are offering empathy.

The client–centred paradigm

The development of the construct of empathy was stimulated by the work of Carl Rogers and others from clinical psychology in the 1950s and 1960s. Rogers[3]

*Bill Reynolds is Reader in Nursing at Turku Polytechnic, Salo, Finland developed an approach to counselling that was at first called non-directive, but is now called client-centred. At first this approach was applied only in one-to-one relationships but in later years Rogers became involved in the group movement and extended his theory to encounter groups and other treatment modalities such as play therapy. He also became interested in the application of his theory to education, and extended it to interpersonal relations in general.

Like all theories, the client-centred approach is built on several, inter-related concepts. One concept is that people are basically rational, socialized, forward moving and realistic. Furthermore the client-centred point of view sees people as being basically co-operative, constructive and trustworthy, when they are free of defensiveness. As individuals, we possess the capacity to experience, and to be aware of, the reality of our psychological maladjustment, and to have the capacity and the tendency to move from a state of maladjustment toward a state of psychological adjustment. These capacities and this tendency will be released in a relationship that has the characteristics of a helping (non-threatening) relationship. This type of relationship may also be described as a therapeutic relationship.

Rogers' view that the relationship should be non-defensive chimes with the suggestion in Chapter 17 that the therapeutic relationship should enable patients to experience freedom to express themselves without fear of censure or rejection. The questions that we need to ask ourselves are: how does a non-defensive relationship occur, or, what are the helping attitudes or behaviours, which create a relationship that enable patients to study the effectiveness of coping strategies? Rogers postulated that three core (facilitative) conditions were necessary, and sufficient to achieve a non-defensive relationship and to enable the patient to learn more satisfactory and productive patterns of behaviour.[4] The facilitative conditions were described as warmth, genuineness and empathy.

Despite his tendency to refer to empathy as an attitude, Rogers' description of the facilitative conditions emphasize the communicative aspect of empathy, and the complexity of empathy.[5] He suggested that the facilitative conditions operative in all effective relationships relate to the helper's attitude, cognition and behaviour. Rogers argues that the patient learns to change when the helper communicates commitment (warmth) and non-defensiveness (genuineness), and is successful in communicating understanding of the patient's current feelings (empathic). He expressed the view that the attitudes and cognitive ability of the helping person are conveyed to the patient through the communication of the helper. This suggests that when attitudes and understanding are shown to the patient, empathy is a skilled interpersonal behaviour.

Many theorists recognize that the core facilitative conditions in therapeutic relationships, postulated by Rogers, are inter-related and that the three conditions have an interlocking nature.[6] By this is meant that they interact in such a way as to increase and compliment each other. For instance, the communication of empathy (the ability to see things from another person's point of view) can be hollow or threatening if the empathizing individual is defensive, and is not genuine. This suggests that warmth and genuineness are part of an empathic response to the patient and are of equal importance to therapeutic outcome. It appears that empathy cannot exist in the absence of the other two conditions. This seems logical since it is difficult to see how a nurse would be able to understand the feelings behind the patient's words (empathic), if external stressors such as dissatisfaction or anger, prevented the nurse from showing commitment (warmth), by seeking clarification when the patient's message is unclear. Putting it another way, a barrier to the exploration of the meaning of the patient's experiences, is a very natural tendency to judge, evaluate or disapprove, when the patient's personal communication is threatening. When this happens the helping person may become defensive, often transmitting this to the patient through unwanted advice or unfriendly voice tone. Unless the helper can work on achieving genuineness, the helper's moment-by-moment empathic grasp of the meaning and significance of the patient's world will be impeded.

THE MEANING AND COMPONENTS OF EMPATHY

For several decades the literature has illustrated that there is disagreement about what empathy means and that there is a need to find a common definition of empathy. The reason for this debate is that while empathy is a complex multidimensional construct involving cognition, behaviour, attitudes, emotions and personality, many writers have viewed it narrowly as a unitary construct.[7]

The components of empathy that are most frequently referred to are cognitive (the helper's intellectual ability to identify and understand another person's feelings and perspectives from an objective stance), and behavioural (a communicative response to convey understanding of another's perspective). A possible explanation is that professionals tend to look for definitions that reflect the aims of the therapeutic relationship. Clinicians, such as nurses, should communicate understanding of the patient's experience (i.e. offer cognitive–behavioural empathy) in order that this can be validated by the patient.[8]

The clinical significance of moral/trait empathy (an internal altruistic force that motivates the practice of empathy), and emotional empathy (the ability to subjectively experience and share in another's psychological state or intrinsic feelings) has not been determined.[9] While it is logical to believe that a predisposition to offer empathy is essential, at the present time, there is little evidence that personality traits are significantly correlated with an actual ability to offer empathy. In other words, the desire to help does not always manifest itself in supportive behaviours. It is reasonable to suggest that emotions can enrich a relationship. Emotion may even play a fundamental role in perceiving the moral dimensions of clinical practice. However, the amount of emotion necessary to respect the perspective of the patient is unknown. Emotional empathy has sometimes been viewed as a synonym for sympathy. Sympathy (an innate biological tendency to react emotionally to the emotions of another) may even block cognitive–behavioural empathy since emotions, such as anxiety, can cause inattention to detail. It has also been reported that high levels of emotional empathy can cause individuals to be sensitive to rejection and to engage in behaviours related to approval seeking tendencies. For those reasons it has been argued that there needs to be fixed (minimum) levels of emotion necessary in a helping relationship.[10]

The relationship of the many components of empathy to each other is poorly understood. Clearly a great deal of work remains to be done in order to understand how all of the variables in the empathic process interact with each other. What is currently understood is that empathy involves several concepts or stages. Several writers have offered the following explanation about the sequence of certain stages and how each of those stages effects the next stage.[11] Firstly, the helper must be receptive to another's communication (the moral component). Secondly, the helper must understand the communication by putting himself in the other's place (the cognitive component). Thirdly, the helper must communicate that understanding to the patient (the behavioural or communicative component). Finally, the patient needs to validate the helper's perception of the patient's world. The final stage has been referred to in the literature as the relational component of empathy, the patients' awareness of how well they are being understood.

The final stage of empathy (the relational component) is important since it offers the patient an opportunity to comment on the accuracy of the helper's perceptions and to experience being understood. The patient's actual awareness of the helper's communication allows him/her to say, 'Yes that is how I see things' or, 'No that is not what I mean.' This assumption is consistent with the Barrett–Lennard multidimensional model of empathy, which he described as

the empathy cycle. He described it in the following manner:

- ❏ **Phase 1**. The inner process of empathic listening to another who is personally expressive in some way, reasoning, and understanding.
- ❏ **Phase 2**. An attempt to convey empathic understanding to the other person's experiences.
- ❏ **Phase 3**. The patient's actual reception/awareness of the helper's communication.

When the process continues, phase 1 is again the core phase and 2 and 3 follow in cyclical mode. The total interactive sequence in which these phases occur begins with one person being self-expressive in the presence of an empathically attending helper and this characteristically leads to further self-expression and feedback to the empathizing helper.

The clients' perception of empathy

An interesting finding from the literature is that most measures of empathy tend to reflect professionals' views rather than patients' views of empathy. Since empathy is closely associated with the client-centred paradigm, the failure to consider patients' views seems paradoxical. If patients are able to observe the amount and nature of empathy existing in a helping relationship, they are in a position to advise professionals about how to offer empathy. Patients are likely to be better judges of the degree of empathy than professionals and their perceptions of helping relationships can contribute to our understanding of empathy.

In the late 1990s an empathy scale was developed that had some of its antecedents in patients' perceptions of their relationships with nurses.[12] The research responsible for the development of that scale revealed that patients knew a great deal about the degree of empathy existing in a relationship. Findings also suggested that patients' experience of the nurse–patient relationship is a fertile source of information about the phases of the empathic relationship, and how it is best brought about. The issues identified from patient reports, when matched with views in the professional literature, formed the basis for an item pool for the Reynold's Empathy Scale.[13]

Twelve items were developed for the empathy scale that were considered to reflect patients' descriptions of helpful and unhelpful interpersonal behaviours. Since the item pool reflected patients' perceptions of their relationships with nurses, the instrument was considered to measure a construct of empathy that was relevant to clinical nurses.

THE REYNOLD'S EMPATHY SCALE AND PATIENTS' VIEWS ABOUT HELPING

The relationship of items on the new empathy scale to patients' views about helping is illustrated by the following patient comments selected from interviews carried out in acute psychiatric admission wards in Scotland.[14] The discussion that follows reveals a relationship between patients' views about effective and ineffective interpersonal behaviour and variables critical to empathy. Positive scale items (effective behaviours) are discussed first.

High empathy items

Item 1 on the empathy scale (**Attempts to explore and clarify feelings**) is an example of the extent to which the nurse is attempting to listen actively. Patients' descriptions of the early phase of their relationship with nurses indicated that sensitive understanding or accurate understanding on the part of the nurse was not happening at that point. However, patients revealed that nurses' attempts to listen determined whether accurate understanding was going to happen at some later point in the relationship. Patient statements supporting this conclusion included:

> It is very hard for her to understand me, but she is trying very hard.

and

> We haven't discussed my problems yet but she is listening and we are getting there.

Item 3 on the scale (**Responds to feelings**) reflects patients' need for nurses to be sensitive to their feelings. For example:

> I don't know her very well, but she is very thoughtful. She doesn't object to my thoughts and tries to understand my feelings.

and

> He tries very hard to understand my feelings. That must be very hard for him because I talk too much.

Responding to feelings enabled nurses to demonstrate that they were willing to journey alongside the patient in an attempt to 'get inside their shoes'. Patients indicated that this was critical during the early stages of a new relationship.

Item 5 (**Explores personal meaning of feeling**) relates to the need for nurses to help patients to clarify their often-confused messages by providing more detail about their emotional experiences. Essentially patients were stating that they found it helpful when nurses sought to investigate feelings that they had been approaching hazily and hesitantly. This is emphasized by the following statements:

> It's not like getting your brains picked. She helps me to let it flow out.

and

> It's like speaking to myself or looking into a mirror. She helps me to explain the reasons for my distress.

Item 7 (**Responds to feelings and meanings**) relates to patients' need for nurses to help them to 'anchor' accounts of problems in the personal time and setting of the problem. When that help was provided patients indicated that they were able to move from the general to the particular, from the past to the present. The following comments illustrate this point:

> He helps me to get to the point and helps me to look at the current situation.

and

> She helps me to move from the past to the present. She is interested in what I am like today.

Item 9 (**Provides the patient with direction**) reflects patients' needs for nurses to help them to focus on solutions to problems. Essentially patients want nurses to assist them to find solutions to personal problems in a manner that reflects their preferences. Patient statements supporting that view included:

> She worked with me on my problems. She helped me to identify how I would like to change my response to family crisis, and to discover what I want to achieve.

and

> We talked about what I would like to happen and how I was going to bring that about.

Item 11 (**Appropriate voice tone**) relates to patients' views that nurses ought to sound committed (warm) and open (genuine). Patients suggested, as Rogers did,[15] that the communication of these attitudes can promote an interpersonal climate of respect, neutrality and trust. Item 11 is a reminder of the fact that the way that a person perceives another is often based on the non-verbal, rather than the verbal communications. The following patient statements illustrate how influential voice tone can be:

> He sounds as if he would rather be in the pub having a pint, rather than listening to my rubbish.

and

> She sounds genuinely interested. This gives you a lot of confidence in yourself.

These statements indicate that item 11 is crucial in determining the extent to which verbal inputs are judged to be warm. Patient statements have also revealed that the empathic cycle, described earlier in this chapter, can be stalled at any stage. The origin of negative items on the Reynold's Empathy Scale (ineffective interpersonal behaviours) stemmed from patients' descriptions of threatening behaviours.

Low empathy items

Item 2 on the scale (**Leads, directs and diverts**) is an example of manipulative communication that is not patient-centred. This is illustrated by the following statement:

> She is very clever. I don't want to talk about myself, but she judges what I say and somehow I find that we are talking about me. This is not comfortable.

Item 4 (Ignores verbal and non-verbal communication) refers to the nurse's inability to listen. Patients suggested that when nurses failed to hear their communicated message, they felt that they did not care. For example:

> She failed to understand what I was trying to explain to her. I felt that she couldn't have cared less.

Item 6 (Judgemental and opinionated) measures the extent to which a nurse is judgemental or neutral. Patients suggested that when the nurse was judgemental, this damaged the emotional quality of the relationship. This is illustrated by the following statement:

> If someone criticizes me or doesn't respect me, I just clam up.

Essentially patients were saying that whenever nurses' communicated attitudes indicated a lack of respect and acceptance, they felt anxious. This had the effect of preventing further self-disclosures.

Item 8 (Interrupts and seems in a hurry) reflects patients' dislike of being interrupted. For example:

> She didn't give me time to explain; it felt as if I didn't matter.

Item 10 (Fails to focus on solutions) reflects a lack of acceptance. Patients suggested that this conveyed an impression that the nurse was not taking them seriously. For example:

> We haven't got around to discussing solutions to my problems yet. I'm not sure if she believes what I am saying.

Item 12 (Inappropriate voice tone, sounds curt) reflects patients' dislike of an unfriendly nurse. The following patient statement illustrates this point:

> I felt defensive because she sounded so hostile.

Patients indicated that nurses needed to select interventions that are appropriate to the phase of the helping relationship and the needs of the individual receiving help. Under some circumstances it might be appropriate to investigate feelings, coping strategies and health goals. The following statement illustrates this point:

> She can be trusted. You can talk to her about things you would be reluctant to talk to other people about.

However, patients have indicated that at a certain phase of the relationship, in-depth probing might threaten them. For example:

> When I don't want to talk about something she recognizes this mood and asks me about it. She wont persist if I am reluctant.

These statements reveal that nurses need to have an empathized awareness of patients' readiness to talk. If a patient signals a reluctance to discuss feelings, the nurse might not find exploration of the personal meaning of feelings (item 5 on the Reynold's Empathy Scale) very productive. An alternative approach would be to say, 'Talk about what is comfortable for you at the moment.' That is an example of helping the patient to clarify the meaning of their communication by providing more detail about their emotional experience (item 1 on the empathy scale). It differs qualitatively from item 5 because it allows patients to continue to feel accepted, but able to make choices.

The findings from the study reported here are similar to research conducted in Canada. The Canadian study[16] reported that patients wanted nurses to respect them, to listen to their (often-confused) stories, and to help them to see things more clearly. Interest in the findings has also been expressed by nurses working in non-psychiatric areas, such as digestive pathology. Since the Reynold's Empathy Scale is now being used as an educational and/or research tool in Scotland, Republic of Ireland, Canada, Spain, Finland and Egypt, the client-centred construct of empathy, that is operationalized by the scale, may have practical utility across several cultural boundaries, and different nursing contexts.

APPLICATION OF EMPATHY IN DIFFERENT NURSING SETTINGS

The cumulative evidence in the research and professional literature provides strong support for the hypothesized relationship of empathy to therapeutic relationships. The papers referred to in this section are only a sample of the available evidence. They have been selected in order to illustrate the clinical usefulness of empathy across a wide range of inpatient and community contexts.

Psychiatric and mental health contexts

The practical utility of empathy to psychiatric and mental health nursing would seem self-evident. In these contexts nurses need to gain understanding of complex behaviours such as withdrawal, anxiety and dysfunctional family systems. They need to understand the purpose of dysfunctional behaviour and what prevents people from giving up patterns of behaviour that reduce satisfaction with living. Nurses who work in psycho-social areas have opportunities to help move the patient in a direction favouring productive social living, and to learn about the purpose of dysfunctional behaviour. The focus should be on the experience of the patient, an outcome that is dependent on empathy. The following papers illustrate this assumption.

Reynolds and Scott[17] summarized several studies carried out between 1970 and 1990. Empathy was shown to be a more important facilitator of a helping relationship than the helper's ideological orientation. For example one study found that behaviour therapists who scored highly in empathy were more potent reinforcers of adaptive behaviour than therapists who were low empathizers. Empathy was shown to be a significant variable influencing improvement among children with learning disabilities in both verbal and behavioural spheres. Similarly empathy was found to be central to clinicians' effectiveness when working with hyperactive and uncontrolled children. With respect to confrontation of unpleasant or maladaptive behaviour, it has been shown that high empathy helpers used approaches which focused on the here-and-now and emphasized the patient's resources. On the other hand, low empathy helpers were found to be more likely to confront patients with pathology rather than with their resources.[18]

In more recent times it has been shown how empathy enables nurses to investigate and understand the individual experience of persons experiencing a state of chaos as a consequence of psychiatric disorder.[19] Additionally, it has been demonstrated that empathy enabled partners of men with AIDS to provide increasingly sensitive care as the clinical course of the disease developed. This illustrates that mental health is not restricted to psychiatric diagnosis *per se*, and that all forms of interpersonal experiences (from lay persons and professionals) can be therapeutic.

Non-psychiatric and mental health contexts

The closeness of nurses to the medical (disease) model may have led some nurses to believe that empathy has no relevance to non-psychiatric clinical areas. It has been argued that empathy is not possible in acute medical/surgical settings because workload does not usually allow a nurse to listen to a patient for 30 minutes or more. However, the development of Psychiatric Liaison Nurses is now starting to reveal that patients in general hospitals have an extensive list of psycho-social needs that are likely to remain unrecognized unless nurses are able to offer empathy to their patients.[20] Furthermore, there is extensive evidence that empathy is an important facilitator of constructive interpersonal relationships across a diverse range of clinical environments. The evidence suggests that patients often experience health needs that have their origin in the medical problem. These health needs are frequently psycho-social in nature, but they are not part of the disease diagnosed and treated by medical doctors. Concerns about body image, sexuality or death are human responses to actual and potential health problems that arise in day-to-day nurse–patient relationships and which call for responsible, helpful nursing actions. This section examines evidence for this assumption across a variety of non-psychiatric clinical areas.[21]

Several studies have emphasized the importance of the nurse understanding the patient's experience of illness and the health care system.[22] For example, it has been shown that women were more likely to experience depressive breakdown following a severe life event, such as mastectomy, if they lacked an opportunity to confide regularly in someone who understood them. In relationship to breast cancer victims, studies indicate the importance of nurses meeting patients' information requirements regarding chemotherapy and breast reconstruction. Evidence exists to support the view that such information is beneficial to the patient's postoperative progress. This suggests that there is a need for nurses to anticipate the information needs of their patients. Apart from the need to use empathy to humanize care, studies have shown that empathy has a positive correlation with relief from pain, improved pulse and respiratory rates, and patients' reports of reduced worry and anxiety.

Furthermore studies have demonstrated[23] that patients with hypertension attributed greater importance to discussing with their care provider their responses to health care, as compared with personal problems and lifestyle matters. Since these patients expressed a need to discuss their responses to health care, nurses need to demonstrate commitment to listening to them. Otherwise, an opportunity for patients to have an active role in problem-solving will be lost and nurses will fail to appreciate patients' individuality.

A study of the effect of nurses' empathy on the anxiety, depression, hostility and satisfaction with care of patients with cancer, is encouraging. Less anxiety, depression and hostility was found in patients being cared for by nurses exhibiting high empathy. An alternative group who are at risk emotionally are the terminally ill. Terminally ill patients have reported that the nurses' empathized awareness of the patient's need to talk about death and dying was very highly valued.[24]

In recent times, the evidence has steadily accumulated in support of the clinical utility of empathy. The following papers illustrate the clinical significance of empathy across a broad spectrum of contexts and clinical issues. For example, a study investigating the psychological distress experienced by patients receiving bone marrow transplants found that psychological distress and life satisfaction could be positively influenced by empathy.[25] Another study[26] illustrated the relevance of empathy to ethical care. This study showed that nurses' ability to make ethical decisions related to the termination of pregnancy requires empathy, respect for human rights and unconditional acceptance of a person. Empathy has also been shown to be a crucial component of care provided during pregnancy.[27] It enables midwives to differentiate between ordinary emotional turbulence, which inevitably accompanied child-bearing and rearing, and experiences of unbearable distress or massive denial requiring psychotherapeutic help. Finally it has been shown that all chronic and progressive problems, including ageing, have emotional and spiritual aspects that demand attention. Grief and shame at growing older and denial of these feelings must be recognized, otherwise patients will ignore or resist direction on lifestyle or medications. A recent paper[28] identified patients with type 2 diabetes as being individuals falling into this category. It was concluded that empathy with these patients' distress can individualize care and strongly influence positive health outcomes for patients.

CONCLUSION

Empathy is essential in order to create an interpersonal climate that is free of defensiveness. This enables individuals to talk about their perceptions of need. This is important since it is unlikely that patients will trust nurses if they do not view them as being helpful and appreciative of their individuality. This may result in a failure to establish patients' needs as seen by them and, as a consequence, a failure to address patients' needs. Additionally, empathy can help move the nurse–patient relationship towards its final objective, patient growth. When nurses assist patients to find solutions to personal problems, in a manner that reflects their preferences, favourable health outcomes occur. Numerous studies have established a correlation between high empathy in helping relationships and improved health. The clinical usefulness of empathy has been demonstrated in a wide range of clinical contexts.

Implications for the Health Service

The relevance of empathic relationships to the goals of health services are suggested by the increasing focus on patient-centred care and the growth of consumerism. The client-centred focus is illustrated by the NHS (Scotland) Patients' Charter which emphasizes that clinicians need to collaborate with users of health services in the prioritizing of clinical needs and the setting of treatment goals. The following standards have been set for clinical care. Patients should:

❑ share in the responsibility for their own health;
❑ tell professionals what they want;
❑ be entitled to be treated as a person, not a case.

While the aims of the Patients' Charter seem desirable, it is difficult to understand how this might be achieved unless professionals are able to offer an empathized awareness of the patient's expectations and needs. This possibility is emphasized by Hogg (1994)[29] who pointed out that users, such as women with HIV, or those with the experience of living in pain, have different expectations and needs of the health service from professionals. Empathy can be learned, but nurses need to be taught how to offer it to patients. Additionally, nurses need uninterrupted time in order to listen to their patients and hear what they want to happen. Otherwise, the aims of the Patients' Charter are likely to remain unfulfilled rhetoric.

REFERENCES

1. Lipps T. Einfühlung, Innere Nachahmung, und Organempfindungen. *Archives of Gestalt Psychology* 1903; **20**: 135–204.
2. Greenson R. Empathy and its vicissitudes. *International Journal of Psychoanalysis* 1960; **41**: 418–24.
3. Rogers C. The necessary and sufficient conditions of therapeutic personality change. *Journal of Consulting Psychology* 1957; **21**: 95–103.
4. Ibid.
5. Rogers C. Empathic: an unappreciated way of being. *The Councelling Psychologist* 1975; **5**: 2–10.
6. Reynolds, W. Roger's client-centred model: principles and general applications. In: Reynolds W, Cormack D (eds). *Psychiatric and mental health nursing: theory and practice.* London: Chapman and Hall, 1990.

7. Reynolds W, Scott A. Nursing, empathy and perception of the normally moral. *Journal of Advanced Nursing* 2000; **32**(1): 235–42.

8. Ibid.

9. Ibid.

10. Ibid.

11. Reynolds W. *The measurement and development of empathy in nursing.* Aldershot: Ashgate Publishing, 2000.

12. Ibid.

13. Ibid.

14. Reynolds W. The influence of clients' perceptions of the helping relationship in the development of an empathy scale. *Journal of Psychiatric and Mental Health Nursing* 1994; **1**(1): 23–30.

15. Ibid.

16. Forchuk C, Reynolds W. Clients' reflections on relationships with nurses: comparisons from Canada and Scotland. *Journal of Psychiatric and Mental Health Nursing* 2001; **8**(1): 45–51.

17. Reynolds W, Scott B. Empathy: a crucial component of the helping relationship. *Journal of Psychiatric and Mental Health Nursing* 1999; **6**(5): 363–70.

18. Ibid.

19. Barker P. The Tidal Model: developing an empowering, person-centred approach to recovery within psychiatric and mental health nursing. *Journal of Psychiatric and Mental Health Nursing* 2001; **8**(3): 233–40.

20. Roberts D. Liaison mental health nursing: origins, definition and prospects. *Journal of Advanced Nursing* 1997; **25**: 101–8.

21. Reynolds W, Scott B. Do nurses and other professional helpers normally display much empathy? *Journal of Advanced Nursing* 2000; **31**(1): 226–34.

22. Ibid.

23. Ibid.

24. Ibid.

25. Murdaugh C, Parsons M, Gryb-Wysocki T, Palmer J, Glasby C, Bonner J, Tavakoli A. Implementing a quality of care model in a restructured hospital environment. *National Academies of Practice Forum; Issues in Interdisciplinary Care* 1999; **1**(3): 219–26.

26. Bates A. Critical thinking by nurses on ethical issues like termination of pregnancies. *Curationis: South African Journal of Nursing* 2000; **23**(3): 26–31.

27. Raphael-Leff J. Professional issues. Psychodynamic understanding: its use and abuse in midwifery. *British Journal of Midwifery* 2000; **8**(11): 686–7.

28. Rappaport W, Cohen R, Riddle M. Diabetes through the life span: psychological ramifications for patients and professionals. *Diabetes Spectrum* 2000; **13**(4): 201–8.

29. Hogg A. *Working with users: beyond the Patients' Charter.* London, Brixton: Health Rights Ltd, 1994.

Chapter 19

GROUPWORK WITH CHILDREN AND ADOLESCENTS

Sue Croom*

INTRODUCTION

There is compelling evidence that responding effectively to Child and Adolescent Mental Health (CAMH) issues represents a critical area for mental health nurses.

❏ One in five children and adolescents suffer from moderate to severe mental health problems.[1]
❏ Links have been established between mental health problems in children and adolescents and issues of public concern such as juvenile crime, alcohol and drug misuse, self-harm and eating disorders.[2]
❏ A significant number of severe problems in child-hood, if not adequately treated can lead to lifelong mental illness in adulthood.[3]
❏ Emotional and behavioural problems in the young not only carry an increased probability of adult mental illness, but may also indicate an increased risk of delinquency as the child grows up and continuing antisocial behaviour in adulthood.[4]
❏ Children with a parent with mental illness are known to be at higher risk of developing a mental health difficulty of their own.[5]

❏ The rate of mental health problems is higher in young offenders, particularly persistent offenders.[6]
❏ Difficult behaviour is the most common reason for children to be excluded from schools and the risk of further mental health problems is high.[7]
❏ Children who do not do well at school are at increased risk of mental health problems. The low self-esteem, and sense of 'in-competence' that this creates, can have an impact on job prospects and relationships leading to a risk of social isolation and difficulties with parenting, which may then affect the next generation.[8]

Some key factors, which appear to protect young people from child and adolescent mental health problems include the development of self-esteem, sociability and autonomy and engagement in social systems, which encourage personal effort and coping.[9] These protective factors can all be promoted through groupwork. For adolescents, such groupwork can improve social and communication skills through role modelling feedback and practice.

Groups can be differentiated according to the devel-

* Sue Croom is a senior lecturer/research fellow/senior clinical practitioner in Child and Adolescent Mental Health (CAMH) with the University of Northumbria where she runs a multi-agency CAMH course, and Newcastle, Northumberland North Tyneside Mental Health Trust where she is developing strategies to work collaboratively with young people and parents to promote their capacity to become part of the solution to responding to CAMH needs.

opmental tasks, which children and young people need to achieve to meet their individual, social, emotional and developmental goals. Younger children can learn *turn taking*, *sharing* and participating in *cooperative play*; middle age range children can use activities and discussion to explore a sense of *who they are*, their *strengths* and *vulnerabilities*, and how to achieve a positive place in their *peer group* and to reflect on their *wider role in society*.

Research supports the efficacy of group therapy and groupwork for children and adolescents. A critical success factor appears to be the relationship of the children to the group therapist. Children seem to get on better with adults, who can develop a warm positive rapport with them, are outgoing, and have a sense of humour.[10]

THERAPEUTIC PRINCIPLES OF GROUPWORK WITH CHILDREN AND ADOLESCENTS

There are some overarching principles, which are essential to successful groups. The following principles have been modified from the work of Yalom[11] and Kolvin *et al.*:[10]

1 **Conveying optimism**: It is crucial that the children and adolescents are helped to see how they have moved on, e.g. 'That's such a good way of looking at things – I don't think you could have done that the last time we met – it's great to see how much you're progressing'. This allows children and young people to see themselves and their peers improve in different ways.

2 **Developing a sense of connection**: All children and adolescents need to feel a sense of belonging. This can help them to appreciate that others can feel or react in similar ways to them – e.g. 'Has anybody else ever felt like that?'

3 **Helping children/young people develop a sense of who they are**: Supporting children/young people in exploring how they think and feel; developing an awareness of their values, e.g. through activities such as art work, discussion and games.

4 **Developing a sense of giving and empathy**: Through adult modelling, and the promotion of supportive, respectful, empathic interactions, children and young people learn to support each other, and thus feel needed and useful. Comforting and supporting a peer can be a mutually rewarding experience.

5 **Recreating a primary family group experience**: Through experiencing the sense of nurture, safety and caring in the group, child/young person can experience alternative patterns to the

maladaptive ones they may have experienced in their families.

6 **Developing of social skills**: Learning skills which promote successful social interactions can increase the likelihood that the young people will be able to experience positive interactions in the group and to transfer these to their everyday lives.

7 **Role modelling by either peers or adults**: Children and young people have the opportunity to observe alternative ways of responding constructively to frustration or embarrassment.

8 **Using the group experiences to explore how the group members relate to each other and the meaning and consequences of these experiences**.

9 **Learning how to discharge distressing feelings or impulses in socially acceptable ways**, e.g. when upset with a peer, attempting to discuss the situation or, if angry, to hit a drum instead of hitting out at a peer or adult.

10 **Acknowledging together some common life experiences**, e.g. sharing situations which may not seem to be fair and particularly for adolescents, recognizing that individuals must take responsibility for the way they live their lives.

GROUPWORK WITH YOUNGER CHILDREN

Groups for young children with emotional or behavioural problems can recreate the experience of a normally developing child from infancy onwards. This can be achieved through the routine and predictability of the group's structure, which is underpinned by a strong nurturing philosophy.[12] Children can build on this safety net of security and trust to meet their developmental tasks, such as the ability to trust, explore, acquire a sense of achievement and begin to develop a sense of internal control.[13] Recreating the nurture of infancy can be achieved through meeting basic needs, e.g. for food. Meal and break times can be informal, enjoyable and very powerful opportunities to express nurture. Meeting emotional needs can be facilitated through studying the child, 'tuning in' to their feelings and needs, e.g. through maintaining proximity to the child, giving eye contact, encouraging activities. The nurses in such groups can model how adults can demonstrate confident, polite and supportive behaviour while engaging in the everyday tasks of living with the children. The nurses thus have the opportunity to use each event in the group as a therapeutic learning experience. As young children cannot be seen in isolation from their family systems, any groupwork needs to be complemented with parallel work and liaison with parents.

Case study 19.1

Tommy, aged 3, has difficulties trusting adults to meet his needs. This tends to manifest itself through aggressive behaviour with adults and peers. His single parent mother, Tracey, is just beginning to get over depression, which started when he was born. This has meant that Tracey has had difficulties tuning in to Tommy's cues, and he has learned that hitting an adult is effective, if he wants their attention.

In the group a nurse, who is allocated to stay close to him, supports him with activities. During the session, he becomes engrossed with building a high tower with a set of wooden bricks, but he finds that it always falls down before he has completed it. Although the nurse is beside him, attempting to engage with him, he ignores her until he fails for the third time, when he charges at her, aiming to hit her. She takes him to one side until he calms down and then suggests they go and build the tower together. She attends closely to Tommy's activity and provides positive encouragement about his progress in order to show her interest and to reinforce his capabilities. She notices that once he starts to find the task difficult, he does not ask her for help, but hits his head hard with the brick. She achieves eye contact with Tommy and comments that they appear to have got to a difficult stage of building. She wonders aloud if the tower needs straightening and when Tommy agrees, she asks if she can help him with it. She continues to subtly support Tommy each time he seems to be getting frustrated until he finally succeeds and she verbalizes her delight at Tommy's achievement. Tommy learns in this session that playing with an adult can be enjoyable if they encourage him, but don't take over his activity. The nurse shares this with his mother, who admits she has been worried about Tommy hitting himself for what she perceived was no reason. The nurse and mother both agree to try to proactively respond to Tommy's ineffectual ways of asking for help. At the next session, Tommy is much more trusting of the nurse and seeks her help through eye contact instead of hitting her. Once she feels Tommy is confident, the nurse introduces another little boy, Andrew, whom Tommy seems to like, to the activity. Andrew is able to verbally ask her for help and Tommy learns how effective this can be, from observing the consequences.

Eventually the nurse moves the boys on from building their own towers to building one together and helps them to take turns. The nurse shares the successful strategies with Tommy's mother, so that there can be generalization of his learning to the home setting. Over time, Tommy and his mother develop a much more trusting and rewarding relationship and Tommy builds on his confidence to begin to interact more spontaneously with other peers in his group.

GROUPWORK WITH CHILDREN AGED 7–11

The developmental task for younger children (7–11) is to build on the sense of trust and initiative[13] they have learned from previous stages of development. This helps them acquire a sense of themselves as competent individuals. Group sessions, which focus on play and activities can be used to develop a sense of achievement and skills with social interactions and peer relationships.[14] Children can be helped to explore relationships and the expression of feelings through the use of play materials, fantasy and conversation. Although the sessions enable children to express themselves, there are clear limits and boundaries, which guide children to behave in socially and developmentally acceptable ways.

Activity groups involving games and exercises can help children to meet their developmental goal of achieving a sense of competence and to explore a range of solutions to cope with issues such as peer relationships, and life event changes such as separation and loss. Structured activities can be particularly useful for children such as those with behaviour problems or impulsivity, who find unstructured time difficult to cope with. The activities can thus facilitate:

❑ The development of *positive group dynamics* such as feeling a sense of cohesion and belonging.
❑ The child to work through *conflicts, hostilities* and *frustration* through games, which can develop and promote their *social adjustment, peer relationships* and *leaderships skills*.

Negative behaviours such as aggression usually elicit a negative response and can set up a cycle of negative feelings – rejection, anger and frustration. Children who have experienced this, need time to develop their trust in the group before they can be helped to give up their well-established defence of rejecting others, as a way of avoiding rejection themselves.

Case study 19.2

During an activity where the children have been making lemonade, Tim accidentally spills some juice onto Annie, who then becomes very angry and tries to throw some juice back at him. The nurse uses a calm tone of voice to convey to the children that she is in control of the situation. (It is crucial that children have the opportunity to observe how adults can resolve situations when they are annoyed or frustrated, so that the child can learn to trust adults to be able to contain difficult feelings. This helps them to internalize alternative ways of successfully managing frustration in everyday life.) The nurse calmly and supportively cleans Annie up, giving eye contact to Tim to reassure him that this can be worked out. Annie is convinced Tim did it on purpose, because her 'world belief' is that 'everyone is out to get me'. The nurse attempts to soothe Annie's distress by empathizing with how upset she must feel in getting wet and in thinking that Tim did it on purpose. At the same time, she reiterates the group rules that throwing things at each other is not allowed. Acknowledging distress while setting limits can be helpful for other children in the group, who may also have experienced similar situations. Once Annie's body posture and voice tone suggests that she is calm enough to be able to listen, the nurse appeals to the rest of the group to think of the possible reasons for why Tim may have spilled the juice and how he could handle this. Using the peer group to generate alternative explanations is helpful in encouraging Annie to consider other interpretations for Tim's behaviour and a range of solutions. The nurse helps the group to develop a solution of Tim apologizing to Annie. She praises Tim when he does this, commenting on his body posture, tone of voice and eye contact. When Annie accepts his apology, she also praises Annie and asks the group to explore how they feel the situation has been managed and how they may use this learning in the future. The situation may only take minutes to deal with, but provides a powerful way of modelling alternative behaviours for children within a group setting.

GROUPWORK WITH ADOLESCENTS

Groups are important for adolescents, whose developmental tasks include developing a positive identity, a confident place among their peers, gradually developing more intimate relationships and finding their role in society.[13] As individuals are born into, live and work in groups throughout their lives, they formulate their identities and learn behaviours associated with their ascribed roles, through dynamic, interactive processes, which often occur in groups. Group therapy can maximize this group interactive process to explore interpersonal fears, fantasies, conflicts and feelings.[15] Adolescents can use the group process to improve their interactive skills, gain acceptance and peer support and give and receive corrective feedback. The group experience can enhance the young persons positive sense of self/identity and their capacity to perform in expected and selected roles. Modelling and role-play can also be used to develop the young person's social skills, coping skills, insight into their problems and strengths and ways of coping through rehearsal, feedback and social reinforcement. Developing these skills can significantly increase the likelihood of eliciting positive responses from significant others such as teachers, parents and peers.

Case study 19.3

Peter is a 14-year-old boy who has a history of somatic complaints. This has led to long absences from school, strained relationships at home and withdrawal from his peer group. He has had intensive investigations, but no physical cause has been found to account for his symptoms. He speaks in a barely audible voice with his head lowered and rarely initiates any interaction. He is initially very reluctant to join the group. The group facilitator strategically organizes the session so that Peter sits next to a 15-year-old, Gary, who is verbal and well-liked by peers because of the kindness and consideration which he often shows them. Gary has a problem with impulsivity and aggression towards adults in the classroom or at home and resents what he perceives as their hostile interference in his life. The facilitator noticed in the first session that Peter appeared able to respond to Gary. She is thus trying to capitalize on the capacity of youths to connect to each other in the groups. After a couple of weeks Peter seems to be enjoying the group activities, the humour and the support of the group. He is able to engage in a role-play where he has to practice asking his parents if he can stay out one hour later than usual because of a special event. The facilitators have previously modelled the use of eye contact, body posture, tone of voice and negotiation skills. Peter receives positive feedback from his peers and the facilitators. He is amazed at how good he feels about doing this and reflects that usually he wouldn't bother trying this with his parents, because it never works. He is encouraged by the group to explore how he feels when he gives up and whether it may be worthwhile giving the skills that have been modelled a try and to reflect on what some of the benefits may be.

Gary also engages in this role-play and reflects that although in real situations he would feel irritated at having to ask, he admits there may be benefits to using these skills. Both young people are able to identify how angry they feel with adults, but the different ways in which they express this. Over time, Peter becomes much more assertive and his reliance on physical symptoms to express his feelings reduce. His parents have needed support to relate to their son, who now has the confidence to express himself and whom they initially perceived as a demanding, 'stroppy teenager'. Gary finds that he can use his innate sense of empathy to begin to explore how adults feel and how to respond assertively rather than aggressively and this has reduced the conflict in his life.

GROUPWORK WITH YOUNG PEOPLE WITH SERIOUS MENTAL HEALTH PROBLEMS

Groupwork can provide an integral component of a holistic treatment programme for young people with serious mental health problems, such as thought disorders. It is essential to identify the exact nature of the thought disorder and the ways it impacts on the young persons experience in order to clarify how to help the young person interpret social and environmental cues. There must therefore be a constant reassessment of the ability of the young person to interact with their environment in order to judge their suitability for groups. After a period of stabilization, group treatment may be beneficial. It is crucial however to assess the other group members level of functioning and the group dynamics relative to the young person with a thought disorder. The group members may scapegoat the young person because of their bizarre behaviour or use it to avoid exploring their own issues. As the young person with thought disorder may find psychotherapeutic exploration too anxiety provoking or over-stimulating, they may need to be present initially for only a part of the time. They will initially be able to tolerate more structured activities and may find that focusing on group activities will help them to orientate themselves to 'reality' whereas the intensity of dealing with past issues and feelings may be too anxiety provoking.

Returning to school or college may be a specific issue for many young people who are experiencing psychosis. Groups which can focus on cognitive strategies such as developing effective study strategies, improving attention and concentration, increasing the use of memory and learning strategies and improving academic performance and coping with social interaction can be critical in helping the young person to achieve their potential.

Groupwork can also be effective for adolescents with eating problems. The emotional support, reality testing and the hope engendered from seeing others improve are important elements of the group experience. The power of peer groups can be particularly useful in challenging dysfunctional cognitive schema and in motivating individuals, e.g. those with bulimia to abstain from vomiting. A number of major issues can be explored. Social skills are important for young people with eating disorders, who often have difficulties establishing close friendships. Assertiveness skills can also be useful for young people with anorexia, who often play a very compliant role and for young people with bulimia who often play a passive role. Their difficulties in acknowledging and expressing anger may underlie their problems.

Need for supervision and support for group facilitators

For nurses to maintain their consistent demonstration of nurture, stimulation, limit setting and facilitation of personal growth, good supervision and support is needed. Nurses may experience the child's transference of the feelings of hate and anger, which they may wish to communicate to their caregiver. Furthermore, children may feel a need to severely test out the nurse to see if she/he will reject him/her as other adults have done. Without support from the rest of the team and the development of insight, the nurse could develop unhealthy counter transference towards the child, feeling for example that this child 'is deliberately trying to wind me up'.

Planning a group

Planning the group is an essential component of the overall group process. Group facilitators need to explore the type of group they wish to run, e.g. for vulnerable young people who are referred to CAMH services or a group, which is universally available to all, e.g. a social skills programme for a particular school year group. The advantage of the former is that it can be focused on the presenting problems. Universal groups have the advantage of being non-stigmatized and are therefore useful in promotion of CAMH and prevention of CAMH problems. Facilitators also need to decide if the group will be 'open' throughout the course of the group or closed once members have been selected in order to build up a group identity.

The venue of the group needs to be carefully considered to ensure it can convey a sense of comfort, safety and confidentiality. The size and organization of the room is important. For discussion groups, sitting too closely together or being in a large open space can be threatening. However, for young children, and children or young people who tend to act out their feelings, there needs to enough room to carry out activities and engage in exercises, which can drain away pent up emotions. The length of the groups, their frequency and the time at which they are scheduled needs to be negotiated with parents, schools and with other relevant organizations. It may be helpful to run a group for children alongside a group for parents in order to maximize the effects.[14]

The mix of the groups for targeted and clinical populations of children or young people also requires careful thought. Much has been written about the contagion effects of acting out children in groups.[15] It can therefore be more productive to have a mixture of acting out children alongside with more socially withdrawn young people. There is also a need to balance gender and cultural needs within groups.[15]

Gaining organizational support for running a group

It is crucial to think how a group fits into an overall CAMH strategy to ensure maximum support for the group's sustainability. For children and young people, developing a sense of trust and consistency is critical to their being able to engage in work, which can help them meet their developmental tasks. Thus, it is important that group facilitators attend each session unless there is an unforeseen circumstance. This provides a powerful message that the group is valued. Contingency arrangements need to be planned in case one of the facilitators is ill to ensure the group goes ahead. The minimum number of facilitators is two, but more may need to be negotiated depending upon the age of the participants, the group mix and the severity of the problems.

Maintaining attendance

Children/young people who have a low self-esteem and a difficulty with developing trusting relationship, may need particular encouragement to attend the group and to maintain attendance. Outreach work involving contacting any young person who did not attend is essential to give the message that they are valued, that their presence was missed by the group and to try to solve any problems related to the following week's attendance.

Managing the group

Children and young people with conduct or behaviour problems can be difficult to work with in a group setting. It is therefore critical to establish ground rules right at the beginning, which the group can refer back to, e.g. only one person speaks at a time, name calling and hitting is not allowed, no criticizing without coming up with a positive solution.

Routines in the group are important in developing a sense of predictability, continuity, consistency, security and group identity, e.g. always starting with an ice breaker and establishing a set time for a break. Food and drinks are essential to convey a sense of nurture and of being valued. It is essential to negotiate the provision of these in advance. At the beginning of the group or with very young children, the group leaders will be in charge of snacks, but as the group develops, members can take more responsibility for the planning of snacks and so reflect the dynamic development of the group and the growing autonomy of the participants.

In the initial *exploration phase*, the members need time to build up a sense of trust and ownership. The group may initially be highly dependent on groupworkers and so compliant to their wishes. As the group progresses, they will probably re-enact their early care-giving relationships and so will need to feel that the groupworkers can contain their feelings and behaviours while providing a consistent flow of nurture and support. This may mean that the children/adolescents engage in varying degrees of 'testing out' to see if the groupworker's limit setting and the group's

ground rules can be manipulated; and if the groupworkers can still like and value them despite being presented with difficult behaviour. Children/young people may be reluctant to reveal very much about themselves because of a fear of rejection and an unwillingness to trust the group, because of situations in the past, where they feel they have been let down. The group leaders need to be in tune with the degree of vulnerability felt by the young people, so that they are not over-exposed to stress before the supportive bonds of the group have emerged. Warm-up sessions can be helpful such as passing around a bowl of sweets and inviting each participant to take as many as they want and then asking them to share information related to the colour. At first the colours may be related to trivia to help the group to relax, e.g. if you have a red sweet, tell the group your favourite pop star. As the group becomes more confident the colours can represent more exploratory issues – such as blue means 'share the best thing that happened in the past week' or orange means 'share with the group what you like about yourself'. Such group exercises also ensure that everyone has the opportunity to participate and learn about each other, and so is useful for developing group cohesion. This early phase provides an opportunity to develop group trust and the group identity/norms, e.g. it's OK not to get it right!

In the *middle phase*, members can learn alternative ways of coping with difficult situations or distressing feelings. Here they can develop a greater rapport with each other and can use the group to discuss/try out ideas rather than constantly needing to check back to the group leaders. This is the most productive stage of the group. Group leaders need to listen actively, checking out and summarizing points, e.g. 'So what I'm hearing is that it can be difficult to negotiate with adults – is that right?' They also need to help the group develop solutions, e.g. 'I wonder how that could be handled?' Positive feedback is crucial for all age ranges. This may take the form of positive comments on activities, positively reinforcing an interesting discussion point or an innovative solution to a problem or pointing out a situation, when one peer has been kind or supportive to another.

In the last stage, there is a need to work through the feelings of loss when the group comes to an end. Group facilitators can liaise with community groups to try to help the children/young people access other groups, when they have completed the therapeutic group, e.g. cubs, youth clubs, football or dance classes. In this way, the young people can continue to use and apply the skills they have learned in other settings.

Managing conflict and scapegoating

If a young person is allowed to monopolize the group, other members may respond with hostility and ridicule.

This increases the potential of scapegoating the young person when the group members project all of their negative feelings onto them. This may also occur towards the most vulnerable members. The response of the group facilitators in modelling a sense of fair play and justice is crucial while simultaneously exploring with the group what they feel is happening and how it can be resolved. In this way, the young people can develop the skills to cope and problem solve in social situations.

Coping with silence in the group

Many children and adolescents can find silence threatening and difficult to cope with. The group facilitators need to be able to sensitively explore with the group what is underlying the silence, e.g. being bored, wanting to avoid the current topic of discussion or simply needing the time to think things through. In this way, the silence can be used productively within the group. Any quiet or withdrawn members may need support to speak in non-threatening ways, e.g. 'You made a very interesting point about this a couple of weeks ago' or 'I guess from your expression that you find this interesting – is there anything you would like to add'.

Case study 19.4

Marylyn stands out in her adolescent group because of her slightly awkward manner and clumsiness. At first the group are tolerant towards each other but as they get to know each other a range of difficuilt emotional and interpersonal issues arise, and Marilyn appears to become their scapegoat. Just before break, she drops the papers she has just collected in following a group exercise. The group get angry saying that she always makes them late for their snack. The group leader reflects back to the group that they seem to be irritated this morning and suggests that it may not be about Marylyn, but about how they are feeling about other things. Through a discussion on how it is possible to project our feelings onto others and an exploration of group experiences related to this, she manages to appeal to the group sense of fair play to explore the impact of their behaviour on Marylyn. Through this, they acknowledge that each person in the group deserves the support of the group. This kind of discussion can help develop a sense of group norms and values, provides an opportunity for the group to explore alternative ways of coping with difficult feelings other than getting angry with someone else and gives them insight into why they may blame others or get the blame themselves and how to deal with this.

EVALUATION

It is crucial to write up the group sessions afterwards in order to:

1 Reflect on the group content.

2 Debrief emotionally laden situations which may arise, e.g. from transference or the group splitting the facilitators into the 'good' leader and 'bad' leader.

3 Document each participant's progress, e.g. their interaction/involvement in the group and their verbal and non-verbal communication.

4 Write notes on the functioning of group as a whole: interactions, mood, body posture, alliance, pairing, power hierarchies, group problem-solving.

The group can thus be evaluated using an analysis of such reports, allowing staff to explore how effective the group has been in helping the members achieve their developmental goals, develop their sense of self-esteem and competence, and gain skills in problem-solving and social interaction. The group can also be evaluated using standard questionnaires, such as the Goodman's Strengths and Difficulties[16] questionnaire. This offers an insight into changes in the profile of the child/young person's strengths and needs, before and after participation in the group.

SUMMARY

Groupwork holds great potential for responding to the needs of younger people of different ages, in CAMH services. Factors which are critical to the successful running of groups include the ability of the group facilitators to convey warmth, a sense of humour, to ensure that safety and integrity of the group members is preserved and to have a good understanding of social, cultural and developmental issues. It is also crucial to ensure that any group is an integral part of the wider strategy for CAMH in order to gain organizational support for implementing the group and networking with the extent systems of the young person and their families. Planning the group in terms of the aims, venue, recruitment and mix of the group together with evaluation and supervision can help to guide the group to be a supportive, learning experience for the young people and an effective component of the overall strategy to reduce the individual, social and community distress arising from child and adolescent mental health problems.

REFERENCES

1. Mental Health Foundation. *Bright futures*. London: Mental Health Foundation, 1999.

2. Audit Commission. *Children in mind*. London: Audit Commission, 1999.

3. Target M, Fonagy P. The psychological treatment of child and adolescent psychiatric disorder. In: Roth A, Fonagy P (eds). *What works for whom? A critical review of psychotherapy research*. New York: Guilford Press, 1996: 263–320.

4. Famington D, Loeber R, Van Kammen WB. Long term criminal outcomes of hyperactivity–impulsivity–attention deficit and conduct disorder in childhood. In: Robins L, Rutter M (eds). *Straight and devious pathways from childhood to adulthood*. Cambridge: Cambridge University Press, 1990: 62–81.

5. Falkov A. *Crossing bridges: training resources for working with mentally ill parents and their children*. London: Department of Health, 1988.

6. Rutter M, Giller H, Hagell A. *Antisocial behaviour by young people*. Cambridge: Cambridge University Press, 1998.

7. Barnes J. Mental health promotion: a developmental perspective. *Psychology, Medicine and Health* 1998; 3(1): 55–69.

8. Graham P. Behavioural and intellectual development in childhood epidemiology. *British Medical Bulletin* 1986; **42**: 155–62.

9. Offord DR. The State of prevention and early intervention. In: Peters RD, McMahon RJ (eds). *Preventing childhood disorders, substance abuse and delinquency*. Thousand Oaks, CA: Sage, 1996: 329–44.

10. Kolvin I, Garside RG, Nicol AR, Macmillan A, Wolstenholme F, Leitch IM. *Help starts here: the maladjusted child in the ordinary school*. London: Tavistock, 1981.

11. Yalom ID. *The theory and practice of group psychotherapy*. New York: Basic Books, 1975.

12. Bennathan M, Boxall M. *Effective interventions in primary schools: nurture groups*. London: David Fulton, 1996.

13. Erikson EH. *Identity and the life cycle*. New York: Norton, 1980.

14. Webster-Stratton C. *How to promote children's social and emotional competence*. London: Paul Chapman, Sage, 1999.

15. Dwivedi, K. *Groupwork with children and adolescents: a handbook*. London: Jessica Kingsley, 1993.

16. Goodman R, Meltzer H, Bailey V. The strengths and difficulties questionnaire: a pilot study on the validity of the self report version. *European Child and Adolescent Psychiatry* 1998; 7: 125–30.

Chapter 20

PSYCHODYNAMIC APPROACHES WITH INDIVIDUALS

Brendan Murphy*

> Upon my word, I think the truth is the hardest missile one can be pelted with.
>
> George Elliot, *Middlemarch*

INTRODUCTION

Models of the mind

Over the past 100 years, the nature of mental health and illness has been widely debated, investigated and disputed. This discussion of the nature of mental health and distress has drawn on a number of influential psychological models of the mind. These include the **behaviourist, cognitive** and **psychodynamic** models.

All these models offer explanations for the development and maintenance of mental distress and propose psychological techniques or psychotherapies that, it is claimed, will ease or remove mental distress.

The psychodynamic model draws upon the insights of Freud and other significant theorists. This approach takes account of unconscious as well as conscious elements of the personality and seeks to resolve unconscious conflicts with the aim of enhancing the overall development of the personality. The psychodynamic approach has developed over a long period, at least 100 years, and it is composed of a number of theories and concepts that can be applied to any therapeutic relationship. It is central to the understanding of psychoanalysis, psychotherapy and counselling. It is perhaps the oldest and most influential approach used in modern talking therapies.

This chapter is about the psychodynamic approach with individuals and aims to outline the development, key concepts and value of the psychodynamic approach with the individual.

Derivation of psychodynamic

A look at the derivation of this word psychodynamic helps to explain some of its meaning. It is composed of two Ancient Greek words, psyche meaning 'mind' and dynamic meaning 'moving force'.[1] The term 'mind' is used here to refer to the sum total of the thoughts, feelings, emotions, impulses and memories that may occur in

*Brendan Murphy MS EMN is currently Clinical Nurse Specialist Psychotherapy with the Derbyshire Mental Health Trust and a trainee on the South Trent Training in Psychotherapy. He worked previously as a Staff Nurse/Charge Nurse at University of Sheffield Department of Psychiatry/Acute Psychiatry and was Charge Nurse at the Norfolk Park Community Mental Health Project and Deputy Co-ordinator of the Leeds City Council Crisis Centre.

an individual, both conscious and unconscious. Mind and 'moving forces' implies that the mind is not a static entity it is in motion, active and has the ability to transform.

Freud[2] took the concept psychodynamic from the then recently invented device, the dynamo. In a dynamo, mechanical energy, pedalling a bicycle for example, is transformed into an electric current through a coil rotating in a magnetic field. If the properties of the magnetic field or the mechanical force varies then the electric current will vary, and perhaps will not flow at all. So we have a variety of elements (coil, mechanical force, magnetic field) and a result that is entirely different, electricity. The result can be seen as a product of the interaction of two or more ingredients. Clearly the analogy between the human mind and an electro-mechanical system like the dynamo is of limited value, because the mind is a much more complicated and subtle system. However paradoxically this analogy does help to capture something of the intricate nature of the mind and its constituents.

THE DEVELOPMENT OF THE PSYCHODYNAMIC APPROACH

It is generally agreed[2, pp.5–12] that psychodynamic theories and interventions evolved from the work of Freud and several of his close colleagues, who developed the theories and practice of psychoanalysis at the beginning of the 20th century in Vienna. It is interesting to note that at about the same time as Freud was producing his psychoanalytic theories in Central Europe the behaviourist theory was developing in the USA.

Ellenberger[3] has shown that many of the key ideas and concepts in psychodynamic thought have a history dating back long before the work of Freud. For example the 'unconscious', elements of the human mind – of which we are unaware – is often thought to be Freud's most important discovery. However, the philosopher Leibenitz had discussed this many centuries before Freud.[3] According to Brown and Pedder at the time that Freud was developing his own theories of the mind 'a work on Aristotle's concept of catharsis was being much talked of in Vienna in the 1880s and may have influenced Freud and his collaborator Breuer.[2]

Freud and his disciples

Freud was born in the same year, 1856, that Charles Darwin finally published the *Origin of Species*. Like Darwin's theory of evolution by natural selection, Freud's psychoanalytical theories had a profound impact on the way that people understood themselves and their place in the world, at least in the Western world. It is dif-

ficult today to understand the impact his new views of humanity had when first produced, because they are such familiar ways of thinking today. For example Masson[4] has claimed that Freud revised his original theory, the trauma theory of the origins of neurosis,[5] because its thesis, that neurosis was often the direct result of the sexual abuse of children by adults, was so unacceptable to his medical colleagues that it threatened his career.

Freud's achievement was to develop a systematic approach to the investigation of the mind. Freud took the insights of earlier philosophers and writers and combined them with his own careful observations as a trained scientist. He used his insight and understanding to synthesize a new account of the human psyche and developed a technique for treating individuals, which he called *psychoanalysis*. This model has been very influential in many areas of medical, cultural and social thought throughout the 20th century.[2] Two of Freud's most influential colleagues, Adler and Jung, had fundamental disagreements with Freud's psychoanalytic theory and went on to develop their own schools of therapy, individual psychology and analytical psychology respectively.[2]

Post-Freudian developments

Since the death of Freud, 1939, his work – and subsequently that of the other pioneers theorists – has undergone a great deal of development and revision, so that today there are a very large number of important theorists who can be described as *psychodynamic*. They include Anna Freud, Reich, Klein, Fairbairn, Horney, Fromm, Erikson, Winnicott, Bowlby, Sullivan, and Kohut. In turn other workers have developed and modified these ideas and techniques so that today many therapists, counsellors and nurses who do not practise psychoanalysis or analytical psychology would acknowledge the pioneering work of Freud and his co-workers. They would argue that they are working in the psychodynamic tradition initiated by Freud. Today, there is a wide variety of psychodynamic practice and theory. There is no one set of theories that is accepted by all therapists and mental health workers using the approach. Having said that, although there is no unchallenged theoretical position in the psychodynamic approach, there are some key psychodynamic principles that are widely discussed and used across the field.[2]

KEY PSYCHODYNAMIC CONCEPTS

This brief, and very selective, account of some of the most important concepts that make up the psychodynamic approach, draws on the works of Freud[6] and Malan.[7]

Hughes describes three important ideas derived from Freud's main theories, which have been influential in the development of the psychodynamic approach:

> That our behaviour is influenced by unconscious thoughts and feelings, and that symptoms may arise because of conflict between conscious thoughts and wishes and unconscious thoughts and wishes. This was part of Freud's Topographical Theory.[8]

> That we are born with innate instincts, which affect our behaviour. This was part of Freud's Structural Theory.[8]

> That early development has an important influence on adult behaviour. This was part of Freud's developmental theory.[8]

These three important areas of psychodynamic theory will now be discussed in turn.

The dynamic unconscious

The Unconscious is defined[9] as, 'an area of mental experience not available to normal awareness'. This is a part of the mind, which is as active as the conscious but of which we have no knowledge. The term may be used to refer to different levels of awareness, from something of which we are 'totally unaware' to that which we do not 'wish to acknowledge'. Freud believed that the conscious and the unconscious opposed each other; so that only through some sort of exploratory effort or work could we succeed in making conscious, that which is unconscious. However the deeper inaccessible regions of the unconscious, that of which we have no knowledge, could find expression by influencing the more accessible regions of the unconscious, that which we do not *wish* to acknowledge. These more accessible regions of the unconscious are called the *preconscious*.

Mental conflict

We are all familiar with the experience of conflicting wishes, which are an inevitable part of all our lives.

Consider the following example:

> Mr E wants a better job with more money yet knows that this entails giving up a home and friends that he loves and moving to another part of the country. Mr E wants more money and a better job *and* wants to keep the home and friends that he loves. In this case he cannot have both.

This is a conflict of which Mr E is aware. Other conflicts may be unconscious. Conflict can be extremely painful and anxiety provoking. Our ability to solve such conscious conflict is often based upon our feeling of personal security and integrity. Those people who have poor sense of personal security, low self-esteem may find the conflict intolerably painful. Conflicts that we meet in adult life may resonate with earlier conflicts, which we encountered as a child and these may become active again if they are still unresolved.

> Mr E is offered a new job with more money. He then develops a series of physical symptoms, particularly pains in his chest near his heart. Mr E describes it as 'heartache', and he feels he is unable take up the job. Concern for his health leads Mr E to turn the job offer down, after which the pains disappear. When he visits his doctor, there does not appear to be any physical cause for the pains in his chest. He is very healthy.

Here only one side of the conflict is obvious. The wish for the new job is conscious. We could suggest that the other side of the conflict is unconscious, but finds some means of expression through the chest pains.

Anxiety?

Human motivation and instincts

Any psychological model needs to explain human motivation: why we do the things that we do. More simply, what is it that makes us get up in the mornings! Freud thought that humans had a particular sort of nature; much like that of other animals, and that most of our behaviour is driven by very basic innate instincts or drives, such as the drive to reproduce and survive. These drives are represented in our minds in the forms of wishes or desires and become associated, from an early age, with the key figures in our life, for example our mothers and fathers.[9]

The drives are tendencies towards or away from certain types of experiences such as pleasure or pain. They are however very mobile and can be affected by the ways in which the outside world reacts to our needs or desires. This is especially important in our early life when the nature of our mind is open and very impressionable. This means that they can become strengthened, blocked, diverted or modified.

In his early theories Freud thought that there were only sexual and aggressive drives. Later modifications to his theory produced two very basic principles or drives, those of life and death. Thus there are the drives associated with life such as the sexual and nurturing aspects of human nature and those associated with death such as the aggressive and destructive aspects of human life.[10]

THE STRUCTURAL MODEL

In 1923 Freud[9] introduced his structural model, suggesting that the mind was made up of three regions the Ego, the Id and the Super Ego. The Ego, the rational thinking part of the mind, is conscious and can be modified through experiences with the outside world. The Id is the instinctual, largely unconscious area of the mind, and is the seat of the basic drives such as sex and aggression. The Super Ego is often described as corresponding to the Conscience, that is, the self-critical aspect of the mind. There are both conscious and unconscious aspects of the Super Ego.

Although the three regions of the mind are clearly separated and easily distinguishable, Freud thought that the division was more like that of the political region known as the Balkans, a complex mix of different races, creeds and languages, often in complex conflicts where borders shift and alliances change.[9]

Later theorists[2] have criticized aspects of Freud's Structural Theory of the mind and pointed out that he had missed out some very important aspects of human nature. A more comprehensive list of the basic drives would include:

❏ Relatedness;
❏ Aggression;
❏ Sexuality;
❏ Hunger;
❏ Curiosity.

Human development

According to the psychodynamic model the individual develops physically and psychologically from childhood, through adolescence and into adulthood. The development of the mind and the body are inextricably linked. There are definite stages of growth and development, which are registered in body and mind. For example, consider the difference in the body and mind of a young infant and an adolescent.

In psychodynamic theory, early childhood relationships mould the individual's mind. The patterns of early relationships, especially with mother or other early carer, are held in the mind. They become a major influence in determining the nature of future relationships. An understanding of the individual's development in the *past* is important for understanding the individual *now*.

Most of us will have suffered shocks, frustrations, rejections and disappointments in the past, especially in our relationships with other people. Many different psychodynamic descriptions have been devised to try to capture the way in which the mind responds to the frustrations inevitable in relationships. All the descriptions agree that past experiences affect the development of personality and exert their influence in the present by contributing to the way we negotiate current relationships.[8]

UNDERSTANDING INDIVIDUAL DISTRESS

According to Malan the psychodynamic model approaches human distress in a specific way:

> As human beings we adopt various defensive mechanisms in order to avoid mental pain or conflict or to control unavoidable impulses. These defences vary from being almost wholly conscious to being completely unconscious. The end product of these mechanisms is often a form of maladaptive behaviour or a neurotic symptom.[7]

Malan offers a basic psychodynamic view of how distress and disturbance are created and maintained by individuals. This can be represented by the Triangle of Conflict[7] (Fig. 20.1).

The Triangle of Conflict refers to the relationship between the *defence*, the *anxiety* and the *hidden feeling*, wish or impulse. It is represented by a triangle that stands on its apex with the defence and anxiety above the hidden feeling. This denotes the idea that the hidden feeling involves the more unconscious of the elements of the triangle.

From surface to depth

In psychodynamic theory it is thought that it is best to work from those elements near the surface and then to gradually reveal more depth or unconscious material. The defences are gradually explored together, with the anxiety and the hidden feeling or impulse, usually being the last element that is approached. This means that as defences are modified, and anxieties are understood and acknowledged, the hidden feeling may safely come into awareness and be expressed.[7]

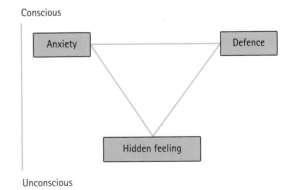

FIGURE 20.1 Triangle of Conflict

The three elements of the triangle will now be considered in more detail starting with the most unconscious aspect of the triangle – the 'hidden feeling'.

Hidden feeling

The psychodynamic model starts from the observation that we suffer mental conflicts, usually conflicting feelings, impulses, 'wishes,' or 'desires'. This conflict causes pain, distress and disturbances within us and we look for ways of removing or escaping from the pain and distress that is caused. Unacceptable impulses, ideas or feelings are rejected and forced into the unconscious area of the mind. This process of making something unconscious is termed *repression*.

Anxiety or mental anguish

The repressed material is active and seeks expression, yet is forcefully kept out of awareness. If there is a danger that the material repressed become conscious, this is experienced as anxiety. Anxiety occurs because the threat of loss, or some other distressing wish or impulse, causes the disturbing aspects of mental life.

Defence mechanisms

Think how common it is when we lose somebody close to us, either in death or through loss of a relationship. We deny what has happened. Denial is the means by which we, albeit temporarily or partially, are able to forget what has happened to us in reality. It can be thought of as a 'defence mechanism'. The defence mechanism removes from our conscious awareness the conflicting impulse, wish or desire, thus rendering it unconscious.

Case study 20.1: A common defence

Jack, who is a Community Mental Health Nurse, attends an early morning referral meeting. At the end of the meeting, while discussing the best referral for a patient whom Jack thinks needs to be seen urgently, his ideas are contradicted and rudely rejected by his manager. The patient is referred to another service with a long waiting list. Jack leaves the meeting feeling angry.

At home, Jack's partner playfully contradicts him. He becomes furious, tells his partner that she does not know what she is talking about and startles himself with the intensity of his reaction.

We might be as puzzled as Jack about his reaction, until we consider that he may be 'displacing' the anger he feels towards his manager, onto his partner. Jack's partner is a safer and more understanding person, with whom Jack can become angry without fear of retaliation.

In this example we can see that the *defence* is a displacement of anger from one person to another.

A hierarchy of defences

The psychodynamic approach thinks of *defence mechanisms* as being the normal human reaction to difficult and impossible situations. There is a view that some defences are more debilitating and constricting to individual development than others.[8] For example, *denial* may be very important at some periods of our life, following the bereavement of a loved one, for example. However if denial becomes a habitual way of dealing with problems, there is a real possibility that this will grossly distort our relationships with other people. Think for instance of the way in which people who drink alcohol, to the extent that it is destroying their relationships with partners, children and friends, may deny that they have any problems or difficulties associated with drinking alcohol. We all use defences, to some degree, to deal with the inevitable pains and frustrations of life.

The psychodynamic approach involves examining *habitual* defence strategies that have developed unconsciously, encouraging the relinquishing of old defences that are no longer necessary, or their substitution by more useful strategies some of which may be thought of as defences.

DEVELOPING THERAPEUTIC RELATIONSHIPS

While it might appear obvious, all mental health work assumes that we are involved in some type of relationship with our patients (see Table 20.1).

Introspection

Introspection involves looking into oneself, or encouraging another person to tune into memories, thoughts,

TABLE 20.1

Nurse and patient	Us and them	You and I
Student and tutor	Mother and baby	Victim and persecutor
Abuser and abused	Lover and beloved	Doctor and nurse

At one time or another we may all be involved in each of the set of relationships outlined above. In reflecting upon these relationships there are a number of useful questions that we might ask.

1 Which of these relationships is important now in your life?
2 How would you describe these relationships if asked?
3 Are there any connections between the relationships? For example do you form the same types of relationships, or are they all very different?
4 Are your earlier relationships in any way like your current relationships?

ideas, motives and feelings. In the psychodynamic approach introspection is thought to be a means of discovering useful information. With the implication that developing the ability to understand and find out about oneself is beneficial. The method of working in the psychodynamic approach is to create the conditions, through a relationship with the patient that allows the patient to talk freely about what is currently on their mind, this is known as free association.[2]

Repetitive patterns of relationship

As was stated earlier the psychodynamic approach asserts that early childhood experiences influence the way in which we subsequently relate to others. We internalize a particular set of relationships and these patterns are stored in our mind. Freud observed that people had a tendency to repeat patterns of relating and behaviour, sometimes at great cost to themselves. Freud termed this the 'compulsion to repeat'.[2, p.115] There is an important implication in this pattern of repeating relationships for any caring relationship, in that the person seeking help is likely to repeat in the relationship with the nurse or helper, important aspects of their habitual relationships.

Transference

Hughes[8] defines *transference* as, 'the transfer of feelings, which belong to a relationship from the past into a present relationship'. These attributions are inappropriate to the present relationship and this process is unconscious. In a general sense we respond to any new situation in terms of our past experience. At times we may respond to people as though they were specific people from our past. This is particularly likely to happen if we are distressed, when regression is more common. Freud saw that transference could be used as a therapeutic agent of change

Counter-transference

Hughes[8] describes the *counter-transference* as; 'the feeling or feelings elicited in the therapist by the patients behaviour and communication.'

It may be understood as a way in which the particular aspects or qualities of the relationship that the patient forges may be experienced by the helper. This will give valuable information about the model of relationship that the patients have internalized.

Case study 20.2a

Carole's early childhood is characterized by strong experiences of rejection. She develops the conviction that she is unwanted and unloved. Carole subsequently has a series of relationships in which she is neglected and rejected. Carole is admitted to the Acute Psychiatric Unit after a serious attempt to kill herself following the break-up of a relationship. On the ward she appears withdrawn and isolated from other people.

Nurse Zeta offers Carole regular time each day to talk about her problems. At first these sessions go well. At the end of the third meeting, however, Carole becomes very angry.

Carole: 'I do not want any more sessions. I cannot believe that you are here to help me; you must be doing it because you have been paid to do it'.

Carole walks out of the room.

Nurse Zeta is left feeling angry, unwanted and rejected.

Carole's transference

Helping relationships often brings to light the particular patterns of relating of the patient through the feelings that the person transfers onto the nurse or therapist. In the example above we can see that Carole has transferred her feelings of anger onto the Nurse Zeta who is trying to help her. Carole has been offered help by Zeta. At first this was acceptable and helpful. After a time, however, Carole appears to have become convinced that the help being offered was not sincere. Zeta could not possibly want to listen to her without having some other motive. Carole is showing us something about her understanding and expectation of relationships.

Nurse Zeta's counter-transference

Nurse Zeta is left feeling unwanted and rejected. These are similar to the feelings that Carole often talks about in her relationships. This may be important information for Nurse Zeta, if she can reflect on the situation, rather than angrily retaliate and reject Carole. This impulse to retaliate might be another important piece of *counter-transference*.

Nurse Zeta's wish to help Carole, is in conflict with her wish to reject her and her feeling of anger. There is, therefore, a danger of repeating Carole's particular pattern of relationship and confirming her belief that she will always be rejected.

Now Nurse Zeta's experience of relating to Carole means that she may be able to avoid the danger of repeating the pattern of rejecting Carole. This could allow Carole to gain a valuable insight into how and why she relates as she does. The therapeutic relationship becomes a means of helping Carole to understand and change her pattern of relationship. Carole and Zeta may be able to construct a different relationship, by using aspects of the knowledge and experience of the way in which Carole relates to her helper.

ANXIETY, DEFENCE AND HIDDEN FEELINGS

We might form a hypothesis using Milan's Triangle of Conflict. Carole fears (**anxiety**) rejection, so she angrily rejects the help offered to her and withdraws (**defence**). It is not yet possible to understand fully what the **hidden feeling** or impulse may be. We could make another hypothesis, that Carole has a lot of unexpressed feelings about the loss of her relationship, and the rejections that she has experienced in the past.

Case study 20.2b

In supervision with a colleague, Zeta is able to express her own feelings of rejection and anger. Her supervisor, while understanding her wish to forget about Carole, urges her to try and use her understanding of the relationship to help her.

They consider that Carole's feeling may, in some ways, be similar to the feelings of rejection and anger experienced by Zeta. They conclude that if Zeta is able to convey this understanding to Carole, it may help to develop the therapeutic relationship and allow Carole to begin to express her feelings of loss.

Zeta asks to meet with Carole again the following day and is surprised when she agrees.

After a short silence:

Carole: 'I am surprised that you want to see me again. Usually people just leave me alone after I have told them that I think like that.'

Zeta: 'Perhaps Carole you are afraid of me getting close to you and then leaving you alone again, as other people have done this in the past. Your anger is a way of protecting yourself when you are afraid that this is happening.'

At this, Carole began to talk about a friend who had spent time with her, and then had abruptly disappeared, taking with her some of Carole's property. Carole spoke about how lonely she felt and how she missed her partner who had left recently and then began to cry.

THE VALUE OF THE PSYCHODYNAMIC APPROACH

In this chapter, the development and key concepts of psychodynamic theory have been outlined. The value of the psychodynamic approach is that it offers a way of thinking about any human relationship, based upon a coherent and flexible understanding of the human mind. The psychodynamic model of mind is based upon direct observations of the development of the human infant, as well as numerous clinical observations of patients suffering emotional distress. These clinical observations have been continuously developed for over 100 years. In turn the observations of infants and adult patients has led to innovations and developments in theory and practice. This approach can offer the nurse or therapist a wealth of understanding of the development of human relationships and how these relationships are maintained.

The psychodynamic approach offers an understanding of the development of mental distress, and how by developing a therapeutic relationship, the patient may be helped to develop new and more fulfilling ways of relating.

REFERENCES

1. *The new Oxford English dictionary*. Oxford: Oxford University Press, 2001.
2. Brown D, Pedder J. *Introduction to psychotherapy*, 2nd edn. London: Routledge, 1991.
3. Ellenberger HF. *The discovery of the unconscious*. London: Allen Lane, 1970.
4. Masson JM. *The assault on truth: Freud's Suppression of the Seduction Theory*. New York: Farrar, Straus and Giroux, 1984.
5. Freud S. The neuro-psychoses of defence. In: Standard edn of *The complete psychological works of Sigmund Freud*, Vol. 3. London: Hogarth Press, 1894.
6. Freud S. *Inhibitions, symptoms and anxiety*, standard edn, Vol. 20. London: Hogarth Press, 1926.
7. Malan DH. *Individual psychotherapy and the science of psychodynamics*. London: Butterworth, 1979.
8. Hughes P. *Dynamic psychotherapy explained*. Oxford: Radcliffe Medical Press, 1999.
9. Freud S. *The Ego and the Id*, standard edn, Vol. 19. London: Hogarth Press, 1923.
10. Freud S. *New introductory lectures*, standard edn, Vol. 22. London: Hogarth Press, 1933.

Chapter 21

PSYCHODYNAMIC APPROACHES TO WORKING IN GROUPS

Phil Luffman*

INTRODUCTION

The psychodynamic approach forms the main component of experiential group treatment. The most essential components, however are the participants themselves, including the groupworker who facilitates or conducts the group. The nurse practitioner is a groupworker, in a dynamic sense, when (s)he views the group as the main instrument of change. The structure of the group may vary, as can the setting, and may include more than one groupworker. However, the purpose of the group, which is to understand better the problems the individual patient faces within a group context, via interpersonal group relations, remains the same.

The patient/member as auxiliary therapist is the most powerful therapeutic factor in making the group an effective medium for change. Giving and receiving of feedback – both supportive and confrontational – and the interventions and interpretations that seek to clarify meaning, are all functions that, when carried out by group participants, promote the self-help culture of the group.

Theory and practice should inform each other whatever model of therapy we adhere to. Within the psycho-dynamic approach these two factors become closely woven together at the point of application, which is focused on the relationships developing in the here and now of the group. The experiences that each group member brings to the attention of others is the operational basis for further exploration and elucidation, and involves all participants in a joint venture. This venture can be difficult and uncomfortable for the participants as thoughts, emotions and hidden wishes that are hard to acknowledge or manage, can surface from the unconscious at any time, and be projected into the group. What can be disclosed and shared will depend on the level of support and cohesion the group has established. The lasting benefits for the effort each individual makes go beyond increased self-understanding to a greater sense of intimacy and belonging based on empathy and respect.

The processes and outcomes of the group are similarly inter-related and are observable in its ongoing development. Even when a group is short-lived or when an individual participates in only a few sessions, processes and outcomes are still evident, as are some of the therapeutic benefits. The group analytic method in

* Phil Luffman is a clinical nurse specialist in psychotherapy with Powys Health Care Trust in Wales. He is a qualified group analyst and is interested in the potential of groups to generate creative ideas and solutions out of human suffering. As a practising Buddhist the nature of suffering and happiness are fundamental concerns that inform his work as a psychotherapist. He lives in Brecon and is married and has a daughter and three sons.

particular utilizes concepts derived from a number of theoretical sources. Central amongst these is classical psychoanalysis and its subsequent developments such as object relations theory. The concept of transference phenomena, which is discussed later, helps to explain how the patient's past comes to be re-activated and remembered in the current relationships between group members.

Freud's hypothesis that our lives and aspects of our behaviour are influenced or sometimes determined by unconscious processes remains an important concept underpinning the psychodynamic approach.[1] Freud described defence mechanisms as operating within a topographical model of Id, Ego and Superego, where the individual unconsciously seeks mastery over primitive impulses and wishes that are in conflict with the higher order aspects of the personality. According to Freud's model this comes under the censorship of the Superego. Object relations theory ushered in a move away from instinct and drive/conflict theory operating within a somewhat sealed off psychic apparatus, to a model that saw humans as essentially relationship seeking from the moment of birth. Winnicott in particular saw the mother–infant relationship as critical in terms of helping the baby differentiate itself from others.[2]

In this chapter I shall also consider groups outside the treatment setting, with some thoughts on naturally occurring groups within a social dimension. Foulkes, the founder of the group analytic method, called these 'life groups'.[3] Any gathering of friends or work colleagues could be described in this way. For the family or primary group, Foulkes gave the name 'root group'. I describe group psychotherapy in terms of its broadest therapeutic factors, which are observable in many group treatment methods. However they become the focus for exploring at the conscious and unconscious level in the analytic group. Therapeutic factors occur in everyday 'life groups'. For example, reducing one's isolation could be achieved by joining a club that meets regularly. What is important to emphasize is that by careful planning and preparation in the setting up of the treatment group, the essential safe boundary provides the conditions whereby therapeutic factors can be realized and exploited as they occur. It is rarely the case, however, that the individual experiences benefits without the necessary working through of their difficulties and conflicts. Similarly when an isolated person joins a club they may initially, at least, experience an increased sense of isolation if they feel unable to fit in.

I shall also consider, briefly, two aspects of the evolving nurse–patient relationship: the transference relationship – an unconsciously derived symbolic relationship – and the personal qualities and attributes of the professional relationship. What has been established in the two-person relationship – especially in the assessment and selection of group members – is the degree of trust and working alliance, which needs to carry over to the group situation.

The specific factors of the analytic group will also be considered alongside the important role of the conductor in preparing individuals for groupwork. Illustrations of these factors are given in a case example from a group session. Finally, I consider the wider applications of the psychodynamic and analytic method. This will consider the problems group psychotherapy can address and the different settings where it might be applied. Sometimes using a psychodynamic approach requires a modification of its methodology. Elsewhere, the method can be used in programmes incorporating large group dynamics such as therapeutic communities, staff groups, or within clinical supervision.[4–6]

WHAT DO WE MEAN BY A PSYCHODYNAMIC APPROACH?

A psychodynamic approach to groupwork covers several well-defined and less well-defined experiential treatment methods in a variety of settings. The small outpatient 'stranger group', of between seven to eight members, meeting once or twice weekly, is one well-defined, well-documented example. It has served as a valuable blueprint by which other applications can be developed, compared and contrasted. As Rutan points out there is no single form of 'psychodynamic group psychotherapy'.[7] Core concepts, however, do exist – such as the influence of unconscious processes, deriving from analytic theory. These provide both a framework and orientation and remain fairly constant for all treatment methods coming under the umbrella of a psychodynamic approach. The analytic framework that helps us understand group processes – and how to work with them – also helps us understand our own experiences and unconscious processes when interacting with others.

The diversity of group psychodynamic treatment methods rests more on the emphasis given to the structure of the group, than to the content process and outcome. For example:

❑ *psychodrama* emphasizes action methods whereby the group, with the directors help, set the stage for the protagonist's internalized drama to be re-enacted. The *audience* – far from passive – fulfills the function of auxiliary egos.
❑ The *group analytic* method, by contrast, emphasizes dialogue and language, to bring into conscious awareness interpersonal conflicts and resistances. This group is not directed, as such, but allowed or encouraged to discover its own meaning and possibilities through communication.

❑ The *therapeutic community*, while incorporating, in most cases, small group therapies, as described above, places more emphasis on large group dynamics within the context of a living, learning environment. Engaging in purposeful community tasks focused on daily living brings to the surface traumas and conflicts from past relationships that become the communities concern. Hinshelwood refers to these processes as unconscious dramatizations occurring between people who are attempting to fulfill their roles and responsibilities within the community.[8]

Although these three methods differ structurally, the common thread is experiential learning of 'self and others' within a group setting. The difficulties this method imposes are matched only by the transformative benefits realized when insight replaces resistance, and when a corrective experience makes sense of past trauma or conflict.

Groups are also structured differently to meet the developmental needs of the patient group to whom they are applied. In the group treatment of young people, for example, a psychodynamic orientation requires certain modifications to make the group environment both safe and comprehensible to its members. Young people will have a shorter concentration span, so therapy time needs to be less than that which might be manageable by an adult or late adolescent group. Refreshment breaks, for example, may be built in mid-way. 'Acting out' may require more input on the conductor's part, to protect the boundary. Dwivedi talks of the 'indigenous peer culture', which the facilitator must join before therapeutic peer culture can be established.[9]

The psychodynamic approach refers to processes of communication, conscious and unconscious *between* people, both verbal and non verbal. From the group perspective we are referring to processes of interpersonal relationships whereby individuals come with their own internal world of past and current relationships, to develop sufficient trust with each other and the group conductor to make the group experience therapeutically meaningful.[10]

Therapeutic factors refer to desirable change outcomes, both immediate – as they occur in the here and now of group exchange – and in the longer term. They are largely dependent on the above processes. For example, being able to talk about an embarrassing or painful feeling or memory is a *process*. Having the experience that ones feelings are acceptable to others is an *outcome*. Group psychotherapy is the method used to explore all communications on a number of different levels, their latent and manifest content, making sense of this for the benefit of both the individual and the group as a whole. More specifically the group conductor, and in turn the group members, become engaged with translating and interpreting those resistances that block communication, and therefore impede the development of the group.

We are talking here of what people find difficult to disclose – for fear of an angry or rejecting response – or difficult to hear, because it is a painful truth. The question is always how can this be resolved and better understood through further exchange by the group? Much will depend on a safe and protected environment, where anxiety can more easily be tolerated. This is a crucial part of the conductor or facilitator's role and is fundamental to his or her dynamic administration of the group.

GROUP RELATIONS IN A SOCIAL CONTEXT

It is difficult to imagine a society or community where groups do not play a significant part in its structure. Governments, councils, work groups, schools and teams are *formal* groups with a specific interest or purpose – such as educating or competing. We gather in groups on special occasions like weddings, birthdays and funerals. By so doing we share in both the joy and sorrow of these events. Through these interpersonal associations – where closer relationships are also formed – people learn about themselves in relationship to others. This will have important implications for self-reliance, self-identity and social well-being. We must add to this the experience and influence of the past, and how this can be re-activated in current relationships. How we manage and convey emotion in our interactions with others is also a significant feature for group and social relatedness.

A group may also reflect an important developmental stage in an individual's life and in meeting the needs appropriate to this stage. For example a nursery or pre-school group represents the need for the young to play and to socialize through play. Especially for the very young, an opportunity is provided to re-enact, through play, ongoing conflicts at home, such as sibling rivalry. A traumatized child exposed over time to conflict and/or emotional neglect could find the co-operative, sharing and rivalrous aspects of play very difficult or impossible to manage. Moving on developmentally, we know that adolescents are particularly concerned with peer group identification. Being able to share with others in these newly formed allegiances is a step away from dependence on the family group. We can see the turmoils of adolescence more clearly – not only from the hormonal and body changes they undergo, but by their membership of multiple groups. These are mainly groupings around home, school and social life, each requiring an adaptation to a different set of norms and expectations.

We need look no further than the family, the primary group, to understand the fundamental nature of our need to belong, relate to, and be identified with others. The long incubation of the infant/child, the transition from complete dependency, to ever increasing self-reliance (under optimal conditions) allows ample time and exposure to a network of interpersonal relationships. The varying forms of communication within these relationships are imprinted on the very young: for example, the way problems and conflicts are dealt with by mechanisms of defence, how affection is given and received. In group therapy we are working with the adversities the patient brings from their current situation. However, it is also relevant to consider the person's background – the shared common ground, from which relationships, and what has disturbed them, originate.

THERAPEUTIC FACTORS

Group psychotherapy is a way of helping people with differing problems and needs, understand their problems and conflicts together. Being able to express and share difficulties in a group can help reduce isolation. Many find it a great relief that their suffering does not have to be borne alone. The group can impart new learning on its members via the diverse feedback available. Yalom extensively researched the therapeutic basis of the group, identifying twelve therapeutic factors from patients self statements following group treatment.[11] These included, *group cohesiveness, universality, catharsis* and *family re-enactment*. By Yalom's own account the high level of subjectivity in the design could not produce hard evidence. However the results have demonstrated the effectiveness of interactive group psychotherapy.

A further factor, *interpersonal learning*, occurs because the person's assumptions, attitudes and beliefs, of self and others, when held up to the scrutiny of the group, can be 'reality tested' by the many points of view now available. New learning or insight can be disturbing. However, it can also be enlightening, as can learning from experience. The image we have, or would like to have, of ourselves is often challenged. For example, a group member who shows much care and concern for others in the group says that he sees his own problems as trivial compared to those of others, to whom he readily seeks to support. A fellow member suggests that perhaps he must work hard supporting others, to justify his place in the group as one with only minor problems. He now takes up the subject of his 'triviality', talking more openly about how his needs are trivialized by his family group. In this way he begins to accept the group's support, for what he now realizes as a profoundly distressing problem. A pattern of relating to others outside the group is re-enacted and repeated within it. His disclosure, having resonated with other members brings about sharing of similar experiences.

Our protagonist in this example provides a reflective space in which others can be put in touch with their own experiences. This process has been likened by Foulkes to a 'hall of mirrors'. One sees oneself reflected in the experience of another. Exchanges, such as this, would typically engage others not only because of similarity but also because of difference. Being able to express how we differ from each other is as important to group cohesion as the experiences we have in common. This factor brings contrast and often tension into the group and prevents it becoming too cosy.

These therapeutic factors are linked with how the group develops over time. Reduced isolation and universality – knowing that we are not alone with our problems – are apparent in exchanges in the early sessions of the group. This is often called the *orientation phase*. Nitsun makes a comparison with our earliest experiences of infancy.[12] He links this phase with the first few months of life when the infant's developmental task is integration with others, in new and unfamiliar surroundings. Like the infant, members of a new group, often strangers to each other, face considerable anxiety if they do not feel that the environment is sufficiently safe and containing. Cohesiveness and catharsis is unlikely, or would be less apparent, unless the group has worked through the orientation phase. This is distinguished by the members' dependency on the conductor to provide answers and solutions to the difficulties the group faces. Taking the patient's point of view, we might ask 'is it not reasonable to expect the conductor to have expert knowledge, and therefore answers and solutions? The conductor, while not rejecting these appeals to his/her expertise can neither gratify them. This can cause frustration as group members are thrown back on their own resources. Because the conductor is an agent in the service of the group, and conveys this by active attention and when necessary participation, neutrality is usually accepted as necessary. The conductor never avoids any issue that is important for group development. The conductor manages and contains the anxiety of the group members by repeatedly drawing attention to what may be happening in the group – whether painful or simply confusing – by interpreting the mood of the group, and sometimes by engaging the group member who has, so far, remained silent. This attitude provides a model for others to emulate.

Mirroring, to which I return later, is not exclusive to the group treatment setting, and it may be an important aspect of empathy. For example, when listening to a friend describe a recent loss we *recognize* something of our own feelings concerning a similar loss. In group treatment mirroring is different, because what passes as being familiar (what Foulkes called the 'foundation matrix'[13] – our common cultural shared experience) is amplified and condensed within the framework which contains all group experience and communication.

TWO ASPECTS OF THE NURSE–PATIENT RELATIONSHIP

Nurses aim to develop therapeutic relationships with patients. Building and maintaining this relationship is central to groupwork. The nurse brings relationship qualities, which are encompassed within the humanistic tradition of therapy, in particular Rogers' client-centred approach.[14] Genuineness, unconditional positive regard, warmth, empathy and understanding are attributes we value in all human relationships. In economic terms they could be described as the emotional 'goods'. Within the clinical setting this composite of professional skills and personal attributes represents an investment the nurse makes to engage patients in their own recovery.

Although the nurse practitioner maintains professional boundaries and neutrality the relationship will always have a number of qualities resembling a personal relationship, especially when the therapeutic work becomes deeper in meaning and resonance. When the patient begins to see the relationship as a resource for change, then we describe this as a *working alliance*. Cognitive and emotional resources are mobilized for learning at this stage. Derlega *et al.* offer a well-researched account of personal relationship theory.[15]

Personal disclosure can be painful and distressing but brings much needed emotional relief (*catharsis*). For some patients this may prove to be unique if they have only experience of traumatic or otherwise uncaring relationships. The positive attributes of a non-judgemental, uncritical supporting relationship, limited as it must be by professional constraints, may put the patient in touch with anxieties concerning closeness and rejection. If the nurse can stay with what is most uncomfortable for the patient then the disturbance becomes more manageable.

The nurse–patient relationship, whether a brief encounter in an acute treatment setting or a longer course of outpatient therapy, will inevitably end. This reality needs to be brought out into open discussion, and its meaning for the patient explored. To some extent it is part of natural loss and mourning that we all face at some point in our lives.

By extension we can now broaden our focus on the individual by locating our attention on what happens between people? We move from the *intrapersonal* to the *interpersonal*. We do not lose sight of the individual but see them more in the context of their relationships, particularly in groups.

The nurse is also an important transference figure for the patient. This means that feelings toward a significant figure from the past, often parental, are transferred onto the nurse and this can provide valuable material for understanding conflicts in the patient's current relationships, including the nurse–patient relationship, as well as making greater sense of what past relationships meant.

GROUP SPECIFIC FACTORS – THE ANALYTIC METHOD

S.H. Foulkes made a major contribution to our understanding of group psychotherapy[16] and the group analytic method is essentially a Foulkesian model. He incorporated ideas and concepts from his own experience of neurology, sociology, gestalt psychology and classical analytic theory. He was influenced also by field and systems theory. Using all these concepts he developed a framework we know now as *group analysis*. Foulkes' own training in psychiatry and psychoanalysis enabled him to create a new paradigm for treating individuals within a shared group context. The standard analytic attitude and reflective stance, whereby unconscious processes are brought into conscious awareness by interpretation, was something that he believed could be facilitated by each group member. Foulkes called this 'analysis *in* the group, *by* the group, including the conductor'.

When we consider the factors below separately, we can find examples of their appearance in many group situations, both clinical and non-clinical. For example scapegoating phenomena occurs when either an individual or subgroup carries the unwanted projections of the majority, or dominant group. The scapegoat may at times offer themselves up for this purpose. The factors acquire therapeutic value when combined in the small carefully selected analytic group; either the 'slow-open' or closed outpatient group, with a recommended attendance of one to three years. The nurse making observations of interpersonal group relations, and the dynamics that unfold, will be familiar with some of the factors that follow. Other central concepts important in group therapy, but not specific to groups and not detailed here, are *counter-transference, resistance* and *acting out*.[17]

The nurse is often ideally placed to observe interactions between patients and the interpersonal dynamics of both the staff and patient subgroups. Where these can be made sense of for the benefit of the patient a psychodynamic culture will emerge, and the nurse will function as a 'nurse therapist'.

Mirroring

Mirroring is probably the most important factor in the process of the experiential group, and promotes further sharing and deepening of the group's commitment and shared sense of purpose. The mirror provides an accurate reflection of what is placed before it. Our thoughts and feelings, our self-image, how we see ourselves, or would like to see ourselves, is not always what is reflected back to us. The individual is confronted with different aspects of their reflection by other group members. Pines describes human mirrors in the group that 'offer us multiple perspectives on ourselves, on how we are seen by others and let us see the many facets of human development, our conflicts and attempts to solve them'.[18]

Through a process of inner assessment the individual gains a more accurate and realistic understanding of themselves and their problems. Foulkes called this 'ego training in action'. In the earlier example given of the man who saw his problems as trivial, the view given back to him – the reflection – was accepted as a more accurate or complete interpretation.

The aspect of mirroring, difficult to convey in words is to do with the multiplicity of cause and effect. One person's disclosure, even a relatively minor comment, can bring about a chain of associations for others that promote further disclosure and in turn further reflecting back of different points of view. It would be misleading to describe mirroring as only of value in the verbal exchanges of the group, when for example two people reflect upon each other's experience. The remainder of the group, silent though they may be at this particular time, will invariably see and hear what there is in this exchange that reflects upon their *own* experience.

Illustration

This is the 5th session in a new outpatient group meeting weekly. There are six members. A seventh left abruptly after announcing in the previous group his intention to take a job offered in another part of the country. During his stay in the group he had been open about several failed relationships where he felt he had given a lot only to get hurt. The remaining members had been split between those who felt his decision was justified given the opportunity presented to him and those who were concerned that his leaving was not in his best interest and were more angry with the lack of notice and planning. There was evidence in his personal relationships that he ended them abruptly. The themes predominating in previous sessions have tended toward trying to manage symptoms and how medication is a mixed blessing. The group is in the *orientation* phase.

A group member (A) is telling others how doubtful she feels that the anti-depressants she takes are having any effect.

A: 'I'm not sure, though, if I can do without them. I don't want to become dependent on this treatment because – well this is a sign of weakness.'

Another member offers an interpretation:

B: 'Perhaps this is about depending on the group which like the medication, is an evening treatment. Feeling that you are weak if you come to depend on the group?'

A: 'I don't know that I agree. The group and medication are two quite different treatments, and anyway the group is new and I don't think I've got that dependent on it.'

Patient A seems uncertain about her answer, then says:

A: 'I suppose I don't know whether either are going to work.'

Other members pick up the theme of 'two treatments'. Views tend to become polarized as members weigh up having one or more treatments to depend on.

C: 'I rely on my medication. I don't have any problem with it. I know what I've been like without it.'

There is ongoing heated discussion on symptom relief as though the members expect this group to be like a medication whose action they do not know.

D: 'I do think we spend a lot of time discussing medication in this group. It's not what I'm here for. I've had a lousy week and maybe others have too, but we are staying with this and not sharing other experiences.'

An awkward silence ensues. The conductor is prepared to wait. Allowing this silence to continue promotes reflection and greater tolerance to anxiety. This has been an important challenge to the rest of the group who seem to be seeking comfortable unity around a subject they have in common. This challenge is far more significant coming from a fellow patient who usually takes a risk by opposing a majority consensus. We will see, by what happens next, that patient 'D' is making another important challenge. The conductor notices that patient 'D' looks tense and uncomfortable and asks if he can say what he is feeling and whether it's to do with the lousy week he's had.

D: 'Well I've had my father and sister staying and they are so wrapped up in their own interests I just think they don't want to know what has been going on for me. I could never tell them I'm coming here. Since my mother left him, no-one wants to look at this loss.'

Conductor: 'I wonder if you are angry with the group as well for not noticing how upset you are?'

D: 'Well it seemed like everyone here was busily discussing things that had nothing to do with me.'

Conductor: 'And you felt shut out?'

D: 'Yes I did, I also feel angry with you because I wanted you to come in and do something to get us away from this preoccupation with medication. During that silence I was thinking about my father who never explained anything to me, and I suppose because you don't explain what's happening here to us I get into all this negative stuff about him.'

The conductor explores further the significance of the transference to him by patient D, then addressing the group as a whole.

Conductor: 'I think the group is also struggling to know whether others can be depended upon, perhaps like a medicine when we don't know the effects.'

Other members contribute at this more personal level having been cast to some extent as the siblings who have the father/conductor to themselves. In the second half of the session members are more at work on the difficulties that underlie symptoms, rather than the symptoms themselves. A further deepening of the intimacy in the group occurs when a member links the departure of patient D's mother to the recently departed patient in the previous session. Issues of loss, particularly of this valued group member, and the real disruption to the group are acknowledged in a way that did not seem possible in the first half of the session.

Mirroring was more apparent in the second half of the session when the more personal disclosures of patient D were mirrored in the experiences others had concerning lack of emotional contact with a parent, unresolved rivalry with siblings, repressed feelings that are never talked about and experiences of loss due to bereavement, divorce and mental illness. Mirroring is an important phenomenon in the group leading to greater cohesiveness, because it promotes the sharing of experiences as a benefit to all rather than a benefit only to the individual. Foulkes tells us that 'the patient sees himself, or part of himself, in particular a repressed part of himself in the other members. He can observe from the outside another member reacting in the way he himself reacts, and can see how conflicts and problems are translated into neurotic behaviour'.

The transference group

Within the dynamic matrix of the group multiples of people significant in the individuals past are transferred onto one or more members of the group, including the conductor. For patient D feelings of jealousy towards his sisters were transferred onto those in the group whose interests excluded him. Similarly the conductor was experienced as the distant father who disappointed him and frustrated his need to engage. Exploring his past relationship, in the light of displaced and projected feelings onto another in the current relationship, helped D make greater sense of his experiences.

Figure–ground relationship

The conductor always sees the individual against the *background* of the group. Depending on what is happening in the group this view may be reversed. The group as a whole is now *foreground* and the conductor will intervene, addressing the group as a single entity. The material each person brings to the attention of the group, and how they bring it, for example patient A not wanting to appear weak and dependant, may be present throughout the group as a sense of helplessness, particularly common in the orientation phase. The conductor needs to shift his point of view, the location between what's happening for the individual and the collective meaning in the group. This does not discount the individual's disclosure but relocates it within a shared context.

Family re-enactment

The group come to represent at different times, for different individuals a re-constituted family of origin. This can be applied to many group structures and it may be apparent at the conscious level. Problems that had no solutions in the past, and are therefore likely to have been forgotten or denied, can be re-worked. For example patient D expressed anger with those in the group who were avoiding an important task. This may not ever have been possible in the past. This is important as a rehearsal for future relationships, and can loosen up defences so that further material can be remembered.

Socialization

The group is a social entity and the membership represent a sample, sometimes a diverse one, of social convention. The less socially skilled can be 'brought on' and the more dominant impatient characters can be held back. The group example above has this socializing factor, as does virtually any formal or informal human gathering. A therapeutic benefit of the structure of the treatment group is the deepening social relatedness and the reduction of isolation. Making valuable connections in the group can inspire similar social behaviour outside the group.

Interpretation/translation

The great value of group treatment following a psychodynamic model is the frequency in which the group develops its own therapeutic agency. The conductor only interprets when analysis fails. We saw how patient B made an interpretation suggesting an unconscious link between dependency on drug treatment and dependency on the group. The conductor participates less when the group works in this way, following rather than leading the group. Interpretation is not an exact science applied by the conductor. Even when it is certain that an interpretation will be accurate it is better to wait and see what group members do before intervening. However, *translation* is somewhat different. Its purpose is to bring into language form unconscious processes of communication whose meaning would remain lost without this translation. In the awkward silence following patient D's challenge the group has suddenly become a difficult place. The conductor will judge when best to intervene to help translate the mood of the group in the light of other factors preceding the silence. In practical terms this may simply mean seeking clarification about what one person says and its impact on others. As with the example of figure–ground configuration, the conductor locates their attention at one moment with the individual and at another with the group.

For example, the fear of dependency on treatment may arise as an issue for one member but it is also an issue for others. The process of translation can help the silent member of the group to participate. This is important for a newly formed group or when a member joins an established group.

Scapegoat phenomena

The *scapegoat* in biblical history carries away the sins of the community from which it is cast out. Similarly, one group member, or a pair, may embody all that is disturbing for others to face in themselves. Though not made explicit in the example given above, there were occasions when one or more members wondered if it were something unbearable about their problems that had 'driven out' the member in the previous session. Issues concerning rejection, and when this becomes acted-out, were taken up during subsequent sessions. A patient who sees their experience as highly singular, or unique, may feel 'outside' the more common experiences of others, and may act out in a way that provokes the very responses they fear. This is a type of self-induced scapegoat phenomena. Much effort is needed to help contain the individual who always feels at odds with the group, and it is quite possible they will drop out in the early sessions of the group.

Pairing and subgroups

Pairing in the group is a commonplace feature. Its significance can be easily over-looked. When two people find they can share an experience they have in common they become a *pair*. This occurs when individuals are the only men in the group, or have experience of an emotionally distant father, which was the case for patient D and A. Sometimes opposite poles attract. Having very contrasting experiences can bring about pair bonding. Often, we are attracted to people for many different reasons. In the therapy group, members share thoughts and feelings toward one another. They sometimes express hitherto forbidden wishes, expressing things that they could not be so open about outside the group. This is an important aspect of developing intimacy, which is held and contained within the boundary of the group. Pairing is not generally problematic, as different associations bring different combinations of people together. Occasionally there is tension in the group if the pair are experienced as excluding the others. Usually this is temporary. When it is not, it can be understood as a form of acting-in and the couple will need help to see the value of integration within a whole group perspective. As mentioned earlier the conductor need only intervene when what happens in the group impedes its development.

Subgroups may arise for equally valid reasons. People who have children form a subgroup as do those without children. A medication subgroup and a non-medication subgroup can at times work hard at not looking at what they have in common. This was the case in the group I have described. The conductor's role here is to draw to the group's attention the value of the pair or subgroup relationship when it is used defensively to avoid a common problem.

The dynamic matrix

Foulkes described the analytic group as a 'hypothetical web of communication', transcending the individual yet still encompassing him/her. Communication at the current conscious level in Foulkes' model is seen as of equal importance to communication at unconscious projective and transference levels. All processes and therapeutic factors belong to this dynamic matrix. Ahlin provides an elegant definition: 'A group matrix is truly a group work creation and its aims and shape bear witness not only to the individual in it but to their ancestors, histories, cultures'.[19]

The conductor's role

How and *when* we use a psychodynamic approach will depend on the setting and resources within which we work. The degree to which we feel able to work in a psychodynamic way is usually related to where we find ourselves during our professional lives. The opportunities available to start working in groups may depend on having like-minded colleagues with whom to share ideas and make plans. Here, I consider our role as group-workers from two opposite ends of the spectrum of group facilitation.

The first focuses on the assessment, selection and preparation of patients for group psychotherapy and our involvement as *boundary keepers* and therapists within such groups. These groups are generally longer-term requiring considerable commitment of time and resources. The less experienced nurse practitioner can gain many useful group skills as co-therapist, working alongside a more experienced conductor. A supportive infrastructure is, however, necessary for this to succeed. The hard work that goes into preparation is never wasted.

The second focus is to consider where less formalized groups are already in place. A daily community meeting on an acute admissions ward, for example, might benefit from a psychodynamic approach, becoming more centred on experiential learning rather than on tasks.

In the assessment and selection of patients for group psychotherapy I usually employ the following procedure.

Having welcomed the patient and explained the purpose and structure of the meeting, I invite them to describe their problems and also to give a *personal history*, starting as far back as possible. The order in which a person brings information into this meeting is not so important. What really matters is the *way* in which the story is told. Weighing up the different selection criteria – for example, psychological mindedness, motivation, curiosity about ones past and how this may link with present difficulties – are at the forefront of the assessment. The patient's capacity, or ego strength, needs to be sufficient to manage the emotional upheaval that the dynamically orientated group process is likely to bring about.

Exclusion criteria

It is easier to consider who would *not* benefit from the group experience and who *should not*, in their own interests, be referred. While there are many types of groups for many types of problems/disorders, the group I have described would not be suitable for people who are addicted to drugs or alcohol, or are paranoid, psychotic or sociopathic. Patients with borderline personalities can be very difficult to hold within a group. Most group therapists agree that the severely depressed patient would be too retarded to use the group and patients who are actively suicidal are too threatening and disruptive. Also unsuitable would be those people in the midst of an acute illness or major crisis. Group psychotherapy is not recommended for people about to embark on major events such as childbirth, marriage or divorce. Their motivation is always worth noting however, and they could be encouraged to return at a later date. People who have had no experience of at least one stable and satisfying relationship in their life will find the group too threatening and would be better directed toward individual therapy/counselling in the first instance.

Inclusion criteria

The most important inclusion criteria is motivation. Patients rarely do well in groups if they have been 'sent'. Uncertainty about the group process can be dealt with along with normal anxieties in pre-group assessment but the patient ultimately must decide that they want to enter the group for themselves. Yalom said that 'an important criterion for inclusion is whether a patient has obvious problems in the interpersonal domain: loneliness, shyness and social withdrawal, inability to be intimate or to love, excessive competitiveness, aggressivity, abrasiveness, or argumenativeness, suspiciousness, problems with authority, narcissism, including an inability to share, to empathise, or to accept criticism and a continuous need for admiration, feelings of unlovability, fears of assertiveness, fears of depending'. He adds that 'patients must be willing to take responsibility for those problems or, at the very least acknowledge them and entertain a desire for change'.[20]

PREPARATION OF THE PATIENT

People suitable for groups need basic information about the treatment on offer. This helps to dispel some anticipatory anxiety and conveys some of the therapists beliefs in the process itself. Practical arrangements may need to be discussed in the light of making an important commitment to treatment. Personal resources are often important, as therapy is an investment in time and often money (travel costs etc). Support of the family or partner may be important and the possible 'postponement' of travel arrangements, moving house etc may be necessary. I mention these issues here only to remind referrers of the typical preoccupations prior to coming into therapy.

At the other end of our spectrum of groupwork are settings where brief group interventions are applied. The aims and service objectives of the departments within which we work determine how a psychodynamic approach can be used, particularly if time is a decisive factor. We have considered in this chapter a broad range of therapeutic factors and processes that can develop over time, especially in longer-term group treatments. How can we now adapt this model to much shorter group interventions while maintaining a psychodynamic perspective? A personal experience comes to mind that may provide at least one of many possible answers. It represents a point on a learning curve to do with being creative with what you have got!

Many years ago I was on a placement in an acute admission department and wanted to provide a time-limited closed psychotherapy group. There was little interest and nothing happened other than me becoming despondent at the thought of a wasted 6-month placement. I took this to my supervisor who invited me to look at what existed in the prevailing culture of the department and to join what ever I could, that involved group relations, and to observe the dynamic processes, which include me. By starting from this point of view I was able to see my own short sightedness. A psychotherapy group of the kind I had in mind would take 6 months to put together. Instead I joined a social worker who conducted a 'leavers group' and this proved to be a very worthwhile experience. The leavers group had two important focuses. It allowed time to look at external issues about going home such as finance, accommodation and work, but it also provided a valuable experiential forum for more interpersonal dynamics to unfold. Patients could share their anxiety about facing the outside world, returning to pick up the pieces of their lives. They could share what the hospital admission had meant to them and much more. The group successfully bridged the often difficult gulf of combining tasks and dynamics. Within these types of groups we begin to see how psychodynamic processes take shape and are incorporated alongside the more obvious theme or occupation of the group which in this example is to do with leaving hospital.

One of the conductor's key functions as administrator and agent of the group is in ensuring a safe and protected environment. This is about boundary maintenance. It is closely linked to confidentiality and containment and is ongoing throughout the life of both brief and longer-term groups. Securing an undisturbed space, arranging chairs so that all participants can see each other, minimizing unnecessary distractions, precise time-keeping are all aspects that help the group focus on the task in hand.

Many groups, it can be argued, do not focus on the dynamic interpersonal relationships as they develop in the group. It may not be of primary importance. For example group treatments may be themed around a particular problem like addiction, or eating disorders or a particular symptom like anxiety. In the example of an anxiety management group, the facilitator is likely to determine objectives for the group from tried and tested procedures. The therapist's role would be to educate and then direct members, much like a teacher, toward achieving these objectives, and so better manage their anxieties. However it is unlikely that when we are involved in such groups we will fail to notice the dynamics between individuals at the interpersonal level. One only has to experience one's own counter-transference feelings of anger toward a silent or vulnerable looking individual, to appreciate this fact.

WIDER APPLICATIONS

The *therapeutic community* employs a combination of group approaches and modifications of the therapeutic community model may be possible in day and inpatient settings. The key purpose is to involve the patient as much as possible in the routine administration of the unit. This returns to the patient a sense of responsibility and empowerment that the more medical treatments take away. Large group dynamics often evoke anxiety and this is increased without tasks and recreational activities to offset them. The therapeutic community frequently manages to combine in a balanced way the more intense 'therapy' groups with the task group. A living and learning environment promotes equal status and valued roles. Even though distinctions must be made between the carers and the cared for and the specific responsibilities each participant carries out, the democratization principle places all members of staff and patients within the same culture of enquiry.

Training and supervision

To process what happens in psychodynamic groups, personal experience of group treatment is invaluable. This is recommended, or built into, many dynamically focused training courses and is mandatory as the personal component on all qualifying courses. This need not discourage the nurse who finds groupwork rewarding, challenging and at times enjoyable, and who may already possess a range of interactive and reflective skills. You will begin to appreciate that it is a lived experience, a personal reality and cannot simply be taught.

A psychodynamic approach to *group supervision* is another application that has value for those nurses interested in extending or developing their thinking about the nurse–patient relationship. In my experience working with community nurses these small groups provide a forum for examining the transference and counter-transference issues that arise in their ongoing work with patients. Like the treatment group a reflective space helps each to share and make sense of their work via a psychodynamic perspective. This is not 'therapy' for staff however. The task is work focused but takes what can be learnt from group dynamics that is common to all.

REFERENCES

1. Freud S. *An outline of psycho-analysis.* Strachey J (ed.) London: The Hogarth Press, 1979.

2. Winnicott DW. The beginning of the individual. *Babies and their mothers.* London: Free Association Books, 1998: 51–8.

3. Foulkes SH. Outline and development of group analysis. *Therapeutic group analysis.* London: Maresfield Reprints, 1984 (first published 1964): 66–82.

4. Wright H. The structure of the supervision seminar. In: *Groupwork: perspectives and practice.* London: Scutari, 1989.

5. Faugier J, Butterworth CA. *Clinical supervision: a position paper.* University of Manchester: School of Nursing Studies, 1993.

6. Lego S. Psychodynamic group psychotherapy. In: *Psychiatric nursing: a comprehensive reference*, 2nd edn. Lippincott: NY, 1996.

7. Rutan JS. Psychodynamic group psychotherapy. *International Journal of Group Psychotherapy* 1992; **42** (1): 19–35.

8. Hinshelwood RD. Resources for unconscious dramatization. *What happens in groups.* London: Free Association Books, 1987: 38–45.

9. Dwivedi KN. Conceptual framework. *Group work with children and adolescents.* London: Jessica Kingsley, 1993: 28–45.

10. Peplau HE. The history of milieu as a treatment modality. In: O'Toole AW, Welt SR (eds). *Hildegard E Peplau: selected works – interpersonal theory in nursing.* London: Macmillan, 1989.

11. Yalom ID. The therapeutic factors. *The theory and practice of group psychotherapy.* New York: Basic Books, 1985: 70–101.

12. Nitsun M. Early development. In: *Linking the individual and the group. Group Analysis.* London: Sage, 1989; **22**: 249–60.

13. Foulkes *op. cit.*

14. Rogers C. The characteristics of a helping relationship. *On becoming a person. The therapist's view of psychotherapy.* London: Constable, 1979: 39–58.

15. Derlega VJ, Hendrick SS, Winstead BA, Berg JH. A social exchange analysis. *Psychotherapy as a personal relationship.* New York: The Guilford Press, 1991: 42–74.

16. Roberts J, Pines M. Group analytic psychotherapy. *International Journal of Group Psychotherapy* 1992; **42**(4): 469–94.

17. Lego *op. cit.*

18. Pines M. Reflections on mirroring. 6th SH Foulkes annual lecture of the Group Analytic Society, 10th May, 1982. *Group Analysis* 1982; (Suppl): **15**.

19. Ahlin G. On thinking about the group matrix. *Group Analysis* 1985; **18**(2): 111–19.

20. Yalom *op. cit.*

Chapter 22

COGNITIVE-BEHAVIOURAL APPROACHES

Paul French*

INTRODUCTION

This chapter explains the framework of cognitive-behavioural therapy (CBT) and highlights the application of this approach with a case illustration. The approach to CBT developed by Aaron T. Beck will be presented, as this is the model in which the author has most experience.

RATIONALE

CBT evolved from the work of Beck[1] and Albert Ellis.[2] This form of therapy has been widely adopted from being a specific treatment for depression, into a treatment option for a diverse range of problems.

Over 20 years ago a treatment manual was developed, which allowed CBT for depression to be taught, replicated, standardized and researched.[3] Since that time a number of research trials have been undertaken to test the efficacy of CBT in treating depression and the evidence clearly points towards CBT being a useful treatment option.[4–7] In fact CBT was found to be as effective as medication in terms of treating the depressive episode but significantly, had specific advantages in that it helped to protect the person against future relapse.[8] This is clearly an important effect in terms of long-term management strategies not only for clients and their families, but it can also offset any cost issues associated with the treatment. CBT aims to teach the person new skills in managing their depressive symptoms whereas medica-

tion merely reinforces the medical model of the illness and the need for further intervention should symptoms occur in the future. Therefore, this skill acquisition is associated with reduced chance of relapse.

These factors have led to the popularity of CBT as a treatment option. The initial treatment manual for depression has been applied to other psychological disorders such as panic disorder,[9] obsessional disorders[10,11] and more latterly psychotic disorders.[12] Despite their diversity each disorder allows a cognitive conceptualization of the problem and identifies specific treatment interventions that apply to it.

Cognitive theory of psychopathology is constructed around information processing[13] where the information processing system is considered to be faulty, thereby maintaining the psychological disorder. This faulty information processing is accessible in the conscious state through *negative automatic thoughts*, which emerge from the *schemas* that have a dysfunctional element to them. Automatic thoughts can be a stream of thoughts that seem to enter our minds. For some people these thoughts can be in the form of mental images. The purpose of the therapy is to assist the client to recognize these thoughts and teach methods to challenge them usually through the *Dysfunctional Thought Record* (DTR).[3,14]

Negative automatic thoughts are, by definition negative in content and pop into our mind spontaneously, hence we have no control over them. They frequently happen at times of uncertainty or stress. Hence when a person is in the midst of a depressive or anxious state

*Paul French has worked in inpatient and community settings since qualifying in 1989, and also as a lecturer practitioner. His main interest is in the development of cognitive models and interventions for individuals at high-risk of developing psychosis in an attempt to develop primary preventative interventions.

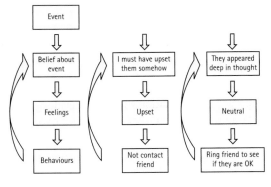

FIGURE 22.1 Thoughts, emotions and behaviour

then their occurrence is generally more frequent. These thoughts trigger certain emotions and subsequently certain patterns of behaviour, which frequently maintain them. This can be seen diagrammatically in Figure 22.1 above.

From this diagram we can see that the event itself does not necessarily result in depression or sadness, rather it is the interpretation of the event, which determines or mediates the subsequent mood. Following from this the mood can determine the behavioural response to the original triggering event and this behaviour can maintain the original belief. What this indicates is that it is not necessarily the events themselves which lead to distress, rather it is how we make sense of these events. Therefore, enabling an individual to recognize patterns of thoughts which may have become distorted is a vital component of CBT. Developing skills to challenge these distorted patterns of thinking in a structured manner, by examining all available evidence, is the next step in assisting the individual to overcome these difficulties.

At this point critics of CBT may point out that an individual may have good reason to feel distress regarding an event, or their belief about an event may be an accurate evaluation. This can be the case in many situations, and it is not the aim of CBT to encourage people to think in a positive manner, contrary to popular belief. The aim of CBT is to enable people to understand how they think about situations, and enhance their ability to evaluate their thoughts based on available evidence, as opposed to a gut reaction based on intuition. If people are evaluating events accurately and they feel upset about these things, they should be encouraged to undertake alternative strategies to manage their distress such as developing problem-solving skills.

THE COMPONENTS OF CBT

CBT is a short-term, structured approach to therapy. A problem list is developed with the individual and these problems are systematically targeted throughout the

therapy process with cognitive formulations developed to understand these problems.

- ❏ **Structure.** CBT is associated with a structured approach to therapy, which can be off-putting at first. However, this structured approach allows a means of maximizing the time spent in therapy and ensures that the individual has their problems prioritized and dealt with in a collaborative manner. This means that there is a set pattern associated with a CBT session, which can be seen below:
- ❏ **Brief review.** This allows the individual to summarize what has been happening to them since the last therapy session without getting bogged down in details which may have little part to play in the problems.
- ❏ **Agenda setting.** This involves developing a collaborative agenda of topics to be covered during the session, which is prioritized and time allocated to each item on the agenda. Factors influencing agenda items will include the stage in therapy; joint prioritization of problems; items put on the agenda from previous sessions and finally any hidden agendas.[2] Setting the agenda allows the session to proceed in a structured manner and without it discussion can often drift with no specific purpose. It can be seen as the first step in socializing the patient to the model.
- ❏ **Feedback.** This allows a process of checking out what was useful or not regarding the previous session. It also ensures that any potential miscommunication is clarified straight away. Feedback should also be utilized throughout the therapy session and each agenda item summarized to ensure understanding.
- ❏ **Homework review.** Homework is set following a therapy session in order to test out or monitor items which have been discussed within session. This is an important part of therapy allowing in-session skills to be transferred and tested in a real world setting. If someone is going to the trouble to undertake homework then there should be a point in the session, which is dedicated to wanting to know the results. If the therapist does not ask about results of homework then the individual may feel what is the point of it.
- ❏ **Main agenda item.** This entails focusing on the main concerns the individual has raised, discussing them in greater detail, developing a cognitive formulation of the problem and collaboratively discussing strategies to overcome these problems.
- ❏ **Set homework.** The process of setting homework to be undertaken between therapy sessions can be quite difficult. This important aspect of therapy should have sufficient time allocated in order to consider what task could be undertaken and a useful strategy is to ask the individual what they think they should do for homework.
- ❏ **Feedback.** This involves checking the content of the

session to ensure that client and therapist understood the things they were discussing.

This structure is vital to the delivery of CBT, however, the process merely allows a framework. There are a number of other skills which need to be integrated into this framework in order to deliver what would be regarded as CBT. Many people assume that the structure of therapy indicates a cold and sterile approach. However, this is not the case and the usual therapeutic skills of warmth, trust and honesty are valued as highly as the other elements of CBT, and they are felt to be a prerequisite to providing the therapy.

The Cognitive Therapy Scale (CTS)[15] provides a check that the structure is being adhered to, but also provides a means of measuring the other skills associated with CBT. This scale defines the 13 core components of cognitive therapy and rates each item between 0 and 6, which can be marked accordingly as the therapist develops in competency. The CTS has been seen to be reliable and valid when measuring therapist competency[16] and is used to rate videotape, audiotape or live observation rather than the therapist's perception of what took place during therapy. It is this ability to rate a therapist's performance which has enabled this type of psychological therapy to be used within research settings, because it is possible to state whether a therapist is doing CBT or not.

One of the major components of CBT is that it should be undertaken in a questioning style, which is termed guided discovery. This means that instead of the therapist providing ready-made solutions to problems, they work with the individual in an attempt to allow them to come to conclusions themselves. This can be particularly challenging for a therapist to undertake especially if they have been brought up in a culture where it is assumed that they have specialist knowledge and know best. However, providing ready-made solutions does not allow the individual the opportunity to learn how to overcome the problems. The process of guided discovery attempts to guide the individual towards an understanding of their difficulties, how they came about and how they are maintained. These processes are drawn up in a formulation describing the individual's problems. Next, potential strategies can be discussed and subsequently tested in order to see whether they work. It is felt that this process of guiding the individual towards coming up with their own solutions means that they hold this information with a great deal more passion than a ready-made solution from someone else. Therefore, through guided discovery, the individual is encouraged to develop a thorough understanding of their problems themselves in order to become their own therapist, which could then impact on future episodes of illness.

Case formulation

A formulation relating to the development and maintenance of problems is a vital aspect of the therapy. Without a clear formulation interventions can be seen as a haphazard application of techniques without any rationale for their use. A formulation should be developed early in therapy generally within sessions one and two, although the formulation should be added to throughout the therapy process and in light of any data generated by experiments. Therapists should be aware of the variety of formulations for individual disorders and utilize these models and the indicated intervention strategies allied to them.

Case example

In this section a case will be presented to enable some understanding of the processes involved in delivering CBT.

Jane was seen following a referral by her GP due to concerns about a postnatal depressive illness. Jane had a 5-week-old baby daughter called Karen. Jane had been in hospital for four days following the birth of Karen during which she felt quite well. However, as soon as she returned home she started to experience overwhelming feelings that Karen would die. Jane was extremely tearful and depressed and had little or no appetite. She was extremely reluctant to let her child out of her sight, due to fears over her safety. Jane was unable to leave Karen alone with anyone, feeling that she was the only person able to look after her properly. This included her mother and the baby's father, Joe. At times Jane felt that Karen got so upset that she would die. Jane had developed a strict routine and was unable to vary from this, e.g. Karen must be woken up at certain times in order to be fed; if this did not happen she felt the baby may not have the energy to wake up and may die.

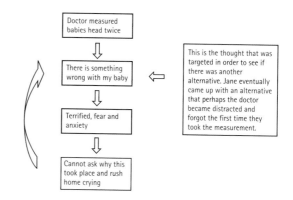

FIGURE 22.2 Targeting Jane's negative thinking

develop relationships with people and understand their problems. However, almost without exception when someone I was working with started to express some concern that things were getting worse, such as hearing more voices or distress regarding their delusions, my intervention was to become a taxi. We would jump in the car and go and see a psychiatrist in order to get their medication reviewed which was frequently altered. I always felt that this was not a particularly good nursing intervention. Since I developed skills in CBT, I now feel as though I have an armoury of tools at my disposal, which we can use before becoming a taxi. These frequently have a positive effect and it has enabled me and the individual to feel empowered to tackle problems without constantly settling for the taxi option. I believe that my nursing background has given me a unique opportunity to deliver these interventions to people in extremely difficult situations and believe that nurses are ideally placed to deliver these interventions.

REFERENCES

1. Beck AT. *Depression: clinical, experimental and theoretical aspects*. New York: Harper and Row, 1967.

2. Ellis A. *Reason and emotion in psychotherapy*. New York: Lyle Stuart, 1962.

3. Beck AT, Rush AJ, Shaw BF, Emery G. *Cognitive therapy of depression*. New York: John Wiley, 1979.

4. Rush AJ, Beck AT, Kovacs M, Hollon SD. Comparative efficacy of cognitive therapy and pharmacotherapy in the treatment of depressed outpatients. *Cognitive Therapy and Research* 1977; **1**: 17–37.

5. Blackburn IM, Bishop S, Glen AIM, Whalley LJ, Christie JE. The efficacy of cognitive therapy in depression: A treatment trial using cognitive therapy and pharmacotherapy, each alone and in combination. *British Journal of Psychiatry* 1981; **139**: 181–9.

6. Simons AD, Murphy GE, Levine JE, Wetzel RD. Cognitive therapy and pharmacotherapy for depression: Sustained improvement over one year. *Archives of General Psychiatry* 1986; **43**: 43–9.

7. Hollon SD, Shelton RC, Loosen PT. Cognitive therapy and pharmacotherapy for depression. *Journal of Consulting and Clinical Psychology* 1991; **59**: 88–99.

8. Blackburn IM, Eunson KM, Bishop S. A two year naturalistic follow up of depressed patients treated with cognitive therapy, pharmacotherapy and a combination of both. *Journal of Affective Disorders* 1986; **10**: 67–75.

9. Clark DM. A cognitive model of panic. *Behaviour Research and Therapy* 1986; **24**: 462–70.

10. Salkovskis PM. Obsessional compulsive problems: a cognitive-behavioural analysis. *Behaviour Research and Therapy* 1985; **23**: 571–83.

11. Wells A. *Cognitive therapy of anxiety disorders: a practice manual and conceptual guide*. Chichester: John Wiley, 1997.

12. Morrison AP. The interpretation of intrusions in psychosis: an integrative cognitive approach to hallucinations and delusions. *Behavioural and Cognitive Psychotherapy* 2001; **29**: 257–76.

13. Beck AT. Cognitive models of depression. *Journal of Cognitive Psychotherapy* 1987; **1**: 5–37.

14. Greenberger D, Padesky CA. *Mind over mood: change how you feel by changing the way you think*. New York: Guilford Press, 1995.

15. Young J, Beck AT. *Cognitive Therapy Scale: rating manual*. Unpublished manuscript, University of Pennsylvania, Philadelphia, 1980.

16. Dobson K, Shaw B, Vallis T. Reliability of a measure of cognitive therapy. *British Journal of Clinical Psychology* 1985; **24**: 295–300.

Chapter 23

USING SOLUTION-FOCUSED APPROACHES

Denise C Webster* and Kay Vaughn**

INTRODUCTION

As the name implies, *solution-focused therapy* (SFT) is focused on solutions and, some would say, does not even have to define the 'presenting problem' in any detail to be effective. At its inception, SFT was seen as a brief therapy and the emphasis was on rapid resolution of a circumscribed problem. Although this is still a valid focus for the therapy, SFT has since been used successfully with people who may require ongoing support or who have multiple problems.

Solution-focused therapy is an approach to working with clients that can be extremely challenging for counsellors who are comfortable with being simply a caring, reflective listener and/or focusing on clients' problems. Although many of the skills necessary to do effective solution-focused therapy are those shared by other schools of therapy, the underlying assumptions about how to help people may be diametrically opposed to other forms of therapy.

As in *cognitive-behavioural therapy*, there is an expectation that the therapist is active, focuses on what is occurring in the present, and recognizes that clients need resources to manage their situation. However, solution-focused therapists do not use programme-based, psychoeducational interventions for specific problems. Nor do they believe that noticing more about the problem is likely to be helpful. They also believe that clients already have most of the resources they need to effectively manage their situation and that both these resources and the way the client views the situation, are likely to be unique. Furthermore, a focus on a specified preferred future is central to a solution-focused approach. The explicit central belief in cognitive-behavioural theory, that faulty thinking is responsible for ineffective coping, and must be challenged is contrary to a solution-focused philosophy that accepts clients' realities as valid for them. Unlike psychodynamic approaches, there is no attempt to determine the source of the situation (not automatically called a 'problem'), either in the client's personal and family history, or in the identification of motives (conscious or unconscious) or defence mechanisms. Although there is an explicit attempt to develop a strong relationship as a client advocate, there is no attempt to discuss the therapeutic relationship itself or to offer theory-based interpretations of material the client presents. The concept of 'resistance' is seen by solution-focused therapists as a problem the therapist has with hearing the client, rather than a client's problem in accepting the therapist's interpretations.

Having evolved from the therapy approaches modelled by Milton Erickson[1] solution-focused therapy has

---

*Denise (Denny) Webster, RN, PhD, CS is a Professor of Nursing, University of Colorado Health Sciences Center. Denny has published widely on issues of women and mental health, self-care for poorly understood conditions and solution-focused therapy. She is co-author of the recent book 'Recrafting a Life: Solutions for chronic pain and illness'.
** Kay Vaughn is a Clinical Nurse Specialist at the University of Colorado Health Sciences Center in Denver. She has published widely on solution-focused work, especially in acute care settings.

been called a form of hypnotic therapy, to the degree that it utilizes a hypothetical preferred future (a form of hypnotic 'crystal-ball gazing'), or a form of strategic therapy, (paradoxical interventions), pattern intervention as well as a 'radical constructivist' therapy[2] because it supports the concept of multiple realities, all of which are dependent on how an individual 'constructs' both problems and solutions to problems. The latter view situates solution-focused therapy as a language-based or narrative therapy that helps clients retell their 'stories' in ways that uncover positive interpretations and possibilities for change.

CORE PRINCIPLES

Assumptions

Solution-focused therapy is not based on explicit theories of personality, psychopathology, or aetiology of pathology. A successful solution-focused therapist has a basically positive philosophy about human potential, the human condition and the inevitability of change as inherent in the lives of humans, as in all life cycles. As a health-oriented, strength-based approach to helping people, the therapist seeks evidence of competency rather than failure or weakness. Because the language of psychiatry tends to be pathologizing, the use of diagnosis or other forms of labelling is avoided. Identifying a client's 'defence mechanisms', whether or not these are interpreted to clients, would be seen as both pathologizing and distorting the client's story, whereas learning about clients' unique ways of coping would be honouring differences that can be built on to facilitate solutions. Clients' worldviews, values and language provide the framework for identifying relevant solutions and ways to achieve them. Realistically, many clients enter therapy with a well-developed language of problems and the therapist has the challenge of using the client's language and helping them shift their language to how they would describe the absence of the problem. For example, clients may label themselves as 'depressed'. In developing a 'picture' of what it's like NOT to be depressed, we may learn one person describes an ability to be in a meaningful relationship, while others may describe having the energy to return to mountain climbing or simply finding daily activities less stressful and more rewarding.

Both the acceptance of clients' realities and language and the search for the language of solutions are grounded in an acceptance of multiple realities or multiple, equally plausible, interpretations of any situation. The presumption that everyone has a unique definition of the situation and reasonable solutions, precludes the use of most problem-based intervention programmes, which rely on the shared dimensions of human experience and generic theories about problem intervention.

The relationship

The development and maintenance of the therapeutic relationship is paramount in solution-focused therapy. The therapist must be active and develop a collaborative, egalitarian relationship with the client. The therapist may define him or herself as an expert at helping people discover solutions. Clients are, however, the most important experts, i.e. they know most about their situation, overall circumstances, resources, and what they think is most likely to be helpful. The therapist practises 'radical acceptance' and respect for the client's expertise and endeavours to frame questions in ways that will communicate understanding of the client's view and support for their efforts.

'Confrontation' in the traditional sense would be seen as non-therapeutic, and 'resistance' is seen as a problem the therapist has in understanding, hearing, or facilitating the client's identification of solutions. There is often an awareness by solution-focused counsellors, that clients can become overly dependent on the counsellor when the therapy process is prolonged, so there may be conscious efforts to identify important relationships outside therapy (family, friends, community resources) and encouragement for clients to develop these 'natural' connections that will be enduring after the immediate need for counselling has been met.

Role of change

'Change' in solution-focused therapy is seen as inevitable, since nothing stays the same, people change in response to changes in circumstance, development, life experience and their perspectives. 'Readiness to change', then, is less about the client's motivation than about having found a goal and approach to a solution that is important to the client. DeShazer's[1] early description of solution-focused therapy identified client's 'relationship to the problem' (and by implication to the therapist) to help counsellors match homework assignments to the client's relationship to the problem and how much clients believe they can influence the situation. For example, if a client is sent for therapy, by a court, to address a problem they believe was not their fault, they would not be motivated to work on remedying that problem. This is not dissimilar from the problem of parents bringing in a child who thinks the parents are unreasonable and don't understand the situation. In both examples, however, the 'identified client' might be motivated to avoid further problems with the law or parents and/or to get them to 'stop picking on' him or her. If the 'client' does not describe having any relationship to the problem, they would be considered a 'visitor' and would be thanked for their time and openness to providing information about their unique perspective. If clients recognize that there is a problem that is affecting them, but feel they have no real role in changing the situation, they would be considered a 'complainant' and would be given homework assignments to help them gather information about the situation (specifically when it does NOT occur, as described below). Clients who believe they can have some influence in changing the situation would be considered 'customers' and would be given homework tasks that would build on their predisposition to 'do' something active, the specifics of which would very likely be unique to the client and situation.

Solution–focused questions

Defining and refining the focus of therapy and unique client-solutions is dependent on the questions posed by the therapist. Questions are generally directed toward real world, present and future-oriented phenomena in the context of real relationships i.e. those occurring outside the therapy session, in everyday circumstances. If time-limitations are part of the reality, then these will be built into the questions. For example, if only eight visits are allowed, goals and solutions will be based on what can be realistically addressed within that time-period, and specific ways to generalize what is being learned to times and situations beyond that period will be explored. The client's past is explored, by the therapist, only for the purpose of identifying forgotten resources and coping strategies or to draw parallels between other times that once felt difficult and were successfully managed or are now seen more positively than they initially were seen.

- ❏ **Presuppositional questions** are routinely asked as part of solution-focused therapy. These questions often utilize 'presuppositional' language – i.e. they imply that a future experience is likely to be successful by using 'when', rather than 'if' when exploring the possible consequences of various solutions.
- ❏ **Presession change questions** build on observations that simply 'doing something', such as making an appointment, is already the beginning of a positive momentum. For example: 'We have noticed that sometimes/often between the time someone makes an appointment [or has sought other help] some things are already better. What have you noticed since [you made the appointment]?
- ❏ **Exceptions questions** focus on what solution-focused therapists call 'when the problem is not occurring'. Avoiding 'problem talk' can be difficult unless alternatives to the problem are identified. There are several approaches to [locating, identifying, unearthing, naming] exceptions. For example, after learning what brought the client to therapy, the therapist might ask: 'Can you tell me about the time when [name for the problem] has either not been

present when it might have been', or 'was not as big a problem' or 'was not so distressing'? 'What was different about those times?' Another way is to begin the first session with the question, 'when you no longer feel the need to [seek therapy or come here] what will be different in your life?'

- ❏ The '**Miracle question**' is another approach to identifying possible exceptions, by projecting a possible future in which the problem no longer exists. When possible, the language used should reflect some awareness of the client's background or beliefs. The generic approach is to ask 'I'd like you to pretend for a moment that when you go to sleep tonight, during the night, a miracle happens and the problems that brought you here today are gone. Since you were asleep you would not know a miracle had happened – and you would notice because things would be different. What is the first thing you will notice, after the miracle occurs?' Although initial responses may be fanciful, it is usually possible for clients to describe in concrete terms, the differences they would observe. For example, someone who has been depressed may say 'I would notice that I woke up without a sense of dread', to which the therapist would reply – 'If you did not feel dread – what would you feel?' The latter step is important for generating positive language and providing increasing amounts of detail to the anticipated solution. The case example that follows provides a sample conversation building on exceptions.
- ❏ **Amplifying differences questions** derive from Gregory Bateson's work, which is often cited by solution-focused therapists. Bateson took the view that 'difference' in and of itself was not important unless it 'made a difference'. In addition to amplifying the exceptions identified by any of the questions posed, it is important to ask, 'and what difference will that make (e.g. when you have the energy to 'organize things around the house?)' [using the client's example]. 'And what difference will it make for you when [the children notice that things seem in better order'?] etc. 'When the children are less critical, what difference will that make?' 'What specific things do you think it would be important to do first?' 'What difference will it make when you can get [e.g. that one small thing] completed?'
- ❏ **Normalizing**. In contrast to identifying differences, clients may find it helpful to learn that their experiences and responses are 'normal' and *not* evidence of inherent pathology. Sometimes counsellors can normalize by indicating they have had similar experiences or would respond similarly. In other cases, looking at problems as normal within a developmental perspective or as part of known trajectory can have a normalizing effect.

❏ **Scaling questions** help people notice that change is a critical part of building hopefulness and reinforces the client's appreciation of the small steps that lead to greater change. Scaling can be done at any point for different purposes. Among the many possibilities, scaling can be done to determine progress toward solutions, commitment to working toward identified solutions, or confidence that progress will be maintained. Generally, scaling involves seeking information about what the scaling represents to the client. For example, if an identified solution is 'taking better care of myself by getting enough exercise' one might ask, 'On scale of 0 to 10 where would you rate the exercise you are getting now?' If "10" is getting enough exercise, what would you be doing to rate a 10? If you are at [a "2"] now, what would you need to be doing to get a 2.5?'

❏ **Coping questions** acknowledge and build on strengths that are not always apparent to the client. Among these are: 'How have you prevented things from getting worse?' 'How did you manage to get yourself up this morning?' 'What keeps you going?'

Other processes

❏ **Compliments**: In contrast to many therapies, active encouragement and enthusiasm for successes (based on progress for the client's goals) is provided whenever it seems the client is open to hearing positive feedback. Statements such as 'that's terrific – how did you do that?' not only support, but can be the 'next questions' for clarifying how best to continue progress toward desired solutions.

❏ **Reframing**: Reframing is a central strategy of all therapies that focuses on what can be controlled, i.e. our interpretations. Since multiple truths are seen as likely, the therapist can explore the acceptability of different plausible content frames based on the therapists' considering what positive meaning the behaviour might hold. Context frames can also be the basis for reframes: e.g. is there a place where this behaviour might have positive value? Negotiation of assumptions must be done cautiously, using questions, rather than statements, if the therapist is to avoid taking the role of the expert and distorting the client's views.

❏ **Homework**: Most solution-focused therapists will take a break (often leaving the room) after getting a picture of the solution and exceptions and prior to assigning 'homework', explaining the need to think for a moment about what has been learned and what might be most helpful. Such assignments are based on the client's own information about what has been working (i.e. sustaining exceptions) and based on the client's relationship to the problem, as described above. Clients then receive feedback that incorporates compliments about coping, a 'bridging statement' linking the proposed homework to what the client has described, and an assignment to be carried out, with the client's approval, before the next meeting. Often clients come to therapy as 'complainants' and will benefit from actively seeking exceptions. If so, they are often given the assignment of 'noticing when the problem does not occur' and what seems to be different about those times. For clients who have already become aware of ways to create exceptions, homework will usually be directed toward continuing that behaviour and noticing what difference it makes to them and others.

❏ **Modelling openness to change**: When clients try a new behaviour that does not work, or repeat old solutions that no longer work, it's time to try 'something different'. Some therapists discuss clients' ideas during the therapy session for doing something different before the next meeting. In other cases, therapists suggest that clients 'do something different' and report what it was and how it worked at the next meeting. Often clients come up with highly original ideas when they are not asked to specify a proposed action during the session.

❏ **Format for solution-focused interviews**: We often start initial sessions asking 'how can I help' and sometimes 'why now' in exploring the client's perspective on the situation. The majority of the session is spent identifying client goals, identifying exceptions and client strengths and steps toward goals. Follow up interviews usually start by asking 'what is better?' and seeking details about any improvement, specifically asking 'how did you do that' and complimenting clients on any progress. Next steps are identified, often using scaling and specifying what difference it makes when the new behaviour is enacted and what difference they think it will make when they continue that behaviour over time.

❏ **Solution-focused nursing process**: For those who find it helpful to translate practice in a nursing process the following chart shows how the elements of the nursing process can be mapped onto the process of solution-focused therapy.

TABLE 23.1 The solution-focused nursing process

Subjective	(Solution)
Objective	(Solution-relationship)
Assessment	(Goal and scaling)
Planning	(Next steps)
Implementation	(Homework)
Evaluation	(Scaling/difference)

Case example

The following example is an abbreviated example of seeking solutions when a client, Greg, has come to therapy at the urging of his sister, who is worried about his being more withdrawn.

Counsellor: 'Hello, Greg. I'm glad you could make it here today. How can I be helpful?'

Greg: 'I'm not really sure you can be. I'm not even sure there is a problem, but my sister insists I talk with someone'.

Counsellor: 'Do you have any idea why she wants you to talk with someone?'

Greg: 'She thinks I'm depressed'.

Counsellor: 'Why would she think that?'

Greg: 'I think I'm just going through a kind of "down" time – I just finished school and don't have a job so I don't really have to be anywhere or do anything – I think it bothers her that I'm not "going anywhere". She's kind of a worrier'.

Counsellor: 'Is it important to you that your sister is not worried about you?'

Greg: 'It's more important to me that she lets me be who I am – but she worries how we'll pay the bills if I'm not working'.

Counsellor: 'So when your sister lets you be who you are, what will you be doing?'

Greg: 'I know what I won't be doing – I won't get a job in an office just to pay the bills'.

Counsellor: 'What will you be doing instead?'

Greg: 'I'm not sure . . . I guess that's really the problem'.

Counsellor: 'Can you remember a time when you felt you really were able to be who you are and your sister was not so worried?'

Greg: 'Yeah, when I was in school, before our dad died, I was taking classes in drama and working at a restaurant as a waiter'.

Counsellor: 'What was different about then and now?'

Greg: 'Well, my sister wasn't so worried about money and she knew how important it was to me to do something creative'.

Counsellor: 'What else was different?'

Greg: 'I really liked what I was studying and the job was as a 'singing waiter' so I got to entertain people while I got paid for waiting tables'.

Counsellor: 'How else was that different from having a job in an office just to pay the bills?'

Greg: 'Well, for one thing I could move around – I have trouble staying still for long – that was always a problem in school until I got into drama. My sister wants me to get a "respectable job" in an office and have a regular income'.

Counsellor: 'If you'd humour me for a moment, I'd like you to imagine that when you go to bed tonight, while you are asleep, a miracle happens and the script of your life story gets rewritten so that you are able to be who you are and your sister isn't so worried. Since you were asleep when this happened, the only way you will know is what you will notice when you awaken. What do you think will be the first thing you will notice?'

Greg: 'Well, for starters, it would be later in the day when I woke up. I've never been a morning person, which is why I liked working in the restaurant at night and doing late rehearsals sometimes'.

Counsellor: 'What else will you notice?'

Greg: 'Well, my sister would not have made breakfast for me; she'd trust that I could fix my own meals – it always makes me feel guilty when she hovers over me'.

Counsellor: 'What else might you notice?'

Greg: 'I would be looking forward to the day – I'd have some plans to meet people and I would have the money to go out'.

Counsellor: 'What difference would that make for you?'

Greg: 'I wouldn't feel like such a loser – I'd be around people who can understand what's important to me'.

Counsellor: 'What difference will it make for your relationship with your sister when you are able to spend more time with people who understand you and you have enough money to be able to go out sometimes?'

Greg: 'Well, realistically, I'd have to be making enough to help pay the bills and go out. I know that would make her less worried and then she might stop complaining about me so much'.

Counsellor: 'So how do you think you might be able to help pay the bills and still have enough money to go out with your friends, so your sister will not complain so much?'

Greg: 'I'm not going to get a job in an office – but maybe I could look for some kind of job that I can move around in, and be around people like me . . . '

After some time spent specifying the requirements he would have for any job he would consider, the counsellor takes a break and returns with a homework assignment:

Counsellor: 'Greg, I'm really impressed that you came here today and that you have some ideas about how you can be who you are and how to help your sister be less worried about you. Between now and next time I see you I'd like you to notice a few things that may help you get a clearer pic-

	ture of how you would like to proceed. First, I'd like you to think about people you know that you think are like you and understand you. Then I'd like you to notice how they spend their time and the ways they are still able to be who they are. Are you OK with that?'
Greg:	'I guess so – I'll have to think about it a bit, but I think I can do that'.
Counsellor:	'Great – and we can discuss what you have noticed the next time I see you'.

In this example, the client and counsellor defined a relationship (one dependent on working within the client's perspective) and developed a direction for future work that is based on the client's preferred future and past successes.

APPLICATIONS

Solution-focused therapy has wide application in mental health and psychiatric care, in both inpatient and outpatient/community settings.[5] It can be incorporated into crisis work with individuals, couples, and families and has been successfully used in family-based services, including child protection, and in school settings with children and adolescents. Solution-focused treatment has also been described for sexual abuse, eating disorders, relationship problems, and depression as well as problems associated with serious mental illness.

Use of SFT also has been described in primary care, to help individuals manage habit problems (such as tobacco cessation, alcohol/drug use) and to facilitate treatment adherence that is consistent with client goals and values. More recently there are examples of working with clients with chronic pain and chronic illness from a solution-focused perspective.[4] Programmes using a group format for clients dealing with similar conditions or problems, can effectively utilize solution-focused principles, often in combination with psychoeducational approaches, as long as the emphasis remains on the centrality of client strengths and goals and is respectful toward clients' idiosyncratic methods of coping and viewing their situation.

Many SFT therapists have developed unique ways to work with younger clients, e.g. they may have them draw pictures or act out with dolls, what they wish there were more of in their lives. Because there are no requirements that all clients express emotions, develop insight, or comply with predetermined goals, SFT provides a flexible approach for working with clients from different socio-cultural and ethnic groups and across the age continuum. When working with clients from different cultural backgrounds it may be important to ascertain what types of questions are considered appropriate and to whom they may be properly addressed. Older clients and those experiencing grief can also benefit from attention to the practices and beliefs that are most important to them in their healing from multiple losses and changing circumstances. Solution-focused reminiscence therapy can help clients recall times and places and people who helped them grow and change in the ways they personally most value. The respect for the individual's worldview can be particularly empowering to women and to clients who may distrust that the 'system' has any concerns about the clients' situation or ability to make decisions on their own behalf.

THERAPY OUTCOMES

One challenge for SFT outcome measurement is that clients with similar problems (or in medical settings, similar diagnoses) may have quite disparate goals as well as many different ways to attain those goals. Outcome assessment of solution-focused therapy can be challenging if therapists or agencies have predefined goals, critical paths, and/or programmes that specify how problems must be resolved. It is possible to measure change in symptom complaints across individuals if reduction of symptoms is a goal shared by clients (and is possible). For example, it may be possible to measure increased ability to function in specified life arenas if a group of clients share the same goal (e.g. regular work attendance among people with substance abuse). For clients who have some debilitating or fluctuating conditions, however, it may be challenging to attribute changes to any specific therapeutic intervention. On the other hand, it may be possible to determine if clients feel they are managing a situation more effectively (if this is a goal clients share).

Client satisfaction is another potentially shared outcome that can be measured; however it's likely that what leads to client satisfaction may be radically different from one client to another. For example, if two depressed women both want to be able to function effectively in their relationships, the ability to identify and express emotions might be the preferred and most effective way for one client to reach her goals, while the ability to act, despite emotional distress, might be the preferred approach for another client with the same goal. Depending on the purpose for assessing outcomes, and the methods used, aggregate results may be differentially useful to counsellors and agencies.

Many agencies have shifted to a more solution-focused philosophy for the purpose of increasing efficiency and improving the economic health of the agency. Unless this type of transition is done with great care and respect for what counsellors believe they do that is helpful, it can lead to counsellor resentment and conscious or unconscious sabotage of the therapeutic approach. The rush to be brief can also be difficult for therapists who derive much of their professional reward from the opportunity to work with clients over time and help them grow and change. Ideally, the same sensitivity to clients' views about 'what works'[3] should be extended to therapists (as long they do not impose those beliefs on unwilling clients). In our experience, counsellors who may be initially unenthusiastic about the approach often become energized by seeing clients rally more quickly than anticipated and find satisfaction in hearing clients' reports of successful 'experiments' using strategies that had been forgotten or trying something 'different'. Realistically, there are those clients who do best with longer-term, often intermittent, therapy for problems that may be continuing and for which a range of changing or different 'solutions' may be appropriate over time. A consultation model of care may be most appropriate for these situations, permitting clients to seek support when they need it without being obligated to spend time and money during times when they are managing effectively.

LIMITATIONS

In addition to the difficulty comparing outcomes there are some populations for whom any verbal therapy may have a limited role. Clients who are acutely psychotic, severely regressed, or have serious cognitive impairments may be unable to benefit from an approach that depends on active client participation in defining goals, strengths, options and progress.

Risk assessment may appear counter to solution-focused principles and must be carefully planned to protect the client without undermining the focus on strengths. In many settings there are required formats and intake information that must be gathered prior to beginning any type of treatment. In such cases, it may be possible to determine risk during an intake procedure and then transition into more strength and resource-based discussion. In cases where safety is a concern we always make it a point to add scaling safety as a therapeutic goal, being careful to label it as the therapist's concern if it is not an identified client goal.

In some circumstances, clients may have either limited life experience or access to information and resources that might be helpful to them. Balancing a need for information with respect for the client's own knowledge and experience can be handled several ways. If clients are working in a group, they will be exposed to a wider range of possible solutions than they might generate individually. 'Modelling and role-modelling' (MRM), a nursing theory consistent with solution-focused therapy, addresses the problem by providing psychoeducation only for issues about which the client

indicates a desire to have additional information.[6] Similarly, MRM looks at clients and their resources from a developmental perspective that nurses usually find helpful and that clients may find normalizing.[7]

SUMMARY

Solution-focused therapy is based on theoretical and practical evidence of 'what works' to help clients identify personally meaningful goals and build on clients' existing strengths and resources. Using a range of questions intended to develop an understanding of the client's perspective and encourage a positive orientation, it can be used with a wide variety of therapeutic concerns in both inpatient and outpatient populations.

Discussion points

❏ Post-modern therapies[8] are often described as avoiding taking ethical positions in the service of accepting clients' views and supporting multicultural perspectives. Can a therapist respect client's world-views and maintain personal integrity?

❏ Accepting clients' reports of problems and possible solutions can reduce a therapist's sense of responsibility for the specifics of therapy outcomes. What are the realistic limitations of therapist responsibility and in what circumstances might other perspectives take precedence over client preferences?

REFERENCES

1. deShazer S. *Clues: investigating solutions in brief therapy*. New York: W.W. Norton, 1988.
2. Barker P. Solution-focused therapies. *Nursing Times* 1988; **94**(19): 53–6.
3. Hubble M, Duncan B, Miller S. *The heart and soul of change: what works in therapy*. Washington, DC: American Psychological Association, 1999.
4. Johnson C, Webster D. *Recrafting a life*. New York: Brunner/Routledge, 2002.
5. Miller S, Hubble M, Duncan B. *Handbook of solution-focused brief therapy*. San Francisco: Jossey-Bass, 1996.
6. Erickson H, Tomlin E, Swain M. *Modeling and role-modeling: a theory and paradigm for nursing*. Englewood-Cliffs: Prentice-Hall, 1983.
7. Webster D, Vaughn K, Webb M, Playter A. Modeling the client's world through solution-focused therapy. *Issues in Mental Health Nursing* 1995; **16**: 505–18.
8. Barker P. The solution-focused therapies. In: *The talking cures* London: NT Books, 1999.

Chapter 24

USING COUNSELLING APPROACHES

Philip Burnard*

INTRODUCTION

The research jury cannot make up its mind about counselling. It is neither easy to define nor easy to research. This chapter considers some of the things that mental health and psychiatric nurses may want to consider before doing counselling. It considers the research evidence and it offers a practical framework for offering counselling to those in emotional distress. Finally, it addresses some cultural issues that need to be considered and closes with some thoughts about integrating these sections.

What is counselling?

In recent years, a range of questions about *what* counselling is, *who* should do it and whether or not it *works* have been asked, both in the literature and in the national newspapers. As consumers become more aware of their rights and more discerning about the nature of the treatments that they are offered, they are – appropriately – asking questions about whether or not counselling is a 'good thing'. The answer to the question remains unanswered, convincingly, at the time of writing this book. All we can surmise is that talking about things seems to help a lot of people. Whether or not 'formal counselling' makes a long-term difference has yet to be clarified. In the meantime, a useful distinction, for nurses, can be made between *counselling* and *using counselling skills*. It is argued that the *latter* are of particular use to the nurse.

There are many published, formal definitions of counselling. Just one is offered here, by Richard Nelson-Jones, a prolific and respected writer in the counselling field, who defined it as follows:

> Essential counselling and therapy skills are communication skills, accompanied by appropriate mental processes, offered by counsellors and therapists in order to develop collaborative working relationships with clients, identify problems, clarify and expand understanding of these problems and, where appropriate, to assist clients to develop and implement strategies for changing how they think, communicate/act and feel so that they can attain more of their human potential.[1]

As with all definitions of this type of activity, it is only *a* definition and not *the* definition. While Nelson-Jones' definition is wide-ranging and inclusive, we might ask questions about what he means by the abstraction 'attain more of their human potential'. Any definition necessarily reflects the authors own belief and value sys-

*Philip Burnard is Professor of Nursing and Vice Dean at the School of Nursing and Midwifery Studies at the University of Wales College of Medicine in Cardiff. He has published widely in the fields of counselling, ethics, research and stress. He is currently Visiting Professor at the Royal Thai Army Nursing College in Bangkok, Thailand and lectures internationally. His current research is into stress in community mental health nursing.

tems and this one is no exception. There are, of course, numerous others in the literature on the topic.[2]

COUNSELLING AND COUNSELLING SKILLS

What, then, are the differences between the two concepts? Counselling, it might be argued, is something that is carried out by people whose job it is to counsel. Such people will be known by the job title 'counsellor' and it seems likely that they will pursue this job on a full-time basis. Counselling skills are part of the things that they use to pursue that job. Such skills, however, are also transferable to other jobs and, in particular, to nursing. Nurses, without being 'counsellors' in the strict sense of the word, can use a range of counselling skills to help their patients talk through problems, express feelings and make decisions. Such nurses do not practise as counsellors but use the skills that are available appropriately and carefully.

Is counselling effective?

The question often arises as to whether or not counselling 'works'. A similar but perhaps clearer question is often asked: 'is counselling effective?' This section offers a short review of some of the current thinking in this area. It is based on the NHS Centre for Reviews and Dissemination, The University of York publication, Vol. 5, Issue 2, August 2001, *Counselling in Primary Care*.

The primary interest of those collating evidence for clinical effectiveness, through systematic reviews of the research literature is the randomized controlled trial or RCT. The use of randomized controlled trials (RCTs) to evaluate counselling and other psychological therapy treatments is contentious.[3–6] However, a number of RCTs of counselling in primary care have been conducted.

Rowland *et al.*[7] published a systematic review of counselling in primary care. The latest update of the review includes seven RCTs of counsellors trained to the standard recommended by the British Association for Counselling and Psychotherapy. The review focused on counsellors meeting these standards as they are increasingly recognized as a useful benchmark in primary care. The counsellors in these trials treated patients with mild to moderate mental health problems (such as anxiety and depression) referred by GPs. In six of the trials, the comparison group was 'usual GP care' including support from the GP within normal consultations, medication and referral to mental health services.

One RCT used a comparison group of 'GP anti-depressant treatment' and was considered separately. The results of six RCTs (with 772 patients) indicated

that counselled patients demonstrated a significantly greater reduction in psychological symptoms such as anxiety and depression than patients receiving usual GP care when followed up in the short term (up to 6 months). Psychological symptoms were measured using validated questionnaires such as the Beck Depression Inventory and General Health Questionnaire. These psychological benefits were modest: the average counselled patient was better off than approximately 60% of patients in usual GP care (if counselling and usual care were equally effective, the proportion would be 50%). There were no significant differences between counselling and usual care in the four RCTs (with 475 patients) reporting long-term outcomes (8–12 months).

Generally, the RCTs reported high levels of patient satisfaction with counselling and that patients were more satisfied with counselling than with usual GP care. However, this comparison of GPs and counsellors is difficult to interpret due to the differences in time each has available to spend with patients.

Two RCTs have compared counselling with other mental health treatments routinely provided in primary care.[8–11] The first compared counselling with cognitive-behaviour therapy provided by qualified psychologists. There were no differences between the two therapies in their overall effectiveness at short- or long-term follow-up. Both therapies were superior to usual GP care in the short term, but provided no significant advantage in the long term.

The second RCT compared counselling with anti-depressant treatment provided by GPs who were given specific guidelines on anti-depressant use. However, the study was designed to reflect anti-depressant prescribing as provided routinely by GPs, and the prescription of medication was not standardized. There were no differences in outcomes between patients receiving counselling and medication at 8 weeks or 12 months follow-up.

HOW DO YOU CHOOSE AN APPROACH TO COUNSELLING?

There are lots of different ways of doing counselling, based on different sorts of philosophical views of people. In this section, I want to explore, in a general way, how our beliefs about people will affect the approach we use in counselling or, indeed, whether we do counselling at all.

One point seems more important than all the others when we consider views of the person. It is simply this: to what degree, if at all, do we feel that people can *change* and to what degree, if at all, can individuals *choose* that change? Presumably, if we do counselling, we must believe that people can change and that they can decide on that change. If we believe that people cannot change then we are unlikely to believe that counselling will be effective. In the paragraphs that follow, I explore the various philosophical points that relate to this idea.

Free will

Philosophically, there are at least three different views we can have about the human condition: free will, determinism and fatalism.[12] Free will involves the idea that we can choose our mental states and, to a greater or lesser degree, our futures. If I consider what choices I have as I write this, I may be led to thinking that all I can do is sit and finish my writing. However, if I think for a bit longer, I will realize that I can choose a huge range of options. Here are just some of them. I can choose to finish this writing task. I can choose not to finish it and to delete everything I have written so far. I can tell the editor that I refuse to write the chapter. I can write complete nonsense and submit it as a chapter. And so on. The point, by extension, is that, arguably, at any point in my life, I can *choose* a considerable range of things to do and not to do. In doing this and in choosing what I do, I am exercising free will. The most extreme statement of this comes in the branch of philosophy known as *existentialism*.[13, 14]

The existentialists argue that, because we have consciousness and because we can reflect on our situation, we are free, psychologically, to choose our lives. This is a mental freedom. We cannot choose to change our physical status in any profound way. I cannot, for instance, choose to wake up tomorrow with blue eyes. But, according to existential theory, I *do* choose my psychological state. I am, according to existentialism, free to choose at any moment in my life – once I have reached an age where I am *aware* of being able to choose. Furthermore, I *must* choose. And in doing so, I become the author of myself. In choosing, I create who I am as a person.

So what is the point of this sort of freedom? Well, simply, perhaps, that many of us deny it. We prefer, instead, to believe that we are controlled either by our pasts or by other people. We sometimes feel *safer* believing that what we do is beyond our control. In that way, we can simply 'give in' to life and accept our lot. Also, in doing this, we do not have to take *responsibility* for who we are. Instead, we can blame our parents, or a 'bad marriage' or any number of other factors for our being in the situation we are in. The evangelizing aspect of existentialism is to convince people of the reality of their freedom to choose and also of their subsequent responsibility. For we

cannot be free and not responsible. If I say, for instance, that I am free to do anything but that I must first check with my wife, I am clearly not free. However, if I *do* exercise my freedom, then I *have* to take responsibility for my actions. For, in choosing, I alone decide what I will do and I must face the consequences of my actions.

All of this fits very well with the notion of counselling as an activity – particularly with the client-centred approaches to counselling in which the counsellor refrains from offering the client advice or ideas or suggestions about how to live but, instead, helps him or her to make his or her own decisions about his or her life. This is completely compatible with the notion of personal free will and with the belief in our ability to choose our lives.

Determinism

An alternative way of thinking about people is to see their mental states as being *determined*. What might this mean? In the physical world – the world that surrounds us – the laws of *causality* are always and everywhere at play. If I consider the computer that I am using to help me write this, I will realize that before this computer existed, it was made up of plastic, metal and some other ingredients. These, in turn, existed in another state (the metal, as ore, for example) before they were used in making the computer. These are facts about the way computers come into being. Any object in the world was, previously, something else. We can always trace, for example, iron, back to its source as ore. This process of things becoming other things is known as a *causal chain*. It is never going to be possible to point to a computer and say 'this never existed as other chemicals and minerals before, it simply came into being in this room!'

Similarly, the argument goes, people's thoughts and actions do not simply spring into being. Instead, they can be traced back to previous events and thoughts. An argument for why I have the personality I have today is that it was in some way *caused* by previous life events. Sigmund Freud, the creator of the psychotherapy known as psychoanalysis referred to all this as *psychic determinism*. He argued that our minds are situated in physical bodies, which themselves, are subject to causal law. Similarly, he argued, our minds are *determined* by previous life events, actions and thoughts. We do not, according to Freud, simply *choose* at any given point but, instead, there is a certain *inevitability* about how we turn out as people. Our thoughts, feelings and actions are not really *chosen* but, instead, *determined* by what has happened to us. This, then, is the counter position to the argument for free will.

Psychoanalysis and determinism

Psychoanalysis, itself, seems to take an interesting line on determinism. While it acknowledges that we are shaped and influenced by our past to the degree that it is our past that makes us who we are, it also argues that *understanding* these links between past and present can *free* us to make life choices. This seems something of a contradiction. It seems that our lives are determined up to a point and then, through the process known as psychoanalysis, we are somehow freed to choose our lives. Again, anyone coming to counselling needs to consider their own position on the free will–determinism axis. Suffice to say, at this point, that there is a middle, compromise position in all of this. It is possible to see people in terms of *relative determinism*. That is to say that at any given time, we have a wide but not limitless array of choices from which we choose. While the existentialist would say that I can choose *anything* and the determinist would say that freedom of choice is a myth, the relative determinist would talk of a limited range of choices, but would also acknowledge that such choices are possible.

Fatalism

For completeness, it is interesting to note a third (or perhaps fourth) position that we might adopt in thinking about the nature of people. Another view is that of *fatalism*. Fatalism is the idea that our lives are, in some way, laid out for us. All we have to do is to *live* our lives, as those lives are already *chosen* for us. There is little we can do to change the ways in which our lives 'work', since a blueprint for them already exists somewhere. This position is usually seen in followers of the sects of certain world religions. However, it can also be found in everyday folk culture. It is not rare to hear people say 'well, if it is meant to be, then it will happen', suggesting that someone, somewhere, has already planned everything. This can, of course, be either a good thing or a bad thing. In cultures where fatalism is pervasive, it is usual to see a quiet acceptance of things as they are and a lack of determination to try to change things.

However, in certain settings, such a position leads to despair and what might be called a loss of the locus of control. In certain depressive states, for example, it is not unusual to find a person believing that nothing they can do will ever change their condition. Sometimes, then, the counsellor's role might be to help a nominally 'fatalistic' person to appreciate that it is the *person* who controls his or her life[15] . . . or is it? Debating and answering this sort of question is at the heart of deciding on an approach to counselling and also in deciding whether or not to counsel at all.

COUNSELLING INTERVENTIONS

All those who take up counselling will have to consider their basic beliefs about the nature of people, as outlined above. After this, it is necessary to consider the degree to which we feel people can make their own decisions, unaided. In counselling terms, there are a range of ways of thinking about this. At one end of the spectrum lies the *client-centred approach* to counselling.[16] This approach involves the view that people can and must choose their own lives and that counsellors should never offer advice or suggestions as to how clients lives might be changed. At the other end of the spectrum is what might be called the *didactic* approach to counselling. This involves the view that it is always worth helping people to *question* their views of the world and to suggest alternative ways of doing things. Thus a cognitive-behavioural approach to counselling would be very different to the client-centred approach in that it would involve the counsellor in being confronting and very assertive in relation to what the client says.[17] For the cognitive-behavioural counsellor, it is not sufficient merely to agree with the client's view of his or her world. Instead, it is the counsellor's job to challenge that view and help to change it with concrete suggestions and instructions. It is also the counsellor's role to help spot faulty and illogical thinking on the part of the client. There is, again, a huge literature on the different approaches to counselling. One useful guide to these is published by the British Association for Counselling.[18]

To enable us to choose the sorts of interventions we make, ranging from client-centred to cognitive-behavioural methods of counselling, it is useful to have a *general framework* that covers all possible effective counselling interventions. Such a general purpose framework is now offered here in the form of Heron's Six Category Intervention Analysis.[19, 20]

This conceptual framework was developed by Heron out of the work of Blake and Mouton.[21] It was offered as a conceptual model for understanding interpersonal relationships, and as an assessment tool for identifying a range of possible therapeutic interactions between two people.

The six categories in Heron's analysis are: prescriptive (offering advice), informative (offering information), confronting (challenging), cathartic (enabling the expression of pent-up emotions), catalytic ('drawing out') and supportive (confirming or encouraging). The word 'intervention' is used to describe any statement that the practitioner may use. The word 'category' is used to denote a range of related interventions.

Heron calls the first three categories of intervention (prescriptive, informative and confronting), 'authoritative' and suggests that in using these categories the practitioner retains control over the relationship. He calls the second three categories of intervention (cathartic, catalytic and supportive), 'facilitative' and suggests that these enable the client to retain control over the relationship. In other words, the first three are 'practitioner-centred' and the second three are 'client-centred'. Another way of describing the difference between the first and second sets of three categories is that the first three are 'I tell you' interventions and the second three are 'You tell me' interventions.

What, then, is the value of such an analysis of therapeutic interventions? First, it identifies the *range* of possible interventions available to the nurse/counsellor. Very often, in day-to-day interactions with others, we stick to repetitive forms of conversation and response, simply because we are not aware that other options are available to us. This analysis identifies an exhaustive range of types of human interventions. Second, by identifying the sorts of interventions we can use, we can act more precisely and with a greater sense of intention. The nurse–patient relationship thus becomes more particular and less haphazard. Since we know *what* we are saying and also *how* we are saying it, we have greater interpersonal choice.

Third, the analysis offers an instrument for training. Once the categories have been identified, they can be used for students and others to identify their weaknesses and strengths across the interpersonal spectrum. Nurses can, in this way, develop a wide range and comprehensive range of interpersonal skills.

It is worth repeating that the skills identified in this chapter as counselling skills are exactly similar to the basic human skills used in day-to-day nursing interactions. Thus an understanding of the full range of the six categories can enhance and enrich the quality of the nurse's approach to care. It should be noted, too, that the analysis does not offer a mechanical approach to interpersonal skills training. This is an important issue. The analysis indicates a *type* of response. The choice of words, the tone of voice, the non-verbal aspects of a particular response must develop out of the individual's belief and value system and out of their life experience. Those aspects of the response are also dependent upon the situation at the time and upon the people involved. All human relationships occur within a particular context. It is impossible to identify what will necessarily be the right thing to do in *this* situation at *this* time. A mechanical, learning-by-heart approach to counselling or interpersonal skills would, therefore, be inappropriate.

One of the great strengths of Heron's analysis is that it allows the mental health and psychiatric nurse to consider *all* types of counselling intervention. Often, in the literature, it is possible to find a description of the client-centred approach OR the cognitive-behavioural approach. Heron's analysis allows the nurse to consider the full range of possible interventions as they relate to helping the patient or client.

The point of the analysis, in this chapter, is to allow nurses to consider what counselling interventions may be appropriate for use with their patients. There is no room, in a chapter of this sort, to offer a detailed account of all aspects of counselling practice and the reader is referred to other chapters in this book about psychotherapy, psychoanalysis and other therapies for further details about what effective interventions may be used with different client groups. More details of this analysis and research undertaken by the present author into it are described elsewhere.[22]

CULTURAL AWARENESS

While counselling is widely recognized as a reasonable practice in so-called Western countries, it is certainly not the only approach to personal problem-solving. In particular, the client-centred approach to counselling, in which the person receiving counselling is encouraged to identify his or her own problems and also their solutions is acceptable only in cultures that value individualism and the primacy of the individual. Anyone working in multicultural settings (and that must surely include most nurses) must remain sensitive to cultural differences among client groups. While it is beyond the scope of this book to highlight particular cultural issues involved in counselling, it is valuable to note the following points, adapted from McLaren's[23] guidelines for multicultural counselling practice, as follows:

❑ There is no single concept of 'normality' that applies across all people, situations and cultures. Mainstream concepts of mental health and illness must be expanded to incorporate religious and spiritual elements. It is important to take a flexible and respectful approach to other therapeutic values, beliefs and traditions: we must each of us assume that our own view is culturally biased.

❑ Individualism is not the only way to view human behaviour, and must be supplemented by collectivism in some situations. Dependency is not a bad characteristic in many cultures.

❑ It is essential to acknowledge the reality of racism and discrimination in the lives of people, and in the therapy process. Power imbalances between therapists and clients may reflect the imbalance of power between the cultural communities in which they belong.

❑ Language use is important: abstract 'middle-class' psychotherapeutic discourse may not be understood by people coming from other cultures. Linear thinking/storytelling is not universal.

❑ It is important to take account of the structures

within the client's community that serve to strengthen and support the client: natural supporting methods are important to the individual. For some clients, traditional healing methods may be more effective than Western forms of counselling.

❏ It is necessary to take history into account when making sense of current experience. The way that someone feels may not only be a response to what is happening now, but in part a response to loss or trauma that occurred in earlier generations.

❏ Be willing to talk about cultural and racial issues and differences in counselling sessions.

Almost all of the above points can be adapted to communication in everyday nursing practice. It is easy, perhaps, for all of us to be ethnocentric – to believe that the way *we* do things is in some way the 'right' way. Only by studying cultures and by listening closely to what clients, patients and colleagues are telling us about other cultures will we begin to avoid this trap.

CONCLUSION

Thus we have come full circle. This chapter started by considering fundamental views we might have of human nature. It outlined the possibilities of *free will, determinism* and *fatalism*. It then explored a *general framework* for considering what we might do as counsellors. Finally, given that we almost all work in culturally mixed settings, it considered the cultural aspects of counselling. Any nurse hoping to help patients and clients through counselling might usefully consider, first, their own beliefs about the nature of people, followed by their views of the cultural contexts of different people. It should be noted, too, that different cultures place different emphases on the issue of free will and determinism. While, as a general rule, many American and Northern European people will value free will, many people in Asian and other cultures will not. The idea that our particular belief system is in some way superior is only one more trap that the would-be counsellor can become ensnared in. We share the world with lots of different sorts of people. It is likely that some will be helped by counselling and others will not. Counselling is usually a fairly non-invasive and inexpensive form of therapy, but it is by no means universally applicable. It should be the aim of every mental health and psychiatric nurse to be able to help select the most helpful therapy for *this* particular patient or client at *this* time. If it is decided that counselling might help, then the framework offered by Heron, in this chapter, can help to shape the counselling experience.

REFERENCES

1. Nelson-Jones, R. *Essential counselling and therapy skills*. London: Sage, 2002.
2. Burnard, P. *Counselling skills for health professionals*, 3rd edn. Gloucester: Stanley Thornes, 1999.
3. Hazzard, A. Measuring outcome in counselling: a brief exploration of the issues. *British Journal of General Practice* 1995; **45**: 118–19.
4. Bower P, Byford S, Sibbald B, *et al*. Randomised controlled trials of non-directive counselling, cognitive-behavioural therapy and usual GP care for patients with depression. II. Cost effectiveness. *British Medical Journal* 2000; **231**: 1389–92.
5. Roth A, Fonagy P. *What works for whom? A critical reader of psychotherapy research*. London: Guilford Press, 1996.
6. Seligman M. The effectiveness of psychotherapy: the consumer reports study. *American Psychologist* 1995; **50**: 965–74.
7. Rowland N, Bower P, Mellor-Clark J, *et al*. Counselling for depression in primary care (Cochrane review). The Cochrane Library, Issue 2, Oxford, Update Software, 2002.
8. Ward E, King M, Lloyd M, *et al*. Randomised controlled trial of non-directive counselling, cognitive behaviour therapy and usual GP care for patients with depression. 1. Clinical effectiveness. *British Medical Journal* 2000; **321**: 1383–8.
9. Sibbald B, Ward E, King M. Randomised controlled trial of non-directive counselling, cognitive behaviour therapy and usual general practitioner care in the management of depression as well as mixed anxiety and depression in primary care. *Health Technology Assessment* 2000; **4**: 19.
10. Bedi N, Chilvers C, Churchill R, *et al*. Assessing effectiveness of treatment of depression in primary care: partially randomised preference trial. *British Journal of Psychiatry* 2000; **177**: 312–18.
11. Chilvers C, Dewey M, Fielding K, *et al*. Anti-depressant drugs and generic counselling for treatment of major depression in primary care: randomised trial with patient preference arms. *British Medical Journal* 2001; **322**: 775.
12. Stevenson L. *Seven theories of human nature*. Oxford: Oxford University Press, 1987.
13. Sartre JP. *Being and nothingness*. New York: Philosophical Library, 1956.
14. Sartre JP. *Humanism and existentialism*. London: Methuen, 1973.
15. Van Deurzen-Smith E. *Existential counselling in practice*. London: Sage, 1988.
16. Nelson-Jones R. *Essential counselling and therapy skills*. London: Sage, 2002.
17. Hawton K, Salkovskis PM, Kirk J, Clark DM (eds).

Cognitive behaviour therapy for psychiatric problems – a practical guide. Oxford: Oxford Medical Publications, 1989.

18. Palmer S, Dainow S, Milner P (eds). *Counselling: The BAC counselling reader*. Rugby: Sage Publications in association with the British Association for Counselling, 1996.

19. Heron J. *Six category intervention analysis*, 3rd edn. Guildford: Human Potential Resource Group, University of Surrey, 1989.

20. Heron J. *A handbook of facilitator style*. London: Kogan Page, 1989.

21. Blake RR, Mouton JS. *Consultation*. New York: Addison Wesley, 1976.

22. Burnard P. *Learning human skills: an experiential and reflective guide for nurses and health care professionals*, 4th edn. Oxford: Butterworth Heinemann, 2002.

23. McClaren MC. *Interpreting cultural differences: the challenge of intercultural communication*. Dereham: Peter Francis, 1998.

Chapter 25

BEREAVEMENT AND GRIEF COUNSELLING

Clare Hopkins*

INTRODUCTION

Bereavement relates to the loss of a person, object or state. *Grief* is the emotion experienced as a result of that loss. *Mourning* is the behaviour that expresses grief at the loss. *Loss* can be said to be part of every human life although the meaning of loss, and responses to it, are unique. Each person's unique feelings of grief and their expressions of mourning will be influenced by the culture and society within which they live.[1] It is from the shared understandings of bereavement and grief that theories about grief and mourning have been formed.

The terms 'bereavement', 'grief' and 'mourning' are most usually connected with loss through death and the accompanying feelings and behaviours. However, bereavement can occur in many other ways. Grief can be experienced through any kind of loss; relationships end without one of the partners dying; people lose their jobs; families break up and move away; pets die; miscarriage and infertility may deprive us of the family we thought we might have. When we cannot fulfil our life plans because of economic circumstances, unemployment,

lack of choice, abuse or deprivation, physical or mental distress or disability, we may be bereaved of our *expectations* and grieve these losses. Receiving a diagnosis of illness – physical or mental – may bring with it pain, loss of expectation, loss of social status, perhaps foreshortening of life expectation and all of these may cause the person (and their family) to grieve. Although this chapter focuses on loss and grief through death, its contents can equally be applied to these other losses.

Grief and loss

Perhaps the experiences of loss and grief are common because people, in general, have positive expectations about life. Many writers[2,3] have suggested that later 20th century and early 21st century society has become obsessed with the healthy body and that illness and the mortality of the individual has become a consideration from which we seek to defend ourselves. Progress in medical interventions during the 20th century has meant that random, mass and untimely deaths through

*Clare Hopkins is a mental health nurse with special interests in working with people who self harm and with people who are in crisis. At present she is a Senior Lecturer in Mental Health Nursing at the University of Northumbria in England.

infection are now less likely in prosperous societies. When deaths do occur in this way, and are not amenable to medical intervention (for example the rise and spread of HIV), it creates widespread fear and alienation of what are seen as susceptible groups.[4] This defence or denial of the prospect of death for every individual may guard against fear, and also serves to fully orientate us towards life. Nevertheless, even when we defend ourselves from death psychologically, we still flirt with death vicariously, through media portrayals of dramatic deaths or near-deaths.[5]

Bowlby[6] wrote extensively about attachment theory and the forming of affectional bonds between people, especially infants and their carers. In his view, attachment behaviour serves as a protection for the growing child together with the development of a sense of security. Affectional bonds also have the complementary function of eliciting 'caregiving' behaviour both from adults to children and between adults. If a sense of 'secure attachment' has been possible for the developing individual then their subsequent acceptance of change, including losses, will determine not only their view of the world but their view of themselves.[7] This is similar to Erick Erikson's concept of 'basic trust'[8] which states that through the formation of bonds with parents or carers, the child comes to believe in her/himself as worthy of help, should difficulties arise.

When a person does not have the ability to maintain a positive style and shows no ability to cope with change, this is often seen as pathological and may be called depression. Because positive expectations and hopefulness appear to be the default position of the human psyche, this opens up the possibility of loss and grief as a response to those losses. If the person has a sense of secure attachment, grief and mourning will be time limited. If the person has not developed a sense of secure attachment, then mourning may be more complex and protracted.

Grief is an emotion expressed in every culture. We all react to loss but the meanings we give to loss will, to some extent, be dictated by the culture in which we live, which will influence the way in which we mourn. Grief can be seen as socially constructed, both in terms of which losses are viewed as bereavement, and which processes of mourning are seen as acceptable. In this way, our culture, in the form of our regional, national, ethnic and religious affiliations will determine how we feel, perceive ourselves and act when faced with losses.[1,9]

We are all affected by our society's understanding of what represents loss and who is, by consequence, entitled to grieve and take part in public mourning and who is denied that right. For example, in Western cultures, which value the sanctity of marriage and the family, the widow's right to show publicly her distress for her dead husband, at his funeral, will be seen as legitimate. A similar expression of grief from his extra-marital lover might be heard with horror and, by consequence, invalidated. Society would expect her to grieve but that her expressions of grief should be muted and private.

Similarly, widespread expressions of grief over the death of well-known public figures such as Princess Diana reinforced culturally acceptable expressions of mourning. However, as the public grieving for Diana was taking place, the media – who had recorded and possibly promoted this display of grieving – debated whether those who mourned so publicly had a 'legitimate' right to do so. This was predicated on the assumption that the lack of personal connection with Diana meant that her death 'should' have had minimal impact on the mourners' lives. It seemed as if these debates about 'legitimacy of mourning' were in some way contravening the 'cultural scripts' about bereavement and grief, and perhaps involved a renegotiation of these scripts.[2]

NURSING AND LOSS

As nurses, we will encounter people who have experienced losses of many kinds. In part this is because family relationships are now more often fragmented and members of families geographically distant from each other. Prior to the middle of the 20th century, families were more likely to be available to support their members at times of loss and this process was made clear through defined religious, funeral and mourning rituals.[10–12] Not only did this allow for expressions of grief by the bereaved but marked out the kind of support which they could expect from others. Now that this framework is less likely to exist, grief is often viewed as a medical responsibility.

Lindemann[13] studied the processes of grief following traumatic bereavement when he studied the responses of survivors of a fire in a nightclub in 1942. This study found that a psychological intervention at the time of the crisis caused by bereavement had a beneficial effect and from this, crisis theory was formed. Crisis theory[14] views a person in crisis as being particularly open to finding new ways of coping, although these may be *either* beneficial *or* destructive. By intervening in the grieving process to provide support throughout the crisis, it was thought that integration of the loss and a speedy return to normal functioning might be facilitated.[13]

20TH CENTURY THEORIES OF BEREAVEMENT AND GRIEF

Throughout the 20th century, many writers studied bereavement. From these studies theories were developed which relate to the process of grief and mourning and the prevention of mental illness.

Elisabeth Kübler Ross[15] described stages in the process of accepting the diagnosis of terminal illness. She identified a series of stages through which the person confronted with their own death may pass, rarely sequentially, often randomly and occasionally simultaneously:

- **Denial and isolation.** A necessary, though usually temporary, stage. Denial acts as a form of protection against overwhelming feelings of powerlessness and loss. Occasionally, it may continue until death.
- **Anger.** Expressions of anger ('why me?') that they are facing death.
- **Bargaining.** Often described as an 'attempt to postpone' – bargaining may be with the person's conception of a Higher Being or with the staff who are treating them.
- **Depression.** A sense of loss and sadness, but perhaps also guilt and hopelessness.
- **Acceptance.** A stage 'almost devoid of feelings' but perhaps characterized by peace and acceptance.
- **Hope.** A complex state which can encompass hope of cure ('a miracle') or hope for a pain-free death or hopefulness gained through a sense of acceptance of death.

Colin Murray Parkes[7] identified related stages in the grieving process which were found in his study of widows bereaved before the age of 65.

- **Searching.** Closely related to 'pangs' of grief which may be experienced spontaneously in the immediate post-bereavement stage but later in response to reminders. The bereaved may have a sense of the lost person being with them or may 'see' them.
- **Mitigation.** Ways in which the bereaved comfort themselves. This may include a sense of the 'presence' of the dead person, a sense of disbelief, avoidance of reminders, a sense of numbness or unreality. The dead person may be 'idealized'.
- **Anger and guilt.** Feelings of anger and irritability addressed either to the deceased or to others are common. Taking the loss as a personal insult and seek to apportion blame: others or themselves.[7]
- **Depression.** Sometimes expressed as apathy and despair.
- **Gaining a new identity.** Taking on roles previously carried out by their dead spouse in practical matters, personal mannerisms, characteristics and interests.

Wolfgang Stroebe and Margaret Stroebe[16] also studied the effect of partner loss. They identified four phases through which the person experiencing such a loss might move.

- Numbness.
- Yearning and protest.
- Despair.
- Recovery and restitution.

All of these theories see grief following bereavement take a broadly similar route, moving from shock and disbelief, through to seeking and yearning for the lost person or object, to a state of abjection and depression. If the grieving process is uncomplicated, the person will gradually regain a sense of stability and will be able to carry on with their lives without the object of their loss.

Accepted theories of loss and grief are being challenged.[1,17,18] There is a growing acceptance that culture influences grief as well as mourning and there is no longer an acceptance that grief is complete once the bereaved person has 'moved on' from their loss and made new links with life. 21st century theories suggest that, through conversations with other people who knew the lost person, the bereaved are able to integrate and experience an 'inner representation' of the deceased as part of the grieving process. There is also an increased acceptance that mourners may not 'get over it' or 'move on' but instead reach a sense of 'accommodation'. Accommodation is not a static phenomenon but 'is a continual activity, related both to others and to shifting self-perceptions as the physical and social environment changes and as individual, family and community developmental processes unfold.'[18]

PHYSICAL RESPONSES TO BEREAVEMENT

The bereaved person may also be at risk of loss of their own health.[7,16] This may be associated with the fact that loss and grief are likely to result in changes in behaviour, for example increased smoking or alcohol consumption, changes in eating patterns, and self-neglect. The grieving person will also be experiencing stress which is related to higher than expected rates of infection, cancer, coronary heart disease as well as disorders of the gastrointestinal system such as ulcerative colitis and peptic ulcers.[16] There may also be an exacerbation of an existing condition.[7] Following the death of a loved one, the bereaved person may develop symptoms which mimic those of the person they are mourning.[19]

WORKING WITH THE BEREAVED

There are many models of counselling which may be used when working with the person suffering from grief because of a bereavement.

Arguably, the most appropriate model is the person-centred approach of Carl Rogers.[20] *Person-centred or non-*

directive counselling aims to develop a 'helping' relationship between counsellor and client, within which the client is encouraged, through talking about whatever they define as the 'problem', to find answers from within themselves. Rogers believed that solutions, and resources, were to be found within the person experiencing the problem. The role of the non-directive or person-centred counsellor is to act as a listener to the 'story' told by the client. By using specific counselling skills, the counsellor 'reflects back' the *essence* of what is said. By doing so the counsellor helps the person to reconsider their story and their perceptions about it, thus finding ways of dealing with 'the problem' from within themselves.

The basic tenet of person-centred counselling is the use of the 'core conditions' within the therapeutic relationship. These core conditions are warmth, empathy, genuineness and unconditional positive regard.[21] Establishment of these core conditions within the therapeutic relationship provides a non-threatening environment in which the person can feel safe and secure and which will provide her/him with the opportunity to carry out the 'work' of grieving. As Barker and Kerr[22] comment, 'therapy is no more than a conversation developed within an extraordinary relationship.'

Grief responses are highly individual and there is no right or wrong way to grieve. A wide spectrum of experiences are 'normal'. However, in the majority of cases the person who is experiencing grief will need to be heard. At each stage of the grief process they will need to speak their thoughts aloud in order to try to make sense of them. Describing events to a sensitive, empathic, non-judgemental listener will help the person who is in the stage of numbness and disbelief to come to a gradual realization of their situation and its implications. Carl Rogers (1980) wrote of empathy:

> It involves being sensitive, moment to moment, to the changing felt meanings which flow in this other person, to the fear or rage or tenderness or confusion or whatever, that he/she is experiencing.[23]

If the person becomes agitated, angry, blaming or guilty, it is important that they are able to express these feelings in safety without the need to fear that they will either overwhelm their listener or that their listener will reject them because they are expressing strong feelings. By *accepting* and tolerating the person's strong feelings, the counsellor will be able to support the grieving person to be less overwhelmed by these feelings. By being *empathic* to the content of what the person is saying and how they are expressing themselves, and being *genuine* in their responses to the person, s/he will have the opportunity to feel valued, at a time when they may be experiencing threats to their life roles.

People who are grieving may be vulnerable to suggestion. Being with someone who is grieving can be stressful. For this reason, family and friends – who may also be grieving or who may be exhausted from the business of supporting the grief-stricken individual – may tend to be directive and prescriptive. Comments such as 'time is a great healer', 'you'll get over it', 'you will find someone else' or 'what you need is … !' will not only have no meaning for the person but may be perceived as insensitive and dismissive. The well-meaning phrase 'I know how you feel' is always inaccurate. Even if the person using the phrase has experienced a similar loss, it will never be the same loss.

In 1982 Wordon[24] published his work on grief counselling and grief therapy which highlighted the 'four tasks of mourning':

- ❏ To accept the reality of the loss.
- ❏ To experience the pain of grief.
- ❏ To adjust to an environment in which the deceased is missing.
- ❏ To withdraw emotional energy and reinvest it in another relationship.

These 'four tasks' provide a framework. Remaining flexible, receptive and reactive to the shifting and changing needs and accepting that 'people do not necessarily pass through the stages smoothly; indeed they may go through all the stages in the space of a few minutes' is vital.[25] Change is an important feature of loss and bereavement – change in roles, in relationships, in view of self and in ways of coping.[26] Following the loss of a loved person, the world has changed for ever and nothing can reverse that change. Adjustment to these changes is central to the grieving process whether the person is accepting their loss and forming new relationships or developing a strong internalized representation of their loved one.

ACCOMPANYING THE GRIEVING PERSON

Hearing the story

People who have experienced a loss will need to tell their story and express their feelings to someone who can comprehend the significance. They may be hurt, angry, despairing, puzzled, uncomprehending but they will all need to talk. Only those who are at the stage of incomprehension and disbelief may find difficulty in testing reality by talking to others. Gently encouraging the person to talk about their loss may be helpful in beginning the grieving process.

Solace can be gained by talking about the person with others who knew her/him, framing an enduring biography for the deceased, creating their ongoing presence in the lives of the living. At such times, the role of the listener is that of a helpful 'editor'. Walter[17] suggests that for this reason funeral rights are important. The British reticence in mentioning the dead, for fear of upsetting the person most intimately connected to them, prevents this healing process. He suggest that bereavement is part of the process of each person's autobiography and that bereavement behaviour – grieving and mourning – are connected to the need to make sense of our own stories of who we are and who we have been.

Supporting

People who have experienced a loss may value practical help during the immediate aftermath of that loss. They will inevitably need to take on new roles and encounter new experiences when their resources and energy are low. They will need help to gain information or encouragement when they are struggling to complete new tasks, solve problems and test reality. This is a subtle process and should not be confused with acting *for* or *giving advice* to the person, rather it involves giving support in the process of liberation and empowerment.

Part of the supportive role could involve literally 'being beside' the person while they accomplish a painful healing task. Similarly, support may include being with the person whilst they undertake a healing ritual, for example attending a specially arranged 'service of remembrance' for a child who was stillborn many years previously.

Nursing hope

Following loss, hope may be absent. Life may seem pointless and hopeless: the person's behaviour may reflect these feelings. Loss of hope may also lead to thoughts about suicide. The person may fantasize about the possibility of being 'reunited' and this will inevitably lead them to ruminate about the possibility of killing themselves.[7,27] This can become a chronic state in which they become 'stuck'. Some may be profoundly shocked to experience such thoughts. They may see it as an indication that they are 'going mad' and feel distressed and ashamed of their thoughts.[28] Exploring these fantasies and establishing the level of risk is important. This is a very delicate process, which requires direct enquiry about thoughts which the person may find frightening and shaming, whilst also assuring her/him that such experiences are not unique to them and may be part of the grieving process.

It is important too that hope is 'grounded in reality'.[29] The use of genuineness/congruence can aid this process. Discussion of the 'hard facts' of a situation may need to be in 'bite size chunks' which can be easily digested.[28,29]

Hope may reappear gradually and will need to be fostered within the helping relationship.[27,30,31] In its emerging state, hope may be different from that which existed before the loss. It may be fragile and subject to many reversals during the process of its reconstitution and needs to develop at its own pace. Asking the person specifically what they hope for and what helps them to maintain hope can help them to focus on positive aspects of their life. The use of warmth, acceptance and respect will also foster hope.

Having one's individual worth affirmed is hope-inspiring.[27]

If the person is to regain hope then they must be able to imagine other possibilities for themselves.[29] By supporting the person in learning new roles or gaining new skills, hope will increase.

People who have experienced a loss may find that they experience feelings of guilt when hopefulness returns. They may feel – or others may imply – that there is something shameful in once more experiencing pleasure in life. Asking what the deceased person would have wanted of them in such situations may help to challenge this sense of guilt and give her/him 'permission' to regain hope.

Many people do not wish to 'forget' or 'move on' from the person who is lost to them. Continuing to grieve may effectively retain the dead person's presence in their life when letting go may feel frightening. This may be especially true of older people.[32] Within Western societies, mourners may be given the message that talking of their loss is only permissible for a defined period of time. If they also experience a sense that their loved one is 'still there' because of a sense of presence or other physical experience they may feel confused and alone until they are reassured that there is nothing wrong or abnormal about these experiences. Costello[32] cites an example of an elderly widow who, four months after her husband's death, experienced the bed 'sag' as if her husband was getting into it. When asked how this felt she said 'Oh once I knew it was him I felt fine, in fact, it felt rather nice.'

NORMAL OR UNCOMPLICATED GRIEVING

There appear to be many similarities between the observed processes of coming to terms with the prospect of loss of one's *own* life and the prospect of life without a *loved person* or a *lost dream*. Grief is necessarily a disorganized and painful process. However, 'normal' grieving will inevitably move towards being able to remember the deceased without discomfort or even with equanimity or pleasure. Estimates for the time it takes for an 'uncomplicated' grief to reach resolution vary considerably from months to years.[25]

COMPLICATED GRIEF

Any form of grieving, which does not lead to resolution of the symptoms of grief and the ability of the person to get on with their lives, can be termed to be 'complicated' grief. The person may resolutely inhibit all signs of their grief or may experience a grief which fails to lessen and is unamenable to consolation over a long period of time. Specific circumstances are implicated:

❑ **The nature of the relationship with the deceased.** The loss of a partner or child is recognized as being especially significant although all losses are significant if the bereaved person identifies them to be so. If a relationship was ambivalent or unresolved at the time of death, if the bereaved person was highly dependent upon the deceased or if they viewed her/him as an extension of themselves, this may complicate mourning.

❑ **Where the loss is sudden, unexpected or untimely.** Although all deaths are 'untimely' to those who mourn, with increasing age and infirmity friends and relatives will come to some expectation of loss before it occurs. When the loss is through accident or sudden illness of a previously healthy person, if it is a child who dies, if the prospect of our own happy and fulfilling life is snatched away without warning, then shock will be intense and the mourning process complex. When accidental death has occurred and for some reason there is no body on which to focus grief this too will present special complications.[7]

❑ **Where many bereavements have occurred together or in quick succession.** If accident or illness has claimed several members of a family, the severity and enormity of the loss will be difficult to comprehend and to mourn.

❑ **How the losses occurred.** The dramatic nature of some deaths complicates the nature of the grieving which follows. The suddenness and often unpredictable nature of suicide, homicide or death in war/terrorist attacks may also bring unanswerable questions and strong sense of 'unfinished business'. Guilt and anger, which are common in bereavement, may be experienced particularly strongly by the survivors of suicide. There may also be strong feelings of rejection and stigma or even a sense of relief.[34,35]

❑ **When a loss re-evokes an insufficiently mourned previous loss.** Sometimes grief may be, what others perceive to be, 'out of proportion' to the loss which they have experienced. When this happens it is very important to explore with the person what losses they have experienced previously and the meaning of those losses. On occasion the person may put their own mourning 'on hold' because they are dealing with the grief of another and delay grieving until forced to mourn by new losses.

❑ **Personal vulnerability of the survivor.** This may include having previous experience of mental illness or existing high levels of anxiety or having a personality which is grief-prone, possibly as a reaction to other bereavements or incomplete grieving of a previous loss.[7]

❑ **Where there is no family or social support network.** Personal and social support provide a buffer against grief.

ANTICIPATORY GRIEF

Anticipatory grief is a complicated issue. Forewarning of loss may allow for adjustment to that loss, but the sense of bereavement which may occur over a protracted period of terminal illness or absence may not only lead to a lessening of emotional intensity as the time of loss approaches, but may also lead to premature withdrawal from the dying person.[13,33]

The link between grief and mental illness

Just as mental illness may be associated with many losses, grief may lead to the experience of mental illness. One of the common experiences of grief is the perception of the person that they are 'going mad'.[7] They may experience strange perceptions – 'seeing' the lost person or experiencing their 'presence'. These experiences can be comforting or distressing. As we have already heard, grief can bring suicidal fantasies – feeling that they want to 'be with' the person they have lost or perhaps such a profound feeling of loss, loneliness and misery that they abandon the wish to carry on alone.[27]

It is common for the grieving person to experience extreme anxiety or episodes of panic. This is understandable. The loss may have robbed the person of the sense of certainty about life that we all take for granted, both their own and that of others. The physical experiences which are often experienced in the early stages of grief – sighing, a sense of hollowness in the abdomen, restlessness, the need to swallow, are clearly linked to anxiety. The author C.S. Lewis writing about the death of his wife describes his experience: 'No one ever told me that grief felt so like fear. I am not afraid, but the sensation is like being afraid.'[36]

On occasions the experience of misery and hopelessness, which are part of the process of grief may fail to remit. At these times, it is important not to consider whether a depressive illness is developing.

Where the death or loss has been traumatic – homicide, suicide, or sudden death to which the person has been witness, then there should be careful monitoring for the symptoms of a post traumatic stress disorder. This can be a complicated process as many of the symptoms are also present in 'ordinary' grieving. Maintaining this awareness and carefully monitoring her/his speech and behaviour will allow referral for specific trauma work if this becomes necessary.[37]

Sometimes a bereavement will bring to light a mental illness which has existed for some time but has been masked. There may be several reasons for this. The lost person or object may have been a crucial element in helping the person in managing the symptoms; the stress of loss may disrupt a fragile coping strategy or the experience of grief may open up the possibility of 'legitimately' requesting help with the problem.

CONCLUSION

Bereavement, loss, grief and mourning are part of *all* our lives although how we experience and act on them will be influenced by the culture in which we live. There are many theories and models of grief and grief counselling. Recent theories do not seek to help the bereaved to 'complete' mourning and 'move on'. Instead they promote the possibility that grief may be never ending without being hopeless as the lost object lives on within the mourner. Nurses have a vital role to play in listening to, supporting and nurturing hope when they encounter grief, whether that grief is because of death, shortening of life expectations or the multitude of other losses, which are part of human existence.

REFERENCES

1. Walter T. *On bereavement. The culture of grief.* Buckingham: Open University Press, 1999.
2. Seale C. *Constructing death. The sociology of dying and bereavement.* Cambridge: Cambridge University Press, 1998.
3. Nettleton S. Governing the risky self: how to become healthy, wealthy and wise. In: Petersen A, Bunton R (eds). *Foucault. Health and medicine.* London: Routledge, 1997: 207–23.
4. Lupton D. *The imperative of health. Public health and the regulated body.* London: Sage, 1995.
5. Walter T, Littlewood J, Pickering M. Death in the news – the public invigilation of private emotion. In: Dickenson D, Johnson M, Samson Katz J. (eds). *Death, dying and bereavement*, 2nd edn. London: Open University/Sage, 2000: 14–27
6. Bowlby J. *Loss, sadness and depression. Attachment and loss*, Vol. 3. London: Penguin, 1980.

7. Parkes CM. *Bereavement. Studies of grief in adult life*, 3rd edn. Harmondsworth: Penguin, 1996.
8. Erikson EH. *Childhood and society*, revised edn. Harmondsworth: Penguin, 1950.
9. Reimers E. Bereavement – a social phenomenon? *European Journal of Palliative Care* 2001; 8(6): 242–4.
10. Clark D. Death in Staithes. In: Dickenson D, Johnson M (eds). *Death, dying and bereavement.* London: Sage, 2000: 4–11.
11. Firth S. Cross-cultural perspectives on bereavement. In: Dickenson D, Johnson M (eds). *Death, dying and bereavement.* London: Sage, 2000: 254–62.
12. O'Gorman S. Death and dying in contemporary society: an evaluation of current attitudes and the rituals associated with death and dying and their relevance to recent understandings of health and healing. *Journal of Advanced Nursing* 1998; 27(6): 1127–35.
13. Lindemann E. Symptomatology and management of acute grief. *American Journal of Psychiatry* 1944; 101: 141–8.
14. Caplan G. *An approach to community mental health.* London: Tavistock, 1964.
15. Kübler Ross E. *On death and dying.* London: Routledge, 1970.
16. Stroebe W, Stroebe MS. *Bereavement and health. The psychological and physical consequences of partner loss.* Cambridge: Cambridge University Press, 1987.
17. Walter T. A new model of grief: bereavement and biography. *Mortality* 1996; 1(1): 7–25.
18. Silvermann PR, Klass D. What's the problem? In: Klass D, Silverman PR, Nickman SL (eds). *Continuing bonds. New understandings of grief.* London: Taylor and Francis, 1996: 3–27.
19. Martocchio BC. Grief and bereavement: healing through hurt. *Nursing Clinics of North America* 1985; 20: 327–41.
20. Rogers C. *Client Centred Therapy.* Boston: Houghton Mifflin, 1965.
21. Means D, Thorne B. *Person-centred counselling in action.* London: Sage, 1988.
22. Barker P, Kerr B. *The process of psychotherapy. A journey of discovery.* Oxford: Butterworth Heinemann, 2001.
23. Rogers CR. *A way of being.* Boston: Houghton Mifflin, 1980.
24. Worden JW. *Grief counselling and grief therapy.* London: Tavistock Publications, 1983.
25. Tschudin V. *Counselling skills for nurses*, 4th edn. London: Baillière Tindall, 1995.
26. Duke S. An exploration of anticipatory grief: the lived experience of people during their spouses' terminal illness and bereavement. *Journal of Advanced Nursing* 1998; 28(4): 829–39.
27. Cutcliffe J. Hope, counselling and complicated bereavement reactions. *Journal of Advanced Nursing* 1998; 28(4): 754–61.

28. Parkes CM. Coping with loss: consequences and implications for care. *International Journal of Palliative Nursing* 1999; **5**(5): 250–54.

29. Hegarty M. The dynamic of hope: hoping in the face of death. *Progress in Palliative Care* 2001: **9**(2): 42–6.

30. Snyder CR. To hope, to lose, and to hope again. *Journal of Personal and Interpersonal Loss* 1996; **1**: 1–16.

31. Gamlin R, Kinghorn S. Using hope to cope with loss and grief. *Nursing Standard* 1995; **9**(48): 33–5.

32. Costello J. Grief and older people: the making and breaking of emotional bonds following partner loss in later life. *Journal of Advanced Nursing* 2000; **32**(6): 1374–82.

33. Costello J. Anticipatory grief: coping with the impending death of a partner. *International Journal of Palliative Nursing* 1999; **5**(5): 223–31.

34. Wertheimer A. *A special scar. The experiences of people bereaved by suicide*. London: Routledge, 1991.

35. Parkes CM. After a terrorist attack. Supporting the bereaved families. *Bereavement Care* 2001; **20**(3): 35–6.

36. Lewis CS. *A grief observed*. London: Faber, 1961.

37. Turnbull G, Gibson M. The aftermath of traumatic incidents. *Bereavement Care* 2001; **20**(1): 3–5.

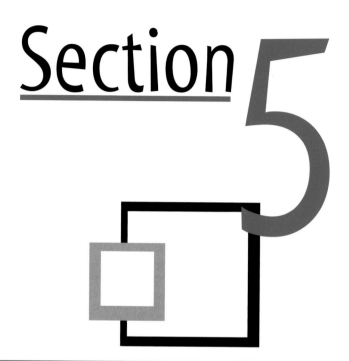

Section 5

Specific needs for nursing

Preface to Section 5

Although ill health can have implications for the family or wider society, it is always, first and foremost, a personal crisis – a personal tragedy.

As the field is increasingly influenced by research and socioeconomic models of service provision, we risk losing sight of the *person* who is the focal point of practice.

In this section, we profile some of the people who present with very different needs for nursing. The psychiastric catalogue contains an increasingly wide range of *disorders, patient types, conditions* and *cases*. We have chosen here some examples of the kind of problems of living, which typically present nurses with most difficulty, or which are viewed as particularly problematic by society at large. We have asked the authors to hold the *person* in sharp focus, using the features of the person's condition or diagnosis as a supporting context, rather than the main item on the caring agenda.

We begin with the person who experiences anxiety – a problem that is understood by everyone, including nurses themselves, and which probably forms a part of many of the other problems of living in the psychiatric canon.

We end with a consideration of the person with dementia, arguably the problem of living most feared in our highly rational society, and which might serve as an icon for much of the anxiety and denial still found in society, when the topic of mental health surfaces.

Chapter 26

THE PERSON WHO EXPERIENCES ANXIETY

Eimear Muir-Cochrane*

... the crushing weight that pressed on my chest and the rapidly beating heart that frequently made me light headed and blanche. Most disabling were the battles for breath that could last for several hours with me eventually locked in some kind of coma-like state where I was barely aware of what was going on around me.[1]

INTRODUCTION

Anxiety is one of the most common treatable mental disorders. Effective treatments include cognitive-behavioural therapy, relaxation techniques and occasionally medication to control muscle tension. Anxiety disorders range from feelings of uneasiness most of the time to immobilizing bouts of terror. Here we shall discuss the most common anxiety disorders: generalized anxiety, phobias, obsessive-compulsive disorder and post-traumatic stress. It is vital that nurses reflect upon their own experience of events that invoke anxiety and learn how to manage these feelings usefully, to be of use to those in their care. Anxiety can be transferred interpersonally. For example, you arrive ready for an examination and find your fellow students extremely anxious. Interestingly,

although you felt quite calm, now you find your anxiety levels increasing dramatically. Today, enough is known about anxiety to develop early intervention and prevention programmes. To that end, this chapter adopts a self-development approach so that nurses can develop their own anxiety management skills, and help patients facilitate their own anxiety management. Remember, if people in your care recognize your anxiety, this will elevate their own.

LEARNING TO RELAX

It seems appropriate to approach the management of anxiety disorders by reflecting on our own anxiety and tension. If, nurses can utilize basic self-relaxation techniques it is likely that they will be more effective in helping people in their care to recognize tension and learn to relax and manage uncomfortable feelings and symptoms that interfere with their normal functioning.[2] Let us begin by thinking about a time when you have felt extremely tense. Make some notes about your thoughts, feelings and sensations at the time. Then think about a time when you were extremely relaxed

---

*Eimear is an academic at the University of South Australia, with current responsibilities for the leadership and management of higher degree students and the program direction of postgraduate mental health nursing courses. Eimear is also the Chair of the University Ethics Committee satisfying her need to promote the ethical conduct of research involving people. Eimear's research interests include the use of seclusion, community mental health and the mental health needs of homeless young people.

and make notes accordingly. What do you notice that is different?

Relaxation training

Relaxation training involves the deliberate letting go of tension, whether *physical* (for example, muscle tension or stomach cramps) or *psychological* (for example, excessive worrying). When someone relaxes, the nerves in the muscles send messages to the brain that are distinctly different to those sent when anxious, tense or stressed. These different signals incur a general feeling of calmness in the person.[3]

Muscle relaxation has an effect on the nervous system, which manifests in physical and psychological ways and is extremely useful in helping deal with feelings and experiences that disrupt everyday living. Relaxation training can help people who have been under stress for long periods of time, and who may have forgotten what it is like to relax and let go of their tension. Daily practice can help restore physical and psychological balance (equilibrium) and reduce tense feelings that include being jumpy, irritable and nervy, as well as physical manifestations of tension (such as stomach complaints, diarrhoea or constipation, and backache). Learning to relax can enable the control of uncomfortable levels of anxiety and tension in stressful situations.

To help people in your care learn to relax it is vital that you examine and assess your own tension and anxiety (see Table 26.1). Tension is *necessary*, physically, to help us move about or to exercise vigorously, and psychologically, to keep us alert to respond to a situation such as a job interview. However a lot of the tension we feel is *unnecessary* and this can be determined by reflecting on the relationship between the level of tension and the activity involved, when the tension is not serving a useful function and where the level of tension remains high after the alerting situation has passed.[4]

TABLE 26.1 Assess your stress

Use the following questions to assess your own stress levels:

- Where do I feel tension? (e.g. in my chest, back jaw etc).
- What are the characteristics of the tension? (e.g. fatigued muscles, soreness).
- Which kinds of things lead to an increase in tension? (e.g. anger, loneliness, impatience, boredom).
- What external factors increase your tension? (e.g. loud noises, having to wait to be served, traffic, your relationships).

TABLE 26.2 Relaxation guide

First of all clear your mind of any worrying thoughts. Let your mind be calm.

Practise breathing in – holding your breath for a few seconds – and breathing out again. Try and control your breathing until it flows smoothly. Imagine that the tension in your body is flowing down and outwards, like water, every time you breathe out.

Now it is time to relax your body, starting with your hands. For each muscle group, tense the muscles for ten seconds, then let go and relax.

Hands: curl your hands into fist and relax.
Arms: tense the muscles in your arms and relax. Be aware of your biceps and the difference between tensing and relaxing them.
Shoulders and neck: shrug your shoulders up to your ears, hold for ten seconds and relax.
Face: raise your eyebrows, hold and relax. Scrunch up your eyes, hold and relax.
Jaw: clench your teeth (not too tightly) hold and relax.
Chest: breathe in deeply – hold and relax.
Back: lean your head and back forward – hold and then relax.
Bottom: tighten your buttock muscles and then relax.
Legs: Push your feet firmly on the floor – hold and then relax. Lift your toes off the ground towards your shins and relax.
Feet: gently curl your toes up – hold and then relax.
Stay sitting quietly for a few minutes enjoying the sensation of being relaxed. Take some slow deep breaths, pay attention to your breathing. Try and practise every day; this will help your body to relearn how to relax and minimize tension building up.

Progressive muscle relaxation

Like most things, relaxation training takes practice to be really effective. Encourage patients to persevere when they say 'I'm too tense to relax' or 'this is not for me, it's not doing me any good' (see Table 26.2).

There are two core components to relaxation training: *recognizing tension* and *relaxing*. Progressive muscle relaxation training involves tensing and relaxing muscles in a repetitious fashion, moving from the hands, to the shoulders, neck and head, and then down through the stomach, and back to the buttocks, legs and feet – tensing and relaxing alternately for about ten seconds each time, usually over a 20–30 minute time period. The best position is sitting comfortably with back straight, feet flat on the floor. It is generally advised not to lie down as there is a good chance of falling asleep. So, sitting upright in a quiet warm place is a good option.

Some people find other ways to achieve the same relaxation effect through exercise, meditation, yoga or tai chi. All these provide an opportunity for self-reflection and letting go of the unnecessary stress we all carry, in varying degrees. If as nurses we can master the art of relaxation, we can model a relaxed and open demeanour to those around us. This, in turn will increase the opportunity to build rapport and trust with our patients to explore how they view their concerns in a practical way and to reduce the amount of unnecessary and uncomfortable anxiety in daily life.

THE NATURE OF ANXIETY

The experience of anxiety is a normal part of the human condition. Everyone experiences anxiety in varying degrees! Anxiety is usually a transitory response to threat or danger. Most people experience a knot in the stomach over mounting bills or just before a job interview at some point in their lives. Certain experiences and memories provoke anxious feelings in everyone, spurring us on, for example, to finish the essay that is due tomorrow. Nervousness in anticipation of an event is normal, yet the experience of anxiety can lead individuals to question the amount of choice and emotional control they have in their lives.[4] If people become preoccupied with unwarranted worries for longer than a short period of time or the feelings cause the person to avoid everyday activities, they may be described as suffering from an anxiety disorder. Anxiety disorders can have an underlying biological cause (e.g. thyrotoxicosis) and frequently run in families. Anxiety is also one of the most treatable mental disorders. It is characterized by a feeling of dread or uncomfortable anticipation with physical, psychological behavioural and cognitive features. Nurses are likely to come across people in their care exhibiting a variety of anxious responses to their situation. In general hospitals, many patients will be anxious about their medical condition, impending surgery or the experience of hospitalization itself. In mental health settings most people receiving care will demonstrate some anxiety with a smaller number being so severely affected that they are unable to function normally in relation to work, family responsibilities, and interpersonal relationships.[5] With such people, specific interventions, including medications are usually required.

Prevalence of anxiety

Between 8% and 12% of the population experience a pervasive level of anxiety that impedes their daily lives with 2–4% of the population experiencing an anxiety disorder. Anxiety is the most prevalent single psychiatric disorder of the modern era. People with anxiety disorders experienced 2.7 million 'days out of role' when they were unable to function fully as a result of a disorder.[6] Loss of productivity from the paid and unpaid workforce has profound implications for the fiscal and social capital of nations. Research in the USA indicates that three of the five most productive things to invest in to reduce lost work productivity are migraine, anxiety and depression.[7] Women were more likely than men to have experienced anxiety disorders (12% compared with 7%). For women, the most common anxiety disorder is post-traumatic stress disorder (4.2% of the 12% of diagnosable women with an anxiety disorder) and the least common being obsessive-compulsive disorder at 0.4%. For the 7% of men diagnosed with anxiety disorders, the most common anxiety disorders are social phobia and generalized anxiety disorders at 2.4%, and the least common being obsessive compulsive disorder at 0.3%.[8] This Australian data is comparable with the incidence of anxiety throughout the Western world.

Aetiology and contemporary treatments

Several theories purport to explain anxiety disorders. The biological view holds that anxiety disorders may have a genetic element, particularly obsessive-compulsive disorder, and are associated with alterations in cerebral serotonin. As with other psychiatric conditions, receptor sites in the brain have now been located for the action of benzodiazepines (anti-anxiety medication), in the medial occipital cortex, supporting the usefulness of these drugs in the reduction of symptoms of anxiety. Learning theory supports the concept that anxiety is a conditioned response to specific environmental stimuli and has a biological survival value. The standard 'flight or fight' response – and the associated increase in heart rate and alertness – prepare the person for danger. Over time, how a person acts in response to a stressful event is often the result of learning. If too many stressors occur in a short time period, the person may experience acute anxiety and exhibit maladaptive behaviour. An example of maladaptive behaviour may be an increase in alcohol consumption after the loss of a loved one through death or separation. Some theorists believe that social and cultural factors will determine how personality develops and how a person responds to stress. For example a person with a low self-image is more likely to have problems coping with an unexpected problem in their daily life than someone with a very positive self-image. Cognitive-behavioural theory embraces a range of learning theories that view the way we feel, think and behave as inextricably linked. Thus a person with a poor self-image may have a disagreement with someone and conclude – 'that person does not like me', feeling anxious and sweaty and deciding to avoid social situations in future. Cognitive behaviour therapy (CBT) is a relatively short-term treatment plan (6–8 weeks) which aims to teach a person how to relax, recognize and cope with their anxious thoughts and feelings. CBT aims to help people become aware of their thinking style, replacing or reframing these with more positive, ways of thinking which can lead to an increase in self-confidence, problem-solving ability, and reduced associated anxiety.[9] The assumption behind CBT is that dysfunctional behaviours are the presumed underlying problem. CBT applies well-established learning principles to eliminate the unwanted behaviour and replace it with more constructive ways of thinking, feeling and acting. The major focus in CBT is to help the person examine and understand the world (their cognitions) and to experiment with new ways of responding (their behaviour). In this way the client can be helped to be future focused and to behave more adaptively.

Much has been learned in the past two decades about the treatment of anxiety disorders. Recent developments in neuro-imaging techniques have led to better understandings of the biology of obsessive-compulsive disorder (OCD) and the brain circuits that may be involved in the production of symptoms. The most effective treatment approach appears to be CBT,[10] consisting of exposure and response prevention and specific medications. Pharmacotherapy for anxiety is recommended usually in combination with CBT in the following circumstances:

❑ where there is co-morbidity such as depression;
❑ when CBT is unsuccessful;
❑ when symptoms are severely disabling.

Recent research has demonstrated a shift in the type of medications being prescribed for the treatment of generalized anxiety disorder (GAD) from exclusive benzodiazepine treatment to a combination of benzodiazepine treatment and antidepressant treatment. In the future more invasive and controversial techniques such as neurosurgical and neurostimulation approaches may hold some promise.

SYMPTOMS OF ANXIETY

Use the material in Table 26.3 to explore the various dimensions of anxiety.

In children, several other symptoms may be observable or reported by their parents who may not recognize these behaviours as anxiety-related. Nurses are frequently in contact with adults and children who are either receiving care or who are family members of the sick person. Children often demonstrate anxiety symptoms as a response to the stress of what is happening around them. Symptoms include irritability, marked self-consciousness, over concern about the future and past events, a constant need for reassurance, unrealistic and excessive worry and distress on separation from parents. Children and adolescents with pervading anxiety require expert assistance through specialist intervention.

TABLE 26.3 Physiological (physical) symptoms of anxiety

Shortness of breath
Dizziness
Choking sensation
Palpitations
Trembling
Sweating
Dry mouth
Decreased appetite
Nausea
Diarrhoea
Elevated blood pressure

> Refer to the notes you made about being tense and anxious. Allocate your thoughts, feelings and sensations to the categories here.

Affective (mood)
Fear
Terror
Dread
Sense of impending doom
Apprehension

Behavioural
Exaggerated startle reflex
Motor tension (foot tapping, restlessness)
Irritability
Nail biting
Altered sleep pattern (too much too little difficulty going to sleep or waking up)

Relief behaviours

Hildegard Peplau[11] identified four relief behaviours commonly occurring as an uncomfortable reaction to the experience of anxiety. These are learned over time and are the physical manifestation of unconscious mechanisms and help the person cope with their feelings. Some of these behaviours prevent us from learning how to manage our emotions usefully and result in a reduced ability to learn new ways of coping. A constructive pattern of relief behaviour such as *realistic problem solving* refers to the individual converting anxiety into useful energies, such as exercising to reduce tension and anxiety, resulting in the development of useful coping skills. The following three relief behaviours are not constructive and once learned are often difficult to unlearn.

❑ **Acting out** refers to impulsive behaviours such as shouting or self-harming in which the person displaces emotions from one situation to another. Acting out often distresses people witnessing the behaviour but the individual may not be as distressed or upset.
❑ **Somatizing** refers to the physical manifestation of anxiety into a condition or sensation such as parasthesia or palpitations.

❑ **Withdrawal** involves removing oneself from situations that are perceived to be threatening.[4]

It is highly likely that these relief behaviours will be manifest when people are under duress. Nurses need to be aware of their function to respond calmly and with compassion.

THE EXPERIENCE OF ANXIETY

At a low to moderate level of anxiety we experience a narrowing of perception. With increased muscle tension (jitters), our speech rate increases, with mixed feelings of challenge, confidence, optimism and fear. At a physiological level anxiety activates the sympathetic nervous system with an increase in blood pressure heart rate and respiration, pupillary dilation and peripheral vascular constriction. Moderate levels of anxiety serve to improve performance, and even high levels of anxiety are often consistent with the demands of the situation. However, high anxiety can disable people to the extent that they find it difficult to perform every-day activities. It is normal to experience anxious thoughts, but it is the extent to which these thoughts render the individual able to carry out their normal activities that determines their disabling effect. Anxious thinking is often distorted thinking: anticipating that things are not going to turn out well and that you won't be able to cope (Table 26.4). This can increase anxiety and lead to depression if it persists. For example if you see someone you know in the supermarket but they do not acknowledge you, an anxious thought may be 'That person does not like me' but a more realistic thought may be 'Oh she has not seen me' or 'She may be preoccupied'. CBT aims to help people understand their negative self talk and to develop more positive and realistic patterns.

ANXIETY DISORDERS

Anxiety can be disabling. The dysfunctional aspects are marked by three major components, behavioural avoidance, catastrophic cognition and autonomic hyper arousal.[14] None of these components differentiates between normal and pathological anxiety. The only criterion is the level of interference in personal, occupational or social functioning. It is also incorrect to say that *abnormal anxiety* is just a matter of being too anxious at a time when others are not. People with anxiety

---

🗔 **TABLE 26.4 Activity**

Think of times when you have been anxious, listing the anxious thoughts you had then. Beside each 'anxious thought' write an 'alternative' thought that might reduce the feeling of anxiety.

---

disorders have recurring irrational and specific fears, they recognize as unrealistic and intrusive.

People suffering from a generalized anxiety disorder experience chronic exaggerated worry and tension that is more intense than the reality of the situation. A diagnosis is made if the person has spent at least six months worrying excessively about everyday problems.

Generalized anxiety disorder

An elderly woman is admitted after her daughter became increasingly concerned about her deteriorating physical activity and social isolation. The patient was bereaved nine months ago. Since then she has become disinterested in activities she previously enjoyed. She says that she has gripping chest pains, often feels as if she cannot catch her breath and that her heart is pounding so loudly that other people can hear it. She is observed wringing her hands constantly and making multiple visits to the toilet.

Panic disorder is characterized by a white-knuckled, heart-pounding terror that strikes with the force of a lightning bolt, without warning. Some people feel like they are going mad, devoured by fear, or dying of a heart attack. Because they cannot predict these attacks, many experience persistent worry that another could overcome them at any time. Most panic attacks last only a few minutes but could last up to an hour in rare cases. With appropriate help between 70% and 90% of this group are helped within 6–8 weeks. CBT, combined with medication – such as high potency anti-anxiety drugs (e.g. alprazolam) and several classes of anti-depressants, such as paroxetine and the older tricyclics and monoamine oxidase inhibitors (MAO inhibitors) are considered 'gold' standards.[10] Sometimes a combination of therapy and medication is the most effective approach to helping people manage their symptoms.

Panic disorder

A 20-year-old student is admitted with a 6-month history of panic attacks. She has become unable to attend university regularly due to overwhelming and disabling feelings of choking, vomiting and difficulty in breathing. She failed her first year of study after she experienced 'blocks' during examinations. Since then her anxiety has worsened to the extent that she is extremely uncomfortable in public places, has difficulty swallowing and thinks she is losing her mind.

Phobias are the most common form of anxiety disorder affecting between 5% and 12% of the adult population worldwide. Phobias occur in specific forms. A specific phobia is an unfounded fear of a particular object or situation, such as being afraid of dogs yet loving to ride horses, or avoiding flying on aeroplanes, but being able to drive on busy highways. There is virtually an unlimited number of objects or situations that a person can be afraid of. Commonly people have phobias of snakes, spiders, open and/or closed spaces, dirt, blood-injuries and needles. Many of the physical symptoms that accompany panic attacks such as sweating, racing heart and trembling also occur with phobias. Formal diagnosis is made when people experience extreme anxiety when exposed to a given situation or object, recognize that the fear is excessive or unreasonable, but are unable to change the feeling, with the result that normal routines, relationships and social activities are significantly disrupted. CBT has the best track record for helping people overcome phobic disorders. The goals of this therapy are to desensitize the person to feared situations and to teach the person to relax, recognize and cope with anxious thoughts and feelings. Anti-anxiety agents or anti-depressants may be also used to minimize symptoms in the short term. There are differing views about the combination of medication and CBT. Some would use a combination but others advocate that the symptoms need to be treated, not suppressed by drugs.

Obsessive-compulsive disorder (OCD) affects almost 3% of the world's population and is a major worldwide health problem. There are two main clinical features to this condition. An obsession is a persistent intrusive and unwanted thought or emotion that the person cannot ignore. A compulsion is a behavioural manifestation of the obsessive thought, resulting in the performance of a repetitious, uncontrollable but seemingly purposeful act. For example a person may have obsessive thoughts about cleanliness and the associated compulsive behaviour of repetitive handwashing, perhaps to the point of having excoriated skin on the hands from excessive washing. The compulsion becomes disabling when the person cannot carry on their normal daily activities due to preoccupation with obsessive thoughts and compulsive acts.

Obsessive–compulsive disorder

A married man, Peter, 35 years old with two children under five is admitted with OCD. Two years ago he developed the obsessive thought that the chemical used to treat his roof was poisoning his children. He began washing his hands and clothes excessively to the extent that he was in danger of losing his job because of the time it took to repeatedly carry out these cleansing rituals. On admission, he was noted to be of low mood with an anxious presentation. He told the nurses that he was on the verge of going mad and was worried his wife would leave him. David was offered a mild anti-depressant and a programme of CBT that involved exposing him gradually (systematic desentization) to stimuli that triggered the anxiety, at the same time helping him to voluntarily refrain from handwashing.

It has only recently been acknowledged that anyone who has experienced a traumatic event may experience *post-traumatic stress disorder* (PTSD), especially if the event was life-threatening. In the past, PTSD most commonly referred to victims of war who had experienced heavy combat. Common PTSD experiences include kidnapping, airplane crashes or other serious crashes, rape, natural disasters and war. If the person is traumatized seriously by the event the resulting psychological damage causes a significant impairment in the ability to maintain previous functioning – such as working or maintaining relationships. Symptoms can range from constantly reliving the event to a general emotional numbing. Persistent anxiety, exaggerated startle reflex, difficulty concentrating, nightmares, and insomnia are common. Typically people with PTSD avoid situations that remind them of a situation as it triggers intense emotion and distress. For example a person trapped on a road during a flood may deliberately avoid driving on that section of the highway.

Research in this area has increased in recent decades as individuals have developed PTSD after being involved in natural disasters such as bushfires in Australia and floods in Europe. Depression is often experienced in PTSD as is the use of prescription and non-prescription drugs and alcohol to dull emotional pain. Psychotherapy, CBT, medication such as anti-depressants and anxiolytics, support from family and friends and relaxation techniques form the basis of treatment programmes with these patients.

NURSING STRATEGIES

Much of the work of nurses involved in the care of people with disabling levels of anxiety involve being with the patient, offering time for the patient to, as Barker[12] calls it 'name their distress' i.e. what meaning the patient places on their experience. The loss of control patients feel due to their disabling anxiety is often an extremely important component of their distress, and therefore gaining control is a common goal. To that end the role of the nurse and structured programmes of therapy such as CBT involves creating a situation in which the patient feels able to exercise choice about their future and how they think and feel about it. The relationship the nurse has with an anxious patient is extremely important if any interaction is to be meaningful. Carl Rogers[13] describes warmth, genuineness, empathy and unconditional positive regard as core dimensions of the nurse–patient relationship. If a nurse does not present a genuine demeanour or exhibits anxiety towards the patient, it is more difficult to be helpful. Nursing strategies can best be related to the level of anxiety a person is experiencing (mild, moderate or severe), rather than the diagnosis of the disorder itself.

TABLE 26.5 Nursing interventions during an episode of panic

- Stay with the person and encourage them to sit down.
- Take some deep breaths yourself and then begin to speak to the person in short sentences.
- Reassure the person that this episode will pass.
- Provide external control by being firm but caring.
- Encourage the person to breathe in and out slowly into a paper bag to reduce hyperventilation.
- Maintain a safe and quiet environment to reduce external stimuli.

The checklist in Table 26.5 illustrates some simple strategies that might be employed if the person is in a state of high anxiety or panic. These emphasize the need to remain with the patient and for the nurse to present a calm demeanour.

Working with anxious patients requires an initial assessment phase to gain a holistic picture of the person's situation and their potential and readiness to make positive changes. Gentle discussion of how the person makes sense of being in hospital or coming to community health services for assistance will provide useful contextual information. Asking 'what brought you here today' can

TABLE 26.6 The value of 'Being with'

Reassure the person that their anxiety will pass. Accept the person without judgement. Be available so that the person can approach you when the need arises.

- Listen attentively to what they are expressing and encourage such ventilation. Answer queries honestly and briefly.
- Meet with the person at the beginning of the day to assist with planning daily activities that are diversional as well as part of the treatment programme.
- Set daily and weekly goals that are agreed by both nurse and patient. Encourage the person to identify what the goals are to be.

TABLE 26.7 Educative interventions

- Relaxation methods: for example controlled deep breathing and relaxation tapes. Group and individual relaxation sessions after visiting time on the ward can be well timed as many patients find this to be a vulnerable time.
- Encourage the use of a reflective journal on a daily basis to share thoughts and feelings.
- Identify the patient's strengths and useful coping strategies and support persons.
- Conduct group and individual sessions about the range of normal physiological response to anxiety and how to identify warning signs of increasing stress.

allow the patient to begin to ventilate and make sense of what is happening for them. From this beginning point the nurse can begin to explore with the patient their coping resources by gentle inquiry into their perceptions of their social supports, economic circumstances, health status, cultural and spiritual beliefs. Particular attention also needs to be paid to the person's interpersonal resources, social skills, positive relationships with family and friends and what Stuart[14] calls intrapsychic resources including positive motivation, drive, and personal and professional ambitions, value systems and self-esteem. The way that people have coped with stress in the past is also a good indicator of their coping mechanisms. As has been previously discussed, people using relief behaviours over time generally find that they are not useful in adapting to expected or unexpected change and result in the person becoming cut off emotionally and often socially isolated. Effective coping skills include tackling the problem in a useful manner by seeking help for example. Stuart[14] also identifies cognitive coping mechanisms of searching for meaning, problem-solving and evaluating how realistic personal expectations may be and readjusting some goals.

For each of the clinical cases cited, brainstorm nursing interventions that can assist these individuals while they undergo treatment. Compare your list with the principles listed in Tables 26.6 and 26.7.

PROBLEMS AND SOLUTIONS

It is not uncommon for people receiving treatment to develop a lowered mood, which prevents them from being able to undertake or complete aspects of their treatment, such as relaxation or CBT activities. The role of the nurse is vital in completing regular holistic assessments to recognize early warning signs of depression. If the person is depressed treatment without medication is more difficult.

Patients with obsessive-compulsive disorders may initially find it very difficult to complete the suggested tasks and to practise relaxation methods they have been encouraged to use. They may complain of being too tense or develop further anxiety about the prospect of changing 'useless' behaviours, such as repetitive counting, checking and handwashing. If the person is admitted to hospital it is not unusual for their compulsions to lessen dramatically in the first few days of hospitalization. However once they have familiarized themselves to their new surroundings the problematic behaviour re-emerges. Further, once the effects of treatment are manifest in a reduction in compulsive acts, different compulsions may emerge as the person's defence against anxiety. Understanding and support are vital to help patients deal with these eventualities.

Being relaxed and having an open and compassionate demeanour are skills that have to be learned over time, and which may not come easily, particularly for nurses who are naturally anxious. Witnessing relief behaviours – such as acting out – can be very stressful and clinical supervision and opportunities to debrief, beyond the immediacy of the event, are important support strategies in the workplace. Often individuals experience more stress some time after experiencing some form of critical incident. Expressing personal judgement about a patient's problems is another potential sign that a nurse is under stress and could benefit from clinical supervision or mentoring. It is also common for health care staff, particularly nurses, to avoid people who are highly anxious. Recognizing the potential for such avoidance and seeking the support of more experienced staff in working through such feelings, can facilitate and enhance personal and professional growth.

SUMMARY

Gaining a personal and professional awareness of stress and anxiety is paramount when caring for people with anxiety disorders. Today, various interventions are helpful in the management of disabling anxiety. Being with anxious patients requires compassion and self-awareness, and understanding of the effect anxiety has on people's lives. Using different strategies nurses, in a variety of health care settings, can help people take control of their problems related to the experience of anxiety and manage them successfully.

REFERENCES

1. Barker P, Kerr B. *The process of psychotherapy: a journey of discovery*. Oxford: Butterworth Heinemann, 2001.
2. Robinson L. The journey threatened by stress and anxiety disorders. In: Carson B, Arnold E (eds). *Mental health nursing: the nurse–patient journey*. Philadelphia: W B Saunders, 1996.
3. Hunt CJ, Andrews, Sumich HJ. *The management of mental disorders, Volume 4. Handbook for the anxiety, stress-related and somatoform disorders*. Glebe: WHO Fast Books in Print, 1997.
4. Horsfall J. Mainstream approaches to mental health and illness. An emphasis on individuals and a de-emphasis of inequalities. *Health* 1998; **2**(2): 217–31.
5. Horsfall J, Stuhmiller C, Champ S. *Interpersonal nursing for mental health*. Sydney: Maclennan and Petty, 2000.
6. *The Mental Health of Australians*. Canberra: Commonwealth Department of Health and Aged Care, Mental Health Branch, 1999.
7. Berndt E, Finkelstein S, Greenberg P, Keith A, Bailit H. *Illness and productivity: objective workplace evidence*. WP # 42–97, Sloan School of Management. Massachusetts: Massachusetts Institute of Technology Cambridge, 1997.
8. Australian Bureau of Statistics. *Mental health and wellbeing profile of adults in Australia*. Canberra: AGPS, 1999.
9. *Beating the blues. An interactive program for people experiencing depression and anxiety*. The Maudsley Page: Mental Health, 2000. www.iop.kcl.ac.uk/main/MHealth/BTB
10. Taylor D, McConnell D, McConnell H, Kerwin R. The South London and Maudsley NHS Trust Prescribing Guidelines, 6th edn. London: Dunitz, 2001.
11. Peplau H. Interpersonal theory in nursing practice. In: O'Toole A, Welt S (eds). *Selected works of Hildegarde Peplau*. New York: Springer, 1989.
12. Barker P. *The philosophy and practice of psychiatric nursing*. London: Churchill Livingstone, London, 1999.
13. Rogers C. *Client-centred therapy*. Boston: Houghton and Mifflin, 1965.
14. Stuart G. Anxiety responses and anxiety disorders. In: Stuart G, Laraia M (eds). *Stuart and Sundeen's principles and practices of psychiatric nursing*, 6th edn. St Louis, MO: Mosby, 1998.

Chapter 27

THE PERSON WHO EXPERIENCES DEPRESSION

Ian Beech*

Depression is awful beyond words or sounds or images; I would not want to go through an extended one again. It bleeds relationships through suspicion, lack of confidence and self-respect, the inability to enjoy life, to walk or talk or think normally, the exhaustion, the night terrors, the day terrors. There is nothing good to be said about it except that it gives you an experience of how it must be to be old, to be old and sick, to be dying; to be slow of mind; to be lacking in grace, polish, and co-ordination; to be ugly; to have no belief in the possibilities of life, the pleasures of sex, the exquisiteness of music, or the ability to make yourself and others laugh.[1]

INTRODUCTION

This quote from Kay Redfield Jamison's book *'The Unquiet Mind'* gives us some idea of what the world is like for someone experiencing depression. This chapter will consider what medicine means when it talks about depression. We shall discuss diagnostic criteria, but it should be borne in mind that it is not the nurse's primary remit to diagnose depression. Neither is it the nurse's role to prescribe anti-depressant medication. These are both primarily medical roles. The nursing role is about 'being with' someone who feels great guilt, shame, hopelessness and worthlessness. It is often about being with that person for much longer than any other professional. At the same time it is not the nurse's role to be the neighbour over the fence or the friend in the pub. People experiencing depression expect nurses to provide something more than a sympathetic shoulder to cry on or an exhortation to 'pull yourself together'.

This chapter is not about how to provide psychotherapy to people experiencing depression. Although I will draw upon some aspects of different psychotherapies (e.g. cognitive therapy[2] and logotherapy[3]), the nursing approach suggested here will not sit exclusively within one theoretical approach. This is for a number of reasons.

❑ The first is that 'therapy' traditionally and culturally (but not of necessity) takes place in a one-hour session under structured conditions. People live their lives 168 hours per week.[4] Nurses working with people experiencing depression come into contact with them (depending on the clinical context) most if not much of those 168 hours, often in unstructured situations and often when emotions are raw. So nurses are primarily doing nursing, not psychotherapy.

❑ Second, in the same way that physical explanations of depression can suggest that the person is, some-

*Ian Beech is a Senior Lecturer in Mental Health Nursing at the University of Glamorgan in South Wales. He works closely with a local NHS trust in working with people experiencing depression and in implementing the Tidal Model. In his spare time he is learning the tenor banjo and vainly trying to gain proficiency in the Tibetan yoga known as sKum-nyé.

how, 'faulty' and needs fixing, so too can many psychotherapeutic approaches.[5]

❑ Third, to work exclusively using a single approach might be appropriate for someone with many years of experience of that particular therapy. However, many readers will be less experienced, and it would be inappropriate to set too daunting a task.

❑ Fourth, when nurses think in terms of a single linear explanation for problems of living, they risk forgetting many other possibly helpful approaches, since such alternatives are not part of the model they learned in whichever therapy class they attended.

When nurses start to work with people experiencing depression there are a number of issues, which can leave them floundering:

❑ 'What if I make things worse?'
❑ 'What if I say something that causes someone to kill him/herself?'
❑ 'What do I say?'

All such questions arise when nurses first encounter depression. Some may adopt the attitude that depression is a physical condition of the brain that can be treated physically and, so as long as nurses prevent the person from committing suicide, the physical treatments will do the trick. Some may pursue a protracted training course to become a nurse therapist and work exclusively within one model of psychotherapy or another. The majority will, however, be somewhere in the middle, especially if relatively inexperienced. You will be involved in the administration of medication and you will be involved in talking to people. This chapter is a journey through some of the theories that try to explain depression and some of the treatments that are given to people. After briefly stopping at these way stations the journey will take us to our most important destination – the nursing approaches that might be helpful to someone experiencing depression and to the nurse who is trying to help that person[a].

What is this thing called depression?

Barker[6] tells us that depression may be thought of in three forms. The first is where the person experiences depression suddenly and for a short period of time following an event such as loss of a job, or loss of belongings. This depression usually lifts as the person begins to rebuild after the event. The second form of depression is short-term but fairly serious in nature following the death of a significant other or the breakdown of a relationship or a traumatic experience. In both of these forms of depression the person may experience a period of abject misery and may require the help of friends, family and possibly professionals to get through the problems. However, the majority of people encountered by nurses belong in Barker's third group: the person whose depression endures and the distress becomes long-term or keeps returning.

Depression may also be thought of as primary or secondary. In *primary depression* the problems associated with the person's mood are the central whereas in *secondary depression* the emotional problems are associated with other problems such as neurological and brain diseases, e.g. Huntington's disease, Parkinson's disease, dementia, endocrine disorders – such as thyroid, parathyroid and diabetes – or a side-effect of medication such as steroids, anti-malarial drugs, phenothiazines.

The American Psychiatric Association in its Diagnostic Statistical Manual IV (DSMIV)[7] provides the medical criteria for the diagnosis of depression. These involve the presence of five or more of the following in a 2-week period, representing a change in 'normal' presentation:

1 Depressed mood most of the day, nearly every day.

2 Diminished interest or pleasure (*anhedonia*) in almost all of the activities of the day, nearly every day.

Numbers 1 and 2 have to be present along with at least four of the following:

3 Significant weight gain or loss when not dieting, and decreased appetite nearly every day.

4 Insomnia (not sleeping) or hypersomnia (sleeping too much) nearly every day.

5 Abnormal restlessness (psychomotor agitation) or a drop in physical activity (psychomotor retardation) nearly every day.

6 Fatigue or loss of energy nearly every day.

7 Feelings of worthlessness or excessive or inappropriate guilt nearly every day.

8 Diminished ability to think, concentrate or make decisions nearly every day.

9 Recurrent thoughts of death, or recurrent suicidal thoughts without a specific plan; or a suicide attempt; or a specific plan for committing suicide.

In a similar vein the World Health Organization[8] provides a list of symptoms and severity to guide diagnosis.

While these criteria give us some indication of the sort of symptoms psychiatrists look for when diagnosing depression, they neither give us an indication of what might be the explanation for a person experiencing depression nor do they tell us what the subjective experience of depression is like for the person.

---

[a] During this chapter I will refer to nurses and *people experiencing depression*. It should not be assumed from this that the two groups are mutually exclusive.

THE QUESTION OF CAUSE

Traditionally[9] nurses learned that depression could be divided into two types:

❑ one with a readily identifiable cause i.e. one or more adverse life-events (reactive and neurotic); and
❑ one which had no readily identifiable cause and which seemed to emanate from within the person (endogenous and psychotic).

This way of thinking about depression has become discredited for two reasons. Firstly people's experiences do no fit such neat stereotypes. Some experience long-term life-threatening depression as an apparent reaction to what might be seen as a fairly mundane life-event, while others might experience a short period of depression with no apparent cause. Secondly both of these ways of thinking about depression present problems for the sufferer. Thinking about depression as reactive encourages people to think of themselves as weak in some way. They are experiencing depression whereas others, when faced with similar life-events, have not become depressed. Thinking about depression as endogenous, on the other hand, is no more helpful because this encourages the idea that the person must have some weakness of character to become depressed for no apparent reason.

Explanations abound for the cause of mental distress. Each theory of psychotherapy puts forward its own formulation of how the mind works and what causes it to work in ways that distress us. Here we consider some common theoretical explanations:

1 Biological
2 Psychodynamic
3 Interpersonal
4 Cognitive
5 Social.

A case illustration might help us appreciate how each explanation conceives of the experience of depression.

Case study 27.1

Joan is a woman who has experienced depression for most of her adult life. She recounts how parents used to beat her. When she left home she got married and had 2 children only to find that her husband had a conviction for child abuse of which she was unaware. She left him and had a number of relationships which resulted in a further 4 children being born. In an accident one night her youngest child was killed.

Over the next few years Joan had attempted suicide on a number of occasions and had undergone a variety of different psychotherapies, had various admissions to hospital with changes to medication but constantly felt guilty about the death of her child, constantly felt worthless, had difficulty sleeping and thought about suicide.

It's all in the brain

The biological theory of depression asserts that the brain's balance of certain chemicals becomes disturbed, perhaps due to stress or genetic predisposition or a combination of factors. As a consequence of the imbalance the person experiences depression. Which chemicals exactly are implicated is subject to some debate.

Whether the same chemicals are implicated in all cases is also subject to discussion among scientists. The usual suspects in such matters are serotonin and noradrenaline. The rationale behind anti-depressant drug therapies is that the drug redresses the imbalance in the brain chemical and therefore alleviates the depression. So in Joan's case a biological explanation might claim that her problems are based in levels of serotonin and/or noradrenaline in her brain, possibly triggered by events in her life and that antidepressant therapy might help to alleviate this.

However, anti-depressant drugs can be inconsistent in their effectiveness. *Different* people experiencing depression respond to *different* drugs in *different* ways. Some people find their depression lifts after taking medication, some find that they have to try a number of drugs or combinations, and some find that the depression remains even after taking medication. Consequently the purely chemical view of depression has some problems associated with it. Could it be that many different things are happening in people's brains that lead to the experiences known as depression? Or perhaps the drugs we presently use are too broad in their focus, and are not 'smart' enough to pinpoint the exact neurochemical nature of depression? In either case people usually find that, while drugs may be helpful to many, they are usually not the whole story of recovery.

It's all in the mind

Psychodynamic explanation

The psychodynamic explanation[10] proposes that, as a child, the person has experienced a highly significant loss and/or developed the belief that being loved was dependent on pleasing others. As a result the child develops a distorted self-image. In adulthood the person experiences a loss or difficulties with relating to events in life and associates this with feelings about the childhood loss or interpersonal relation. This association of feelings about the current situation and the childhood memories often includes anger. The anger is internalized back into the person and this increases and intensifies feeling of guilt and lack of self-worth. In Joan's case the abuse suffered at the hands of her parents and the loss of her child could be explained as the dynamic processes, which have led to her depression.

Interpersonal explanation

Interpersonal theory[11] puts forward the view that a person develops a depressive way of being as a result of negative interpersonal relationships and the lack of positive reinforcement in life. Again, for Joan, the criticism and hostility shown by her parents may have led to her depressive way of being.

Cognitive explanation

The cognitive explanation[12] of depression considers that depression results not from what is happening in the world of the person but in how the person thinks about what is happening in the world. In other words the person interprets events in a negative way, this brings about negative responses and depressive feelings, which cause events to become more negative and a spiral of depression ensues. In Joan's case a cognitive explanation would focus on her schemata (ways of thinking) about herself in negative ways i.e. her feelings of guilt and worthlessness.

Social explanation

The social model[13] holds the view that depression in women arises out of social vulnerability particularly in four areas: early loss of a mother; involvement in care of young children; absence of a confiding relationship; lack of a job. When stresses occur, depression arises as a result of vulnerability in these areas failing to shore up the person. Joan did not physically lose her mother in early life but lost the nurturing relationship, which was replaced with abuse. She has no significant relationship, is involved in caring for children, is female and has no job. In other words, she shows patterns of vulnerability that the social model would expect to find in a woman experiencing depression. Although such 'social' explanations emphasize the importance of the 'world outside', it also acknowledges how the world of experience is internalized, if you like, in what we call 'the mind'.

The fact that Joan's case could be viewed in terms of any of the theories outlined above shows that these theories are not *the* truth about depression. They are useful frameworks, which professionals may find helpful in approaching their work with people.

TREATING THE PERSON EXPERIENCING DEPRESSION

Medication

The drugs used in depression can be thought of in terms of groupings:

❑ Drugs that inhibit the reuptake of serotonin into nerve cells.

❑ Drugs that inhibit the reuptake of serotonin and noradrenaline into cells.
❑ Tricyclic anti-depressants.
❑ Monoamine oxidase inhibitors (MAOIs).
❑ Others.

All drugs are chemicals that have effects on the body. When the effect is desirable, we call it a *therapeutic* effect. When it is undesirable we call it a side-effect. In some cases the side-effect can become the therapeutic effect and vice versa depending on circumstances. For example the tricyclic anti-depressant amitryptiline can have a side-effect of causing urine retention, and is sometimes given to 'treat' difficulty in controlling the bladder at night (nocturnal enuresis). One of the balancing acts to be achieved with anti-depressant medication is that of preparing people for the side-effects that can appear *before* the therapeutic effect. Each of the above groups has particular side-effects. Comprehensive information cannot be provided here on all of the drugs available so pointers for good practice, only, are suggested.

Although most nurses do not, as yet, prescribe anti-depressant medication, they do administer such medication and monitor its effects. As such it is important for nurses to be up-to-date with the medication in common usage, in terms of:

❑ recommended dosages;
❑ likely side-effects;
❑ how long the drug might take before the person might expect to experience any effect;
❑ any special precautions, or contraindications (where the drug would be inappropriate, or dangerous); and
❑ the answers to any common questions which might be asked.

This knowledge should be kept constantly under review. It is not sufficient, for example, to purchase a book on pharmacology for nurses during pre-registration training and consider that to be the end-word on medications. Drugs are constantly being developed. New drugs come on the market and older ones fall out of favour or are removed from common usage. New precautions and instructions often appear after a drug has long been in use and nurses need to be up-to-date on these issues, as well as aware of where to access information, and where to point people who take the drugs for information. A good point of reference for both nurses and people prescribed anti-depressant medication is the Norfolk Mental Health Care NHS Trust website at http://www.nmhct.nhs.uk/pharmacy/ which provides information in readily accessible language about drugs in common usage in mental health.

Other physical approaches

Further physical methods of treating depression are electroconvulsive therapy (ECT) and transcranial magnetic stimulation (TMS). ECT is a well-known treatment for depression involving the administration of a controlled current of electricity across the skull of the person who has been anaesthetized and had a muscle relaxant administered. The aim of the treatment is to induce a seizure. It is not clear how this treatment might improve symptoms for someone experiencing depression, but many psychiatrists (and some patients) do still consider it to be a useful weapon in their armoury against depression. TMS is a newer treatment that is not widely used at time of writing. The treatment involves the application of controlled bursts of an electromagnetic field around the head of the person. This is thought to stimulate the activity of neurones and alleviate some of the problems of depression. Given the questions posed at the use of mobile phones and their ability to induce an electromagnetic field in the vicinity of the head and possible associated side-effects it will be interesting to see how this form of treatment develops.

ECT has been a contentious subject for many nurses with some taking the view that they would not wish to be involved in the treatment. The ethics of ECT is beyond the remit of this chapter (see Chapter 56). As the law stands in the UK, the only treatment from which a nurse may lawfully abstain is abortion and so many nurses may find themselves working with people who are about to receive or have received ECT. However, the responsibilities of the nurse are similar whether patients are being treated with ECT, or with other medications. The person's questions and fears should be addressed, and information given regarding what the person might expect on waking after the procedure – for example headache and some memory loss.

Psychological therapies

Psychological therapies provided to help people experiencing depression are based on the psychological theories discussed previously. Depending on availability, people may be offered one or more of psychodynamic, cognitive, interpersonal, behavioural and marital therapies. In the current system of psychiatry in the UK it is rare for someone to be offered such therapies in the absence of medication. In spite of the public perception of the psychiatrist as a latter-day Freud using psychotherapeutic techniques in a purpose built surgery, most psychiatrists operate within a biological mindset which recourses to medication as a first resort.[14]

Nevertheless there are some tools developed in psychotherapy that nurses can use. For instance the Beck Depression Inventory (BDI) is a self-rating scale that covers 21 areas of a person's life and scores each of these between 0 and 3. The scores are totalled and scores over 16 in total are indicative of depression. Unfortunately it is often merely used to obtain a baseline score on admission to hospital and then filed and repeated after three weeks to evaluate anti-depressant drug therapy. In fact the BDI is a useful tool for nurses to use because it enables focus on the particular areas that the person is experiencing as problematic. In other words it enables the nurse to discuss things with the person in a focused way rather than just general conversation.

NURSING APPROACHES

The nursing care of someone experiencing depression is a skilled activity that is neither medicine nor psychotherapy, but might take from these and other disciplines to help people. On meeting the person for the first time it is worth considering the work of Peplau[15] who considered roles in the relationship between nurses and people in care. She reminded us that the first role the nurse fulfils for the person is that of *stranger*. 'Trust me I'm a nurse' would probably not be a very successful chat up line, yet there is an assumption that just because we approach someone wearing a badge saying 'Nurse' then people must not only trust us but pour out their innermost feelings to us. When they don't we often regard them as unco-operative.[16]

Curiosity skilled the nurse

It can often be difficult for us to remember that we are strangers to people because we assume that we *know* them. Wherever people enter the psychiatric system they are accompanied by copious amounts of medical, nursing and other professionals' notes. While notes are necessary for communication between professionals there is always the danger that they can become *the* story about a person's life. This can have negative consequences.

❏ Because of the nature of the problem-solving approach employed by health professionals, people's lives get to be seen in terms of their problems rather than strengths.
❏ Professionals risk losing all curiosity about people, assuming that they know *the* story. Consider the 'man who throws refrigerators'. Dick, who had been resident in a large psychiatric hospital for many years, was known as the man who threw refrigerators. He was thus known because he had *once* thrown a refrigerator across the kitchen of the ward in 1973. His

notes recorded, however, that 'when he gets angry he throws refrigerators'.

Building relationships

One of the first principles of psychiatric nursing should be *curiosity*. Nurses should be interested in people's stories. To allow people to tell their story we need to create conditions where this might happen. When a person is experiencing depression s/he often feels worthless and boring. Often friends and relatives will have given up the arduous task of trying to 'cheer up' the person. That someone might be willing to spend time with the person, without the expectation that the person comes up with a full unexpurgated story of his/her life, can help to reassure the person. You may need to sit with the person for a while *not* talking and *or* asking lots of questions, but simply being there. This can be difficult. There is often a temptation to fill the silence or to talk to the more lively person or to find something else to do. At the same time a balance has to be achieved. Altschul[17] has described her wish to both feel safe in a ward environment but also to have her own space.

People experiencing depression can develop a hostile way of relating to others, as a way of maintaining their ideas of worthlessness: i.e. 'people have no time for me because I'm worthless so I won't have any time for them'. In Joan's case, she had developed a disdain for many health professionals because they hadn't helped her. Invariably, she entered into what the professional thought was a 'therapeutic session', but Joan had no intention of allowing anything 'therapeutic' to develop. As a result the professionals had quickly changed from what Watkins[18] describes as 'rescuer role' into the 'persecutor role'. Rescuers see people as in need of rescuing. Nurses often want to help people in distress by fixing their problems. Once the problem will not be fixed the rescuer can turn into the persecutor, blaming the person with the problem for not getting mended. Where people do not 'mend' quickly we need to develop the skill of being neutral towards hostility and also not having expectations that the person can be fixed like some broken washing machine.

Nurses need to begin to build the relationship with the person by using the active listening skills and open questioning described in Chapters 10 and 17.

Here is a snippet of my early conversation with Joan.

> ### Process illustration
>
> **Ian:** 'Joan can you tell me a bit about how you feel just now?'
> **Joan:** 'I feel everything is hopeless, everything is just black'.
> **Ian:** 'Black?'
> **Joan:** 'I'm just going through the motions. I can't do anything and no-one can help me'.
> **Ian:** 'You say no-one can help you, can you say a bit more about that?'
> **Joan:** 'Yes well, I've been to see psychologists, the last one I saw I ended up getting her to tell me all about her children (laugh); it was easier than talking about my problems'.
> **Ian:** 'So you have found that you could move the conversation away from discussing your problems. Does that help?'
> **Joan:** 'Laugh ... well it makes me feel better in the short-term but it doesn't get me anywhere'.

By using simple questioning techniques I was able to listen to her and find out more about her feelings and experiences without putting words in her mouth. As our conversation developed it became clear that other professionals had begun their work with Joan, assuming that she had to change before establishing where (within Joan) this change might take place.

> ### Process illustration
>
> **Ian:** Can you tell me a bit more about what you see as the problem with therapy?
> **Joan:** Well I've had loads of people sitting with me telling me that I've got to change to get better and there they are, every time I see them they wear the same clothes, they come to work at 9 o'clock and go home at 5 o'clock and do the same things every day. Where do they get off telling me I've got to change?

Despite having seen a number of different therapists Joan felt that they were all too busy trying to 'cure' her to ever begin to know her as a person. By adopting these simple techniques I was able to get to a point where, when I summarized what Joan had told me about herself, she responded by saying that no-one had ever understood how she felt in the way that I did.

Despite being strangers people do generally expect nurses to be doing something in clinical settings. People generally expect nurses to have a plan and also for that plan to be focused on some of the problems that they are experiencing. Case study 27.2 indicates how much people expect there to be a plan even in the face of contradictory evidence.

Case study 27.2

Jeff was admitted to an acute psychiatric ward experiencing depression and found that he was placed in the day room of the ward while the nurses spent a lot of time in the office.

Three years after his discharge from the ward Jeff remained convinced that the nurses' plan must have been to check out his mental state by observing him from a distance and seeing how he behaved.

Negative statements

People experiencing depression may very often talk in very negative ways about their lives, their families, and their futures. This can often be disconcerting. It can be very easy to get into confrontation with the person by arguing, 'of course you are not worthless.' The nurse's 'advocacy' merely confirms (paradoxically) that the nurse believes him/her to be worthless. One way to address this is to use the 'friend technique'.

Person experiencing depression: 'I'm a useless mother. I can't get anything right'.
Nurse: 'If you had your best friend sat next to you and your best friend said "I'm a useless mother, I can't get anything right!" What would you say to your friend?'

The friend technique usually elicits one of three responses:

1   'I know just how you feel!'
2   'Pull yourself together, of course you're not useless!'
3   Some sort of helpful suggestion.

The first response – 'I know just how you feel' – seems, at first sight, to undermine the whole purpose of the technique, which is to try to elicit a more helpful way of thinking about the situation. If the person responds in this way it is worth pursuing the feelings she is referring to. 'OK, so you know just how your friend feels, so what might you be able to say to your friend that might help her at the moment?'

If the response is something of the nature of 'pull yourself together!' the nurse might say, 'OK, so has anyone ever said something like that to you?' 'Did it help you?' 'What else might you say?' On rare occasions the person may say something quite helpful straight away.

In each scenario notice that the nurse's response is *not* to enter into argument, but to try to elicit a more helpful response. The nurse aims to help the person address and deal with her/his negative way of thinking. However, this will not happen by attacking the person's beliefs. Generally speaking when our beliefs are attacked we hold on to them more strongly.

Discussing suicide

People experiencing depression often consider suicide. Nurses need to assess the risk that this poses to the person. We can only do this by talking to people *about* suicide. Joan had made several suicide attempts and it was important to assess the risk of another attempt. People expect nurses to be interested in their problems so it would be strange for someone who is feeling suicidal, to discover that no-one wanted to talk about it. In Joan's case this is how the subject was discussed.

Ian: 'Anyone who had not met you before might say that, given you have tried to kill yourself on a number of occasions and you are still alive, you didn't really intend to die. What would you say to that?'
Joan: 'Well the last time I took an overdose was late at night in the winter and I went up the mountain where I didn't think anyone would find me. You don't expect a group of soldiers to be out on exercise at that time. And you don't know that the cold slows down your metabolism so the tablets don't work so quickly do you? … but I'll remember next time!'
Ian: 'OK so on a day-to-day basis what is it that stops you from killing yourself?'

At no point did I say to Joan that I did not believe she was serious in her attempts at suicide. At the same time however I was able to ascertain the seriousness of her intentions. I could then move on to discussing with her reasons why she may not have killed herself already. Frankl[19] took the view that the drive behind existence was our desire to find meaning in our lives. If a life has meaning then it will endure. When working with someone who is depressed this means that it is important to find out what positives there are in life. This can sometimes seem to be contrary to the way in which nurses are trained to think. After all nurses seek to assess people's problems and then plan care based on what those problems are deemed to be. If we simply concentrate on people's problems we get a very strange view of people's lives. We define people in terms of problems and we see depression as a discreet entity that we can treat. Frankl teaches us that people have strengths. For example they do not come into contact with services the moment they start to feel down; they adopt their own strategies for getting by. It is only when these strategies appear not to work that people seek help from others.

In Joan's case she often talked at length about her children and how the thought of them being without a mother prevented her from harming herself. One of the strategies that could therefore be developed was to discuss her children with her and to develop plans for how she might keep herself safe from harming herself. Barker[20] terms this the security plan. For Joan this included not drinking alcohol when she was alone in the house because this made her feel more depressed and for her to go round to her daughter's house when she felt particularly low.

Discussion that enables people to think in terms of taking some control of their situations create the conditions for them to start to think about themselves in a more positive light and not simply to rely on the professional to put things right. It also validates the person's own solutions as opposed to the received wisdom from the professional. In Joan's case, she was able to move on to some extent after her dead child appeared to her in a dream and told her she had experienced enough guilt and that she should get on with her life.

SUMMARY

Nursing involves the skilled relationship with the person experiencing depression to enable the person to develop ways of making sense of the experiences in his/her life. To do this the nurse employs a variety of theoretical approaches to ensure that the relationship is purposeful and focused on the concerns of person in care.

REFERENCES

1. Redfield-Jamison K. *The unquiet mind: a memoir of moods and madness*. London: Picador, 1995.
2. Gilbert P. *Counselling for depression*. London: Sage, 1992.
3. Frankl V. *The doctor and the soul: from psychotherapy to logotherapy*. New York: Vintage, 1986.
4. Barker P, Kerr B. *The process of psychotherapy: a journey of discovery*. Oxford: Butterworth Heinemann, 2001.
5. Nelson-Jones R. *Six key approaches to counselling and therapy*. London: Continuum, 2000.
6. Barker P. *Severe depression: the practitioner's guide*. London: Chapman and Hall, 1992.
7. American Psychiatric Association. *Diagnostic and statistical manual of mental disorders*, 4th edn, text revision. Washington: American Psychiatric Association, 1994.
8. World Health Organization. *ICD-10: The ICD-10 classification of mental and behavioural disorders: clinical descriptions and diagnostic guidelines*. London: Gaskell/Royal College of Psychiatrists, 1992.
9. Ackner B. *Handbook for psychiatric nurses*, 9th edn. London: Baillière Tindall/Cassell, 1964.
10. Beeber L. *The client who is depressed*. In: Lego S. Psychiatric nursing: a comprehensive reference, 2nd edn. Philadelphia: Lippincott, 1996: 201–7.
11. Barker P, *op. cit.*
12. Gilbert P, *op. cit.*
13. Brown G, Harris T. *The social origins of depression: a study of psychiatric disorder in women*. London: Tavistock, 1978.
14. Barker P. Psychiatric Lara Crofts? Forget it. *Nursing Times* 2001; 97(33): 31.
15. Peplau H. *Interpersonal relations in nursing*. Basingstoke: Macmillan, 1988.
16. O'Hagan M. Two accounts of mental distress. In: Read J, Reynolds J (eds). *Speaking our minds: an anthology*. Basingstoke: Macmillan, 1996.
17. Altschul A. There won't be a next time. In: Rippere V, Williams R (eds). *Wounded healers: mental health workers' experiences of depression*. Chichester: John Wiley, 1985: 167–75.
18. Watkins P. *Mental health nursing: the art of compassionate care*. Oxford: Butterworth Heinemann, 2001.
19. Frankl V, *op. cit.*
20. Barker P. *The Tidal Model: theory and practice*. Unpublished, 2000.

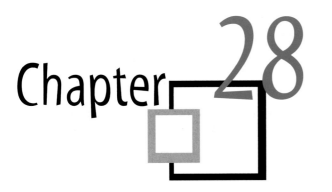

Chapter 28

THE PERSON WHO IS SUICIDAL

Ruth Gallop* and Elaine Stamina**

INTRODUCTION

A psychiatric-mental health nurse will inevitably care for persons who try to harm themselves or express feelings such as 'I wish I were dead' or 'there is nothing worth living for'. The act of self-harm is a *behaviour* – an expression of an internal feeling state. Being suicidal is not a disease – it is not a disorder. While we are compelled to try to prevent people from killing themselves we will not always succeed. More importantly we need to put most of our energy into *understanding* the internal state of the person and trying to help him or her deal with the feelings. Hopefully over time and with appropriate support the person will begin to feel life is worth living.

Suicidal and self-harm behaviours can be found in clients who receive many different diagnoses Suicidal behaviour is not restricted to patients diagnosed with some form of depression. Patients with diagnoses of schizophrenia, bipolar affective disorder, personality disorder, eating disorders and post-traumatic stress disorders, all can be at risk for self-harm. Everyone in the mental health system may be, at one time or another, at risk for self-harm. It is the responsibility of the nurse to

be alert to the possibility of this behaviour, to have the knowledge to assess for suicide and to have the basic skills needed to support and care for the suicidal patient.

The term suicidal behaviour is often used to cover many different behaviours:

❑ completed suicides;
❑ non-fatal self-harm behaviours (including suicide attempts and self-harm without suicidal intent); and
❑ suicide threats.

Sometimes self-harm reflects the wish to die, and sometimes it does not. Trying to sort this out requires substantial knowledge and understanding plus clinical acumen Here, we shall focus on the person who has the wish to be dead.

PREVALENCE OF SUICIDE

Death by suicide continues to be a serious problem. Table 28.1 shows the most recent suicide rates per 100,000 for a number of countries. In the last decade the rate of attempted suicide has risen. Completed sui-

*Ruth Gallop is Professor, Faculty of Nursing and Department of Psychiatry University of Toronto, Toronto, Canada. Her research, clinical work and writing focus on clients' perceived as treatment and management challenges. These clients often receive diagnoses of borderline personality disorders; have histories of severe early trauma and current self-harm behaviours.
**Elaine Stamina is Clinical Leader Manager, St Michael's Hospital, Toronto, Canada.

TABLE 28.1 Death rates for suicide in 1999 (deaths per 100,000 residents)

Country	All	Male	Female
England	12	18	6
Northern Ireland	12	20	4
Republic of Ireland	15	24	6
Scotland	21	33	10
Wales	14	23	5
Canada (1997)	12	19.5	5
USA 10.7		17.6	4.1

Adapted from: Suicide Statistics, http://www.samaritans. org.uk/know/statistics_suicide.html , 23 November 2001; Statistics Canada's Internet Site – Selected leading causes of death by sex, http://www.statcan.ca/english/Pgdb/ People/Health/health36.htm , 4 April 2001; and from Deaths: Leading Causes for 1999, http://www.cdc.gov/nchs/ data/nvsr/nvsr49/nvsr49–11.pdf , 23 November 2001.

cide rates are higher for men than women. Rates for *parasuicide* (acts of self-harm without the apparent intent to die) are documented as high as 466 per 100,000 per year for persons greater than 15 years of age.

The female-to-male ratio is 1.6:1, which indicates that more females than males attempt suicide, and more males than females complete suicide.[1]

There is a link between self-harm behaviour and suicide. Thirty to 47% of persons who complete suicide have a history of self-harm behaviour. In the UK, 1% of persons who engage in self-harm complete suicide within one year and 3–5% complete suicide in 5–10 years.[2]

THE NATURE OF SUICIDE

The novice clinician is often reluctant to ask about suicide. Often this is because of a lack of understanding about the feelings and dynamics surrounding suicide. First of all we shall list a few basic facts about suicide and then follow this with some of the theoretical and conceptual explanations that make suicidal behaviour understandable.

- ❏ **Asking about suicide does not make a person suicidal.** If you think a person is suicidal, then ask them! This is, quite literally, a *vital* question to ask, and should be part of all assessments (see below for assessment guidelines).

- ❏ **Most people who commit suicide have a previous history of self-harm.** Previous self-harm is always a cause for concern. Unfortunately people who self-harm can be viewed as 'attention-seeking', or seen as a distraction from people in 'real need'. Given that research shows many people who self-harm go on to complete suicide, each incidence of self-harm needs careful assessment for risk.

- ❏ **Most people who are considering suicide have mixed feelings.** It is extremely important to understand the role of ambivalence in suicide. A patient who tells you s/he wants to die, or telephones you, saying that she is about to take an overdose, or leaves a message that she has harmed herself, may be indicating that she is not sure that she really wants to die. She may *feel* like dying but some small part of her is unsure. However, communication about suicidal ideation or suicidal behaviour can be an expression of the ambivalence between the wish-to-live and the wish-to-die; and a means to reach out for help.[3] If the clinician recognizes this ambivalence, then s/he can capitalize on it as a way of helping the person to stay alive and to receive the needed help.

- ❏ **Many people who attempt or complete suicide give out warnings or clues.**[4] It is a misconception that people who talk about attempting suicide never do it. The opposite is actually true. Most people who have attempted or completed suicide have given warnings or clues of their intent. Although suicide may appear impulsive in many cases, as we shall discuss and illustrate below, it is not. People give out clues directly and indirectly:
  - (a) personal items may be given away;
  - (b) a sense of calm may indicate that the final plan is in place;
  - (c) wills may be completed or letters sent.

All such warnings need to be received seriously.

- ❏ **Most people who commit suicide have a plan.** Suicide is often a carefully thought out plan. Many people 'feel' suicidal and experience suicidal thoughts or wishes to die but may not act on it. However, others move from thinking about suicide to creating and executing a plan. The plan or method of choice is often one which has a social context.[5] For example, more men than women use violent means such as firearms and more women than men use overdoses. Many people do not change methods. If access to one method is removed, then the person may not choose another method. For example, if pills are removed from cupboards then the person may not choose a method other than overdose.

WHY PEOPLE COMMIT SUICIDE

Many different theories attempt to explain the motivations for people who engage in suicidal behaviour. Different disciplines have developed their respective theories. A competent clinician will use the knowledge from different theories to understand the complexity of suicide. Suicide occurs within a complex set of individual and social circumstances. Multiple risk factors, occurring simultaneously, are indicative of a higher risk for suicidal behaviour.[6]

❑ **Social theories.** Various factors are thought to contribute to increased suicidality across specific population groups. People who experience a lack of social support are more prone to suicide (for example divorced, separated or widowed people, or those who live alone); more men than women complete suicide (specifically men over 65 years of age); people who experience sudden losses, stressors, crises or unexpected change in economic circumstances (either wealth or poverty) are also at increased risk.

❑ **Biological theories.** It is suggested that some people may have genetic predisposition towards chemical disturbances, such as depression or psychotic disorders, which make them more vulnerable to suicide. Studies have indicated that people with low levels of serotonin in the brain (as measured by the level of a main metabolite 5-HIAA [5 hydroxyindoleacetic acid]), are more prone to depression and suicide.[7,8] Alteration of biochemical states through substance misuse such as alcohol or cocaine, also can distort a person's perspectives, increasing a sense of hopelessness or distorting reality.

❑ **Psychodynamic or internal personal theories.** The loss of an important relationship or attachment (actual or perceived) is thought to precipitate tremendous psychological pain. Often childhood experiences leave an individual vulnerable to the experience of loss. The person may experience overwhelming distress and despair. Life may seem hopeless and suicide the only option.

❑ **Learning theories.** Suicide is also seen as a mechanism by which people 'cope' with problems of living. As such, suicidal behaviour can become a part of a person's repertoire of coping skills.

Hopelessness

One concept appears to be of particular importance in understanding suicide intent and suicide behaviour. Psychological research indicates that a sense of hopelessness may be an important catalyst for the catastrophic event of suicide.

Hopelessness is a manner of thinking and feeling which frames life with negative perceptions of the present and bleak expectations about the future.[9] Current and future situations, relationships, and views about oneself are interpreted with pessimism. The person anticipates that life will never become better and that s/he is unable to effect any positive change.

People who experience hopelessness tend to think in a very narrow manner. This constriction in cognitive processes limits the range of understanding of situations and potential choices that may be available for problem resolution. When presented with a situational problem to solve, a person whose thoughts are hopeless and rigid, may conclude that suicide is the only choice. Death is an escape from the pain of life.

Circumstances generating hopelessness and depression

Crisis

A suicide attempt is often preceded by some form of crisis. This may be an extreme life-event – death of a partner or child, loss of a job or divorce – or it can be a less extreme life-event that has significant meaning for the individual

> Kim, a 15-year-old boy, jumped off a high bridge. The boy, of Asian heritage, was the only son of an immigrant family. The family had worked hard so that their son could get the best education. The boy had been caught and humiliated in a school prank. His parents were about to be informed. The shame was unbearable.

Loss and abandonment

Some people are exquisitely sensitive to loss and abandonment, whether real or imagined. When forming successful relationships is difficult for a person, disruption of an existing relationship can feel catastrophic. Sometimes, in the eyes of the observer, the relationship is seen as transient or not very substantial. However, for the individual the loss can re-evoke earlier feelings of being alone. It is not unusual for people with histories of childhood abuse or neglect to be highly sensitive to loss.

> Jane was hospitalized after taking an overdose. During her stay she formed a friendship with a male patient. After he was discharged she spent her time off the unit visiting him. After two meetings he told her he was too busy to see her and anyway had a girlfriend. Jane was angry and then upset. She left the unit and took a large overdose.

Social isolation

Humans are by nature interpersonal creatures. We all need connection with others. To be in the world without any others who know or care about us can be devastating. Having difficulty forming relationships can lead to isolation, as can certain illnesses, such as schizophrenia and depression. People may feel so unworthy that they isolate themselves from others.

> John had lived for years with his outgoing brother. After his brother died, John who was naturally quite shy, gradually withdrew from activities and contacts. He rejected the visits of the community nurse. One night he turned on the gas and died.

Internal motivations

The reason for the suicide attempt is not always apparent. It may be driven by internal events – such as voices or other psychotic thoughts. Occasionally the motivation is revenge or punishment of another – leaving a legacy of guilt in the survivor. For people with a history of severe abuse, the intense internal pain generated can lead to suicide.

> Mary experienced severe sexual abuse as a child and lived a chaotic life. When her father (the perpetrator) was nominated for a community award, she sent her diaries to the newspapers and then took an overdose.

> Jane had been hearing voices for several months and was diagnosed with schizophrenia. There were many voices in her head and they were all telling her to kill herself to rid the world of the devil within her. During hospitalization she tried to leave the unit. She was found walking through drifts of snow in subzero weather, in bare feet, to go to the train tracks to lie down and end her life, as the voices had commanded.

Chronic depression, constricted thinking

Despite the best efforts of clinicians, depression can remain chronic and debilitating. Years of hopelessness, different medications without success and a feeling that this will never get better, can lead to increased risk for suicide.

> After years of treatment for depression: medication, psychotherapy and ECT, Susan still felt she had not been helped. She was unsuccessful in attaining her teaching certificate and could see no reason for living. Apart from this she denied any other problem. She said that her husband and children would be better off without her. She was found in the lake.

THE NURSING ROLE

The role of the nurse in caring for the suicidal person is grounded in the therapeutic role. All the principles outlined in earlier chapters on therapeutic practice are relevant Treating each person with respect, dignity and empathy is essential for persons who often view the self as bad or worthless. However working with a person who is suicidal requires additional knowledge. The nurse must be able to:

1 Assess for *suicidal risk*.

2 Assess the *mental status*.
3 Promote *safety*.
4 Explore *precipitants*.
5 Promote *alternative* coping strategies.

Using a case study, we shall demonstrate the application of this necessary knowledge.

> ## Case study 28.1
>
> Fred is a middle aged, divorced man and father of three teenagers. He recently lost his job due to drinking and is now facing eviction from his flat for financial reasons. He has been treated with anti-depressants for 6 months and feels no better. He attempted suicide previously after his divorce. His father committed suicide when he was ten. Last night, he took an overdose of sleeping pills 'to end it all'. He has been admitted to hospital because he says he is useless and worth more dead than alive.

Assessment for suicidal risk

Rationale

A suicide attempt is very difficult to predict. However, assessment of a patient's risk for suicide will direct the provision of an appropriate level of protection and guide interventions. Risk for suicide is re-evaluated throughout the course of care to assess the patient's response to personal situational changes and clinical interventions. A suicide risk assessment is discussed with members of the health care team, incorporated into the care plan and documented in the clinical record. A careful review of the risk is critical for discharge planning.

> On admission, Fred appears downcast and is curled up in bed. As part of your assessment you have explained to him that it is important to explore his wish to die.

The following outline reflects the broad areas to include in your assessment with examples of how questions might be posed. Remember, asking someone about his/her thoughts of suicide will not cause the person to attempt it.

Suicidal ideation

Nurse: 'Since you have been admitted to hospital do you continue to think about harming yourself or taking your life'?

Fred: 'Well, may be a little less so at the moment but I still think everyone would be better off without me'.

Nurse: 'Are you able to control these thoughts or do they occur spontaneously'?

Fred: 'If I am distracted with other people around then

the thoughts seem to go away, but when I am alone, I can only think about dying'.

Suicidal plan

Nurse: 'If you were to make another attempt, how might you try it'?

Fred: 'They took all my pills from me in the emergency department, but that's what I would do'.

Nurse: 'Apart from this current overdose have you made other attempts in the past'?

Fred: 'Once before, when my wife ended our marriage, I got drunk and took a handful of pain pills'.

Nurse: 'During this current attempt, how did you arrive at the hospital'?

Fred: 'I called my brother and told him what I had done. I wanted to say goodbye and ask him to keep an eye on my kids for me. He called the ambulance'.

Nurse: 'Did you make any other preparations for your death such as writing a note or leave a will'?

Fred: 'Yes, I wrote my sons'.

Nurse: 'Fred, you have told me about your thoughts and plans to die. However, is there anything that would prevent you from taking your life'?

Fred: 'I think about my sons. I remember how alone I felt when my father died and I worry that they might feel the same way'.

Nurse: 'Do you think your concerns about them may be helpful in stopping you from carrying out your plan'.

Fred: 'I don't know. They are my only reason for living but I still think they might be better off if I were gone'.

You recognize that several risk factors exist for this patient. Although he says he thinks less about suicide you know that *ambivalence* between the wish to live and the wish to die is common in people who are suicidal. His thoughts can be distracted when in the presence of others. However, the suicidal thoughts are intrusive and relatively continuous when he is alone and continue to put him at risk.

Fred also has a plan to end his life and has used it in the past. You are also aware that a history of previous attempts, especially within one year of the current attempt, are more likely to result in a completed attempt within the next year. In his previous attempt he combined the pills with alcohol. His history of substance misuse creates a potential for impulsive and lethal choices.

The circumstances around his current attempt are of concern. He was alone at the time of his attempt and wrote a note to his sons. This indicates that he was anticipating life for others after his death. However, he reached out and called his brother. He was able to tell someone of his attempt, which initiated a rescue. His ability to reach out and notify someone of his feelings

and his actions will also be important information to help him to protect himself in the future. He identifies reasons to live, his sons, but is unsure if this reason would help him to stay alive. Fred also has a family history of completed suicide, which is an additional risk factor.

Recent stressors

Nurse: 'Have you experienced any recent problems or losses in your life'?

Fred: 'I was fired from my job 2 months ago. They caught me drinking on the job again so I was let go. Now I can't afford my child support payments and my flat. I can't seem to do anything right. I'll never get out of this mess. My children don't want to see me. The only answer for everyone is for me to be dead'.

Nurse: 'Things seem pretty hopeless to you now. When problems are overwhelming, it can be difficult to find ways to manage and work through them, one step at a time. Later on, we can explore options that you may want to consider trying'.

Fred's recent losses and a lack of social support increase his risk for suicide. Each person's response to stress and loss is highly individual. Events that overwhelm one person do not necessarily overwhelm everyone. However, some people, such as Fred, feel desperate, alone and hopeless in the midst of surmounting problems. Acknowledging a state of hopelessness confirms for Fred that you accept his current feelings and do not try to falsely 'cheer him up'. However, you prepare him for future discussions about his coping strategies, and how you might support him to find alternative solutions to his problems. Validation of current and future supports, for example his brother will be important to help the patient maintain and build on relationships which are protective and provide a sense of belonging.

Impulsivity and substance use

Nurse: 'You mentioned that you were fired for drinking. How much do you drink in a day on a regular basis'?

Fred: 'I don't drink daily. I only drink when I'm worried or upset. Sometimes I'll go for weeks and not drink. Then a problem will come along and I drink until I fall asleep'.

Fred is using alcohol as a means of coping. His use of chemicals adds to his suicide risk by impairment of judgement and perception and increasing lethality when mixed with medications. During another meeting with him you will explore this further. What recent problems triggered this episode of drinking, which resulted in his employment termination? Had he ever received treatment for alcohol use? In a similar manner to your assessment of alcohol misuse, you also understand that other street drugs will add to potential impulsivity and increase suicidality and therefore, you assess for drug use.

Mental status assessment

Rationale

It is important for the nurse to assess the patient's mental status and level of suicidality *frequently* and *repeatedly* during an episode of care, to be sensitive to alterations in the person's current mental state. Assessment of the patient's mental status provides the nurse with clinical information about the patient's thoughts, feelings and behaviours beyond the aspect of suicide. This provides important clinical data to determine competency and an ability to engage with the treatment team. Elsewhere in this text detailed assessment information is provided (see Chapter 52) A suicidal patient's mental status can change in response to external events, internal biochemical changes. This may be indicative of mental and/or organic illness, or in response to medications or ingested chemicals. The severity of a depression can also be reflected in reduction or cessation of activities associated with daily living. Therefore, a mental status assessment needs to be frequently repeated. Also, a current assessment will ensure that the clinician alters the treatment approaches to be appropriate for the clinical status and requirements.

> After a few days of admission you have observed that Fred is spending almost all of his time in bed, sleeping. He is refusing to get up for meals. He is isolating himself and rarely interacts with other patients.
>
> You meet with him to assess his mental status and revise his care according to his altered state and subsequent needs.

Assessment of affect

Nurse: 'Fred, you seem to be sleeping most of the day and I noticed that you were not up for meals. How have you been feeling today'?

Fred: (He is slow to answer and keeps his face turned away from you.) 'I have nothing to get up for and I'm not hungry. Please go away and leave me alone'.

Nurse: 'You seem very sad at the moment'.

Fred: 'I have no life and I don't want your help'.

You recognize the features of despair and hopelessness. He does not feel motivated even to eat.

Assessment of behaviour

Fred's non-verbal communication – his face and body turned away from you and no eye contact – is a further indication of the severity of his feelings of despair. He is unable to connect with others and participate in life sustaining activities such as eating.

Assessment of cognition

Nurse: 'What are you thinking of while you lie there'?

Fred: 'I try not to think. I try to block out these voices in my head'.

Nurse: 'Sometimes when a person feels so awful, thoughts in the form of voices can occur. They sound very real and can be very disturbing. Is this sort of experience happening to you'?

Fred: 'One voice in my head continually tells me to die, to kill myself, I am no good. If I don't eat, I'll die and that is what I should do'.

Fred is hearing 'voices' which command him to take his life. You are aware that these voices can be very powerful and frightening and may indicate that the person is experiencing a distortion in reality. He is unable to consider other options for his life. His thoughts about himself are negative and intrusive with the presence of psychotic, self-destructive content that may put him at further risk for suicide. His refusal to eat has become a passive manner to end his life. His plan of care will need to incorporate a nutritional assessment and assistance with nutritional requirements, an increased frequency in observation and assistance with hygiene.

The components of this mental status assessment demonstrate that Fred is still severely depressed. He has a hopeless mood with rigid thinking and intrusive commands to end life. His behaviours are not life-sustaining. Based on these observations you believe Fred is at risk for attempting suicide. You increase the level of observation for Fred and convey your concern to the clinical team.

Promoting safety

Rationale

The balance between the maintenance of safety for a patient and the assurance of her/his integrity as a human being can be a challenge for nurses. Safety and integrity seem to be mutually enhancing ideals rather than conflicting values. However, in the care for someone who attempts to end his life the measures necessary to protect a patient from himself may inherently diminish individual choice and freedoms. Although individual suicides are difficult to predict, the clinician's responsibility is to assess foreseeable risk and to plan for safe measures.[10]

Patients who attempt suicide may resist protective efforts from clinicians and families. If the patient is either not competent to make treatment decisions or unable to develop an alliance with staff then the risk for suicide is higher and the need to ensure safety is enhanced in situations of uncertainty.

By its very nature, a hospital environment has numerous potential hazards. A psychiatric unit may have more than one suicidal client, with more than one preferred method. Therefore, most psychiatric environments consider the majority of suicide methods in the planning and development of the environmental structure. Mental health units frequently incorporate construction features to protect patients from suicide: all medications and patient belongings may be locked in cupboards which can be accessed only by nurses; all environmental finishes – which could be used as a means for suicide – may be constructed to counter self-destructive actions (e.g. collapsible curtain rods, shatter proof plexiglas windows and mirrors; and locks that secure the environment yet enable rapid response from staff).

Although immediate protection may be essential, it should neither be more extensive nor of greater duration than the patient clinically requires. The clinician must perform a careful balancing act – maintaining the dignity and self-responsibility of the person as much as possible while insuring safety. Excessive containment or coercion may at the very least foster a maladaptive dependency. Worse, it can be punitive and an infringement of patient rights. If a patient feels punished and violated through excessive force then, any ambivalence that s/he may have about suicide may be eroded and the person may feel more determined to die. These negative outcomes counter the therapeutic goal to help the patient to a healthy life through the development of constructive adaptive skills and choices.

Although physical measures are important for safety, no measure is a replacement for being with the patient and providing human connection. Human interaction and responsiveness may itself convey a sense of belonging and hope. Also, frequent, direct observation and presence by a skilled clinician provides timely awareness of subtle and overt changes in a patient's mental status and associated behaviours. An observant nurse can respond to subtle patient cues and intervene at a time of increased distress. In the event of an actual attempt, the nurse can intervene immediately and provide emergency care to the patient who is frequently or constantly observed, and thereby diminish potential lethality. In a non-hospitalized scenario, the observation may be provided by a friend or family member who stays at home with the patient or by asking the patient to stay at a temporary residence in a crisis centre.

Example

You have increased your observation of Fred to every 15 minutes based upon your previous assessment. During one of your observations you notice someone visiting Fred and handing him a plastic bag of items. You introduce yourself to the visitor.

Nurse: 'I notice that your friend has brought you some items, Fred. It's very helpful to have a friend who cares about your needs. Our concern is also for your need for safety. Would you and your friend show me the articles that have been brought for you, then if necessary, we can find safe places to store them for your future use'?

Fred: 'I feel like a child if you check everything. The articles are mine and I don't want to give them over to anyone'.

Friend: 'I would never do anything that would harm Fred. Why are you suggesting that I would'?

Nurse: 'We know friends want to be helpful and caring, but sometimes items you may not recognize as risky are brought in. We can help to ensure your continued safety by identifying items that can pose a risk to you. This is something we can do together'.

Among some toiletry items, there was a bottle of non-prescription pain pills for headache.

Fred: 'I need those pills for headaches. I want them at my bedside'.

Nurse: 'If you are having headaches I want to hear about it, how frequently you have them and what medication you have found helpful. We will work with you to find safe ways to provide pain relief for you. These pain pills can either be sent home with your friend, or labelled and locked for your security'.

You recognize the need for choice in adult decision-making. Although Fred initially expresses a loss in adult integrity, you have provided him with choices that he can make which are congruent with ensuring his safety. You acknowledge the headaches are not viewed exclusively within the context of suicide.

Exploring precipitants to suicidal thoughts and plans

Rationale

Suicide is an expression of feelings and thoughts. As a nurse it is useful to gain some understanding of what was going on in the person's life that precipitated suicidal intent or behaviour. Asking about suicide does not 'put the idea in the patient's head'. Honesty and trust are the core of the nature of the therapeutic relationship. Openness about the possibility of ending one's life facilitates discussion about the circumstances that can contribute to despair. When a person feels listened to, s/he may be able to tell the clinician if the distress has reached an intolerable point such that suicide feels imminent. Then a clinician can intervene. Careful listening can help the patient learn to identify the triggers behind the thoughts and behaviours. Being able to identify triggering events and feelings, associated with suicidal thoughts and behaviours, can lead to more adaptive problem-solving.

Example

Nurse: 'Fred you have been saying you have no future and you sound very hopeless about everything. I know its very hard to talk about what has been going on in your life but it might be possible that as we talk about what has been going on, together we can look at some ways to find some relief and move forward. For example, it might be helpful to talk about what was happening that led you to start drinking at work'.

Alternative coping strategies

Rationale

Suicide is often seen as the only solution to a problem. It can be the permanent solution to a temporary problem. The overwhelming despair of a crisis can impede rational decision-making. Working with a patient to reframe situations more fully or realistically can be a challenge. However, gradual, and continued assistance to consider alternative, meaningful coping strategies can be helpful.

Example

Nurse: 'You told me that when you are under stress you drink alcohol to excess and this adds to your problems. What other things have you done in the past to solve problems that have not created more difficulties for you'?

At this point you are trying to build on the person's strengths and identify effective coping strategies. Problem-solving needs to be in *small* increments with positive reinforcement for each achievement. Even as you try to move forward you continue to monitor for risk and safety.

NURSE RESPONSES AND REACTIONS TO SUICIDE

A nurse may experience many feelings in the event of a patient's suicide attempt or completed suicide. A sense of helplessness, anger, sadness, a need to rescue, self-blame, frustration, and rejection often leaves the nurse feeling 'manipulated' or 'victimized' by the patient. Clinician's also have their own values regarding suicide, which are grounded in personal, social and cultural history. For example, a nurse who is a young mother may be bewildered and angry at a mother who tries to take her own life, risking leaving her children motherless. Or the nurse's religious beliefs make lead her to judge people who attempt suicide to be morally weak. The occurrence of suicide in a clinical setting can be very distressing for staff and patients. Both groups will need opportunities to talk about their feelings (see below). For patients issues of safety may be foremost. Many clinicians will feel that somehow they did not do enough to save the patient. Despite our best vigilance and assessment, some people will be so determined to die that we cannot stop them. Responses to suicide have been compared to grief responses and post-traumatic stress with clinician's reporting flashbacks, hyper vigilance, insomnia, fear and confusion. It is important for the nurse to be aware of and manage his/her own feelings and responses to the suicidal patient so that therapeutic care is not impeded by the nurse's own internal distress.

After a suicide: caring for the care-giver

Nurses, as individual clinicians and as members of a health care team, require attention to their responses to suicide. Critical stress debriefing sessions are frequently offered to teams who have been affected by this type of trauma. These sessions provide confidential, non-judgemental opportunities for staff to explore their feelings about the event and scenarios leading up to it. Facilitated by a professional who is not a member of the team it provides a forum for sharing and support. Individual nurse supervision and counselling may also play an important role to help the nurse restore clinical confidence and prevent burnout.

CONCLUSION

This chapter has focused on the nursing role of the person who is suicidal. The critical interventions outlined here emphasize the clinical knowledge required to keep the person alive and to start the process of recovery. These interventions are only a part of a longer journey directed at helping the person develop a more positive sense of self or find ways to create meaning and relationships in his or her life.

REFERENCES

1. Bland RC, Newman SC, Dyck RJ. The epidemiology of parasuicide in Edmonton. *Canadian Journal of Psychiatry* 1994; **39**(2): 391–6.

2. Hawton K, Arensman E, Townsend E, *et al.* Deliberate self-harm: systematic review of efficacy of psycho-social and pharmacological treatments in preventing repetition. *British Medical Journal* 1998; **317**: 441–7.

3. Shneidman E. Classifications and approaches. In: *Definition of suicide*. New York: Wiley, 1985: 23–40.

4. Linehan MM. A social-behavioral analysis of suicide and parasuicide: implications for clinical assessment and treatment. In: Clarkin JF, Glazer HI (eds). *Depression, behavioral and directive intervention strategies.* New York: Garland STPM Press, 1981.

5. Kral MJ. Suicide as social logic. *Suicide and life-threatening behavior* 1994; **24**(3): 245–55.

6. Fuse T. *Suicide, individual and society.* Toronto: Canadian Scholars Press, 1997.

7. Asberg M, Traskman L, Thoren P. 5-HIAA in the cerebrospinal fluid: a biochemical suicide predictor? *Archives of General Psychiatry* 1976; **33**: 1193–5.

8. Mann JJ. Psychobiological predictors of suicide. *Journal of Clinical Psychiatry* 1987; **48**(12): 39–43.

9. Beck RW, Morris JB, Beck AT. Cross-validation of the suicidal intent scale *Psychological Reports* 1974; **34**: 445–6.

10. Jacobson G. The inpatient management of suicidality. In: Jacobs D (ed.) *The Harvard Medical School guide to suicide assessment and intervention.* San Francisco: Jossey-Bass Publishers, 1999.

Chapter 29

THE PERSON WHO SELF-HARMS

Ruth Gallop* and Tracey Tully**

INTRODUCTION

Although self-harm is often confused with suicide attempts or suicidal gesturing, survivors cognitively distinguish these activities from attempts to kill themselves, and may in fact self-injure in order to avoid suicide.[1-4] Self-harm can take many forms ranging from intentional self-poisoning to severe body mutilation. This chapter we will focus on self-harm that involves bodily self-injury. Bodily self-injury includes cutting, burning, abrading or hitting oneself, inserting sharp objects in the anus or vagina, pulling out body hair or other self-attacking behaviours that are idiosyncratic to the individual. In the general population, the prevalence of self-harm is in the range of 0.75–4%[5-8] and in clinical populations, 20–40%.[4,5,9,10] In the UK, cutting is the second commonest form of self-harm after overdose.[11] The majority of people who injure their bodies in the ways considered here are women.[12]

Self-injury is often an attempt to communicate distress, relieve pain and maintain connection to oneself and others. Suicide attempts, on the other hand, are directed at discontinuing all connections and ending consciousness (see Chapter 28) However, it is important for nurses not to view self-injury as less serious than a suicide attempt and therefore respond to self-harm with less concern. A history of self-harm is a key predictor for repetition of self-harm and a subsequent completed suicide.[11]

Unfortunately, people who self-harm are often seen in a negative light by health care professionals, including nurses. These individuals may be viewed as attention seeking, manipulative 'bad' patients undeserving of taking up time in an overburdened health care system. Caring for people who self-harm can be very stressful and difficult work. Because our role as mental health nurses is to help people grow and make sense of life events, it is often frightening and frustrating when people, in spite of our best efforts, continue to self-harm. The risk of working with these individuals is that we respond to our frustration and seeming lack of ability to help with anger and rejection.

For the nurse to retain a balanced caring view of these patients so the nurse can engage in a therapeutic relationship requires an understanding of the function of self-harm and the skill to engage in a relationship that is neither too caring nor too rejecting. Acquiring that knowledge and finding the balance that enables appro-

*Ruth Gallop is Professor, Faculty of Nursing and Department of Psychiatry, University of Toronto, Toronto, Canada. Her research, clinical work and writing focus on clients' perceived as treatment and management challenges. These clients often receive diagnoses of borderline personality disorders, have histories of severe early trauma and current self-harm behaviours.

**Tracey Tully is a Clinical Nurse Specialist in the Women Recovering from Abuse Program (WRAP) at the Women's College Ambulatory Care Centre of Sunnybrook and Women's College Health Sciences Centre in Toronto, Canada, and a doctoral candidate in the Faculty of Nursing at the University of Toronto.

priate boundaries in the nurse–patient relationship to be maintained will be the focus of this chapter.

EARLY TRAUMA AND SELF-INJURY

Recent studies indicate that the overwhelming majority of individuals who self-injure have a history of childhood trauma. Childhood trauma can include neglect, emotional, physical, or sexual abuse, or experiences such as prolonged separation from parents for reasons such as serious illness or war. It is estimated that between 79% and 96% of individuals who cut themselves were victims of childhood abuse or neglect.[4,5,13,14] Within the mental health system, the research has shown that certain diagnoses are strongly associated with trauma and self-harm (see Chapter 35). These include *borderline personality disorder*, and *dissociative identity disorder*. As research about self-injury remains in its early stages, the particular nature of the relationship between trauma and self-harm has not yet been fully determined. However, it is thought that one possible link between early trauma and self-injury lies in the set of fundamental beliefs about oneself and others that arise from a history of trauma. We do know that the earlier the age of abuse, the closer the relationship of the abuser and the longer the duration of abuse, the worse the self-harm.[15] What is clear is that people who self-harm have a negative view of themselves. They think they are bad, worthless and powerless. Feelings about their badness and awfulness are overwhelming and experienced as never-ending. Emotions are viewed as dangerous and potentially engulfing, and the individual does not trust their capacity to pass through intense emotions safely. Further, the self-injuring individual often lacks the words to name or describe the emotional experiences, thus adding to the distress. Action becomes the way to deal with overwhelming emotions and the body becomes the place for attack.

FUNCTIONS OF SELF-INJURY

Recently, several authors have proposed a number of psychological functions that self-injury may serve for an individual.[1,2,12,16,17] Self-injury may serve the purpose of re-enacting early trauma or abuse-related experiences and can render one powerless. Therefore, the act of inflicting harm on oneself may be a way to exert control, mastery, personal agency, and autonomy in a life that seems otherwise chaotic and uncontrollable. One self-injuring woman commented:

> When I cut myself, I am the only one who has a say over how badly I am treated. I get to choose for myself how

severely I hurt myself and when I want to stop. I wish I could have said this about the abuse I got from my father.

The self-loathing that many traumatized women experience may generalize into thinking of both the self and the body as bad and ugly. In physical and sexual abuse, the body was violated and this abuse included both emotional and physical boundary violation. These boundary violations may lead to self-injury that temporarily helps define the body boundaries. Cutting the external body symbolically attacks the internal badness. Because of boundary confusion this represents (symbolically) an attack on the abuser.

Self-harm may also function to regain equilibrium, both emotionally and physiologically, when ability to self-soothe or sense of control is impaired. Self-harm is often a means to soothe oneself or create a sense of calm and equilibrium in overwhelming situations. In their early development, comforting experiences by nurturing care-givers have, generally, been absent in the lives of people who self-harm. As such, they did not acquire the internal ability to comfort themselves when in distress, and are unable to rely on more sophisticated means of coping in adulthood.[18] As one woman poignantly stated:

> When I'm feeling all alone, like nobody in the world cares about me, I have a very strong urge to cut myself. Some people are able to ask for a hug during a time like this. Other people can listen to a favorite piece of music, or eat comforting foods. I only know how to be calmed by cutting myself. My parents never showed me any love, only pain and suffering, so now I have no way of showing myself love.

Another woman said:

> Before I cut I feel like a volcano about to erupt. The feeling is so overwhelming that I literally feel like I will explode if I don't self-injure. As soon as I do it's like all that is built up inside is released.

Management and maintenance of dissociative processes may also be a function of self-injury. Dissociation is the compartmentalizing of experiences so they can be split off from consciousness. The act of harming oneself may move one into a dissociative state when escape from painful emotions or memories is needed. In this way, self-injury may provide needed distance and numbness. Conversely, self-harm may be a way to return one to a sense of reality, to remind oneself that one is alive after being stuck in a state of numbness. Another woman said:

> When I cut myself and see the blood flow out of me I know that I am alive. I spend so much of my life feeling nothing, feeling detached from the body I live in. I desperately want to feel something, anything, other than nothingness.

Self-injury may also serve to express feelings, such as guilt, shame, rage, or communicate needs. People who self-injure may not know the words, or trust the power of their words, to convey their pain. As a consequence, they may rely on their injuries as a way to speak for them, or as a means of having their needs met. As one person explained:

> I don't know how to talk about what I'm feeling, I only know how to act on it. I realize this is a big problem because lots of people think I'm trying to get attention. Just because I got somebody's attention when I cut, it doesn't mean that I was trying to get their attention.

It is also important to consider when self-harm occurs. Cutting rarely occurs in the presence of others – whether family, friends or clinicians. It may occur minutes, hours or days *after* being in the presence of another. The benefit of being in the presence of another can drain away very quickly. Being alone invites the overwhelming pain and affect associated with the trauma and self-badness to start to be experienced.

Finally as we consider the functions of self-harm it is apparent that self-harm is used to deal with intense, often overwhelming emotional states. In all of the quotations above self-harm is experienced as an effective, reliable although problematic, means by which to decrease the intensity of one's distress. The critical feature is that the feelings are intolerable and must be stopped and cutting serves a self-soothing capacity to relieve this distress.

Although an external activity, cutting shares some features with an internalized sense of soothing and object constancy, cutting can be relied upon to be available on demand to comfort and diminish pain. Cutting unlike the childhood trauma is within the control of the individual. Of course the relief it brings is short-lived and often leads to shame and guilt at the activity and so the cycle of pain, relief, shame starts again.

SELF-INJURY IN OTHER POPULATIONS

Mental health nurses need to be aware of other populations in which self-harm may occur.

❑ **Psychotic populations.** While self-injury among individuals with a negative sense of self and/or trauma history generally follows a pattern of high frequency and low severity, psychotic individuals who self-harm may do so infrequently and sustain serious injuries. The most severe acts of self-injury are to be found in the psychotic population. Self-injury may take the form of limb amputation, autocastration, or removal of eyes. These extreme acts are generally performed in response to disturbances in thoughts or perceptions such as persecutory or somatic delusions or command hallucinations.

❑ **Forensic populations.** As many as 50% of incarcerated individuals exhibit self-injurious behaviours. However, only about 10% pose a serious threat to themselves. However, due to the nature of the prison system, all attempts are treated as potentially life-threatening, which means that prisoners are transferred to the medical wing for treatment, an environment that is more tolerable than the general prison population. This has led some to suggest that self-injury among prisoners is motivated by secondary gain. Further research needs to be done in this area to gain knowledge of all possible functions of this behaviour. Given that many individuals in the forensic system have experienced violence, the functions of their self-injury may be similar to those seen in traumatized women. In addition, one must consider that self-injury among prisoners may be a form of stimulating oneself in a monotonous environment.

❑ **Developmentally or physiologically impaired populations.** Individuals who suffer from Lesch–Nyan syndrome, autism, deLange syndrome, and Tourette's syndrome generally exhibit self-injurious behaviours. The type of self-injurious behaviour that may be observed in these individuals includes self-directed head banging, biting, hitting, or slapping. The behaviour is generally repetitive and rhythmic in nature and occurs with much higher frequency, often for several hours daily, than in the population of traumatized women who self-injure. It is generally accepted that the behaviour provides sensory stimulation, or is consistent with obsessionality, impulsivity, compulsivity, or motor tics.

❑ **Socially sanctioned self-injury.** The anthropology, theology, and sociology literature offer several accounts of self-injury. Generally these self-injurious acts are performed as rites of passage, or as a way of joining, remaining part of, or demonstrating one's commitment to a group.[19] Injuries may include self-flagellation, facial scarification, insertion of objects under the skin, or other self-mutilative acts that are consistent with cultural or religious practices.

THE NURSING ROLE

Case study 29.1

Jane is a young woman with a long history of abuse perpetrated by various family members. Throughout most of her life she has told herself that she is a terrible, evil, dirty person for what happened to her. She believes that she deserves nothing good in her life and that she will achieve very little. Jane attempts to cope with her overwhelming sense of badness and worthlessness and her intense feelings of shame, fear and anger by cutting her forearms, thighs and breasts. She is requesting help at this time because her self-injury is worsening in both frequency and severity and is beginning to affect her work performance.

Establishing and maintaining clear and consistent boundaries

Rationale

Providing clear, reliable, consistent expectations of the relationship are essential. During your first meeting it is very important to establish a framework for working within the therapeutic relationship. This is important for work with all clients, but especially critical for trauma survivors who self-injure because their boundaries have been violated so severely. They have not known safe, reliable people and therefore have no expectations that someone will be safe and reliable.

> **Example:** You first meet Jane when she arrives at an outpatient mental health clinic requesting to talk to someone about her self-injury. Near the end of the first session Jane asks if she can have a hug from you.

You recognize this request could be potentially a boundary transgression, and should be considered carefully. Many survivors of childhood trauma have confusing reactions around physical touch. Touch may have been sexualized or associated with physical violence. As such, many mental health professionals develop a guideline around the use of touch so as not to re-play an earlier dynamic. This becomes your first opportunity to put into action the words you communicated about boundaries and conveys the importance of consistency in your message. It is critical that the discussion that follows her request does not have a punitive or rejecting tone, to which she will already be sensitive. Instead, ensure the discussion conveys your empathy and an openness to discuss her request. The following is one way that you *might* proceed with this request.

Nurse: 'Thank you for asking, Jane, however, a hug is something that I feel we need to talk about. As we are coming to the end of our time together today we can talk about this for a few minutes [adhering to the time frame is another way of maintaining consistent boundaries]. It seems that you have experienced some strong feelings today. Part of the work that we'll be doing together is putting into words what you feel inside of your body. Do you have an awareness of what you were feeling about

me or about our time together today when you asked for a hug'?

Jane: 'Nobody has ever listened to me like you did today. Most people think I'm crazy for what I do and they just tell me to stop or they won't see me any more. I felt that you cared about me. I wanted to see if that was really true because when people care for each other they hug'.

Nurse: 'So is it fair to say that you were feeling close to me and you were curious about how I was feeling about you'?

Jane: 'Yes'.

Nurse: 'I also felt that we had a nice connection today and I would agree with you that many close relationships involve physical touch and intimacy. However, this relationship is unlike others that you may have in your life, therefore many of the social norms you are used to will be quite different in our relationship. Hugging is one of those areas that is different in this relationship. A hug can seem like a simple gesture to communicate caring, but I am more comfortable using my words to express how I'm feeling. This is also one of the goals that we will be working on – to help you move away from using actions to express feelings and towards using your words. I appreciate your courage for asking me for a hug. You may leave today and have some more feelings about this conversation. I encourage you to take note of what you may be thinking and feeling and I invite you to raise these thoughts and feelings with me when we meet next week'.

Note how the nurse *supported* Jane and *confirmed* her connection to Jane. This will help to comfort and soothe her. Many nurses might feel the urge to hug Jane because her life has been so painful and to deny her could feel cruel and rejecting for a nurse. Further it can be very rewarding to know that a client experienced you as caring and you want to maintain that feeling. However, it is also important for the nurse to realize that Jane's emptiness cannot be filled in the short term by hugs or creating dependencies. Instead, she requires your help with developing the internal capacity to comfort herself so that she can begin to care for her own needs.

Boundary-related issues can take many forms with clients who self-harm. Below are three further examples of situations that require the nurse to be able to reflect on her own needs in the relationship. These situations can be the basis for further discussion of boundaries. After each we have given one of many possible explanations for conflict in the nurse as s/he responds. Nurses need to be aware of their own responses and seek help and supervision when confused about reactions and actions.

Vignettes illustrating boundary issues:

1 A client asks you if you self-injure or if you have a history of trauma; you may think that revealing your own history will make the client feel more understood.

2 A client asks you to place a brief call to him/her every day. You believe you really understand this person and by being available can effect real change.

3 A client asks if he/she can extend his/her appointments with you by 15 minutes. You don't have anything planned so this request feels reasonable.

Ensuring responsibility for change lies with the client

Rationale

Communicating the message that you believe a client is capable of keeping him/herself safe minimizes the potential for power struggles and offers an opportunity for the client to reflect on internal resources that can be called upon when making changes.

> **Example:** Jane asks if you require her to sign a contract stating that she will not engage in self-injury.

Nurse: 'It is our belief that contracts aren't a useful way for you to learn how to keep yourself safe. Instead, we are going to work together to build your belief that you can cope with distress by not self-injuring'.

As nurses, we cannot be anyone's constant protector. Rather, we need to work towards helping clients keep themselves safe. Clients may have difficulty maintaining a contract and then feel shameful that they have betrayed the contract. One client said:

> I've signed lots of papers saying I won't cut, but when I really want to cut and I'm in that dark place I don't care that I signed my name to something. It's just a piece of paper that doesn't mean anything. I can find lots of places on my body where I can cut and nobody will know about it.

Asking a client to sign a 'no-harm contract' is likely serving the nurse's, rather than the client's needs. It may help the nurse to feel less anxious and protected from litigation, but it does little to encourage responsibility and empowerment.

Exploring the functions that self-injury serves for the individual

Rationale

Early in the therapeutic relationship it is important to explore the various ways in which self-injury has been helpful as well as the ways in which it has been unhelpful. Acknowledging the adaptive qualities of the behaviour communicates a message of non-judgement and non-blame. This serves to strengthen your alliance. In addition, it provides important clinical information for both of you.

> **Example:** On Jane's second appointment with you she tells you that yesterday she overheard two women in a shop commenting on the scars to her forearms. One woman wondered if she had been in an accident. The other woman disagreed and stated, 'I heard about this from my friend who works in a hospital. These people are total freaks. They're absolutely nuts. They can't control themselves and need to be locked up in psych wards and even tied to the bed'.

Jane: 'I must be your craziest patient. I'm sure you tell all of your friends about the freak who hacks at herself. I almost didn't come back to see you because I'm afraid you'll have me locked away'.

Nurse: 'This sounds as if this was a very powerful experience for you. It seems that you are wondering if I judge you in a similar way'.

Jane: 'Yeah'.

Nurse: 'I want to be clear that I do not believe that you are crazy. I think it's also important for you to know that hospitalization for self-injury is not a recommended form of treatment. I see you as doing your very best to cope with what life has thrown you [acknowledging the adaptive quality of self-injury]. From what you have already told me about your early life, it makes sense that you chose self-injury as a way of coping with distress. Self-harm can be a very effective, although ultimately destructive way of dealing with pain. As with all ways of coping that are not beneficial in the long run, eventually they stop working as effectively, or they get in the way of living the life you want. Because you have come for help with your self-injury you have already acknowledged that your self-injury is no longer working for you in the way it once did. Perhaps we can use this as an opportunity to talk about the various ways that self-harm has helped to get though life. We can also talk about the ways that it gets in the way of your life. This may give you some insights into the reaction that you had with the women in the shop'.

At the end of this discussion, it may be useful to engage in a teaching piece around the functions of self-injury that have been previously identified. A reading list of books or articles can be very useful. This may serve to normalize her experience. Also encourage Jane to consider the ways in which her self-injury is no longer serving her well. What are the areas in her life that are affected by this way of coping? Examining the drawbacks of self-injury may assist with motivation for change.

Informing a client that inpatient admission is not ideal may also reassure her. After a careful assessment in Accident and Emergency where suicidality is ruled out, inpatient admission should be avoided, as it is often a hothouse for regression and re-enactment of previous conflictual relationships in this population.

Openness to engage in dialogue about self–injury

Rationale

Openness functions to decrease shame, stigma, and secrecy of the act. It also communicates that you can tolerate all of who they are and not reject or abandon them. For those women whose self-injury occasionally functions to communicate an aspect of themselves, open dialogue and acceptance of the behaviour (not to be confused with condoning) encourages verbal forms of expression, rather than merely physical means. Finally, it can provide a means of gathering further information about her self-injury that is essential to consider when preparing for changing behaviour.

> **Example:**
>
> Nurse: 'We have spent some time talking about the ways that self-injury serves you well. We have also talked about some of the drawbacks. Before we talk about how you might change your self-injury, we need to have more information about other aspects of your self-injury'.

Let this be an opportunity to explore and gather information about the following areas:

❑ Interpersonal stressors related to self-injury.
❑ Situational triggers to self-injury, both internal and external.
❑ The thought process that accompanies self-injury, both before and after the episode.
❑ The overwhelming affect that is associated with self-injury, both before and after the episode.
❑ The confusing and threatening physiological responses that are experienced.
❑ The role of flashbacks and dissociation.

Goal setting

Rationale

While it is essential that we be empathic when working with individuals who self-injure, empathy alone is not sufficient. We need to convey to people who self-harm that if they want to, together we can work to change things. Goals need to be modest, attainable and mutually agreed upon.

Nurse: 'As a way to plan the remainder of the time, it is important that we focus on what you would like to achieve by the end of our time together. Have you thought about this'?

Jane: 'Last time we met I thought a lot about all the parts of my self-injury that we talked about. I never thought much about my triggers, my feelings, my thoughts and the other aspects of my self-injury. I might like to work on decreasing the amount that I self-harm'.

Nurse: 'That sounds like a goal that would be reasonable to work on in the time frame we have. You told me that you are cutting yourself weekly at present. When you say you want to decrease the frequency, do you have a sense of by how much you would like to decrease'? [Ask Jane to get very specific and break down her goal into something measurable.]

Jane: 'I would feel a lot better if I cut down to once a month'.

In addition to identifying her goal, there are also other areas to consider when working towards change. The following area should also be explored with Jane:

❑ Why does she think this is an important goal to work on?
❑ Who does she need to have on her side to achieve this goal? What supports are essential?
❑ Who will not be helpful to have in her life when she is working toward this change?
❑ What might get in the way of achieving this goal and how will she manage this potential barrier?

Self-care of injuries

Rationale

A client you have a relationship with may come to you having self-injured. While you are concerned about the self-injury, your primary concern once you have established that urgent care is not needed is to focus on understanding triggers and developing alternative coping methods. Avoid turning excessive focus to the actual injury.

> Jane arrives for her appointment and she informs you that she cut her arm 2 hours ago. You can see through her shirt sleeve that the wound is bleeding.

It is important that you remain calm and do not respond as if the injury is a crisis. Remember that most cutting can be tended to with basic first aid. Ask Jane to reveal the injury. Assess the severity of the cut and establish the need for sutures. If you establish that she does not require medical intervention, encourage Jane to tend to her own wounds, that is, direct her to the first aid kit at your clinic and invite her to use the washroom or an unoccupied private space. Since she has been self-injuring for many years, she is well aware of the appropriate intervention. If she is not, suggest that she apply pressure, irrigate the wound, dress the wound, keep it clean, and monitor for infection.

Once Jane has returned from tending to her cut, invite her to talk about what triggered the self-injury, that is, encourage her to put into words what she enacted on her body. At this time it is important not to focus the details of the act of injuring or the wound itself.

Use of distraction techniques

Rationale

The nature of the distraction activity may reduce its benefit. Maintaining a focus on immediate action to cope with overwhelming emotions reinforces a sense of urgency. Finding activities that reduce tension and reduce the urge rather than distract from the urge are more useful.

> Jane arrives for her appointment and tells you that she was surfing the Internet for self-harm websites. She tells you that several of the websites suggest using techniques such as rubbing ice on one's forearm, snapping elastic bands on wrists. She tells you that these techniques are apparently good because they distract from the urge to self-harm. She wants to know what you think about this.

While this is a relatively common technique that is suggested, we do not recommend this approach as it sends the message that one still needs to take immediate action when the urge to self-harm presents itself. If an individual responds to the urge to self-injure with another action (e.g. applying ice) s/he has already started to follow a similar pattern which may lead to self-injuring. Instead, we encourage working towards a place where action is not needed. That is, where she can sit with distressing thoughts, sensations, feelings without experiencing this as intolerable. As one woman stated:

> In the last group I was in I learned a lot about distracting myself when I wanted to cut. This did not work for me at all. It was like a band-aid that covered up the real problem that was going on. They would tell me to use an ice cube or rubber band on my wrist when I want to cut. I thought this was a bunch of crap. It's like they don't get it that I want to stop doing destructive things to myself. Besides, by the time I get to the point of wanting to hurt myself, it's too late, the train is already going 100 mph and I can't stop it. I need to learn how to not let the train out of the station.

The development of alternative methods of comforting oneself, or dealing with affect is an important part of the work. This will happen over time. For example, you can work together to develop a list of activities that make a person feel less agitated, e.g. bathing, music, writing a diary.

CONCLUSION

Working with a person who self-harms is demanding work. In addition to her responsibilities towards the person in care, the nurse needs to look after herself, through maintaining supportive networks, engaging in pleasurable activities, and finding a balance between personal and professional pursuits. Clinical supervision should be available to all psychiatric-mental health nurses. However, for nurses engaged in work with people who self-harm, supervision is essential (see Chapter 64). Like other areas of psychiatric-mental health nursing, this work is grounded in the therapeutic relationship (see Chapter 17). The specific knowledge about self-harm is layered upon this fundamental therapeutic use of self.

REFERENCES

1. Babiker G, Arnold L. *The language of injury: comprehending self-mutilation.* Leicester: The British Psychological Press, 1997.
2. Connors R. Self-injury in trauma survivors: 1. Functions and meanings. *American Journal of Orthopsychiatry* 1996; **66**: 197–206.
3. Himber J. Blood rituals: self-cutting in female psychiatric inpatients. *Psychotherapy* 1994; **31**: 620–31.
4. van der Kolk B, Perry JC, Herman JL. Childhood origins of self-destructive behaviour. *American Journal of Psychiatry* 1991; **148**: 1665–71.
5. Briere J, Gil E. Self-mutilation in clinical and general population samples: Prevalence, correlates, and functions. *American Journal of Orthopsychiatry* 1998; **68**: 609–20.
6. Favazza AR, Conterio K. The plight of chronic self-mutilators. *Community Mental Health Journal* 1988; **24**: 22–30.
7. Pattison EM, Kahan J. The deliberate self-harm syn-

drome. *American Journal of Psychiatry* 1983; **140**: 867–72.

8. Whitehead PC, Johnson FG, Ferrence R. Measuring the incidence of self-injury: Some methodological and design considerations. *American Journal of Orthopsychiatry* 1973; **43**: 142–8.

9. Evans C, Lacey JH. Multiple self-damaging behaviour among alcoholic women: a prevalence study. *British Journal of Psychiatry*, **161**: 643–7.

10. Zlotnick C, Mattia JL, Zimmerman M. Clinical correlates of self-mutilation in a sample of general psychiatric patients. *Journal of Nervous and Mental Diseases* 1999; **187**: 296–301.

11. NHS Centre for Reviews and Dissemination. Deliberate self-harm. *Effective Health Care*, 1998; **4**: 1–12. University of York.

12. Conterio K, Lader W. *Bodily harm: the breakthrough healing program for self-injurers*. New York: Hyperion, 1998.

13. Romans SE, Martin JL, Anderson JC, Herbison GP, Mullen PE. Sexual abuse in childhood and deliberate self-harm. *American Journal of Psychiatry* 1995; **152**: 1336–42.

14. Zlotnick C, Shea MT, Pearlstein T, Simpson E, Costello E, Begin A. The relationship between dissociate symptoms, alexithymia, impulsivity, sexual abuse, and self-mutilation. *Comprehensive Psychiatry* 1996; **37**: 12–16.

15. Stone MH. Some thoughts on the dynamics and therapy of self-mutilating borderline patients. *Journal of Personality Disorders* 1987; **1**: 347–9.

16. Miller D. *Women who hurt themselves*. New York: Basic Books, 1994.

17. Suyemoto KL. The functions of self-mutilation. *Clinical Psychology Review* 1998; **18**: 531–54.

18. Gallop R. The failure of the capacity for self-soothing in women who have a history of abuse and self-harm. Journal of American Psychiatric Nurses Association, 2002; **8**: 20–26.

19. Favazza AR. *Bodies under siege: self-mutilation and body modification in culture and psychiatry*. Baltimore, MD: Johns Hopkins University Press, 1996.

Chapter 30

THE PERSON WHO HEARS DISTURBING VOICES

Cheryl Forchuk* and Elsabeth Jensen**

---

1 Michael sat alone in the TV room on the inpatient psychiatric ward. 'NO, NO, NO! I will not do THAT! Now you leave me alone! Shut up! Get out of here!'

A student nurse, Donovan, stood in the doorway. Michael was his assigned patient for the day. How should he approach him?

2 Sally greeted the community nurse, Suchita with a smile and a cup of tea. 'Sometimes, I think you and St Georgette are the only two true friends I have in the world'.

After a few minutes of conversation, Suchita inquired: 'So, how are you finding that new medication?'

'Terrible!' replied Sally, 'It was drowning St Georgette so I could barely hear her – so I had to stop taking it right away'.

3 'I'm really loving this "Women in History" course. It really has me thinking', Ngozi explained to her room-mate. 'But after today's class, one thing keeps coming back to me. If Joan of Arc were alive today – wouldn't we just say she was hallucinating and drug her up or lock her up?'

'Well', replied Nadine, 'how do we know she didn't have schizophrenia?'

VOICES AS AN EXAMPLE OF HALLUCINATIONS

Nurses will frequently encounter people who are hearing disturbing voices. 'Hearing voices' is frequently described as an auditory hallucination. Hallucinations can involve any sense. For example, in addition to auditory hallucinations there are visual hallucinations, olfactory hallucinations, taste hallucinations and tactile hallucinations. Something is generally described as a hallucination if others cannot perceive it.

Different kinds of situations may make different kinds of hallucinations more likely. For example, hearing voices or auditory hallucinations is quite common in people with a diagnosis of schizophrenia. It is therefore a phenomenon encountered quite regularly by psychiatric/mental health nurses. Visual hallucinations are more likely in a drug-induced situation, for example someone who has taken street drugs such as PCP or LSD, or someone on opiates for pain control. Tactile hallucinations are common during drug withdrawal. For example, someone suffering from alcoholism may complain it feels like 'bugs are crawling all over' during withdrawal. Taste hallucinations are more rare but, in our experience, have occasionally been noted with a drug-induced psychosis. All of these depictions are generalizations. For example, although people diagnosed with schizophrenia typically have auditory hallucinations hearing voices, they can also sometimes report visual hallucinations (seeing things).

*Cheryl Forchuk is a Professor in the School of Nursing, University of Western Ontario Canada, with a cross appointment in the Department of Psychiatry, Faculty of Medicine and Dentistry. She is a Scientist at the Lawson Health Research Institute/London Health Sciences Centre.

**Elsabeth Jensen is a Research Coordinator in mental health nursing research, an Adjunct Assistant Professor in the School of Nursing, Faculty of Health Sciences, University of Western Ontario, a Lecturer in the Continuing Education Department of Fanshawe College, and has a private practice in health counselling in London, Ontario.

Another distinction sometimes made is the distinction between a hallucination and an illusion. Both phenomena involve perceiving something that is not perceived by others. However, an illusion is based on the apparent misperception of something that can be seen by others. For example, a person may see something more sinister in a shadow – but others can, at least, see the shadow. Or, people may hear a ringing bell, but not that the bell is calling out a name.

As the scenario with Suchita and Sally illustrates, not all auditory hallucinations are disturbing. An early study[1] found that the relationship one had with the 'voice' was often an indicator of chronicity. People who had lived with their voices for a long time would sometimes develop a positive relationship with them. Miller, O'Connor and DiPasquale[2] found that the majority of patients who were hallucinating reported some positive effects of hallucinations. These attitudes did not change after treatment, but those people with more positive experiences of hallucinations were more likely to continue hallucinating after treatment. Romme[3] compared 'patients' who heard voices to those that had not been identified as patients and found that non-patients were more likely to report a positive experience with the voices. They concluded that hearing voices lay on a continuum with normal functioning.

In a previous study[4] Forchuk asked individuals with chronic mental illnesses about their social support. Almost all of the 124 clients in the study reported very small social networks (friends to whom they could turn for help). In two situations, the clients reported that their only supports were the community nurse and their 'voices'. In another two situations the only supports were the community nurse and a pet. When one has a very small social network, each individual in the network is very important. So, although the nurse or others may perceive the auditory hallucination as a *symptom*, the client may perceive it as a close friend. Obviously, these things need to be discussed and understood for nurses to be able to work with clients on their goals and not simply on their own assumptions of what constitutes a problem.

Interestingly, the idea that someone would have a relationship with a hallucination is not new to nursing. Nursing theorist Hildegard Peplau[5,6] adopted Harry Stacks Sullivan's[7] definition of interpersonal relationships. Interpersonal relationships are defined as any relationship involving two or more people. All but one of the people may be illusory.

Clearly, not all auditory hallucinations are disturbing. Does that mean they are not a problem? This is also a complex issue, and begs the question, a problem for whom? A client of mine would spend all day in her room. It was difficult to encourage her to get her off her bed for meals or even to go to the washroom. In discussing the issue with her, she described why she spent so much time in bed. She was listening to a centuries old conversation among several angels, and sometimes if she was lucky she would hear God as well. They were discussing plans for the great flood. Details about the animals and the geography kept her fascinated for hours on end. How could she leave for lunch and miss the possibility of hearing God's input to the conversation? Were these voices a problem? She had lost contact with almost all her family and her level of functioning on a day-to-day basis was dramatically reduced by her constant focus on the voices. On the other hand, she saw herself as an important person, and involved in an important process. She felt that without her voices she would be 'nothing'. Not all auditory hallucinations interfere with functioning or the person's activities of daily living. These things need careful evaluation together with the client.

Some hallucinations are horrifically disturbing. Clients have described hearing screaming, tortured voices pleading with them for relief. Others have described taunting, insulting voices that can issue commands (called command hallucinations) such as to jump off a bridge or strangle a friend. Frequently, disturbing voices list every fault of the client before them and tell them that they are worthless or evil.

Clients have experienced multiple disturbing voices that make contact with another human being very difficult to even sort out among the other voices. Sometimes, in these situations, there are insulting voices and friendly voices all speaking at once, clamouring to be heard. The nurse trying to speak is simply one more voice competing for attention.

WHY DO SOME PEOPLE HEAR VOICES?

Beyerstein[8] stated that: 'Anything that prompts a move from word based thinking to imagistic or pictorial thinking predisposes a person to hallucinating'. He further states that things which bias 'the brain's representational system towards memory images at the expense of sensory information can also predispose to hallucinating'.

Voices as a symptom of psychosis

Hearing voices is most commonly considered a symptom of psychosis. Psychosis is a break with reality. Psychosis may accompany many different kinds of situations. People may experience psychosis as part of an illness experience (e.g. schizophrenia, a manic or depressive phase of a bi-polar disorder, Wernicke's syndrome, high fever, or a brain tumour); it may be experienced with extremely stressful situations, e.g. Intensive Care Unit/ICU psychosis, post-traumatic stress syndrome, massive losses, culture shock, a medication side-effect (e.g. disulfaram/antabuse, opiates), illicit drug use (hallucinogens such as LSD, PCP), or a symptom of withdrawal from an addictive drug (e.g. alcohol, barbiturates). Delusions and disorganized thinking are other symptoms of psychosis.

Auditory hallucinations as a common symptom of schizophrenia

Although there are many causes of psychosis, mental health nurses will encounter this symptom most commonly among people who have been diagnosed with schizophrenia. Someone with schizophrenia is generally not psychotic all the time. They typically have periods of wellness between acute psychotic episodes. The pattern of psychosis and wellness varies considerably among individuals. For a few people, the symptoms of psychosis are chronic in nature and are unremitting, that is, the symptoms do not fluctuate with acute periods followed by periods of wellness.

Hallucinations are considered to be a 'positive' symptom of schizophrenia. This means that they are present in schizophrenia, but not present in the 'normal' population. Other positive symptoms are delusions (unusual belief symptoms, described more fully in Chapter 31), and disorganized thinking. The 'negative' symptoms of schizophrenia are symptoms that reflect something is 'missing'. These include a lack of energy, a lack of motivation, emotional withdrawal, and difficulty in abstract thinking. The experience of psychosis also varies considerably among individuals with schizophrenia. Some people may be more troubled by the positive symptoms, others by negative symptoms or a combination of both.

Men typically develop symptoms of schizophrenia in their late teens, while women typically develop the first symptoms in their early twenties. This means that men may be less likely to have completed vocational training or become independent from their family of orientation before developing the illness. Women are more likely to have completed their schooling and may have started families of their own, when the symptoms first strike. This difference in age of onset can create very different treatment and rehabilitation issues. For example, someone who has had the symptoms at a young age may need a lot of assistance to meet educational and vocational goals. Someone who developed the illness at a later age may have completed more developmental tasks and have additional strengths to draw on. On the other hand, there may be issues related to coping within the family of procreation. It must be understood, that these are generalizations and the specific issues still need exploring with each individual.

Auditory hallucinations as a symptom of dissociative identity disorder

Disturbing voices are also experienced by people diagnosed with dissociative identity disorder (also known as multiple personality disorder).[9,10] This condition is usually a consequence of serious, life-threatening sexual abuse early in life. During periods when one personality is in charge, the voices of one or more other personalities are talking, sometimes to each other. These voices are experienced as being inside the head. Some voices can be frightening. The person may hear the voice(s) suggesting self-harm or suicide. The person hearing the voices will often believe they are 'going crazy'. As a result, they are often reluctant to disclose that they hear voices for fear they will be locked away.

In cases of dissociative identity disorder, medication is usually ineffective. The intervention of choice is psychotherapy with a therapist sensitive to the issues of childhood sexual abuse, and skilled in working with people with personality disorders.

Biological reasons

The biology of actual perceptions and imagined perceptions appear to be the same.[8] This has been demonstrated with studies using EEG recordings and PET scans.[11-13] Beyerstein[8] states:

> Because functionally equivalent states of the central awareness system can arise from either memory or sensory sources, it is possible for dreams, perceptual memories, fantasies and hallucinations to become indistinguishable from real events. Hallucinations result whenever internal events trigger a pattern of brain activity equivalent to that normally generated when sense organs respond to a publicly observable event.

Spiritual and cultural reasons

There may also be reasons for hearing voices that are spiritual/religious or cultural reasons. Within many traditions, it is considered normal to be able to communicate with the dead including friends, relatives or even strangers. Similarly, many cultures would value communication with a spiritual power, spiritual guide, angel or higher being that may not have been previously alive on earth. Also, many people believe in a sixth sense that allows them to see or hear things that others do not. It is extremely important in these situations to be aware of cultural and family norms and not pathologize a spiritual situation. Often, involving other community members or family members can help to understand what kind of process is occurring. For example, in North America, many first nations (indigenous) people would be expected to communicate with a spirit guide. In the Northwest Territories of Canada the mental health legislation includes consultation with a first nations elder, to determine if an involuntary admission status is appropriate if the potential patient is native. The assessment is complex and includes both a mental health specialist and a native elder since just because one has a spirit guide, it does not mean that one cannot suffer a psychosis or auditory hallucination.

Interpersonal reasons

Hildegard Peplau also described the potential interpersonal development of auditory hallucinations. She believed that hallucinations could develop to avoid anxiety and to mitigate loneliness. She describes this as developing through four stages.[6,14] These stages were further elaborated by Clack.[15]

The stages of hallucinations are:

1 **Comforting** – The individual feels lonely and/or anxious and finds that focusing on comforting thoughts relieves the discomfort. At this stage the thoughts are clearly understood to be one's own.

2 **Condemning** – The person continues to court similar relief and increasing reliance on illusory figures to meet needs. The individuals gradually put themselves into a 'listening' mode and are unable to control their own awareness.

3 **Controlling** – There is a marked loss of ability to focus awareness, indicated by withdrawal from others in order to interact with the hallucination, the person gives up trying to combat the hallucination and may feel lonely when the voices leave.

4 **Conquering** – The voices become increasingly threatening, particularly when commands are not followed. There is a failure of strategies to conceal ongoing interactions with hallucinations. There is a continued loss of control over concentration and awareness.

INTERVENTIONS TO ASSIST WITH HEARING PROBLEMATIC VOICES

Assessing problematic voices

Before any intervention can be planned an assessment is needed. The nurse may simply ask the individual if they are hearing any unusual voices. It also needs to be ascertained as to whether or not the individual considers experiencing such voices to be a problem or not. Occasionally, a person who is experiencing problematic voices will deny this, or be unable to confirm this due to language or cognitive difficulties. Behaviours to note would include looking at a specific area where nothing is obviously present, talking to someone that others do not see, or giggling/laughing to oneself. Obviously, any of these behaviours can have other explanations, so one must be careful to observe and try to confirm but not to jump to conclusions.

Medical approaches

The primary medical approach to treat psychosis is with the use of anti-psychotic medications (also called neuroleptics, or major tranquillizers). Nurses are involved in administering the medications, observing for the effectiveness of the medications, and monitoring for side-effects.

Anti-psychotic or neuroleptic medications are used mainly to treat schizophrenia but can also be used in manic states and delirium.[16] These medications are not curative and thus do not eliminate the underlying thought disorder. Rather they may allow the patient to function in a supportive environment.[16]

Neuroleptic medications fall into two broad categories. The traditional agents (e.g. haloperidol, chlorpromazine) function by primarily blocking dopamine receptors. They are most effective in treating positive symptoms of schizophrenia such as delusions, hallucinations, and thought disorders. The newer neuroleptics (e.g. clozapine, olanzapine) function by blocking serotonin receptors. They are most effective with patients resistant to traditional anti-psychotics and are especially useful in treating negative symptoms of schizophrenia such as withdrawal, blunted emotions, and a reduced ability to relate to people.[16]

Side-effects from the use of neuroleptic drugs occur in almost all patients. These are significant in up to 80% of patients.[16] The major side-effects of traditional neuroleptics are parkinsonian effects, tardive dyskinesia, dystonia/dyskinesia and akathisia. Parkinsonian effects are characterized by akinesia, rigidity, shuffling gait, drooling and tremors.[16]

Tardive dyskinesia can occur from long-term treatment. Symptoms include lateral jaw movements and 'fly-catching' motions of the tongue.[16] A prolonged holiday from neuroleptic may diminish symptoms or cause them to disappear after 3 months. However, in many individuals, the effects are irreversible and continue even after medication is stopped.[16] Other side-effects include drowsiness (which usually occurs in the first 2 weeks of treatment), confusion, dry mouth, urinary retention, constipation and orthostatic hypotension. They can also result in the depression of the hypothalamus causing amenorrhoea, galactorrhoea, infertility and impotence.[16]

The newer antipsychotics also have potential side-effects. Most serious are blood dyskrasias, including agranulocytosis, which are potentially fatal. Clients on clozapine require regular blood monitoring of white blood cell counts to ensure the count is within normal limits. Such clients need to be taught to report symptoms such as lethargy, malaise, and sore throat immediately. Other potential side-effects include CNS symptoms (e.g. seizures, drowsiness), orthostatic hypotension, cardiac abnormalities, GI symptoms (e.g. constipation, diarrhoea), musculoskeletal effects (e.g. muscle weakness, pain) and respiratory (throat discomfort, nasal congestion).[17] Weight gain is a common complaint with these medications. Depending on the particular medication, one study reported that between 9.8% and 29.0% of patients had a greater than 7% increase in body weight.[18] In particular, clozapine and olanzapine were reported to produce a weight gain of between 4 and 4.5 kg after 10 weeks of standard dose treatment.[18] Weight gain can have serious clinical implications. It can negatively impact on compliance, compound the stigma associated with mental illness, and it can increase the risk of physical diseases associated with obesity such as diabetes and cardiovascular disease.[18,19]

The nurses role is to monitor and document side-effects and therapeutic effects, educate the client and family on the medication so as to promote compliance and minimize the impact of side-effects, and to provide support for clients experiencing adverse effects of the medication. In particular, nurses can play an important role in the early detection of tardive dyskinesia and in counselling clients and families so as to reduce the embarrassment associated with these symptoms.[17,20]

Cultural/spiritual approaches

Cultural and spiritual approaches begin with the recognition that a cultural or spiritual issue may be present. Family members or other members of the cultural/religious group will need to be consulted to understand the issue and to assist in identifying appropriate strategies. The nurse may facilitate referral to an appropriate healer/Spiritual leader and assist in coordinating the traditional healing with the treatment plan.

Interpersonal approaches

The primary nursing role related to hallucinations relate to interpersonal approaches. The primary intervention is always to establish a therapeutic trusting relationship (see Chapter 17). To do this, it is essential to be patient and listen to what the individual is saying.

Peplau[6,14] suggests that nursing interventions reverse the process that occurred when the hallucinations developed. To do this, it is first important to identify the phase of hallucination development. The nurse then helps the individual identify and name the anxiety. The nurse provides regular opportunities to interact with real people to mitigate the loneliness the individual may be experiencing.

Clack[15] in her classic paper on hallucinations, suggests several strategies to assist people with hallucinations:

1 The first step is always to establish a therapeutic relationship, show acceptance and listen.

2 Next, look and listen for cues or symptoms of the hallucination. Focus on the cue and elicit the individual's observation and description.

3 Then, identify if the hallucination is emotionally or toxically based (e.g. street drugs). Clack suggests that if asked, the nurse should acknowledge that he or she is not experiencing the hallucination.

4 Clack suggests that the nurse next follow the direction of the individuals and help them observe and describe the hallucination. Eliciting observations of current and past hallucinations is part of the process of establishing trust, as well as assisting in understanding what the person is experiencing. This helps the person in determining why the hallucinations are occurring. The individual is to be encouraged to observe and describe thoughts, feelings and actions. Clack suggests the person should observe or describe needs that may be underlying the hallucinations in order to see what needs it may be serving.

5 The nurse would then suggest and reinforce meeting needs through interpersonal relationships and to explore other behaviour concerns.

Since Clack's paper was written we now have many more medications to assist the individual. This means a person may recover from the symptoms much more quickly than the early paper would suggest. Some nurses may even believe that their role can therefore be restricted to administering the appropriate medication. However, Clack's interventions are still useful. The importance of listening, accepting and being patient is still very important. Also, if the individual is obtaining a lot of secondary gains from the hallucinations, that person may be unwilling to continue the medication. Therefore, understanding whether additional needs are being met by the hallucination is as important today as in 1962.

STRATEGIES TO ASSIST WITH COPING

People who continue to experience hearing problematic voices often develop specific coping strategies to deal with the problem. Finding out the pattern of when the voices occur may help in identifying appropriate coping strategies. For example, many people report that the voices are worse when they are alone. They may need to carefully structure their time to include ample opportunity for interacting with others. Some people have found that listening to something else helps to block out the voices. For this reason some people will use headphones and a portable CD player or radio to help block out problematic voices. It is useful to explore with each individual the pattern of when the voices are most problematic and when they seem to fade away. This can be used to strategize specific coping approaches.

Buccheri and others[21] summarized several strategies that had been reported in the literature to manage auditory hallucinations. These strategies include: self monitoring of the hallucinations; reading aloud and summarizing; talking with someone; watching and listening to television; saying 'stop' and naming objects; listening to music with headphones; listening to relaxation tapes with headphones; wearing a unilateral ear plug; and humming a single note. In testing whether these strategies were useful, they found all study participants found at least one strategy assist to relieve the distress associated with auditory hallucinations. In a later study, Buccheri and others[22] found that 82% of the participants continued to use at least one strategy.

Frederick and Cotanch[23] asked research participants to report self-help techniques they had found useful for coping with auditory hallucinations. The responses were grouped into physiological approaches to reduce arousal (relax, lie down, sleep, calm music, alcohol, extra medication); physiological approaches to increase arousal (loud music, walk, pace, jog); cognitive approaches (acceptance of voices, reduced attention to voices); and behavioural changes (leisure or work activity, seek interaction, isolate self). The findings highlighted the variety of different techniques that different people find useful.

Consider again the people introduced at the beginning of the chapter:

---

1 Michael sat alone in the TV room on the inpatient psychiatric ward. 'NO, NO, NO! I will not do THAT! Now you leave me alone! Shut up! Get out of here!'

A student nurse, Donovan, stood in the doorway. Michael was his assigned patient for the day. How should he approach him?

Donovan needs to remember that the first steps are always to listen and to work on establishing a therapeutic relationship. Since this is a new patient assignment, it would be unlikely that Michael would trust Donovan immediately. So patience is required. Donovan would need to introduce himself and let Michael know he is available.

'Michael, my name is Donovan. I am a student nurse and will be with you today … I heard you talking a moment ago and you sounded pretty upset. Perhaps you could tell me about that …'.

2 Sally greeted the community nurse, Suchita with a smile and a cup of tea. 'Sometimes, I think you and St Georgette are the only two true friends I have in the world'.

After a few minutes of conversation, Suchita inquired: 'So, how are you finding that new medication?'

'Terrible!' replied Sally, 'it was drowning St Georgette so I could barely hear her – so I had to stop taking it right away'.

Suchita might explore with Sally the relationship with her auditory hallucination. Sally and Suchita could work together to explore ways to expand Sally's social network. For example, Sally may join a recreational programme or a consumer/survivor self-help group that facilitates making new friends. When Sally has more social supports she may be less reliant on St Georgette as her only friend.

3 'I'm really loving this "Women in History" course. It really has me thinking'. Ngozi explained to her room-mate. 'But after today's class, one thing keeps coming back to me. If Joan of Arc were alive today – wouldn't we just say she was hallucinating and drug her up or lock her up?'

'Well', replied Nadine, 'How do we know she didn't have schizophrenia?'

As nurses we need to be open-minded in our understanding of the experience of hearing voices. The experience may be considered part of a normal occurrence within various cultures and spiritual belief systems. The experience of hearing voices may or may not be indicative of a mental illness such as schizophrenia. We need to consider whether or not the experience is creating any problems for the person. We need to listen carefully to the person to work on their goals, rather than simply considering hearing voices as a symptom to be controlled.

REFERENCES

1. Benjamin L. Is chronicity a function of the relationship between the person and the auditory hallucination? *Schizophrenia Bulletin* 1989; **15**: 291–310.

2. Miller L, O'Connor E, DisPasquale T. Patients' attitudes towards hallucinations. *American Journal of Psychiatry* 1993; **150**: 584–8.

3. Romme M. Listening to the voice hearers. *Journal of Psychosocial Nursing and Mental Health Services* 1998; **36**: 40–44.

4. Forchuk C. The orientation phase of the nurse-client relationship: Testing Peplau's theory. *Journal of Advanced Nursing Practice* 1994; **20**: 532–7.

5. Peplau HE. *Interpersonal relations in nursing*. New York: JP Putnam, 1952.

6. Peplau HE. Anxiety, self and hallucinations. In: O'Toole AW, Welt SR (eds). *Interpersonal theory in nursing practice: selected works of Hildegard E. Peplau*. New York: Springer, 1989: 270–326.

7. Sullivan HS. *The interpersonal theory of psychiatry*. New York: WW Norton, 1952.

8. Beyerstein B. Believing is seeing: organic and psychological reasons for hallucinations and other anomalous psychiatric symptoms. *Medscape Mental Health* 1996; **1**(11): 1–10.

9. Putnam FW. *Diagnosis and treatment of multiple personality disorder*. New York: Guilford Press, 1989.

10. Stafford LL. Dissociation and multiple personality disorder: a challenge for psycho-social nurses. *Journal of Psychosocial Nursing and Mental Health Services* 1993; **31**: 15–20.

11. Bentall RP. The illusion of reality: a review of psychological research on hallucinations. *Psychology Bulletin* 1990; **107**: 82–95.

12. Tiihonen J, *et al*. Modified activity of the human auditory cortex during auditory hallucinations. *American Journal of Psychiatry* 1992; **149**: 255–7.

13. Cleghorn JM, *et al*. Regional brain metabolism during auditory hallucinations in chronic schizophrenia. *British Journal of Psychiatry* 1990; **157**: 562–70.

14. Peplau HE. Interpersonal relations and the process of adaptation. *Nursing Science* 1963; **1**(4): 272–9.

15. Clack J. An interpersonal technique for handling hallucinations, in nursing care of the disoriented patient [Monograph 13]. *American Nurses Association Publication* 1962; 16–29.

16. Mycek M, Harvey RA, Champe PC, Fisher B, Cooper C. *Pharmacology*. Philadelphia: Lippincott-Raven, 1997.

17. Spratto G, Woods A. *PDR nurse's drug handbook*. Montvale, NJ: Medical Economics Company, 2001.

18. Allison DB, Casey DE. Antipsychotic-induced weight gain: a review of the literature. *Journal of Clinical Psychiatry* 2001; **62** (Suppl 7): 22–31.

19. Blin O, Micallef J. Antipsychotic-associated weight gain and clinical outcome parameters. *Journal of Clinical Psychiatry* 2001; **62**: 11–21.

20. Johnson BS. *Psychiatric nursing*. Philadelphia: J.B. Lippincott, 1986: 251–3.

21. Buccheri R, Trystad L, Kanas N, Waldron B, Dowling G. Auditory hallucinations in schizophrenia: Group experience in examining symptom management and behavioural strategies. *Journal of Psychosocial Nursing and Mental Health Services* 1996; **34**: 12–25.

22. Buccheri R, Trystad L, Kanas N, Dowling G. Symptom management of auditory hallucinations in schizophrenia: Results of 1-year follow-up. *Journal of Psychosocial Nursing and Mental Health Services* 1997; **35**: 20–28.

23. Fredrick JA, Cotanch P. Self-help techniques for auditory hallucinations in schizophrenia. *Issues in Mental Health Nursing* 1994; **16**: 213–24.

Chapter 31

THE PERSON WHO EXPERIENCES DISTURBING BELIEFS

Elsabeth Jensen* and Cheryl Forchuk**

INTRODUCTION

Alcock[1] contracted a sore throat while in the orient. He was offered an antibiotic and a Chinese herbal remedy based on snake bile. He accepted the antibiotic but declined the snake bile. Within a few days he was better, concluding that the antibiotic had worked. Later he learned his infection was viral, and that it had simply run its course. He struggled with the fact that he believed the antibiotic was responsible for his recovery. Like so many others, he had faith that the antibiotic would help, in spite of evidence to the contrary. Had he chosen the snake bile, he could as easily believe in its effectiveness, as the infection would have cleared in the same number of days.

Beliefs, simply defined, are convictions or opinions held as truths in the mind of the believer.[2] Many beliefs are supported by facts, many are held on faith. The common feature is that the believer holds their beliefs to be true. Even healthy people hold beliefs that may not hold up against facts and scientific evidence. Spiritual beliefs are based on faith and may be quite contrary to facts and evidence based on science. They are, however, considered valid and are known to contribute to good health.

History provides a long list of stories involving beliefs. When Columbus sailed west in 1492, he challenged the prevailing belief that the world was flat. However, despite his success, there are still people who believe the world is flat. Even in the presence of evidence, strong beliefs may not be given up easily. There are other, more ordinary, examples of beliefs that are held strongly in current times. How often have you heard someone say, 'I have no friends', 'I don't have a thing to wear', or 'I am so overweight', when the evidence is quite contrary? Superstitions provide another example of strongly held beliefs. Have you ever avoided walking under a ladder, or thrown salt over your shoulder after spilling it? Even educated people behave in ways that respect superstitions from time to time.

HOW DO BELIEFS DEVELOP?

Alcock[1] describes beliefs as our 'expectations about our world'. They derive from four sources: direct experience; observation; logical thought; and authority. Beliefs are developed out of direct experience. These are based on the patterns we observe in our world from the moment of birth. If two events occur together, they set up an

*Elsabeth Jensen is a Research Coordinator in mental health nursing research, an Adjunct Assistant Professor in the School of Nursing, Faculty of Health Sciences, University of Western Ontario, a Lecturer in the Continuing Education Department of Fanshawe College, and has a private practice in health counselling in London, Ontario.
**Cheryl Forchuk is a Professor in the School of Nursing, University of Western Ontario, Canada, with a cross appointment in the Department of Psychiatry, Faculty of Medicine and Dentistry. She is a Scientist at the Lawson Health Research Institute/London Health Sciences Centre.

association in the brain. The feeling of hunger is associated with unpleasantness. Mother providing milk leads to feeling satisfied. This leads to associating food with feeling good. Touching a hot stove causes pain, so stoves are associated with pain. Watching siblings cry from falling off the bicycle can lead to a fear of bicycles. Observing mother apply butter to the burn leads to believing that burns are helped by applying butter. Logical thought applied to reading about burn treatment later in life, leads to the belief that it is best to apply cold water, and not butter, to the burn. Being taught by parents and teachers to wash hands after playing with something dirty, leads to believing that one must always wash hands after touching anything that is dirty. Being told by parents that we are bright or stupid creates beliefs about self: 'I have the ability, I can do this', or 'I'm stupid, I'll never be any good'. We also learn about the world from authority figures. We are told, 'Don't trust strangers,' 'This is how we do (don't do) it in our family'. These, and many other lessons are combined to create our belief system about the world and how it works.

How do beliefs become disturbing?

Since many people hold false beliefs about themselves, their health, and the world, why is this of interest to nurses? There are times when false, or groundless, beliefs can interfere with health and functioning. When a person's beliefs have the potential to cause them to do harm to themselves, or to another person, by commission or by omission, the beliefs come to be defined as disturbing. The beliefs may not disturb the person holding them, but they disturb other people. In such cases, the term 'delusions' is used. A delusion is a rigidly held, irrational belief that persists in spite of evidence that it is not true. Usually people will have a cluster of beliefs that are groundless and extreme. This is referred to as a 'delusional system'.

Muse[3] observed however that, 'The same type of delusion has caused certain persons to be canonized as saints in the early Christian period, persecuted as witches in the middle ages, and confined in an institution in the 20th century'. This observation is important as it alerts us to the social context of beliefs. What may be seen as a problem in one situation may not be seen the same way in another. In fact, culture can be a powerful influence on ideas and beliefs. Cultural ignorance in health care providers can result in misunderstandings and incorrect assessments. The following definition is helpful in understanding how to be clear that what is observed is a delusion, and not something else.

The *Diagnostic and Statistical Manual of Mental Disorders*[4] provides the definition most often used in mental health care. According to this authority:

A delusion is a false belief based on an incorrect inference about reality that is firmly held, despite the beliefs of almost everyone else, despite obvious proof or evidence to the contrary. The person holds a belief that is not ordinarily accepted by other members of the person's culture or subculture.

The belief is not an article of religious faith. A value judgement is only considered to be a delusion when the judgement is so extreme as to defy credibility. The person may talk about their delusion, or may infer it from their behaviour, for example, eyeing other people with suspicion and mistrust. Delusions can occur on a continuum. Delusions can interfere with relationships, with work, and with self-care. They are of particular concern when they jeopardize the person's safety, or the safety of others. When they do, the person will often come to the attention of the mental health care system.

Delusions can occur alone or in combination with other signs and symptoms of mental illness. They are a known feature of several psychiatric diagnostic categories including, but not limited to, schizophrenia, depression, psychotic depression, mania, schizo-affective disorder, anorexia nervosa, bulimia, delusional disorder, psychosomatic disorder, paranoid personality disorder, schizotypal personality disorder, and a variety of substance abuse disorders.[4] The experience of abuse in childhood is also a factor in the development of delusions in adults with mental illness. In studying people with delusions, Read and Argyle[5] found that 50% of the people had a history of childhood sexual abuse or a history of childhood physical abuse, and an additional 29% had experienced both forms of abuse. This means that 79% of these people were abused as children.

Beliefs form in the brain where they serve the purpose of reducing anxiety, and increasing structure and consistency, in the person's day-to-day dealings with the world. They result from the processing of information in both hemispheres. There is some evidence that false beliefs, or delusions, can result when the left hemisphere receives incomplete information from the right, or if the interpreter function of the left hemisphere is malfunctioning. Brain research provides some evidence that disturbing beliefs, or delusions, are at least modestly associated with impairment of the central nervous system.[6]

Delusions have been reported to be a feature of disorders of the central nervous system. Examples of this include Capgras syndrome, and dementias resulting from substance abuse. Capgras syndrome causes the person to believe that people close to them have been replaced by identical doubles or robots. This condition has been linked to diffuse or localized lesions, especially of the right hemisphere.[7]

Understanding delusions can be difficult for a beginning practitioner. They may or may not be a feature of many different mental health diagnoses. While delusions are a feature of these many conditions, not every person with that diagnosis will suffer from delusions. It is important to assess the person, to identify the presence or absence of delusions. If they are present, they are not all the same. Depending on their characteristics, they may require different interventions.

NURSING THE PERSON WITH DISTURBING BELIEFS

The task of the nurse is to observe, from the perspective of a participant-observer. Based on the nursing assessment, the nurse makes inferences through identifying themes and forming hypotheses. Finally, the nurse experiments with interventions in the nurse-client relationship that will effect changes favourable to the client.[8]

Peplau[9] defined delusions as one of several possible responses to repeated frustration. Fixed responses, such as delusions, occur after repeated frustrations that require reorganization of the personality in order to deal with the anxiety resulting from the frustration. The beliefs cannot be given up, as this would cause overwhelming insecurity in the person. In this sense, delusions are a defence against long-standing anxiety and insecurity. This view has support from others.[6]

It is easier to provide nursing care based on the type of delusion being suffered, rather than the psychiatric diagnosis. The different types of delusions cut across the different diagnostic categories. A person may suffer from more than one type of delusion. The client may also be suffering from more than disturbing beliefs. People with schizophrenia, for example, often experience both disturbing beliefs and disturbing voices, or other forms of hallucination. When this is the case, Chapter 32 will provide helpful guidance.

It is important to know that there is often a thread of truth at the core of most delusions, and that these often serve as a way of dealing with underlying anxiety.[10,11] This last fact is very important as delusions can be challenging for the beginning nurse. By their nature, delusions are bizarre and irrational. They challenge common sense. It is imperative, however, that one avoids challenging the belief. The nurse should, however, assess carefully.

When beliefs are suspected to be delusional, it is important to gather as much information from other sources as possible. This includes talking to family and friends. A colleague recently discovered, to her amazement, that the young man she had admitted *was* indeed a successful rock star, with a Porsche, a mansion, and a large bank account, even though he was poorly dressed, penniless, and dishevelled on admission. In this case, family members had been available to validate his story.

Had they not been available, he might easily have found himself under treatment for delusions!

Three major types of delusions are encountered in nursing practice.[3,11] These are delusions of *persecution*, delusions of *grandeur*, and *negative delusions*. Other categories may be encountered, including sexual delusions, somatic delusions, and delusions that are difficult to understand. Case examples will be used to illustrate the major types.

Delusions of persecution

Delusions of persecution involve the belief that others are after the person, and that he or she is at risk of being harmed by these persecutors. These delusions can be dangerous. People may try to defend themselves from the danger that they believe is present. In the process, they can harm or even kill others. These occur more commonly in people who may have experienced danger from others at a point in their life, and in abusers of some drugs, such as amphetamines.

Case study 31.1

Mikel is a 25-year-old man admitted for assaulting the postman. He is under close observation as he is still potentially violent. As he speaks, his eyes move about, scanning his environment constantly. He sits forward on a chair in the dayroom, talking in a low voice.

Mikel: 'I don't know why I am here. I am not crazy. I don't like to be locked up'.

Nurse: 'Can you tell me what happened just before you came here?'

Mikel: 'A policeman came. He said he wasn't, but he had the uniform on. I know them. I tried to protect myself, then, others came. They took me here. What will happen to me?'

Nurse: 'You say you "know them"; have you had other experiences with the police?'

Mikel: 'They came after me. The police, I don't trust them. They take people, and you never see them again. They beat me, left me for dead. I came to this country. I thought I would be safe here, but they are everywhere. Now they found me, and brought me here'.

He continues to look anxiously about the room as they talk.

In Mikel's delusion, people wearing any kind of uniform are police, and they are the enemy. He sees his efforts to protect himself as legitimate. In his case, he had been a victim of the horrors of war. His beliefs about danger were formed in the past, but are out of place in the present. His belief that he needs to protect himself from the non-existent threat makes him dangerous to others. His beliefs are disturbing as they threaten the safety of other people, especially those wearing a uniform.

Delusions of grandeur

The person with delusions of grandeur holds exaggerated beliefs about their abilities, status, worth or accomplishments. The content is boastful or egotistical. Others who know the individual do not substantiate the contents of the belief system. The behaviour resulting from the delusions, is disturbing to others around the individual.

Case study 31.2

Dr Fairchild is a 59-year-old physicist, admitted after his wife had taken him to the family doctor for an evaluation of strange behaviour. She discovered he had spent a large amount of money on laboratory equipment for the basement. When she asked him about this, he had told her that he had discovered time travel. She was told not to worry, as he had access to unlimited wealth through his discovery. On checking with his Dean, she confirmed that her husband had suffered a number of grant rejections, had been reported by a number of his students for bizarre grading of exam papers, and as a result, the University was considering suggesting early retirement. The Dean had spoken repeatedly with Dr Fairchild about these concerns.

Dr Fairchild carried his briefcase around on the ward. It was filled with papers with equations and strange symbols. 'My work will solve the great mysteries of the ages. I will be able to talk to the greatest scientists as they make their discoveries. The University is very fortunate to have my work based here. I can show you my work, but it is very complex and requires a genius to comprehend it. You should be grateful I am even sharing this information with you. Not everyone is worthy, you know'.

Dr Fairchild's beliefs are not disturbing to him. They are disturbing to his wife, who sees the family resources dwindling. They are also disturbing to his Dean, who is concerned about productivity and performance. He is at risk of squandering his resources and of damaging the relationships he has with his wife and his employer.

Negative delusions

Negative delusions usually occur in people who are depressed. They are mood congruent and involve themes of despair, inadequacy, and hopelessness. These beliefs are disturbing as they can result in self-harm or suicide. The delusions also interfere with the person's ability to get on with his/her life tasks.

Case study 31.3

Willow is a 15-year-old student, admitted for depression and delusions involving snakes. Her schoolwork has deteriorated over the past six months and she has gained weight. She looks downward, avoiding eye contact. Her clothes are plain and very baggy.

Willow: 'The snake is eating me. I am going to die'.
Nurse: 'Can you tell me more about the snake?'
Willow: 'It's inside me. It's eating everything'. Tears flow. 'The monster put a snake in me because I was bad. He said it was my fault. He said the snake would eat me and I would die because I was bad. I'm not supposed to tell. But I'm scared, I don't want to die, but I'm bad. I have to die. The snake will kill me by eating me from the inside'.
Nurse: 'You sound afraid'.
Willow: 'I'm scared. I don't want to die. I wish I could get it out'. Her head is low. Her voice is barely audible.

Willow is depressed and believes she is dying. Obviously no snake could survive inside the human body, yet this is her belief. She is clearly troubled. By stating she wishes she could get the snake out, Willow alerts the nurse to the possibility that she might do something that would result in self-harm. The content of the delusion should also alert the nurse to the possibility of sexual abuse. The nurse should not introduce the topic, but should it arise, it will be important for her be empathic and non-judgemental.

As with other delusions, it will take time for the individual to feel safe enough to begin to share the issues that are at the core of their beliefs. Although it may be tempting to simply point out the seemingly obvious, this action will only aggravate the individual and raise their anxiety even higher.

The two main approaches to helping people with disturbing beliefs are the interpersonal nurse–client relationship, and appropriate medical evaluation and treatment.

INTERPERSONAL APPROACHES

The development of a therapeutic relationship with the client (Chapter 17) provides the necessary context for dealing with the underlying issues. Delusions are a way of coping with repeated frustration and the anxiety they cause, and there is usually a core of truth, or fact, at the base of them. As Donner[10] points out, the underlying core of the delusion must be decoded before the underlying need can be understood. Only when the underlying need is met in a healthier way can the delusion be given up. This can only happen in the context of a safe and trusting relationship. Donner cautions that the delusion should never be interpreted directly to the client. Neither should it be confronted, as this will only escalate the client's anxiety.

The *orientation phase* is the beginning of the therapeutic relationship. During this phase the nurse and the client are getting to know each other, and are contracting as to the focus of the therapeutic relationship. When the client is believed to be suffering from delusions, it is important to find out as much as possible from the client, family, friends, associates, and any other source of information.

The nurse also needs to consider her or his comfort and confidence in working with people with delusions. Depending on the nature of the delusions, nurses have found that extended contact can lead to impatience and anger on the part of the nurse.[11] If the particular beliefs, or underlying issues, cause anxiety in the nurse, this must be examined. Peer consultation, or consultation with the multidisciplinary team can be an important source of support for the nurse.

Given the nature of delusions, safety is always a concern. The clients may be on close or intensive observation for their safety or to protect others. The content of the delusion is an important consideration. For a person such as Mikel, who fears people in uniforms, it would be unwise to have a uniformed person provide close observation. In Willow's case, her 'monster' is a 'he'. She will experience less anxiety if observed by a woman. These suggestions may seem so obvious that the reader wonders why they are made explicit, yet there are many examples in the real world of problems arising from failure to consider the obvious.

Rosenthal and McGuiness[11] have clear recommendations for nursing the person with delusions. They caution against agreeing with delusions, suggesting the nurse tactfully avoid agreement. Agreement is as unhelpful as disagreement. At the same time, logic and debate are inappropriate, as this frustrates the client and escalates their anxiety, which is already overwhelming. That is why the client is suffering from delusions in the first place. Instead, it is recommended that the nurse focus on the client's feelings as this validates the client's reality.

To avoid both agreeing *or* disagreeing with the delusional content, and yet enter into a dialogue, may seem to be a confusing set of guidelines to follow. One approach is to look for what is *true to the listener* about what is said, and then support or agree with that piece. For example, when Willow says she is frightened of the snake, the nurse can agree that she (Willow) is frightened. For example, 'It sounds like you are feeling very afraid of what is happening'. The nurse would not say, 'It sounds like that snake in you is really frightening', since that would reinforce the delusion. Similarly, a statement like, 'Don't you realize a snake would be killed by the acid in your stomach' would be seen as argumentative and would risk the establishment of trust in the nurse. At times, a patient will directly ask the nurse whether or not the nurse believes the client. Again, the nurse walks a tightrope to agree with truth

while not reinforcing nor confronting the delusion. An example might be, 'I don't feel or see the snake, but I believe it is real to you'.

It can be tempting at times to try and use logic to talk someone out of a delusion. This tends to result in either the person not trusting the nurse's motivation or coming up with a more elaborate explanation to account for the logic presented by the nurse. An example from the clinical experience of one of the authors illustrates this problem.

Case study 31.4

I had been providing clinical supervision, with the use of a one-way mirror, to a nurse who was pregnant while I was also pregnant. The patient appeared to be less and less willing to be open about his concerns as our pregnancies became more obvious. In discussing this with him the nurse discovered he was concerned that his 'crazy talk' might harm the unborn children. After further exploration he felt that if the unborn children were disturbed they would begin to kick and make the mothers uncomfortable. An agreement was made that he would discuss what was truly bothering him if we both agreed to let him know immediately if we experienced extreme kicking. This seemed to work well and he returned to his usual frankness in discussing his concerns during counselling sessions. Months later, on the first day I returned from maternity leave, this patient was waiting at the door of the hospital for my return, and demanding to know if the baby was alright. He wanted to see a baby picture 'for proof'. I told him the baby was fine, but did not share a picture. Every day for the next week this patient waited at the hospital door and again asked if the baby was alright. I thought his concern was related to the earlier issue of his 'crazy talk' potentially harming the baby. I decided to show him a picture to prove the baby was fine and allay his concern. Much to my surprise, he said, 'Just as I thought, that is my baby'. I asked him why he thought that and he replied, 'See – the baby is bald just like me – that is my baby'. I foolishly argued the point by saying that there are many bald babies to which he replied, 'Yes, I have many children'.

When working with a client over a long period of time the nurse will observe both periods of wellness and difficulty. In these situations it may be possible to discuss the delusional content while it is not being currently experienced. It is often helpful for clients to learn to recognize early signs of difficulty to prevent relapse. For example, a nurse case manager had been working with a particular client for three years. During this time the client had several relapses. When this client was psychotic he always had a delusion that his food was poisoned. He would eventually refuse all food and drink and be hospitalized for 4–6 weeks in order to recover both physically and mentally. The nurse case manager and client were able to establish that the early signs of trouble were finding that his food seemed to have a metallic taste. This client learned to alert the case manager to when this occurred, so he could have an early assessment and readjustment of medication. This strategy was successful in breaking the pattern of regular re-hospitalizations.

MEDICAL APPROACHES

When strong beliefs are sufficiently disturbing, and interfere with health and functioning, they often result in admission to hospital. This allows the physician to evaluate the case, to test which medication will be of best benefit, and to titrate the dosage. Hospitalization also provides intensive nursing care in support of the medical plan of care. As Nightingale observed: '. . . I would go further, and state that to the experienced eye of a careful observing nurse, the daily, I had almost said hourly, changes which take place in patients, and which changes rarely come under the cognisance of the periodical medical visitor, afford a still more important class of data . . .'[12]

Nurses are responsible for communicating their observations to the other members of the team. Nurses are also responsible for administering prescribed medications and reporting the person's responses to these. It is necessary for the nurse to have a good knowledge base of the classes of medications usually prescribed for persons with disturbing beliefs. It is only through careful observation that benefits and side-effects can be identified. Some side-effects are minor, while others may be transient. Still others can cause disability or even death. The nurse's role includes educating the person about the medication. The lessons should include information about the benefits of the medication, the importance of taking it as prescribed, and the common side-effects. Knowledge of strategies for dealing with side-effects such as dry mouth, and blurred vision, can be very reassuring to the person.

One of the nurse's roles is that of teacher. Information about the medication is given as part of health teaching. It is important for the person to understand that the medications are intended to help them get better. Information should be given verbally and in written form, for the person to keep. Written materials should be in lay language for easy comprehension, and should be typed in size 14 or larger font. This is to compensate for the visual effects of the medication. The information should be succinct. Keeping it to one page per medication allows the person to post it in the medicine cabinet at home. The written material should always have contact information, should the person have

any questions or concerns after discharge. More details about antipsychotics medication are provided in the chapter on the person who hears disturbing voices.

Having a working stage therapeutic relationship provides an easy vehicle for discussing concerns or questions the person may have. It will also allow the nurse to be fully aware of how the medication is affecting the person. This information will be essential to the physician making decisions about the medical plan of care.

CONCLUSION

We all hold some beliefs that others would disagree with. An extreme example of this would be a delusion. While some delusions may be innocuous, others may be very disturbing and can place the individual at risk. The nurse needs to help the person feel as comfortable as possible, to be honest about concerns, to listen carefully to what is being said, assess for severity of problems and response to treatment, and work with the client on mutually agreed goals. The particular challenge in communicating with the person with disturbing beliefs, is to support and listen to the client without reinforcing or directly confronting the delusions.

REFERENCES

1. Alcock JE. Alternative medicine and the psychology of belief. *Medscape* 1999 [cited 2000 Mar 6]; Available from: http://psychiatry.medscape.com/prometheus. . . ram0302.04.alco/pnt-sram0302.04.alco.html
2. *Webster's encyclopedic unabridged dictionary of the English language*. New York, NY: Gramercy Books, 1989.
3. Muse MB. *Psychology for nurses*. Philadelphia: WB Saunders, 1926.
4. American Psychiatric Association. *Diagnostic and statistical manual of mental disorders*, 4th edn. Washington, DC: APA, 1994: DSM IV.
5. Read J, Argyle N. Hallucinations, delusions, and thought disorder among adult psychiatric inpatients with a history of child abuse. *Psychiatric Services* 1999; **50**(11): 1467–72.
6. Butler RW, Braft DL. Delusions: a review and integration. *Schizophrenia Bulletin* 1991; **17**(4): 633–47.
7. Buckwalter KC. Are you really my nurse, or are you a snake sheriff? *Journal of Psychosocial and Nursing Mental Health Services* 1993; **31**: 33–4.
8. Peplau HE. Themes in nursing-safety. In: Mereness D (ed.) *Psychiatric nursing: developing psychiatric nursing skills*, 2nd edn. Dubuque (IW): WC Brown, 1971: 142–7.

9. Peplau HE. *Interpersonal relations in nursing.* New York: GP Putnam, 1952.

10. Donner G. Treatment of a delusional patient. *American Journal of Nursing* 1969; **69**: 2642–4.

11. Rosenthal TT, McGuinness TM. Dealing with delusional patients: discovering the distorted truth. *Journal Mental Health Nursing* 1986; **8**: 143–54.

12. Nightingale F. Notes on hospitals. In: Rosenberg CE (ed.) *Florence Nightingale on hospital reform.* London: Garland Publishing, 1989 (original work published in 1863).

Chapter 32

THE PERSON WITH SCHIZOPHRENIA

Tom Keen*

If I am mad I let you see
When I laugh I am looking at me
While I talk of hope you will understand
Why look at me I'm just another hand.

My brain is like a big unpaid bill
What's the good when my fancies can't fulfil
Those who keep me I am keeping all them
How many points ponder this pen.

From what I write if my righting is wrong
If you hark to its lilt you might make a song
Those who know me please treat me as not mad
That's good of you when you know you're not bad.

You ask me where I put my pill
I digest it that's why I'm not ill
I put my thoughts before me and direct them after
Look there's a lot to learn from laughter.[1]

DIAGNOSIS AND SYMPTOMATOLOGY

The diagnosis of schizophrenia refers to a complex and controversial[2] cluster of conditions occurring in roughly 1% of people worldwide, and affecting about 250,000 individuals in the UK.[3] There are no diagnostic tests for the multi-faceted condition, and aetiology remains uncertain, despite significant recent clarification of genetic and neurological factors.[4] Instead the diagnosis is made on the evidence of a variety of subjective experiences (symptoms) and observable behaviours (signs) which commonly include:

❑ holding apparently false or incredible beliefs that seem at odds with one's cultural or educational background (*delusional thinking*);
❑ hearing sounds, thoughts-out-loud or voices (often making critical or abusive comments and threats) in the absence of any actual external stimuli or speakers (*auditory hallucinations, thought-echo*);
❑ experiencing one's thoughts, feelings, speech or bodily functions being controlled, interfered with or manipulated by some external force (*thought broadcasting, withdrawal or insertion; passivity phenomena; 'made' actions*);
❑ believing that neutral, outside events and people or insignificant objects have special meaning for or about oneself (*ideas of reference, delusional perception*);

*Tom Keen lectures in mental health at the University of Plymouth, England. He previously worked as a nurse, therapist or manager in various situations including acute admission wards, adolescent psychotherapy, therapeutic community and community mental health centres. Previous teaching experience includes sharing responsibility for staff development in Torbay Mental Health Unit.

❑ speaking (and therefore presumably thinking) idiosyncratically or unintelligibly, with unusual patterns of expression, disjointed sentences, repetitiveness or coining novel words and phrases (*thought disorder, loosened association, word salad, neologisms*);

❑ becoming unusually withdrawn, both socially and emotionally, or obsessively preoccupied with fantasy and esoteric ideas (*autism*);

❑ showing less interest, emotion or enthusiasm than usual (*impaired volition, anhedonia, blunt or flattened affect*);

❑ seeming to others to behave or feel differently to their normal expectations (*inappropriate behaviour, incongruous affect*).

All, some or none of these may persuade a psychiatrist to diagnose schizophrenia. Sufferers also complain of anxiety, agitation, depression, moodiness, lack of concentration and memory problems. These are all common experiences not only as schizophrenia develops, but also during critical life-periods such as adolescence or mid-life, and make early psychiatric diagnosis difficult. Standardized diagnostic manuals recognize many other behavioural idiosyncrasies and experiential oddities as signs or symptoms of various schizophrenia subtypes and provide clear guidelines to psychiatrists, researchers or others needing to establish a diagnosis.[5,6]

Schizophrenia encompasses such a wide range of diverse presentations that evidence from countless incompatible clinical cases could contradict almost any generalized statement about the diagnosis. Schizophrenia has no typical course and no typical underlying gross pathology. Since its initial formulation, arguments about the validity of the diagnosis and its nature, causes and treatment have abounded and continue.[7] People unfamiliar with schizophrenia see nothing in common between the apparently spontaneous breakdown, dramatic imagery, persuasively surreal fears or frantically poetic outpourings of a 20-year-old student, and the chronic torpor, expressionless features and superficially stagnant life of an unkempt middle-aged vagrant who seems to spend time and money on nothing but smoking. Schizophrenia disables people in innumerable ways, and almost anything that nurses do could be a valid intervention at some point in someone's diagnostic career. This chapter will of necessity miss out much that is important, and probably include much that is disputed, but presents a variety of perspectives on an intriguingly complex and continuously controversial diagnosis.

Categories and classification

The core features of schizophrenia can be divided into three blurred categories:[8]

❑ **Positive symptoms** – so-called because they represent qualitatively different experiences than normal, or behavioural exaggerations of conventional social conduct. They include apparent exaggerations or distortions of thinking (delusional thought); perception (hallucinations); communication and language (incomprehensible speech, incongruous affect); and behaviour (catatonic posturing and impulsivity).

❑ **Negative symptoms** – which by contrast represent an apparent loss of normal function or a diminution from social norms. People diagnosed as schizophrenic sometimes seem unemotional or avoid intimate contact with others. They may become withdrawn and speak little, or seem inactive and apathetic with apparently little purpose or energy.

❑ **Schizophrenic thinking** – subtle changes in perceptual analysis and reasoning, that psychiatrists construe as 'formal thought disorder' and 'loosened associations'. These cognitive patterns may be analogous with, if not identical to the kinds of thought patterns that cognitive psychologists call 'divergent thinking' and 'loosened constructs'.[9] Schizophrenic people often analyse reality from unusual perspectives and classify experiences or objects in innovative or surreal ways. Schizophrenic thinking seems sometimes unnecessarily complex, unconventionally abstract, or strangely literal and concrete.[10]

Although schizotypal thought-patterns are sometimes subsumed within the category of 'positive symptoms', it is useful to consider them separately, not only because they are also found in 'ordinary', undiagnosed people (as are many of the negative and positive symptoms) but also because the three symptom-clusters seem to respond differently to psychiatric treatments.

Positive symptoms tend to occur or predominate during acutely disturbed periods in sufferers' lives. Breakdowns tend to occur more frequently and with greater severity after stressful life-events, such as accidents or illness, natural disasters, economic changes, celebrations, anniversaries etc. Positive symptoms are especially likely to recur or intensify when a sufferer's socio-emotional environment becomes tense or fraught with *communication deviance* – unclear or disguised meanings; denied or deviously articulated feelings; or high levels of *expressed emotion* (q.v.).[11] Neuroleptic drugs, the mainstay of mainstream psychiatric treatment, target and often effectively suppress positive symptoms, but are less successful in banishing sufferers' subjective unease or less florid symptoms.[3]

Negative symptoms are not so readily ameliorated by anti-psychotic medication. Indeed, sedation and other side-effects of injudiciously prescribed neuroleptic drugs may worsen them.[12] Apathy, withdrawal, self-neglect, uncommunicativeness etc. may develop before the onset, or continue in the absence of more dramatic positive symptoms. These symptoms are not only compounded or mimicked by the effects of drugs (both psychiatric and recreational, e.g. cannabis) but are also worsened by impoverished economic, cultural or social circumstances.[7] Concerned others (e.g. relatives, friends, naïve professionals) often critically attribute negative symptoms to someone's personality and react by rejection, silent judgement, criticism or antagonism. Such responses by carers and staff have been shown to compromise sufferers' fragile personal integrity, aggravate their symptoms and increase pathological behaviour.[13,14]

The third category of schizophrenic phenomenology – the tendency to use heavily concrete, highly abstract or bafflingly divergent forms of thinking – tends to pre-date initial breakdowns and also persists as a stable part of sufferers' personalities, even after effective neuroleptic suppression of positive symptoms. Schizotypal thinking is commonly found in relatives and friends of diagnosed schizophrenics, as well as many people who have no connection at all with the diagnosis. Negative symptoms and schizotypal thinking are not solely diagnostic of schizophrenia, but occur throughout populations. Extremely indolent and mildly to moderately depressed people superficially display the equivalent of negative symptoms. Many creative people and social innovators score highly in schizotypal thinking.[8,10] Recently it has also been persuasively demonstrated that even hallucinations and delusional thought are much more ordinarily distributed than may appear the case to many professionals,[15,16] who risk becoming blinkered or glamoured by constant exposure to the extreme pathologies encountered in clinical work.[17]

Schizophrenia subtypes

The various characteristics used to diagnose schizophrenia tend to occur in loosely segregated clusters, and clearly many different conditions nestle beneath the single diagnostic umbrella. Both official diagnostic manuals classify schizophrenia into subtypes, while independent researchers have applied statistical factor-analysis to symptom clusters and found three core syndromes that loosely conform to traditional diagnostic subtypes, and also fit emerging neurological knowledge[18,19] (see Table 32.1).

Psychiatrists commonly attribute the various symptoms and unusual behaviour of diagnosed schizophrenics to the consequences of subtle defects in brain structure and function, that may respond to carefully targeted psychological and pharmacological treatments. Sharing

TABLE 32.1

Symptom-cluster	DSM-IV	ICD-10
Reality–distortion Hallucinations; delusions	**Paranoid** Preoccupation with delusions or frequent hallucinosis	**Paranoid** Delusions usually with hallucinations predominate
Disorganized Incoherent speech; incongruous affect; thought disorder	**Disorganized** Disorganized speech or behaviour; flat or inappropriate affect	**Hebephrenic** Inappropriate mood; incoherent speech; negative symptoms
	Catatonic Motor immobility with waxy flexibility of limbs or stupor; or excessive purposeless activity not externally influenced; or extreme negativism – resistance to instructions, rigid stereotypical posturing, mutism; repetitive imitation of someone else's speech or movement	**Catatonic** Prominent psychomotor disturbances; either catatonic excitement, stupor or posturing
Psychomotor poverty Lack of responsiveness; flat affect; poverty of speech; inactivity; anhedonia	**Residual** Absence of prominent delusions, hallucinations, disorganized speech and grossly disorganized behaviour; negative symptoms or continuing but attenuated positive symptoms, e.g. odd beliefs or unusual perceptions	

this clinical perspective facilitates close cooperation between nurses, psychiatrists and the medical canon of diagnosis, treatment and cure. It can reassure those who crave diagnostic certainty and the potential security of professional harmony about medical treatment. It also risks invalidating the personal hypotheses of other sufferers, and constructing too big a knowledge-and-power imbalance between professionals and some service users, leading to either unwarranted dependence or negativistic resistance. Some psychiatrists have expressed concern about becoming too dogmatically entrenched in biomedical explanations, and propose more balanced approaches that acknowledge peoples' holistic integrity.[7,20] Clinical symptoms of schizophrenia can also (not necessarily *instead*) be thought of as valid, if often miserable or misunderstood aspects of people's experiences, thus enabling the establishment of strong therapeutic alliances between sufferers and professional carers.[21] Problematic behaviour or psychotic experiences can be therapeutically construed as individuals' attempted solutions to other more deeply lying, vaguely troubling or intensely difficult problems. Withdrawal may represent an individual's constructive response to unexpressed fear of others' judgement or opinion of himself; an attempt to reduce the undifferentiated torrent of stimuli pouring into his consciousness; or an admittedly lonely or self-defeating solution to extreme shyness or feelings of low-worth. Shouting, talking to oneself or playing bad music loudly may help an individual to express feelings, avoid troubling conversations or sort out thinking, but it may also silence the chattery background or frightening foreground of hallucinosis. Hallucinations themselves may be symbolic residues of past abuses; dramatically serving to disguise pain, shift blame, maintain threat and shout a warning; all in one elegant neuropsychological synthesis.[22]

To develop effective clinical relationships with people, nurses should share their professional conceptual frameworks with sufferers. Once both parties are psychoeducationally initiated into each other's world-views, a more effective partnership can be established by pooling both formal psychiatric nomenclature and subjective, personal phenomenology. In such a shared enterprise, diagnoses, symptoms and personal beliefs become equal partners in a joint problem-solving approach. Symptom clusters become potential frameworks for helping people to clarify their experiences, and collaborate with care planning. *Coping strategy enhancement* is the jargon term for therapeutic strategies based on identifying what people do that actually helps them, and working out ways of doing that even more effectively or frequently.[23] If shouting helps silence voices, but attracts unwanted public attention, how about singing, or whistling?

The course and outcome of schizophrenic experience varies widely. Some people only ever have one breakdown (22% of diagnoses); others recover completely between recurrent attacks (35%); while about 40% of diagnosed people either remain permanently affected or show progressive personal and social deterioration.[4] Despite decades of research, psychiatrists have been unable to establish clear patterns of biological, psychological or social causes[12] although expectations are increasingly expressed that rapidly evolving brain-imaging technologies, advances in genetic understanding and epidemiological studies will soon clarify the causes and underlying nature of schizophrenia.[24]

The lack of a consistent symptomatology, widely variant prognoses and continuing difficulty to identify definite aetiologies has led many people to condemn the diagnosis as at best flawed,[7] or at worst prejudicial and in itself delusional.[25–27] However, mainstream psychiatry remains unmoved by such criticisms. When tightly defined using standardized diagnostic procedures, the incidence of schizophrenia is found to be remarkably similar worldwide, however culturally and economically dissimilar the populations studied.[11] This is an epidemiological rarity, and suggests not only a profoundly widespread genetic basis for the condition, but also that the genetic differences involved may be evolutionary in origin and derive from complex human psychological and anthropological characteristics, such as language development and social group diffusion, rather than simple individual pathology.[8,10] While people continue to suffer intensely from the distressing and socially disabling emotional, intellectual and interpersonal experiences associated with schizophrenia, mental health nurses will be needed to provide care, compassion and sensitive understanding, whatever the nature of this complex diagnosis eventually proves to be.

SCHIZOPHRENIA: A MENU OF INTERVENTIONS

Clinicians and researchers have recently evolved a package of reasonably well-evidenced psychiatric interventions for the various forms of schizophrenia. Estimations of the effectiveness of this treatment package vary, partly according to whether outcome studies concentrate on measuring formal reductions in clinical symptoms, or focus upon overall social recovery and subjective increase in personal well-being.[28] Nevertheless, current policies dictate that mental health services should be able to offer the following menu:

1   Community-based teams to ensure early intervention in the course of the illness, prevent prolonged periods of non-treatment and provide support during crises.

2   Monitored anti-psychotic medication and flexible compliance strategies.

3 Applied cognitive-behavioural therapy.

4 Therapeutic support for families.

5 Social, occupational and vocational support and skills training.

6 Targeted health promotion, and attention to sufferers' physical health.

COMMUNITY–BASED TEAMWORK

The UK Department of Health has published clear guidelines for the kinds of service structures needed for the effective integration of interventions.[29] As well as improved residential services such as acute admission wards[30] and hostel accommodation, local services should include a range of alternative provisions:

❏ **Early intervention services** are intended to help people when they first develop schizophrenic symptoms, and for the first few years of any subsequent illness. Because of the complexity of both adolescence and schizophrenia, services should focus on specific symptoms and preferred solutions, rather than strict diagnostic protocols. They need to be conscious of the risk of stigmatization and social censure, and focus on people's social integration and normal developmental process, not simply their pathology and clinical status. Staff must be family-oriented yet also aware of the importance of separation and identity issues in people's lives. There should be seamless connections between children's, adolescent, family and adult mental health services; and firm partnerships with all other relevant agencies, including primary care, education, employment and social services.

❏ **Crisis resolution teams** provide 24-hour rapid response, with intensive but time-limited support to individuals, families or social networks early in the development of crises. Crisis resolution work stresses engagement with sufferers and carers, and strives for the active involvement of all protagonists within the situation. Interventions need to be pragmatic, and factually focused. CR teams reduce immediate emotional heat by: effective containment of emotions and catastrophic fantasies; systemic engagement, empathic calmness, explorative clarity; and an emphasis on solution-focused problem-solving approaches, rather than custodial or medical interventions. They function as gatekeepers, referring people on as soon as the protagonists feel back in control of themselves or their situation.

❏ **Intensive home treatment** is linked to crisis intervention, and ensures the provision of close contact, active support and therapeutic interventions to individuals and families to prevent further crises. Interventions may include whatever is needed: sleeves-rolled-up practical help and instruction; liaison with other agencies; shared recreational or social activity; family management and therapeutic work; systemic or individual psychotherapy; medication management etc.

❏ **Assertive outreach teams** establish and maintain contact with people who have complex needs, and are difficult to engage, or repeatedly withdraw from contact with services. Teams should communicate intensively with each other, users, social networks and agencies. They should be self-contained, well-led and mutually supportive; oriented to long-term treatment and continuity of care; highly creative, flexible and imaginative in building, maintaining and repairing their relationships with users; and focused on risk management and physical health needs as well as psycho-social welfare.

❏ **Primary care liaison teams** epitomize the future integrated provision of mental health services based on the dissolution of rigid boundaries between agencies and artificial categories, such as *health* versus *social* needs. PCLTs should establish better partnership arrangements between social care agencies, mental health specialists and primary care staff; and enhanced mental health education and training for the latter. Teams can grow from pre-existing generic community mental health teams by professionals detaching from bases in specialist centres, and moving fully into primary care situations or giving much more attention to inter-agency liaison.[31]

Such a comprehensive set of services reflects the logical implications of the 'stress-vulnerability' model of schizophrenia first propounded by Zubin and Spring.[32] Services should respond not only clinically to the individual who carries the diagnosis (i.e. to their *vulnerability*) but also preventatively by targeting resources and practical interventions at the very real social, economic and interpersonal *stressors* that can precipitate schizophrenic relapse in vulnerable individuals.

ANTI-PSYCHOTIC MEDICATION AND COMPLIANCE

Psychiatric treatment for people with schizophrenia almost always involves drug therapy to stabilize psychotic symptoms and reduce people's chances of relapse. Successful treatment should also improve people's ability to resume ordinary life and live independently; but although current medication relieves some symptoms for many people, there remains a need for more effective, better-tolerated drugs. Some people avoid medication entirely, preferring their symptoms to side-effects; others try to manage their symptoms by flexible use of medication and other remedies, including dietary supplements.[12] Evidence of the prophylactic effectiveness of fish-oil-based preparations is accumulating. These contain concentrated doses of two fatty-acids that are essential for building and maintaining healthy brain tissue. Clinical trials of eicosapentaenoic and docosahexaenoic acids (EPA and DHA) are underway;[3] meanwhile many users are responding to anecdotal reports and adding the capsules to their shopping lists. Horrobin[10] provides a fascinating and full account of the significance of fatty acids in brain structure and function, and the evolution of schizophrenia.

Compliance – or informed choice?

The severe side-effects of anti-psychotic drugs discourage many sufferers. Estimates of non-compliance vary, and professionals may often be quite mistaken in guessing how compliant people are,[33,34] but surveys suggest up to 80% of people fail to follow prescriptions.[35] Other reasons suggested for non-compliance include:[36]

❑ universal reluctance (detected by general physicians and others) for patients to adhere long-term to medical prescriptions;
❑ poor therapeutic relationship; lack of trust, empathy, mutual respect etc;
❑ personal health-beliefs that conflict with the illness-models advanced by professionals;
❑ disagreements between sufferers and professionals about the predicted likelihood of relapse;
❑ recovered patients often recollect only slight or tolerable symptom severity and social handicap when unwell, while professionals dispute their evaluation.

Evidence suggests that people who avoid pharmaceutical treatment increase their risk of relapse; and subsequent hospitalization is extremely expensive relative to the cost of medication.[3] This has motivated professionals to develop effective systems of convincing people to take medication. Strategies vary, but generally emphasize:[37]

❑ the importance of maintaining good collaborative relationships;
❑ careful dosage titration and monitoring of medication;
❑ not trivializing people's reports of side-effects, and regular assessment of them, using tests such as LUNSERS;[38]
❑ pragmatic, flexible, solution-focused approaches and compromise;

❑ shared exploration of health-beliefs and resistances to treatment;
❑ objective evaluations of relapse-risk and symptom-severity;
❑ motivational interviewing techniques which help people to analyse the potential costs and benefits of specific decisions.

Depot preparations slowly release their active component over several days or weeks after intramuscular injection and represent another way of increasing compliance. People receiving such preparations require especial sensitivity and attention to their willing cooperation if they are not to relapse; or become treatment dropouts or service avoiders. The term 'compliance' has been challenged for perceived authoritarian connotations, and more collaborative language proposed:[39]

> Anyone faced with … serious mental health problems has … difficult decisions to make. Anyone in such a situation might value an ally who could help them … to come to decisions that are right for them … the person may then require assistance … to carry through their chosen course, and help to review their decision … in the light of events. But that is not *compliance*, rather *collaborative alliance*.[40]

Psychiatric medication for schizophrenia

The drugs used for schizophrenia are collectively described as *anti-psychotic* or *neuroleptic* and comprise a mixture of pharmacological subgroups, including the commonly distinguished *typical* and *atypical* anti-psychotics. This distinction is based upon the observation that many older drugs cause a *typical* range of side-effects, including especially movement disorders. In fact the picture is more complicated. While many newer drugs appear not to produce such severe side-effects, some older drugs were also *atypical*, and the newer drugs have their own emerging drawbacks. There is some equivocal evidence that the effects of standard anti-psychotic drugs may be enhanced by supplementing them with other medicines, particularly carbamazepine and beta-blockers.[3]

It is difficult to establish the truth about the relative merits and demerits of psychiatric drugs for various reasons. Experimental trials vary in their methodology and may use incompatible, bafflingly complex or obscure statistical analyses. They often feature patients, treatment outcomes or prescription schedules that match awkwardly with everyday clinical practice. Comparisons are not always made with realistic or relevant alternative treatment regimes. Most trials are funded by organizations that have specific financial or political interests in the outcome.

Drop-out rates are often very high, making final results difficult to interpret. Publication and reporting biases may make less favourable or more critical findings difficult to access. Even relatively uncontroversial findings of effectiveness cannot guarantee that a specific medication will be efficacious for any one individual sufferer.[3]

Typical anti-psychotics

Haloperidol and chlorpromazine are among the most common classic anti-psychotics. They seem both more effective and more harmful than placebo in reducing positive symptoms, but not significantly different to each other in overall effect. Some (e.g. flupenthixol, fluspirilene, haloperidol) are available as long-lasting 'depot' injections. Despite manufacturers claims and counter-claims, there seems little convincing evidence that any one preparation is generally more efficacious than another.[3]

Sedation often occurs early in treatment, frequently accompanied by a vague, dreamlike sense of oddness and anxiety. Dose reduction, drug-switching or night-time single-dose administration may help people accommodate to these effects.

Dry mouth, blurred vision, flushing, urinary retention, constipation, ejaculatory inhibition and impotence result from a specific neurochemical characteristic shared by many psycho-pharmacological agents. Dizziness and unsteadiness can result from lowered blood pressure. If people persist with the medicine, these effects often diminish and become more tolerable, but for many others constitute the insufferable last straws that lead to non-compliance. Unfortunately many professionals construe these as minor irritations that should be endured for the greater good of fewer psychotic symptoms.[41]

Movement disorders are perhaps the most distressing neuroleptic side-effects. Termed *extra-pyramidal* effects, after the neuronal tract that generates them, these variously affect many patients and include:

❏ generalized muscle spasms and stiffness (*dyskinesia, dystonia*);
❏ muscle spasms in the head and neck that may be accompanied by rolling of eyeballs (*torticollis, oculogyric crises*);
❏ a syndrome resembling Parkinson's disease – limb rigidity, tremor, expressionless face and shuffling gait (*Parkinsonism*);
❏ restlessness and agitated movements, accompanied by an inner sense of unease and urgency – often misconstrued by professionals as symptomatic worsening requiring increased medication (*akathisia*).

Extra-pyramidal effects are generally treated by anti-muscarinic drugs such as orphenadrine or procyclidine that can be given orally (or intramuscularly in emergencies) but may cause an increase in dry mouth etc. The anti-muscarinics are less effective against akathisia, which responds best to dose reduction or drug switching.

The most severe and distressing movement disorder is *tardive dyskinesia*. This consists of repetitive, involuntary movements of the face, tongue and neck muscles and sometimes of the arms and legs. People feel unable to control their lip-smacking tongue-protrusion, chewing, blowing and sucking movements. They cross and uncross their legs, flap their hands; or march on the spot. Tardive dyskinesia develops most commonly in people over 40 who have been on typical anti-psychotics for three months or more. It is usually irreversible, even when anti-psychotics are discontinued. Paradoxically, withdrawing established neuroleptics may even worsen the side-effect. Switching to one of the newer atypicals may be the only available pharmacological course of action.[3]

The movement abnormalities caused by extra-pyramidal side-effects are difficult to endure. As well as being distressing, uncomfortable and often painful, they are also a source of stigma, being highly visible, and commonly portrayed as an aspect of madness or a sign of disease, rather than a consequence of treatment. It is difficult for people to rehabilitate themselves after a breakdown and integrate successfully into work and community when they feel so uncomfortable and can readily convince themselves that they are as odd as they may look to others. Users' groups report that alternative self-help remedies to these problems include the recreational drug cannabis, and dietary supplements such as vitamin E and vitamin B6. Evidence for these treatments remains both controversial and largely anecdotal.

Interference with metabolism of the hormone prolactin causes other distressing and embarrassing side-effects such as menstrual difficulties, breast enlargement and milk-production in women, or impotence and breast enlargement in men. These effects generally respond to either dose reduction, or neuroleptic discontinuation, and replacement with another atypical preparation. Some anti-psychotics (especially chlorpromazine) also affect people's skins, causing sunburn and sensitivity to sunlight, pigment changes, rashes and granular deposits in the cornea. Patients should avoid sunbathing and use blocking lotions. Medication in liquid form should be handled carefully. Skin effects usually disappear after stopping treatment.

Blood disorders leading to loss of white cells (*agranulocytosis*) and susceptibility to serious infection are rare but important side-effects. Blood counts help to monitor this possibility, but nurses should be alert to signs of infection, such as sore throats and general discomfort.

Body temperature is an unreliable indicator, as anti-psychotics can lower it. If serious infection is suspected, medication should be stopped. *Neuroleptic malignant syndrome* is manifested by sudden onset of muscle stiffness and worsened extra-pyramidal symptoms, accompanied by a fast pulse, high, low or variable blood pressure and a very high temperature. The sufferer may seem drowsy, drooling or delirious, or become very frightened and agitated. Medication should be stopped immediately, and urgent medical aid summoned, as the condition is potentially fatal (in 20% of cases) due to possible failure of the heart, kidney or respiratory functions. Rest and rehydration are the first priorities if there is any delay in admission to an emergency treatment facility. Thankfully, the condition is extremely rare.

Atypical anti-psychotics

Atypical anti-psychotics include clozapine, risperidone, olanzapine and quetiapine. Others are actively being produced but have either yet to complete laboratory and clinical trials (e.g. zotepine, aripiprazole) or have given grounds for concern after initially enthusiastic claims for their safety and effectiveness (e.g. sertindole, ziprasidone). Side-effects, especially extra-pyramidal movement disorders, are supposedly much milder than typical anti-psychotics, but they are generally more expensive, leading to ambivalent prescribing policies.[3] The most commonly prescribed atypicals are clozapine, risperidone and olanzapine. Clozapine is particularly effective in people who have failed to respond to other neuroleptics, but because it can cause *agranulocytosis*, clozapine is often regarded as a last resort. Prescription must always be accompanied by stringent blood monitoring.

Many clinicians recommend that atypicals (except clozapine) should be given to people when first diagnosed, not only because of any increased efficacy, but also as fewer, less severe side-effects would increase compliance. This would reduce the risks of relapse and subsequent expensive residential or intensive community treatment. Others disagree, claiming that atypicals anti-psychotics are not significantly different enough from conventional neuroleptics in either their efficacy or side-effects. The most balanced view seems to be that atypicals represent a refinement of available treatments for schizophrenia, but not a revolution.[3] In the UK, prescribing guidelines from the National Institute for Clinical Excellence should clarify this issue. Further research and development will continue, and the latest drug to be announced, aripiprazole, has a different, more subtle mode of action than its predecessors, stimulating renewed excitement among both professionals and sufferers.

Atypical anti-psychotics seem less severe than the older neuroleptics, but are not entirely free of side-effects. Some, including clozapine, may lower the epileptic threshold, causing seizures in vulnerable individuals. People may prefer to take preventative anti-convulsants if continued anti-psychotic medication is advised. As clinical experience of these drugs grows, evidence of possible heart effects such as myocarditis is accumulating and causing concern. Diabetes is both a complicating factor (especially with olanzapine) and a possible side-effect. Weight gain is an obvious side-effect of atypicals as well as earlier neuroleptics. It may be due to metabolic changes, but could also be secondary to either increased well-being and appetite, or decreased activity due to sedation and drug-induced lethargy. Either way, weight-gain has knock-on psychological and physical health problems, including lower self-esteem, tiredness, cardiovascular disease and an increased risk of diabetes. In common with such effects as reduced sexual desire and breast enlargement, weight-gain can be extremely upsetting and make people reluctant to continue with medication.

PSYCHO-SOCIAL INTERVENTIONS FOR SCHIZOPHRENIA

Psychiatric treatment has traditionally focused on the neurobiological nature of schizophrenia. Developmental, interpersonal and social facets have received relatively less attention in devising clinical responses, despite featuring strongly in research. Users however have repeatedly asserted the value of various psycho-social interventions, often from nurses who spend large amounts of time in social contact with diagnosed schizophrenics; or clinical psychologists whose therapeutic orientation differs from medically trained psychiatrists.[42,43] Comprehensive care for schizophrenia comprises a holistic package which should include cognitive-behavioural therapy, family interventions, supportive education, and life-, social- and vocational skills training.[44] Many of these interventions have been incorporated into the Thorn[45] and PSI[46] training courses, and should be integrated into basic mental health nurse education programmes.

Psycho-social help is usually offered in conjunction with medication, although some sufferers prefer social support and psychological therapies as mainstay alternatives to drug treatment, either throughout their care, or during their less disturbed periods.[12] Psychiatrists usually consider the clinical and social risks too high to base care upon non-pharmaceutical treatments, although some professionals believe they offer effective alternatives to drug-based treatment for many users. Therapeutic Community, psychodynamic and other non-pharmaceutical approaches have reportedly helped people with their schizophrenic symptoms, but although these approaches continue to develop,[47–50] psychiatrists generally consider them insufficiently evidenced, and therefore unsound as sole foundations for clinical treatment.

APPLIED COGNITIVE–BEHAVIOURAL THERAPY

CBT, like some psychodynamic formulations, emphasizes the meanings that experiences have for individuals, and the consequences of their subsequent behavioural responses. CBT helps people become aware of connections made unconsciously between experiences, patterns of thinking and subsequent feelings and behaviour. Therapist and client collaborate to explore the meanings that sufferers attribute to events. They examine the evidence for and against specific beliefs, meanings or attributions; devise challenges to habitual patterns of thinking and reacting; and employ logical reasoning and other, neglected personal experiences to develop more rational and effective alternative responses. CBT is effective when expertly applied to symptoms of schizophrenia,[12,51] but could become more valuable if its principles could be absorbed, generalized and applied by nurses in everyday working situations. Sufferers should benefit from working within cognitive-behavioural therapeutic milieux, where supportive reality-testing and modification of symptoms could occur early in someone's breakdown process, before pathology becomes deep-rooted, chronic or confrontationally defended.[52]

For such therapeutic environments to become effective, staff should revise residual, traditional psychiatric thinking about psychotic symptoms. Delusions and hallucinations have traditionally been understood as simply abnormal phenomena, which are either present or absent, and vary significantly in only one dimension – severity. Nurses intending to engage people in therapeutic conversation need to regard delusions and hallucinations as multi-dimensional. Delusions vary in intensity of conviction; degree of preoccupation; nature and depth of distress caused; and their motivational power.[53] They are not fixed, but alter with new experiences and collaborative analysis of evidence or logical basis. Hallucinations similarly vary in intensity, frequency, abusiveness and controllability.[54] Schizophrenic people's emotions are not merely flattened; rather their symptoms are often accompanied by significant emotion that can be empathically engaged. Hallucinatory and delusional content or themes can have both direct and metaphorical meaning derived from people's often long-neglected experiences. Nurses should not regard psychotic symptoms as simply meaningless pathologies, thereby running the risk of invalidating sufferers' experiences, and provoking further alienation. Delusions and hallucinations can be meaningfully construed as complex psychological phenomena actively generated from the interaction of people's personalities with past and current experience.

Nurses working from this perspective can suggest normalizing rationales for psychotic symptoms, whereby peoples' pathological experiences and behaviours are interpreted as valid expressions of their vulnerability. Nurses have been enjoined to make more use of formal assessment measures[55] and many are now available.[45] Semi-structured interview formats (e.g. the KGV[28] comprising detailed questions about every aspect of schizophrenia) enable closer, more attentive conversations about the individual's personal experiences of illness. *Time–life diagrams* are simple parallel line diagrams that encourage people to reminiscence about ordinary life-events occurring along a narrative thread of well-being, often discarded in favour of preoccupation with illness-events, and a life-story based upon treatment. Collaboratively devising time–life diagrams helps people to unpick the rich non-clinical threads of their experiences and re-stitch their narrative tapestry to incorporate less pathologically pessimistic possibilities. *Externalizing questions* explore the impact of illness as an outside intruder into personal life. They can help people to detach from preoccupation with internal defectiveness and devise coping strategies that deal more effectively with the intrusion of schizophrenia into their lives.[56]

Meta–representation

The clinical and academic discipline of cognitive neuropsychology attempts to integrate psychological and biological explanations of behaviour by developing insights into how electrochemical, hard-wired brain processes mediate mental phenomena like thoughts and feelings, and how these intangible phenomena are behaviourally operationalized. One such explanation is that the failure of a neurocognitive function called *meta-representation* causes schizophrenic cognitive pathology.[57] Meta-representation underlies two other important cognitive functions: *theory of mind* and *self-monitoring*. Humans develop both faculties while wiring-up our plastic brains during the primary attachment phase of infancy.[58]

Theory of mind refers firstly to the realization that other people have minds too, but that they may well be different from our own; and secondly to our ability to form theories about other people's minds: to create accurate impressions of others' intentions or feelings; to make sense of their actions and communications; and to successfully predict or anticipate their behaviour. Effective communication and social activity require shared implicit understanding that others have thoughts, feelings and intentions similar or dissimilar to our own; that their behaviour is governed by discernible motives; and that attentive interpersonal observation provides reliable clues to others' states of mind. Schizophrenics often report or display difficulty with these abilities.

Self-monitoring is an essential function for conscious intention and regulated action. The brain requires continuous feedback about thoughts or intentions in order to successfully maintain cognitive processes or actions until their purpose is accomplished. We need to remind ourselves whether the thought we are generating is a memory, wish, hope, plan or fantasy. Without such self-monitoring we would 'forget' that we are imagining, pretending, fearing or hoping that something is the case (e.g. 'I'm *pretending* that I'm rich' or 'I'm *afraid* he won't like me' or '*What if* the fire alarm is a bugging device?') and believe it to be so: 'I'm rich, he doesn't like me and the fire alarm is a bug!'

Meta-representation is the means by which the brain continuously checks the context for each representation of reality or intention. During cognition and action, meta-representation 'remembers' our purposes and intentions, our self-monitoring and our reading of others' minds. In its absence, we would not only fail to 'know our own minds', we would also 'forget' that we are thinking about something that someone else said or thinks, and feel confused as to how we find ourselves thinking about such stuff at all. The hypothetical mechanism has been tentatively mapped onto known brain organization, and could help to construct intervention strategies for specific cognitive and communication anomalies.

WORKING FROM FAMILY PERSPECTIVES

The relationship between schizophrenia and family life has been contentiously debated for decades, and the various controversies are far too complex to be dealt with here. Two broadly different approaches to working with families exist – family therapy and family management – and while both claim effectiveness, one (family management) dominates conventional psychiatric practice.[59] Family therapists, frequently from non-psychiatric backgrounds, base their interventions upon a theoretical proposition: that families function as complex organic social systems; and an assessed judgement: that some aspects of a family's organization are less than optimally effective and are disabling its functional capabilities. This dysfunction creates internal stress which impacts hardest on the most vulnerable individual or role within the family, and causes breakdown. Changes made to functional subsystems like problem-solving, communication, family roles, affective responsiveness, affective involvement and behaviour control can enable the whole family to cope better with internal stress or external pressures and ease the strain on individuals.[60] Family management practitioners adopt similar rationales, but emphasize that schizophrenia is a serious organic disease which engenders a shared need for education and support to cope with the consequences of diagnosis. However, even family management interventions remain underused, despite evidence of their effectiveness.[44]

Professional interventions into the normally private environment of family life are usually justified in one of two inter-related ways:

❑ family members are stressed by burdens, e.g. caring for an unwell member, or economic distress and need support to manage responsibilities, resolve concerns or prevent further functional deterioration;
❑ the family system itself does not operate as effectively as it might, and consequently individual members are subjected to stressful interactive processes that can be eased by changes in family functions and relationships.

Families with a schizophrenic member experience considerable stress. There is often pain and puzzlement about their vulnerable relative's behaviour and obvious distress; grief over lost hopes and fear for future possibilities; anger and guilt about recrimination and self-blame. Equally, people with schizophrenia often experience aspects of family life as stressful, and relapse more often and more severely where there is an intense atmosphere of criticism, hostility or emotional over-involvement. These behaviours can be measured to assess a family's quotient of *expressed emotion*, and it has been established that high expressed emotion environments constitute serious stress for individuals vulnerable to a range of physical and psychological disorders, including schizophrenia. Research suggests that reducing the intensity and frequency of high expressed emotion as a precipitating stressor helps, as also does limiting the time spent in overall interaction.[11]

The proposition that defective interpersonal family functioning prior to the onset of symptoms may precipitate initial conversion to active schizophrenia has been hotly disputed.[2] It remains a matter of contention[61] and has historically fuelled the development of some forms of family therapy.[59] Most family interventions for schizophrenia however are based upon relatives' needs for support with their caring responsibilities; or aim to reduce stressful interactions, so that the diagnosed individual relapses less and the welfare of other family members is not so compromised.[62]

Potentially effective interventions derived from various schools of thought and practice include:

❑ education about schizophrenia: symptoms, vulnerability and stressors;
❑ facilitating discussions about each other's perspectives on specific problems and favoured solutions;
❑ validating and positively reframing family members' intentions and behaviours;
❑ support for family members' efforts to tolerate and appreciate individual differences and interpersonal boundaries;
❑ recognizing and finding ways of increasing the frequency of effective interpersonal behaviours;
❑ identifying and reducing the frequency and intensity of excessive emotional resonance, critical comments and hostile reactions;
❑ training and support in problem-solving strategies;
❑ reinforcing clear, direct communication and reducing less transparent, more evasive or ambivalent messages;
❑ clarifying expectations about roles, responsibilities and personal accountability;
❑ helping to adjust expectations of each other's behaviours to attainable standards;
❑ encouraging interaction between estranged or uncommunicative members;
❑ supportive collaboration with caring relatives, especially in acute crises;
❑ modified bereavement counselling for (especially parents') grief-like reactions to loss of idealized expectations for their child;
❑ planned respite and recuperative activity for all vulnerable members, both patient and carers;
❑ structuring activities and rationing time spent together.

Schizophrenia impacts not simply on the individual sufferer, but also on family, friends, colleagues, neighbours and even wider social networks. Emotional reactions such as grief, anger, shame and fear are common, as are unhelpful responses such as rejection or infantilization. All may respond to supportive interventions, and family-based approaches are relevant to whatever social matrix is involved.[63]

SOCIAL, VOCATIONAL AND LIFE SKILLS

Because of its impact on cognitive and communication processes, schizophrenia often disables people's abilities to conduct effective interpersonal relationships and to perform ordinary domestic or vocational tasks. Preoccupation with internal mental states; memory and attention difficulties; and the cumulative effect of negative symptoms and neuroleptic induced deficits compli-

cate everyday interactions. After several years of breakdown, withdrawal, treatment and relapse, people may lose technical skills and social abilities they once took for granted. If severely affected at adolescence, some sufferers may never have acquired the social confidence and practical skills necessary to survive independently. Skills training programmes use a variety of techniques, including role-play, video-recording and behaviour modification, and can be classified into three types:[44]

❑ **Life skills, or daily-living programmes** provide group or individual training in ordinary social survival and include teaching and supervised practice in: financial management and budgeting; personal self-care; domestic skills like cooking and cleaning; shopping and allied consumer skills like complaining; civic skills such as voting.
❑ **Social skills training** aims to enhance people's abilities to perform well in social and interactive relationships. Training includes: assessment of trainees interpersonal skill deficits and excesses (i.e. not looking at people, or staring too intently; speaking too loudly, quietly or monotonously); analysis of how well people pick-up and cognitively process interpersonal cues; and graded practice of specific verbal and non-verbal communication skills.
❑ **Vocational skills** are needed to obtain and retain employment. Specific skills for particular jobs need to be learnt, but also people sometimes need help with their orientation towards work and fundamental issues like time-keeping, rule-observance, taking orders etc. Many services have developed their own supported employment programmes or industrial therapy units where sensitive support and training can be provided. Ultimately the aim should be for people to be as fully integrated as possible into ordinary working life.

Skills training programmes offer nurses the opportunity to work closely not only with users, but also with occupational therapists, whose professional preparation includes intensive experience of skills development techniques. However, skills training may be more effective when integrated into everyday life in supportive residential, outreach or daycare services. Benefits from formal training sessions alone may not endure long outside, or generalize poorly into ordinary situations.[64]

PHYSICAL ILLNESS AND HEALTH PROMOTION

An unfortunate percentage of sufferers go on to develop chronically relapsing or deteriorating forms of schizophrenia. Their needs for nursing care shift as negative symptoms dominate their clinical profile, and increasingly inactive or impoverished lifestyles begin to take their toll. Mortality from all causes is higher in the psychiatric population than the general public. Even when figures for suicide and accidents are excluded, the severely mentally ill population has an excessively high death rate. Long-term schizophrenia puts people in increased jeopardy from cardiovascular conditions, respiratory problems, infectious diseases and endocrine disorders.[65] Iatrogenic illness from cardiovascular, metabolic and endocrine side-effects of neuroleptics may explain some of these discrepancies. Lifestyle causes (which may also be secondary to neuroleptic-induced deficits) include increased tobacco use, reduced exercise and poor diet. People may also use street-drugs or drink alcohol excessively. In addition, primary care and mental health professionals often fail to assess, recognize or treat physical illness in psychiatric patients. They may wrongly attribute reported symptoms to psychological causes, and interpret patients' physical problems as aspects of psychiatric illness. Some primary care professionals may be unfamiliar with and feel uncomfortable dealing with psychiatric patients. Patients may themselves not communicate their difficulties to professionals, through social skill deficiencies, fear of stigmatization, embarrassment or because of the effects of delusional beliefs, high anxiety etc.

The UK Department of Health now requires primary care services to monitor the physical health of people with schizophrenia and provide effective health care. Sufferers should at least receive annual medical checks of blood pressure and urinalysis, be vaccinated against influenza and have help to reduce smoking.[66] Strategic interventions by mental health services include:

❑ liaison with accommodation, employment and benefit agencies;
❑ regular meetings between primary health care and specialist mental health teams;
❑ effective integration of health and social care agencies;
❑ greater involvement of patients or their advocates in health and social care decisions.

Mental health nurses and social care staff in whatever setting should ensure that they collaborate with long-term sufferers and liaise with physicians to focus on physical health as well as psychological and social welfare. Within therapeutic alliances, or as part of assertive outreach, nurses could help sufferers to:

❑ enjoy more exercise and stimulating recreational lifestyles;
❑ maintain healthy accommodation and hygienic living standards;
❑ limit the amount they smoke;

❑ avoid excess alcohol and drug-use;
❑ eat well, as personal taste and finances allow;
❑ monitor any damaging side-effects from medication.

Nurses' physical health promotion work should be characterized by the same empathic attitudes that prevent them becoming high-expressed emotion carers in relation to people's psycho-social needs. If nurses strive too zealously to manipulate, persuade or coerce people into pure, healthy lifestyles, they run the risk of being experienced as health fascists. Sufferers may feel misunderstood or threatened and label their supposed helpers as the enemy; do-gooding types with little knowledge or understanding of alienation, isolation or poverty; uncaring, punitive straitlaced or interfering critics. People are more likely to value their own health and well-being if nurses validate them as adult personalities with the right to some peccadilloes and even venial sins. The keynotes should be harm-limitation and a 'motivational interviewing' emphasis on the benefits of feeling more lively, being comfortable, eating well and having some spending money not ear-marked for next day's nicotine.

THERAPEUTIC RELATIONSHIPS WITH PEOPLE WITH A DIAGNOSIS OF SCHIZOPHRENIA

While treatment schedules and care plans consisting of various combinations of technical interventions are potentially clinically effective, they don't help nurses and sufferers to determine how best to establish and maintain trusting relationships, nor how to communicate positively with each other. One of the earlier accounts in the modern era of nursing people with schizophrenia contains some retrospectively interesting advice:

> We need careful re-thinking about our nursing methods; and about nurses' attitudes; and any tendency to institutionalized reactions; for such reactions are far more common than one would imagine, and inevitably the patient suffers. I can remember early on in my psychiatric training, I was playing a card game with a schizophrenic patient and endeavouring to make light conversation with her. She rarely spoke, but after an hour she put down her cards and said wonderingly "You treat me as if I were normal". I shall never forget the look on that patient's face as she said this. I believe it sums up what should be our attitude at all times to those suffering from schizophrenia.[67]

Nearly 30 years later, this quotation may seem quaintly platitudinous, but it also innocently throws into relief some recent criticisms of psychiatric services. The poem quoted at the beginning of this chapter expresses similar sentiments. One unintended consequence of nurses becoming increasingly associated with the psychiatric treatment of the biological basis of schizophrenia, rather than collaborative allies and advocates, is the risk of people feeling objectified or 'othered'.[68] 'Othering' attitudes can be benign, albeit infantilizing or dependence-inducing, as well as malign perverse, or degenerate. An attitude of superior difference can be conveyed para-linguistically by tone of voice; by using technical, managerial or authoritarian language; by being purposely unclear and indirect in everyday or formal interactions; and invalidating in various other ways – by closed office doors; non-collaborative care; imposition of rules and strictures; thoughtlessly worded signs; casual unexplained use of psychiatric or legalistic jargon; and by thinking, however unconsciously and however people may behave, that schizophrenic patients are childlike, dull, dangerous, or incomprehensible.

There are many ways in which staff can become unhelpful in their relationships with schizophrenic patients. Sufferers can be puzzled, frustrated or dismayed by unclear, indirect, ambivalent ambiguous or disguised communications. People who experience schizophrenic symptoms often speak and behave in apparently incomprehensible or simply unusual or challenging ways. When nurses or others respond in patronizing, dismissive, authoritarian or otherwise invalidating fashion, sufferers naturally feel even more confused, disturbed, distressed or angry.

The noxious effect of high expressed emotion within family life is replicated in studies of staff cultures. Criticism, hostility and emotional over-involvement are just as potent precipitators of illness when portrayed by staff as they are when performed within the closer bounds of family life. Emotional over-involvement in this context does not mean caring about, but rather uncontrolled emotional resonance – of whatever hue – in staff responses to patients' behaviours. If professionals are not to create a psycho-noxious, un-therapeutic environment then individual therapeutic supervision and team support and sensitivity meetings are essential adjuncts to collaborative care-planning.[14]

In reaction to the unhelpful impact of what they perceive as uncomprehending, uncaring or hostile attitudes within professional service organizations, sufferers and carers have recently developed self-help and user-led alternatives, such as Crisis Houses, Drop-In Centres and Hearing Voices groups. These less medically driven, non-prescriptive and more democratic resources are judged by many sufferers to match their needs more sensitively and have led to many professionals adopting similar attitudes and strategies as traditional service are evaluated and improved to accommodate users' and carers' expressed wishes.[69]

Nurses should engage fully with the ordinariness (however unexceptional or extraordinary) of people diagnosed as schizophrenic, as well as be interested in or sympathetic to them as sufferers from clinical illness. Thus, care plans should take account of the importance of enjoying the company of persons diagnosed as schizophrenic; initiating and holding normal conversations; and sharing recreational, purposeful social activities. Nurses should be warm, empathic and positive. They should be fascinated companions, supportively encouraging people to clarify and make constructive sense of their experiences.

However, the diagnosis of schizophrenia often entails a fragile sense of self. People develop vulnerable identities, with weakness and potential erosion of normally secure personal boundaries.[70] Sufferers are exposed to potential flooding by or fusion with their socio-cultural environments. People, objects, events, ideas or emotions from outside can invasively pollute highly susceptible inner selves. In developing companionable relationships, nurses need to be aware of this heightened sensitivity. Feeling constantly under threat, many schizophrenics develop exquisitely delicate sensory antennae, and become subliminally aware of minute stimuli and implicit messages normally masked behind disguised verbal communication. This perception of an invasive, inexplicable and uncontrollable outside world leads not only to high anxiety and social withdrawal, but also to mistrust of outside influences and uneasiness about social intercourse.[70] Thus nurses' fascination and warmth should not only be genuine, it should also be carefully modulated. Watzlawick suggested 'the meaning of any communication is the response you get'.[71,72] When in therapeutic interaction with people, nurses should carefully notice their companions' reactions, and engage no more closely than they seem ready to tolerate. There may be no intention to invade, invalidate or otherwise abuse. Nevertheless, because of differences in sensitivity and reliability of schizophrenic 'theory of mind' compared with most non-schizophrenic clinical staff, empathy will not be easily accurate. Basically, if people seem hurt by your communication, think of it as a hurtful communication; if they seem pleased, then score it as pleasant.

Because of anxiety and difficulties in controlling sensory input, people diagnosed as schizophrenic are potentially vulnerable to invasive intrusion from aspects of 'the outside world'. This vulnerability complicates their more ordinary needs for social communion and companionship. The conflict exposes sufferers to twin fears: of alternately being engulfed by over-intimate outsiders; or disregarded and abandoned in isolation.[73] Nurses need to constantly monitor people's behavioural and emotional responses to maintain the most helpful, least threatening social distance. Interacting through shared activity may help to counteract relationship and communication difficulties. Incorporating a third point into the relationship, such as a physical activity, chore or creative project, helps triangulate or neutralize the struggle to achieve unthreatening empathy and engagement. Apart from the simple fact that people appreciate nurses' practical assistance and interested involvement,[74] painting and sculpture,[75] cooking, repairs, maintenance, gardening and other ordinary activities of everyday life offer unemotional absorption and neutral escape from interpersonal tension.[76,77]

Case study 32.1

Jim Limber was a middle-aged Irishman who was diagnosed as paranoid schizophrenic and formally detained in a psychiatric hospital after frequent attacks on strangers whilst he was working as a labourer. Jim claimed they were homosexuals who had stolen his ideas and money, and also intended to abuse him. Jim knew that he'd invented rocket propulsion, hovercraft and jet engines, amongst other things, but a conspiracy of homosexual men removed his brilliant ideas before he could patent them, and stored the profit in a docklands warehouse. Wandering around after a hard night's drinking, he'd seen the golden glow from his treasure gleaming through the pre-dawn mist.

One day a nurse suggested that Jim get involved in preparing the small garden being rehabilitated outside the ward. Once outside, Jim started furiously digging over a flower-bed. 'That'll be a well prepared bit of soil! What would you like to plant there, Jim?' 'Pansies!' Jim grinned as he replied. 'Forgive and forget, eh Jim?' thought the nurse, and dared to share the joke. 'I wish I could'. Jim responded. 'Well, I suppose there's lots you'd like to forget', replied the nurse 'but then there's a lot we don't remember – like when we're small'. 'I remember Ireland, and the smoke of peat'.

For the rest of the morning, Jim told whimsical stories about childhood – poverty, drunkenness, abuse, and a deep sense of nostalgia. 'It's strange, Jim. There's so much difference between life as it was, and the life you feel you should have been entitled to'. 'Strange to miss so much misery – there's no point getting nowhere I suppose'. Jim mused quietly, and there was no hint of madness in his conversation from then on, but there was a very well dug-over garden.

REFERENCES

1. Jim Limber. One of many poems written by a man diagnosed with paranoid schizophrenia, who lived for several years on a 72-bedded locked ward.
2. Keen T. Schizophrenia: orthodoxy and heresies: a review of some alternative perspectives. *Journal of Psychiatric and Mental Health Nursing* 1999; **6**(6): 415–24.
3. NHS Centre for Reviews and Dissemination. Drug treatments for schizophrenia. *Effective Health Care* 1999; **5**(6).
4. Frangou S, Murray RM. *Schizophrenia*, 2nd edn. London: Martin Dunitz, 2000.
5. American Psychiatric Association. *Diagnostic and statistical manual of mental disorders*, 4th edn – revised. Washington DC: APA, 1994.
6. World Health Organization. *Classification of mental and behavioural disorders: clinical conditions and diagnostic guidelines*: ICD-10. Geneva: WHO, 1992.
7. Thomas P. *The dialectics of schizophrenia*. London: Free Association Books, 1997.
8. Nettle D. *Strong imagination: madness, creativity and human nature.* Oxford: Oxford University Press, 2001.
9. Bannister D, Fransella F. *Inquiring man*, 2nd edn. Harmondsworth: Penguin, 1980.
10. Horrobin D. *The madness of Adam and Eve: how schizophrenia shaped humanity.* London: Bantam Press, 2001.
11. Leff J. *The unbalanced mind.* London: Weidenfeld and Nicolson, 2001.
12. Kinderman P, Cooke A (eds). *Recent advances in understanding mental illness and psychotic experiences.* British Psychological Society Division of Clinical Psychology, 2000.
13. Atkinson J, Coia DA. *Families coping with schizophrenia.* Chichester: Wiley, 1995.
14. Kuipers E. Working with carers: interventions for relatives and staff carers of those who have psychosis. In: Wykes T, Tarrier N, Lewis S. *Outcome and innovation in psychological treatment of schizophrenia.* Chichester: John Wiley, 1998.
15. Leudar I, Thomas P. *Voices of reason, voices of insanity.* London: Routledge, 2000.
16. Romme M, Escher S. *Accepting voices.* London: MIND, 1993.
17. Jenner A, Monteiro ACD, Zagalo-Cardoso JA, Cunha-Oliveira JA. *Schizophrenia: a disease or some ways of being human.* Sheffield: Sheffield Academic Press, 1993.
18. Liddle P. The symptoms of chronic schizophrenia: a re-examination of the positive–negative dichotomy. *British Journal of Psychiatry* 1987; **151**: 145–51.
19. Liddle P, Friston K, Frith C. Patterns of cerebral blood-flow in schizophrenia. *British Journal of Psychiatry* 1992; **160**: 179–86.
20. Clare A. Psychiatry's future: psychological medicine or biological psychiatry? *Journal of Mental Health* 1999; **8**: 109–111.
21. Repper J. Adjusting the focus of mental health nursing: incorporating service users' experience of recovery. *Journal of Mental Health* 2000; **9**: 575–87.
22. Coleman R, Smith M. *Working with voices: victim to victor.* Newton-le-Willows: Handsell Publications, 1997.

23. Nelson H. *Cognitive-behavioural therapy with schizophrenia: a practice manual.* Cheltenham: Stanley Thornes, 1997.

24. Sharma T, Chitnis X. *Brain imaging in schizophrenia.* London: ReMEDICA, 2000.

25. Boyle M. *Schizophrenia: a scientific delusion?* London: Routledge, 1990.

26. Johnstone L. *Users and abusers of psychiatry*, 2nd edn. London: Routledge, 2000.

27. Bentall R. Why there will never be a convincing theory of schizophrenia. In: Rose S. *From brains to consciousness? Essays on the new sciences of the mind.* London: Penguin, 1998.

28. Drake R, Haddock G, Hopkins R, Lewis S. The measurement of outcome in schizophrenia. In: Wykes T, Tarrier N, Lewis S. *Outcome and innovation in psychological treatment of schizophrenia.* Chichester: John Wiley, 1998.

29. Department of Health. *The mental health policy implementation guide.* London: Department of Health, 2001.

30. Department of Health. *The mental health policy implementation guide: adult acute inpatient care provision.* London: Department of Health, 2002.

31. Regel S, Roberts D. *Mental health liaison: a handbook for nurses and health professionals.* Edinburgh: Baillière-Tindall, 2002.

32. Zubin J, Spring B. Vulnerability: A new view of schizophrenia. *Journal of Abnormal Psychology* 1997; **86**: 260–66.

33. Hughes I, Hill B, Budd R. Compliance with antipsychotic medication: From theory to practice. *Journal of Mental Health* 1997; **6**: 473–89.

34. Smith JA, Hughes I, Budd R. Non-compliance with anti-psychotic medication: Users' views on advantages and disadvantages. *Journal of Mental Health* 1999; **8**: 287–96.

35. Bebbington P. The content and context of compliance. *International Clinical Psychopharmacology* 1995; **9**(Suppl. 5): 41–50.

36. McPhillips M, Sensky T. Coercion, adherence or collaboration? Influences on compliance with medication. In: Wykes T, Tarrier N, Lewis S. *Outcome and innovation in psychological treatment of schizophrenia.* Chichester: John Wiley, 1998.

37. Kemp R, *et al. Compliance therapy manual.* London: Bethlem and Maudsley NHS Trust, 1997.

38. Day J, Wood G, Dewer M, Bertall R. A self-rating scale for measuring neuroleptic side-effects. *British Journal of Psychiatry* 1995; **166**: 650–53.

39. Perkins R, Repper J. Compliance or informed choice? *Journal of Mental Health* 1999; **8**: 117–29.

40. Perkins R, Repper J. *Dilemmas in community mental health practice: choice or control?* Oxford: Radcliffe Medical Press, 1998: p. 64.

41. Healy D. *Psychiatric drugs explained*, 2nd edn. London: Mosby, 1997.

42. Rose D. *Users' voices.* London, Sainsbury Centre for Mental Health, 2001.

43. Rogers A, Pilgrim D, Lacey R. *Experiencing psychiatry: users' views of services.* Macmillan: London, 1993.

44. NHS Centre for Reviews and Dissemination. Psycho-social interventions for schizophrenia. *Effective Health Care* 2000; **6**(3).

45. Gamble C, Brennan G. *Working with serious mental illness: a manual for clinical practice.* London: Baillière Tindall, 2000.

46. Fahy K, Dudley M. An introduction to psycho-social interventions in services. In: Thompson T, Mathias P (eds). *Lyttle's mental health and disorder*, 3rd edn. Edinburgh: Baillière Tindall, 2000.

47. Breggin P, Cohen D. *Your drug may be your problem: how and why to stop taking psychiatric medication.* New York: Perseus Books, 2000.

48. Kuipers E. The management of difficult to treat patients with schizophrenia, using non-drug therapies. *British Journal of Psychiatry* (Suppl.) 1996; (31): 41–51.

49. Mosher L, Burti L. Is psychotropic drug dependence really necessary? In: *Community mental health: a practical guide*, Chapter 5. New York: Norton, 1994.

50. Alanen YO. *Schizophrenia: its origins and need-adapted treatment.* London: Karnac Books, 1997.

51. Tarrier N, Yusupoff L, Kinney C, *et al.* Randomised controlled trial of intensive cognitive behaviour therapy for patients with chronic schizophrenia. *British Medical Journal* 1998; **317**: 303–7.

52. Drury V. Recovery from acute psychosis. In: Birchwood M, Tarrier N. *Psychological management of schizophrenia.* Chichester: Wiley, 1994.

53. Garety P, Hemsley D. *Delusions: investigations into the psychology of delusional reasoning.* Hove: Psychology Press, 1997.

54. Haddock G, Slade PD (eds). *Cognitive-behavioural interventions with psychotic disorders.* London: Routledge, 1996.

55. Standing Nursing and Midwifery Advisory Committee. *Addressing acute concerns.* London: Department of Health, 1999.

56. White M, Epston D. *Narrative means to therapeutic ends.* New York: WW Norton, 1990.

57. Frith CD. *The cognitive neuropsychology of schizophrenia.* Hove: Lawrence Erlbaum, 1992.

58. Siegel DJ. *The developing mind: toward a neurobiology of interpersonal experience.* New York: Guilford Press, 1999.

59. Burbach F. Family-based interventions in psychosis – An overview of, and comparison between, family therapy and family management approaches. *Journal of Mental Health* 1996; **5**: 111–34.

60. Epstein NB, Bishop D, Ryan C, Miller IW, Keitner GI. The McMaster model view of healthy family functioning. In: Walsh F (ed.) *Normal family processes*. New York: The Guilford Press, 1993: 138–60.

61. Johnstone L. Do families cause schizophrenia? Revisiting a taboo subject. In: Newnes C, Holmes G, Dunn C (eds). *This is madness: a critical look at psychiatry and the future of mental health services*. Ross-on-Wye: PCCS Books, 1999.

62. Kuipers L, Leff J, Lam D. *Family work for schizophrenia*. London: Royal College of Psychiatrists/Gaskell, 1992.

63. Jones DW. *Myths, madness and the family: the impact of mental illness on families*. Brighton: Palgrave Publishers, 2002.

64. Benton M, Schroeder H. Social skills training with schizophrenics: a meta-analytic evaluation. *Journal of Consulting and Clinical Psychology* 1990; **58**: 741–7.

65. Osborn DPJ. The poor physical health of mentally ill people. *Western Journal of Medicine* 2001; **175**: 329–34.

66. Cohen A, Hove M. *Physical health of the severe and enduring mentally ill*. London: Sainsbury Centre for Mental Health, 2001.

67. Frost M. *Nursing care of the schizophrenic patient*. London: Henry Kimpton, 1974: p. 8.

68. MacCallum EJ. Othering and psychiatric nursing. *Journal of Psychiatric and Mental Health Nursing* 2002; **9**: 87–94.

69. Newnes C, Holmes G, Dunn C (eds). *This is madness too: a further critical look at mental health services*. Ross-on-Wye: PCCS Books, 2000.

70. Chadwick PK. *Schizophrenia: the positive perspective*. London: Routledge, 1997.

71. Watzlawick P, Beavin J, Jackson D. *Pragmatics of human communication*. New York: Norton, 1967.

72. Watzlawick P, Beavin J, Jackson D. Some tentative axioms of communication. In: Morse BW, Phelps LA (eds). *Interpersonal communication: a relational perspective*. Minneapolis, MD: Burgess Publishing Company, 1980: 32–42.

73. May R. *The courage to create*. New York: Norton, 1994.

74. Perkins R, Repper J. *Working alongside people with long-term mental health problems*. Cheltenham: Stanley Thornes, 1997.

75. Killick K, Shaverien J (eds). *Art, psychotherapy and psychosis*. London: Routledge, 1997.

76. Wilson M. *Occupational therapy in short-term psychiatry*. London: Churchill Livingstone, 1996.

77. Wilson M. *Occupational therapy in long-term psychiatry*. London: Churchill Livingstone, 1996.

Chapter 33

THE PERSON WHO IS AGGRESSIVE OR VIOLENT

Eimear Muir-Cochrane*

INTRODUCTION

This chapter explores anger, aggression and violence in the workplace. Adopting a reflective practice, personal understandings of aggression are explored in the context of the challenges that face mental health professionals working in hospital settings. Nursing interventions that focus on prevention, de-escalation and management are discussed using case studies and reflective exercises. The chapter aims to develop the reader's personal awareness of aggression and violence by:

❏ exploring personal understandings of anger and frustration;
❏ defining and differentiating between anger, aggression and violence;
❏ increasing knowledge of the dynamics of aggression;
❏ describing physical and physiological approaches to anger and aggression;
❏ identifying predisposing factors to the expression of anger and aggression;
❏ discussing different nursing interventions for clients exhibiting aggression;
❏ identifying ways of reducing the potential for aggression and violence in the workplace.

Definitions

❏ **Anger**: an emotion aroused to real or perceived threat to self, others or possessions.
❏ **Aggression**: a disposition that may lead to constructive or destructive actions but that usually has long-term negative consequences.
❏ **Violence**: the harmful and unlawful use of force or strength. The violent person is generally understood to refer to someone who attacks another.[1]

Violence and aggression in society and the workplace

Violence and aggression are universal phenomena and occur in all cultures in society, although some societies are perceived as more violent than others. In a book on the management of violence and aggression, Mason and Chandley refer to issues concerned with the contemporary nature of violence in society. The amount of reporting of violence from around the world television, the press, Internet and radio, has dramatically increased over the last few decades. This influences how people perceive its prevalence. In the Western world, concerns for personal safety have generated the associated 'industry of protec-

---

*Eimear is an academic at the University of South Australia, with current responsibilities for the leadership and management of higher degree students and the program direction of postgraduate mental health nursing courses. Eimear is also the Chair of the University Ethics Committee satisfying her need to promote the ethical conduct of research involving people. Eimear's research interests include the use of seclusion, community mental health and the mental health needs of homeless young people.

tionism'.[1] This can be seen in the growth of sales of personal alarms, as well as home security systems. Sensationalist reporting is increasing, including images of *mentally ill people as violent*. Although there is little evidence to support such a view, the public often construe disorganized and agitated behaviour in people with mental illness as examples of antisocial conduct and hostility. Thus, the public, health professionals and psychiatric patients are often fearful of other psychiatric patients, believing them to be potentially aggressive and violent. It is generally assumed that aggressive and violent behaviour occurs more in psychiatric settings than in other health care settings, but this is not the case.[2] All health care settings have the potential for aggression since the experience of anger is a normal adaptive reaction. However, it is the intensity of the experience of anger, its duration and expression that causes people problems.

The frequency of aggression towards nurses in health care settings is increasing and well-documented, posing a major occupational health and safety hazard.[3,4] In mental health between 40–80% of staff are assaulted while at work.[5] Nurses now work in a diverse range of health care settings: home, hostels, health centres, police stations, as well as inpatient hospital units. The first week of hospitalization is recognized as a period in which the incidence of aggression or violence is higher than at any other time of inpatient care,[6] suggesting that the time around the admission of an individual ought to receive special attention by the mental health care team.

A recent UK study reported that NHS staff are four times more likely to be victims of violence during the course of their work than other workers.[7] It is a sad reality that nurses need to prepare themselves with skill and knowledge to deal with aggression and violence in the workplace. The increasing risk of aggression and violence ranges from verbal abuse through to assault with violence.[8] It is vital that evidenced-based policies, procedures and training have a high profile in the management of aggression in all health care organizations. In Australia, in 2001 the New South Wales (NSW) Nurses Association adopted a 'no tolerance' approach to violence in health care settings after an inpatient psychiatric patient bludgeoned an elderly resident to death. Unfortunately, the necessity of anger management practices for patients (particularly in those health care settings where patients reside for long periods) received little attention. Instead, the commitment of the NSW government to increase the number of security guards in health care settings suggests a containment focus rather than a therapeutic approach to the problem of workplace aggression and violence.

It is also of concern that many aggressive incidents go unreported, perhaps because nurses see aggression as a frequent but unfortunate reality, because they become accustomed to such experiences, and perhaps because of the paperwork required to report incidents. Although aggression cannot be avoided altogether, the incidence of aggression can be reduced through prediction measures and prevention strategies. While it would seem reasonable to suggest that the characteristics of the human environment have a powerful effect in mitigating or precipitating aggression and violence, research cannot yet demonstrate this. There is some evidence that training and experience in aggression management are useful tools to reduce injuries to staff but it has not yet been proven that this leads to a reduction in the overall incidence of violence.[6]

Anger

As the song goes, anger is an energy. Anger is a normal and powerful human emotion that people may experience several times a week. It is an under-researched emotion and a satisfactory definition of anger is difficult to achieve. Although on an individual basis, we can all understand what it is to be angry, it is more difficult to define what anger means for other people.

Mental health nurses recognize that making judgements about those in our care is unhelpful for the patient.[8] Yet, if someone is angry and we do not make a judgement about the appropriateness of their anger how are we to help them? Thus it is not always inappropriate or unhelpful to make a judgement about someone's anger to assist in the resolution of the situation.[9] However, making generalizations about people (e.g. people who are angry have no self-control) is to be avoided.

> ### Reflection
>
> Think of a time when you have witnessed violence or aggression but were not directly involved. How did you feel? What were your thoughts about what was happening?

> ### Reflection
>
> Think about a time when you have spoken to someone who was angry about something. What conclusions did you make about the strength of their feelings? How would you define anger in your own words?

The difference between anger and aggression

Anger and aggression differ. Anger can be understood to be an immediate emotional arousal whereas aggression is an enduring negative attitude. We can be angry without becoming aggressive and we can be aggressive without being angry (e.g. during war).[10] It is generally accepted that anger can be conceptualized as having three core components.[10] *Physiological arousal* occurs due to stimulation of the cardiovascular and endocrine systems and results in physical tension and irritability; *cognitive arousal* shows in antagonistic thought patterns, suspicious and negative thinking; and *behavioural arousal* is manifested by verbal aggression and impulsive reactions. This model proposes that exposure to stressors in their environment can cause irritability and tension, which over time can result in distorted and angry thinking patterns and ultimately aggressive behaviour. Generally speaking, this kind of aggression is interpreted as a maladaptive coping strategy and frequently causes problems for the person in daily living and interacting with others.[11]

For newly qualified health professionals, working with people who are potentially violent may be their biggest fear. There is no evidence to suggest that the sex of staff of their gender is associated with the risk of assault in the workplace.[12] However, women and homosexuals often perceive themselves to be in a vulnerable position and at most risk of becoming victims of violence. It is vital that such perceptions are recognized and dealt with appropriately so that staff can feel confident and empowered in the workplace.

Reflection

Think about a time when you have been aggressive. This may have been when you were very young or as an adolescent. Try and remember what you were feeling and thinking and how you behaved. Such personal reflections can cause feelings of discomfort, fear, shame and regret as we acknowledge that we may have lost control over a situation. Hold on to this feeling of discomfort as this may be exactly how patients feel when they become aggressive or violent.

Theories of violence

Common themes in the study of theories of violence include fear, frustration, manipulation, intimidation and pain or altered state of consciousness.[1] The various assumptions that underpin theories of aggression include whether or not aggression was learned, whether processes were cognitive or affective and whether determinants were internal or external.[1] *Trait* anger is attributed to individual differences in personality whereas *state* anger refers to the temporary emotional state that arises from stress frustration or irritation. Each act of aggression depends on the person's values, personality and attitude. There are many evolutionary theories that stem from the perspective that aggression is a universal instinct. From a psychoanalytic perspective, Freud saw aggression as a response to frustration and/or pain. Aggression is conceptualized as an instinct, balanced by Thanatos (the death instinct) and Eros (the representation of love and self-preservation). Other behavioural and cognitive perspectives focus on the tenet that

aggression is learned. At the neurophysiological level research has indicated that damage to the amygdaloid nucleus in the brain may be associated with violence. There is some evidence to suggest that temporal lobe epilepsy has been associated with episodic aggression and violence. Other implications for the manifestation of aggression and violence are trauma to the brain that has resulted in cerebral changes and diseases such as encephalitis, tumours in the brain, particularly the limbic system and the temporal lobes. Medical conditions such as chronic obstructive pulmonary disease, stroke, dementia, polypharmacy and urinary tract infection have roles to play in the increase of anxiety and aggression they cause, due to frustration and cognitive confusion.

Biochemical factors such as hormonal dysfunction, for example Cushing's disease or hyperthyroidism may contribute to the expression of aggression. There is anecdotal evidence, but no proven correlation yet, between the experience of premenstrual syndrome and violence. Research is continuing to attempt to identify which neurotransmitters, for example dopamine, serotonin, adrenaline, noradrenaline and acetylcholine may be linked with the manifestation of aggressive and violent behaviour.

Socioeconomic and environmental factors

As noted, violence and the expression of aggression in all Western societies is increasing. Explanations for increase include the lack of infrastructure in the community for health, housing and education; increasing casual employment; the experience of alienation in individuals due to family break-up; race, sexual and religious discrimination; and poverty. Alcohol, street drugs and firearm use are all associated with the incidence of violent behaviour. Physical overcrowding in housing or institutions such as prisons and lack of recreational facilities to expend energy and natural aggression also contribute to an increased potential for violence in the community and have been recognized as proximal factors.[1]

Aggression scales

The assessment of risk of aggression is notoriously difficult. Nevertheless, several tools have been used to assist in the detection and rating of aggression, for example the Nurses' Observation Scale for Inpatient Evaluations (NOSIE) and the Modified Overt Aggression Scale (MOAS). Self-rating scales are of limited use as their utility depends on the person having insight, self-understanding and good communication skills. Other scales involve the nurse or other health professional completing them during an observation period of the patient. Most scales involve the rating of aggressive behaviour as verbal, physical, aggression against property or self-harm with items within these categories on a five-point ordinal scale. Other behavioural and affective components may be included.

The experience of the nurse in working with potential aggression and violence

Without education, skills training and clinical supervision, nurses tend to respond to inappropriate or aggressive behaviours as they would outside the work environment. Because of the powerful nature of anger as an emotion, people exposed to anger may feel fearful and intimidated. It is generally accepted that nurses will avoid patients if they are fearful of them. Patients experiencing paranoia are often neglected by nurses in this way and the avoidant behaviour reinforces their suspicious thinking and may increase the potential for aggression. Clearly this is not therapeutic for either the nurse or the patient. A number of other common, but unhelpful responses have also been identified as reasons why nurses might avoid patients.[11] Wishing to punish or humiliate the patient is a response that counters the patient threat. This is a *reaction*, not a considered response and is inappropriate when working with people who are aggressive regardless of their diagnosis.

Condoning or approving of violence, either among patients or between nurse and patient, is serious and destructive. Many such practices have existed up until recently in mental health institutions and have reportedly included the sexual assault of female patients[12] by health professionals. Such behaviour contravenes codes of ethics and professional conduct. Another negative response involves the adoption of a passive attitude or the use of professional verbal cliches in response to the aggressive behaviour by patients. For example, imagine that you discovered that a friend had disclosed confidential information about you, to someone you did not know very well. Imagine how you may feel when on confronting your friend in an angry and upset manner, they replied 'I understand that you are very angry right now' or 'I know how you feel'. You are likely to feel enraged and certainly not appeased by such responses!

Genuinely helpful responses by nurses involve reflection of issues such as 'What was the aggressive patient thinking at the time?' and 'What is the context of their anger?' These can serve to work through the situation in a therapeutic way. Self-management of our own anger and frustration is necessary to develop effective skills in working with aggressive patients.

Individual responses by staff to aggression and violence in the workplace will be influenced by childhood experiences, and the adults who were our role models. Working with aggressive patients can evoke feelings of frustration, exasperation, irritation and distress. Nurses need to recognize the need for clinical supervision to process feelings and reflect on their practice.

❑ Consider a situation in which you observed the demonstration of anger either by a patient or relative.
❑ Write a list of what you think indicated that the person was angry.
❑ Compare your list with Table 33.1.

These defining characteristics are signals for nursing staff to continue close assessment and observation of the patient and to plan care that might maintain emotional and physical safety for all in the immediate environs.

Patients with mental health problems may exhibit behaviours that may lead to an aggressive or violent incident and being alert to these behaviours and early interventions can assist in the prevention of escalation of angry behaviour. Patients who are sarcastic in conversation, who express ideas of self-harm or harm to others, who are experiencing paranoid thoughts or general suspiciousness, or who have difficulty concentrating due to disturbances of thought or perception, may also be at risk of becoming aggressive.

Indicators of biologically based aggression are useful in identifying the possibility of an organic basis to aggressive or violent behaviour. Where the aggressive incident is unprovoked, if the episode involves a sudden shift in emotion to aggression from calm,[13] if the episode is out of character for the individual, or where the person shows no remorse, nurses ought to be alerted to the possibility of pathophysiological causation and advise the multidisciplinary team of the need for further investigation.

TABLE 33.1 Observable characteristics of anger

- Intense distress
- Pacing
- Gritting or grinding teeth
- Increased energy
- Agitation
- Change in tone of voice (raised or lowered)
- Raised or lowered eyebrows
- Flushed face
- Withdrawal
- Staring
- Fatigue
- Clenched fists

KEY CONCEPTS IN AGGRESSION MANAGEMENT

Prevention

In most areas of practice aggressive behaviour can be expected. Staff must be adequately prepared to identify types and levels of aggression, to communicate problems among themselves simply and clearly, and to confront aggression directly. Appropriate training will decrease fear and hostility and will also help staff maintain a therapeutic environment. The prevention and management of aggression and violence is an interdisciplinary function, facilitating a multi-faceted approach involving individualized interventions to minimize aggressive episodes. Aggression management has cognitive, behavioural and social components. Management should begin with those measures that have the least possibility of causing harm.[13] Behavioural and environmental strategies are fundamental in maintaining a therapeutic atmosphere and are used as preventive measures with the careful use of PRN medication in consultation with the multidisciplinary team (see Table 33.2). Decision-making with regard to restraint and seclusion lie with the most senior staff. This involves a balance of the individual's personal freedom and their physical safety, and that of other patients and staff.

Limiting choices may be useful when cognitive impairment is a factor. For example ask if the person would like to go for a walk or watch television, rather than asking an open-ended question such as 'What would you like to do?' For patients who have difficulties thinking, concentrating and carrying out activities independently, an increased level of structure to their day can reduce anxiety and thus the potential for frustrated or agitated behaviour. For patients who are medicated and experiencing side-effects of neuroleptic drugs, or

🖵 **TABLE 33.2** Behavioural approaches to help maintain control on a psychiatric inpatient ward

- Maintain quiet and calm staff demeanour as role models
- Increase staff presence in patient areas to imbue calm
- Regulate interaction patterns
- Separate groups or individuals that 'do not get along'
- Divide large groups into smaller ones
- Reduce noise
- Dim bright lights
- Limit choices and create environmental cues
- Allow the most effective staff to take the lead
- Identify and suppress trigger events (lunch times visiting times)
- Maintain activity schedules that include diversional, physical, intellectual and relaxation activities for patients to engage in.

lethargy, a rest time after lunch can help maintain a sense of calm in both staff and patients. Identification of trigger events (meal times, before and after visiting time, weekends) that may contribute to patient's outbursts, and careful assessment at these times, can reduce the opportunity for the escalation of aggression.

Nursing management of aggression and violence

In aggressive situations the aggressor is often agitated, may be sweating, talking quickly or shouting and pacing around. Nursing interventions that can 'slow down' and ease the overstimulated individual can be extremely useful in preventing aggression turn to actual violence.

If you were extremely angry about something, to the point of feeling that you were losing control, what interactions or behaviours might help you calm down? Make a list and compare with the list in Table 33.3.

Illustration

A 25-year-old man, Simon, was admitted to an acute in-patient psychiatric ward following a period of increasingly disorganized behaviour. Simon complains of other people reading and hearing his thoughts, is easily distracted, appears suspicious and has great difficulty concentrating on everyday tasks. After being visited by his girlfriend, he becomes increasingly agitated and tearful, demanding cigarettes and requesting to go home. Simon begins to pace around the day room and kicks a chair over in anger.

Illustration

A middle-aged relative has been visiting his daughter, a 14-year-old patient in a child and adolescent unit. His daughter becomes distressed during the visit and the father becomes increasingly agitated, shouting at the senior nurse in charge that he wants to see the consultant psychiatrist. The nurse in charge smells alcohol on his breath.

While senior nursing staff manage the situation, continuous assessment, observation and documentation by other team members is important. Monitor how other patients are reacting to the situation. Witnessing aggression is potentially stressful and distressing.

Remaining calm when dealing with an angry person sounds simple but is a skill to be learnt. Setting verbal limits and clearly distinguishing between acceptable and unacceptable behaviour, whilst negotiating with the distressed relative can prevent further escalation. As a rule of thumb avoid touching patients and relatives when they are aroused. Although comments made to nurses by patients and relatives may be derogatory, personal and

TABLE 33.3 Principles of de-escalation: 'Act don't react!'

- Take a deep breath: prepare yourself; don't simply jump in
- Adopt a comfortable and relaxed but not passive demeanour
- Continuously assess your safety and that of others
- Be genuine and warm
- Take your time, do not attempt to rush things along
- Be respectful
- Listen actively
- Speak clearly and slowly in short sentences
- Maintain a large personal space
- Encourage the patient to talk and to identify how they view the problem
- Do not argue and do not tell the patient that you know how they feel (you don't)
- Describe what has been happening to the patient (stressors and antecedents)
- Identify potential strategies with the patient if possible
- Provide a number of ways of resolving the situation if possible
- If in doubt call out for assistance[1]

hurtful, they are merely words and the best course of action is to ignore them. Do not argue with the person as this is most likely to make matters worse. Approximately 3% of the general population use alcohol harmfully but as a socially endorsed activity in society, alcohol is readily available to people in times of distress. Close assessment of signs of drug or alcohol intoxication or withdrawal can prevent associated aggressive events.

Restraint and seclusion

In some cases it is necessary to physically restrain an individual when preventive and de-escalation measures have failed to calm the patient. For some nursing interventions – such as the giving of intramuscular tranquillizing medication – it may be necessary to physically restrain the patient, if they are unwilling to take the medication. In the past, formalized staff development and training in self-defence and physical restraint was uncommon in health organizations. However, current standards of practice require staff have mandatory preparation in the general principles of physical restraint. The English National Board (for example) now recommends that all pre-registration courses for nurses and midwives contain material on aggression and violence.[14] For staff working in areas of potential aggression and violence, two basic rules apply:

- ❑ never attempt to restrain someone on your own, unless life is in immediate danger; and

- ❑ call for help if you cannot reach alarm systems.

Each organization should have its own policies and procedures regarding types of physical restraint and self-defence strategies, including breakaway techniques.

As noted, decision-making with regard to the use of restraint, lies with the most senior staff and involves a delicate balance of individual's personal freedom and the safety of others. The use of reasonable force and the patient's removal of freedom can be justified to take control *for* the patient, for the time they are 'out of control'. In some cases a patient may be physically restrained so that they can be placed in seclusion. Seclusion involves the confinement of an individual in a secured room, from which they cannot leave of their own volition.[15] Seclusion is a last resort, used when other nursing interventions have failed or are unavailable. The literature suggests that patients often associate seclusion with punishment[16] emphasizing the importance of open communication between staff and patients, when someone is secluded, to reduce anxiety and fears associated with confinement. Seclusion can offer physical and emotional safety for both patients and staff and the opportunity for counselling interventions.

Open and ongoing communication between all members of the multidisciplinary team is necessary to alert staff to changes in the individual's mental state and to plan care accordingly. This is not to say that all violent incidents can be foreseen or even prevented, but that safety concerns for staff and patients can be maximized. Debriefing of all incidents of aggression and violence for staff as well as patients is an important component of aggression management. Individuals need opportunities to work through their own feelings and to evaluate the efficacy of nursing interventions, to reduce burn-out and enhance personal and professional growth.

Illustration

A social worker is approached and verbally threatened by a female patient after a one-to-one session discussing social security benefits. Nursing staff intervene, and the patient eventually calms down. In the debriefing session that follows the social worker explains that the patient had been expressing paranoid thoughts about the staff, thinking that they were conspiring to steal her money and possessions.

TEACHING MANAGEMENT OF AGGRESSION

On a one-to-one basis, nurses have an important role in assisting patients to manage their anger and aggression. Keeping a diary and recording negative feelings on a daily basis can identify personal triggers for anger and frustration. Exploring alternative ways of coping with stress such as physical outlets (exercise) and seeking out staff when feeling angry or agitated can also reduce the potential for aggression and help the patient feel more in control of their emotions. The use of activities that include mental and physical stimulation (regular exercise and relaxation strategies) can offer routine and structure to a patient's daily activities. Token economies are contractual agreements that identify target behaviours and reward patients with tokens for good conduct. Rules ought to be pre-determined and these programmes require expert psychology assistance in their establishment within a prescribed care plan. Non-aggressive behaviour can be successfully rewarded through verbal reinforcement although a consistent staff response is required for this to be effective. Assertiveness training helps patients express their needs and wishes and helps them get the attention they need. This kind of training in one-to-one and group settings can also help patients deal with the frustration of activities of daily living in the community such as standing in queues and being on hold on the telephone for periods of time.

Common mistakes

In stressful situations it is not uncommon for individuals to react in a way that at the time appears to be of use but that is ultimately counterproductive.

❑ Disagreeing or raising your voice (unless it is to be heard) with people who are angry, is of no value and will cause the situation to escalate.
❑ In a similar way demonstrating emotions such as frustration, distress or anger yourself is likely to increase the tension of the situation.
❑ Never approach an angry person without backup. Continuous assessment of safety is important as the situation may deteriorate quickly.
❑ Do not attempt to use humour, sarcasm or to touch the patient.
❑ Above all learn by observing those who have successfully managed such situations, learn by your mistakes and the insights gained from debriefing critical incidents.

CONCLUSION

Working with patients who are angry and frustrated arouses a range of emotions in those who care for them. Aggression and violence are not symptomatic of mental illness, but reflect the general expression of these emotions and behaviours in mainstream society as well as the powerlessness and frustration patients often experience when patients within the health care system. Nurses need special personal attributes, skills, education and training to manage difficult situations safely and therapeutically. This chapter has explored personal and professional strategies for exploring the experience of anger and aggression in the workplace. Ongoing reflection and critique of personal and team practices are significant elements in maintaining therapeutic environments for patients under duress.

REFERENCES

1. Mason T, Chandley M. *Managing violence and aggression*. London: Churchill Livingstone, 1999.
2. Morrall PA. *Madness and murder*. London: Whurr, 2000.
3. Bain E. Assessing for occupational hazards. *American Journal of Nursing* 2000; **100**(1): 96.
4. Slattery M. The epidemic hazards of nursing. *American Journal of Nursing* 1998; **98**(11): 50–53.
5. Royal College of Nursing. *Dealing with violence against nursing staff*. London: RCN, 1998.
6. Delaney J, Cleary M, Jordan R, Horsfall J. *An exploratory investigation into the nursing management of aggression in acute psychiatric settings*. Central Sydney Area Health Service, Sydney Australia, 1999.
7. Royal College of Psychiatry. *Management of imminent violence clinical practice. Guidelines to support mental health services*. London: College Research Unit, 1998.
8. Rogers P, Vigden A. Working with people with serious mental illness who are angry. In: Gamble C, Brennan G (eds). Working with serious mental illness. A manual for clinical practice. London: Ballière-Tindall, 2000.
9. Novaco R. *Anger control*. Toronto: Lexington, 1975.
10. Binder RL, McNeil DE. Staff gender and risk of assault on doctors and nurses. *Bulletin of the American Academy of Psychiatry and the Law* 1994; **22**(4): 545–50.
11. Horsfall J, Stuhmiller C, Champ S. *Interpersonal nursing for mental health*. Sydney: Maclennan and Petty, 2000.
12. Davidson J. *Every boundary broken. Sexual abuse of women patients in psychiatric institutions*. Sydney: Women and Mental Health, 1997.
13. Wick J. Non-drug management of aggression in nursing facilities. *Consulting Pharmacy* 1998; **13**: 9–16.
14. Beech B. Sign of the times or the shape of things to come? A 3 day unit of instruction on 'aggression and violence in health settings for all students during pre-registration nurse training'. *Accident and Emergency Nursing* 2001; **9**: 204–211.
15. Muir-Cochrane EC, Holmes CA. Legal and ethical aspects of seclusion: An Australian perspective. *Journal of Psychiatric and Mental Health Nursing* 2001; **8**: 501–6.
16. Meehan T, Vermeer C, Windsor C. Patient's perceptions of seclusion: a qualitative investigation. *Journal of Advanced Nursing* 2001; **31**(2): 370–77.

Chapter 34

THE PERSON WITH A DIAGNOSIS OF MANIC DEPRESSION

Ian Beech*

INTRODUCTION

This chapter considers the nursing care of the person diagnosed as manic-depressive. Although nurses' primary responsibility is not to diagnose or prescribe treatment, they do have a role in treatment regimes and need to understand the diagnosis and medical responses to manic depression.

The chapter will focus on the care of the *person* who is experiencing manic depression and the alliance nurses need to build to enable the person to recognize and take control of mood swings.

DIAGNOSTIC CRITERIA

Although the condition has long been known as manic depression both the *World Health Organization*[1] and the *American Psychiatric Association*[2] now use the term 'bipolar disorder' to indicate the fluctuation of the person's mood between the two poles of depression and mania. The American Psychiatric Association divides bipolar disorder into two types. *Type I* is characterized by the person having experienced one or more manic episodes. *Type II* is characterized by the experience of one hypomanic episode and one major depressive episode. The difference between mania and hypomania is considered to be the length of time that the episode lasts, with mania lasting for one week or longer and hypomania lasting for 4 days.

The experience of mania

The experience of mania or hypomania is not simply that of being a little over-excited. There is an important qualitative difference between being happy or full of the joys of spring, and experiencing mania. A manic episode involves the person showing some or all of the characteristic changes in *emotion, cognition, behaviour* and *physicality* (Table 34.1):

Table 34.1 indicates the possible signs and symptoms of mania but does not help us understand what the experience might be like for the person. Let us consider the case of Mary.

In Mary's case she believes that her manic depression was the result of the stresses caused by a difficult marriage and the birth of her son. However, she also believes that there may also be a genetic component to her condition. This view of the 'cause' of manic depression is not unusual, as it is often seen to 'run in families'. However, at present no specific gene has been identified. Sufferers

*Ian Beech works as a Senior Lecturer in Mental Health Nursing at the University of Glamorgan in South Wales. He works closely with a local NHS trust in working with people experiencing depression and in implementing the Tidal Model. In his spare time he is learning the tenor banjo and vainly trying to gain proficiency in the Tibetan yoga known as sKum-nyé.

TABLE 34.1 Symptoms of manic/hypomanic episode[3]

Emotional changes	■ Mood swings between euphoria and elation to anger and irritability ■ Switches of affect from happy to depressed and hostile ■ Uncritical self-confidence ■ Wish to be gratified in whatever the person does
Cognitive changes	■ Racing thoughts ■ Distractible ■ Rapid and loud speech that is difficult to interrupt ■ Flight of ideas ■ Impaired judgement ■ Ideas of reference, delusions and hallucinations
Behavioural changes	■ Dramatic mannerisms, flamboyant dress and makeup ■ Increase in goal-directed activity ■ Intrusive, demanding, domineering and sometimes aggressive ■ Resists efforts to treat ■ Dislikes having wishes thwarted ■ Impulsive ■ Acts in sexual ways that are unusual for the person, e.g. hypersexuality
Physical changes	■ Full of energy, doesn't easily tire ■ Extreme motor activity leading to exhaustion ■ Insomnia with decreased need for sleep ■ Change in appetite ■ Lack of attention to personal hygiene, appearance and general health

often describe a stressful event or events in their lives to which they believe they can trace back the onset of their problems. The well-known comedian and writer Spike Milligan,[4] for example, traced his problems back to having been caught in a shell blast in the Second World War. However, his father also was someone who was prone to mood swings.

Kay Redfield Jamison[5] describes her experiences thus:

> When I am high I couldn't worry about money if I tried. So I don't. The money will come from somewhere; I am entitled; God will provide. Credit cards are disastrous, personal cheques worse. Unfortunately, for manics anyway, mania is a natural extension of the economy. What with credit cards and bank accounts there is little

Case study 34.1

Mary is in her fifties and used to be a primary school teacher. After the birth of her son she found that she started to have difficulty sleeping. She used to lie awake and mull over the ideas that were going through her mind. Although she could still carry out her job she found that she was having difficulty concentrating and also that she could get by on less and less sleep. She became increasingly more irritated with her husband because he was trying to restrict the things that she wanted to do such as going shopping and spending. One day she went out shopping for food in the local shops and, seeing a car that she liked in a nearby showroom, she bought it.

She became increasingly convinced that her husband was determined to have her 'put away' and after a few more days she was admitted to the local psychiatric hospital under the 1959 Mental Health Act. Thirty years later she can vividly remember four male nurses holding her down and injecting her with something (she doesn't know what) in her backside.

Because of her feelings towards her husband at the time she was viewed as paranoid and was diagnosed as suffering from schizophrenia. She received treatment for this for over ten years before a new consultant psychiatrist decided that she was probably suffering from manic depression and began to treat her with lithium carbonate.

Mary now no longer teaches but gives talks to students and school children about manic depression and is involved in various voluntary organizations working to raise awareness and reduce stigma of mental illness. She has developed various strategies to help her to control her own swings in mood.

beyond reach. So I bought twelve snakebite kits, with a sense of urgency and importance. I bought precious stones, elegant and unnecessary furniture, and three watches within an hour of one another (in the Rolex rather than Timex class: champagne tastes bubble to the surface, are the surface, in mania), and totally inappropriate siren-like clothes. During one spree in London I spent several hundred pounds on books having titles or covers that somehow caught my fancy: books on the natural history of the mole, twenty sundry Penguin books because I thought it could be nice if penguins could form a colony.

At first sight it may seem that to feel so full of energy, to have no worries about finances, to be sexually active must be a wonderful feeling that many people might aspire to. However this is not the case. People often find that they feel great as a manic episode commences but soon the fall-out both for themselves physically and mentally and their relationships is immense. Mary Ellen Copeland, for example, describes her experience as one in which:

> I feel unable to stay physically still or to quiet my brain. My body hurts all over. Every cell says I want to rest, but the body and mind cannot and will not cooperate.[6]

It is important therefore for nurses to be aware that what the person is experiencing is not merely exuberance or being full of the joys of spring but a feeling of moving beyond this to being out of control and likely to perform actions that the person would not usually wish to perform.

NURSING APPROACH

The nursing approach to someone diagnosed with manic depression has three dimensions.

❑ The first approach is adopted for someone in the acute manic phase. Here, the main considerations are to address the physical, psychological and social consequences of behaviour carried out while manic.

❑ The second involves ensuring that, if a mood-stabilizing drug is prescribed, the person experiences no major problems with the drug and can maintain a therapeutic level in the body.

❑ The third approach involves working with the person when the manic phase has abated, aiming to develop the person's awareness of possible trigger factors so that self-management strategies may be developed.

The manic phase

An often-underestimated complication of an acute phase of mania is that the person does not rest and is on the move continually resulting in a very rapid use of calories. This can be coupled with an excitability that prevents the person concentrating on mundane matters like eating and drinking. It is easy, therefore, for the person to become physically exhausted and dehydrated. With this in mind the nurse should consider ways of providing food and drink in ways that do not require the person to sit for prolonged mealtimes. It is unprofitable to argue with the person about sitting in communal eating areas for long periods of time at mealtimes. This will result only in the creation of tension between the nurse and the person, so undermining the relationship.

Mania is often characterized by excitability and distractibility and consequently the person often reacts quickly and excitably to environmental stimuli. Therefore it is a helpful nursing approach to try to aim to promote a quiet and relaxed environment for the person. This is not always possible in an acute admission ward, given the distractions provided by the audience of other people. Given that some people in mania can often be amusing and entertaining, there is a risk that nurses, and other patients, might provide an 'audience' for the person (wittingly or unwittingly) as a means of providing light relief from the everyday humdrum of the ward.

Wherever possible nurses should be relaxed and quiet in their approach and avoid getting into protracted arguments and conflict with people as this provides distraction and further, unhelpful, stimulation.

People in manic phases are often given high doses of medication to try to lower the mood and control behaviour. If this is the case there are a number of considerations that have to be taken into account. Anybody subjected to high doses of drugs such as haloperidol and acuphase (clopixol) may experience drowsiness and blurred vision, Therefore, it is important for nurses to be aware of a possible lack of co-ordination and the risk of falling over objects or spilling hot drinks.

People in mania can sometimes be argumentative and apparently difficult to take issue with. Again, in such situations it is important to maintain a calm approach and to avoid entering into protracted argument with the person since this will merely stimulate further argument.

The person should, rather, be encouraged, gently, to attend to dress and personal hygiene issues. Again it is important that this does not become a battleground in which there are seen to be winners and losers.

Another common feature of mania is hypersexuality (heightened sexual activity). Nurses often find it difficult to strike a balance between not wishing to interfere in the private matters of people in care and not wishing to abdicate responsibility under their duty to care for people. Ron Coleman[7] distinguishes between nurses caring *for* people and caring *about* people. He considers that when nurses care for people they try to wrap them in cotton wool and not allow any personal freedom, whereas when nurses care about people they take risks and allow people personal autonomy. With the issue of hypersexuality the nurse must consider whether or not the activity of the person is consistent with mania. It should be remembered that if a person's mood swings into depression after a manic episode there could be considerable feelings of guilt associated with actions that were carried out while the person was suffering from mania.

Mood-stabilizing medication

People who are diagnosed with manic depression are often prescribed mood-stabilizing medication. These drugs fall into two types: the first is lithium compounds; the second are anti-convulsant medications (drugs often used to treat epilepsy). These have been found to have some beneficial effect in mood stabilization.

In either case the nurse should remember the need to give the person comprehensive and detailed information about the drug, before asking the person to take the medication. Very often people taking mood stabilizers are expected to take them for quite long periods of their lives, often for years. To expect someone to comply with a long-term prescription of any medication without giving full information is asking for the conflict between professionals and people in care. In Mary's case, when she was first prescribed lithium carbonate she was told that it wasn't really a proper medication at all, it was a salt. This is technically true if one is a pharmacist. However, Mary's impression was that lithium was no more dangerous, or effective, than the salt she put on her food. As a result, she took it only when she remembered, rather than according to the necessary therapeutic pattern. She only discovered that lithium was different when she was talking to someone at a dinner one evening who happened to also be prescribed lithium and had been given a card with fuller information about the drug.

People should be given full information about what to expect from the medication in terms of both therapeutic effects, side-effects, special precautions they should take, especially in terms of eating and drinking. The necessary blood tests while on the drug, should also be clearly described. Again Mary was once told that if she took lithium she wouldn't have to have injections, but wasn't told that she would need blood tests, with the use of needles.

There are many useful sources of information about medication management. One such resource, for nurses and people in care, is the Norfolk Mental Health Care NHS Trust pharmacy website at http://www.nmhct.nhs.uk/pharmacy/[8]. There are, however, a number of specific points that need to be considered here.

Lithium products

Lithium is produced in two forms – lithium carbonate and lithium citrate. Both are thought to produce an effect by balancing the sodium and potassium ions found at nerve synapses. It has a narrow therapeutic blood level range of 0.4–1.2 mmol per litre of blood. Lower than these limits is generally considered to be non-therapeutic and higher is moving towards toxicity. It is therefore important that people prescribed lithium have regular blood tests to both assess levels in the blood and to monitor the function of the thyroid gland which can be adversely affected by lithium.

Because of the fairly narrow therapeutic range, and because of the relative ease with which people can slip into toxicity, nurses need to both be aware of the signs and likely causes of toxicity, and also to inform people of this risk. People should be informed that, should they begin to experience blurred vision, unsteadiness in walking and standing, diarrhoea and vomiting, slurred speech, a bad hand tremor, clumsiness, increased thirst

or passing urine, and/or drowsiness/confusion, they should seek medical advice.

There can be a number of causes of toxicity but common factors can be anything which causes dehydration, as this increases the lithium concentration in the body (e.g. drinking large amounts of tea, coffee or cola drinks as these contain caffeine which increases urine production), sweating in hot weather, drinking alcohol (alcohol is a diuretic), vomiting or diarrhoea, and taking aerobic exercise.

Problems can also develop if the person chews the tablet rather than swallows it whole, as this causes a surge of lithium to be absorbed rather than a steady slow absorption.

It may seem that giving people all of this information when they may never experience such side-effects, is playing hostage to fortune, especially if the person appears in any way reluctant to take medication. However given the potential physical dangers of not informing people, nurses have no option but to provide detailed and appropriate information. In addition, we need to remember that, if a person experiences side-effects, after the nurse has given the impression that no

---

Case study 34.2

Bob has had a number of manic episodes over the last few years and during these he sometimes finds that when he becomes agitated he suffers from nocturnal enuresis.

When he was admitted to a new unit for the first time Bob wet the bed on his first night. Following this it was decided by the nursing staff to limit Bob's fluid intake to try to stop him wetting the bed at night.

Unfortunately Bob was prescribed lithium carbonate and began to suffer from toxic symptoms brought on by dehydration.

---

such effects are likely to occur, the patient's trust in the nurse may be seriously undermined.

Anti-convulsant medication used to control mood

Carbemazepine, sodium valproate and lamotrigine are all used to try to stabilize mood swings, alone or in conjunction with lithium products. These products have various possible side-effects and interactions with other drugs, which require a detailed knowledge on the part of the nurse. Carbemazepine, for example, can reduce the effectiveness of the contraceptive pill, while sodium valproate can cause weight gain. Such possible side-effects need to be discussed, to ensure that the person is aware of such problems, and acknowledges the possible influence on lifestyle.

Other medication

People with a diagnosis of manic depression may sometimes be offered major tranquillizers (e.g. chlorpromazine) or anti-depressants.

Again, given nurses responsibility for the administration of such medication, they need to be fully conversant with appropriate dosages, effects and side-effects etc., and also need to be creative in their approach to communicating such information to the person for whom the drugs have been prescribed.

SELF-MANAGEMENT

Copeland[9] encouraged people with manic depression to develop a personalized chart that might help them build up a profile of the type of mood swings to which they may be subject. From this people can become more aware of the things in their lives that might trigger swings into mania and/or depression. Nurses can play an important role in this process by providing people with information about monitoring of moods, providing people with contacts with organizations such as the *Manic Depression Fellowship*, which runs courses on self-management, and providing encouragement that, although it may take a while to gain some sense of mastery over moods that the task is possible. Barker[10] indicates that people susceptible to manic phases may feel powerless in the face of apparently inevitable mood swings. By beginning to address likely precursors to mood changes not only do people begin to identify triggers but also gain a sense of ownership of the problem so that rather than passively accepting the latest wonder drug from professionals they enter into a collaborative approach to finding a way of living their lives that doesn't result in life being constantly defined in terms of problems rather in terms of strengths.[11]

Copeland[12] suggests that people should try to identify early warning signs of *depression* (e.g. lethargy, sleep problems, negative thought patterns), and early warning signs of *mania* (e.g. thrill seeking, increased sexual activity, being argumentative), alongside a series of things to do every day (e.g. eat well, exercise). In so doing and by reviewing their charts regularly, people can establish patterns in their lives of what causes them problems and what helps. In this process it is important that nurses do *not* suggest what people should be charting. To be effective, such a chart should be personal, and potentially, meaningful as an educational vehicle for self-management.

Nurses should also avoid being judgemental about people in terms of their diagnosis. For example Mary can remember going to see a nurse about a project

---

Process

Mary trusted a nurse on her ward, chiefly for his faith in her. Rather than dismissing how she felt about her mood, and focusing on PRN medication, he sat and listened as she told him about her thoughts about what was bothering her.

He encouraged her to keep a diary about how she felt on a day-to-day basis charting how she felt, how she had slept, and what appeared to have helped her.

After her discharge from hospital he made himself available to her if she phoned or visited the ward to answer her questions or simply to reassure her that she was coping.

Many years later Mary is still subject to mood swings but has accurately identified likely contributory factors and strategies that she employs to maintain balance. Building on that original trusting relationship, she has developed a network of professionals whom she feels she can trust and she has also identified those whom she would rather avoid.

---

she wanted to set up in the community. Many years after the meeting she was able to see her medical notes and found a letter from the nurse to her consultant saying that Mary had been enthusiastic, happy and forceful (and) perhaps needed her medication reviewing!

Advanced directives

One of the ways that people are enabled to feel ownership of their lives is by the use of advanced directives.[13] These are documents within which people have considered the possibility of suffering mood swings in the future and have laid out in clear terms the issues that are important with the view that should decisions have to be made about care in the future the advanced directive might inform the process when the person is deemed to be incapable of making decisions at the time.

The advanced directive has no current legal status in UK law. This is also the case in other countries such as Australia and New Zealand and in the majority of states in the USA. Nevertheless in all of these countries there appears to be increasing evidence of advanced directives gaining increasing moral force.[14] Minnesota in the United States authorized advanced directives in 1991 and since then Alaska, Hawaii, Idaho, Illinois, Maine, North Carolina, Oklahoma, Oregon, South Dakota, Texas and Utah.[15] In England and Wales the white paper reviewing the 1983 Mental Health Act[16] has suggested that advanced agreements become best practice. Advanced agreements are different from advanced directives in that an agreement requires negotiation and agreement whereas a directive can simply set out the wishes of the individual It seems therefore that in countries such as the UK, Australia, New Zealand and USA there is a groundswell of opinion gathering that is in favour of adopting more consensual approaches to care planning and treatment, giving advanced directives moral if not legal force. As Coleman says:

> We do not want you to work on us any more. We want you to work with us and that means on our terms not your terms. And we don't want you to perceive our needs because this is what professionals do, they are wonderful at it: 'This person needs this, this, this and this'. You never ask us what we need.[17]

Advanced directives may be as brief or as detailed as the person wishes. For example the person may simply state a preference for a certain type of medication, given the bad side-effects in the past of other drugs. Or there could be a statement that the person would or would not willingly accept ECT (given the legal fact that a person may be given ECT against his/her will if detained under Section 3 of the Mental Health Act 1983 and subject to a second opinion). On the other hand an advanced directive might be very detailed, setting out everything from power over the person's post and money to who looks after the dog and the goldfish.

Although an advanced directive carries no legal force it certainly carries a moral force, especially if professionals have been involved in the process of empowerment and in developing such directives. Nurses can play an important part in helping the person to formulate such a directive with other members of the multidisciplinary team. The key issue is that such directives should be meaningful. In particular, they should be taken into account if the person is, for example, admitted to hospital.

PROVIDING INFORMATION

In the process of learning to take control of their changes in mood, people usually find that the support of significant others in their lives is important. This support is more likely to be forthcoming, and lasting, if it is predicated on sound up-to-date information about the diagnosis.

There now exists a wealth of information about manic depression, in the publications of organizations such as the MDF, in libraries and on the Internet. However, people often expect that nurses will be knowledgeable about their diagnosis and treatment, and will provide them with reliable and meaningful information to extend their knowledge and understanding.[18] Secondly, nurses attempt to engender trust in the people for whom they care. This is extremely difficult if all the information to which the person has access comes from sources other than the nurse. Third, people often worry about whether or not their children might develop manic depression at a later date. Nurses need to be honest and reassuring – neither overstating nor dismissing these fears.

In conclusion the person with a diagnosis of manic depression presents in different ways to the nurse. When the person is in a manic state the nurse needs to address this in a calm, rational way to promote a calming environment and an avoidance of harm. If the person has become depressed then equally the nurse needs to address this (see Chapter 27, The person who experiences depression). When the person is prescribed mood-stabilizing medication the nurse should be sufficiently knowledgeable to avoid complications of medication and to negotiate a medical approach that the person can live with. When the person feels that his/her mood is stable the role of the nurse is to help the person to develop mechanisms to begin to control his/her moods and to feel empowered in the decision-making process.

The nurse's role in helping the person who is diagnosed with manic depression involves a complex of skills and knowledge – from physical considerations such as hydration to complicated interpersonal processes involved in negotiation and facilitating empowerment.

REFERENCES

1. World Health Organization, *ICD-10: The ICD-10 classification of mental and behavioural disorders: clinical descriptions and diagnostic guidelines.* London: Gaskell/Royal College of Psychiatrists, 1992.
2. American Psychiatric Association. *Diagnostic and statistical manual of mental disorders*, 4th edn, text revision. Washington: APA, 1994.
3. Lego S. The client who is diagnosed bipolar. In: Lego S (ed.) *Psychiatric nursing: a comprehensive reference*, 2nd edn. Philadelphia: Lippincott, 1996: 213–17.
4. Milligan S, Clare A. *Depression and how to survive it.* London: Arrow, 1994.
5. Redfield-Jamison K. *The unquiet mind: a memoir of moods and madness.* London: Picador, 1995.
6. Copeland M. *The depression workbook: a guide for living with depression and manic depression.* Oakland: New Harbinger, 1992.
7. Coleman R. The politics of the illness. In: Barker P, Stevenson C (eds). *The Construction of power and authority in psychiatry.* London: Butterworth Heinemann, 2000: 59–66.
8. Norfolk Mental Health Care NHS Trust Pharmacy Web Site at http://www.nmhct.nhs.uk/pharmacy/ accessed November 24th 2001.
9. Copeland M, *op. cit.*

10. Barker P. Locus of control in women with a diagnosis of manic-depressive psychosis. *Journal of Psychiatric and Mental Health Nursing* 1994; **1**: 9–14.

11. Watkins P. *Mental health nursing: the art of compassionate care.* Oxford: Butterworth Heinemann, 2001.

12. Copeland M, *op. cit.*

13. Manic Depression Fellowship. *Planning ahead for people with manic depression.* London: MDF, 2001.

14. National Alliance for the Mentally Ill at http://www.nami.org accessed January 24th 2002.

15. National Alliance for the Mentally Ill, ibid.

16. Department of Health. *Reforming the Mental Health Act.* London: HMSO, 2000.

17. Coleman R, *op. cit.*

18. Jackson S, Stevenson C. What do people need psychiatric and mental health nurses for? *Journal of Advanced Nursing* 2000; **31**: 378–88.

Chapter 35

THE PERSON WITH A DIAGNOSIS OF BORDERLINE PERSONALITY DISORDER

Shaun Parsons*

INTRODUCTION

Borderline personality disorder (BPD) is perhaps the most well-known of all personality disorder diagnoses and the one with the most preconceptions attached to it. Mention BPD and words such as hopeless, destructive and pointless are often heard. I hope to challenge some of these views and show that nurses can approach BPD in a constructive and collaborative manner.

First of all I shall examine the history of personality disorder, defining BPD. The treatment options will then be explored before finally offering some practical points on working with people with BPD.

PERSONALITY DISORDER: A BRIEF HISTORY

The concept of personality disorder is relatively recent; however, descriptions of individuals who would now be described as personality disordered are ancient. Mack *et al.*[1] report that the ancient Greeks recognized individuals with impulsive and dysfunctional traits who, nevertheless, were not mentally disordered. The first modern description of personality disorder was made by

Pritchard who observed a pattern of asocial and damaging behaviour in criminals and concluded that the criminals were not insane in the sense that the term was used at the time, but that they had a significant abnormality of behaviour that was equivalent to, but not the same as, mental disorders. The differences were that the symptoms were long-standing and pervasive and appeared to be part of the individual's character. Pritchard named this new entity moral insanity and this became the forerunner of the modern concepts of psychopathy, antisocial personality disorder and dyssocial personality disorder. He described a disorder that consisted of considerable disturbance in social behaviour, a loss of moral sense and difficulty in self-control. These symptoms were not accompanied by any apparent impairment in mental state. Livesley *et al.*[2] marked the development of moral insanity as the beginning of the current idea of personality disorders: a distinct and enduring group of disorders separate from mental disorder. Schneider introduced the important concept that for a personality to be described as disordered there must be evidence of a degree of dysfunction and disruption to either the patient or society. He used this principle to provide the first workable definition of people with psychopathic

*Shaun Parsons is a Lecturer in Clinical Psychology at the University of Newcastle and he practises as a Forensic Psychologist in the NHS. His research interests include the monitoring and treatment of sex offenders in community and prison settings and the interaction between the police and people with mental health problems.

personality as abnormal personalities who either suffer personally because of their abnormality, or make a community suffer because of it. Schneider also described abnormal personality as an extreme variant of normal personality, viewing personality as a continuum or dimension rather than a categorical dichotomy (either one thing or another). However, Schneider's dimensional view of personality did not prevail within psychiatry, although it echoed the ideas of psychologists exploring normal personality such as Allport[3] who saw personality as trait-based and dimensional.

The idea of personality disorders as distinct entities continued to dominate psychiatric classification throughout the 20th century. However, there was some dissent. For example, Kraepelin did not agree with the hypothesis that personality disorders were separate from other mental state disorders but saw personality disorders as related to the major psychoses. Kretschmer developed Kraepelin's idea[4] hypothesizing a continuum between the schizophrenic spectrum disorders and personality disorder. This led to Hoch and Polatain[5] describing pseudoneurotic schizophrenia, which is the predecessor of the current concepts of borderline and schizotypal personality disorders.

Personality disorder in current psychiatric classifications

Personality disorder as used in current psychology/psychiatry was first defined in the American Psychiatric Association's Diagnostic and Statistical Manual second edition (DSM II). In DSM II the concept of disordered personality trait and disordered personality pattern were combined to form the modern concept of personality disorder. The third revision of DSM, DSM III,[6] developed the concept further by introducing a number of important innovations. Firstly, DSM III placed personality disorders on a separate Axis (II) from the mental state disorders, which were located on Axis I. This innovation formally acknowledged Pritchard's idea that personality disorder caused equivalent problems and distress to mental disorder, yet was quite different. It also allowed a diagnosis of personality disorder to be made when a mental state disorder was present, something that theoretically had not been possible in earlier systems.[7] Further, the concept of personality disorder – as outlined in DSM III – incorporated Schneider's view that there must be some degree of dysfunction of daily activity for personality disorder to be present. Finally, DSM III[8] was a categorical as opposed to a dimensional system continuing the prevailing theme in 20th century psychiatric classification regarding personality disorder as a distinct diagnosis rather than an extreme variant of normal personality as originally proposed by Schneider.

DSM III was revised in 1987, although the personality disorders remained largely unchanged[8]. The DSM was again revised in 1994 with the publication of DSM IV.[9] Again, the personality disorders remained largely unchanged although they were reduced in number to 10, with the relegation of passive–aggressive personality disorder to a research disorder and the deletion of the research disorders of sadistic, self-defeating and depressive personality disorders. A further innovation of DSM IV has been the close collaboration between the World Health Organization (WHO) and the American Psychiatric Association working parties so that DSM IV and the International Classification of Diseases 10th edition (ICD-10)[10] are broadly similar, although not identical. This concept remained a feature of DSM IV and its adoption by the WHO in ICD-10, in their definition of personality disorders as inflexible and maladaptive traits, aligns the two classification systems closely. Schneider's dimensional concept of personality disorders as an extreme of normal personality has not, however, been adopted by DSM IV or ICD-10. Instead Pritchard's view of personality disorder as a separate, distinct phenomenon from mental state disorders has been utilized by the authors of DSM with the creation of a separate Axis, Axis II for personality disorders. ICD-10 recognizes the distinction implicitly by using broadly similar descriptive terms for the criteria of personality disorders as DSM IV.

Current tensions in the classification of personality disorder

The diagnosis of personality disorder remains controversial and at times problematic. However, the debate surrounding the diagnosis and classification of personality disorders embraces a vast literature and a proper review would require a book in its own right. Therefore what is offered here can be no more than a summary.

Since the formulation of DSM III there has been considerable debate about the nature of personality disorder. One key is the continuation of the current dichotomous categorical system of diagnosis, or its replacement with a dimensional, continuum based system. Also, there continues to be criticism of the number of personality disorders currently in both classification systems (ICD and DSM) with many researchers and clinicians arguing for a reduction in the number of personality disorders due to the high level of co-morbidity, or co-occurrence, between the disorders. Clark *et al.*[11] for example, argue that it is very rare to have a personality disorder diagnosed in isolation, and that they are almost always diagnosed with another personality disorder. They argued that the co-occurrence of personality disorders was evidence that they were not discrete entities but rather represented a continuum of distress based upon personality dimensions.

Proponents of the current system argue that categorical systems allow the clear identification of a disorder and that this leads to clear treatment pathways based upon evidence of effectiveness (see for example, Frances *et al.*[1]). However, proponents of the dimensional system argue that personality disorder is an illusion and that what is being observed are in fact operationalized personality dimensions.[12]

The DSM IV Axis II personality disorders

The ten personality disorders on DSM IV's Axis II are listed below. A further diagnosis of personality disorder 'not otherwise specified' (personality disorder NOS) is also possible. The personality disorders are organized in three clusters.

1 **Cluster A:** Paranoid personality disorder; schizoid personality disorder; schizotypal personality disorder.

2 **Cluster B**: Antisocial personality disorder; borderline personality disorder; histrionic personality disorder; narcissistic personality disorder.

3 **Cluster C**: Avoidant personality disorder; dependent personality disorder; obsessive–compulsive personality disorder.

BORDERLINE PERSONALITY DISORDER

As can be seen above, BPD is one of the Cluster B group of personality disorders. This group consists of personality traits which underpin behaviours such as impulsivity, affective instability, antisocial behaviour and cognitive disturbance. BPD is said to be present if five of the following criteria are present.

Diagnostic criteria for 301.83 borderline personality disorder[9]

A pervasive pattern of instability of interpersonal relationships, self-image, and affects, and marked impulsivity beginning by early adulthood and present in a variety of contexts, as indicated by five (or more) of the following:

1 Frantic efforts to avoid real or imagined abandonment. (Note: do not include suicidal or self-mutilating behaviour covered in Criterion 5.)

2 A pattern of unstable and intense interpersonal relationships characterized by alternating between extremes of idealization and devaluation.

3 Identity disturbance: markedly and persistently unstable self-image or sense of self.

4 Impulsivity in at least two areas that are potentially self-damaging (e.g. spending, sex, substance abuse, reckless driving, binge eating). (Note: Do not include suicidal or self-mutilating behaviour covered in Criterion 5.)

5 Recurrent suicidal behaviour, gestures, or threats, or self-mutilating behaviour.

6 Affective instability due to a marked reactive of mood (e.g. intense episodic dysphoria, irritability, or anxiety usually lasting a few hours and only rarely more than a few days).

7 Chronic feelings of emptiness.

8 Inappropriate, intense anger or difficulty controlling anger (e.g. frequent displays of temper, constant anger, recurrent physical fights).

9 Transient, stress-related paranoid ideation or severe dissociative symptoms.

As can be seen, several different kinds of BPD 'patient' are possible, depending upon which diagnostic criteria are selected. A person may be diagnosed with BPD whose behaviour is characterized by impulsivity, anger control problems and feelings of emptiness. Alternatively, another person with the same BPD diagnosis may be characterized by self-harm, affective instability and paranoid ideation. This makes the diagnosis of BPD wide ranging, with many different individuals, with very individual problems characterized as having BPD. From a nursing perspective this highlights the need to focus less upon the diagnosis of BPD and more upon the individual presentation and the needs and problems of the individual when considering nursing care.

NURSING THE PERSON WITH BPD

As noted, the term BPD is often associated by clinicians with many negative stereotypes. Such people are often described as difficult, challenging, demanding and hopeless. Although BPD individuals do exhibit a range of behaviours which may be challenging and difficult to treat perhaps the most difficult thing they have to cope with is the label of BPD itself. Being labelled 'borderline' often slams the doors of psychiatric services in their faces as they are described as hopeless and intractable 'cases'. In the following section many of the stereotypes of 'borderline' behaviour will be expanded. However, it cannot be stressed highly enough that any nursing judgement must be based upon an assessment of the individual not the 'borderline' label that the individual has been given. The individual's problems and challenges are just that – individual. They deserve to be dealt with individually. Nevertheless patients with BPD may exhibit a number of common behaviours, which may be problematic in clinical situations. These include:

❏ Self-harm.
❏ Dichotomous thinking and inability to sustain relationships.
❏ Manipulative behaviour and promotion of interpersonal conflicts.

This list is by no means exhaustive. Although many of the problems listed above are closely connected these are the behaviours which, in my view, are most challenging for nurses. These are the manifestations of the loneliness, fear of loss, desire for attention and impulsivity which underpins the borderline diagnosis. Perhaps one of the greatest paradoxes of BPD is that patients experiencing the disorder often feel great interpersonal loneliness and are terrified of abandonment. Yet, because of their dichotomous thinking, impulsive violent behaviour and interpersonal instability, they cause relationships to break down and are often unable to maintain a stable close relationship. This creates what they fear most, abandonment and being alone.

Faced with interpersonal loneliness, people with BPD will go to great lengths to avoid being alone. In treatment settings they soon become aware of behaviours that result in attention – such as violence or self-harm – and will engage in these behaviours, in part, to avoid feeling lonely. However, they are also aware of the emptiness of such gestures and often feel considerable worthlessness and lack of self-esteem as a result. Therefore, although we shall address each of the key behaviours in turn, it is important to remember that they are not separate but part of the whole person that you are nursing.

Self-harm

Self-harm is one of the most challenging behaviours for any clinician to deal with. In the case of BPD the nurse is invariably in the front line. Individuals with BPD often self-harm to a prodigious degree as the case study below demonstrates.

Self-harming in people with BPD has many causes but is perhaps best conceptualized as having two main themes:

❏ Feelings of worthlessness.
❏ Manipulative behaviour.

As discussed above, BPD is associated with feelings of worthlessness and low self-esteem, and some self-harm in BPD patients is related to this. After engaging in self-harm individuals often report feelings of release, sometimes

---

Case study 35.1

June is a 29-year-old woman who has had contact with psychiatric services since she was 19 years old when, as a university student, she took an overdose following the breakdown of a relationship. She has been in contact with psychiatric services since this time and 7 years ago was diagnosed as having BPD. She has self-harmed 72 times over the last 10 years, initially these were small cutting injuries to her arms, legs and abdomen but she has also taken three serious overdoses, one of which has resulted in serious damage to her liver. Over the past year she has escalated her self-harm attempts and a recent cutting event required extensive surgery to repair the damage.

---

feeling they have provided an outlet for their feelings of worthlessness or a visible manifestation of their pain. Although this may be difficult to understand the deep sense of loneliness and worthlessness is often described as being like an intense pain. Creating a physical pain is a release, and another feeling upon which to focus.

However, much self-harm in individuals with BPD stems from manipulative behaviour. Here the person uses self-harm to achieve a desired goal. It is important to note that the goal may not appear beneficial or desirable to an observer but is perceived as beneficial to the person with BPD. For example, in June's case her first episode in self-harm followed the breakdown of a relationship with her boyfriend. When her boyfriend told her he was terminating the relationship because of her unpredictable behaviour, June became frantic. At first she pleaded with her boyfriend to stay and promised to 'behave better'. When this strategy was unsuccessful, June threatened to take an overdose of paracetamol. When her boyfriend left, June took 35 paracetamol tablets and telephoned him to tell him what she had done. She also told him he was responsible for her forthcoming death and that she hated him. Fortunately her boyfriend telephoned the emergency services and June was successfully treated. In a further example June's recent severe cutting incident followed from a telephone conversation in which she was told that she could not be seen by a member of the emergency community psychiatric response team. This was because of an agreed care contract with June, which meant that she would not seek out of hours service but would engage in telephone counselling. June terminated the telephone call, went into the kitchen and cut her wrist so badly that she severed three of her tendons and cut an artery. Only then did she call the emergency services. As a result of this she nearly bled to death and is likely to be left with some permanent disability in her hand.

In both of the examples discussed above the self-harm behaviour is a direct attempt to manipulate the situation so that June achieves her own goals. The example also demonstrates another important consideration, that of escalation. Escalation refers to the level of self-harm required to produce the desired response from the BPD individual's point of view. The first time an individual ever cuts themselves deliberately there is likely to be a significant response from friends, family and psychiatric services. However, if this is the 25th cutting incident then there is likely to be less of a response; after all it has happened before, and the individual has survived. Therefore, to generate the same level of response the person with BPD is forced to carry out a more dramatic and often more serious self-harm attempt. As the seriousness increases so does the risk of serious injury or death. This need to escalate combined with feelings of worthlessness and emptiness is one of the reasons why BPD has a high mortality rate.

Dichotomous thinking and promotion of interpersonal conflicts

As these two topics are closely intertwined they will be discussed together. Dichotomous thinking, describes a way of thinking that is not unique to BPD, but is a pervasive feature of the thinking of the majority of individuals with BPD. Dichotomous thinking is essentially seeing the world in black and white terms, without any shades of grey in between. For example, in a relationship, a BPD individual's partner may be seen as either completely perfect, and loved unconditionally, or equally as useless and totally hated. This form of thinking is also applied to the person her or himself. Most of us recognize that we have both good and bad aspects to our character and behaviour. Individuals with BPD often see themselves as wholly good and wholly bad. Although dichotomous thinking is problematic it would be possible to devise a treatment strategy in order to help the individual think in less rigid terms; however, what makes dichotomous thinking so problematic in BPD individuals is that they tend to alternate between the two poles with bewildering speed. One day, or even hour, a relationship, individual or object will be perfect – the next useless, hated and to be despised. Often these changes in mood and view point occur with only trivial causes or often with no obvious cause. It is this alternating dichotomous thinking which makes sustaining a personal or clinical relationship with an individual with BPD so exhausting and difficult. Comments and behaviours which yesterday resulted in a calm and reasoned discussion today result in rage and contempt. In personal relationships, dichotomous thinking combined with the other features of BPD, cause relationships to breakdown therefore exacerbating the interpersonal loneliness felt by the individual.

In clinical relationships – particularly inpatient settings – dichotomous thinking causes particular problems for the nurse. Firstly, it is difficult to undertake care planning in a collaborative and meaningful way. A care plan agreed one day may suddenly be completely unacceptable the next. Reminding the individual that they agreed, often wholeheartedly, earlier, results in denial, anger and even violence. This denial is often accompanied by a sudden change in attitude toward the nurse who is now an object of scorn and dislike. For the nurse this process can be personally demoralizing and hurtful, however, it also leads to the second problem, that of the promotion of interpersonal conflict. When one nurse becomes unacceptable the individual with BPD may turn to another staff member. At first this new nurse is considered wonderful and showered with praise whilst the original nurse is described in uncomplimentary terms. Such situations have the potential to result in staff disagreement and conflicting care approaches in an unprepared team. Junior staff and non-clinical staff are often particularly vulnerable to this process. However, the same process also happens between other people resident in the inpatient unit with individuals with BPD engaging in short friendships with others, which then break down for the reasons described above. New friendships are formed, often with previous friends being described in uncomplimentary terms and the process is repeated. In a very short time an unsatisfactory atmosphere of hurt, anger and distress can result. The methods for managing this behaviour in clinical situations are discussed later.

Although working with people with BPD can be problematic there is no need to be overly negative. There are methods of working with individuals with BPD that are at least partly successful and these are explored below. Firstly a brief review of treatment approaches for BPD will be given and secondly a suggested approach for nursing BPD individuals in other inpatient and community situations will be discussed.

TREATMENT OF BPD

Two treatment approaches for BPD have been shown to be effective in randomized controlled trials (RCTs).

One of the most popular and effective approaches is dialectical behaviour therapy (DBT).[13] The goal of the therapy is to teach individuals with BPD how to manage their stress and emotional trauma instead of trying to solve their problems by removing them from situations of crisis and placing them in inpatient situations. Therefore it is a community-based therapy. DBT involves using skills training to address maladaptive behaviours such as self-harm, behaviours which may interfere with therapy and the quality of life while at the same time countering the isolation and interpersonal loneliness experienced by people with BPD by helping them to build supportive relationships, which are characterized by reflection, empathy and acceptance. These approaches are balanced with dialectic strategies that involve the acceptance of change and the validating of experience with problem-solving and the use of paradox and metaphor.

The above strategies are accomplished through both group and individual work and also a therapist led telephone support service, which provides an alternative to damaging behaviours in crisis situations. The clinical effectiveness of DBT has been examined in randomized controlled trials (RCTs). These trials have shown that DBT is more effective than other therapies in reducing self-harm, length of hospital admission, dropout from treatment, inappropriate anger and also in improving social adjustment.[14]

A second approach is pharmacological, using serotonin reuptake inhibitors (SSRIs) such as fluoxetine. This approach is based upon the theory that low levels of a neurotransmitter in the brain called serotonin may result in irritable, impulsive and self-harming behaviour.[14] These are characteristics of BPD. There has been some evidence that this approach may be an effective treatment for BPD. Cornelius *et al*.[15] found that the impulsive and depressive symptoms of BPD were reduced by the administration of fluoxetine, and Markovitz and Wagner[16] found that venlafaxine (another SSRI) was effective in treating BPD. In a RCT, Salzman *et al*.[17] found that the administration of fluoxetine significantly reduced anger, independently of a reduction in depressive symptoms in BPD patients, when compared to BPD controls. There would, therefore, seem to be strong evidence that SSRIs may be a useful and effective intervention for BPD.

PRINCIPLES OF CARING FOR THE PERSON WITH BPD

As can be seen above there are at least two potentially successful treatment approaches to BPD. However, there are also a number of basic principles which can be used in both community and inpatient settings.

Setting and agreeing boundaries

Perhaps the most important element in nursing people with BPD in both inpatient and outpatient settings is negotiating and setting boundaries. Boundaries are agreed limits to behaviours engaged in by the person with BPD and the responses to these behaviours by

the care team. For example using the case study presented earlier when Julie was an inpatient she would often demand the immediate attention of nursing staff whenever even when all the staff were busy with other people. When Julie did not get immediate attention she would damage an item of furniture. Staff negotiated a care plan with Julie which stated that if she asked to see a member of staff for anything other than a brief enquiry the nursing staff would do their best to ensure that her key worker would spend time with her within 2 hours. It was also agreed that if Julie damaged furniture she would be charged for the damage. The staff then agreed that this approach would be applied by all staff and that if Julie did damage furniture she would still be seen within two hours of her request, and she would be presented with a bill at a later date. This ensured that Julie knew that one-to-one time with her key worker was available, at her request, but also acknowledged that staff resources were limited and that Julie had a responsibility for the damage she caused. A further key point is that the boundaries were realistic. They took account of staffing levels and also Julie's ability to pay for the damage she caused. It would be pointless issuing bills which everyone knew would not be paid. A further point is that there is no element of punishment in the procedure, even if Julie did damage furniture she would still be seen, although not any faster, but she was only being asked to repair the damage she caused; she was not being fined.

Consistency

The above example also emphasizes the importance of consistency. In the example described above the approach only worked if all staff responded in an agreed way in all circumstances. Therefore effective communication and education of all staff, including non-clinical staff is essential. However, consistency needs to be balanced with flexibility. If staff felt that Julie's need for individual work was urgent then Julie would be seen as soon as possible.

Supporting staff

Working with people with BPD is demanding and at times demoralizing. It is essential that effective support and clinical supervision arrangements are in place. Staff should have the opportunity to discuss problems and progress in supportive team meetings and all staff should remember the potential for the promotion of interpersonal conflict that people with BPD can engender.

Supporting other people in care

As noted earlier, staff should be aware of the potential for BPD individuals to promote interpersonal conflict amongst their peers. Staff need to be aware of the potential for these situations to arise and to try to prevent them developing into major sources of distress. However, it is often impossible to manage these situations on an inpatient unit and is one of the main reasons why whenever possible people with BPD should be treated in outpatient situations.

Risk taking

Finally, the most ethically and professionally difficult issue to be faced when working with people with BPD, is risk taking. This is particularly the case in community settings. Recently Julie telephoned her key worker and demanded to be admitted to hospital, as she felt unwell. A recent multidisciplinary team meeting had agreed that Julie should only be admitted as a last resort and that all other treatment and support options should be tried first. Julie's community psychiatric nurse (CPN) called to see Julie and after seeing her thought that Julie should not be admitted, but instead offered more support in the community. Julie appeared reluctantly to agree, but later telephoned again and said that unless she was admitted she would self-harm. Julie's CPN is now in an impossible position. If Julie is admitted into hospital then the care plan is undermined and Julie has learned how to manipulate staff to achieve her aims. Conversely if Julie is not admitted she will probably self-harm. It is essential that the multidisciplinary team have a strategy in place to deal with such a situation. There is a clear tension between the clinical need for consistency and the ethical, professional and legal requirements to keep her safe. These also need to be balanced by the need to allow Julie to make her own decisions and take responsibility for them. There are massive ethical problems with allowing Julie to self-harm, but admitting Julie may prejudice Julie's long-term improvement and prospects. There is no easy answer in this situation and any decision of what risks might be taken, should be discussed with the multidisciplinary team and most importantly with Julie. It cannot be a nursing decision alone.

CONCLUSION

We can see that BPD is a controversial diagnosis and, as a label, may actually hinder an individual's contact with psychiatric services. However, some treatments have been shown to be effective and nurses play a key role in delivering these options. Consistency of approach, team working and above all an individual tailored care plan are the only way to work with this challenging group of people.

REFERENCES

1. Mack AH, Forman L, Brown R, Frances A. A brief history of psychiatric classification. *Psychiatric Clinics of North America* 1994; **17**: 515–23.
2. Livesley WJ, Schroede RML, Jackson DN, Jang KL. Categorical distinctions in the study of personality disorder: implications for classification. *Journal of Abnormal Psychology* 1994; **103**: 6–17.
3. Allport GW. *Pattern and growth in personality*. New York: Holt, Rinehart and Winston, 1961.
4. Kretschmer E. *Physique and character*. New York: Harcourt Brace, 1925.
5. Hoch P, Polatin P. Pseudoneurotic forms of schizophrenia. *Psychiatric Quarterly* 1949; **23**: 248–76.
6. American Psychiatric Association. *Diagnostic and statistical manual of mental disorders*, 3rd edn. Washington DC: APA, 1980.
7. Kroll J. *The challenge of the borderline patient: competency in diagnosis and treatment*. New York: Norton, 1988.
8. American Psychiatric Association. *Diagnostic and statistical manual of mental disorders*, 3rd edn, revised. Washington DC: APA, 1987.
9. American Psychiatric Association. *Diagnostic and statistical manual of mental disorders*, 4th edn. Washington DC: APA, 1994.
10. World Health Organization. *The ICD-10 classification of mental and behavioural disorders*. Geneva: WHO, 1993.
11. Clark LA, Livesley WJ, Morey L. Special feature: personality disorder assessment: the challenge of construct validity. *Journal of Personality Disorders* 1997; **11**: 205–31.
12. Livesley J. Past achievements and future directions. In: Livesley WJ (ed.) *The DSM-IV personality disorders*. New York: Guilford, 1995: 497–506.
13. Linehan MM. *Cognitive-behavioural treatment of borderline personality disorder*. New York: Guilford, 1993.
14. Coccaro EF, Kavoussi RJ. Neurotransmitter correlates of impulsive aggression. In: Stoff DM, Cairns RB (eds). *Aggression and violence, genetic, neurobiological and biosocial perspectives*. Mahwah, NJ: Laurence Earlbaum, 1996: 67–85.
15. Cornelius JR, Soloff MD, Perel JM, Ulrich MS. A preliminary trial of fluoxetine in refectory borderline patients. *Journal of Clinical Pharmacology* 1991; **11**(2): 116–20.
16. Markovitz PJ, Wagner SC. Venlafaxine in the treat-

ment of borderline personality disorder. *Pharmacological Bulletin* 1995; **31**(4): 773–7.

17. Salzman C, Wolfson AN, Schatzberg A, *et al.* Effect of fluoxetine on anger in symptomatic volunteers with borderline personality disorders. *Journal of Clinical Psychopharmacology* 1995; **15**(1): 23–9.

Chapter 36

THE PERSON WHO USES SUBSTANCES

David B Cooper*

Pre-reading exercise

Before you begin this chapter, complete this short exercise:

1   Pick a favourite substance or activity that you enjoy regularly (e.g. drinking tea, coffee or alcohol, eating chocolate, a regular spliff or that special pack of daily biscuits or crisps). It could even be jogging, or going for fast food meals. Whatever you *really* like to do regularly.

2   *Do not* take any of your choice substance or activity for one week.

3   Record how you feel throughout the week (happy, sad, angry?). Did you cheat, if so why? What were the prompts? Or, just as important, why didn't you start? What excuses did you give yourself for *not* doing this exercise?

It will become apparent that we all crave the loss of substances, and/or activities, that we do regularly, and take for granted, if access is restricted. This exercise was designed to stimulate your thinking about harmful substance use and how the nurse[a] may perceive his or her role. Once aware of one's position, it is possible to move forward.

INTRODUCTION

This chapter offers an introduction to harmful substance use, and emphasizes the important role of nurses in the preventions and identification of people whose substance use is harmful to themselves or others. The term 'substance' is used to refer to the legal substance (alcohol) and illegal substances (such as: cannabis, cocaine, opiates and opioids, ecstasy).

Whatever the nature of substance use, it should be considered in the context of the individual's personal history and circumstances. Stereotypes of the substance user

*David B. Cooper has been involved in the substance use and health profession for 23 years working as a practitioner, researcher, lecturer, consultant, manager, author, editor and writer. David is former editor of *The Drug and Alcohol Professional*, founder member and former chairperson of the Nursing Council on Alcohol, author of *Alcohol Home Detoxification and Assessment* and edited *Alcohol Use*.

[a] Nurses includes midwives and health visitors.

should be abandoned in favour of a more individualized, eclectic and holistic understanding of the person. Interventions on behalf of the person whose substance use is harmful to themselves or others should be based on thorough assessment and should involve the individual.

Because harmful substance use can have physical, mental, emotional, social and economic implications for the individual it is important that all dimensions of the person's situation are considered as the individual makes the difficult adjustments necessary to resolve a substance use problem.[1]

The importance of prevention, early identification and brief intervention cannot be overemphasized. To assist the nurse in recognizing the signs of, and in understanding the short- and long-term effects of, harmful substance use, this chapter aims to offer the first steps on which the nurse can build knowledge and awareness.

Harmful alcohol use is discussed at length in recognition of the high impact on health and social care professionals and services.

Because illicit drug use is criminal activity, the advice/guidance to the harmful users is to stop. However, realistically, the approach should be one of harm reduction.

This chapter will use the term 'substance use' for the following reasons:

❏ Acknowledgement that not all substance use is harmful.
❏ You will have contact with the individual whose substance use is harmful but who has yet to acknowledge this.
❏ Prevention and early identification and brief intervention are more effective.
❏ One needs to talk in the language of the user.
❏ The nurse plays a primary role in preventions, early identification and brief intervention.
❏ Dependence/addiction, addicts, alcohol related problems, tolerance, withdrawal and treatment can be covered in more depth once a basic understanding of substance use, and its place in society, is understood.
❏ The terms misuse and abuse have been exchanged for harmful use in recognition that not all substance use leads to physical, social or psychological damage and that the nurse should be alerted to the harm the substance may have caused or can causes the individual presenting for treatment.
❏ Licit or illicit substance use does not always lead to chronic substance use.

SUBSTANCE USE IN PERSPECTIVE

The use of a substance to stimulate and/or alter the state of one's mind is as old as the first time that fruit, fer-

menting as part of the decaying process were sampled by man and woman. Depending on the country and or region, in which you live, the substance of choice, and its legal status, varies. In most Western countries, alcohol is the mind-altering substance of choice.

While illicit substances use makes good headlines, the actual impact on health, in comparison to harmful alcohol use is low. The World Health Organization[2] suggests worldwide, 140 million individuals are dependent on alcohol and over 400 million have alcohol related problems. This is in comparison with 5 million persons injecting drugs in 136 countries.

According to the Department of Health,[3] of the substance users presenting to drug misuse agencies to March 2001, 67% accounted for heroin use. The most frequently reported main drugs were cannabis (9%), methadone (8%), cocaine (7%) and amphetamine (3%). The primary cause of harm from illicit drug use comes from the supply of adulterated drugs, lack of regulation to assure a standard purity of the substance or hazardous experiment use.

When comparing harmful illicit drug use with harmful alcohol use, and the impact on all health and social services sectors, one can begin to put the impact of harmful alcohol use into perspective.

It is acknowledged that nurses are reluctant to include screening and intervention for harmful alcohol use. Several studies have concluded that:

❏ Nurses are uncertain as to whether, or how far, harmful alcohol use comes in to their remit (*role legitimacy*).
❏ Nurses feel that they do not have sufficient knowledge and skill to recognize and respond to harmful drinkers (*role adequacy*).
❏ Nurses feel that if a harmful drinker were identified they would not have sufficient access or support from specialist alcohol services[4,5] (*role support*).

Also, there is anecdotal evidence to suggest that the nurse's reluctance extends to substance use *per se*.

Because of the widespread consequences of harmful substance use, the impact on the role of the nurse is considerable. Nurses are ideally placed to provide brief information and advice indicated to be effective in reducing harmful alcohol use.[6] A number of randomized control trials, looking at harmful alcohol use have demonstrated that, in comparison with controls, harmful drinkers receiving 5–10 minutes of brief structured advice plus a self-help booklet from a primary health care worker can reduce alcohol consumption by around 25%.[7]

Various signs that may alert the nurse to the existence of a substance-using client

❏ Physical health problem, e.g. vitamin deficiency, gastritis, infections, ulcers.

❑ Mental health problem, e.g. anxiety, depression, suicide attempts.
❑ Symptoms of substance use, e.g. tremor, shakes, sweating, constipation, diarrhoea.
❑ Problem at work, e.g. lateness, absenteeism, accidents.
❑ Criminal offences.
❑ Family problems, e.g. neglect, child disturbance, marital disharmony.
❑ Requests for help, e.g. from the client, family or other professional.
❑ Evidence of substance use, e.g. smell, used paraphernalia.
❑ Known history of substance use.
❑ Family history of substance use.
❑ Other, e.g. complaints of fatigue, lethargy, insomnia, restlessness.

ALCOHOL USE

Traditionally, alcohol studies have concentrated on how much is consumed over the 'sensible limits'. However, this does not offer a clear picture of alcohol use. Closer examination of patterns of consumption and drinking behaviour, such as type of beverage consumed, amount consumed in one sitting, rate of heavy drinking, how people drink and why people drink is required.[8] Our Healthier Nation[9] asserts that:

Drinking too much is an important factor in accidents and domestic violence and can impair people's ability to cope with everyday life ...' It acknowledges that 'people's health is affected by their circumstances' and that 'whether people drink sensibly can dramatically affect their physical and mental health and that of others ...

A single drinking occasion can also have health consequences. Binge drinking, and the stress of returning to work has been associated with Monday deaths from heart attacks.[10] Road casualty figures indicate that 35% of pedestrians were registering alcohol levels of 100 mg/100 ml, when they met their death.[11]

It is estimated that 6 billion pounds per annum is spent on alcohol misuse. £3 billion accounts for the total NHS spending (12%) on hospital treatment for harmful alcohol use and £3 billion in costs of sickness absence, unemployment, premature death, alcohol related crime and accidents.[12]

The most significant costs to the NHS arise not from the treatment of chronic long-term alcohol use but from the often hidden or unexplored harmful use that results in physical, social or psychological consequences, accidents at home or workplace, drink driving related trauma, or from violence. In mental health terms, evi-

dence suggests that in 54% of psychiatric admissions, drug or alcohol use was implicated. This figure rose to 73% when the patients also had a diagnosis of schizophrenia.[13]

Two recent reports have significance for the nursing profession. The first relates to foetal alcohol syndrome, and suggests that even small amounts of alcohol can be problematic in terms of the health impact on the foetus and child.[14] This follows closely on recent reports indicating that women are more likely to suffer liver damage because of harmful alcohol use.

The second report emphasizes the important impact the nurses can have on the identification of harmful alcohol use. The study showed that:

❑ Nurses are interested in screening and brief intervention and many are willing to incorporate this approach into practice.
❑ Skills-based training in practice was the most effective, and cost-effective, implementation strategy.

The results should provide direction for future planning of health promotion programmes and policies ... which could contribute to decreasing the health and social costs of excessive alcohol consumption in the population.[15]

Alcohol use: some facts

Alcohol is the most popular psychoactive substance used in modern society. When used in moderation, it does little more than act as a social 'lubricant', lowering inhibitions and facilitating social interaction. Excessive, heavy and prolonged use, however, can have serious consequences for health.

Alcoholic drinks are mainly comprised of water and ethanol (alcohol) and are produced by fermentation of fruits, vegetables or grain. Congeners are added to give the drink its distinctive flavour, taste and smell.

One standard drink (SD) of alcohol contains approximately 15 mg of pure ethanol. This is based on a standard measure of one average-strength drink, i.e. half a pint of beer, lager or cider, a single measure of spirits (e.g. whisky, gin, vodka), a small glass of wine, a small glass of sherry, or a measure of vermouth (or aperitif).

It has been suggested that the following SDs represent maximum levels for 'safe' weekly/daily consumption. Consumption above this level can be expected to lead to health problems.

❑ for men: up to 21 SDs. Not exceeding 4 SDs per day.
❑ for women: up to 14 SDs. Not exceeding 3 SDs per day.

However, since many varieties of alcoholic drinks of varying strengths are available, and there are very few average weight, height, healthy men or women, it can be very difficult to estimate how much alcohol one has consumed, and how safe one is.

Alcohol absorption and elimination

Key points in alcohol use are:

❑ Alcohol is one of the quickest-acting orally administered substances.
❑ It is a toxic substance.
❑ The only organ capable of eliminating it from the body is the liver.
❑ Alcohol passes chemically unchanged from the stomach into the blood supply within 5 minutes.
❑ Adding carbonated drinks, alternating alcohol with carbonated drinks, drinking on an empty stomach and drinking quickly may speed up absorption.
❑ It takes approximately 30 minutes for alcohol levels to peak in the blood and one hour for the liver to eliminate one SD.
❑ Any other alcohol taken during this time will accumulate in the blood, waiting processing.

Health consequences of excessive alcohol use

Harmful alcohol use can lead to a wide range of health problems affecting virtually all parts of the body and can interfere with the effects of many prescribed drugs such as oral contraceptives, antibiotics, anti-inflammatory agents, tranquillizers, anti-depressants and diuretics. The habitual over-use of alcohol is associated with a number of psycho-social problems.

Sudden withdrawal, even at low levels of consumption can be accompanied by unpleasant symptoms such as sweating, increased anxiety, tremor, headache, thirst, nausea and occasional vomiting.

ILLEGAL SUBSTANCES

It is time to step back and take a common-sense look at substance use *per se*. The message should now be about reducing the harmful consequences of substance use, about safe use – sensible use. A former Ambassador in Columbia in his 'personal view' paper, presents a sound case for the legalization of illicit drug use.[16] Within the lifetime of this publication it is likely that cannabis will be reclassified to a class C drug, paving the way for medicinal use for physical illnesses such a multiple scle-rosis. Thankfully, this action will take the user out of the criminal system.

The reader is directed to Mathre ML, Cannabis Series: the whole story. This series in The Drug and Alcohol Professional, *1:1 (2001) through to 3:3 (2003) dispels the myths surrounding the use of cannabis and explores the medicinal and recreational use of this drug.*

Politicians and judges are now muting the possibility of legalization of illicit drugs:

> Legalizing doesn't mean approval, it means control. It brings [the problem] into the open . . . [The legalization of drugs would reduce drug-related problems by] saving money on law enforcement, unblocking courts and reducing prison overcrowding . . . [It would also] improve civil liberties and reduce the spread of HIV/AIDS. [We should abolish] all offences related to cannabis. If this works it should be followed by other drugs . . . If consumption increases, [we should] stop and rethink the strategies. The sale of drugs to children should remain an offence, as it is with alcohol and tobacco . . . If someone becomes so addicted to a drug that he becomes a harm to others or his or her self, then the courts should be able to send him or her for treatment.[17]

It is conceivable that the legalization of all illicit substances will follow within the lifetime of most readers.

OPIATES AND OPIOIDS

Opiates are narcotic analgesics, derived from the sap of the opium poppy (*Papaver somniferum*). Their synthetic equivalents are collectively known as opioids.

Heroin

Heroin, a narcotic made from morphine, can be sniffed, injected or smoked. The purity of the drug is often unknown, and consequently accidental overdose or death can easily occur. Heroin users who share needles and syringes are at risk of septicaemia, hepatitis and HIV/AIDS.

The effects of heroin include euphoria, drowsiness, and a sense of well-being and raised self-esteem. Tolerance develops quickly, demanding increased intake to achieve the desired effect. Physical and psychological dependence may follow. Contamination of the substance often leads to severe allergic reactions, which may be exacerbated by poor diet and self-neglect. This degenerative process may lead to death if medical intervention is not available. Withdrawal is unpleasant, and is often described as being 'like a severe dose of flu'. Other problems include constipation and vomiting. Complaints of diarrhoea, abdominal cramps and muscle spasm are common. Although it has been suggested that withdrawal from heroin is easier than withdrawal from nicotine or methadone, it should be attempted gradually, using reducing doses of methadone as a heroin substitute.

STIMULANTS

Amphetamines

Amphetamines can be sniffed, injected or taken in tablet form. The effects can last for up to 5 hours and include an increase in pulse and respiration, reduced fatigue and increased muscular activity. The individual becomes restless and over-talkative. Weight loss and excessive body fluid loss are potential complications.

The user may complain of headache, tiredness and lack of social interest. During intoxication accidental injury and death may occur as a consequence of irrational behaviour. Amphetamine overdose may cause fever, paranoid psychosis, respiratory failure, hallucinations, seizures, coma, disorientation and cardiovascular collapse.

There are no specific withdrawal symptoms, although the user may complain of lethargy, prolonged sleep and excessive hunger. Psychological dependence is a major obstacle to successful withdrawal and much individual support and counselling will be needed.

Cocaine

Cocaine is an alkaloid derived from the coca plant. This white crystal-like powder is a powerful but short-acting stimulant. It can be sniffed, injected or smoked. Occasionally it is mixed with heroin to maximize the effect. When cocaine is treated with baking powder and water it forms into tiny chalk-like lumps or 'rocks' and is referred to as 'crack'.

The effects of cocaine peak within 30 minutes and then gradually decrease. The user experiences a tremendous feeling of physical and mental power. This physiological arousal and euphoria lead to an indifference to pain and fatigue. Normal requirements for food are decreased. Large doses may lead to agitation, anxiety, hallucinations and erratic behaviour.

Dependence is usually psychological. The individual may complain of depression, fatigue and inability to cope. Chronic use may cause restlessness, nausea, sleeplessness, paranoid psychosis, hyper excitability and severe depression. Repeated sniffing also leads to erosion of the nasal membrane.

HALLUCINOGENS

Hallucinogens (psychedelics, psychotomimetics or psychotogens) include LSD (lysergic acid diethylamide), hallucinogenic mushrooms and cannabis. The prime effect of these substances is the alteration of perceptual functions of the brain.

Cannabis

When used recreationally, cannabis has no long-lasting effects and is safer than alcohol. Cannabis, a preparation of the hemp plant, is available in three forms:

❏ 'Grass', a dried leaf (marijuana).
❏ Resin, a compact block ('hash').
❏ Oil, the most highly concentrated form.

It has been suggested that cannabis may play an important role in pain and symptom relief in multiple sclerosis suffers and some cancers.[18] Cannabis is usually mixed with tobacco and smoked, although occasionally it is eaten or baked. The immediate effect is one of relaxation, talkativeness and hilarity. Intensification of sound and colour may also be experienced. There is a reduction in short-term memory function and in motor skill. Concentration is poor. These effects last up to one hour after social use.

High doses of cannabis can lead to confusion. However, the main health hazard appears to derive from the inhalation of tobacco smoke. The use of cannabis is often transient.

Lysergic acid diethylamide (LSD)

LSD is a derivative of ergot, a fungus commonly found on rye and other grasses. An exceedingly potent substance, only minute doses of LSD are required to achieve a hallucinogenic effect.

The short-term user experiences a 'trip', in which hallucinations, disturbance of perception, increases in awareness, disorientation and disassociation from the body may occur. These experiences commence within 30 minutes following ingestion and peak 2–6 hours later, gradually fading after 10 hours.

Excessive and long-term use can cause prolonged psychological reactions and re-experiencing of past 'trips'. However, LSD is not known to cause physical dependence.

'Magic' mushrooms

There are approximately 12 varieties of mushrooms,

which contain hallucinogenic chemicals. The most common of these is *Psilocybe semilanceata* ('liberty cap').

'Magic' mushrooms contain two active ingredients, psilocybin and psilocin. The mushrooms may be crushed, eaten fresh, brewed in a tea or cooked in soup. The user experiences effects similar to those of LSD, along with euphoria, hilarity, increased heart rate and blood pressure, and dilated pupils. Commencing within 30 minutes, the effects peak at approximately 3 hours and last 4–10 hours.

Dependence, withdrawal and overdose are unlikely, the primary danger to health lying in the possibility that the individual may pick and consume a poisonous mushroom by mistake.

Ecstasy

Ecstasy is like heroin and cocaine, a class A substance. There are many debates about Ecstasy's recreational drug use with much publicized material following the death of an individual. The impact on the long-term health of the regular user has yet to be determined.

THE ROLE OF THE NURSE

Although our understanding of substance use has improved in recent years, there is still a tendency for nurses to shy away from interaction and intervention with substance-using individuals. During one's interactions with substance-using individuals, it is important to realize that the substance use may merely form a small part of the presenting problem. Each individual presents with a unique set of concerns, which may have caused, contributed to, or interacted with the development of the overall problem.

Those individuals whose substance use is harmful often change their behaviour as a direct result of a major life-event, such as a change in an important relationship, an accident or illness, redundancy, a birth or a death. Such events can curtail, neutralize or enhance the nurse's endeavours with an individual[19] and must be taken into account in the formulation of treatment programmes. Therefore, an individualized, eclectic and holistic approach to prevention, identification and treatment, in which all-relevant professionals should intervene as necessary.[19]

To provide effective intervention the nurse should be prepared to:

1 Identify the individual at risk.
2 Recognize the types of problems that are likely to be experienced by the individual.

3 Assist the individual in the process of acknowledging, exploring and understanding the substance use.
4 Appreciate the individual's own perception of the substance use.
5 Consider with the individual the personal action and or treatment options.
6 Facilitate the individual's achievement of the chosen goal(s).
7 Acquaint the individual with the services and facilities available to assist.
8 Act non-judgementally.
9 Provide nursing interventions in withdrawal.
10 Provide understanding and support should relapse occur.

THE PERSON WHOSE SUBSTANCE USE IS HARMFUL

The question of substance use should be raised in a non-threatening manner. While the individual may be evasive or defensive at first, at least the nurse will have demonstrated concern and made the first approach. The subject should not be laboured, but tactfully and sensitively progressed at each contact. The nurse is not a judge, but a facilitator, educator and carer.

Assessment

Nursing assessments should include investigations of substance use. While nurses become accustomed to asking about the most intimate details of bowel action or sexual function, many feel uncomfortable about broaching the subject of substance use. This may reflect a lack of basic knowledge, as well as a need to make such questioning routine.

Intervention and treatment can be undertaken following a full and systematic assessment of the needs of the individual and family. If treatment is to have a favourable outcome, a complete picture of the individual's substance use should be obtained. Moreover, clear understandings of the individual's own actions and treatment goal(s) are essential: are they reduction in use, a change to a less harmful substance, controlled use, withdrawal, or total abstinence?

Many individuals with substance use problems 'sound out' a service before committing themselves to care. Therefore, any information given on treatment options should be clear and to the point, and should be communicated both verbally and in written form.

Assessment should include details of past and present substance use and the following factors should always be considered:

- ❑ Psychological state.
- ❑ Work, social and cultural factors.
- ❑ Problematic effects of use.
- ❑ Motivation for treatment.
- ❑ Family psychodynamics.
- ❑ Relevant personal factors.
- ❑ Physical state and complications.

BRIEF INTERVENTION

Brief or minimal intervention implies a form of treatment typically less intensive in terms of time than traditional treatment methods. It involves providing the individual with information regarding the risks to health associated with harmful substance use. The nurse can provide guidance or advice, verbally or in the form of an information leaflet. Research suggests that the use of brief interventions are as effective as more intensive interventions for those who are not severely dependent,[20] and that such interventions are more effective than none.[21] The individual should be asked in a 'sensitive, but matter of fact way', when undertaking an assessment and should be encouraged to look not only at the amount used but also when and who with.[22]

A prerequisite, for the individual and the nurse, is the correct identification of the amount of the substance of use and amount consumed to correctly assess any health risks. It is important that the professional reassures individual that the advice given is not necessarily to stop but to facilitate that individual to conclude that a reduction or change to drug use behaviour will be beneficial to that person's health and social circumstances.

It is important to consider the significance of effective, timely interventions and communication between the individual and the nurse and how one's own values, attitudes and beliefs can have impact upon the quality of care provided.[23] In order to offer effective intervention the nurse needs to build a relationship with the patient or client based upon acceptance, respect and trust.[24] This does not mean the relationship has to be long term; the nurse can also convey these feelings in a relationship that lasts only a few minutes. It is essential for the nurse to be self-aware in relation to the presentation of emotion, feeling, and presentation of self and aware of his or her own attitudes to substance use. What is considered 'harmful use' is often dependent upon individual interpretation. One's own substance use may be greater than that of the person presenting and consequently assumed by the nurse to be 'normal'. This will influence the quality standard of care, dismissing the patient's problem as menial or insignificant.

The central theme underpinning all intervention is effective communication. Information should be neither patronizing nor jargonistic. The patient can then be encouraged to reflect on key themes in order to assess the level of understanding or to clarify any questions and make an informed choice.

Prevention

Whether or not an individual develops a substance use problem, often depends on the social resources available. It is vital that the problems and experiences that can set the stage for harmful substance use are recognized by the caring professions and that the relevant agencies persevere in improving and developing preventive strategies both at the local and national level.

Most health districts now have a drug and or alcohol advisory service, as well as a health promotion officer dealing with HIV/AIDS-related issues who offer an advisory resource to the nurse. The introduction of such initiatives as outreach programmes and needle exchange schemes has also proved valuable in the early identification of substance users.

HARM MINIMIZATION

Harm minimization is a practice by which substance users are advised on safe methods of substance use, rather than being urged to abstain. The user is offered blood tests and health checks, is given advice on safer using practices, and is supplied with clean 'works' and condoms. The underlying philosophy is that while it may be impossible to eradicate altogether the illegal use of substances, it is nonetheless beneficial for individuals and society to make existing substance use as safe as possible.

Needle exchange schemes aim to distribute clean needles, syringes and containers with a view to preventing the sharing of equipment and thus reducing the spread of infection. These schemes allow for access to this paraphernalia as well as to health promotion materials and advice.

CONCLUSION

There is little public and professional understanding of the effects of harmful substance use. Anyone can experience the consequences of harmful substance use without understanding that his or her use has harmed or may harm themselves or others. The image of self-inflicted harm from substance use still exists. The intention to self-harm may not be deliberate; the circumstances of the use may merely be inappropriate.

Harmful substance use occurs not only at high but also low levels of usage. The emphasis lies with harm reduction with accurate identification, brief interventions, education and health promotion, that can be routinely employed by the nurse. Therefore, the focus is not solely on the quantity but also in the way or circumstances surrounding the use, how it affects mood and how this in turn affects the individual, family and others, and the environment.

This chapter has offered an introduction to the many issues surrounding the care of individuals whose substances use may or may not be harmful. While treatment with chronic substance users has become an area of specialist practice, nurses in every field need to be aware of the signs and the consequences of substance use.[25–27]

Substance use problems occur in every age group and social class. Within the family, substance use problems may have serious implications not only for the individual directly affected, but also for his or her spouse, partner and children. Indeed, the nurse may first detect the existence of harmful substance use not through contact with the substance user, but in interactions with family members. Therefore, it is vital that nursing interventions undertaken in response to harmful substance use are based on an assessment not only of the individuals but the family.

As professionals, we need to be aware of the complications and effects that alcohol can have upon the individual and society. There is an identified need for an emphasis in raising the awareness of both the nurse and the public to the potential dangers of the 'safe drug', alcohol. In our interactions with individuals using alcohol harmfully, the starting point must be the recognition that alcohol use forms only a small part of the problem but that identification and brief intervention for those consuming alcohol harmfully may be integral to that individual's future health.

We will never know all there is to know about substance use. There will always be surprises. What intervention one offers depends on the knowledge, and the ability to use one's own and other people's knowledge. As professionals one has a responsibility to offer the best that is known, to the best of one's ability, at that time.

Knowledge and understanding of substance use is constantly changing. The challenge is to remain open to the information that will help provide:

❑ appropriate therapeutic intervention;
❑ at the appropriate level;
❑ at the appropriate time;
❑ at the appropriate cost; and
❑ with the appropriate understanding of the individual presenting with the problem.[28]

REFERENCES

1. Department of Health. *Tackling drugs together: a strategy for England 1995–1998*. London: HMSO, 1995.

2. World Health Organization. *Management of substance dependence fact sheet*, 2002. www.who.int/mental.health/topics.html

3. Department of Health. *Statistical bulletin: statistics from the regional drug misuse database. Use of drug misuse services in England – October 01, 2000 to March 31, 2001*. London: Department of Health, 2002.

4. Shaw W, Cartwright A, Spratley T, Harwin J. *Responding to drinking problems*. London: Croom Helm, 1978.

5. Cooper D. Problem drinking: alcohol survey results. *Nursing Times* 1994; **90**(14): 36–8.

6. Watson HE. Prevention, intervention, education and health promotion. In: Cooper DB (ed.) *Alcohol use*, Chapter 12. Oxford: Radcliffe Medical Press, 2000.

7. Freemantle N, Paramjit G, Godfrey C, *et al*. Brief interventions and alcohol use. *Effective Health Care Bulletin* 1993; **7**. Extracted from: Heather N, McAvoy B, Kaner E. *Phase IV: Implementing countrywide screening and brief alcohol intervention strategies in primary health care, England*. WHO Collaborative Project on Identification and management of alcohol-related problems in primary health care. Geneva: World Health Organization, 2000.

8. Smart RG. Trends in drinking and patterns of drinking. In: Grant, M (ed.) *Drinking patterns and their consequences*, Chapter 2. Philadelphia: Brunner/Mazel, 1997: 25–41.

9. Department of Health. *White Paper: Our healthier nation: a contract for health*, Chapter 2. London: The Stationery Office, 1998.

10. Evans C, Chalmers J, Capewell S, *et al*. 'I don't like Mondays' – day of the week coronary heart disease deaths in Scotland: study of routinely collected data. *British Medical Journal* 2000; **320**: 281–9.

11. Alcohol Concern. *Press Release: Drink–walk warning to pedestrians*. London: Alcohol Concern, 1999.

12. Alcohol Concern. *Press Release: Alcohol misuse costing country £6 billion*. London: Alcohol Concern, 2002.

13. Smith J, Frazer S, Bower H. Dual diagnosis in patients. *Hospital and Community Psychiatry* 1994; **45**: 280–81.

14. Little J, Hepper P. *Alcohol insight: Report number 8, Maternal alcohol consumption and the behaviour of the foetus*. London: Alcohol Education and Research Council, 2001. www.aerc.org.uk

15. Kaner E, Lock C, Bond S, McAvoy B, Heather N, Gilvary E. *Alcohol insight: Report number 12, A randomised controlled trial of training and support strategies to*

encourage screening and brief intervention by primary care nurses. London: Alcohol Education and Research Council, 2002. www.aerc.org.uk

16. Morris K. The failure of prohibition: a personal view. *The Drug and Alcohol Professional* 2001; **1**(2): 12–17.

17. Pickles Judge J. *A futile war.* 'Byline', BBC 1, 1991.

18. Stimmel B. *Pain and its relief without addiction.* New York: Haworth Medical Press, 1997.

19. Davidson R. Facilitating change in problem drinkers. In: Davidson R, Rollnick S, MacEwan I (eds). *Counselling problem drinkers.* London: Tavistock, 1991: 3–20.

20. Heather N. *Brief intervention strategies.* In: Hester RK, Miller WR (eds). *Handbook of alcoholism treatment approaches: effective alternatives.* Needham Height: Allyn and Bacon, 1996.

21. Bein T, Miller W, Tonigan S. Brief interventions for alcohol problems: a review. *Addiction* 1993; **88**: 315–36.

22. Watson HE. Minimal intervention for problem drinkers. *Journal of Substance Misuse* 1996; **1**(2): 107–10.

23. Cooper DB. *Conclusion: entering the room.* In: Cooper DB (ed.) *Alcohol use,* Chapter 19. Oxford: Radcliffe Medical Press, 2000.

24. Tschudin V. *Counselling skills for nurses,* 4th edn. London: Ballière Tindall, 1995.

25. ENB. *Training needs analysis.* London: English National Board for Nursing, Midwifery and Health Visiting, 1995.

26. ENB. *Substance misuse – guidelines for good practice in education and training of nurses, midwives and health visitors.* London: English National Board for Nursing, Midwifery and Health Visiting, 1996.

27. ENB. *Curriculum guidelines for education programmes for substance misuse.* London: English National Board for Nursing, Midwifery and Health Visiting, 1996.

28. Cooper DB. The need for professional communication. In: Cooper DB. *Alcohol use,* Chapter 18. Oxford: Radcliffe Medical Press, 2000.

Chapter 37

THE PERSON WHO IS PARANOID OR SUSPICIOUS

Denis Ryan*

INTRODUCTION

The term *paranoia* has a long history, predating contemporary understandings and being synonymous with the concept of insanity.[1] It is one that over time, has moved through a complete cycle of change. In its earliest understanding it was a generic and broadly understood term, which implied a general state of madness. It also had a variety of descriptive as well as diagnostic understandings in professional circles. More recently, it has acquired a shared professional and lay meaning. In much the same way as terms such as 'stress' have become popular in non-professional circles, paranoia or paranoid have become widely used but often poorly understood.

From an assessment, diagnostic and treatment perspective, the use of language and accuracy of definition is obviously important, although it can have potentially negative consequences in terms of labelling and stigmatization. In many ways, much of the popular misconception of the true meaning of paranoia has added to the stigmatization of people who receive this psychiatric diagnosis. For this reason, it is worth reconsidering the aims of diagnosis in relation to people who might be viewed as paranoid or suspicious.

While there may be a range of benefits which may emanate from the use of a system of diagnostic classification in relation to either clinical or administrative practice, diagnostic classification systems serve three main purposes.[2] These relate essentially to the standardization of language across disciplines; to the study of the natural history of particular disorders and the development of effective treatments; and finally to the development of an understanding of the causes of the various mental disorders.

The inconsistencies of definition

While the requirement for adequate definition may be well served by ascribing an appropriate diagnostic label, one of the main difficulties in usage is their dynamic nature. The changing nature of the diagnosis of paranoid conditions has been an issue of debate within the literature. To some extent, it may be argued that the paranoia debate has persisted since the time of Kraepelin and Bleuler, a period from when many of the debates on classification can be dated.[3]

Differences have existed in relation to symptomatology and presentation and at a more fundamental level, have revolved around the issue of whether or not paranoia could be considered a distinct diagnostic entity. Some authors have argued that paranoid conditions

*Denis Ryan is a Lecturer in Nursing at the Department of Nursing, University of Limerick in Ireland. Prior to that he was a Nursing Tutor with the Mid Western Health Board and Nursing Practice Development Co-ordinator for the South Eastern Health Board. He was Assistant Chief Nursing Officer in both the South Eastern and Mid Western Health Boards and has worked mainly in acute inpatient, community care and Addiction Services.

became subsumed into the concept of schizophrenia because of the dominance of the Bleulerian concept of schizophrenia, which was extremely loose.[4]

The origins of the term paranoia date from at least the early 1800s, when the terms 'paranoia' and 'madness' effectively had a shared meaning.[1] However, the identification and acceptance of paranoia as a distinct entity has evolved since Kraepelin's work. In his original categorization of mental disorders, he distinguished between paranoia and dementia praecox. While Bleuler subsequently disagreed with Kraepelin in terms of specific diagnostic criteria, he agreed that paranoid disorders should in fact be seen as a separate entity. Kraepelin originally described individuals with paranoid disorders as people who would present with systematized delusions, but would not present with hallucinations. In this conceptualization, paranoid disorders were characterized by their prolonged course without recovery, but not at the same time leading to mental deterioration.[5] Bleuler disagreed insofar as he believed that hallucinations could be a feature in some patients.[6]

The insufficiency of definition became highlighted in the 1960s when it was acknowledged that despite the established existence of the phenomenon there were 'no reliable statistics concerning the incidence of paranoia and paranoid reactions'.[7] While both major international classification systems (DSM and ICD) have established diagnostic criteria and ongoing refinements over time, there remain inconsistencies between them which do not inspire confidence. In the more recent editions of both the DSM and ICD classification systems, while the distinct classification of paranoid conditions within schizophrenic disorders has continued, paranoid reactions have been largely subsumed within the broader categorization of delusional disorder. Within that distinct classification some authors[8] argue that by the end of the 20th century, the accuracy of diagnosis remained complicated by the fact that many people who suffered from the condition often either present with differing complaints, or may in fact have co-morbid conditions and do not necessarily present to mental health services.

Paranoia is not, of course, only associated exclusively with schizophrenia or delusional disorder. It is also associated with other conditions such as substance abuse and mood disorder. In relation to substance abuse, a number of authors have reported that paranoia is associated with cocaine abuse,[9] although the nature of that paranoia has been described as being a transient feature said mainly to manifest itself when individuals are in a cocaine intoxicated state and marked by 'hypervigilance' relating to potential environmental threats.[10,11] However, it would seem that paranoia is most associated with three categories of disorder – namely, paranoid personality disorder; delusional (paranoid) disorder; and paranoid schizophrenia.

PARANOID IDEAS AND THEIR PRESENTATION

Paranoia, in both lay and medical circles, describes exaggerated suspiciousness or mistrust, or suspiciousness not warranted in the first instance. A key misunderstanding in relation to paranoia is its relationship to suspicion.

Suspiciousness, in its own right, does not necessarily constitute paranoia. It may be justifiable based on past experience or earlier learning. The most obvious feature which distinguishes suspiciousness and paranoia is that the level of mistrust is either out of keeping with the past experience or wholly unjustified. Another important distinguishing feature of paranoid ideas is their ongoing and persistent nature. While exaggerated or unjustifiable suspicion are key indicators of paranoid conditions, it is probably the fact that they persist on an ongoing basis which clearly distinguishes paranoid ideas from normal suspicion. There is also a tendency for individuals with paranoid conditions to persistently seek out supportive evidence to confirm their beliefs while ignoring objective and factual, if contradictory, evidence. Another important feature of paranoid ideas is that the level of severity may vary from person to person. The level of impact on functioning can vary to such an extent that whereas some individuals function relatively well in the normal social environment, others become sorely incapacitated.

When examining the concept, one should remember that paranoia is best understood in terms of its presentation. In that regard, paranoia is likely to manifest itself with either cognitive and behavioural manifestations or both. Paranoid ideation, which may present itself in verbal expression or behavioural responses is essentially a manifestation of a health condition, rather than a disease itself. Most frequently, the paranoid person manifests delusions of importance or persecution.[1] While it is important to remember that ideas of exaggerated importance or persecution may be associated with various disorders, the delusional nature of the ideas is very specific to paranoia.

A complicating factor is that paranoid delusions may often co-exist with other disorders. Some individuals present to caring professionals with depression or anxiety while denying the existence of delusional ideation.[12] The need to distinguish the delusional nature of paranoid ideas was highlighted in a study of risk factors for depressive episodes, which identified sub-clinical suspiciousness as a risk factor for new episodes of depression.[13] This highlighted the importance – from both a diagnostic and intervention perspective – of clearly differentiating suspiciousness from paranoia.

To assist with appropriate identification of paranoia, it is also important for mental health nurses to be aware that there are a range of 'at risk' people. While not exclusively the case, it is reported that paranoia is more likely to manifest itself in middle or later life, more among women than men.[6] Those who present are also more likely to either be currently or formerly partnered with variable rates of presentation among married, separated, widowed and divorced persons. Overall, partnered people have higher rates than unattached persons.[6]

Because of the widespread use of the word paranoia in the vernacular to denote people who either are or believe they are experiencing a threat, the technical and professional understanding of the concept may have in some way become somewhat unclear. These issues can hinder adequate assessment and treatment.

PEOPLE DIAGNOSED AS PARANOID

The International Council of Nursing defines nursing as an occupation which:

> encompasses autonomous and collaborative care of individuals of all ages, families, groups and communities, sick or well and in all settings. Nursing includes the promotion of health, prevention of illness and the care of ill, disabled and dying people. Advocacy, promotion of a safe environment, research, participation in shaping health policy and inpatient and health systems management, and education are also key nursing roles.[14]

While this definition refers to all nurses, in relation to paranoia, the care and management of such individuals is invariably an area of special concern for psychiatric-mental health (PMH) nurses. To fulfil the requirements of this definition, there are a number of implications for mental health nursing practice.

As with other branches of nursing, PMH nursing practice has tended to concentrate on care of the ill. While treatment is vital, little attention has been paid to health promotion and illness prevention. The matter of definition may, in this context, seem somewhat unnecessary at first glance. However, the issue of adequate and proper definition does help practitioners and consumers alike to identify the legitimate areas of concern for mental health nurses.

There is little doubt that there is still a range of difficulties and obstacles which hamper the process of arriving at an adequate definition of the primary function of the mental health nurse.[15] The principal difficulties seem to relate largely to the ongoing debate as to whether or not mental health nursing is a form of creative human expertise, or whether it is, or should be, more scientific in nature. Confounding this debate is the issue of autonomous and collaborative practice between various disciplines and professions within psychiatry. While there are clear arguments that the core function

of nursing, irrespective of the individual branch of the discipline, deals with the manifestations of illness, it is also a reality that psychiatric-mental health nursing has distinctive features and that at least part of the role of the mental health nurse is to work collaboratively with other professions – especially psychiatrists.[16]

Assessment and diagnostic issues

People who present for treatment are likely to have concerns and fears. Frequently these may manifest themselves or may be misinterpreted as suspiciousness, irritability or negativity. It is also important to remember that paranoid ideas are a manifestation of a range of disorders. This highlights the importance of adequate assessment and screening to distinguish (for example) paranoid ideation and paranoid delusions, which in turn, may lead to a distinction between psychotic and non-psychotic disorders. As previously acknowledged, collaborative care is increasingly the norm in mental health care practice. Rigorous attention to the distinction of symptomatology may also help in the collaborative process of arriving at a diagnosis of the particular condition of which paranoia is a feature.

While paranoid delusions may occasionally present as an isolated feature, more frequently they will present in association with:

❑ different kinds of delusions;
❑ hallucinations;
❑ changes in speech content or form;
❑ alterations in affect and level of orientation;
❑ agitation; or
❑ aggressive behaviour.[17]

In addition, paranoid ideation or delusions should also be considered in the context of an individual's physical health status and substance use. The levels of impairment and the range of areas of impairment also need consideration. Such considerations point to the necessity for accurate and comprehensive assessment. While it may be relatively easy to identify severe forms of paranoia,[1] it is quite a different issue to distinguish between clinical paranoid states and understandable levels of suspicion.

Probably the most profound complicating factor is the fact that much of the assessment must rely on interview methods with both the individual as well as family or concerned others. In that regard it is likely that the interview process itself will be complicated by the nature of the paranoid ideas or delusions, if present.

To arrive at an accurate diagnosis, it is vital that an adequate history of a range of areas is obtained. This will include such issues as psychiatric, psychological, social and medical histories. A wide range of conditions are associated with paranoia:

- neurological disorders;
- metabolic and endocrine disorders;
- vitamin deficiencies;
- sex chromosome disorders;
- infections;
- alcohol and drug abuse disorders;
- toxic disorders;
- pharmacological disorders;
- delusional (paranoid) disorder;
- mood disorders;
- schizophrenia;
- schizo-affective disorder;
- schizophreniform disorder;
- paranoid personality disorder;
- brief reactive psychosis;
- induced psychotic disorder;
- primary degenerative dementia (Alzheimer's type);
- organic personality disorder.[17]

It is extremely important for subsequent treatment that any associated conditions, of which paranoia may be a feature, are identified. For example, the DSM-IV suggests that paranoid schizophrenia will be characterized by a preoccupation with one or more delusions, but is also frequently associated with auditory hallucinations, unfocused anger, anxiety, argumentativeness, or violence.[18] In addition, interpersonal interactions tend to be very stilted and quite formal or extremely intense. The presentation of paranoia in delusional disorders differs from that in schizophrenic disorders, insofar as the delusions described are systematized, encapsulated and non-bizarre in nature.[6] Essentially, the nature of the delusions in delusional disorders are such that they are characterized by connectedness and being part of an overall theme.[1] The fact that they tend to be non-bizarre in nature means that the situations, which are the subject of the delusions, could occur in real life, such as being followed by another person[6] and the condition is not generally associated with significant impairment in most areas of living.

One of the most frequent ways in which paranoia is understood both in lay and health care circles, is in relation to personality characteristics or traits. Paranoia tends to include self-consciousness, hypersensitivity, mistrust and fear.[11] However, paranoid personality disorder needs to be distinguished as a distinct disorder in terms of its level of persistence, pervasiveness and inappropriateness. Individuals with paranoid personality disorder tend to be suspicious of the motivations of other people. This is not only inappropriate, but ongoing and pervasive. People with paranoid personality disorder are likely to present as tense, guarded and hypervigilant and will frequently question, without reason or justification, the motives, trustworthiness or loyalty of people with whom they are involved – frequently either friends or family. They have a tendency to be solitary and frequently

invest significant energy and time in interpreting ordinary events or interactions as 'evidence' of malevolent intent. In addition, they frequently misinterpret completely benign events or actions as ones which are intended, or have the effect of being demeaning or threatening to them personally. The DSM-IV distinguishes paranoid personality disorder from other disorders such as paranoid schizophrenia and delusional disorder in that delusions or other perceptual distortions and eccentric behaviour are not dominant features of paranoid personality disorder.[18]

TREATMENT AND THE NURSE'S ROLE

There are considerable difficulties in accurately defining paranoia as well as the various meanings and conditions in which paranoia may be a feature. It is hardly surprising therefore, that these difficulties are reflected in the role of the mental health nurse. Nurses should be aware that in dealing with paranoia, the range of conditions and presentations – from personality disorder and paranoid reactions to delusional and schizophrenic disorders – need to be considered.[1] Also, manifestations of suspiciousness and paranoia exist on a continuum – ranging from normal caution and vigilance in the face of threat, to transitory beliefs and/or expressions of pathological suspiciousness (or manifestations of a psychotic disorder) in the absence of any objective threat or potential harm.

Irrespective of the point on this continuum where the level of paranoia occurs, the central feature relates to the issue of trust, or more appropriately mistrust. Another key feature is that of being misunderstood. Individuals with a paranoid presentation may believe they are victims. However, it is possible that they have been victims of mistreatment with experience of being wronged.

Specifically in relation to paranoid personality disorder some core beliefs are likely to influence how they perceive themselves and subsequently behave.[19] These would include beliefs:

- of impending disaster (a continuing sense of foreboding);
- that the world is full of enemies;
- that accidents are doubtful, and that negative events are initiated by others with hostile intent;
- that all events relate to the person themselves;
- that they are never to blame and that guilt is not attributable to them but to others;
- that they are in some way different from the rest of humanity, and possess unique awareness or insight, which is not shared by others.

Consistent with these core beliefs, people who are paranoid are likely to believe others either exploit or deceive them. They are likely to demonstrate a strong sense of hurt and express beliefs that they have been deeply and irreversibly injured, despite objective evidence to the contrary. Especially in the initial period of contact with health care professionals, interaction with the paranoid person is likely to be characterized by difficulty in forming and/or maintaining a therapeutic relationship. From the nursing perspective, the therapeutic engagement must of course, be understood in the context of the person's core beliefs, and especially related to mistrust and suspiciousness. It is likely that great difficulty will be encountered in obtaining an accurate history through direct interview with the person. The paranoid individual will likely be reluctant to share information, and will withhold personal information for reasons of 'self-protection'.[18]

This tendency should be interpreted within the context of an understanding of the paranoia itself. In the case of paranoid delusions, people with paranoid delusions are more likely to jump to conclusions on the basis of less information,[20] than those who are not paranoid. It is also likely that patients with paranoia will attribute negative events to external sources or causes, and will do the exact opposite in relation to positive events – attributing the source of positive events to some internal cause, related directly to themselves.[21,22]

The interpersonal relationship is the core medium through which mental health nurses practice.[16] The DSM-IV[18] notes that paranoid individuals have consistent difficulties in interpersonal behaviour. The mistrust and suspiciousness, which are core features of paranoia, may manifest in hostility, argumentativeness, guarded behaviour, secretiveness, aloofness or deviousness. Further, paranoid individuals may be quick to take offence, reluctant to forgive and ever willing to counter-attack.[23] While it may be argued that such behaviour is understandable because paranoid people believe they are vulnerable to shame and humiliation at the hands of others – especially those in authority[24] – understanding why interpersonal difficulties arise will not of necessity automatically reduce the difficulties that arise between paranoid patients and others on a unit, or significant others in their own lives.

In addition to seeing themselves as victims, paranoid individuals are also likely to see themselves as blameless in conflict situations, and are likely to explain, legitimize and understand aggression on their part as a justified counter-attack.[19]

It is ironic that the symptomatology of paranoid conditions is the very issue that can impede treatment. The suspiciousness and mistrust, which are central to paranoid conditions, mean that it is less likely that people with paranoia will present for treatment – or at least to do so on a voluntary basis. The often involuntary nature of treatment services is likely to be interpreted as evidence (either new or confirmatory) of persecution or harm – directed at the person themselves. The imagined source of that harm or further persecution may be the person's family or significant others, or indeed the health care professionals involved in the provision of care.

It is important, therefore, that full consideration is given to the issues of suspiciousness, fear, sense of threat or persecution in terms of the overall approach to care and treatment, which will require a multidisciplinary and collaborative focus. One of the greatest challenges when dealing with paranoid patients is to persuade them of the need for treatment. The initial phase of treatment will concentrate on the establishment and development of a trusting and therapeutic relationship. Above all groups of patients, it is extremely important to emphasize confidentiality and to be conscious that guarantees of confidentiality are likely to be tested on an ongoing, and sometimes unreasonable, basis.

Many individuals with paranoid conditions may never fully reject the delusional system or ideas which they hold, despite achieving improvements in their level of functioning.[25] This has implications for the level and type of support necessary or the nature of intervention required of the mental health nurse. While medication has been a consistent feature in the overall management of paranoid conditions, there is a lack of consensus in relation to its efficacy. The use of anti-psychotic medication has never been properly evaluated in relation to delusional (paranoid) disorder.[6] The dominant, orthodox, view argues that anti-psychotic medication has a role to play in the management of paranoid personality disorder, while others[17] caution that medication will have limited (if any) use in patients whose paranoia is non-delusional in nature. Where medication forms a part of the overall treatment approach, the nurse will have a vital role in helping to ensure compliance. This may involve the direct administration of medication, and psycho-educational approaches involving explaining usage, management and unwanted side-effects to both the individual and their families. It may also involve teaching self-medication management techniques as well as monitoring compliance.

Much of the debate on treatment approaches for a range of mental health conditions has revolved around somewhat polarized views of whether or not they have a biological or a psychological or social genesis. There is no doubt that there is a value to such a debate. For example, there are likely, to be very clear benefits from the perspective of the development of phenotypic descriptions, which in turn may lead to the discovery of definite pathologies.[4] However, at a more immediate and clinical level, the utility of such debates seem somewhat more irrelevant. In the absence of clear and unambiguous evidence, there is some validity in acknowledging that biological factors are likely to have an important influence on psychotic disorders, while at the same time, recognizing that psychological processes are the principal factors related to understanding how people make sense of the experience of such disorders.[26] While pharmacological treatment may be important to the management of paranoia, the use of psycho-social interventions such as cognitive behaviour therapy, seem to offer a more pragmatic approach to understanding the issues involved.[27,28] Reference has already been made to the difficulties related to late access to treatment and non-compliance. These issues, either in isolation or combined, can make treatment more difficult. A further complication is that people with paranoid conditions have extremely complex forms of presentation[17] often in the context of co-morbid conditions.[29]

Despite these complications, the essence of the challenge for the mental health nurse is to help the person manage the manifestations of their illness in the best way possible. This will involve forging an alliance with the client, in spite of, and within the limits of their paranoid ideation. This will involve ascertaining the level of 'investment' the person has in their own paranoid experience or ideas.[25] This will also mean combining the apparently conflicting, though complementary roles, of building trust – accepting the person without being drawn into, or validating, their particular worldview. This is likely to involve challenging falsely held assumptions, as well as re-structuring thoughts or re-framing their meanings. In many instances this will also involve bridging the gap between the patient and significant others in their lives – especially those seen as the source of persecution or threat. Therapies such as cognitive behaviour therapy are likely to have a role in this regard, both with the individuals themselves and significant others in their lives.

A distinction needs to be drawn between causal theories and models of care and treatment that help people to live with, understand, or manage manifestations or symptoms of illnesses. In many instances, the core belief or idea may never go away completely, but there is some evidence that irrational ideas, even of delusional proportions, may be altered in terms of their intensity, becoming less 'fixed' in the sense traditionally understood concerning delusions.[30] In addition, significant others, as well as clients, need to arrive at an understanding of the condition and perhaps ultimately an accommodation with each other, as to how best to manage their lives. This will require at minimum a psycho-educational input.

The nurse has a central role in the care and management of people who present with paranoia.[1] This draws on the work of early nursing theorists such as Travelbee[31] and Peplau.[32] The core arguments of these nurse theorists suggest that the central role of nursing in the care of such people lies in the practice of 'active' listening and therapeutic engagement. Barker has argued that Travelbee's proposal of the techniques of active listening, and de-construction of the validity of irrational beliefs[31] is an historical forerunner of cognitive approaches in current use.[1] Such assertions are consistent with more recent definitions of psychiatric-mental health nursing, which propose that the process of therapeutic engagement relies heavily on the personal and professional characteristics and experiences of the nurse. Such an understanding of the interpersonal process of the therapeutic relationship – between nurse, patient, family and indeed the broader community – is particularly important when dealing with complex presentations such as paranoia.

REFERENCES

1. Barker P. Persecution complex: the enigma of paranoid disorders. *Nursing Times* 1997; **93**(2): 30–32.
2. Williams JBW. Psychiatric classification. In: Hales RE and Yudofsky SC (eds). *Synopsis of Neuropsychiatry*. Washington, DC: The American Psychiatric Press, 1996.
3. Adityanjee AYA, Theodoridis D, Vieweg VR. Dementia praecox to schizophrenia: The first 100 years. *Psychiatry and Clinical Neurosciences* 1999; **53**: 437–48.
4. Fear CF, McMonagle T, Healy D. Delusional disorders: boundaries of a concept. *European Psychiatry* 1998; **13**: 210–18.
5. Kendler KS. Kraeplin and the diagnostic concept of paranoia. *Comprehensive Psychiatry* 1988; **29**(4): 4–11.
6. Black DW, Andreason NC. Schizophrenia, schizophreniform disorder and delusional disorder. In: Hales RE and Yudofsky SC (eds). *Synopsis of psychiatry*. Washington, DC: The American Psychiatric Press, 1996.
7. Cameron N. Paranoid reaction. In: Freedman AM and Kaplan HI (eds). *Comprehensive textbook of psychiatry*. Baltimore: Williams and Watkins, 1967: 666–7.
8. Hsiao HC, Liu CY, Yang YY, Yeh EK. Delusional disorder: retrospective analysis of 86 Chinese outpatients. *Psychiatry and Clinical Neurosciences* 1999; **53**(6): 673–6.
9. Rosse RB, Fay-McCarthy M, Collins JPJ, Alim TN, Deutsch SI. The relationship between cocaine-induced paranoia and compulsive foraging: a preliminary report. *Addiction* 1994; **89**(9): 1097–105.
10. Satel SL, Southwick SM, Gawin FH. Clinical features of cocaine-induced paranoia. *American Journal of Psychiatry* 1991; **148**: 495–8.
11. Brady KT, Lydiard RB, Malcolm R, Ballenger JC. Cocaine-induced psychosis. *Journal of Clinical Psychiatry* 1991; **52**: 509–12.
12. Kendler KS. The nosologic validity of paranoia

(simple delusional disorder). A review. *Archive of General Psychiatry* 1980; **37**: 699–706.

13. Messias R. Suspiciousness as a specific risk factor for major depressive episodes in schizophrenia. *Schizophrenia Research* 2001; **47**(2–3): 159–65.

14. International Council of Nursing, The ICN Definition of Nursing. In: http://www.icn.ch/definition.htm.2002.

15. Hamblet C. Obstacles to defining the role of the mental health nurse. *Nursing Standard* 2000; **14**(51): 34–7.

16. Peplau HE. Psychiatric nursing: challenge and change. *Journal of Psychiatric and Mental Health Nursing* 1994; **1**(1): 3–7.

17. Bloch B, Pristach CA. Diagnosis and management of the paranoid patient. *American Family Physician* 1992; **45**(6): 2634–41.

18. American Psychiatric Association. *Diagnostic and statistical manual of mental disorders*, 4th edn. Washington DC: APA, 1994.

19. Kantor M. *Diagnosis and treatment of the personality disorders*. St Louis, Tokyo: Ishiyaku EuroAmerica, 1992.

20. Bentall RP, Corcoran R, Howard R, Blackwood N, Kinderman P. Persecutory delusions: a review and theoretical integration. *Clinical Psychology Review* 2001; **21**(8): 1143–92.

21. Bentall RP, Haddock G, Slade PD. Cognitive behavior therapy for persistent auditory hallucinations: from theory to therapy. *Behavior Therapy* 1994; **25**: 51–66.

22. Bentall RP, Kaney S. Content specific information processing and persucotary delusions: an investigation using the Emotional Stroop Test. *British Journal of Medical Psychology* 1989; **62**: 355–64.

23. Fenigstein A. The paranoid personality. In: Costello CG (ed.) *Personality characteristics of the personality disordered*. New York: Wiley, 1996: 242–75.

24. McWilliams N. *Psychoanalytic diagnosis, understanding personality structure in the clinical process*. New York: The Guilford Press, 1994.

25. Botman JA. Paranoid patients benefit from alliance with therapist. *Behavioural Health Treatment* 1997; **2**(10): 8.

26. Fowler D, Garety P, Kuipers E. *Cognitive behaviour therapy for psychosis: theory and practice*. Chichester: Wiley, 1995.

27. Cormac I, Jones C, Campbell C. *Cognitive behaviour therapy for schizophrenia (Cochrane Review)*. The Cochrane Library, 2002.

28. Sullivan J, Rogers P. Cognitive-behavioural nursing therapy in paranoid psychosis. *Nursing Times* 1997; **93**(2): 28–30.

29. Maina G, Badá AA, Bogetto F. Occurrence and clinical correlates of psychiatric co-morbidity in delusional disorder. *European Psychiatry* 2001; **16**: 222–8.

30. Garety PA, Hemsley DR, Wessely S. Reasoning in deluded schizophrenic and paranoid patients: biases in performance on a probabilistic inference task. *Journal of Nervous and Mental Disease* 1991; **179**: 194–201.

31. Travelbee J. *Interpersonal aspects of nursing*, 2nd edn. Philadelphia, PA: FA Davis, 1971.

32. Peplau H. *Interpersonal relations in nursing*. New York: Putnam, 1952.

Chapter 38

THE PERSON WHO HAS BEEN SEXUALLY ABUSED

Mike Smith*

INTRODUCTION

This chapter deals with some simple principles of working with adult survivors of childhood abuse. The principles used in dealing with abuse in young people are similar, however the legal framework is quite different.

I receive referrals from other nurses because they do not feel confident or competent to work with sexual abuse. Indeed some professionals are afraid to work with people's stories and narratives when they include sexual abuse. My understanding of sexual abuse is based on both personal and professional experience. My knowledge is, therefore, the result of an exploration of those twin experiences and their results on the person as an adult. I believe in a very simple approach to people with an experience of sexual abuse. All that you need to help most people is a warm, interested and caring human approach. If they are able to explore their experiences, own them and then make decisions in their life about how they wish to move on and thrive, the person has the necessary knowledge to do the rest. It is the *technician* who is important, not the technique, when it comes to helping people come to terms with their abuse. Many

therapies are touted and some of them undoubtedly help the abused person. However, people's experience of their survival and recovery tells us that it is the therapist rather than the therapy that is most important in these days of evidence-based practice.

I hope to outline here the nature and scope of the problem, its effects upon the person, along with some ways of helping people who have been abused to move on in their lives.

SEXUAL ABUSE – A DEFINITION

> The sexual molestation of a child by an older person seen as a figure of trust or authority such as parents, relatives, family friends, youth leader and teachers etc.

Sexual abuse can be any sexual act with a child/young person that is performed by an adult or an older child. Such acts include fondling the child's genitals, getting the child to fondle an adult's genitals, mouth to genital contact, rubbing an adult's genitals on the child, or actually penetrating the child's vagina or anus. There are other, often

---

*Mike Smith was overall winner of the RCN nurse of the year in 1997 and is known for his campaigning approach to change beliefs about the nature of psychotic experiences and the 'treatments' offered. Mike has written many practical books about working with psychotic experiences and now works freelance.

overlooked, forms of abuse. These include an adult showing his or her genitals to a child, showing the child obscene pictures or videotapes, or using the child to make obscene materials. The definition and interpretation of *molestation* is probably the most debated concept, i.e. what constitutes molestation. If the person believes that they have been abused then they have. However this is *not* a legal definition and some cases of abuse, when explored by the victim, have little recourse to legal satisfaction.

The term sexual abuse in psychiatric practice most commonly refers to the involvement of a young person below the age of 16 in sexual activity with a significantly older and/or powerful person. It is referred to as *abuse* since it is assumed in Western society that the older person must, by definition, be taking advantage of the younger one, since a person under 16 cannot give informed consent (in law) to sexual activity. As with many things this legal framework for what is and is not abuse, differs from country to country and may be radically different from continent to continent.

Usually the victim of the abuse cannot understand fully the implications of what is happening at the time. Therefore, although he or she may appear to consent to the activity, the consent is not truly *informed* in the legal sense. Although the abuser may also be young, there is usually a significant age and status difference between the parties, which puts the abuser in a position of power. This power difference means that even where there is apparent acquiescence, this is usually based on fear of the consequences of refusal and so is not true consent.

Sexual abuse can be an isolated or a recurrent event and may be disclosed or hidden. There are however vast differences not just in the physical way in which a person is abused, but also the social and emotional circumstances in which the abuse takes place.

Abuse can range from inappropriate or unwanted touching to sexual penetration. It may be perpetrated with 'love' or with violence. The abuse can be disguised as play or it may be a more overt assault. The abuser may be a relative, an acquaintance or a stranger. Abuse can be limited in its occurrence, happening only a few times to the person, or it may be a part of everyday life for the person. Some abused people may only realize they have been abused much later on in life when they talk with other adolescents or adults and realize that their experiences were 'different'. For some people, abuse may be related to one specific person. Others may be abused on a number of occasions by different adults. This further reinforces their feelings that it was their fault or destiny. A small proportion of people may be victims of organized circles of sexual abuse for the gratification of paedophiles.

The way people experience abuse, and its subjective meaning to the abused person, is critical to how they respond as adults. Some of these responses, be they coping strategies or survival techniques, may even become pathologized. The person then may find themselves diagnosed with a mental disorder such as schizophrenia or borderline personality disorder (BPD). Some studies of people in general psychiatric populations, have found that a large number of people with a variety of diagnostic labels attribute the origin of their psychotic experiences to life-events,[1,2] especially those with histories of abuse.

Commonly those who are currently experiencing abuse, are referred to as *victims* of sexual abuse; those whose experience of abuse is in the past are referred to as *adult survivors* of sexual abuse.

How abuse may be perpetrated: some examples

- A girl was sexually abused by her father until her teens. She eventually reported what was happening to the authorities as an adult, with the result that her father was tried and imprisoned.
- A girl was involved in the making of pornographic material by her stepfather until her teens, when she eventually reported what was happening. She was removed, along with her younger sister, from the family home and was brought up by the state as a 'looked after' child.
- A 9-year-old boy was touched by a teacher while showering after Physical Education, under the pretence that he was helping him wash. He thought he was alone in this experience until a number of boys reported similar abuse several years later.
- An altar boy was touched during prayer by a priest and told that he was an evil filthy heathen that needed the priest's help to prevent him from going to hell.
- A teenager living in care was befriended by a policeman and his family, treated as a member of the family and then sexually assaulted. She didn't wish to lose the affection of the family so tolerated the sexual molestation, eventually blaming herself when it was discovered because she had enjoyed and indeed encouraged the abuse.
- A young girl's teenage stepbrother used to play games with her at an early age that she later realized (at puberty) had been sexually abusive.
- A boy was regularly abused by an aunt with the knowledge of his uncle, with whom he was often sent to stay. This abuse took place over several years during which he was unable to say why he did not wish to visit these relatives.
- A young girl was recruited to work as a prostitute from the age of thirteen by a much older man whom she says she loved.

matic experiences in early life, especially abuse in its many forms. It is most commonly associated with the diagnosis of BPD; however other authors have suggested it is a *logical* consequence of abuse, rather than a symptom of a disorder. Splitting occurs when the person appears to swing between idealizing and devaluing people in relationships. The person pits people against one another, making allies of one group and enemies of the other. When the person engages in 'splitting' they perceive a person is either good or bad, and the person is unable to accept that there is both good and bad within a person. Such 'categorization' is extremely changeable, shifting from day to day. One day the person is good and bad the next. Splitting presents the survivor of abuse with particular difficulties in forming and maintaining long-term relationships, especially therapeutic relationships.

OTHER PRACTICAL CONSEQUENCES

❑ **Intense feelings.** Memories of abuse and surrounding events can bring intense feelings and other experiences, which can be very intrusive to the extent of becoming flashbacks.

❑ **Flashbacks and nightmares.** Recollections of the abusive experience may intrude into the person's waking thoughts, or may recur in dreams. These are often triggered by subtle events that the person can begin to recognize over time. With support the person can learn to live with these disturbing experiences, by anticipating them or avoiding the situations that 'trigger' them.

❑ **Shame and guilt.** Survivors frequently blame themselves, suffer from low self-esteem or feel deeply embarrassed about seeking help. They may become depressed, harm themselves and have thoughts of suicide. Mental health workers are very positive and well intentioned when they tell the person they are not to blame. However, victims who have disclosed abuse, accept that this is what everyone else thinks, but they still know that they are to blame. This is one result of how the abuser made the person feel at the time of the abuse, and when they were groomed for the abuse. Consequently, they find it hard to come to terms with their shame and guilt.

❑ **Intense anger.** This may be directed at the abuser, and may be linked with a wish to confront or to completely avoid them. It may also be directed at others who seem to have colluded with the abuse or may be directed at people in general. Often people find it hard to understand their anger and this further reinforces their view that they are a bad person.

❑ **Self-harm and self-injury.** People who have been sexually abused are far more likely to demonstrate self-destructive activity.[4] This may be because of anger, internalization of shame, or may be a symbolic way of cutting out the filth, dissociating and reintegrating. The literature contains many examples of 'why' a person who has been abused may go on to self-harm. I developed a workbook for people who self-harm, to explore how their life experiences resulted in them self-harming and how they might cope with their feelings and so reclaim their lives.[7]

❑ **Internalized feelings of shame.** Harrison[8] wrote about how female survivors of sexual abuse internalized their shame and anger, resulting in self-harm, self-loathing, poor self-esteem and alternative ways of displaying distress.

❑ **Disrupted relational patterns.** Some survivors tend to avoid intimate relationships and are distrustful of the motives of all other people. Others may find they tend to form very intense intimate relationships, which can be emotionally draining. It is interesting to note that these are also features of borderline personality disorder, a label often attached to abused people who find themselves in the psychiatric system. This raises the question: is BPD a biological entity caused by difference, a genetic vulnerability as some medical theories point out, or is it a description of some people's coping strategies for dealing with abusive experiences? If the latter is true then pathologizing people's distress and coping, by attributing pathological diagnoses, further reinforces their distress by increasing their shame and sense of self-blame.

❑ **Coping and adjustment.** Sigmon *et al.*[9] found that coping and adjustment were seriously affected among both men and women survivors. In response to sexual abuse experienced during childhood, avoidance coping emerged as the most frequently used strategy by both sexes. Although there were no gender differences in current use of problem-focused and avoidance strategies, males described greater use of acceptance whereas females utilized more emotion-focused coping. In general, women reported significantly greater trauma-related distress than men, including higher levels of anxiety, depression, and post-trauma symptoms.

❑ **Using substances to assist in coping.** Men who have suffered sexual abuse are more likely to suffer from psychological problems than the general population, including alcohol misuse and self-harm.

❑ **Sexual identity, emotional and sexual relationships.** In their study of 10 adult men survivors, Gill and Tutty[10] found that the men described the abuse as having significantly affected their sexual identity, as well as their emotional and sexual relationships as adults.

❑ **Sexual difficulty or dysfunction.** People often report difficulties in enjoying normal sexual activities, which further increases their feelings of abnormality and shame, and reinforces, for them, the experience of grooming by their abuser.

❑ **Fear of the consequences of the abuse.** Survivors may wonder whether they will ever be able to form normal relationships or whether they might become abusers themselves. This can lead to people ruminating to a degree that is further damaging to them. For some people this fear can have dissociative consequences. I have worked with a number of men and women who hear voices telling them that they will abuse children, become a paedophile or a rapist, as a direct consequence of their own childhood abuse. In a lesser, but equally damaging way, these fears can also take the form of intrusive thoughts when not dissociative, and can lead to the person being labelled as having an obsessive–compulsive disorder, and can also identify the person as being a 'high risk' on a risk assessment because of the nature of the intrusive thoughts.

❑ **Isolation and stigmatization.** Survivors may feel they are totally alone with their experience. They can feel that they have been marked out and that somehow others know of their history, even without being told, and so treat them differently.

As with any human response to trauma, the degree of the person's reaction can vary widely between individuals. Some people apparently come to terms with very severe abuse comparatively easily; others find the abuse has a lasting effect on them.

THE VICTIM'S EXPERIENCE

Victims often report feeling very alone with the experience of abuse. Often they are afraid of telling others, because of the fear of retribution or the consequences for their family.

Victims frequently feel they will not be believed or taken seriously if they tell others what has happened. Often this fear is confirmed when they do try to raise the matter. The social conditions in which people are abused, and how disclosure is mitigated against, are important when the person reflects on their experience, as they seek greater understanding of their abuse.

Victims frequently feel guilty. The abuser may suggest they are to blame for the abuse or they may take responsibility upon themselves. Children naturally tend to assume responsibility for events that are not of their making, and this is particularly true in the case of abuse. I have seen this phenomena extended into a 'delusional disorder' where a person comes to believe that they are responsible for all the evil in the world.

The guilt and shame is increased if the child has

found any aspect of the abuse gratifying. In this context it is important to note that the sexual response of many people, at the time of abuse, is normal.

Victims commonly report feeling extremely scared and confused by the abusive experience. They are often alone, or groomed into feeling alone, by the abuser. For some people fear is used to prevent disclosure.

Abusers often control their victims with threats that may be real or psychological. Living for long periods in fear can affect people's development. A number of victims have told me that all they can remember abut their childhood is being scared.

Perhaps the most personally damaging effect, at the time of abuse and later, is when the victim feels responsible for the abuse of others: friends or siblings or their other parent. Many abused people have been prepared to take the abuse to spare a brother or sister. Some young children are encouraged to bring other friends into the circle of abuse. Later, this is something they find very difficult to live with and often is more difficult to manage than their own experience of abuse.

HELPING THE ABUSED PERSON

Some general principles underpin the help that might be offered survivors of sexual abuse. *Talking* about abuse, *being believed* and being helped to come to your own conclusions are all intrinsically helpful for the abused person.

Here I shall describe the structure, which I use to work with sexually abused people. This is based on my own research with people who had recovered from mental illnesses, which focused on 'how' the person managed their recovery. This is not a panacea for sexual abuse, but merely describes the mental processes that many people follow in reclaiming their experiences, so that they might move on from the mad times of their life.

In general, people describe *reaching a*:

❑ **Turning point** in their lives, where they experience a resolve to move on from their current situation, and to reclaim their life, so that they might move beyond that to enjoy their life again. *People do this by*:

❑ **Identifying** what they are recovering *from*: i.e. their life experiences to date, and the practical manifestations of their abuse in their current life – relationships, feelings of shame and blame, and being clear about *how* they were abused, groomed and its effects on their early life. *They then need to*:

❑ **Explore** in depth, the meaning, symbolism, metaphor and consequences of these experiences, how they were perpetrated, how they felt about them then, and how they feel about them now. *Then they begin to*:

- ❏ **Understand** their abuse, its links to their life, some of the more subtle consequences of the abuse, how they cope with their feelings, their beliefs about their abuse and their abuser and what they want to do about that. *For some people this leads to:*
- ❏ **Accepting** and resolving to move on with their life, and growing again. This may include acknowledging their experience of abuse but doing nothing overtly about it, or developing less harmful ways of coping. Exploring their experiences, in greater depth with someone the person trusts, is perhaps the final step towards reclaiming their life.

This approach is a structure for helping address their experience of abuse and perhaps reclaim their lives through the recovery process. This structure leads the person and the helper to ask a great number of questions of each other, and provides a framework within which to ask the questions that might help. I believe this is a natural process that most people eventually arrive at in their lives, even if left alone. If recovery is a journey however, then there must be some short cuts or a route map. Nurses can be guides along this journey, and can offer expert advice on the most appropriate way to get to a destination. The person sets the destination, but the nurse can advise the person, from their experience, as to what might be the best way to get there.

It is important to remember, however, that for some people looking back at their life is not practical, or possible, or perhaps something they want to do. What a nurse can do is to adopt Florence Nightingale's approach: placing them in the best position for nature to take its course.

In other words if the person does not want to do all the above things, this is OK. It is not compulsory. The nurse needs to help the person to be in a position where they aren't disadvantaged or stopped from recovering, when they feel the time is right. Generally I do this by dealing with practical problems, teaching ways of coping with distressing consequences of the abuse – such as the feelings of shame – and letting the person know that its okay not to do anything about the abuse. This is handled far better when the person feels ready.[11]

Case study 38.1: Mia's story

I was asked to work with Mia, a 17-year-old woman, by a colleague who did not feel confident to deal with her recently disclosed sexual abuse, nor her severe self-harm that had increased since she had finally disclosed her sexual abuse. When I met Mia she was very labile, angry and very unclear about her feelings. Yet she wanted to talk about her abuse. I told her we could do that, in her own time. However, she also told me some things that concerned me more. She was in hospital in an intensive care unit because of the degree of her

cutting. She had been using crack cocaine to cope with her feelings of shame, and owed her dealer £1500. She said that the only person who loved her was her dog, who was in care because she was in hospital. I explained to her that with so many adverse things going on in her life, in my experience looking at her abuse might not be a priority either for her alone or for us. Instead, I suggested that this might be done alongside getting her discharged, finding her a decent home, getting her dog back, and regaining access to someone she trusted in her life (her community nurse). This she did over time as she developed trust with her nurse, who became a friend and ally. Eventually, she was able to examine her experience of abuse with the nurse, following the process outlined above.

This process is outlined in greater detail in my book on psychiatric first aid.[11]

Case study 38.2: Paul's story of recovery

Paul was a 30-year-old man referred to me as a schizophrenic. He had been treated with a number of traditional and atypical neuroleptics and was now thought to be suffering from a personality disorder of the borderline type (BPD). Paul had been in an intensive care unit for 13 months and was compulsorily detained. I was informed that Paul had sabotaged attempts to help him leave hospital by burning himself or attacking staff after reasonable periods of stability. Paul told me he was desperate to leave hospital. He had no contact with any friends or relatives (i.e. having no social network outside of the mental health arena was an obvious hurdle to reclaiming his life). However, he had one strong relationship with a nursing assistant Ricky. This relationship in itself was questioned as some staff felt that Paul 'manipulated' the staff and was using Ricky to get what he wanted. Ricky felt that they had a common interest in the same football team, were a similar age and he understood him (it later transpired that Ricky also had similar life experiences to Paul).

At first, we met on an ad hoc basis over three weeks, as Paul and Ricky began to trust me a little more and I focused on telling them that I was not a therapist, but a resource for them to use to bounce some ideas off about why Paul harmed himself. As a first step, Paul agreed to write his life history over a two-week period with Ricky's support in typing it up in the evenings and at night (Ricky was working nights at the time).

Paul told of a disturbing account that had been unknown to the people supporting him. He recalled a number of incidents in his life that he felt had influenced him as an adult:

- ■ His father had killed himself when Paul was six. He had argued with his mother and hung himself from the shower above the bath. Paul found his father and had vivid flashbacks of his father hanging and himself and his mother trying to lift him and also his baby sister crying in the background.

- Paul's mother began a new relationship when he was eight and married again when he was nine. This stepfather occasionally sexually assaulted Paul, but more frequently physically punished him. This included severe beatings and locking him in a cupboard for long periods. Paul's sister was sexually abused far more often by this person and he twice recalls his mother being beaten by this man with vivid memories of her crying.
- Paul began to absent from school at about 11 and became involved in sniffing solvents and petty crime. He also ran away from home after being locked up for three days by his stepfather. He received more frequent beatings and ran away from home more only to be returned. He did tell a police officer once about being locked up but was told by them 'well you deserve it; I'd lock you up'. He left the family home aged 14 and entered the care system as a 'looked after child' as his mother and stepfather felt he was uncontrollable after he had set fire to the family home when he was locked in a room.
- Paul's sister committed suicide by overdose when he was 17; she was aged 13.
- Paul went to prison for a long catalogue of crime – mostly violent assaults, including racially motivated assaults – until the age of about 25 when he entered psychiatric hospital for the first time. He did not return to prison, neither was he prosecuted for a crime after that point.

Paul wrote a 25-page typed life history, which he felt was, in itself, therapeutic and gave people a picture of him as he believed he was. We then began to explore two specific things: the voices that he heard and his self-harm behaviour. Paul heard several voices. Six of these predominated, but two were significant. He was terrified of a man's voice, which reminded him of his dead father. He also heard a supportive voice of a friend he met in prison, called Leroy. His stepfather's voice commanded him to 'do it' which he believed meant to kill himself. However, he didn't want to kill himself. He found in prison that harming himself helped him in a number of ways:

1. He felt clean.
2. He felt that he had bargained with the voice.
3. He was left alone by the voice when in pain.
4. He could see his hurt in the burns and showed it to others, 'they respond to that', he said 'and not the pain inside'.

We agreed to do two things: to agree a plan with his team that would help him return to his flat. This relied on working closely and honestly together. This was almost spoiled, Paul told me later, when unreliable staff (not regular staff) tried to make him fail. Secondly we agreed that he wanted to explore his feelings about the death of his sister, the beating of his mother and finally his own physical and sexual abuse with someone independent of his care (at that time, this was myself).

We followed a loose framework, which allowed us to explore what his life experiences meant to him now; how he felt to blame for the death of his sister and the pain of his mother; and how he had always felt that he was a bad person who had to be punished. Paul eventually decided that he was continuing his own abuse by punishing himself and that he had to do something about it by resolving to move on.

To help him to do this I taught him some coping strategies to deal with his voices and the desire to self-harm.[11] He set limits, structured the time spent with his voices, learned to say no to his voices and reduced the power of his powerful voice by renaming it the 'coward' and the 'pervert'. He also focused upon the voice of Leroy and chatted with him when he felt down. Leroy was a powerful man in real life and he asked Leroy's voice to protect him from the coward, which it mostly did. When he thought about harming himself he used a variety of techniques to interrupt his thoughts and would have a range of things to do that he liked doing: having a hot bath, watching football and running continuously around a set track.

Paul eventually left the hospital after three months, moving back into his flat. Ricky spent two days working closely with him, transferring his care to a person introduced some weeks earlier from an assertive community team. Ricky continued to see Paul as a friend. Paul has not been back to hospital, although once he set fire to his legs with lighter fuel 'as a bargain', after two days spent listening to his voices. Paul felt he was relapsing and was terrified of going mad. His voices reinforced this. I visited him once then and explained that he was in control, wasn't going mad and that sometimes we all just have bad patches. He was, however, afraid of his voice, so again we explored what had already been agreed: that the voice (of itself) was not the problem but rather it was its identity, and its meaning in his life, which gave it the power.

Paul's fear of this voice was the issue that he needed, again, to surmount – not the idea that he had 'relapsed'. We explored again the reasons why his voice had appeared again, so powerfully. Paul had experienced a series of flashbacks after seeing (although not meeting) his abuser in a supermarket. Having clarified what was the real problem this then enabled Paul to regain control in his life.

REFERENCES

1. Romme M, Escher S. *Accepting voices*. England: Mind Publications, 1993.

2. Ensink B. Trauma: a study of childhood abuse and hallucinations. In: Romme M, Escher S (eds). *Accepting voices*. England: Mind Publications, 1993.

3. Warner S. *Understanding child sexual abuse – making the tactics visible*. Gloucester: Handsell, 2000.

4 Shapiro S. Self mutilation and self blame in incest victims. *American Journal of Psychotherapy* 1987; **61**:(1).

5. Diclemente R, Ponton L, Hartley D. Prevalence and correlates of cutting behaviour. *Journal of the American Academy of Child and Adolescent Psychiatry* 1991; **30**: 735–9.

6. Lefevre S. *Killing me softly. Self-harm, survival not suicide*. Gloucester: Handsell, 1996.

7. Smith M. *Working with self-harm a workbook*. Gloucester: Handsell, 1998.

8. Harrison D. *Vicious circles. An exploration of women and self harm in society*. London: GPMH, 1994.

9. Sigmon M, Green R, Nicholls K. Coping and adjustment in male and female survivors of childhood sexual abuse. *Journal of Child Sexual Abuse* 1996; **6**: 57–75.

10. Gill M, Tutty L. Male survivors of childhood sexual abuse: qualitative study and issues for clinical consideration. *Journal of Child Sexual Abuse* 1996; **6**: 19–33.

11 Smith M (ed.) *Psychiatric first aid in psychosis*. Gloucester: Handsell, 2002.

FURTHER READING

Browne A, Finkelhor D. Impact of child sexual abuse: a review of the research. In: Donnelly AC, Oates K (eds). *Classic papers in child abuse*. Thousand Oaks, CA: Sage, 2000: 217–82.

Finkelhor D. *Child sexual abuse: new theory and research*. New York, NY: The Free Press, 1984.

Finkelhor D, Browne A. The traumatic impact of child sexual abuse: a conceptualization. *American Journal of Orthopsychiatry* 1985; **55**: 530–41.

Jones DPH, McGraw JM. Reliable and fictitious accounts of sexual abuse in children. *Journal of Interpersonal Violence* 1987; **2**: 27–45.

Mullen P, Martin J, Anderson J, Romans S. The effect of child sexual abuse on social, interpersonal and sexual function in adult life. *British Journal of Psychiatry* 1994; **165**: 35–47.

Ryan G. The sexual abuser. In: Helfer ME, Kempe RS, Krugman RD (eds). *The battered child*, 5th edn, Chapter 14. The University of Chicago Press, 1997: 329–46.

Chapter 39

THE PERSON WITH AN EATING DISORDER

Elaine Fletcher*

INTRODUCTION

Food plays a significant part in most peoples lives in Western society. Mealtimes are a social time where families or friends can meet, be nourished by way of food, company and interpersonal fulfilment. However, not all family systems function in this way.

Babies cry to demonstrate their need to be fed and in this way will usually form their first relationship. Early parent–child relationships that are unsatisfactory may lead to the child missing out the pleasurable and comforting associations many of us have with food and nutrition. As children progress through life, food may be used as a reward, or its withdrawal as a punishment. Food can become the vehicle for powerful transactions that represent or mirror relationships; whether those that exist, or those that are missing.[1] This may be akin to the power struggle the child is encountering within their personal relationships.

When children reach puberty many changes begin to occur within them, and they will see themselves appear physically different. They will be more curvatious and aware of their sexual organs. For girls it is probably more noticeable. Boys are more likely to take pride in a stronger, larger physique, whereas girls will see their body becoming rounder and fatter, women having a higher proportion of body fat to that of men.

A child will reach puberty at a certain weight (usually 40–45 kg),[2] although this varies from child to child. A young person who has stress in their lives at this point may experience these changes as stressful and very unwelcome.

Young people who develop an eating disorder have often experienced separation from family, or tense relationships within the family. Often they find it difficult to express their feelings (especially anger) appropriately. The person may have conflicts over their sexuality and be unable to achieve mature relationships, or may be living within an abusive family system. Invariably, the person is highly self-critical and perfectionist, with a drive to please others, often failing to see the importance of having their own needs met.

A child, especially a female, may be disturbed and feel out of control by the onset of puberty. In recalling

*Elaine Fletcher qualified as an RMN in 1980 and has worked in Adult Acute care, a Regional Eating Disorder Unit and most recently in Research and Training around the Tidal Model. Elaine has a wide range of both clinical and academic experience and has much work published. She has a Diploma in Nursing Science and is presently undertaking a Masters in Advanced Practice.

an often idealized and far less traumatic, stress-free childhood, the person often experiences an overwhelming desire to return to this more secure place. Orbach[3] describes how this stage can involve a major split between the body and the self.

As noted, in the West food is high on both social and leisure agendas: cookery programmes occupy a large part of television viewing time, cafés and coffee shops dominate city malls and high streets; and advertising for recipe books, diets and catering services feature in a wide range of media. At the same time the media have, for many years, bombarded society with images of the 'ideal' women, possessing the 'perfect' body – someone who, presumably, has not succumbed to the pressure of advertising and has managed to resist the many foods dangled in front of our eyes.

EATING DISORDERS

Around 0.5% of young women experience anorexia nervosa and 2% bulimia nervosa.[4] It would be simplistic and misleading to apportion all blame for the development of eating disorders at the door of the media. However, many women express a desire to lose weight and to be slimmer than they are. The messages seem very clear:

- ❑ be in control of what you eat;
- ❑ do not to listen to your body when it tells you that you are hungry;
- ❑ to be thin means to be happy;
- ❑ be on guard against fatness at all times.

People who develop an eating disorder are not the few who take the pursuit of thinness to the extreme, but rather are people who use food as a way of managing the reality of a life which is (or at least is perceived to be) in constant turmoil, riddled with great unhappiness, anxiety and fear.

Anorexia nervosa and *bulimia nervosa* affect both men and women but are nine times more common in women than in men.[5] People with eating disorders spend much of their time preoccupied with weight, body shape, food and meals. They often exercise to the exclusion of other activities. They are often terrified of what is happening in their lives, their families, work or education. People with a diagnosis of anorexia nervosa have described painful, overwhelming fear of their situation and an intense drive to 'turn back the clock' in terms of their physical development, which they imagine in some way will restore a sense of order and control or manageability.

The media frenzy around eating disorders serves to undermine the seriousness of the condition.[6] Anorexia nervosa has a morbidity rate of 8–18% when indexed cases are monitored for 10–20 years.[7]

ANOREXIA NERVOSA

In anorexia there is a marked avoidance of high calorie, usually fatty food. This avoidance is often accompanied by a variety of behaviours, such as excessive exercise, abuse of laxatives, diuretics, purging as well as eating minimal amounts of foods. This results in the sufferer being abnormally thin – below 85% of the body weight expected for their age and height. The person will be preoccupied with recipes and often will cook elaborate meals for others, gaining a sense of achievement or control by eating nothing or very little themselves. Often in the early stages of the illness the person's family or friends will praise them for looking slim, this serving to reinforce the self-starvation.

Sometimes the person will hide food, and will vomit following a meal or wear several layers of clothing so that those close to them are unaware of their rigid avoidance of food. The person will usually develop a strict routine, upon which they become increasingly dependant as a means of control over their situation or their lives.

The person will sometimes, but not always, see himself or herself as much bigger than they are, thus perpetuating the reduction of calories, self-hatred and distancing themselves from the reality of their lives.

The medical complications in anorexia nervosa are complex and multiple, in a condition that is often secret. The sufferer is so driven in their aim to avoid detection that their difficulties may reach a serious level before anyone becomes aware of it. By asking for help with emotional or physical elements of their condition, the person may fear that their maladaptive coping strategies will be uncovered, thus leading to complete vulnerability and chaos.

Physical complications

- ❑ Cardiac arrhythmia (abnormal heart rate).
- ❑ Sudden cardiac failure (heart failure with little or no warning).
- ❑ Bradycardia (slow heart contraction, resulting in slow pulse rate).
- ❑ Oedema (abnormal infiltration of the tissue with fluid).
- ❑ Metabolic disorders (an interruption of the chemical changes necessary for life maintenance).
- ❑ Gastrointestinal difficulties (stomach and intestinal abnormalities).
- ❑ Hypothermia (abnormally low body temperature).
- ❑ Endocrine systems disruption (interruption of the function of endocrine glands).
- ❑ Amenorrhoea (absence of menstruation).
- ❑ Osteoporosis (loss of bone density).

❑ Haematological disturbance (disturbance of the formation, composition and functions of the blood).
❑ Dermatological disturbance (problems with the structure and functions of the skin).

Anorexia nervosa usually affects young women within a few years of menarche (median onset of 17 years). While there is an association with educational achievement, it is not found solely among the higher social classes, as once was thought.[8]

The DSM-IV diagnostic criteria

The DSM-IV defines anorexia as follows:

1 Refusal to maintain body weight at or above a minimally normal weight for age and height (e.g. weight leading to maintenance of body weight less than 85% of that expected).
2 Intense fear of gaining weight or becoming fat, even though underweight.
3 Disturbance in the way in which one's body or shape is experienced, undue influence of body weight and weight on self-evaluation, or denial of the seriousness of current low body weight.
4 In post-menarchal females, amenorrhoea, i.e. the absence of at least three consecutive menstrual cycles.

BULIMIA NERVOSA

The onset of bulimia nervosa is on average slightly later than in anorexia (about 18 years). Once again it is most prevalent in women. In Western societies 1–3% are affected.[9]

People with bulimia nervosa are less likely than those with anorexia to be 'avoidant' of their life. They are more likely to work and have relationships; however these relationships may be chaotic or unsatisfactory. They may feel that their eating patterns reflect the disturbance in their lives. Often having suffered anorexia in the past (30%), people with bulimia nervosa may restrict their dietary intake for a period of time then binge on what they consider to be and usually are large amounts of food. People will describe the binge as a response to a life event or a way of expressing their feelings. Binges may be totally frenzied and food consumed in massive quantities; the person then often feels disgusted and filled with self-loathing. The person usually panics and feels compelled to purge and cleanse themselves of food. They will then induce vomiting, take laxatives or diuretics and excessive exercise in an attempt to regain control and remove the calories from their body. Most people are very ashamed and are driven to secrecy. The person may become entrenched in a secret life that revolves around planning a binge, buying food, preparing the binge, then organizing ways to ensure that they are able to purge without being discovered.

The individual is usually of normal body weight for their age and height; however they can see themselves as bigger. They will describe an intense hatred for their bodies and fear of weight gain.

DSM-IV criteria

The DSM-IV defines bulimia as:

1 Recurrent episodes of binge eating. An episode of binge eating is characterized by both of the following:
   ■ Eating in a discrete period of time an amount of food that is definitely larger than most people would eat in a similar period of time and under similar circumstances.
   ■ A sense of lack of control during the episode (e.g. a feeling that one cannot stop eating or control what or how much one is eating).
2 Recurrent inappropriate compensatory behaviour in order to prevent weight gain, such as self-induced vomiting, misuse of laxatives.
3 The binge eating and inappropriate compensatory behaviours both occur on average, at least twice a week for 3 months.
4 Self-evaluation is unduly influenced by body shape and weight.
5 The disturbance does not occur exclusively during episodes of anorexia.

TREATMENT FOR ANOREXIA

Nursing people with anorexia nervosa is frequently perceived as emotionally stressful. Often, patients cannot bear to 'give up' a way of living, which they consider to be their main life support, their way of adding safety to their turbulent world. Often, the person believes that to relinquish anorexia will result in family disruption, or in pressure to achieve academically, or relationship intimacy, any of which may be too frightening to imagine.

The person is usually 'sent' to hospital and feel they are there to please others rather than because they need care or treatment. Engagement is often very difficult and takes some considerable time to establish. The relationship is very much dependent on honesty and effective working relationships.

If the person is under the age of 16 years, or the onset of anorexia began at an early age, the person's emotional development will be delayed, thus rendering them child-like emotionally, despite their chronological age. If this is the case, it is important to involve the person's family as much as possible. The family needs to be helped to understand the cause of the sufferer's distress and need of support to help them to relinquish the anorexia.[10] This often takes the form of traditional family therapy or parent counselling. This is obviously very much dependent on the family members' participation and their willingness to engage in the process.

Sometimes the nurse's role is to help the person understand the nature of their eating disorder and to explore how they can come to terms with family issues, even if the family is unwilling to be involved.

Treatment can be offered in outpatients in less severe cases (i.e. when weight loss is less than 25% of total body weight). The philosophical orientation of the treatment centre will influence the method of therapy offered. However, focused forms of psychotherapy, such as cognitive analytical or brief dynamic therapy are more effective than supportive therapy.[11]

The person with an eating disorder lives a tortured existence, and often feels as if their disorder is their only companion. The person will gradually lose any sense of their own value as a person, with their own strengths and resources. They will find making or maintaining relationships too intense and demanding and the emotional commitment, however small, frequently becomes unmanageable.

Practitioners working in the eating disorder field encounter people who have suffered severe emotional pain and who, as a result, are leading a life, which may, literally, be a slow death.

Nurses need to remember that the eating disorder is a function of emotional distress; the person is usually trapped in the cycle described earlier. It is essential to get to know the person and understand why there is a need for the disorder. Each person will have a very different understanding of their eating disorder and the purpose that it serves. Looking after the person with an eating disorder is usually a nursing role in an inpatient setting; thus the person is at a very severe stage of emotional and physical ill health.

There is a need for the nurse to be very aware of their own sense of self and a strong supervision structure is necessary to explore emotional issues and the general meaning of their work.

The person will usually be very physically weak, may be emotionally labile and extremely mistrustful. Building those relationships may cause the nurse some dilemmas. How does the nurse build rapport with someone who needs to gain weight to survive (physically), yet who feels unable to relinquish his or her maladaptive control over food intake? Nurses often need to support people while they painstakingly chew very small amounts of food, or they may need to take them to the toilet, as they are physically too weak to walk. It is vital that this does not become a power struggle, which may mirror other problematic relationships or situations in the person's life. The nurse needs to help the person gain self-esteem, develop alternative methods of coping with stress and to 'practice' forming constructive relationships. Goals need to be negotiated around both physical and emotional needs.

When people are below a certain weight this limits their cognitive functioning, and psychological support may have little impact. As the person's weight increases they will be much more 'in tune' with their emotions. Consequently, their anxiety about the weight gained, and also their distress about the issues in their lives, will increase dramatically. Group, family and individual therapy should begin at this point.

It is important to explain care plans honestly, involving the person as much as possible, ensuring goals are small achievable steps. The person's dignity needs to be maintained and outmoded and damaging practices, such as removing personal possessions, should be avoided at all costs. However walks outdoors, and trips to the cinema etc., may be negotiated as the person engages more fully in their therapy, and has the physical strength to do them safely. People value structure when they are at a very low weight. They need to know that everyone in the team is aware of the care plan and that no-one will deviate from it. The person will feel compelled to ask an individual nurse to give them a little longer to finish a meal or agree to overlook them leaving some of it. Here it is important to explain the reasons behind the plan as well as its necessity. Structure is helpful in the early stages of treatment when cognitive functioning is poor and the person's life has been governed by rigid rules for some time. This helps the person to reduce some of the eating routines, as they allow themselves to feel that they aren't so much giving up the anorexia, as that the care system is taking responsibility. Once the person is out of immediate danger of death, the responsibility needs to be gradually returned. The nurse should support the development of alternative coping strategies, participate in individual psychological therapy and family therapy and, most of all, explore with the person what needs to change and how they could begin to effect these changes.

TREATMENT FOR BULIMIA

People with bulimia are less likely to require hospital admission and treatment can be provided as an outpatient in most cases.

Treatment packages such as focused cognitive therapy or brief psychotherapy (10–15 sessions) have been found to be of most use to sufferers. About 40–60% of patients became symptom-free following a course of therapy.[12] The treatment needs to be highly collaborative and homework goals need to be set to take place between the sessions. People need to become aware of, and discuss, the events that 'trigger' a binge and be helped to identify alternative ways of coping with them. In particular, the person needs to develop ways of 'buying time' so that they can think about alternatives to bingeing. They need help to plan regular meals that incorporate the major food groups, and should avoid lengthy periods between meals (5 hours should be the maximum). If they are physically hungry they are less likely to be able to resist the binge. Specific discussion around how they will ward off bingeing is particularly useful (e.g. not keeping 'binge' food in the house, buying food for only one day at a time, or leaving the house for a walk or to meet friends, immediately following a meal). It is also useful to ask the person to record all food intake and daily activity, so they may be helped to see connections between ways in which they use food and ways they deal with life issues.

People are likely also to have low self-esteem and over valued concerns about their shape, which will also need to be addressed separately.

If bulimia co-exists with other difficulties, such as depression, personality disorder or alcohol dependence, treatment may need to be longer term. It is important to help the person relearn ways of functioning and address their ways of thinking about the past (often disturbing life events), as overcoming the bulimia may lead to other destructive behaviour, such as drinking binges, cutting or promiscuity.

CONCLUSION

The nursing care of people with an eating disorder is complex and not without emotional stress. It is important that the nurse is clear about and understands the psychological characteristics of the disorders and is prepared to work hard to establish a trusting relationship with the person.

There is a multitude of evidence that suggests that a person with an eating disorder, especially anorexia nervosa, has difficulty in maintaining a sense of power or control in their lives.[13–15] It can be the role of the nurse to work with the person on perceived low self-control and to explore with them and where appropriate their family's ways of creating greater independence. It is important as nurses that we support the person in regaining or developing their sense of self-control and do not create a dependency that may deplete it further. The relationship should be one of trust, empathy, growth and empowerment.

The importance of the nurse–patient relationship as a vehicle for achieving health was first highlighted by Hildegard Peplau.[15] Like Peplau, other writers describe how vital the formulation of a therapeutic relationship is when nursing people with an eating disorder.[16–18] The quality of the relationship is determinate on a number of factors: positive regard, acceptance, trust, confidentiality and consistency. Nursing researchers have found that if a person experiences a lack of empathy and genuineness from the nurse their recovery will be hindered.[19,20]

It is imperative that nurses manage their own anxiety and do not become overwhelmed by the anxiety of the patient.

Good communication structures and continuity of care help to lessen the problems and anxiety conflicting information and practice can cause. It is vital that nurses understand that the suffer will feel a compulsion to dispose of food, drink large amounts of water prior to being weighed or exercise excessively; these behaviours are as a result of extreme distress and not a personal attack on the nurse. These actions need to be addressed in a non-punitive manner conveying to the person that while the nurse is not condoning these ways of managing fear, they can understand them. Nurses need to use clinical supervision, staff meetings and discussion forums to maintain support, consistency and self-awareness. Continuing education is also important so that knowledge is updated and standards can be evaluated and improved.

REFERENCES

1. Buckroyd J. *Eating your heart out*. London: Optima, 1989.

2. Crisp AH. *Anorexia nervosa: let me be*. London: Academic Press, 1980.

3. Orbach S. *Hunger strike*. London: Faber and Faber, 1986.

4. American Psychiatric Association. *Diagnostic and statistical manual disorders (DSM-IV)*, 4th edn. Washington, DC: APA, 1994.

5. Hsu LK, Crisp AH, Callender JS. Psychiatric diagnoses in recovered and unrecovered anorectics 22 years after onset of illness: a pilot study. *Comprehensive Psychiatry* 1992; **33**: 123–7.

6. Bloom C, Gitter A, Gutwill S, *et al.* Eating problems: a feminist psychoanalytic treatment model. New York: Basic Books, 1994.

7. Zerbe KJ. *Women's mental health in primary care*. London: WB Saunders, 1999: 109–37.

8. Turnbull S, Ward A, Treasure J, Jick H, Derby L. The demand for eating disorder care: an epidemiological

study using the general practice research database. *British Journal of Psychiatry* 1996; **169**: 705–12.

9. Vanhoeken D, Lucas AR, Hoek HW. Epidemiology. In: Hoek HW, Treasure JL, Katzman MA (eds). *Neurobiology in the treatment of eating disorders*. Chichester: John Wiley, 1998.

10. Russell GFM, Szmukler G, Dare C, Eisler I. An evaluation of family therapy in anorexia nervosa and bulimia nervosa. *Archives or General Psychiatry* 1987; **44**: 1047–56.

11. Troop NA, Treasure JL. Setting the scene for eating disorders. II: Childhood helplessness and mastery. *Psychological Medicine* 1997; **27**: 531–8.

12. Fairburn CG, Norman PA, O'Connor ME, Doll HA, Peveler RC. A prospective study of outcome in bulimia nervosa and the long-term effects of three psychological treatment. *Archives of General Psychiatry* 1995; **52**: 304–12.

13. Williams GJ, Chamore AS, Millar R. Eating disorders, perceived control, assertiveness and honesty. *British Journal of Clinical Psychology* 1990; **29**(3): 327–35.

14. Williams GJ, Power KG, Millar HR, *et al.* Comparison of eating disorders and other dietary/weight groups on measures of perceived control, assertiveness, self-esteem and self-directed hostility. *International Journal of Eating Disorders* 1993; **14**(1): 27–32.

15. Peplau HE. *Interpersonal relationships in nursing*. New York: Putmans, 1952.

16. Dexter GC, Wash M. *Psychiatric nursing skills: a patient-centred approach*. London: Chapman and Hall, 1990.

17. Martin P. *Psychiatric nursing – a therapeutic approach*. London: Macmillan Education, 1987.

18. Ironbar NO, Hooper A. *Self instruction in mental health nursing*. London: Baillière Tindall, 1989.

19. Varcarolis EM. *Foundations of psychiatric mental health nursing*. London: WB Saunders, 1990.

20. Altschul A. *Patient–nurse interaction*. Edinburgh: Churchill-Livingstone, 1972.

APPENDIX 39.1

EATING DISORDER: A PERSONAL ACCOUNT

Jane Noble

After having suffered from a restricting anorexia for over 20 years, all of a sudden I developed bulimia. Until the beginning of the 1990s, little was understood about this particular eating problem. Unlike anorexia, there was no physical sign that something was wrong. However, it is a very serious illness and has one of the highest mortality rates. I soon found myself trying to restrain myself from eating everything in sight.

I remember the first time I binged. This was due to a deep emotional issue, where I felt so rejected. I couldn't cope with my feelings. I 'snapped', and went around shops, newsagents, and petrol stations so I could binge. I always convinced myself that this would be the last time. The evening was spent eating non-stop, vomiting and then repeating the same actions. I was like an animal. I would buy lots of chocolate, bread, sandwiches, cereal, margarine, milk for cereal, ice-cream, chocolate bars. The list is endless. Sometimes before I even got back to my flat, I had eaten half the food in the car. I just never knew when I felt full or hungry. My pattern was not to eat all day, so everybody, I believed, thought I wasn't eating. I would binge in secret, so start my evening ritual at 6 p.m. Physically I had begun to put weight on. My glands would become so swollen, looking in a mirror was a nightmare, for my face looked so fat. My body chemicals became out of balance and I was prone to fainting a lot more. I had no energy left in me, and so became very apathetic. It felt like I had been in a boxing match, where my whole body ached.

Mentally there was nothing but repulsion and disgust towards myself. I was embarrassed to go out, for I believed everyone *knew* I was like an animal. I was terrified of people making a comment on how well I looked, for that would mean I looked fat. And I did. My face was more filled out and I looked less emaciated. I walked around with shame, disgust and repulsion at what I had done. It felt like I'd been abused, so misunderstood. When I was receiving cognitive therapy, even my consultant thought that it was 'brilliant' that I was gaining weight. I was 'recovering' from anorexia. If only I dared to say those words of repulsion, to admit that I was bingeing. The feeling of loneliness, isolation, and the fact that my psychiatrist was pleased, made me seriously think about ending my life. I felt I had no control over my actions: that this wasn't me. I would go through the next day in self-denial of what had happened the night before. I would spend the day believing that it wouldn't happen again. But it always did. In fact my bingeing was getting worse. I couldn't believe I would engage in such a disgusting behaviour.

When a new Eating Disorder Unit was set up in the city, more and more insight was gained as to the various ways people used food to abuse themselves. Personally, I have yet to meet anyone who suffers an eating disorder who has not come from a dysfunctional family, or had some traumatic ordeal in life, so knocking their self-esteem, self-worth and confidence.

For me, and for other sufferers I know, using a psychodynamic approach has proved the most effective treatment. Working with a therapist, who looks at the underlying emotional chaos, actually helped to alleviate my bingeing. This approach also requires a lot of nurse input, where the sufferer can work in a trusting relationship. Nursing staff helped me by being aware of the times I was most vulnerable to bingeing (which was supper time). If needed, I would talk to a member of staff. Neither was my eating a taboo subject in the one-to-one nursing sessions. Honesty is the only way forward. While on occasions nursing staff used practical resources to support me, my emotions were never forgotten.

It seems appropriate to say that I was admitted to hospital, just over 7 months ago, when a new nursing model had been implemented – the *Tidal Model*. I really feel the Tidal Model complements the psychodynamic approach, by advocating care that is client-centred, and empowering. It has enabled me to identify what my problems are, and what I think might be the best way to move forward. I must say, I don't always like that, for often I would much prefer that decisions were made for me. But I'm learning. Although the Tidal Model has been shown to be effective on acute admissions wards, I can see how excellent it will be for eating disorder sufferers of every nature. Those of us who suffer bulimia can hopefully feel confident that bulimia can be effectively treated, with psychotherapy working alongside the Nursing Tidal Model, as well as other disciplines, like occupational therapy, voluntary work, liaising with dietitians and any other facilities that are available.

I won't even begin to say I am over bulimia, for I am not. However, with the various treatments in place, I can at last begin to try and understand myself, why I behave the way I do and why I always feel the need to abuse myself. At the end of the day the only person suffering is me. How logical! But true.

Chapter 40

THE PERSON WHO IS HOMELESS

Paul Veitch* and Jon Wigmore**

INTRODUCTION

This chapter offers the reader an introduction to the problems facing homeless people and to the practice implications for the psychiatric and mental health nurse (PMHN) working in acute and community settings. We will explore who the homeless are, before focusing on a subgroup of the homeless population in the UK defined as 'single homeless people'. This focus is shared with the chapter looking at specialist services for homeless people (see Chapter 47). Most of the issues and related nursing approaches we outline will have a UK focus, but will be applicable to the many other mental health service users who are insecurely housed, living in poverty, and facing restricted access to health care in other countries.

Homeless people provide a graphic illustration of both the enmeshed nature of social and health problems, and the structural deficiencies of the services attempting to address them. The range and intensity of health and social problems faced by homeless people are often daunting to professionals. We consider that the PMHN has a valuable set of skills to offer and is well placed to address the multiple needs of homeless people who suffer from mental health difficulties. To be helpful to homeless people, we need to address issues of poverty, stigma, and social exclusion. This calls for a varied knowledge base, encompassing mental illness, drug and alcohol use, physical health, housing, the social security systems and an awareness of the agencies addressing them, as well as the underlying ethical dilemmas produced.[1] The 'inverse care law' is evident here, where homelessness is an extreme form of social exclusion with huge health problems, yet homeless people have great difficulty accessing and utilizing health care.

For the growing number of specialist practitioners who work in homelessness teams in particular, this work demands an ability to work outside the familiar clinically orientated multidisciplinary setting, and in partnership with a network of providers, some of whom may be philosophically at odds with traditional mental health services.

WHAT IS HOMELESSNESS?

Absolutes and universal truths relating to homelessness and homeless people do not exist.[2]

*Paul Veitch has worked as a psychiatric nurse in the North East of England for over 20 years. He has a Masters in Psychiatric Nursing and has specialized in working with people who are homeless.
**Jon Wigmore has worked in hostels for homeless people since 1983, in Glasgow, Bristol, Bradford and London. He qualified as a psychiatric nurse in 1996. He is currently employed as an Investigations Manager for the Health Service Ombudsman.

There has never been a consensus about what homelessness means or who homeless people are, and we would advise our readers to exercise caution when confronted by generalizations about the needs of 'homeless people' in the literature and media. What is true of one subgroup of homeless people may be the opposite for another. Attempts at quantification usually reflect the professional and political interests of those framing them, and are additionally problematic as even people generally agreed to be homeless at a given point in time are notoriously hard to count and easy to discount. Definitions are particularly critical however because they determine the moral agenda, shape and extent of the services available.[3]

In the UK homelessness is simply defined (by legislation) as having no accommodation which one might 'reasonably' occupy. This includes the following groups:

❑ People 'sleeping rough' or rooflessness.
❑ People living in direct access hostels and shelters aimed at homeless people.
❑ People (and families) using temporary accommodation – hostels, bed and breakfast hotels or occupying empty buildings.
❑ People in prison, hospital or care, without access to move-on housing.
❑ People staying with family and friends (often called the 'hidden homeless').

The demographic and health profiles of the subgroups of homeless people moving between those forms of non-tenure vary considerably. Homeless people include asylum seekers and refugees, young people, older people, children, families, people from ethnic minorities, single people, and couples. We will be concentrating on the subgroup known as 'single homeless people' here and in Chapter 47, because they experience considerably poorer physical and mental health than any other section of society, and arguably of any other homeless subgroup. They are the most likely to experience physical and mental health problems as a direct result of their lack of tenure. We define the single homeless broadly as adults who usually sleep rough or in institutional settings (prisons, hostels, shelters and squats), who no statutory authority has accepted a responsibility to re-house.[4]

More holistic conceptions of homelessness attempt to encompass processes people experience in losing access to housing – perhaps the single most important component of health. Brant's[5] definition attempts a synthesis between housing status (the quality and tenure of accommodation), and features of structural and personal social relationships:

A person is homeless when he or she does not have a place to live that can be considered to be stable, permanent and of a reasonable housing standard. At the same time, this person is not able to make use of society's relations and institutions (understood in the broadest sense, such as family networks and private and public institutions of all kinds) due to either apparent or hidden causes relating to the individual or to the way in which society functions.

One of the people we work with was recently asked about why when they had a place to call their own, they still regularly 'slept rough'. Their answer illustrates the difficulty in 'defining' homelessness; 'You can take the man off the streets but you can't take the streets out of the man'. This man had been found what most would describe as 'suitable' accommodation. It was warm, safe and secure, offered a variety of support systems and was well integrated with the health care and social systems the man otherwise utilized. However what it did not provide was the camaraderie and sense of place, which he had found over a number of years living in street locations. To experience this he regularly slept rough with groups of drinkers in a disused cemetery. Belonging to the 'homeless family' and the social support it provides can be central to why many remain homeless or do not succeed in what from the outside appears to be a suitable abode. Qualitative research allows us some insights into this world.[6,7]

In the UK approximately 90% of the single homeless are men aged between 25 and 50 years old, with a recognized recent increase in youth homelessness. It is problematic to determine the degree to which ethnicity is a factor, but black people are over-represented in overall homelessness figures, while being less so in hostels and shelters. Particularly in the London boroughs, Irish people are over-represented. London has about half the single homeless people in UK. Military and institutional occupational backgrounds are over-represented as are young people leaving the care of statutory social services. The single homeless are generally estranged from their birth and extended family with high divorce rates.

Some experiences such as a history of childhood parental abuse and unemployment appear to make people vulnerable to homelessness. Specific crisis points often precede an episode of homelessness (such as prison discharge or relationship breakdown). In the UK discharge from long-stay psychiatric hospital does not appear to have been a major cause of homelessness so much as the closure of large scale hostels and lodging houses in the 1980s and 1990s.

Homelessness and mental health problems

A strong body of evidence points to markedly higher rates of psychiatric problems in populations of homeless adults than among the securely domiciled.[8–10] Most studies support the finding that unusually high rates of psychosis and substance misuse are a common feature of homeless populations. That mental health problems exist for young homeless people,[11] homeless children and families,[12] homeless mothers,[13] and homeless people from ethnic minorities[14] have also been reported. A relationship between homelessness and offending behaviour is identified in the literature.[15] The difficulties of addressing combined substance misuse and mental illness, which exists in this group, has long been acknowledged.[16] A consistent criticism of health research on homeless people has been of methodological flaws

The physical health of homeless people has also been investigated. Those at the most extreme end of the homeless continuum (the roofless) are more at risk from poor physical health with high rates of trauma, skin conditions, respiratory conditions and venereal infections. Chronic problems with hypertension, obstructive pulmonary disease, diabetes and dental problems are also a feature. There is a likelihood that previously non-existent disorders will develop with a prolonged period of homelessness.[18] Homeless children are a group with whom primary preventative strategies could be aimed. Many of the behavioural consequences of substance misuse may appear superficially to be presentations of mental illness, and sometimes substance misuse (either acute or long term) can cause mental illness. Being able to distinguish between presentations of intoxication, overdose, delirium and withdrawal are important as all can have serious medical and psychiatric consequences requiring careful assessment and sometimes hospitalization.

As well as combinations of substance misuse and mental illness homeless people also suffer from physical illness, which requires treatment and impacts upon psychiatric management, e.g. epilepsy. Trauma is frequently encountered often secondary to substance misuse, injecting injuries/infections and falls during drinking sessions. Cognitive impairment can prevent people utilizing some psychotherapeutic interventions. Because of the above we recommend the PMHN give the assessment of the physical state a high priority when working with people who are homeless.

High rates of alcohol and street drug use are also found in single homeless populations and companionship (within a group of fellow drug users) is recognized as a factor in sustaining drug use.

Mental disorder plays a role for some in becoming homeless although these individuals tend to have a preexisting heavy loading of poverty and familial instability. For those who become homeless following an episode of mental ill health, alcohol and substance misuse are often a major factor.[19]

WORKING WITH PEOPLE WHO ARE HOMELESS

Addressing powerlessness

Of fundamental importance in understanding why many homeless people do not readily utilize health services is an awareness of power differentials. Acknowledging the particular powerlessness of homeless people within services, particularly mental health services, is important. Without an awareness and understanding of this powerlessness, which adds to that intrinsic to the experience of mental illness, the standard clinical repertoire is unlikely to suffice and will fail to meet the needs of homeless people. What makes homeless people different in the first instance is what they typically present *without*. There will rarely be family, next of kin, or people who will attract the status of carers in the eyes of clinicians.

Out of the hospital setting, homeless people face severely restricted access to facilities that will sustain mental and physical health. Timms[20] terms such personal infrastructure 'a substrate for health'. This substrate – which mental health services (and most statutory agencies) generally assume exists for all people – includes the basic foundations 'that make possible health and treatment'. These include adequate housing, a reasonable diet, family and friends, and a hygienic and safe domicile. The absence of these gives rise to a range of dilemmas for clinicians, but regarding a formal address as the resolution of a person's difficulties is also problematic. Upon discussing hospital discharge arrangements a homeless man pointedly informed a colleague 'There is one place you have not thought about where I would happily be discharged to … and that is the place I was sleeping before you brought me here'.

The powerlessness of homeless people stands in even greater relief when they deal with psychiatric services, where even benign staff attitudes may give rise to what has been termed 'therapeutic nihilism'; a 'justification for neglect'.[21] This mindset arises in the first instance from an awareness of how little power therapeutic interventions have, to redress the considerable deficits in the resources available to homeless people. Acknowledging that marginalization and discrimination are a part of the homeless experience is therefore of importance. Our services are often complex and can appear unnecessarily fragmented. Often homeless people lack social and network negotiation skills and do not have the family or social supports of the domiciled people services are orientated toward. Many are skilled at survival in the harsh conditions of street living and this often goes without acknowledgement. Assessment from a strengths perspective rather than a deficit-based approach can help redress power differentials.

Frustrations arise from still-prevalent value-laden stereotypes of homeless people. These include the idea that homeless people move around a great deal (and are therefore rightly someone else's problem), and are likely to be 'alcoholic, personality disordered, as having chosen to live in this way, and as not appreciating the help that they are given'.[22]

Case study 40.1

Simon, a 50-year-old man who had been successful in business was made homeless following a series of disastrous losses. Depression and alcohol use had contributed to his downfall and he came to live in a hostel. He had to ask permission to leave the building, was unable to find a satisfactory degree of privacy and felt humiliated by his lack of financial independence. Although not seeking psychiatric help, Simon spoke to the PMHN who visited the hostel. The PMHN was able to convey an understanding of Simon's frustration, which enabled Simon to decide to find a less restrictive hostel.

Engagement toward assessment skills

Here there is an emphasis on the development of rapport before 'therapeutic' work can begin. Some people resent homeless hostels where, as mental health workers become more prevalent in such settings, staff begin to request information about past psychiatric histories. One man with such experience wrote, 'The reason so many homeless reject hostels in preference to sleeping rough is because in ever more hostels today the homeless individual, as a condition of staying in the hostel, is forced to see a psychiatrist, who after a very brief interview diagnoses, as often as not, mental illness – a stigma for life'.[23]

Before being able to carry out a nursing assessment there is an important phase we call 'pre-assessment' (or engagement toward assessment) which is necessary for some individuals. It would be wrong however to regard all homeless people with mental health problems as 'difficult to engage'. Many workers in this field use self-referral as an important aspect of their work because they acknowledge that *the services are difficult to engage* (or navigate) rather than patients. This pre-assessment/engagement phase is an acknowledgement that people who are homeless often have had poor prior experience of institutional authority, that psychiatric contact is stigmatizing and that premature attempts to address mental health problems may serve to reinforce earlier negative experiences with services. Usually this

work is carried out in the community as part of outreach work (see Chapter 47).

Consider what value there is for the individual in talking with you, for example are there any tangible benefits from such a conversation and how does it promote trust? Becoming familiar with places homeless people frequent (free food outlets for example) and by spending time, sharing space and resources can help to establish your credibility. These are time-consuming activities out of keeping with usual practice in the discipline. Working this way requires innovation, resourcefulness and an ability to adapt to changing circumstances.

Being 'culturally competent' across gender, lifestyle and age spectrums means learning about the ethnographic context you are working with and should lead to a broad knowledge of local service utilization patterns among homeless people. Such activities can be a necessary precursor towards understanding the potential harshness of the homelessness experience. This means being non-intrusive by using verbal or non-verbal cues which consent an approach, and taking care not to overwhelm with information. Try to become attuned to cues (anxiety or irritability) that your presence might be causing difficulties such as paranoia. Listening to the peers of people who are homeless and their concerns about individual behaviour can help you to pick up on changes in functioning or otherwise unidentified risks.

As trust is developed help can be offered in more goal-directed areas with a health orientation, offering information, escorts to hospital appointments or providing letters of support/references leading to direct referral to health or personal social services (particularly those which help to maximize income). Specialized groupwork interventions have been described in the literature aimed at the process of engagement.[24] There is a need to be overt in describing the rationale for any assessment process or interview, 'The hostel worker was concerned that you appeared alone and distressed, I wanted to discuss this with you. Might there be something I can help with?'

The ability to engage with homeless individuals is an important initial step in reconnecting people to using ordinary, non-homelessness services. It is a process aimed at people who do not utilize services either through a lack of awareness of what services exist and especially those who are active service avoiders. The balance between delaying treatment for longer-term gain in rapport, needs careful consideration. Such initial pre-assessment does allow for a screening process to take place whereby overt evidence of psychiatric problems such as extreme over-activity or active suicidality will usually be apparent. These will invariably lead to emergency measures.

Case study 40.2

Alan was for the first time willing to share time with the PMHN over a cup of tea at the day centre. However he was tearful and unable to concentrate on the simple conversation. He soon left the building, but tolerated the company of the nurse on a walk. When crossing the bridge he talked of feeling compelled to jump but was agreeable to a formal interview in the emergency room where his active suicidal intent led to a hospital admission.

The right 'level' of assessment is necessary. Many individuals have the experience of being interviewed by numerous professionals and the danger of unnecessary assessment, especially in crisis, should be borne in mind. Relevant background information may be available elsewhere and unnecessary repetition can damage a fragile and vital rapport. The PMHN should empower the person toward self-determination while presenting options for change (or the potential consequences of not changing) in the least restrictive circumstances. Maintain awareness that the healing or recovery process takes time and may only be achieved in small steps.

Case study 40.3

Police arrested Alf because of threatening behaviour toward a man walking his dog in the park where Alf had been sleeping rough. This led to a compulsory psychiatric admission to hospital when Alf was considered to be mentally unwell. At the first opportunity Alf absconded from the ward and has never been seen since. Opportunities to engage with Alf prior to this episode may have led to an improved outcome.

The adaptation of nursing interventions

An important principle when working with homeless people is to provide for basic requirements before attempting more sophisticated interventions. By helping people to achieve a route to shelter, nourishment and finances we are underpinning any later psychotherapeutic work with a perception by the patient that we are capable, oriented to their needs and trustworthy. Linear models of service delivery (assessment – treatment – resolution) are unlikely to be helpful where the nurse needs to remain responsive and accept that cyclical or intermittent patient contact, sometimes by way of casual encounters on the street, are an aspect of work in the homeless field. However, programmes of case management (some of the principles of which have informed assertive outreach) have been developed and some specific homeless services use adaptations especially for homeless people[25, 26] (see Chapter 47).

Although psychotic, depressive and psychoactive substance use disorders predominate in homeless populations there are no distinct disorders peculiar to the homeless. The implication of this is that the PMHN's psychiatric knowledge base and associated repertoire of assessment and therapeutic skills, will equip him or her to address the *psychiatric illnesses* presented by homeless people. These are amenable to classification and treatment programmes. However PMHNs do not treat mental illness *per se*. Rather they address the *human responses* to mental health problems and the social factors which impact on the presenting difficulty. Single homeless people using psychiatric services present human expressions of distress and of being overwhelmed by multiple inter-related difficulties and it is the human responses to these difficulties which are addressed by the PMHN. Nurses have articulated how the issue of homelessness has impacted on their thinking.[27–29]

The successful nurse will therefore be able to acknowledge the aspects of being homeless which impinge on the mental health problems encountered and be able to adopt clinical practices that take this into account. The wide range of difficulties which are faced by homeless people are a challenge to nurses who need a sound knowledge of substance misuse problems and of serious mental illness which are often combined, sometimes with offending behaviour as an issue. Using a team approach with systematic communication, supervision and support structures helps nurses to be flexible in assessing priorities.

Case study 40.4

Eddie was living in some woods 12 miles from the primary care centre. The PMHN was unable to engage him in formal assessment despite concerns expressed about his obvious distress, as he was more concerned with attending to his personal hygiene and finding dry clothes. Following team discussion the PMHN was able to obtain a good local supply of the necessary items as well as some emergency cash for Eddie. Following the assessment which Eddie now participated in a suitable hostel was found and Eddie accepted treatment and support for a depressive illness.

STRUCTURAL INTERVENTIONS FOR THE HOMELESS PERSON IN HOSPITAL

Our experience suggests that the lifestyles and usage of inpatient hospital facilities by homeless people still attracts a disproportionate scrutiny and 'moral evaluation' by many staff. When homeless people are inpatients of psychiatric units there is rarely a day-to-day critical audience (someone with an awareness of their powerlessness) to challenge clinical decision-making. The first task of the PMHN working with a homeless patient, particularly in the inpatient setting, is to understand the structural powerlessness of the person and to address this with concrete strategies. A reliance on experience with securely domiciled populations can lead to false assumptions about the appropriateness of behavioural or nursing interventions.

- **Talk to the patient about the services they use in the community.** For example hostels vary hugely in terms of philosophy, staffing levels, and ability to manage challenging behaviour. Some hostels allow for alcohol use on the premises while others do not. If the person agrees, initiate contact – the hostel staff may be an important resource when planning leave and discharge.
- **Recognize that homeless people have 'carers' and offer them a role in the clinical process.** These may include peers, partners, and staff of voluntary organizations, housing workers, outreach workers or advocates. A hospital admission may provide an opportunity for family reconciliation. The families of homeless people may be excluded from local initiatives to meet the needs of families and carers in the locality (such families are stigmatized too).
- **If the patient has no access to temporary accommodation, get them housing advice quickly.** Many homeless people are referred unnecessarily to high care mental health hostels because alternatives have not been considered. Statutory authorities usually have an obligation to assess the needs of homeless people.
- **Homeless people need advocates more than any other section of society.** You may have to explain what an advocate is and take extra steps to engage the patient with them. Workers (who may have been trying to manage difficult behaviour for some time) sometimes have an interest in extended hospital stays for their clients. Homeless people need *independent* advocates where these are available.
- **Ensuring linkage with Community Mental Health Services.** Specialist homeless services themselves may not be ideal and can carry a stigma of their own. Linkage into 'ordinary' local mental health and primary care services (which may be more comprehensive than the specialist homeless team) is important and needs careful negotiation. This is often more than simply referral and involves ensuring people can utilize such resources thus preventing a breakdown in continuity. A period of 'shared care' is often necessary with support to the workers who might have limited experience of working with homeless people.
- **Discharge arrangements** for people who are homeless should involve enhanced aftercare packages.

THE ASSESSMENT OF RISK

Personal safety

Settings that the PMHN may need to access such as day centres may not have the safe interviewing facilities many PMHNs are accustomed to and patients are interviewed sometimes without the kind of information usually available from referrers such as primary care staff. Due to the complexities of need and the variety of agencies attempting to help, fragmentation can occur and clinical notes are often unavailable.

Seeing patients accompanied by other staff members or in a joint assessment can sometimes compromise an assessment due to the effect of inhibiting the patient. A balance needs to be found whereby the advantages of a multidisciplinary assessment are acknowledged and may outweigh any disadvantages. Some facilities search people for weapons (especially in the USA) but a more subtle approach may be to have a high index of suspicion that any person may be potentially carrying an offensive weapon (usually for personal protection). Where people report a previous use of weapons it is important to ascertain if the patient is currently armed. Patients may be intoxicated with drugs or alcohol leading to an increased possibility of impulsive violence.

If people are visited in a domiciliary setting, e.g. a squat or shared house, then the possibility of individual patients being accompanied by an unknown person makes precautions necessary. Consider the use of joint visits (including Police accompaniment) and reserve the right not to visit the temporary domicile.

Suicidality and homelessness

The homeless are a group often unpopular with workers because of the perception or expectation that such persons will present with multiple needs, causing difficulty in assessment and clinical management. An inquiry into suicide and homicide by people suffering from mental illness[30] makes special mention of homelessness with 3% of suicides in England and Wales, 2% in Scotland and 1% in Northern Ireland being suicides of homeless individuals. Some 71% of these suicides in England and Wales occurred when homeless people were psychiatric inpatients or within three months of hospital discharge. Half of these were being formally followed up and yet two-thirds were out of contact with care providers at the time of death.

These findings led the inquiry team to recommend that all homeless patients who had received inpatient care should receive the most enhanced aftercare packages. Reliable evidence about rates of self-harm and attempted suicide in homeless populations is subject to even more complex epidemiological difficulties than diagnosable mental disorder. However research with young people in the North West of England which was concerned with service utilization found 43% of their sample reported previous suicidal intent. The most important protective factors identified (social support of family or partners) are often absent in the case of many single homeless people.[31] This focus on suicide and self-harm belies the fact that many homeless people are themselves at risk of violence from others.

Exploitation and victimization of the homeless mentally ill

The homeless mentally ill are particularly at risk of exploitation from others. Such persons can potentially have relatively high incomes (from social security) and are more likely to carry cash and possessions with them at all times. They can be 'obvious' victims because of their appearance and the places they frequent. Hiday and colleagues[32] found a substantial rate of violent criminal victimization among a homeless mentally ill sample, finding the combination of substance misuse and homelessness more likely to put an individual at risk. Careful assessment of interpersonal relations is necessary as what from the outside appears to be an exploitative relationship may provide a person with companionship and protection. Providing a third party payee who takes charge of an individual's finances has not been shown to benefit such people and may be perceived as an unwanted intrusion.[33] Helping people find an address to which they can receive mail or store possessions is a helpful and less intrusive strategy.

The sharing of confidential data concerning an individual's welfare is necessarily done within disciplinary expectations concerning professional practice, as well as with regard to Human Rights legislation. Information made available to agencies providing care can also be used to an individual's detriment if such information is misunderstood, for example some psychiatric diagnoses are treated pejoratively and can prejudice an individual's chances of housing or another benefit.

CONCLUSION

People who are mentally ill and homeless are some of the most socially excluded and vulnerable persons in often-prosperous modern societies. PMHNs have the potential to fulfil a role as the champions of these people as they have the right blend of skills and flexibility of role (across clinical and social domains) to meet the multiple needs of people who are homeless. The need is to develop and adopt nursing practice to the services which homeless people use.

RECOMMENDED READING AND WEBSITE

Bhugra D (ed.) *Homelessness and mental health – studies in social and community psychiatry.* Cambridge University Press, 1998.

Health Advisory Service. *People who are homeless – mental health services. Commissioning and providing mental health services for people who are homeless.* London: HMSO, 1995.

Orwell G. *Down and out in Paris and London.* In: Davison P (ed.) *The complete works of George Orwell.* London: Secker and Warburg, 1933.

www.gla.ac.uk/homelessness

REFERENCES

1. Timms P, Borrell T. Doing the right thing. – ethical and practical dilemmas in working with homeless mentally ill people. *Journal of Mental Health* 2001; **10**(4): 419–26.

2. Neale J. Homelessness and theory reconsidered. *Housing Studies* 1997; **12**(1): 47–61.

3. Scott J. Homelessness and mental illness. *British Journal of Psychiatry* 1993; **162**: 314–24.

4. Pleace N, Burrows R, Quilgars D. Homelessness in contemporary Britain: conceptualisation and measurement. In: Burrows R, Pleace N, Quilgars D (eds). *Homelessness and social policy.* London: Routledge, 1997.

5. Brandt P. Reflections on homelessness as seen from an institution for the homeless in Copenhagen. In: Avramov D (ed.). *Coping with homelessness: issues to be tackled and best practices in Europe.* Aldershot: Ashgate, 1999: 529.

6. Payne J. An action research project in a night shelter for rough sleepers. *Journal of Psychiatric and Mental Health Nursing* 2002; **9**: 95–101.

7. Baumann SL. The meaning of being homeless. *Scholarly Inquiry for Nursing Practice: An International Journal* 1993; **7**(1): 59–73.

8. Dennis DL, Buckner JC, Lipton FR, Levin IS. A decade of research and services for homeless mentally ill persons: where do we stand? *American Psychologist* 1991: **46**: 1129–38.

9. Munoz M, Vasquez C, Koegel P, Sanz J, Burnam MA. Differential patterns of mental disorders among the homeless in Madrid (Spain) and Los Angeles (USA). *Social Psychiatry and Psychiatric Epidemiology* 1998; **33**: 514–20.

10. McAuley A, McKenna HP. Mental disorder among a homeless population in Belfast: an exploratory survey. *Journal of Psychiatric and Mental Health Nursing* 1995; **2**: 335–42.

11. Sleegers J, Spijker J, van Limbeck J, van Engeland H. Mental health problems among homeless adolescents. *Acta Psychiatrica Scandinavica* 1998: **97**: 253–9.

12. Herth K. Hope as seen through the eyes of homeless children. *Journal of Advanced Nursing* 1998; **25**(5): 1053–62.

13. Zima BT, Wells KB, Benjamin B, Duan N. Mental health problems among homeless mothers. *Archives of General Psychiatry* 1996; **53**: 332–8.

14. Leda C, Rosenheck R. Race in the treatment of homeless mentally ill veterans. *Journal of Nervous and Mental Disease* 1995; **183** (8): 529–37.

15. Gelberg L, Linn S, Leake BD. Mental health, alcohol and drug use, and criminal history among homeless adults. *American Journal of Psychiatry* 1988; **145**(2): 191–6.

16. Drake R, Osher F, Wallach M. Homelessness and the dual diagnosis. *American Psychologist* 1991: **46**: 1149–58.

17. Susser E, Conover S, Struering E. Mental illness in the homeless: problems in epidemiological method in surveys of the 1980s. *Community Mental Health Journal* 1990; **26**: 387–410.

18. Gerlberg L, Linn LS. Assessing the physical health of homeless adults. *Journal of the American Medical Association* 1989; **262**(14): 1973–9.

19. Sullivan G, Burnham A, Koegal P. Pathways to homelessness among the mentally ill. *Social Psychiatry and Psychiatric Epidemiology* 2000; **35**: 444–50.

20. Timms P. Management aspects of care for the homeless mentally ill. *Advances in Psychiatric Treatment* 1996; **2**(4): 158–65.

21. Watts D, Morgan HG. Malignant alienation. *British Journal of Psychiatry* 1994; **164**: 11–15.

22. Timms P, Balazs J. ABC of mental health: mental health on the margins. *British Medical Journal* 1997; **315**: 536–9.

23. Blue A. Clarke cuts a blow to homeless. *The Independent* 16th January, 1997.

24. Veitch P. Checkmates. *Mental Health Practice* 2000; **4**(4): 26–7.

25. Rosenheck RA, Dennis D. Time limited assertive community treatment for homeless persons with severe mental illness. *Archives of General Psychiatry* 2001; **58** (11): 1073–80.

26. Susser E, Valencia E, Conover S, Felix A, Tsai W, Wyatt RJ. Preventing recurrent homelessness among mentally ill men: a 'critical time' intervention after discharge from a shelter. *American Journal of Public Health* 1997; **87**: 256–62.

27. Rasmusson DL, Jonas CM, Mitchell GJ. The eye of the beholder: Parse's theory with homeless individuals. *Clinical Nurse Specialist* 1991; **5**(3): 139–43.

28. Strehlow AJ, Amos-Jones T. The homeless as a vulnerable population. *Nursing Clinics of North America* 1999; **34**(2): 261–74.

29. Taylor CS, Warren BJ. What goals and interventions are important for psychiatric nurses to use when working with homeless chronically mentally ill? *Journal of Psycho-social Nursing* 1993; **31**(4): 35–9.

30. Department of Health. *Safety first: five-year report of the national confidential inquiry into suicide and homicide by people with mental illness.* London: DOH, 2001.

31. Reid P, Klee H. Young homeless people and service provision. *Health and Social Care in the Community* 1999; **7**(1): 17–24.

32. Hiday VA, Swartz MS, Swanson JW, Borum R, Wagner HR. Criminal victimisation of persons with severe mental illness. *Psychiatric Services* 1999; **50**(1): 62–8.

33. Rosenheck R, Lam J, Randolph F. Impact of representative payees on substance use by homeless persons with serious mental illness. *Psychiatric Services* 1997; **48**(6): 800–806.

Chapter

THE PERSON WITH DEMENTIA

Trevor Adams*

INTRODUCTION

Over the past 15 years, there has been a considerable interest in psychiatric nursing of people with dementia. This is due to the increase in the number of older people in Western society and their greater likelihood of developing dementia. Butterworth[1] has noted that people with dementia have often been a marginal concern within psychiatric nursing and have frequently been seen as an undesirable area of clinical practice. The situation is now very different and dementia care has become a dynamic, progressive and exciting area of practice within psychiatric nursing.

Until recently, people in the early stages of dementia were often placed in mental hospitals.[2] People with dementia, like other patients, were managed and controlled by psychiatric nurses through a regimen of nursing tasks such as feeding and dressing.[3] This regimen shared many characteristics typically found in institutional settings in which preference is given to the needs of the staff, rather than the people with dementia.[4] The culture of institutionalization within mental hospitals had a harmful effect on both patients and psychiatric nurses. This was a repeated and consistent finding of numerous reports on mental hospitals in the 1960s and 1970s, notably *Sans Everything*,[5] which dealt specifically with older people. In *Sans Everything*, an acting chief male nurse reported that '[A]fter six months in certain hospitals, there are ways in which psychiatric nurses are no longer like ordinary people. Their attitude to mental illness changes – as it does to old age, to cruelty, to people's needs, and to dying. It is as if they become numbed to these things'.[6] In this way, people with dementia often found themselves placed in difficult and even humiliating situations, in which they were devalued, disempowered and marginalized by psychiatric nurses.

More recently, newer discourses relating to personhood and the voice of people with dementia have entered psychiatric nursing. These discourses have reconstructed people with dementia and their care. In many dementia care placements, these newer discourses exist alongside residual medical–custodial discourses that identify people with dementia as having impaired or no ability to make worthwhile choices about their own care. This latter way of constructing people with dementia can be convenient to psychiatric nurses and other care staff, positioning themselves as having no moral obligation to ask people with dementia what they actually want. The newer discourses, however, portray people with dementia as people who, like everyone else, make sense of the world, experience selfhood and display identity.[7,8] The emergence of these alternative perspectives has done much to lessen discriminatory and

*Trevor Adams, PhD MSc RMN Cert Ed CPN Cert has worked in dementia care nursing for over twenty years. During this time he has been involved in developing dementia care through practice, education and research. He is Lecturer in Mental Health, European Institute of Health and Medical Sciences, University of Surrey, UK and is currently Mental Health Pathway Leader for the MSc in Advanced Practice.

oppressive practices towards people with dementia, and has started to bring about a new culture of dementia care.[9] However, it would be complacent to think that this has totally eradicated bad practice. In many clinical areas, the care of people with dementia still lacks the resources and prestige to make the new culture of dementia a reality.

This chapter draws on these innovative discourses to construct a sensitive and politically aware approach to psychiatric nursing with people who have dementia. A common thread running through the chapter is that psychiatric nursing should be underpinned by a partnership between the person with dementia, their family, and the psychiatric nurse.[10,11] This approach supports contemporary trends in health and social policy that relate to the importance of informal care as a means of delivering community care.[12,13] In addition, the idea of partnership helps us recognize that psychiatric nurses also have emotional needs that have been incurred within clinical practice, that may be addressed by clinical supervision.[14,15]

It should be recognized that the notion of partnership challenges models of informal care such as that developed by Nolan *et al.*[16] that construct the 'carer as expert' and privileges the carer, in the case of dementia care, at the expense of the person with dementia.[17] Within this context, Nolan *et al.* establish the professional carer as 'the senior partner'[18] and thus set up a hierarchy that subordinates the person with dementia. Moreover, forms of nursing that focus on the needs of informal carers, such as the Admiral Nursing Service run by the Dementia Care Trust in the UK, fail to take account of the systemic nature of dementia care within the family, and similarly privileges the needs of the informal carer over those of the person with dementia.[19,20]

Moreover, people with dementia may, through geographical and social isolation, have little contact with other people, including members of their own family. There may therefore be no-one available to take on the role of 'carer as expert' and would lead to the exclusion of people with dementia who are out of contact with a potential informal carer. Secondly, various studies have pointed out that the perspective of informal carers may be different, not only from health and social care providers but also from the person with dementia.[21] The construction of dementia care in terms of partnership should never allow the interests of informal carers to take precedence over, and obscure the interests of the person with dementia. Lloyd makes this point clear in the title of her paper 'Caring about carers: only half the picture?'[22] In this way, the 'carer as expert' approach may be seen as a further way of disabling people with dementia and perpetuating their oppression.

THE EXPERIENCE OF PEOPLE WITH DEMENTIA AND THEIR FAMILIES

People can develop dementia at any age, although its likelihood increases with age. Various studies have described the subjective experience of people with dementia as they come to realize that they are getting forgetful.[23,24] Keady and Gilliard[25] describe nine stages that people go through as they develop dementia (Fig. 41.1). Their work provides worthwhile insights into the subjective experience of people in the early stages of dementia.

However, it is not just the person who is diagnosed that suffers from dementia. In a very real way their relatives, friends and work colleagues all suffer from the effects of dementia. For various reasons, such as denial and a lack of knowledge about dementia, close family members and friends may take some time before realizing the full implications of their relative or friend's behaviour. Eventually though, often as the result of a crisis, one or more family members or friends will come to realize that someone close to them has a serious, though at this stage undiagnosed, mental disorder. Then, family members often seek help from a local medical practitioner. The amount of help and support they receive will depend partly on the doctor's view of the situation, their sensitivity and willingness to involve the relative, and their decision about whether to refer the case to a specialist agency. The person with dementia should receive from the medical practitioner a physical examination, an assessment of their mental state and should have investigations that clarify the diagnosis and exclude other possible causes.

The medical assessment should include an interview with someone who knows the person with dementia well, such as a close family member who can give their

---

Slipping: The person gradually becomes aware of trivial slips and lapses in memory and/or behaviour.

Suspecting: Increased number of slips, which the person cannot 'explain away'. The person begins to suspect that there may be something seriously wrong. By 'covering up' the person makes a deliberate effort to compensate for these slips and hides them from other people.

Revealing: The person reveals to close friends and relatives that they are having problems.

Confirming: The person openly acknowledges that they have a problem.

Maximizing: The person uses strategies to adjust to the dementia.

Disorganization: Cognitive and behavioural difficulties increasingly dominate the person with dementia.

Decline: Semblance of normality and reciprocal relationships with other people is gradually lost. Meeting the person's bodily needs become the prominent feature.

Death: Finally the person with dementia dies.

FIGURE 41.1 The development of dementia.

In addition, psychiatric nurses have an important role to play in maintaining a positive and humanitarian attitude towards people with dementia within contemporary society (Fig 41.3). One has only to think of the holocaust in the 1930s and 1940s to see the extent to which a society can construct mentally impaired people as worthless. The ethical framework that any psychiatric nurse chooses to underpin their practice must assert the essential value of people with dementia. Due to the relocation of psychiatric nursing education within higher education, psychiatric nurses are now in a better position to make, and articulate, the ethical basis of their practice.

ASSESSMENT

To ensure the validity of the assessment, a number of features should be displayed.

❏ Firstly, assessments should not be based solely upon one 'assessment meeting' but rather information should be gained over the course of a number of visits.
❏ Assessments should take place in a setting in which the person with dementia feels most comfortable.

❏ Psychiatric nurses should do their best to get the person with dementia and their carer(s) to relax by facilitating an informal and sociable relationship.
❏ Psychiatric nurses should do everything they can to help the person with dementia talk about their views and preferences.
❏ The assessment should be based on what the person with dementia and their relatives can do, rather than, as is often the case, what they can not do.
❏ Psychiatric nurses should collect additional and supplementary data from people such as family members and friends, and other members of the multidisciplinary team.
❏ Case notes should be written as soon as possible after the assessment meeting so that as little as possible is forgotten or misremembered. It is easy to put off writing-up an assessment especially after a long day!
❏ Finally, the assessment should be written up on appropriately designed documentation. The written assessment should be available to any member of the multiprofessional team as well as informal carers and the person with dementia.

The primary focus of the assessment should be the person with dementia. The psychiatric nurse must make

Skill \ Context	With the person who has dementia	With family carers	Within the multidisciplinary team
Information–giving	Talking about the diagnosis with the person with dementia. Describing services that are available to the person with dementia	Describing dementia to carers. Providing information about giving care	Talking about the person with dementia and their context to other members of the multidisciplinary team
Communication	Eliciting the views of people with dementia	Helping carers give an account of what has been happening	Talking to other members of the multidisciplinary team on an equal basis
Supportive counselling	Reassuring someone with dementia who is anxious about what is happening	Enabling a stressed-out carer to feel more relaxed	Talking to other members of the multidisciplinary team about mutual problems relating to working with clients
Networking	Putting the person with dementia in touch with various caregiving agencies	Putting carers in contact with supportive agencies	Putting other members of the multidisciplinary team in touch with other appropriate agencies
Advocacy	Eliciting the views of people with dementia	Representing the views of the person with dementia to carers	Explaining the views of people with dementia to the multidisciplinary team
Care planning	Involving people with dementia in making decisions about their care Planning the care with the person who has dementia	Involving carers in care planning	Developing care plans with other members of the multidisciplinary team
Physical care	Feeding someone with dementia Therapeutic touch to reassure the person with dementia	Describing to carers issues about their relative's physical care	Discussing physical care issues with members of the multidisciplinary team

FIGURE 41.3 Use of psychiatric nursing skills in specific dementia care contexts.

sure that family members do not act as interlocutors and speak on behalf of, or perhaps instead of, the person with dementia. This denies the person with dementia the right to talk about what they want and to feel that they have a sense of ownership about the decisions they make. It is essential though that information is not only taken from just one informal carer but the whole family. Psychiatric nurses can use a variety of assessment schedules when assessing the person with dementia, such as the Mini-Mental Test.[73] The assessment, and for that matter the intervention, should be sensitive to the cultural background and social context of the person with dementia. Most of all, the assessment should not disable and should be directed at identifying the strengths that the person with dementia possess, not their shortcomings.

INTERVENTION

Psychiatric nurses working with people who have dementia need to employ a range of skills similar to those used by nurses in other areas of mental health care. These skills are focused on communication and include information-giving, communication, supportive, networking, advocacy, care planning and physical care. Moreover, psychiatric nurses can use these skills with (i) the person with dementia; (ii) family carers; and (iii) the multidisciplinary team.

Until recently psychiatric nursing of people with dementia has typically been constructed by biomedical discourses. I have tried to reconstruct the speciality through the use of newer discourses, which construct people with dementia and their care within a psychosocial and sociopolitical framework. By constructing dementia care in this way, psychiatric nurses will not only focus on biomedical features of people with dementia that give rise to their being seen and treated as objects, but will emphasize their status as people, with preferences and rights like anyone else. When psychiatric nursing was constructed in terms of the biomedical discourse, it was largely oblivious to the ethical and political consequences of its practice. However, psychosocial and sociopolitical discourses have enabled psychiatric nursing to emphasize the subjective and interpersonal context of caring for people with dementia.

REFERENCES

1. Butterworth T. Breaking the boundaries. *Nursing Times* 1988; **34**: 36–9.
2. Payne S. Outside the walls of the asylum? psychiatric treatments in the 1980s and 1990s. In: Bartlett P, Wright D (eds). *Outside the walls of the asylum*. London: The Athlone Press, 1999: 244–65.
3. Robb B. *Sans everything: a case to answer.* London: Nelson, 1967.
4. Barton R. Forward. In: Robb B (ed.) *Sans everything: a case to answer.* London: Nelson, 1967: ix–xi.
5. Robb B. *Sans everything: a case to answer.* London: Nelson, 1967.
6. Osbaldeston M. Nobody wants to know. In: Robb N (ed.) *Sans everything: a case to answer.* London: Nelson, 1967: 13–18.
7. Kitwood T. *Dementia reconsidered: the person comes first.* Buckingham: Open University Press, 1997.
8. Sabat SR. *The experience of Alzheimer's disease: like through a tangled veil.* Oxford: Blackwell Publishers, 2001.
9. Kitwood T, Benson S. *The new culture of dementia care.* London: Hawker, 1995.
10. Adams T. Developing partnership in dementia care: a discursive model of practice. In: Adams T, Clarke C (eds). *Dementia care: developing partnerships in practice.* London: Baillière Tindall, 1999: 37–56.
11. Fortinsky RH. Health triads and dementia care: integrative framework and future directions. *Aging and Mental Health* 2001; **5** (Suppl 1): S35–S48.
12. Nolan M, Davies S, Grant G. *Working with older people and their families: key issues in policy and practice.* Buckingham: Open University Press, 2001.
13. National Health Service. *National service framework for older people.* London: NHS, 2001.
14. Carradice A, Keady J, Hahn S. Clinical supervision and dementia care: issues for community mental nursing practice. In: Keady J, Clarke CL, Adams T (eds). *Community Mental Health Nursing and Dementia Care: Practice Perspectives.* Open University Press Buckinghamshire, 2003, pp. 215–35.
15. Holman M. Supporting and Supervising in Dementia Care. In: Adams T, Manthorpe J (eds). *Dementia Care,* Arnold, London, 2003 pp. 213–24.
16. Nolan M, Davies S, Grant G. *Working with older people and their families: key issues in policy and practice.* Buckingham: Open University Press, 2001.
17. Nolan M, Keady J. Working with carers. In: Cantley C. (ed.) The handbook of dementia care. Buckingham: Open University Press, 2001: 160–72.
18. Nolan M, Davies S, Grant G. *Working with older people and their families: key issues in policy and practice.* Buckingham: Open University Press, 2001.
19. Meredith H. Nursing support for carers. *Elderly Care* 1997; **9**: 10–11.
20. Eaton L. Admirable service. *Nursing Times* 1995, **91**: 16–17.
21. Clarke CL, Heyman B. Risk management for people with dementia. In: Heyman B (ed.) *Health and*

health care: a qualitative approach. London: Arnold, 1997.

22. Lloyd L. Caring about carers: only half the picture? *Critical Social Policy* 2000; **62**: 136–50.

23. Bender M, Cheston R. Inhabitants of a lost kingdom: a model of the subjective experiences of dementia. *Ageing and Society* 1997, **17**: 513–32.

24. Mills M. Narrative identity and dementia: a study of emotion and narrative in older people with dementia. *Ageing and Society* **17**: 673–86.

25. Keady J, Gilliard J. The early experience of Alzheimer's disease: implications for partnership and practice. In: Adams T, Clarke C (eds). *Dementia care: developing partnerships in practice*. London: Baillière Tindal, 1999: 227–56.

26. National Health Service. *National Service framework for older people*. London: NHS, 2001: 23.

27. Kovach CR. *Late-stage dementia care*. Washington: Taylor and Francis, 1997.

28. Goldsmith M. *Hearing the voice of people with dementia*. London: Jessica Kingsley, 1996.

29. Barnett E. *Including the person with dementia in designing and delivering care*. London: Jessica Kingsley, 2000.

30. Allen K. *Communication and consultation; exploring ways for staff to involve people with dementia in developing services*. Bristol: Policy Press, 2001.

31. National Health Service. *National Service framework for older people*. London: NHS, 2001: 23.

32. Bamford C, Bruce E. Defining the outcomes of community care: the perspectives of older people with dementia and their carers. *Ageing and Society* 2000; **20**: 543–70.

33. Barker PJ, Reynolds W, Stevenson C. The human science basis of psychiatric nursing: theory and practice. *Journal of Advanced Nursing* 1997; **25**: 660–67.

34. Butterworth CA. *Psychiatric nursing in the community, the application of new technologies to an organisation in transition*. Birmingham: Aston University, Management Centre, 1986.

35. Menzies I. *The functioning of social systems as a defence against anxiety*. London: Tavistock Institute, 1972.

36. Kitwood T. *Dementia reconsidered: the person comes first*. Buckingham: Open University Press, 1997.

37. Kitwood T, Benson S. *The new culture of dementia care*. London: Hawker Publications, 1995.

38. Adams T, Keady J. Why we need dementia care nursing. *Nursing Standard* 2001; **13**: 2–3.

39. Lawton J. *The dying process: patients' experience of palliative care*. London: Routledge, 2000.

40. Hughes EC. *Men and their work*. Westport, CN: Greenwood Press, 1958.

41. Merleau-Ponty M. *Phenomenology of perception*. London: Routledge, 1962.

42. Page S. Dementia care and cholinesterase inhibitors. *Professional Nurse* 2001; **16**: 1421–4.

43. Keltner NL, Zielinski AL, Hardin MS. Drugs used for cognitive symptoms of Alzheimer's disease. *Perspectives in Psychiatric Care* **37**: 31–4.

44. Holden U, Woods R. *Positive approaches to dementia care*. Edinburgh: Churchill Livingstone, 1995.

45. Grainger K. Reality orientation in institutions for the elderly: the perspective from interactional sociolinguistics. *Journal of Aging Studies* 1998; **12**: 39–56.

46. Feil N. *The validation breakthrough*. Baltimore: Health Professions Press, 1993.

47. Bornat J. Approaches to reminiscence. In: Norman IJ, Redfern SJ (eds). *Mental health care for elderly people*. Edinburgh: Churchill Livingstone, 1997.

48. Kitwood T. *Dementia reconsidered: the person comes first*. Buckingham: Open University Press, 1997.

49. Fox L. Mapping the advance of the new culture in dementia care. In: Kitwood T, Benson S (eds). *The new culture of dementia care*. London: Hawker Publications, 1995.

50. Adams T. Kitwood's approach to dementia and dementia care: a critical but appreciative review. *Journal of Advanced Nursing* 1996; **23**: 946–53.

51. Harding N, Palfrey C. *The social construction of dementia: confused professionals?* London: Jessica Kingsley Publications, 1997.

52. Cheston R. Stories and metaphors: talking about the past in a psychotherapy group for people with dementia. *Ageing and Society* 1996; **16**: 579–602.

53. Gillies BA. A memory like clockwork: accounts of living through dementia. *Journal of Aging and Mental Health* 2000; **4**: 366–74.

54. Sabat S. Intact social, cognitive ability, and selfhood: a case study of Alzheimer's disease. *American Journal of Alzheimer's Disease* **1**: 11–19.

55. Miesen BML. Attachment theory and dementia. In: Jones G, Miesen B (eds). *Caregiving in dementia*. London: Routledge/Tavistock, 1992: 454–69.

56. Goldsmith M. *Hearing the voice of people with dementia*. London: Jessica Kingsley, 1996.

57. Harding N, Palfrey C. *The social construction of dementia: confused professionals?* London: Jessica Kingsley, 1997.

58. Armstrong D. Surveillance medicine. *Sociology of Health and Illness* 1995; **17**: 393–404.

59. Dean H, Thompson D. Fetishizing the family: the construction of the informal carer. In: Jones H, Millar J (eds). *The politics of the family*. Aldershot: Avebury, 1996.

60. Heaton J. The gaze and visibility of the carer: a Foucauldian analysis of the discourse of informal care. *Sociology of Health and Illness* 1999; **21**: 759–77.

61. Gilleard C, Higgs P. *Cultures of ageing: self, citizen and the body*. Harlow: Prentice Hall, 2000.

62. Adams T. The social construction of identity by

community psychiatric nurses and family members caring for people with dementia. *Journal of Advanced Nursing* 2000; **32**: 791–8.

63. Adams T. The conversational and discursive construction of community psychiatric nursing for chronically confused people and their families. *Nursing Inquiry* 2001; **8**: 98–107.

64. Adams T. The social construction of risk by community psychiatric nurses and family carers for people with dementia. *Health Risk and Society* 2001; **3**: 307–19.

65. Irving K. *Case studies in restraint in an acute teaching hospital: a Foucauldian approach.* Perth, Western Australia: Curtin University of Technology, 2001.

66. Tilley S. The mental health nurse as rhetorician. In: Tilley S (ed.) *The mental health nurse.* Oxford: Blackwell Science, 1997: 152–71.

67. Crowe M. An analysis of the sociopolitical context of mental health nursing practice. *Australian and New Zealand Journal of Mental Health Nursing* 1997; **6**: 59–65.

68. Crowe M. Psychiatric diagnosis: some implications for mental health nursing care. *Journal of Advanced Nursing* 2000; **31**: 583–9.

69. Cheek J, Rudge T. The panopticon revisited? An exploration of the social and political dimensions of contemporary health care and nursing practice. *International Journal of Nursing Studies* 1994; **3**: 583–91.

70. Manthorpe J. Ethical ideals and practice. In: Cantley C (ed.) *A handbook of dementia care.* Buckingham: Open University Press, 2001: 186–98.

71. Hope T, Oppenheimer C. Ethics: politics, principles and practice. In: Jacoby R, Oppenheimer C (eds). *Psychiatry in the elderly.* Oxford: Oxford University Press, 1997: 709–35.

72. International Council of Nurses. *Code for nurses,* 1973.

73. Folstein MF, Folstein SE, McHugh P. Mini-mental state: A practical method for grading the cognitive state of patients for the clinician. *Journal of Psychiatric Research* 1975; **12**: 189–98.

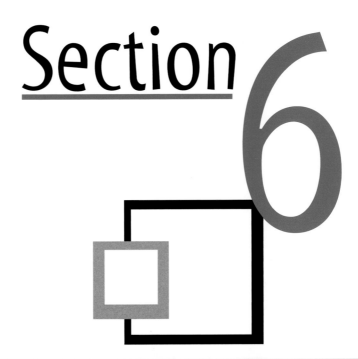

Section 6

The organization of care

Preface to Section 6

Nursing does not take place in a vacuum, but is framed by some broader conceptualization of care and treatment provision. These wider models of mental health care serve as media within which nursing can express itself and can also help others to make their own distinct contribution to the care and treatment process.

In this section we illustrate some of the commoner forms of organized care, beginning with acute hospital services, which remains the traditional focus for mental health services, at least in the Western world. We end with a consideration of early intervention services focused on people with an experience of psychosis. Hopefully, the future will see the growth of early intervention services, for all kinds of significant problems of living, and the gradual diminishment of emphasis on hospitalization, which dislocates people from their natural habitat, often a potential source of healing, and certainly the ultimate destination on the recovery journey.

This section illustrates how many of the philosophical values and principles of practice, already covered in previous sections, find expression in the development of new services – like crisis teams, assertive outreach or intensive care – and also remain at the heart of the ongoing development of more established services – like community teams, family support, homeless support and the secure environment.

Chapter 42

ACUTE INPATIENT NURSING CARE

Angela Simpson* and Peter Dodds**

> If you really want to help somebody, first you must find
> him where he is and start there. This is the secret of caring.
> Kierkegaard.

INTRODUCTION

Acute inpatient wards provide short-term admission to hospital for psychiatric assessment, treatment and care. Acute inpatient care is distinguished from other psychiatric support in that the person in crisis urgently requires admission to hospital, where intensive support is provided and the person's changing condition closely observed. On admission the person is usually highly distressed and requires a more intensive form of support than that available in community settings. The primary aim of hospital admission is to assess the person's con-

dition, providing the human support, environmental conditions and treatment, needed to re-establish emotional stability. In hospital, the person is involved in a collaborative helping process. Individual care needs are jointly identified and constructive helping relationships developed. On discharge, responsibility for providing care at home is transferred to a mental health worker based in the community, who continues to work with the person and his/her family or supporters.

Psychiatric nurses in acute wards are members of a wider multiprofessional team including psychiatrists, occupational therapists, social workers and members of community mental health teams. Links with other support agencies (e.g. voluntary sector organizations and service user groups) are well established. Acute care is highly team focused; this multiprofessional approach

*Angela Simpson is Lecturer in Mental Health Nursing at the University of York. Her interests include Mental Health Service User and Carer Collaboration and Nursing Practice Development. She maintains a fervent interest in developing nursing practice in practice having led an acute psychiatric inpatient nursing team to accreditation as a Nursing Development Unit.

**Peter Dodds is Senior Nurse for Oakburn ward, an acute inner city admissions unit based in Bradford, England. Peter led his team to gain a national reputation by abandoning formal observations and replacing this with high levels of structured service user engagement. These nurse led changes discredited the 'controlling' interventions commonly experienced by many service users and has liberated the nursing team on Oakburn to offer genuine care.

allowing timely medical treatment, nursing and social care to be provided.

Although psychiatric nurses are the key providers of therapeutic care in acute inpatient settings, they are also the primary administrators of medically prescribed treatment. It is important to distinguish between these two distinct dimensions of the nursing role.

PSYCHIATRIC TREATMENT AND CARE

The biomedical model often dominates the way that nurses think about their role.[1] However, this can limit greatly the role of caring *with* people in acute distress. The biomedical model emphasizes diagnosis and the need for treatment. Psychiatric 'disorders' are understood in biological terms and planned interventions are primarily physiological. Where nurses frame nursing interventions around the medical model, nursing shifts away from its primary focus of human caring, featuring instead the need to observe *patients* for signs and symptoms of *illness* primarily in response to *treatment* (medication). This aligns nursing to medicine, limiting unnecessarily the focus of nursing practice – long recognized as having the capacity to be therapeutic in its own right.[2,3]

Where the medical model governs nursing practice, the experience of care becomes technical rather than character building in orientation. Opportunities are lost to develop human caring that emphasize the strengths of the individual as well as empowerment through recognizing people as 'experts of the self'. Opportunities to develop nursing practice also become limited, leaving nurses and nursing fundamentally disempowered and therefore disadvantaged within the multiprofessional team. Mental health service users understand the limitations of the biomedical approach and make a clear distinction between psychiatric treatment and psychiatric care.[4]

> Professionals look for outward signs of illness, inappropriate statements, the speed, the content, the volume of speech, tremors or drug side-effects. Patients on the other hand are concerned with how they feel – how worthwhile their life seems to them.[4]

Psychiatric care is the counter-balance to psychiatric treatment. Without adequate emphasis on psychiatric caring the person in acute distress is a mere recipient of treatment, which is 'being done' impersonally to them. Psychiatric caring nurtures the prospect of personal transformation through active participation in a helping process that involves the person as an equal partner. Although caring is not a nursing monopoly, given the close proximity of the nurse to the person in crisis and the core aim of developing close interpersonal relationships, caring is a very strong feature of the nursing role and, as Clarke notes[5] nurses have a *moral responsibility to care*.

For nurses in acute settings placing emphasis on psychiatric caring involves working purposefully with people in crisis, recognizing the value of each person but also the fundamental value of nursing itself. This involves developing a vision of nursing that is *distinct* from, yet *complementary to*, the biomedical model. Nurses may well incorporate some of the skills associated with diagnosis and cure like carefully monitoring reactions to medication. However, such interventions are a very small part of the nurses' role, better characterized by the human caring elements of practice. Wright[6] notes that the 'high-tech' treatment orientated elements of nursing practice, may make little sense without the counterbalance 'high-touch' interactive human skills. Without these:

> the patient may be treated but is not healed and feels alone and abandoned as a person.[6]

Here we explore *person-centred* nursing in acute inpatient settings. This is a 'high-touch' approach, in which purposeful *care* is distinguished from *treatment*. This style of practice views the human focus of nursing as a fundamental priority and challenges nurses to structure supportive interventions around the core aim of maximizing human contact, individually and in groups. Interpersonal relationships are best constructed through wholehearted participation in caring, so it is necessary for nurses to consider the human experience of acute distress.

EXPERIENCING ACUTE DISTRESS

For the person on the brink of admission to hospital, acute crisis is characterized by significant, often overwhelming, personal distress. This manifests itself in many different ways, but typically people in acute breakdown talk of an experience that includes a profound sense of unease and isolation. While relationships with relatives, friends and key workers often become fractured in crisis, the fragmentation of relationships in acute distress extends beyond the person's external world to include the relationship that the person has with the *self*. It is not unusual for the person to withdraw, or develop an overly critical relationship with the self, which can reduce self-esteem and introduce profound self-doubt. So the experience of acute distress may be experienced as bewildering and frustrating.

The experience of acute distress is life-changing. Acute distress commonly highlights a person's sense of identity and the value of personal relationships, as well as their sense of 'future self'. Consequently, the sense of personal instability can often seem overwhelming. *Crisis* literally means 'decisive moment'. This raises the prospect that people in acute distress might learn something of value from the experience, transforming what might initially be perceived as a dispiriting or seemingly hopeless experience, to their positive advantage. In Chinese, the same character means 'crisis' *and* 'opportunity'. In this respect, the experience of acute breakdown holds the potential of a constructive emotional turning point. The destabilizing and all consuming human experience of acute distress requires a fundamentally *human* response. Typically, the person needs:

- ❑ To feel safe.
- ❑ To be encouraged – sometimes assisted – to maintain basic everyday living.
- ❑ To be encouraged to find the words to articulate distress.
- ❑ To explore distress, recognizing its inherent value.
- ❑ To be placed at the centre of his/her own care.

To meet these needs, nurses must construct personable relationships with people in crisis.[7] Given their close relations with people in care, nurses might be regarded as the *human* face of psychiatry. By developing a nursing focus that instils a collaborative *person-centred* approach to practice, nurses develop the human focus of their work. However, unless this *caring* emphasis is clearly acknowledged, understood and prioritized in practice it can easily be forgotten and as a consequence becomes devalued.

DEVELOPING ACUTE NURSING PRACTICE

The practice of psychiatric nursing is best *developed* in practice. *Managing* the nursing resource isn't enough. When nurses resolve to develop the focus of nursing work, especially in teams, they are doing important work, nurses might be said to be 'creating the future rather than simply encountering it'.[8] The necessary shift towards developing nursing practice in practice is more a question of emphasis, attitude and belief than simply a matter of resources.[9] A Chinese proverb 'better to light a candle than curse the darkness' aptly captures the need for nurses to abandon the culture of cynicism that often infects team morale in favour of an optimistic approach toward the development of psychiatric nursing in acute care.

Recognizing that nursing can and should determine and drive its own agenda in acute psychiatric care is liberating, but it is also very important to note that in seeking to develop nursing practice, nurses are not seeking greater power. Rather, the nursing focus involves becoming increasingly person and family centred, nurturing a style of practice that narrows the gap between the fun-

damental human care needs of the person in crisis and what it is that nurses provide (the human focus of care).

Developing nursing practice in acute settings might at first appear an overwhelmingly difficult task. However, this focus hinges more on a switch of nursing emphasis, developing approaches to nursing intervention that embody close person to person contact. Changes are small scale, but purposefully tailored towards making a significant impact on the *experience* of care.[9] This does not necessarily involve working harder, but it does involve working smarter, adopting a more considered and thoughtful approach to nursing the person. Nursing teams that identify with the need to develop nursing practice in practice tend to be identifiable as those that:

- ❑ Develop an inquiry culture in which nurses take keen interest and ask open-ended questions.
- ❑ Openly discuss the possibilities of different approaches to care.
- ❑ Develop formal and informal 'on the job' ways to reflect on practice.
- ❑ Look beyond the traditional parameters of nursing work, establishing structures and modes of working that support close interpersonal contact.

In the next section of this chapter we follow the story of Suzy, Ward Manager of Cherry Ward as she seeks to develop nursing practice on a busy acute psychiatric admission unit.

Suzy's story

Suzy is Ward Manager of Cherry Ward an acute psychiatric admission ward. Since being promoted, she has developed managerial competence and undertakes routine ward management responsibilities with ease. Most days, routine administrative and managerial tasks occupy her working day. The ward is frequently busy. Suzy is dissatisfied with some elements of her work. Her management role, with all the 'monitoring' activities this entails, has resulted in a growing sense of distance between Suzy and the wider nursing team. This 'monitoring' function seems to contribute to a culture in which Suzy is constantly checking what the team is doing rather than focusing on what the team has the potential to become. Although Suzy won promotion on the back of her reputation as an excellent clinical nurse, her nursing skills are not routinely applied in practice. She is aware that she 'manages' at a distance and is not closely 'involved' with the team of nurses she is responsible for or the people admitted to the ward. Since being promoted, Suzy has made few inroads into developing nursing practice on Cherry Ward. Nursing practice has an increasingly defensive flavour; emphasizing controlling elements of practice with reduced interpersonal contact between nurses and 'patients'.

Improving the quality of nursing care on Cherry Ward will involve the nursing team collectively re-thinking their approach to nursing practice. This is a practice development *process* in which the nursing team is invited to reconsider the role and function of nursing. As Ward Manager, Suzy is lynch pin. Ward Managers are cultural architects of nursing practice; they are able to influence the style of nursing practised and also set the tone of the ward atmosphere.[10] Developing nursing practice in practice hinges on effective teamwork.

EFFECTIVE TEAMWORKING

Effective teams are cohesive, self-supporting, and are very clear about their core purpose, or 'what it is that they are in business to do'. Douglas McGregor[11] described features of effective teamworking and the environment in which teams best function:

1 The atmosphere tends to be relaxed, comfortable and informal.

2 There is a great deal of open discussion regarding core team tasks.

3 The tasks and objectives of the team are well understood and accepted. Open discussion of core tasks has occurred and team members feel able to commit to them.

4 Team members listen to each other and are not afraid of looking foolish, because the team is supportive of new ideas/new approaches to work, even if new ideas seem extreme.

5 Disagreements are not surpressed, but rather are examined collectively with team members seeking to resolve problems constructively.

6 Decisions are made through consensus.

7 Criticism is frequent but comfortable.

8 Members of the team are able to openly express their feelings and ideas.

9 Clear direction is given.

10 The leader does not dominate the group. Team members are empowered to undertake tasks consistent with core team values.

Suzy recognizes that the 'relaxed open and informal' conditions that nurture effective teamworking also reflect the climate that best supports a therapeutic care environment. By developing a clinical leadership style that promotes these conditions she might empower the nursing team whilst also facilitating an improvement in the 'therapeutic atmosphere' on Cherry Ward.

Creating these supportive conditions will require Suzy to re-think her ward management role, seeking to reduce the 'distance' between herself and the nursing team, whilst also engaging more directly with the 'core business' of therapeutic caring at ward level. To achieve this Suzy will need to consider:

❑ Decentralizing her role within the team allowing responsibility for decision-making to be devolved to nurses working directly and more intimately with people in care.

❑ Adopting a style of leading that seeks to empower others.

❑ Developing a facilitative, involved and interactive style of communicating with the nursing team in order to promote an 'open' ward learning culture.

❑ Accepting that people make mistakes, but can learn and grow through these when well supported.

❑ Becoming an active role model of the style of therapeutic care she proposes for implementation on Cherry Ward.

❑ Recognizing that she is also learning and will also make mistakes from which she will learn and develop.

❑ Promoting the transition towards this new style of working in a collaborative spirit of 'adventure and fun'.

Central to the process of improving teamworking and developing therapeutic caring on Cherry Ward is the need for the nursing team to clearly identify, articulate and act on the 'core tasks' required to meet the human care needs of people in acute distress. This level of awareness is best facilitated through open team discussion.

CLARIFYING AND ACTING ON HUMAN CARE NEEDS

In order to establish the core tasks associated with nursing the person in acute distress, Suzy will facilitate a team away day. Unlike other managerially driven 'time out' days that have focused on 'What's not going right', 'What is going to happen as a consequence' and 'Rule reiteration' Suzy recognizes that this team away day will offer something different and is an opportunity for:

❑ Open 'whole team' discussion.

❑ Allowing the team to focus on what it might mean in *human* terms to be an inpatient on Cherry Ward.

❑ Identifying what people in acute distress *need nurses to do*.

❑ Allowing the team to propose the actions that need to be taken to meet the human care needs of the person in acute distress.

❑ Suzy to positively acknowledge the nursing team – saying thank you for the efforts routinely made by the team.

In order to achieve this agenda, Suzy will facilitate team discussion that centres on what it might be like to be a 'patient' on Cherry Ward. In order to address the gap between what nurses currently provide and what service users commonly remark that they need[12] Suzy will encourage discussion from the point of view of the person in distress and their family. It is important that this discussion is grounded in the 'everyday experience of the person in crisis'. Case examples can be used to track the everyday nature of the experience of the person in distress, the point being to illustrate what *actions* nurses routinely take to provide therapeutic care. Again it is important not to dwell on the 'philosophical underpinnings of practice' i.e. 'how nurses justify what they think they are doing' – rather the focus must be maintained on *what actions nurses can take* to best support the person in acute crisis.

One way of encouraging the team to focus on caring from the perspective of the person in crisis is to encourage discussion about what nurses routinely *do*. For example when admitting a person to hospital. Allow the team to write down what they currently do and explain why. Following on from this ask the team to write down what they would want to see *done* if a family member or close friend were admitted to the ward. Teams will usually employ 'softer' certainly less 'professional' language when describing the kind of supportive and collaborative care they would like to see offered to family or friends. This allows discussion to focus on the need to provide a more personable service, designed to meet the fundamental *human* care needs of the person in crisis. The key question to be addressed by the Cherry Ward Nursing Team is 'What actions can nurses take to translate this softer caring focus into everyday practice?' This practical focus allows nurses to identify with the person in crisis as a person who has fundamental care needs such as:

❑ Someone to listen to me.
❑ Someone to understand me.
❑ Someone to tell me what I might expect to happen and when.
❑ Friendly contact with someone that I can talk to and begin to trust.
❑ A safe, warm, stable and predictable environment.
❑ To get some rest.
❑ For there to be a sense of purpose to my admission to hospital.

The nursing team must work together to address these issues and might best address these concerns by:

❑ Creating a culture of *listening to* and where possible *acting on* what people in acute distress say that they need.
❑ Work in a way that is consistent with reducing the 'professional' barriers between the nurse and the person in crisis.
❑ Take action to develop 'professional friendships' with people in crisis, characterized by equality and mutual respect.
❑ Work in partnership with people on the ward to provide a stable, clean, warm and supportive care environment.
❑ Develop the person's sense of purpose through providing therapeutic structure to every day life on the ward.

STRUCTURING CARE TO ENABLE RECOVERY

Annie Altschul[13] recognized that the care environment is best organized when it is flexible enough to incorporate all needs. She also observed that people help each other where the supportive conditions exist for them to do so. The healing potential of the social environment has long been recognized and utilized by service users who commonly find value in meeting and talking with other people in distress.[12] The atmosphere and social surroundings of the ward is known as the milieu. Creative development of the milieu helps to provide the social conditions in which it becomes possible for people in care to undertake purposeful work, learning from each other, whilst living with and through individual experiences of distress. Within this supportive milieu the person in acute distress is able to:

❑ Undertake individual work to develop an understanding of the experience of distress.
❑ Share experiences with others in a similar situation both informally on the ward and through structured groupwork.
❑ Contribute towards helping others through shared experience.

The milieu is best developed through a combined sense of purpose, which helps to facilitate an inclusive 'spirit of collective togetherness'. To achieve this, the nursing team must provide therapeutic structure to ward based activity supporting both individual and groupworking. This structure is used to facilitate a milieu in which people can share their common experiences of distress, but remains flexible and responsive enough to cater for individual needs. This *therapeutic* structure is essential as it represents the counter-balance to the dominant *treatment* structure of the medical model. It is important to recognize that structuring care effectively brings a sense of purpose and organization to acute care. Without this nurses offer a service that is reactive rather than purposefully proactive.

Here, Jane's story is used to illustrate how the

key nurse works *with* the person to structure and organize care. The key nurse recognizes the need to work flexibly, responding to Jane's changing needs. This process involves working individually with Jane, involving other members of the team as supports in the key nurse's absence. This individualized care programme is augmented by inputs from the multiprofessional team and leads, ultimately, towards the development of the discharge planning process. The admission process is addressed in Chapter 51; here we focus on how nurses might provide individual and groupwork whilst recognizing the role of the wider multiprofessional team.

Jane's story

A concerned local shopkeeper telephones the police. He recognizes Jane as a regular customer who is usually very chatty and well presented. Today he sees her wandering round the town centre in the early morning well before the shops are due to open. She seems perplexed and somewhat dishevelled. On talking to her, she cannot account for what it is that she is doing. At the police station a doctor sees Jane. She appears profoundly worried and seems suspicious of people around her. Reluctantly, she agrees to admission to hospital.

On admission, Jane is provided with an environment in which she can begin to feel safe and emotionally supported. Nurses are best placed to provide this as the nursing team has continual presence in the ward environment. The 'key-nurse', (responsible for developing a close relationship with Jane and co-ordinating her care) becomes the lynchpin for meeting Jane's needs. Typically, nursing teams regard the process of 'admission' as pivotal to relationship building and also establishing the comfort of the person in their new surroundings. To achieve this, other nurses on the ward, support the nurse conducting the admission by allowing her sufficient time to complete the process. Beyond the process of admission however, the way things are organized on the ward is typically much looser and has less structure. This can result in confusion or lack of clarity about which nurse is doing what and when. Each nurse needs to function as key nurse to several people and needs to be 'free' to work individually with them on a regular basis, and to be involved in groupwork.

PRIORITIZING THE CARING PROCESS

Nurses structure short periods of direct contact time into every shift to help develop the helping relationship with Jane and to assess further her condition. This approach is likely to instil a growing sense of trust, purpose and increasing emotional attachment between Jane and the key nurse. This is the best way for nurses to get to know Jane. The ward manager or team leader will actively foster the expectation that people will have dedicated therapeutic sessions, perhaps lasting an hour,

twice a day. To prioritize this time for direct patient contact the ward manager might need to employ a few simple strategies like:

- ❏ Using a telephone answering machine.
- ❏ Restricting visiting for specific periods of time.
- ❏ Employing notices to tell others that important therapeutic work is in progress.
- ❏ Notifying other occupational groups that appointments need to be booked outside of these times to undertake specific procedures or assessment.

INDIVIDUAL SESSIONS

Using Barker's *Tidal Model*[14] Jane's individual sessions would focus on what was happening for Jane *here-and-now*, what she believed was *important* (in terms of her needs), and what personal knowledge or understanding she was gaining from the experience about 'what needs to happen next'. Individual sessions should emphasize collaboration. Nurses provide individual ring-fenced time for each person, but then allow the person in care to guide how 'collaborative working' might best be developed. Nurses might ask:

- ❏ What do you want from this time together now?
- ❏ How can *we* work together?
- ❏ What shall *we do*?

In the *Tidal Model* the record of the session is written 'live' rather than as a nursing report, after the event. This confirms the person's active role in the whole process of caring and being-in-care.

GROUPWORK

The value of sharing experience should not be underestimated as a medium for promoting shared learning and understanding. Groupwork can be very simple – organizing a venue for people to talk through issues like:

- ❏ 'What is going on for me today';
- ❏ 'How I am coping'; and
- ❏ 'What I will do if things start to go off course'.

In the Tidal Model Barker has identified three core forms of groupwork, which he believes are central to the recovery process. These have a particular application in an acute setting.

The Recovery Group usually is held in the morning when people may feel at a low ebb, and may lack the motivation to engage in anything too demanding. The group is held in a relaxed atmosphere, where people have a chance to identify and discuss positive aspects of themselves, which are often overlooked in the focus on their problems. A set of questions is often used to stimulate discussion:

❑ What is your favourite book, film or TV show and *why?*
❑ What would you do if you won the lottery?
❑ How do you think your pets (cat or dog) would describe you?
❑ What is the hardest thing you have ever done … and how did you do it?

The *Solutions Group* is usually held in the afternoon and focuses on developing the participants' awareness of what positive change would mean for them. Usually, one person is encouraged to be the 'model' for difficulties that might be common to the group, which helps the 'model' identify possible solutions that already may be part of the person's repertoire, albeit perhaps at a low level.

The *Information Group* is usually held in the evening and focuses on providing people with information about their ongoing care and treatment or supporting services. Common topics include:

❑ Medication – effects, side-effects and contraindications.
❑ Support in the community following discharge.
❑ Self-help groups – their form and function.
❑ Financial matters.

A genuine 'expert' should lead this group. In the case of community-based support, often a former user of psychiatric services will lead the discussion on mutual support or self-help groups.

POWER AND MULTIPROFESSIONAL TEAM MEETINGS

Team meetings are a well-established means of reviewing progress as well as planning future care in acute settings. Often, meetings are led by a consultant psychiatrist and involve a wide range of other professional groups such as social workers, occupational therapists and members of community mental health teams. In Jane's, it would not be unusual for 6–8 professional staff (most of whom will have little direct contact with Jane), to be involved in discussing and making important decisions about ongoing care. It goes without saying that Jane's involvement in this process is essential. However, meetings are commonly structured in a way that risks intimidating anyone, far less someone who is mentally distressed.

There is an absolute requirement to plan and structure Jane's future care and treatment efficiently and this needs to involve team-wide discussion. However, traditional 'reviews' and 'ward rounds' are unlikely to allow Jane the best opportunity to express herself. Recognizing this, the key nurse must support Jane through the multiprofessional team meeting ensuring that one way or another Jane's point of view is heard. The nurse might:

❑ Identify Jane's view of her progress and the support she needs in advance of the meeting.
❑ Arrange for Jane to see the doctor outside the larger meeting if she prefers to do so.
❑ Encourage Jane to make a list of what needs to be said in her own words.
❑ Agree with Jane that the nurse will talk through 'Jane's issues' on her behalf if she feels unable to do so.

PACING THE PERSON

For Jane, re-establishing emotional stability is a *process*, a significant element of which involves allowing sufficient time within a supportive environment for her to adjust to her changing life circumstances. Only where these features of recovery become comfortably established does it realistically become desirable for her to face the important next step of returning home. Barker has argued that the most important question that needs to be asked in acute care is 'what needs to change for the person to return home?'[15] For many people the problems that were part of their admission to hospital are still awaiting them – at home or in the community. The process of discharging the person from hospital is likely to involve the key nurse in:

❑ Discussing individual concerns with Jane.
❑ Supporting her in discussions with the wider multiprofessional team regarding her individual care needs on discharge.
❑ Supported visits home.
❑ Trial periods of leave at home prior to discharge to test out common assumptions regarding Jane's ability to cope.
❑ Introducing Jane to the community-based key worker who takes over responsibility for co-ordinating care for Jane on discharge.
❑ Working with Jane and the multiprofessional team to determine a discharge plan and agreed discharge date.

Length of stay in hospital is often viewed as a measure of best practice and the desire to somehow speed up the process of caring is a seemingly constant feature of modern health care policy. Nurses must remain vigilant to ensure that the process of managing care does not distract nurses from the core work of providing therapeutic care. It is not unusual for people to change their 'presentation' when in hospital. The key question is, to what extent does this reflect the kind of change needed to allow the person to return home, *and* return to ordinary living? People in care need to be treated as 'people' rather than impersonal objects, processed by the health care system. Nurses have an absolute responsibility to remain true to the individual care needs of the person in crisis. They might best do this by acknowledging that recovery has its own pace, a tempo that is individual to the person

CONCLUSION

The primary focus of psychiatric nursing in acute settings is to establish close interpersonal relationships that focus on relating with the person in acute distress, attempting to understand the person's experience and the effects this has on their ability to live everyday life.[15] Psychiatric mental health nurses must also consider how to organize and structure nursing care to support this degree of human contact, inside ward environments that offer a responsive crisis service. This is best achieved when nurses work toward creating a milieu that is purposeful and structured in order that the person in care might begin to learn individually and in groups about their experience of acute distress.

Acute inpatient nursing is highly team focused. Team nursing in acute settings becomes strengthened when nurses identify with nursing as a practice of equal value and standing within the multiprofessional team. From this vantage point nurses might re-think their practice recognizing the value and purpose of structuring ward-based activity to enable close human contact with people in crisis. It has long been recognized that nursing has the potential to be therapeutic in its own right.[19] If nurses fail to recognize and utilize their own 'natural' therapeutic potential, they might always be likened to a caterpillar, who on observing a butterfly proclaims 'You'd never get me up in one of those!'

REFERENCES

1. McMahon R. Therapeutic nursing: theory, issues and practice. In: McMahon R, Pearson A (eds). *Nursing as therapy*, 2nd edn. Cheltenham: Stanley Thornes, 1998.
2. Peplau H. *Interpersonal relations in nursing*. London: Macmillan, 1988.
3. Barker PJ. *The philosophy and practice of psychiatric nursing*. Edinburgh: Churchill-Livingstone, 1999.
4. Barchard C. Patient perspectives on mental health-care delivery. *Community Mental Health* 1998; Summer: 17–19.
5. Clarke L. *Challenging ideas in psychiatric nursing*. London: Routledge, 1999.
6. Wright S. Facilitating therapeutic nursing and independent practice. In: McMahon R, Pearson A (eds). *Nursing as therapy*, 2nd edn. Cheltenham: Stanley Thornes, 1998.
7. Jackson S, Stevenson C. What do people need psychiatric and mental health nurses for? *Journal of Advanced Nursing* 2000; **31**(2): 378–88.
8. Barker PJ. *The Tidal Model*. Newcastle: University of Newcastle, 2000.
9. Bowles AE. *Getting extraordinary things done in a mental health service: reflections on a transformational journey*. Unpublished Conference Presentation: Valuing Mental Health Nursing, 3rd European Mental Health Nursing Conference, Belfast, 1998.
10. Fretwell JE. *Freedom to change: the creation of a ward learning environment*. London: Royal College of Nursing, 1985.
11. McGregor D. *The human side of enterprise*. New York: McGraw-Hill, 1960.
12. Rogers A, Pilgrim D, Lacey R. *Experiencing psychiatry*. London: Macmillan, 1993.
13. Altschul AT. *Patient–nurse interaction*. Edinburgh: University of Edinburgh/Churchill Livingstone, 1972.
14. Barker P. The Tidal Model: developing an empowering, person-centred approach to recovery within psychiatric and mental health nursing. *Journal of Psychiatric and Mental Health Nursing* 2001; 8(3): 233–40.
15. Barker PJ. *Assessment in psychiatric and mental health nursing*. Cheltenham: Stanley Thornes, 1997.

Chapter 43

COMMUNITY MENTAL HEALTH CARE

Denis Ryan*

INTRODUCTION

The development and expansion of community mental health services in the second half of the 20th century and the expansion of primary health care poses challenges for traditional mental health care. This chapter will concentrate on the role of mental health nurses as key stakeholders in that development and considers nursing within the evolving community mental health and the necessary partnerships involved.

CONTEXT

Health and illness prevention have been the subject of intense debate and reappraisal in the latter half of the 20th century. Traditional understandings of health were underpinned by the 'medical model', which dominated the practice of health service providers for over two centuries. Although beneficial to our understanding of biological functioning, this approach has hindered appreciation of the relationship between various facets of human functioning as well as the relationships between man and the broader environment.

The influence of the medical model also had a profound impact on the organization and delivery of care,

especially the development of specialities, which concentrated on individual human 'systems' or 'subsystems'. Nursing has tended to follow medicine, organizing itself along similar lines as medical practitioners, developing areas of specialist practice, which distinguished between adult (general) nursing, paediatric (sick children's) nursing, mental handicap and mental health nursing, as well as midwifery. This separation between mental health and general nursing has existed since the 1860s, when psychiatric or mental health nursing (as we know it today) evolved in Great Britain and Ireland.[1] Since then, these branches of nursing have remained separate.

Since at least the early 1950s there has been an evolving and significant debate in the literature around the issue of the development of generic mental health workers and integrated or collaborative working. Early theorists such as Hildegard Peplau argued that one of the key roles of the mental health nurse was to support (on a voluntary basis) the work of psychiatrists. This perspective seems to argue for the legitimacy of the complementary role of psychiatric-mental health nurses and psychiatrists. Conversely, much of the debate around the issue of the professionalization of nursing has centred on the *distinctive* nature of nursing practice, the *autonomy* of nurses and the *development of unique knowledge*. On superficial inspection, it would seem somewhat

*Denis Ryan is a Lecturer in Nursing at the Department of Nursing, University of Limerick in Ireland. Prior to that he was a Nursing Tutor with the Mid Western Health Board and Nursing Practice Development Co-ordinator for the South Eastern Health Board. He was Assistant Chief Nursing Officer in both the South Eastern and Mid Western Health Boards and has worked mainly in acute inpatient, community care and addiction services.

contradictory to be involved in a supportive role of another profession, while at the same time developing autonomous practice. However, the reality of care practice settings, which involve a range of health care professionals, means that collaborative care is both a reality and a necessity. It is also important to note that collaborative care does not or should not imply superiority or conversely subordinate roles.

EVOLUTION OF COMMUNITY MENTAL HEALTH NURSING

The second half of the 20th century witnessed a sustained period of change in the organization and delivery of mental health services. As the negative effects of institutional living became recognized, institutional care, internationally, increasingly became politically, professionally and socially unacceptable. From the 1950s onward, there was a marked decrease in the overall population of traditional psychiatric hospitals. In tandem with this reduction, outpatient, day-care and community-based services developed. Despite the parallel evolution of services, there was not a proportionate increase in, or transfer of, resources to community-based services. However, today, it is estimated that most mental health treatment and care is in community settings.[2]

Despite the fact that care in the community has been evolving for over 50 years, there still is no consensus as to the proper role and function of mental health nurses who work in community settings.[3] Much of the debate centres on the issue of whether or not community mental health nurses should work with those who have severe and enduring mental illnesses, or those with less disabling mental disturbances. These debates are a function of various ideological and professional concerns, resource considerations, and boundary debates, which will be addressed in this chapter.

Whatever about the distinctions between 'serious' and 'less-serious' mental health conditions, the importance of mental health issues to the overall health agenda in the foreseeable future has been highlighted by the World Health Organization.[4,5] The burden of mental illness has been a growing cause of concern at both the global and local levels, and trends in care and treatment have mirrored trends towards greater emphasis on provision of mental health services in primary care settings.

The extent to which national governments emphasize the importance of mental health is reflected in health policies and strategies (e.g. in Ireland – *Quality and Fairness; A Health System for You*).[6] It is notable that in most Western countries such national and local strategy documents reflect the development and enhancement of primary care, as well as a move towards more integrated care. This has distinct implications for the future development of community-based psychiatric/mental health nursing practice.

From the establishment of the asylum system, mental health care has evolved as a specialist area of practice, both physically and metaphorically segregated from the mainstream of health and social services as well as society. The influence of this historical development cannot be overstated and has contributed to the view among members of the public, as well as other professionals, that mental health nursing requires special characteristics of its practitioners.[7] While this may be flattering, it may act as a disincentive for those wishing to choose nursing as a career.[8] In addition, viewing mental health nursing as a specialist area may add to the stigma of mental health difficulties, when most other health matters can be addressed at a primary care level.

These are some of the factors that have contributed to the difficulty of defining the future role of the community psychiatric-mental health nurse.[3] In addition, the difficulty of prescribing future roles cannot be unrelated to the fact that there had been a variety of systems of community mental health nursing practice. These seem to have evolved organically, directly related to service need and existing organizational models, rather than being strategically planned. In addition, they have evolved differently within different jurisdictions. By way of illustration, the development of community mental health nursing in the UK and the Republic of Ireland might be considered.

Both have cultural, geographical and historical ties and mental health services and practice evolved from shared historical origins. However, there are clear distinctions between both systems. For example, the most usual model of community mental health teams in the UK is multidisciplinary, located in the community within which they operate. While this system is similar to that in the Republic of Ireland, there are distinct differences. In the UK system, community mental health teams normally do not have access to their own dedicated inpatient services,[10] while the Irish system has and remains (in most cases) directly a part of specialist mental health services, which provide both inpatient and community care. Both systems are, however, based on principles of sectorization.

It has been argued that community mental health teams will play a major role in developing a future framework for mental health services.[11] While there is little doubt that this will be the case, the current diverse nature of definitions of the 'community mental health team' means that a clear understanding of its contribution to care and treatment remains poorly understood and certainly is not universal in nature. Many teams have evolved in response to local circumstances and while ostensibly following a common model, their development has occurred in an unstructured and fragmented manner.

Fragmentation may relate to the fact that community mental health nurses, while increasingly recognized as specialist practitioners, have attempted to establish themselves as a distinct professional group. The distinctions relate to other groups within community mental health teams as well as within other services. Therefore, while both the traditional focus of community mental health nurses was similar in nature, organization and design to that of public health nurses or health visitors – based mainly on a model of domiciliary care and support – community mental health nurses also try to highlight distinctions between themselves and other community nurses. At the same time, community mental health nurses have also tried to distinguish their work from that of hospital-based psychiatric-mental health nurses[12] and social workers, clinical psychologists, occupational therapists, psychiatrists, who may be their team colleagues.

One of the most important reasons for this concern with role and function relates to the atmosphere of change and uncertainty which has permeated health service provision over the past 20-odd years. Clear roles, relationships and boundaries were features of hospital-based care and were not entirely eroded with the change to community-based care. However, the variety of emergent models and the dynamic nature of the change which has ensued, may well have destabilized nurses, encouraging the search for professional meaning which has become a feature of the development of community mental health nursing.

DEVELOPMENTS IN COMMUNITY MENTAL HEALTH CARE

Since the beginning of the deinstitutionalization programme in the 1950s, emphasis has been given to the care in the community and the prevention of inappropriate admissions to hospital-based care. The evolution of community mental health nursing has been closely aligned to such policies. Two core models of community nursing have evolved which, while separate, can be seen as developmentally interlinked and likely to influence future developments of this area of practice.

In the first model community mental health nursing developed as part of a *secondary level* care initiative, segregated from other forms of nursing, established within specialist mental health teams.

The second model involves integrated service provision as part of *primary care* teams. The recent debates concerning the merits and demerits of nurses' work with people with severe and enduring mental illnesses, or more extended roles, is linked inextricably to these two models of care. The broader model of collaborative/integrated care at primary care level has been advocated as a desirable approach in such diverse jurisdictions as Australia[13] and Ireland.[6] In these settings emphasis is placed on the provision of mental health care within a primary care framework, although the specific operational models may differ.

The specialist team approach

Traditionally, mental health services have been specialist *and* separate, provided mainly as a secondary or tertiary service. The separateness of psychiatric services was evident in the situation of asylums, which were built geographically remote and separate from other medical services. This distinction was also evident historically when early nurse leaders vehemently opposed the use of the title 'Nurse' by asylum attendants.[1] While there is little doubt that the integration of acute inpatient services within large general hospitals has helped bring about a greater acceptance of mental illnesses, perceptions of professional difference continue among and between health care professionals involved in mental health care practice.[7]

With the increasing demand for non-institutional mental health care alternatives from the 1950s onwards, it is unsurprising that specialist practitioners in mental health nursing emerged to meet this need. However, they were drawn from a background and ethos of institutionally based care. Current day hospital and day centre services evolved from models of domiciliary care and outpatient clinics, which were literally extensions of hospital programmes. However, nurses figured strongly in all such developments.

Much of the emphasis of the specialist team approach was based on a philosophy of supporting individuals following discharge from hospital and providing care aimed at preventing inappropriate readmission. Much of this concentrated on developing a supportive network for people. The change in the location of the service from hospital to home, or at least within the patient's local community, involved not just a change of site, but also involved a change in professional mindset. It also required a change in the 'power' relationship[14] between service provider and the user.

The predominant feature of nurse–patient relationships in hospital was one in which the locus of control and power rested firmly with the nurse. This relationship has significantly altered in community care practice where the nurse is effectively a 'guest' in the services user's home. Domiciliary and outpatient care is distinguished from hospital care in the level of negotiation required. While the clearly defined role of the hospital nurse means that their function is explicitly and implicitly understood, the authority and credibility of the nurse in community-based care systems must be established and maintained on an individual basis.

In addition to the altered power relationships, the setting of care is important. With increasing emphasis being placed on holistic approaches to care, access to the natural living environment is recognized as central to an understanding of the person's normal world. This has benefits from the perspective of assessment and intervention planning. This access also provides opportunities for long-term care initiatives.

A natural extension of the type of support and interventions undertaken in domiciliary care was the expansion of day hospital and day-centre care. These were developed within specialist multidisciplinary teams, aimed at making care available at a site as close as possible to the person's own home. Most centres were developed to serve designated geographic locations or particular populations, and were underpinned by principles of service sectorization. In an organizational context, most day hospitals and day-centres were developed as part of dedicated and specialist mental health services. Within such structures, mental health nurses provide counselling, psycho-social interventions, liaison services, depot injection clinics, psycho-educational initiatives, among other services. In addition they may also fulfil the role of care co-ordinators.

Specialist services that remain organizationally segregated from primary care have often been accused of merely translating the traditional hospital care into an extra-mural service. One function of the asylum system was to act as an agency of 'social control'. The obligation of mental health services to detain individuals was enshrined in legislation. In some jurisdictions, such as the UK, although the asylum system has been dismantled, recent legislation implies that particular groups still require 'policing' in relation to their continued care.[9] While such roles have been legitimized, and largely fall within the remit of community mental health nurses, the ethos of community care within specialist care teams is based, at least in part, on a social control ethic deriving from its asylum origins, and illustrated through reliance on chemical methods of control, such as depot injections or major tranquillizers. The administration of such injections was a major feature of early community mental health nursing and in some instances continue to remain so.

The role of the community mental health nurse in medication administration and management has been contentious from the perspectives of professional development and autonomy. The early development of community mental health nursing was strongly associated with post-discharge care, in which medication management played a predominant role. The role of mental health nurses in medication management, and issues of compliance with the treatment regimes can be viewed from two perspectives. On the one hand, the role of nurses is seen as vital, with increasing calls for an enhanced role in relation to prescribing medication. On the other hand, broadening the role of the nurse to include such traditional medical functions can also be interpreted a reassertion of the dominance of the medical model of care,[9] thereby retaining nursing in a subservient relationship to medical practitioners. Such moves have been welcomed by many,[15] perhaps because they can be seen as a logical conclusion to the blurring of roles and the merging of skills, which may occur in multidisciplinary work.

Generally speaking, multidisciplinary work has evolved as the norm in specialist mental health care teams. Despite the obvious attractions of such an approach for clinically based nurses with (by implication) the removal of middle-management grades, for mental health nursing there is a greater reliance on other disciplines, a consequent diminution of professional autonomy and arguably, decreased efficiency through inappropriate utilization of specialist skills.[16] Indeed this form of working has been blamed for generating role confusion and uncertainty, culminating in increased pressure on staff working within such arrangements.[17]

The seriously mentally ill and the 'worried well'

The concentration on medication must also be understood within the context of the client group using the services. Perhaps because specialist mental health services and community mental health teams provide a second level service, especially to people following discharge from acute or rehabilitation programmes, the focus was on the most severely mentally ill, who require the highest levels of support. Within the more recent history of community mental health nursing there has been a shift in emphasis, and a tendency in some instances at least, for community mental health nurses to work with the 'worried well'. This trend can be understood as a natural progression to meet the needs of the largest number of people who use primary care services, who may have underlying or co-morbid mental health conditions. It is also a move that has been severely criticized.

It can, for example, be argued that the level of dependency of those with serious and enduring mental health illnesses requires specialist intervention from highly competent professionals. In some countries at least, it has been argued that this population (from a policy perspective) is the group towards which community mental health nursing resources should be directed.[18,19] However, adequate operational definitions of the concept of severe and enduring mental illness have not yet emerged. This has hindered research initiatives and clinical practice. Despite conceptual confusion, it is clear that most definitions deal with the illnesses which are persistent, ongoing and are associated with a significant burden within either personal, interpersonal, family or social domains. People with such illness, including schizophrenia, require social support as well as other forms of 'clinical' support. In the case of schizophrenia, social support is assumed to be associated with caring and competence.[20] However, it is not just the *level* of social support which is important, it is also the *type* of support available which must be considered.[21]

EVOLVING ROLES IN SPECIALIST COMMUNITY CARE TEAMS

Within the broad model of specialist community mental health teams, several different approaches have developed, which have expanded the nurse's role from its origins. There has been increasing recognition that the original model of community mental health care, which operated within normal business hours, was insufficient within a care system that had decreased reliance on inpatient care. Where community services were effectively an extension of institutionally based care, operation within normal business hours remained a sustainable model of practice. In such situations, a pool of staff from hospital services could supplement demands for 'out of hours' requirements. However, as this model developed, and as access to inpatient care became increasingly difficult, the requirement for out of hours arrangements increased. While the emergence of concepts such as crisis intervention teams, as well as assertive outreach programmes were generally welcomed as initiatives that are necessary to support individuals to manage manifestations of their illness, there has also been criticism of the expansion of such services, primarily on the basis that such an expansion effectively replaces the model of supervision and control which were the hallmark of the old asylum system.[22]

Integrated care models

Much of the debate around where community nurses should be based and their legitimate role, revolves around the issue of the organization of care and the utilization of scarce resources. In most countries there is agreement that community mental health nurses are specialist practitioners and some of the debate has focused on whether or not such specialist practitioners should be a support and training provider for non-mental health specialists, such as primary care teams and other hospital-based staff or should themselves, be part of those teams. In practice, community mental health nurses combine both functions in many instances.

In addition it can be argued that the organizational context in which community mental health teams (and by association community mental health nurses) evolved, no longer makes organizational sense. Community mental health nursing was largely born out of deinstitutionalization. It has since been shaped by the influence of the user/consumer movement, which can be credited with increasing accountability and transparency in the traditional health services. These combined issues were linked, notably, to the work of institutionally based services that were required to act as an agency of social control while at the same time being shrouded in secrecy.

While there has been a protracted debate about the best organizational arrangements and base for community mental health nursing, public health policy has encouraged the view that health care provision should be focused on primary health care provision. Internationally, models of community mental health nursing have been based in primary care services. Many of the mental health nursing services in such arrangements have concentrated their therapeutic engagements on the so-called 'worried well'. Conversely, there have been repeated calls in nursing literature for the concentration of the valuable expertise of expert nurse practitioners on with the most seriously mentally ill. These calls seem logical, but in some instances have followed negative media attention on scandals and crimes related to former mental health service users, thereby emphasizing the potential for violence or neglect associated with serious mental disorders. However, it can equally be argued that responses of this nature are reactionary and only represent one facet of mental health nursing. If community mental health nursing services are limited in such an artificial manner, other service users are deprived of a valuable service.[23]

Primary care services provide care for a wide range of psychological and social problems that often require psycho-social interventions that can be delivered appropriately by mental health nurses. Currently, some of the arguments surrounding the use of mental health nursing in primary care services relate to the issue of the legitimate roles of health care professionals and the blurring of boundaries. While interdisciplinary working requires the natural blurring of roles, the use of community mental health nurses to treat people with less serious disorders (the worried well) may have more to do with the desire of overworked general practitioners to divert such demanding patients to others, than appropriate utilization of specialized practitioners within a team context.

Another confounding factor in primary health care settings in some jurisdictions – such as the UK – is the often arbitrary and arguably artificial distinction between 'health' and 'social' care. In other jurisdictions, such as the Republic of Ireland, health policies, incorporated the notion of 'health and social gain' as an index of measurement – thus integrating these concepts in a health framework with consequent implications for practice.

THE COMMUNITY MENTAL HEALTH NURSE AND INTERDISCIPLINARY WORKING

A consensus is emerging that community mental health nurses play a valuable role in service delivery. When considering the roles and functions of community mental health nurses in interdisciplinary work, it is helpful to consider the care groups with whom nurses most frequently work. National health strategies commonly express the belief that community mental health nurses are a highly qualified and skilled professional group that should work with those with serious and enduring mental health difficulties. This seems to enjoy widespread support among health care professionals.[27] However, there is also some support for community mental health nurses acting as resource agents or in a consultancy role for primary care teams[27] as a source of specialist referral.[28] There also is support for roles in the care and treatment of people with Anxiety disorders; who need to develop problem-solving skills; who present with depression as well as psychotic disorders[28] – in other words a range of mental health difficulties.[23]

Traditionally, community mental health nurses were accessed through a referral system. In most instances, this was through another health care professional – most commonly a consultant psychiatrist, another member of the specialist multidisciplinary team or the general practitioner. While this may have meant that scarce resources were likely to be used for those with greatest need, it also meant that integrated work with other non-mental health care professionals was extremely limited. The move towards integrated models of care has been progressively advanced from the 1980s onwards and an important feature of that progression has been the move to develop new team structures – liaison mental health (psychiatric) teams, assertive outreach programmes and crisis teams – as well as care programme approaches in which community mental health nurses could play a prominent role.

The role of the community mental health nurse is evolving and developing. A complicating factor, which inhibits adequate definition of the distinct attributes of the community mental health nurse, is that professional boundaries were expected to become somewhat blurred through interdisciplinary work. However, there is some indication that professional boundaries remain a feature of interdisciplinary work.[16] While there is evidence that the community mental health nurses are valued by stakeholders it is also clear that these teams are frequently inadequately resourced.[29]

The debates over nurses' exclusive focus on people with serious and enduring mental illness, coupled with the demise of traditional psychiatric hospitals, has highlighted the need for specialized services for a wide range of people in primary care. It has also generated debate over who should provide these services and the skills, knowledge and background they should have. Primary care teams are increasingly faced with complex mental health issues for which they are not always adequately prepared.[30] This raises the issue of the community mental health nurse acting as a skills or training resource to non-mental health practitioners, which has also been widely advocated.

Community mental health nurses are in an excellent position to provide a wide range of services to people in the community.[23] Their roles might include those of therapist, consultant/advisor, liaison agent and assessor[2] either on their own or in combination. It is likely that these roles will form the basis for a practice model in future primary health care teams. To facilitate the removal of the often false and arbitrary distinction between physical, psychological and social problems, the role of health educator/promoter could perhaps be added to this list. However, to fulfil these roles to the highest level, the educational preparation and training of future practitioners will need to reflect these roles, while the needs of those moving from traditional hospital-based services and training need also to be identified and addressed.[24] Specialist training and further education, while desirable, are not an essential requirement for community mental health nursing practice in all circumstances.

While adequate educational and training preparation are essential for the development and enhancement of community mental health nursing services, it is equally essential to recognize that the essential components of the psycho-educational and therapeutic roles are fulfilled. The relationship between service users and health care professionals is the single most valued component of care as reported by patients.[25] Community mental health nurses are in a position to support service users through the creation or maintenance of the therapeutic milieu. To provide support, the environment in which care is given should be characterized by an ethos of acceptance; the creation and maintenance of a positive atmosphere; expectation of change; responsiveness; normalization; and an educative component.[26] While these features are likely to require greater empirical validation, they provide an initial framework, through which the requirements of community mental health nursing might best be understood.

REFERENCES

1. Nolan P. *A history of mental health nursing.* London: Chapman and Hall, 1993.

2. Walker L, Barker P, Pearson P. The required role of the psychiatric-mental health nurse in primary health-care: an augmented Delphi study. *Nursing Inquiry* 2000; 7: 91–102.

3. O'Brien LM. Nurse–client relationships: The experience of community psychiatric nurses. *Journal of the Australian and New Zealand College of Mental Health Nurses* 2000; 9: 184–94.

4. World Health Organization (2001). *The World Health Report 2001. Mental health: new understanding, new hope.* Geneva: WHO, 2001.

5. World Health Organization (2000) *WHO guide to mental health in primary care.* London: Royal Society of Medicine, 2000.

6. Department of Health and Children. *Quality and fairness: a health system for you.* Dublin: Stationery Office, 2001.

7. Wells JSG, Ryan D, McElwee CN. 'I don't want to be a psychiatric nurse': an exploration of factors inhibiting recruitment to psychiatric nursing in Ireland. *Journal of Psychiatric and Mental Health Nursing* 2000; 7: 79–87.

8. Wells JSG, Ryan D, McElwee CN, Boyce M, Forkan CJ. *Worthy not worthwhile?: choosing careers in caring occupations.* Waterford: Waterford Institute of Technology, 2000.

9. Wells JSG. Severe mental illness, statutory supervision and mental health nursing in the United Kingdom: meeting the challenge. *Journal of Advanced Nursing* 1998; 27(4): 698–706.

10. Barr W, Hukley P. The impact of community mental health reform on service users: a cohort study. *Health and Social Care in the Community* 1999; 7(2): 129–39.

11. McKenna H, Keeney S, Bannon D, Finn A. An exploration of community psychiatric nursing: a Northern Ireland perspective. *Journal of Psychiatric and Mental Health Nursing* 2000; 7(5): 455–61.

12. Morall P. *Mental health nursing and social control.* London: Whurr, 1988.

13. Australian Health Ministers' Conference. *Second National Mental Health Plan.* Canberra: Australian Government Publishing Service, 1988.

14. Muir-Cochrane E. The context of care: Issues of power and control between patients and community mental health nurses. *International Journal of Nursing Practice* 2000; 6(6): 292–300.

15. Snelgrove S, Hughes D. Interprofessional relations between doctors and nurses: Perspectives from South Wales. *Journal of Advanced Nursing* 2000; 31 (3): 661–7.

16. Brown B, Crawford P, Darongkamas J. Blurred roles and permeable boundaries: the experience of multidisciplinary working in community mental health. *Health and Social Care in the Community* 2000; 8 (6): 425–35.

17. Sainsbury Centre for Mental Health. *Pulling together: The future role and training of mental health staff.* London: Sainsbury Centre for Mental Health, 1997.

18. Gournay K. Schizophrenia: a review of the contemporary literature and implications for mental health nursing theory, practice and education. *Journal of Psychiatric and Mental Nursing* 1996; 3: 7–12.

19. Audit Commission. *Finding a place: a review of mental health services for adults.* London: HMSO, 1994.

20. Buchanan J. Social support and schizophrenia: a review of the literature. *Archives of Psychiatric Nursing* 1995; 9(2): 68–76.

21. Clinton M, Lunney P, Edwards H, Wei D, Barr J. Perceived social support and community adaptation in schizophrenia. *Journal of Advanced Nursing* 1998; 27(5): 955–65.

22. Godin P. A dirty business: caring for people who are a nuisance or a danger. *Journal of Advanced Nursing* 2000; 32(6): 1396–402.

23. Bowers L. Community psychiatric nurse caseloads and the 'worried well': mis-spent time or vital work? *Journal of Advanced Nursing* 1997; 26(5): 930–36.

24. Bugge C, Smith LN, Shanley E. A descriptive study of multidisciplinary mental health staff moving to the community: the demographic and educational issues. *Journal of Psychiatric and Mental Health Nursing* 1997; 4: 45–54.

25. Solomon P, Draine J. Satisfaction with mental health treatment in a randomised trial of consumer case management. *Journal of Nervous and Mental Disease* 1994; 182: 179–84.

26. Evans IM, Moltzen NL. Defining effective community support for long-term psychiatric patients according to behavioural principles. *Australian and New Zealand Journal of Psychiatry* 2000; 34: 637–44.

27. Bruce J, Watson D, vanTeijlingen ER, Lawton K, Watson MS, Palin AN. Dedicated psychiatric care within general practice: health outcome and service providers' views. *Journal of Advanced Nursing* 1999; 29(5): 1060–67.

28. Badger F, Nolan P. General practitioners' perceptions of community psychiatric nurses in primary care. *Journal of Psychiatric and Mental Health Nursing* 1999; 6: 453–9.

29. Shanley E, Watson G, Cole A. Survey of stakeholders' opinions of community psychiatric nursing services. *Australian and New Zealand Journal of Mental Health Nursing* 2001; 10: 77–86.

30. Russell G, Potter L. Mental health issues in primary healthcare. *Journal of Clinical Nursing* 2002; 11: 118–25.

Chapter 44

CRISIS ASSESSMENT AND INTERVENTION*

Clare Hopkins**

INTRODUCTION

We all know what it is to be in crisis. We are faced with a problem for which we do not have a solution and that is not responsive to any of our usual coping strategies. For example, you miss the last bus home and are stranded in an area where you feel at risk. You have no money for a taxi and no means of contacting friends or relatives (your usual coping strategies). The reader will be able to think of many similar examples of being in crisis. Crises of this sort may be very distressing but are often self-limiting, even if no action is taken. If you are attacked and your personal belongings are stolen this then becomes an *emergency*, but morning will eventually come, or someone will offer you help. There are various factors that distinguish this kind of crisis from a mental health/psychiatric crisis.

When people experience a mental health crisis:

❏ They may be having feelings and experiences that are completely new to them and which may be extremely frightening.
❏ They and those around them may perceive the person as being 'different' not only from their usual self but also from most other people.

❏ This sense of difference can be isolating, or may even evoke anxiety fear, guilt and hostility in others. It may also leave those who are usually the person's friends and supporters feeling baffled and helpless. This in turn may mean that they keep their distance and withdraw their support. They too may be in crisis.
❏ If this is their first experience of such a crisis, they may have limited ways of coping. If they have experienced this kind of crisis before and were unable to find a way to cope, they may feel helpless.

Mental health crises take many forms and can be seen by professionals as having differing degrees of severity. However, if the person and their family are in crisis because of a mental health problem, these differing degrees will be irrelevant, they will simply be in crisis and in need of help. Much will depend upon their previous experience of mental health problems and their own coping styles.

CRISIS THEORY AND THE PERSON IN MENTAL HEALTH CRISIS

In November 1942 there was a fire at the Coconut Grove nightclub in Boston where nearly 500 people

*The advice and support of Stephen Niemiec, Nurse Consultant at the Newcastle Crisis Assessment and Treatment Team, is acknowledged in the development of this chapter.
**Clare Hopkins is a mental health nurse with special interests in working with people who self-harm and with people who are in crisis. At present she is a Senior Lecturer in Mental Health Nursing at the University of Northumbria in England.

died. Erich Lindemann and his colleagues worked with the survivors and relatives of the dead to help them come to terms with their grief. Lindemann[1] proposed theories about the grief process and how people who were experiencing this process might be helped to come to terms with their loss, and so avoid the possibility of longer-term psychological difficulties. Lindemann and Caplan[2] set up a community programme in Boston based on crisis theory and using crisis intervention techniques. For the time, this was highly unusual, since it focused on short-term therapy with the aim of avoiding longer-term distress and psychological pathology.

According to Caplan[2] the experience of crisis is universal. People face crisis when they encounter an 'obstacle to important life goals'; one that is not amenable to the person's usual coping strategies. 'A period of disorganization ensues, a period of upset during which many abortive attempts at solution are made'. Caplan identified three phases of crisis:

1 **'Onset'**: The immediate increase in tension as the individual realizes that the problem cannot be resolved quickly.

2 **'Breakdown'/'disorganization'**: Tension and anxiety quickly rise to intolerable levels and all of the person's coping strategies become exhausted. It is at this point that the person may turn to others for help. This is often the point at which the person's behaviour may change – they may stop meeting their responsibilities or cease caring for themselves.

3 **'Resolution'**: Because crises are often passing events, a resolution of some kind may occur. However, this resolution may be positive or negative. If the outcome is positive then the person may have learned new, positive, ways to help themselves in the future, or they may develop ways of coping, that are harmful.

The aim of crisis intervention is to help the person during the phases of 'breakdown' or 'disorganization,' when they may be amenable to finding or learning new ways of coping with difficulties. The term crisis has a range of different meanings and derivations. The original Greek term for crisis meant *decision*. In Chinese the word is represented by two symbols, one meaning *danger* and the other *opportunity*.[3] The Shorter Oxford English Dictionary[4] defines crisis as:

A turning point in the course of anything; also, a state of affairs in that a decisive change for better or worse is imminent.

Crine[5] sums up the aims of crisis intervention:

In times of crisis people tend to be more dependent, more open to suggestion and advice, than they usually are. Crisis intervention aims to capitalize on this psychological state to achieve the maximum impact on the individual and his family with the minimum of medical intervention.

Although crisis theory was built around the experiences of people who are normally psychologically healthy but exposed to extraordinary events, it has been successfully applied to people in mental health crisis. However, it is important to stress the difference between a mental health crisis and a psychiatric emergency. Crompton[6] uses Caplan's model to describe a psychiatric emergency:

A psychiatric emergency is when the person has gone beyond the breakdown phase, and has adopted a maladaptive solution.

A psychiatric emergency may require a more formal response if the maladaptive strategy involves risk to the person or to those around them and these formal responses may include invoking mental health legislation or involving the police.

EVOLUTION OF CRISIS SERVICES IN THE UK

The evolution of teams using crisis theory in the UK has been slow and erratic and there has been no consistent approach to providing services. Allen[3] and Orme[7] suggest that this is due to the lack of consensus on what is actually meant by the term 'crisis' and how such events might best be resolved. The trend towards community-based care began in the 1950s when there were approximately 150,000 psychiatric beds. By 1996/7 the number of beds had reduced to 38,780.[8] Deinstitutionalization is often attributed to the introduction of anti-psychotic medication, however this does not explain the general trend towards treating all forms of mental illness outside the large psychiatric hospitals.[9] More significant may have been a growing acceptance among psychiatrists that incarcerating people in institutions often had a negative effect, was extremely expensive and was influenced by the growing public awareness of human rights.[10] An evolution in medical education to include a larger psychiatric component gave general practitioners greater confidence to manage people with mental health problems within primary services.

Initially, the service provided by community psychiatric nurses was largely during 'office' hours. However, innovative teams set up at Napsbury Hospital and in the London Borough of Barnet[11,12] aimed to offer a multidisciplinary assessment and follow-up care.

During the 1980s and 1990s the crisis intervention

and home treatment model became increasingly popular, in one form or another, partly due to reports of the success of crisis teams in the USA[13] and in parts of Australia and New Zealand.[14,15]

The British Government's *'Spectrum of Care – Local services for people with mental health problems'*[16] recommended 'intensive home support' and the Department of Health[17] Report *'Modernizing Mental Health Services – safe sound and supportive'*, describes the new vision for mental health services to provide 'access to help 365 days a year and 24 hours a day'. The National Service Framework[18] demanded 'timely access to specialist assessment and treatment' as well as 'evidence that services respond to mental health needs quickly, effectively and consistently 24 hours a day 365 days a year (p. 12). The National Health Service Plan[19] promised that:

> By 2004, all people in contact with specialist mental health services will be able to access crisis resolution services at any time. The teams will treat around 100,000 people a year who would otherwise have to be admitted to hospital including black and South Asian service users for whom this type of service has been shown to be particularly beneficial. Pressure on acute inpatient units will be reduced by 30% and there will generally be no out of area admissions that are not clinically indicated.

This legislation mirrors the demands of users of mental health services who have identified the need for access to 24-hour crisis telephone lines as well as access to home treatment services.[28]

However, in a questionnaire survey of trusts, to identify the number of home treatment teams, only 16% of services had such a team.[20] A similar questionnaire survey[7] carried out in 1997 focused on the number of services providing specific home-based treatment to clients. Of those who replied to her questionnaire the researcher found that only 48 (32%) provided such a service.

The diversity of crisis team service provision is reflected in a variety of factors, which include:

❑ **Hours of availability.** Some offer a 24-hour, seven day a week service, while others operate restricted hours with perhaps 'on call' support at night.
❑ **Style of team title,** e.g. Crisis Assessment Team, Crisis Resolution Services, Psychiatric Emergency Team, Early Intervention Service.
❑ **Service aims,** e.g. assessment of all people referred to mental illness services, provision of home treatment services, reducing the number of admissions to hospital, acting as 'gate-keeper' for the available acute hospital beds, facilitating early discharge from hospital.

❑ **Composition of teams,** e.g. nurses only,[21] support workers, social workers, psychiatrists, psychologists[22] occupational therapists, and service user development workers.[23]
❑ **Inclusion and exclusion criteria,** e.g. only people under 65, only people known to mental health services, only people who are classified as having a 'serious mental illness'. Some exclude anyone with a primary drug and alcohol problem, organic illness or those not previously known to the service.

Although crisis assessment and crisis intervention/home treatment can be seen as separate services, they are in fact interdependent. Without an assessment of the person in crisis and their resources within their community, it would not be possible to make a decision about whether they can be treated within their home environment or whether they should be offered admission to hospital. Equally, the process of assessment of the person in crisis, if conducted skilfully, and with reference to the principles of crisis theory, may provide a sufficient intervention to prevent further treatment being necessary.

ASSESSMENT AND TREATMENT

Working with people in crisis offers very special opportunities, but also represents very special responsibilities. Crisis theory holds that at the point when crisis occurs, the person is more than usually open/vulnerable to change – either positive or negative and this opportunity should be used to its maximum positive effect. The process of crisis assessment may be divided into five phases. However, this is not to suggest that they necessarily occur neatly or sequentially:

❑ Speedy assessment.
❑ Assessment of risk.
❑ Helping the person and their family/carers to describe and examine the crisis.
❑ Seeking opportunities and solutions.
❑ Negotiating a plan.

Speedy assessment

Crises merit a speedy and timely response. Once the team has accepted the referral, assessment will occur rapidly.[24] If there are no indicators of risk to staff this assessment will probably take place in the person's home. Members of their family, friends or perhaps other professional carers may be present when members of the team arrive. Nurses in crisis situations need to be calm, responsive and thoughtful, enabling them to gather information from multiple sources to permit them to make knowledgeable judgements about the situation and the level of risk it presents.

Offering a full and clear explanation of their role, the reason for the visit as well as an explanation of the alternatives which the team can offer will help to diffuse tensions caused by assumptions about contact with mental health workers. It is also important to be aware of public beliefs that such contact signals that the person is 'mad' and may therefore be forcibly removed to hospital.

A respectful, warm, empathic but professional manner is essential as is a keen awareness and observation of social and cultural etiquette, which is congruent with being in another person's home. As Brimblecombe notes:

> For staff, the non-institutional setting of home treatment provides an opportunity for creativeness in working practices, but also demands a willingness to negotiate from a position where the client has authority in their own home, as opposed to having little or none as in the traditional hospital setting.[10]

As well as establishing rapport and trust, the initial phase offers opportunities for noticing things about the client and their environment in a way that will be less obvious once the nurse has become accustomed and familiar with them.

- **Observation of the person** – Does the person appear malnourished, dehydrated, dirty, dishevelled? Do they smell of alcohol? Are they behaving in an unusual way – are they guarded, suspicious, fearful, anxious, agitated, restless, elated, grandiose, angry, depressed or perhaps confused, disorientated, sedated? Do they behave in a manner suggestive of unusual thought processes?
- **Observation of the environment** – Does the environment give any clues to the person's state of mind – is it untidy and chaotic? Is it obsessionally neat, suggesting compulsive traits? Does the person's home suggest that they have financial difficulties? (little furniture, no evidence of any food or drinks). Is there physical evidence of alcohol or drugs? Is there anything about the environment that might betray unusual thought patterns (notices pinned up, windows/doors sealed up and curtains permanently drawn, unusual decoration, unwillingness to use electricity or gas).
- **What evidence is there of the person's mood state?** What does their body language betray – agitation, euphoria, irritability, hopelessness or helplessness? What do they say? Can they concentrate on the interview? Is their speech accelerated, disjointed or slowed, affectless, preoccupied, obsessional? Is there evidence of rhyming, punning,

loosening of association or any other evidence of a psychotic process? Do they describe disturbance in sleep, appetite, thought, libido and energy levels? Are they experiencing thoughts of harming themselves or others?
- **Does the person have any physical difficulties?** Do they need attention and do they impact negatively on their mental health or level of risk?
- **If other people are present, how does the person relate to them?** And how do the others present relate to the person identified as being in crisis. Are there tensions, anger, threats of violence between them or to others?

Assessment of risk

In the context of crisis care, the following factors are important:

- Do the client and her/his family accept the feasibility of treatment at home?
- Has it been possible to establish a high level of rapport and trust with the person in crisis? This will give an indication of whether the client would feel able to contact the team for support at times of (increased) risk.
- Are there any aspects of the client's behaviour (including drug and alcohol use), which indicate that they could act impulsively to harm themselves or others.
- Will the client and her/his family take part in negotiating a safety plan?
- Do members of the client's family feel confident in their ability to offer support? Has the client's family become exhausted or lost empathy with the client, because of high levels of stress?

Direct, though sensitive questioning, in the context of an established rapport can be used to establish the level of risk.

Client:	'I just don't see the point of anything anymore, now there is just me'.
Nurse:	'Sometimes when people say that they "can't see the point" what they are saying is that they would rather be dead, that they are thinking of killing themselves, have you ever thought about killing yourself?'
Client:	'Yes, well I have ... '
Nurse:	'And when you have thought like that, have you ever thought how you would do it?'
Client:	'I did wonder about taking all of Ian's tablets that are still in the cupboard, at least I think they are still there'.

This short exchange enables the nurse to ascertain that suicidal thoughts exist, that there is a plan, but that this plan is vague and untested, and opens up the opportunity for further exploration of the subject.

Helping the person to describe and examine the crisis

Helping people tell their story is one of the basic skills for nurses working in crisis services. The following skills are particularly important:

❑ Listening.
❑ Asking questions.
❑ Helping the person identify the difficulty.
❑ Developing problem-solving skills, identifying strengths and supports, generating solutions and maintaining hope.

Listening

Listening is not a passive activity. If you, as a stranger, are to be trusted with the intimate details of another person's life it is vital that a trusting relationship be built quickly. Active listening demonstrates not only attention but also respect for the story that is unfolding but can help the person to 'discharge' uncomfortable feelings and is a vital part of crisis intervention.[25]

Asking questions

Asking the right questions is very important. The nurse conducting an interview with the person in crisis will have a clear idea of what information needs to be gathered. However, an ability to work flexibly around this structure, constantly seeking opportunities to ask questions which assist the person to express themselves and ventilate their feelings as well as the opportunity to show that the thoughts and feelings which have been expressed are heard and valued is essential. This can also help with the development of rapport and safe containment of feelings.

Helping the person identify the difficulty

By recounting the details of their crisis, the person can often come to a new or clearer understanding of what is causing the difficulty. It may be that they have been so wrapped up in their thoughts that they have become overwhelmed by the enormity of their problems. Perhaps their thoughts have been so accelerated that they have been unable to make any coherent sense of them. As a (professional) stranger, you can help them to make the supreme effort to express their thoughts. It may be that their thoughts are in such disarray that this

is impossible. Having a member of the crisis team present may also help the person discuss their difficulties with the family, and how this makes them feel.

Client:	'I've just felt I have nothing to go on for …'
Daughter:	'But Mum, what about me and your grandchildren. We need you'.
Client:	'Do you? I just thought I was a burden'.
Daughter:	'You're not a burden Mum, we love you'.
Nurse:	'It sounds as if you didn't realize that Mrs Jones'.
Client:	'No, I didn't'.

Developing problem-solving skills, identifying strengths and supports, generating solutions and maintaining hope

People in mental health crisis have often lost contact with their skills in solving problems. The symptoms they are experiencing may be new to them or they may be facing a situation that they have faced before when the 'solution' to their dilemma was that other people intervened and took control of their lives. This may have been seen to be the only course of action that was possible at that time. Crisis intervention – especially when linked to the possibility of home treatment – offers the opportunity to help the client and their family to find positive ways of coping with the crisis, that include remaining in the 'least restrictive environment' of their home.[18]

Seeking opportunities and solutions – how do we assist?

Working with people in crisis often involves flexibility, ingenuity and the ability to think laterally about possible solutions. The following represents some ways of helping the person find positive solutions:

❑ Helping them to remember ways in that they have coped with difficulties in the past and applying this knowledge to their current crisis. Where the crisis represents a totally new experience then an exploration of coping strategies used successfully in other circumstances is helpful.
❑ Remaining solution-focused rather than problem-focused, during discussions about the crisis and ways of dealing with it. There is a fine balance to be kept in doing this, avoiding becoming a 'Pollyanna', or being captured by the client's sense of despair.
❑ Giving information that is sufficient, reliable, timely and hope-mediating.
❑ Being sensitive to the possibility that the person (or their family) might come to view the person as the problem, and blame them, be hostile to them, or encourage them to be self-blaming. For example, if a family member is in crisis because they have become

depressed, 'Mum's depression' might be used to make sense of events within the family, thus making Mum the focus for blame. The crisis worker needs to model the use of non-judgemental language – showing that they are aware of the person and not the label.

❏ Fostering collaboration between the team, the person in crisis and their support network, offering help in a respectful manner and offering the opportunity for the development of coping strategies which might involve gaining support from friends or family.

❏ Negotiating ways of managing the crisis situation between all involved parties and, if the person is to be offered home treatment, negotiating what the input of the team will be, stressing the availability of the team to both the client and their family.

❏ Remaining aware of the issues of power, dominance and potential oppression that has traditionally existed between nurses and people classified as mentally ill, crisis team workers can actively work to prevent the risk of 'bringing the institution into the community'.[26]

NEGOTIATING A PLAN

Negotiating with the client and carers is essential if home treatment is to be offered. The key areas of negotiation are:

❏ The willingness of both client and carers to engage in home treatment.

❏ A plan to manage risk, which is negotiated jointly between the person, their family or friends and the team.

❏ The accessibility of the team by telephone.

❏ Arrangements for visits to the client at home, identifying who will be visiting and who may (or may not) be present.

❏ The length of the involvement of the team (usually short-term).

❏ The fact that the nurse will be liaising with other professionals/helping agencies involved in that person's care and negotiation around what information may be discussed with others.

Home treatment

Once the person in crisis has been accepted for home treatment it is important that the multidisciplinary team discusses and reflects upon the particulars of the crisis. A case manager should be appointed who will co-ordinate the progress of their care, involving other professionals both within the Crisis Team and also from the wider network of services, both statutory and voluntary.

Case study 44.1

As Mrs Jones's mood begins to lift, her Case Manager within the Crisis Team begins to realize that since the death of Mr Jones a year ago, she has not allowed herself to grieve his loss. However, she is now beginning to talk about her feelings and, as home treatment is inevitably short term, after discussion with Mrs Jones and Caroline, she is referred to a bereavement counsellor at the GP surgery. It also becomes noticeable that Mrs Jones's sole activity when she is not at work is housework. With her agreement, Pam arranges for one of the team's occupational therapists to see her to help her decide what other activities she would like to do and to give her some understanding of how activity can help to lift mood.

Functions of a home treatment team

Home treatment services offer the opportunity for treatment of a mental health crisis in an environment which is familiar and among people who are supportive. Lack of home or support may represent an obstacle to treatment at home although such difficulties can be overcome creatively. Intensive support to family and friends may help them in their support of the person in crisis; short periods of respite away from home with other family members or perhaps in a mental health hostel can provide everyone with sanctuary from the crisis, after which the person may be successfully returned to their home. Home treatment services aim to help the person in crisis by:

❏ Reducing stigma and increasing the person's level of autonomy.

❏ Monitoring mood, mental state and level of suicide risk.

❏ Offering case management including monitoring a care pathway with involvement of other relevant professionals, both from within and outside of the team including agencies in the voluntary sector.

❏ Offering the opportunity for the person to ventilate their feelings within a safe, therapeutic relationship and to find creative solutions to problems.

❏ Acting as a source of support, encouragement and knowledge (including modelling skills) for the family and friends of people who are identified as being in crisis.

❏ Managing and administering medication, monitoring for possible side-effects.

❏ Helping the person to devise a crisis management plan for use should further episodes of crisis occur, thus enabling them to utilize knowledge gained through their current experiences and to acknowledge that they have power to take back some control in a situation where events had seemed outside their control.

Advantages of crisis management/home treatment

Home treatment offers a humane response to mental health crises, allowing the person the opportunity to foster their strengths and those of their family. It causes less disruption in the lives of the person in crisis and their family and has been identified as being the preferred option of users and carers.[27,28] It can provide an effective response to first episodes of psychotic illness and possibly prevent recurrent admissions to hospital[2] It is cheaper than admission to hospital,[30-33] is less likely to cause chronicity or institutionalization and reduces the associated stigma for both client and their family.[13,29] Reducing the number of admissions to hospital reduces pressure on beds.[23,33] It also offers the opportunity for clients to feel empowered by offering them the opportunity to take control of their recovery.

CONCLUSION

Crisis assessment and intervention services represent a response to political and economic factors[16-19] and the demands of users and carers.[27] As yet there is little consistency between teams and much diversity exists in ways of responding to local need. Crisis theory[2] suggests that the person who has reached the stage of 'breakdown/disorganization' will seek help and will be at the point where interventions (be they good or bad) will have the optimum effect. This offers nurses both a golden opportunity and an onerous responsibility. Teams that offer crisis intervention within the client's home can also assist both client and their carers to develop effective coping strategies for use should the crisis reoccur. The role of case manager within the crisis service is vital in linking clients with services in a timely and responsive manner. This may include admissions to hospital. Although crisis intervention can be offered to many clients, for some there will always remain the need for true 'asylum' of admission to hospital.

REFERENCES

1. Lindemann E. Symptomatology and management of acute grief. *American Journal of Psychiatry* 1944; **101**: 141–8.

2. Caplan G. *An approach to community mental health.* London: Tavistock, 1964.

3. Allen K. What are crisis services? In: Tomlinson D, Allen K (eds). *Crisis services and hospital crises: mental health at a turning point.* Aldershot: Ashgate, 1999: 1–11.

4. *The shorter Oxford English dictionary*, Volume 1. Oxford: Oxford University Press, 1984.

5. Crine A. How crisis intervention can help change people's lives. *Mind Out* 1981; April 7.

6. Crompton N. Crisis theory and crisis management: the way forward. *Mental Health Nursing* 1996; **16**(5):16–18.

7. Orme S. Intensive home treatment services: the current position in the UK. In: Brimblecombe N (ed.) *Acute mental health care in the community. Intensive home treatment.* London: Whurr, 2001: 29–54.

8. Department of Health. *Health and personal social services statistics for England* 1997. London: HMSO, 1998.

9. Eisenberg L. Is psychiatry more mindful or brainier than it was a decade ago? (Editorial). *The British Journal of Psychiatry* 2000; **176**: 1–5.

10. Brimblecombe N. Community care and the development of intensive home treatment services. In: Brimblecombe N (ed.) *Acute mental health care in the community. Intensive home treatment.* London: Whurr, 2001: 5–28.

11. Scott RD. A family oriented psychiatric service to the London Borough of Barnet. *Health Trends* 1980; **12**: 65–8.

12. Ratna L. Crisis intervention: the Barnet Experience. *Alternative Health International* 1998; **1**(1): 1–10.

13. Ramon S. Exemplary crisis services in Europe and the USA. In: Tomlinson D, Allen K (eds). *Crisis services and hospital crises: mental health at a turning point.* Aldershot: Ashgate, 1999: 138–60.

14. Hoult J, Rosen A, Reynolds I. Community orientated treatment compared to psychiatric hospital orientated treatment. *Social Science and Medicine* 1984; **11**: 1005–1010.

15. Carrol A, Pickworth J, Protheroe D. Service innovations: an Australian approach to community care – Northern Crisis Assessment and Treatment Team. *Psychiatric Bulletin*, 2001; **25**: 439–441.

16. Department of Health. *The spectrum of care. Local services for people with mental health problems.* London: HMSO, 1996.

17. Department of Health. *Modernising Mental Health Services – safe, sound and supportive.* HMSO: London, 1999.

18. Department of Health. *National Service Framework.* HMSO: London, 1999.

19. Department of Health. *NHS Plan.* HMSO: London, 2000.

20. Andrew J, Owen S, Sashidharan P, Edwards LJ. Availability and acceptability of home treatment for acute psychiatric disorders. *Psychiatric Bulletin* 2000; **24**: 169–71.

21. Slinger P. Fast action. *Nursing Times* 1996; **92**(1): 36–7.

22. Minghella E. Home based emergency treatment. *Mental Health Practice* 1998; **2**(1): 10–14.

23. Bracken P, Cohen B. Home treatment in Bradford. *Psychiatric Bulletin* 1999; **23**: 349–52.

24. Brimblecombe N. Assessment in crisis/home treatment services. In: Brimblecombe N (ed.) *Acute mental health care in the community. Intensive home treatment.* London: Whurr, 2001: 78–102.

25. Szmukler G. The place of crisis intervention in psychiatry. *Australian and New Zealand Journal of Psychiatry* 1987; **21**: 24–34.

26. Bracken P, Thomas P. Home treatment in Bradford. *Open Mind* 1999; **95**: 17.

27. Bailey S. Bradford crisis services: where are they? *Open Mind* 1994; **72**: 15.

28. Reynolds I, Hoult J. The relatives of the mentally ill. *The Journal of Nervous and Mental Disease* 1984; **172**: 480–89.

29. Joy C, Adams C, Rice K. Crisis intervention for people with severe mental illnesses. *The Cochrane Database of Systematic Reviews*, 2001.

30. Bengelsdorf H, Church JO, Kaye R, Orlowski B, Alden D. The cost effectiveness of crisis intervention. *The Journal of Nervous and Mental Disease* 1993; **181**: 757–62.

31. Knapp M, Beecham J, Koutsogeorgopoulou V, *et al.* Service use and costs of home-based versus hospital-based care for people with serious mental illness. *British Journal of Psychiatry* 1994; **165**: 195–203.

32. McCrone P, Chisholm D, Bould M. Costing different models of mental health service provision. *Mental Health Research Review* 1999; **6**: 14–17.

33. Ford R, Minghella E, Chalmers C, Hoult J, Raftery J, Muijen M. Cost consequences of home-based and in-patient-based acute psychiatric treatment: Results of an implementation study. *Journal of Mental Health* 2001; **10**: 467–76.

Chapter 45

ASSERTIVE OUTREACH

Mike Smith* and Mervyn Morris**

INTRODUCTION

Mental health services aim to provide a holistic approach to care, combining biomedical, social and psychological models of intervention, to facilitate and support the person in difficulty toward recovery. This requires effective integration across professions and agencies, as well as resources and time. Each of these factors presents a significant challenge for services, and much depends on the ability and willingness of service users to engage with the mental health team.

While for many people the level of service received may be regarded as satisfactory, for a variety of reasons a significant number of people have overwhelming problems and, on the strength of their relationship with services, providers fail to help. This may be in part due to their symptom experience, but it is much more likely due to lifestyle or lack of community supports, as well as having bad experiences of services, which may include cultural insensitivity and even institutional racism. Whatever the cause a typical pattern emerges; the less engaged is the person in difficulty, the more difficult it is for services to identify and co-ordinate meeting their needs; and the more likely that problems and emergency admissions are likely to occur. Medication often becomes the only (and often contentious) option. More critically, the service user's needs are no longer at the centre of care, as professionals attempt to take control of the situation.

Assertive outreach services are not so much a new form of therapy, but a more intensive arrangement of resources for people who, due to choice or circumstances, have not developed a helpful relationship with services, often resulting in greater distress and frequent re-hospitalization. Assertive outreach provides an opportunity to break this pattern and move beyond focusing on monitoring and medication compliance. Assertive outreach teams have the resources and time to

*Mike Smith was overall winner of the RCN nurse of the year in 1997 and is known for his campaigning approach to change beliefs about the nature of psychotic experiences and the 'treatments' offered. Mike has written many practical books about working with psychotic experiences and now works freelance.
**Mervyn Morris, trained in the 1970s, with further training and experience in teaching, therapeutic communities, community nursing, psychodynamic and family interventions. He currently works at University of Central England, developing training programmes including EU projects and WHO consultancy. Mervyn's research focus is on alternative approaches to psychosis.

rise above the low expectations services often have of 'difficult to engage' people with complex needs. *Recovery* is a possibility for all.

For nurses, assertive outreach services provide the resources for the highest standards of practice, with opportunities to be creative and innovative. Nursing philosophy and practice can be seen at the heart of this approach, where attention is paid to *people* rather than their pathology; where relationships are the key to success; and where the focus is achieving personally meaningful change for those individuals. Working as part of an assertive outreach team is an ideal situation for nurses who want to make a difference. Where it works well, there is a very low staff turnover because of high levels of job satisfaction.

The policy context

Assertive outreach services can be seen as a culmination of policy development in mental health, where greater emphasis has been placed increasingly on effective multiprofessional and inter-agency working. In the UK the 1995 report 'Building Bridges'[1] brought in to sharp focus the problems of services for people with 'severe mental illness' in the community. The needs of a small number of service users within this broader group have driven the implementation of assertive outreach.

This smaller group of service users can be understood in two ways: Firstly, the service recipients are perceived by service providers as possessing at least some of the following characteristics:

❑ Experiencing a particularly disruptive and enduring illness, resulting in severe functional impairments.
❑ A history of psychiatric services having difficulty sustaining engagement, reflected by a pattern of regular and compulsory admission to hospital.
❑ Reluctance to comply with treatment plans, primarily medication.
❑ 'Co-morbid' presentation of a drug or substance misuse problem, homelessness and involvement with criminal justice systems.
❑ Multiprofessional and multi-agency interventions in their lives.

Secondly, assertive outreach (AO) is viewed as a better way of meeting the needs of both society and care providers. There have been a number of events involving tragic deaths of professionals,[2] members of the public (notably the death of Jonathan Zito in 1992)[3] as well as service users (most notably Ben Silcock, who was mauled by Lions in London Zoo in 1992). These and many similar incidents created significant press interest

and political lobbying related to the community treatment of people with 'severe mental illness'. Resulting inquiries, reports and the formation of 'pressure groups' have highlighted failures in the co-ordination of assessment for and provision of services, and also raised the question of compulsory treatment extending beyond the hospital setting.

The political agenda is a significant issue for AO, as we believe that compulsory treatment in the community mitigates against sustainable engagement and a therapeutic relationship. While such legislation may be forthcoming (human rights legislation notwithstanding!), assertive outreach offers an alternative, in the form of a comprehensive, more intensive, consistent, personalized and sustaining relationship with services, which aims to minimize the events that lead to compulsory treatment. From a service user perspective, this should mean a reduced need for compulsory (and costly and unhelpful) hospital admission and, as part of a negotiated care package, better treatment compliance. Additionally, service users value such a service. If provided in such a way that the relationship offers choice and empowerment, AO enhances personal well-being and goal attainment, and as a result minimizes circumstances that lead to avoidable tragic events.

History

Assertive outreach in the UK developed from assertive community treatment (ACT) or programme of assertive community treatment (PACT), which was developed by Marx, Stein and Test in the USA in the 1970s.[4] This programme evolved from the closure and retraction of state facilities in the deinstitutionalization era of the 1970s in America and was the first systematic move to re-provide more appropriate new services in a community, rather than just withdrawing or re-locating established services.

Discharge from long-stay hospitals was based on the idea that many people's illness had become 'stable' or 'manageable' and thus could be returned to the community if 'rehabilitated'. However it became clear that successful rehabilitation in hospital was a poor predictor of success after discharge. The lack of community support for many led to the repetitive cycle of hospital admission and discharge; the so-called 'revolving door'. ACT was developed as both a more cost-effective way of intervening as well as a humane attempt to respond to people whose lives were obviously unsatisfactory. Stein and Test's work is seen as seminal in the field and essential reading for the background of assertive outreach.[5–7]

ACT is the most extensively evaluated model of community care for the severely mentally ill and has become state policy for many states in the USA, as well as national policy in many other countries including England, where it is now a standard required component of services as part of the National Service Framework for Mental Health.[8] In the USA the National Alliance for the Mentally Ill has campaigned to ensure its provision across the whole of the USA, reflecting the perception of many who believe mental health services have not focused their resources on the most needy and most difficult group. As outlined above, reports on service failures in the UK have created similar perceptions.

The development of ACT has also raised concerns about creating circumstances where at least some services see their primary function as surveillance and medication compliance, with the potential of becoming an 'aggressive' treatment programme. The primary aim of ACT is to develop a care package that enables the potential for recovery, and usually includes medication as one component. The user-centred focus provides the grounds upon which the professional can engage and negotiate the best decision where compliance becomes an issue.

In developing assertive outreach in the UK, many began by studying the ingredients of the typical assertive outreach team in the USA. The concept of fidelity to the key elements of the AO model provides a valuable reference point.[9,10] AO services contrast with previous psychiatric community services in many ways, most notably in that they have much smaller staff–service user ratios, and actively involve the whole team rather than a single professional key worker, enabling intensive engagement and the development of more complex care packages.

Assertive outreach teams provide support to generic community mental health teams by taking over the care of people who may be regarded variously as 'difficult', 'disruptive', 'exhausting', 'morale sapping' and also perceived as people who 'drag important and useful time and attention from other service users'. However these are not the acceptance criteria for an assertive outreach team. Part of the role of assertive outreach services is to ensure they make their boundaries fair but clear, and ensure good working relationships with those teams with whom they relate.

In some services, including Northern Birmingham Mental Health Trust, the development of assertive outreach has been part of a wider reconfiguration of community services. This has included the development of home treatment teams, a move from *generic* community psychiatric nurse caseloads to separate teams for primary care liaison (offering mainly short-term working with people), and longer-term 'rehabilitation and recovery' teams for people with more enduring

problems, but who have relatively stable lifestyles and health.

WHAT ASSERTIVE OUTREACH DOES

Assertive outreach services are provided by a team of professionals with a range of skills. In the UK context this includes nurses, doctors, psychologists, social workers and occupational therapists.

Many teams find that, in time, they need to include employment/vocational workers, sports/recreation specialists, befrienders, advisors/counsellors, community activists and also 'experts by experience' – people who have recovered from psychiatric illness and who can share their experiences of recovery.

AO aims not only to maximize access to co-ordinated and consistent professional resources, but also to act as a gateway for the wider network of community services and supports, which in the longer term will provide the more permanent relationships necessary for personal development and achievement. The importance of connecting people to non-professional relationships and away from mental health services cannot be overemphasized. Relationships between service users and professionals are limited both in terms of the extent to which they can become personally involved, and the risks that they can take with people. Other supports – particularly other service users – can say and do things that are helpful precisely because they are not professionals.

AO teams provide a wide range of services:

- ❏ A single point for case management (hence the necessary range of skills in a team);
- ❏ initial and ongoing assessments;
- ❏ discrete psychiatric services;
- ❏ employment and housing assistance;
- ❏ family support and education;
- ❏ substance abuse services;
- ❏ and other services and supports critical to an individual's ability to live successfully in the community.

Ideally, AO services are available 24 hours a day, every day, to minimize potential distress for the person and disruption to relationships and plans, should a crisis develop.

AO teams are more effective if they can communicate a belief in *recovery*, and then facilitate this by working creatively with the person both when they are well and when they are in difficulty. In our experience AO works best where it offers and supports the belief that a person can accommodate their experiences and play a valuable role in their community. This takes time and a commitment, both from the nurse and the person who uses the service.

CHARACTERISTICS OF AN ASSERTIVE OUTREACH TEAM

Several characteristics of an AO team distinguish it from other community mental health teams. Only by demonstrating these features, can a team be said to be achieving fidelity to the AO models that have been shown to be effective and efficient. The following are perceived to be the essential components:

❑ The **core team** comprises a breadth of skill to address all of a service user's needs in a timely (prompt) way, thus minimizing the risks posed by having separate teams involved in supporting the person. As the main **provider** of services, multidisciplinary representation is required in each team (psychiatrist, nurses, social workers, occupational therapists, employment workers, etc.) with a small service user–staff ratio to minimize the need for referral to other mental health service providers.

❑ The AO team shares a single base, and acknowledges that **staff members are interchangeable** across roles, thus ensuring that services are not disrupted by staff turnover or illness.

❑ **Engagement** is an essential part of the team's work, although this may take many years to fully establish. This involves developing rapport, building trust, and demonstrating a consistent and persistent desire to work with the person. Positive relationships are more likely to develop if the service demonstrates willingness to address the service user's agenda, to work flexibly, to demonstrate integrity, and to remain supportive when problems or conflict arises.

❑ **Team rather than individual engagement** is a paramount aim, although team members will have differing relationships and thus have potentially different opportunities for helping the person.

❑ AO is an **'in-vivo' service**, taking place in the service user's community. Services are not provided in offices (outpatient or in day-centres), but in community facilities, the service users own home, at a friend's house, the pub, or their place of employment. Community participation, access and networking, maximizes the service's ability to match intervention to the actual situation of the service user, and the service user's potential to maintain and develop their identity in the community. Should someone be admitted to hospital, the team remains fully engaged and involved, and facilitates discharge at the earliest opportunity.

❑ Treatment is **highly individualized**, recognizing that people and relationships change over time, emphasizing a flexible and dynamic approach, and engaging with the person in such a way that allows them to enable personal responsibility. Nurses in assertive outreach teams report that this is the greatest focus of their work, creating team relationships with people that can help through respect, maximizing choice and self-advocacy, and working through disagreement without coercion or rejection. *Hope* is a fundamental component of any therapeutic relationship, and all interventions should encompass the possibility of recovery; helping the person reclaim their lives, rather than maintain them as ill people in perpetuity.

❑ Treatment and support are **ongoing** rather than time-limited. AO is not a curative process but a form of support which enables the person to maintain their community links when they are unwell and to be in the best position to grow and recover when they are well.

❑ If the service user moves out of area then the team strives to maintain contact, maintains contact, and continues to provide and co-ordinate care. If a move is more permanent the team continues to be responsible until a care transfer to another team has been agreed jointly and enacted upon fully.

❑ A focus upon **meaningful occupation and employment**. The team encourages and facilitates service users to pursue interests and gain employment, providing 'vocational rehabilitation' services directly without referral to other teams. This is beneficial in terms of independence and de-stigmatizing people, but requires significant support to deal with issues of confidence as well as shifting often long-established negative self-perceptions.

❑ Many of the people using the service have **substance use and misuse problems**. The AO leads on these interventions, and co-ordinates the substance abuse component of care.[11] Consequently, services should include at least one team member with expertise in dual diagnosis working.

❑ An **educational approach** is taken that allows service users to become collaborative partners in their treatment. Service users are encouraged to reflect upon and learn about themselves and their illness, and also develop skills in managing symptoms and also better coping strategies in areas of difficulty. This is a two way process and requires the staff to have a broad view of how service users make sense of and bring meaning to their lives, and to work with rather than enforcing just one (biomedical) view of psychosis. Employing 'experts by experience' (i.e. recovered service users) is particularly valuable in this area, including helping staff to challenge their views of the origin and nature of mental distress.

❑ **Family support and education with the active involvement of the service user:** AO staff include the service user's support systems (family, 'significant others') in discussions about goals, strategies and interventions, facilitating better understanding of illness experience, their ability to help, and including them as part of the recipients of an AO service. Families are no less important to service users than anyone else, and often more important where there is a need to improve negative and emotionally charged relationships, particularly to reduce conflict, increase autonomy, and restore a more positive role.

❑ **Community participation:** AO staff support and, where appropriate, facilitate service users to be more integrated into their local community through the use and membership of community facilities and organizations of their choice.

❑ The team pays attention to meeting all **health care needs**, offering support and guidance on health matters that improve well-being, as well as encourage and facilitate access to health education and other related services in the local community. Mental health service users have some of the highest rates of untreated physical disease morbidity, which can not only increase psychiatric symptom experience, but also undermine any sense of hope and aims for personal achievement.[12]

❑ To ensure their continued fidelity and success AO teams must have clearly stated **values that are evident in practice**. These normally include relationship building, personal recovery and individualization of services, and a commitment to evaluating and responding to service users experiences of the service.

CAPACITY OF AN ASSERTIVE OUTREACH SERVICE

Studies suggest a target professional–user ratio of 1:10 is ideal. Experience suggests that assertive outreach teams should slowly build up their caseloads, as the early stages of engagement with services are more intensive and thus more time consuming.

AO services recognize that overall capacity is limited by team dynamics and the amount of people a whole team can effectively engage with. Experience suggests there should certainly be no more than 10 case-managers serving 100 service users. Beyond this number, another team becomes necessary. In largely rural areas like Wisconsin USA where Stein and Test's model originated, the need for a smaller service is recognized focused differently in more sparsely populated areas.[13]

While rural areas have relatively few people requiring an AO approach, large cities (especially with multi-ethnic/cultural populations) can develop specific services with a focus on working with younger people in early intervention or with specific communities such as the African–Caribbean population. However services are configured, it is essential that the team composition reflects the community within which it works, to ensure a full grasp of social and cultural issues for service users, as well as enabling effective community networking.

Doctors and administrative staff are 'supernumerary' and rarely case manage. A dedicated psychiatrist (full or part-time) is needed for a minimum of 16 hours per week for every 50 service users. The psychiatrist provides clinical services to all service users, works as part of the team to monitor each service user's clinical status and response to treatment, contributes to supervision of staff delivery of services, but leads in consultation with the team on psychopharmacologic and other medical treatment.

TARGET GROUP FOR ASSERTIVE OUTREACH

The service user group who require AO are people with a history of severe and disruptive mental illness who have not benefited from treatment to date, have a history of difficulty with or resistance to engaging with treatment and complying with programmes and often have a secondary substance abuse problem or forensic history.

Clinical criteria suggested for selection are:

1 Service users between the age of 16 and 65 with a severe and persistent mental illness, invariably experiencing symptoms within the range of psychotic illness diagnoses (individuals with a primary diagnosis of a substance use disorder, personality disorder or learning disability are not appropriate).

2 Service users with significant 'functional impairments' as demonstrated by at least one of the following criteria:

■ Inability to consistently perform the range of practical daily living tasks required for basic adult functioning in the community (e.g. maintaining personal hygiene; meeting nutritional needs; caring for personal business affairs; obtaining medical, legal, and housing services; recognizing and avoiding common dangers or hazards to self and possessions) or persistent or recurrent failure to perform daily living tasks except with significant support or assistance from others such as friends, family, or relatives.

■ Inability to be consistently working at a self-sustaining level or inability to consistently carry out a role at home (e.g. household meal preparation, washing clothes, budgeting, or child-care tasks and responsibilities).

- Inability to maintain a safe living situation (e.g. repeated evictions or loss of housing).

3 Service users with histories of high use and demand for psychiatric services characterized by:
  - High use of acute psychiatric hospitals (e.g. two or more admissions per year, or a hospital stay of more than six months, or detention under the mental health act at least once in previous two years) or psychiatric crisis resolution services such as home-based treatment.
  - Intractable and severe major symptoms (e.g. affective, psychotic, suicidal).
  - Co-existing substance use of significant duration (e.g. greater than six months).
  - High risk or recent history of criminal justice involvement (e.g. frequent arrests and imprisonment).
  - Inability to meet basic survival needs or residing in substandard housing, homeless, or at imminent risk of becoming homeless.
  - Residing in an inpatient bed or in a supported community residence, but considered able to live more independently if intensive services are provided, or requiring a residential or institutional placement if more intensive services are not available.
  - Inability or unwillingness to participate in residential or traditional office-based services.

TEAM ORGANIZATION

The team ethos is fundamental to AO, where close working overcomes the many professional and agency boundaries. The team structure is a flattened hierarchy, where each member has a valuable role. While there are legal aspects to the responsibility of the medical consultant, the most effective decision-making is based on a shared responsibility for care. However the team leader's role (often a nurse) is crucial in facilitating a strong team ethos and promoting the philosophy of consistent care necessary, as service users will engage to some degree with the whole team. Expert opinion highlights that services work best where the manager is an integral member of the care providing team, ideally contributing 50% of their time as an active practitioner.

Another core fidelity criterion is that all members of the team meet every day, to share information, agree visiting and intervention arrangements, and maintain morale through mutual support and team supervision. The team also needs to reflect more expansively on the care provided to each service user, and the overall service expectations. This includes regular client reviews, the development of the team's engagement strategies and interventions, team dynamics, inter-team and inter-agency working, community relationships and networks.

Each team should be able to identify a strategic plan against which it can measure its effectiveness, and through formal reporting identify measurable areas of success but also limitations, both of which are essential to identifying future resource issues and priorities. A service's focus shifts as it develops, so for example, a team that is in the early stages of development, will have a very different agenda to more established services running at capacity.

Optimally, the service is available 24 hours/day every day, although routine hours of operation involve two 'shifts' per day with some services more limited at weekends. As a minimum services should be active 12 hours per day on weekdays and eight hours each weekend day and every holiday.

Various arrangements exist for an after-hours, on-call system, with the ideal being where staff are contactable by telephone or in person, and medical support is also available during all out of hours periods. Where teams do not work seven days or over 24 hours, it is crucial to have an effective operational policy and close relationship with Home Treatment or residential (crisis, hospital) services.

The AO team has the ability and capacity to provide multiple contacts per week to service users. These may be as frequent as two to three times per day, every day, depending on need. Many, if not all, staff shall share the responsibility for addressing the transient needs of service users requiring frequent contacts. The AO team has the capacity to rapidly increase service intensity when required. On average the mean yearly number of visits for each service user should be three per week.

INTERVENTIONS IN ASSERTIVE OUTREACH

AO associations recommend that teams should offer the following interventions.[14]

The team revolves around a *case management* approach. Each service user is allocated a case manager (often referred to as key worker or lead worker). Allocation of the case manager is dependent on several factors, but most significantly is determined by the relationship with the service user. This person is responsible for the co-ordination of the assessments and care plans for each service user, and takes the lead in the engagement and treatment process. Case managers are also responsible for the prompt review of treatment plans and the timeliness and accuracy of information gathered and held, and must also ensure that service users rights and desires are advocated for within the team, and that access to independent advocacy and representation is available, wherever possible.

The case manager should also be responsible for any crisis plan and should be the lead person in working with the service users social support and family.

ASSESSMENT

Initial assessment

The AO team leader or the psychiatrist (with participation of designated team members), completes an assessment and treatment plan on admission to the service.

Comprehensive assessment

A comprehensive assessment is completed within one month of admission according to the following requirements:

1 Each assessment area is completed by the most appropriate AO team member and will include self-reports, reports of family members and other significant parties, and written summaries from other agencies – including police, courts, and outpatient and inpatient facilities, where applicable.

2 The assessment includes an evaluation of :
   - Psychiatric symptomatology and mental state.
   - Psychiatric history, including adherence to and response to prescribed medical and psychiatric treatment.
   - Medical, dental, and other health needs.
   - Extent and effect of drugs or alcohol use.
   - Housing situation and activities of daily living (ADL).
   - Vocational and educational experience.
   - Extent and effect of criminal justice involvement.
   - Social functioning.
   - Recent life-events.

Although most, if not all, team members, are involved in the assessment, the service user's psychiatrist, case manager, and individual treatment team members, assume responsibility for preparing the written assessment and ensuring that a comprehensive treatment plan is developed.

Recovery planning

The team aims to encourage hope by an ongoing commitment to support the person towards his or her own recovery. This begins from day one with the formation of a care plan that aims to meet or clarify the person's own aspirations and desires to recover.

Crisis assessment and intervention

Crisis assessment and intervention is provided continuously. This includes telephone and face-to-face contact, provided in conjunction with the local mental health crisis service as appropriate. This also includes responding to any previously developed crisis plan. For example, this might include identifying who needs to be informed, who is willing to become involved as a support, what places provide safety and comfort, as well as medication preferences.

Symptom assessment, management and intervention

Symptom assessment, management, and individual supportive therapy help service users cope, and gain ownership and accommodation of their symptom experiences. This should include the following:

1 Ongoing assessment of the service user's mental illness symptoms and response to interventions.

2 Education regarding his or her illness and the effects and side-effects of prescribed medications, where appropriate.

3 Symptom-management efforts directed to help each service user identify the symptoms and occurrence patterns including early warning signs of becoming unwell and develop a range of strategies to cope and help lessen their influence. This information also forms the basis for drawing up a crisis plan as outlined above.

4 A full range of psychological interventions, both on a planned and as-needed basis, to help resolve life events that have triggered symptoms, adjust to secondary problems of involvement with mental health services, as well as developing and accomplishing personal goals and coping strategies for successful day-to-day living.

Medication prescription, administration, monitoring and documentation

The team psychiatrist and medical team role includes:

- ❑ Assessing each service user's symptom experiences and related behaviour, and prescription of appropriate medication.
- ❑ Monitoring general health, particularly where users are not engaged with primary care services.
- ❑ Regularly reviewing and documenting the service user's symptom experiences as well as his or her response to prescribed medication treatment.

❑ Educating the service user about illness from a medical perspective, and the effects and side-effects of medication prescribed to regulate it.

All team members are involved in the assessment and documentation the service user's symptom experiences and responses to medication, including monitoring for medication side-effects.

SERVICES

Substance abuse services

Substance use and misuse is particularly complex with people who have severe mental illness, particularly when used to help manage symptoms. The complex relationship between these two problems requires time, resources and experience beyond that available to substance misuse services, and are thus provided by a dual diagnosis specialist 'in-house'. The substance abuse service includes:

❑ Identifying substance use, effects, and patterns.
❑ Recognizing and evaluating the relationship between substances used, symptoms and psychotropic medications.
❑ Developing motivation for stopping or decreasing substance use.
❑ Developing coping skills and alternatives to minimize substance use.
❑ Achieving sustainable periods of abstinence or stability in use.

Even where specialist dual diagnosis services exist the management and intervention work remains the responsibility of the AO team.

Work-related services

Service users are helped to find and maintain employment in their community. This will include:

❑ Assessment of job-related interests and abilities, through a complete education and work history assessment as well as on-the-job assessments in community-based jobs.
❑ Assessment of the effect of the service user's mental illness on employment, with identification of specific behaviours that interfere with the service user's work performance and development of interventions to reduce or eliminate those behaviours.
❑ Development of an ongoing job plan to help each service user establish the skills necessary to find and maintain work.

❑ Individual supportive therapy to assist service users to identify and cope with the symptoms of mental illness that may interfere with their work performance.
❑ On-the-job or work-related crisis plan.
❑ Work-related supportive services, such as assistance with grooming and personal hygiene, securing of appropriate clothing, wake-up calls, and transportation.

Activities of daily living

AO services provide support to help service users gain or use the skills required to:

❑ Carry out personal care to an agreed level.
❑ Perform household activities – including cleaning, cooking, shopping, and laundry to their own standard.
❑ Find and maintain housing which is safe and affordable (including finding someone to lodge with), dealing with landlords, cleaning, furnishing and decorating, procuring necessities (such as telephone, furnishings, linens), getting services connected, e.g. gas, electricity.
❑ Develop or improve money-management skills.
❑ Use available local transport (usually public).
❑ Register with primary care services and obtain treatment, e.g. GP, dentist, diabetes or asthma specialist, cardiac rehab services as necessary.

Social, interpersonal relationship, and leisure-time experience

Many people who use AO services are also excluded or alienated from social networks that provide the opportunities and experiences necessary for personal development and achievement. A critical part of care is reintroducing people to everyday activities and relationships so that they can make friends, meet people and enjoy themselves. Practical skills may be developed in a variety of ways to help people in this aspect of their lives, particularly building confidence and personal responsibility.

The aims of these experiences should be to:

❑ Improve communication skills, develop assertiveness, and increase self-esteem.
❑ Develop social skills, increase social experiences, and where appropriate, develop meaningful and reciprocal personal relationships.
❑ Plan appropriate and productive use of leisure time.
❑ Relate positively to landlords, neighbours, professionals and other service providers.

❑ Familiarize themselves with available social and recreational opportunities and increase their use of such opportunities.

Support services

Support services aim to ensure that service users obtain the basic necessities of daily life. These include:

❑ Medical and dental services.
❑ Safe, clean, affordable housing.
❑ Financial support.
❑ Social services.
❑ Transport.
❑ Legal advice and representation.

Education, support and consultation with service users' families and other major supports

The service user's family and 'significant others' may also require support. If it meets with the service user's agreement this may include:

❑ Education about the service user's symptoms, illness, and the role of the family in providing support through allowing personal responsibility and offering hope through recognizing potential for recovery.
❑ Interventions to resolve areas of day-to-day problems, family conflict, and crisis.
❑ Ongoing communication and collaboration, face-to-face and by telephone, between the team and the family, particularly to deal with personal difficulties of family members where these are problematic for the service user, or where the service user can be helpful.

DISCHARGE FROM ASSERTIVE OUTREACH TEAMS

Discharge criteria

Discharge from assertive outreach occurs when the service user and staff mutually agree to the termination of services. Discharge occurs when service users:

❑ Move permanently (or for an extended period) outside the geographic area of AO responsibility. In such cases, the AO team transfer their service responsibility to a provider in the new locality. The AO team maintains contact until the transfer is complete and engagement with the new service established.

❑ Demonstrate an ability to function in all major role areas (i.e. work, social, self-care) without requiring significant assistance from the team for an extended time period (usually not less than two years).
❑ Request discharge, despite the team's best efforts to develop an acceptable treatment plan. Where discharge is requested the option of returning to the AO service is maintained.

Documentation of discharge includes:

❑ The reasons for discharge.
❑ The service user's status and condition at discharge.
❑ A written final evaluation summary of the service user's progress toward the goals set forth in the treatment plan.
❑ A plan developed in conjunction with the service user for treatment after discharge and for follow-up.
❑ The signature of the service user's primary case manager, team manager, and psychiatrist.

CRITICISMS

AO has been extensively evaluated with clear evidence of its effectiveness in reducing readmission rates, improving quality of life for service users, reducing offending and maintaining engagement. However questions remain, concerning the validity of the evidence[15] and the ability to generalize the original model from the mid-west of the USA to other settings, such as inner city UK.[16] Although the model is said to be preferred by families and service users, there have been criticisms from service users in the UK, regarding the 'aggressive' use of the model and its singularity of approach in assertively providing medical treatment.[16,17] Most of these concerns are about implementation rather than the model itself, and could be addressed by adhering to basic principles. This is why assertive programme associations try to ensure a degree of fidelity to team composition, organization and interventions outlined in this chapter.

There are real concerns where services and team membership do not reflect the population they serve, particularly in terms of cultural competence, and this is compounded where there is ineffective building of bridges with community leaders and resources. However this is not unique to assertive outreach.

CONCLUSION

This chapter has offered two perspectives to understanding assertive outreach – the needs of the individual and the wider expectations of the community. Dealing with people who are vulnerable, and who may also present as a risk to themselves or others, presents dilemmas for practitioners, and the team philosophy often focuses on decision-making in this area. It is axiomatic that people can only recover by being allowed to make decisions wherever and whenever possible, and of course this includes consideration of others. For professionals a balance needs to be struck between giving the person the opportunity to move on, test themselves and learn through taking risks and making mistakes, and avoiding situations that can very rapidly and seriously change to crisis.

Close and supportive teams who skilfully and meaningfully engage with service users, explore the potential of each service user to take responsibility for her or his life. Assertive outreach is ultimately about a climate of hope, respecting individuality, finding potential and facilitating opportunity for people where these essentials for recovery are least likely to exist.

REFERENCES

1. Department of Health. *Building bridges; a guide to arrangements for inter-agency working for the care and protection of severely mentally ill people.* London: Department of Health, 1995.
2. Blom-Cooper L. *The falling shadow: one patients care in the mental health system.* London: Duckworth, 1995.
3. Ritchie JD, Lingham R. *The report of the inquiry into the care and treatment of Christopher Clunis.* London: HMSO, 1994.
4. Marx AJ, Test MA, Stein L. Extrohospital management of severe mental illness. *Archives of General Psychiatry* 1973; **29**: 505–11.
5. Stein LI, Test MA. Retraining hospital staff for work in a community programme in Wisconsin. *Hospital and Community Psychiatry* 1976; **27**: 266–8.
6. Test MA, Stein L. The clinical rationale for community treatment: a review of the literature. In: *Alternatives to mental hospital treatment.* New York: Plenum, 1978.
7. Stein LI, Test MA. Alternatives to mental hospital treatment:1. Conceptual model, treatment programme and clinical evaluation. *Archives of General Psychiatry* 1980; **37**: 392–7.
8. Department of Health. *National service framework for mental health.* London: The Stationary Office, 1999.
9. Teague GB, Bond GR, Drake RE. Programme fidelity in assertive community treatment. *American Journal of Orthopsychiatry* 1998; **68**: 233–45.
10. McGrew JH, Bond GR. Critical ingredients of assertive community treatment: judgement of experts. *Journal of Mental Health Administration* 1995; **22**: 113–25.
11. Department of Health. *Mental health policy implementation guide: dual diagnosis good practice guide.* London: DOH, 2002.
12. Cooley C, Morris M. Mental health and cancer: is there a missing link? *British Journal of Nursing* 1999; **8**: 1478.
13. Stein LI, Santos AB. Assertive community treatment of persons with severe mental illness. Pavillion: Norton, 1998.
14. Northern Birmingham Mental Health Trust. A model operational policy for assertive outreach services. Birmingham: Northern Birmingham Mental Health Trust, 2001.
15. Gomory T. *Programmes of assertive community treatment (PACT): a critical review.* Tallahassee FL: School of Social Work, FSU, 1998.
16. Smith M, Coleman R, Allott P, Koberstein J. Assertive outreach: a step backwards. *Nursing Times* 1999; **95**: 46–7.
17. Spindel P, Nugent JA. *Questioning the increasing use of assertive community treatment teams in community mental health.* http://www.humberc.on.ca. Accessed 21/10/1999.

FURTHER READING

Department of Health. *The mental health policy implementation guide.* London: The Stationery Office, 2001.
Sainsbury Centre for Mental Health. *Mental health topics: assertive outreach.* London: Sainsbury Centre for Mental Health, 2001.
Stein LI, Santos AB. *Assertive community treatment of persons with severe mental illness.* Pavillion: Norton, 1998.

Chapter 46

FAMILY SUPPORT

Chris Stevenson*

FROM INDIVIDUAL TO SYSTEM

Western society tends to locate problems within the individual because of certain beliefs about mental illness. Simultaneously, there is a lack of regard for the perspective of other people who have been involved in the process of moving towards being a patient for the first time, or when people are re-involved with the psychiatric system. Often people are stripped of their existing connections when being admitted to hospital. A sense of closure arises as the person loses her/his connectedness with her/his social world.

> Closure does not usually lead to family members abandoning one another in a physical sense, but rather a kind of dehumanizing process may follow. When a crisis is developing the family may be faced with an unbearable sense of hurt and pain. In the face of this, family members may cut off from the person who is ill.[1]

> Closure can be a point of no return. A symptom ... represents a partial death of that person as a social being. Being in the psychiatric space makes this death official'.[2]

The process of closure constitutes a treatment barrier,[3] which I argue can be broken down by engaging with a person's social network. In the first instance,

working with families (relatives and any significant others, including professionals) requires a different approach to organizing meetings and starting off on the 'right foot'. This is addressed in the sections on convening, engaging and joining, which offer practical ideas[a].

CONVENING FAMILY MEETINGS

When people begin to think about working with families, it can be daunting to think about inviting them to a meeting. For example:

❑ To whom should a letter be addressed?
❑ Is it better to write or phone?
❑ What needs to be said?
❑ Where is it best to meet with families?
❑ Who *should* attend to carry out 'proper' family work?

Fortunately, there is much guidance in relation to making such 'opening moves', although each family is necessarily different. For example, although some early family therapists refused to undertake therapy unless all family members were present, this is a less rigidly held position today. Currently, there is more attachment to thinking systemically when working with individuals. Finally, there is a growing interest in seeing families in

*Chris Stevenson is Reader in Nursing at the University of Teeside, England. Previously she was a Lecturer at the University of Newcastle. Her doctoral research focused on the processes inherent in family work.

[a] The guideline is offered for the new family workers, but with the assumption that s/he will be supported by a more experienced worker/team.

their 'natural' milieu, rather than in the unreal context of the professional's domain. Carpenter and Treacher provide more detail on these issues,[4] but some 'rules of thumb' are noted below.

1 **Who should the letter be addressed to?** Sometimes it is sensible to send a letter to 'The Jones Family', especially in situations where there is already a sense of commitment from the family members about attending. For instance, on admission, some family members will say to staff that they want to be involved as much as possible. A more personalized address is needed when you are requesting attendance of someone less 'known'. This allows you to include specific information relevant to each person. For example, 'I understand from Joe that you have particular concerns about how he will manage at school since he has been having problems'. You will need to contact people in the wider network separately.

2 **Is it better to write or phone?** There is no conclusive answer to this one. Sometimes it is easier to make a call, but you are then only communicating with one family member. A phone call involves a two-way exchange, space for questions about the meeting to be asked and answered.

3 **What should you say in a letter or on the phone?** Box 46.1 shows a letter that I would have as a 'standard', although I would always think about what needed to be included for each family/family member. For example, I would need to know if a particular family member was aware that their relative was receiving care for a problem.

A phone call would have a similar content, although the discussion could take place immediately. An information leaflet can be included which sets out the reasons a family meeting might be useful, how it is conducted etc.

4 **Where is it best to meet with families?** Overall, choose somewhere the family members are comfortable with. There are times when a health service facility is useful, for example, of video recording and viewing technology are wanted. It can be important to choose somewhere that is non-stigmatizing – not everyone wants to be seen entering or leaving a psychiatric clinic. It is sometimes good to see family members in their own living circumstances, gaining a flavour of family life, although more creativity can be needed in facilitating the meeting. Family life is a rich ecology, but that very richness can get in the way of talking.

5 **Who should attend in order to carry out 'proper' family work?** As mentioned earlier, there are ongoing debates about what constitutes a family system or social network. As a general rule, speak to the person in distress about whom s/he thinks it would be helpful to involve. There may be very good reasons why someone is not wanted, and/or very good reasons why someone does not think it useful to attend. Early family therapy work worked on the principle that therapeutic work could only occur in the session or outside the meeting by people who are regular attendees. More recently, there has been recognition that families can communicate with people who do not attend, taking the story of the meeting back home. Practically, it may be better to meet with part of a network than not meeting at all.

> ### Box 46.1 Standard convening letter
>
> Dear
>
> Since I have been involved with Joe, I have become very aware of how important you, his family (and/or named friends and professionals), are/is to him, and I guess that there is much concern for you around how his situation arose, what is happening now and what the future holds.
>
> I have found that it is often useful to get together the important people when someone's life is interrupted in order to discuss how we might move forward. With this in mind, I want to invite you to a 'family' meeting on...... at...... I enclose some information about the venue, and how to get there.
>
> The meeting would involve the family team. This is made up of a group of people who work for ...... and who have a special interest in the wider context of people's problems. Having a team makes it easier to hear all the information people have to offer and allows more ideas to be generated about what might be helpful. Of course, everything discussed is treated as strictly confidential.
>
> I would like to offer you the opportunity to discuss my invitation in more detail. I am contactable on ...... The best time to reach me is usually ......, or you can leave a message with ...... and I will get back to you. I look forward to speaking and to meeting with you.
>
> Yours sincerely,

ENGAGING

Once you have successfully invited family members to attend a meeting it is important to make them feel sufficiently attached to the event. Remember that most families will not have any understanding of what they might contribute to the meeting. They may feel vulnerable, for example fearing that they will be blamed for the problem, or that they will be given responsibilities that they are unable to enact. In my own study, a family member said:[5]

> ... because I think we both (parents) came here both of us before we came, came with a preconceived idea that, as I say, we were in some way being made to feel guilty, the guilty party. It was quite a relief ... to be told that we weren't to blame ourselves ... I think it's nice to voice our opinions and not feel under any pressure ...

Engaging with families is like being a good host. For example, offer to shake hands with everyone; invite people to come in and find a comfortable seat; inquire about how they found the journey to the meeting; offer drinks; use 'small talk' (which is big in its effect of relaxing people).

At this point you will need to explain to the family members how the session is to unfold so that they know what to expect. You may have already sent out an information leaflet, but it is still worth re-iterating important aspects of the process. You may want to ask the family's permission to audio or video record the meeting, in which case you will need to follow the consent procedure that the organization has in place. In this phase, you must be careful not to make the family members feel uncomfortable or coerced. It is best to try and accommodate their particular needs. For instance, some families are happy to have the meeting taped if they have the opportunity to review the tape and if they can ask for tapes to be wiped at any time. Family members may prefer to meet the team who are positioned behind a one-way mirror before the meeting begins.

JOINING

It is often argued by family therapists that if you want to effect change in families, then the therapist and family need to be joined. For example, Minuchin and Fishman state:[6]

> Joining is more an attitude than a technique, and it is the umbrella under which all therapeutic transactions occur. Joining is letting the family know that the therapist understands them and is working with them and for them ... under her protection ... the family [can] have the security to explore alternatives, try the unusual, and change. Joining is the glue that holds the therapeutic system together'.

These authors identify three joining positions that can be taken by the therapist:

❑ In the *proximal* position, the therapist relates closely to the family, at times making alliances with some family members. The therapist uses positive ways of looking at the family's functioning. Carpenter and Treacher see this as particularly advantageous when working with families where blame and negativism are plentiful.[4] The (male) therapist might say, 'It is particularly good to see you here today Mr Brown. It is not always easy for us men to talk about family issues'.

❑ In the *median* position, the therapist listens actively but tries to stay neutral. The therapist does not enter into alliances, but prompts the family to tell their story. The therapist might say, 'Who would like to begin to tell me how come we are meeting here today?'

❑ In the *disengaged* position, the therapist takes the stance of an expert fixer, whilst trying to create a sense of competence or hope of change with the family. The therapist is a gatherer of information, finding out about how families explain their experiences, and about patterns of communication. There is a strong leadership role for the therapist in this position. The therapist might ask, 'When the problem is around, who is the most able to ignore it?'

How the nurse positions her/himself depends greatly on the school of family therapy that s/he prefers. In the first cluster of examples from practice that follow, the interviewer is distant from the family and takes the role of leading the family to new understandings and insights about the problem that has beset them with the support of the expert team. In the second cluster, the interviewer and team are close to the family and are involved in a two-way exchange (dialogue).

Cluster 1

Reframing

'To change the conceptual and/or emotional setting or viewpoint in relation to which a situation is experienced and to place it in another frame which fits the "facts" of the same concrete situation equally well or even better, and thereby changes its entire meaning'.[7] For example, when a person characterized as depressed says she is struggling to spend time with her children the nurse might respond, 'So the children have some space to develop their own independent playing'. This can have the effect of releasing the mother figure from feeling guilty, because the meaning of 'mothering' has been altered. There are many powerful examples of re-framing. One of the best reviews is given by Richard Bandler and his colleagues.[8]

Messages/task setting

Sometimes it is useful to give the family a message that is prepared by the team. For example, the team may choose to convey its respect for the way in which the family has been trying to deal with the problem. Messages can be given informally or the interviewing therapist may read from a script. Messages may contain a task-setting component. For example, the family team may tell the family that they have to complete some task within or between the sessions. For example, a family who are 'at verbal war' with one another may be told by the therapist to find some time each day when they can 'debate' (re-frame) the family issues. They must not discuss those issues at any other time and must be prepared to report back during the next family meeting.

Paradoxical intervention

Some strategic family therapists have developed 'paradoxical intervention'.[9] In relation to systems theory, some family therapy approaches take the view that symptoms in one (or more) family member are a means to keep the family in a steady state. This state is safe, if unfulfilling. For example, the young person who begins to eat differently does not have to face the prospect of leaving home, her/his parents do not have to face an 'empty nest' and the prospect of relating to each other as partners rather than parents. Consequently, strategic therapists recognize that encouraging families to change may lead to resistance. The fear of change is greater than the desire for change. This allows an argument for paradoxical intervention – the person wants to change and gives messages to this effect, for example, 'I am sick of being unable to go out'. This is taken as permission for the therapist to work covertly without contravening ethical codes. In order to push the family in a 'therapeutic' direction, the therapist uses the family resistance that is directed at her/him as the energy for change. The therapist gives a message that is seen as paradoxical by the family. That is the therapist directs the family to continue with the very behaviour that is problematic, hoping the family members will resist the prescription and in so doing establish a different pattern of relating and behaving. The following nursing case study illustrates the use of paradoxical intervention.

Case study 46.1

Jean has been an inpatient on an acute, psychiatric admission ward for six months. Recently, there have been discussions about alternative accommodation for her. The options have ranged from going back to her own flat to supported hostel accommodation or group living. From a systemic perspective, Jean has become part of the ward system. She has a function there, e.g. organizing shopping for staff and other patients, and feels that the nursing staff are, in her words, 'like family'.

Contemporaneously to the discussions about accommodation, Jean has begun to scream for periods of time ranging from a few minutes to half an hour. This occurs both in the main ward area and at the ward entrance. The screaming is loud and is clearly distressing for the other patients as well as for Jean herself. The nursing staff has engaged her in conversations about the meaning of the screaming, but these have not allowed Jean to act differently. She says that she cannot control the screaming at all, but is concerned that it upsets others. The symptom can be seen as a way of keeping the system in balance as the screaming means that Jean is less likely to be discharged to alternative living and the ward staff are obliged to focus on Jean's needs, making her feel more attached.

Following a case discussion with the ward-nursing team, a paradoxical intervention was chosen. Although the team was sceptical about whether such an approach would work, they were aware that the behaviour they were trying to treat was very entrenched. A message was prepared. Jean was to be advised that the ward team had been very concerned about her and decided that the screaming was obviously very important and a way in which she could release her feelings. Therefore, she should try to scream even more, even if she does not feel like it. For the next four days she would have access to a room where she could go to scream in private without disturbing others. She should do this four times a day at 09.00, 12.00, 15.00 and 18.00 hours. She was advised that she must scream as loud as possible for at least 20 minutes. Of course, the screaming might occur outside these times, but that was to be expected.

For the first day, Jean followed the prescription. There was no screaming outside. Then she approached staff to say that she would be unable to scream any more because her throat was too sore. At this point it is important to reinforce the paradoxical message. The staff advised Jean that it was even more important that she should scream, as her feelings would be bottling up by the minute. Therefore, she should continue to go into the room and practice screaming silently. She should adopt the position for screaming and open her mouth and scream without making any noise. This led to a cessation of the screaming. This illustrates an important facet of paradoxical prescription. There must be no room for the patient/family to escape from the paradox.

In this case study, if the nursing staff had not followed through with the idea of screaming silently, Jean would have avoided the prescription by adding another dimension (the lost voice). As Watzlawick and colleagues put it:[10]

The choice of an appropriate paradoxical injunction is extremely difficult and ... if the slightest loophole is left, the patient will usually have little difficulty in spotting it and thereby escaping the supposedly untenable situation planned by the therapist.

For this reason, and because the intervention is covert, it is always better to take a team approach in using paradoxical intervention.

Cluster 2

Reflecting team process

Andersen developed reflecting team process,[11] which is characterized by everything that is said during meetings being out in the open. Clients hear what professionals say about the client's situation, rather than the professional network being secretive. The openness is achieved by various methods. One way is for clients to meet with a team of professionals. One professional talks with the family for a while with the team listening to that talk. At an appropriate moment, the listening members of the team talk about what they saw, heard and thought when they listened to the family talk. Thereafter, the family members have a turn in responding by talking about what they were thinking when they listened to the team's talk.[12] In relation to interviewing, there are some guiding principles:

❑ **Adoption of a not-knowing approach.** The interviewer does not presume that s/he has the expertise in relation to the situation. For example, Anderson and Goolishian describe the case of a 40-year-old man who chronically felt that he had a contagious disease and was perpetually infecting others, even killing them with it.[13] Multiple negative medical consultations and psychotherapies had failed to relieve the man of his conviction and fear about his infectious disease. Although he talked of difficulties in his marriage (his wife didn't understand him) and his inability to work, his primary concern was his disease and the ever-spreading contamination. He was frightened, distraught, and unable to be at peace because of the harm and destruction that he knew he was spreading. Early in his story, wringing his hands, he told about being diseased and infectious. The consultant (Goolishian) asked him, 'How long have you had this disease?' Looking astonished and after a long pause, the man began to tell his story. He had sought help for his problem, but had always been told that he was in excellent health. These negative reports convinced him that his disease was much worse because it was unknown to medical science ... He continued to consult physicians, but the physical and laboratory examinations were always negative. By now he was being told that he did not have a disease but that he did have a mental condition, and he was referred on several occasions for psychiatric consultation. Over time he became convinced that no-one understood the seriousness of his contamination, the extent of his disease, nor the destruction he was causing. As the consultant continued to show an interest in his dilemma, the man became more relaxed ... he elaborated his story ... The consultant did not simply take a history or re-collect events of the static past. His curiosity remained with the man's reality (the disease and contamination problem). The intent was not to challenge the man's reality or the man's story, but rather to learn about it, and to let it be re-told in a way that allowed new meaning and new narrative to emerge. In other words, the consultant's intent was not to talk or manipulate the man away from his ideas, but rather through not-knowing (non-negation and non-judgement) to provide a starting point for dialogue and the opening of conversational space. Colleagues viewing the interview were quite critical of this collaborative position and of questions like 'How long *have you had* this disease?' They feared that such questions have the effect of reinforcing the patient's 'hypochondriacal delusions'. Many suggested that a safer question would have been, 'How long *have you thought* you had this disease?' ... to have asked [this] question would only have served to impose the consultant's predetermined or 'knowing' and 'paradigmatic' view that the disease was a figment of the man's imagination or a delusion or distortion in need of correction ... most likely, the man would have felt misunderstood and alienated.

❑ **Radical listening.** The interviewer and reflecting team listen attentively. They try to hear what the person says without reference to their preferred ways of understanding. This radical listening can open up possibilities for creative reflection. For example, as reflecting team member, I have said, 'When I heard Sylvia say that she is the Duchess of Kent, I imagined how she might walk and talk and dress differently, and I wondered how other people might respond to her then'.

❑ **Use of systemic/relational questions.** See Chapter 10 on questioning.

❑ **Reflective formats for the session.** The interviewer, family and team can move between speaking and listening positions. As there is no desire to uncover the 'real truth' about a problem, it is possible to construct layers of meaning through reflection upon reflection upon reflection. Deciding when to change position, from talking to listening and vice versa, is negotiable. There may be a pause in the flow of conversation that invites a change, or a family member, interviewer or team may request it, although it is never demanded.

❑ **Attention to our own personal and professional beliefs/prejudices.** What is offered as a reflection is often accompanied by the reflector's own consideration of why they have offered the particular reflection rather than another. For example, I encountered a couple when working as part of a family team as part of the observing/listening system. The couple had been on the brink of divorce and this was attributed to the husband's long-standing depression. However, he had strong negative beliefs about marital breakdown, thinking that the couple would have to grin and bear the situation for the sake of the children. He was obviously uncomfortable at being in the meeting and was vocal in his dislike of feminists and social scientists who made claims that divorce was often a humane alternative to inharmonious family life. Behind the screen, I felt that I was being personally attacked by a chauvinist with a vested interest in keeping the status quo within the family. However, since working in a reflecting team I had become accustomed to listening attentively to what people say and examining my own prejudices alongside that. As the meeting unfolded, I discovered that the man's father had died when he was a boy and he had struggled to gain an identity in the context of a female household. He interpreted 'evidence' from social science and feminism through the lens of his own experience and found it wanting. His antagonism to such theory was *understandable* once the broader context of his life was included. By the end of the meeting I found myself in admiration of someone who would sacrifice himself for the sake of providing a role model for his sons.

Generating ideas to reflect back to family/interviewer can be difficult especially when you first begin to work in this way. While there are some general guidelines for producing feedback, it is important to remember that sometimes intuition gives us ideas about what to offer. The 'helpful ideas', shown in Box 46.2, encourage us to think about what was *actually* said and different possible versions.

Having thought about what was said, by whom, to whom, the range of ideas and the nature of silence, about how things could be interpreted differently, the opportunity to feedback to the family needs to be sensitively handled. Some guidance is given in Box 46.3.

Box 46.2 Helpful ideas when reflecting – guidelines

Content:

- How were things described? For example, I noticed that when Mary refers to herself she always says 'just' – like 'It's just my opinion'.
- How could things be described? For example, I wondered whether when John says he is tired of living it could be that he is tired of fighting the problem?
- How were things explained? For example, it caught my attention that there was a lot of talk about how tablets work or don't work.
- How could things be explained? For example, I know that a lot of people make sense of what's happening for them in relation to changes in their physical body. I have a different idea that how we talk about problems can make them grow smaller or larger.
- What relationships seemed to exist between issues? For example, I noticed at several points in the session that when Joan becomes tearful Jean looks away.
- What relationships may exist between issues? For example, I found myself making connections between Gail's angry outbursts and Neil's needs to have a bit of space.
- What may have happened if something else was attempted? For example, I heard the family say that when Harry has a drink they all start to nag at him. I was wondering what would happen if someone in the family asked him whether there was anything upsetting him?

Process:

- Who talked?
- Who talked with whom?
- How many different ideas were expressed?
- Silences?

Narrative: Theory, principles and practice

When we understand someone, we understand his or her stories.

Narrative is a different mode of understanding, one less concerned with objective understanding. Narrative carries the weight of context and so, for Bruner, it is a more suitable medium for relating human experience.[14] It is through the fictions and stories that we tell ourselves and others that we live our lives. Stories allow us self-protection, to find a way to be with others, but also can create tangles and interrupt the flow of life.

Box 46.3 Ideas about reflecting back

- Use of language (non-prejudicial, not jargon laden). For example, I noticed that being a person described as having alternative ways of thinking has meant that Don has had to put his life on hold.
- Use of metaphor/imagery. For example, I wondered whether this family know the story of Alice in Wonderland – Alice is asked by the Caterpillar 'Who are you?' and Alice can hardly answer for she has undergone so many changes since being in Wonderland.
- Conversational style. The reflecting space is not about scoring points off one another as practitioners, i.e. seeing who can come up with the best reflection which mirrors some reality of the family's distress. Rather it is about opening up different versions of how life is or can be played out.
- Remain positive. For example, I was impressed that Hilary was able to share her tears with the rest of her family and the team.
- Remain within the context set by the conversation listened to. For example, I heard Frank say that he was 'horrified' by what has been happening at his work.
- Tentative advice in third person. For example, I just wondered whether it would be worthwhile to try …
- 5–10 minutes uninterrupted, a longer period of reflection risks losing the listeners' attention.

There is a growing interest in narrative in health disciplines. In a recent series in the *British Medical Journal*, Greenhalgh and Hurwitz offer the following summary points in relation to narrative based medicine:[15]

- ❑ The process of getting ill, being ill, getting better (or getting worse), and coping (or failing to cope) with illness, can all be thought of as enacted narratives within the wider narratives (stories) of people's lives.
- ❑ Narratives of illness provide a framework for approaching a patient's problems holistically, and may uncover diagnostic and therapeutic options.
- ❑ Taking a history is an interpretive act; interpretation (the discernment of meaning) is central to the analysis of narratives (for example, in literary criticism).
- ❑ Narratives offer a method for addressing existential qualities such as inner hurt, despair, grief, and moral pain which frequently accompany, and may even constitute, people's illnesses.

Launer offers some case material of a narrative approach in action.[16] When a narrative approach is favoured within family therapy the members of the team remember that there are many versions of the family's story, authored by each member.

Box 46.4 indicates the principles that guide interviewing when taking a narrative approach.

In the field of family therapy, David Epston and Michael White have used narrative approaches extensively.[17] These authors state that stories are created to make our life experiences meaningful and, in turn, such stories shape our lives. Sometimes a particular story becomes so well rehearsed that it is difficult to step outside of the text and act in a more productive, creative or less pathologizing way. In therapy, there is a space for revising (revisioning) stories and the life practice that follows from them. For Epston and White, the therapist and family member(s) can work to re-author family events and co-create an alternative story. They describe a client, Rose, who had been struggling with a demanding job in advertising and was insecure in her sense of self.[17] She met with Epston who invited her to tell her story. He followed this up with a letter that re-storied her life experience as an odyssey involving overcoming the legacy of neglect and oppression through her special wisdom, determination, and ability to self-protect. She was described as having 'grit' and a 'survival instinct'. A month after receiving the letter, Rose had found a job in her ideal career, felt her life was on the right track, had renewed her relationship with her mother, established the validity of her abusive experience through checking with her siblings. 'Rose was radiant and witty as she contemplated the future she was now anticipating'.[17]

Social network meetings

Often when people come into hospital, there is a sense of relief from relatives and sometimes from psychiatric and non-psychiatric professionals who have been struggling to find an appropriate way to help the person in distress. The social network will have generated a variety of accounts (sometimes conflicting) about the problem

Box 46.4 Principles that guide interviewing within a narrative approach

- Adoption of a not-knowing approach. The therapist does not believe and/or act as if s/he has all the answers. Rather the family members are seen as the experts in relation to their predicament.
- Radical listening. The therapist attends to channels of communication that are not routinely followed, e.g. the use of a particular grammatical style, the use of metaphor, etc.
- The use of systemic/relational questions (see Chapter 12).
- Reflective formats for the sessions (see above).
- Attention to personal and professional beliefs and prejudices.

and how it should be addressed. There may be a feeling that there can be a cooling off period during which the person admitted can 'settle down' on the ward. However, coming into hospital can be an awkward experience for first timers and old hands alike. When individuals and relatives are asked about the process of coming into hospital they tend to identify several problems. Patients have to find a way to relate to the ward staff and understand how they operate personally and in terms of the ward routine. They state the need to feel some sense of control about what is happening and what is going to happen. They are concerned that they will never 'get out of hospital'. The relatives state that they feel excluded from decisions and that the valuable information they have is not gathered and/or used. Given this sense of confusion and lost opportunity, what is the evidence for engaging with the social network around crisis and admission?

Finnish colleagues have been working with people in crisis and at risk of hospital admission and with people newly admitted.[18] The team found that it was worthwhile to make the boundary between hospital and community more open. They convened a meeting of the key people to create a space in which treatment can be discussed openly. In other words all decisions are made with respect for the opinions of the patient and her/his family and the professional network. The aim is to come to a consensus about the way forward which all parties sign up to. This has the benefit of circumventing the possibility of different agendas being played out. The evaluation of the Finnish team's approach is summarized as follows: In a sample of 30 people with a psychotic diagnosis, only 9/30 had more than 31 hospital days in two years follow-up; 9/30 used neuroleptics, but six out of these nine discontinued without detriment; 20/30 patients had no psychotic symptoms at follow-up, 7/30 had mild symptoms and three severe symptoms.

Alex Reed and members of the North Shields Family Team have developed these ideas and instigated meetings on an acute psychiatric admission ward in North Tyneside, with support from the inpatient staff.[19] The meetings are called reception meetings. Everyone who is admitted to the ward has the opportunity to have a meeting. There is a standard letter that is given to every patient that explains something of why the meetings are offered, who can attend and so on. Box 46.5 shows the letter as it is currently used.

The meetings are organized to be as warm and welcoming as possible. For example, participants are always offered a drink. The professionals concerned actively try to avoid using professional jargon that is exclusive and to adopt a more conversational style. The people who convene and the facilitator have to be careful that the family members are not made to feel that they are being called

---

Box 46.5 Reception meeting invitation letter

Dear Mr Jones

Ward 21 Reception Meeting Invitation

This letter provides some information about a service that is offered to people when they come to Ward 21, and they may wish to make use of:

What is a reception meeting?

Entering hospital may be a stressful or worrying experience, both for the person coming in, and also possibly for any relatives or friends who are close to them. For this reason, we believe that it can be very useful to arrange a meeting in which you or your family or close friends can talk with members of the staff team about your recent experiences; any worries or concerns you may have or information you might need about our service; and also any ideas or suggestions about what might be most helpful to you at this point in time.

Who will be invited to the meeting?

As well as your family and close friends, a member of the nursing team from the ward will also attend. If there are any other professionals who have been working with you before you came into hospital, it may also be helpful to invite them, so that they too can share their thoughts and ideas.

When will the meetings take place?

We believe that these meetings are most helpful when they occur within a short time after entering hospital, so a reception meeting has been *provisionally* arranged for you on ...., at .... here on the ward. The discussion is likely to last between an hour and an hour and a half.

How to get more information about the reception meeting

The reception meeting will only take place if you wish it to do so, and if you would like the opportunity to discuss the idea in more detail, please do not hesitate to approach a member of the nursing staff. If you are happy for the meeting to take place, a copy of this invitation will also be sent to those relative friends and professionals who it is agrees should attend.

Yours sincerely

---

to account for something. Nor is the agenda to make the family aware of what is medically best for their relative, or to arrive at and convey a diagnosis. The meetings are organized around the idea that families are agents of change and not objects of change. The family member, including the member in distress, are seen as the experts about their own family life and lives in general. Their ideas and support are invaluable within the therapeutic process. The meetings do not follow a set agenda, as the preference is to work with the concerns that people bring. The staff hosting the meeting positively encourage the expression of views, even though this may be difficult for some people who have been silent previously. The meetings are organized in such a way that people are encouraged both to speak and listen, much as in reflecting process described above.

CONCLUSION

Research, theory and personal practice experience support the idea that involving families in meetings can open up possibilities for creating change. This chapter has given some practical advice about how meetings with families can be organized and conducted. A word of warning, however; it is important to acknowledge that different families are made up of different individuals, in varied personal and emotional circumstances. Whilst the guidance offered here is a starting point for family work, the particular context will inform how family meetings proceed. Therapeutic recipes can be fruitfully adapted.

REFERENCES

1. Reed A. Manufacturing a human drama from a psychiatric crisis: crisis intervention, family therapy and the work of RD Scott. In: Barker P, Stevenson C (eds). *The construction of power and authority in psychiatry*. Oxford: Butterworth Heineman, 2000: 154.

2. Scott RD, Starr I. A 24-hour family orientated psychiatric and crisis service. *Journal of Family Therapy* 1981; **3**: 177–86.

3. Scott RD. The treatment barrier: Part I. *British Journal of Medical Psychology* 1973; **46**: 45–55.

4. Carpenter J, Treacher A. *Marital and family therapy*. Oxford: Blackwell, 1989.

5. Stevenson C. *Negotiating a therapeutic context in family therapy*. Unpublished Ph.D. thesis, University of Northumbria, 1995.

6. Minuchin S, Fishman C. *Family therapy techniques*. Cambridge, MA: Harvard University Press, 1981: 31–2.

7. Watzlawick P, Weakland J, Fisch R. *Change*. New York: Norton, 1974: 95.

8. Bandler R, Grinder J, Andreas S. *Frogs into princes: neuro-linguistic programming*. Moab, Utah: Real People Press, 1979.

9. Cade B. The use of paradox in therapy. In: Walrond-Skinner S (ed.) *Family and marital psychotherapy: a critical approach*. Routledge and Kegan Paul: Boston, 1979.

10. Watzlawick P, Beavin AB, Jackson DD. *Pragmatics of human communication*. New York: Norton, 1967: 242.

11. Andersen T. The reflecting team. *Family Process* 1987; **26**: 415–28.

12. Andersen T. Reflections on reflecting with families. In: McNamee S, Gergen K (eds). *Therapy as social construction*. London: Sage, 1992: 54–68.

13. Anderson H, Goolishian H. The client is the expert: a not-knowing approach to therapy. In: McNamee S, Gergen K (eds). *Therapy as social construction*. London: Sage, 1992: 25–39.

14. Bruner J. *Acts of meaning*. Cambridge, MA: Harvard University Press, 1990.

15. Greenhalgh T, Hurwitz B. Why study narrative? *British Medical Journal* 1999; **318**: 48–51.

16. Launer JA. Narrative approach to mental health in general practice. *British Medical Journal* 1999; **318**: 117–19.

17. Epston D, White M, Murray K. A proposal for re-authoring therapy. In: McNamee S, Gergen K (eds). *Therapy as social construction*. London: Sage, 1992: 96–115.

18. Seikkula J, Sutela M. Co-evolution of the family and the hospital: the system of boundary. *Journal of Strategic and Systemic Therapies* 1990; **9**: 34–42.

19. Reed A, Wilson M, Stevenson C. Social network meetings ease trauma of psychiatric admission. *Nursing Times* 1998; **94**(42): 52–3.

Chapter 47

SPECIALIST SERVICES FOR HOMELESS PEOPLE

Jon Wigmore* and Paul Veitch**

The whole issue of access needs a lot more thought. Homeless people face huge resistance from many mainstream health professionals ... most services are facing in the wrong direction to help'.[1]

INTRODUCTION

If the psychiatric-mental health (PMH) nurse is to work creatively within specialist programmes, it is essential to recognize that mental health services are idiosyncratic obstacle courses, which homeless people are particularly ill-resourced to negotiate. The well-documented features of mainstream health care systems that keep homeless people out[2,3] have provided an inverse template for the development of targeted services. Here, outreach into the places single homeless people choose to go, is the key function that makes engagement possible.[4]

Mental health programmes targeted at homeless people – probably uniquely within the field of psychiatry – focus on nursing casework, occurring almost exclusively within non-clinical 'host' homelessness services, staffed in the main by generic support workers. Consequently, we shall emphasize the knowledge and skills required to work effectively with such services. The success of nursing interventions depends on it.

Engagement with people experiencing multiple deprivations and alienation from service providers requires the ability and the humility to make available 'a broad bandwidth of roles and functions'.[5] Another major focus of this chapter will be upon engagement and assessment within the case management paradigm. In our view this is the only approach that encompasses the multi-dimensional range of interventions, which this work demands.[6,7]

OVERVIEW

The extent to which voluntary sector homelessness services vary in purpose, staffing, ethos and structure cannot be overstated.[4] Specialist mental health services for single homeless people generally operate within *direct access* homelessness services, because these are the services that make the least demands on their users in terms of conditions of usage. They are therefore very accessible to people with severe mental health and drug and alcohol problems, particularly rough sleepers who endure

---

*Jon Wigmore has worked in hostels for homeless people since 1983, in Glasgow, Bristol, Bradford and London. He qualified as a psychiatric nurse in 1996. He is currently employed as an Investigations Manager for the Health Service Ombudsman.

**Paul Veitch has worked as a psychiatric nurse in the North East of England for over 20 years. He has a Masters in Psychiatric Nursing and has specialized in working with people who are homeless.

the greatest physical and mental illhealth of all homeless people and are the furthest away from mainstream services.[3] Our focus will therefore be on PMH nursing approaches applicable to day-centres, direct access hostels, shelters, and street outreach services.

Day-centres

In 1996 over 200 day-centres in the UK were being used by an average number of 10,000 people a day, a third of whom were under 25 years old.[8] Most offer basic services: cheap or free food and facilities (e.g. laundry, showers), animal care, access to donated items, opportunities to socialize with others, and a variety of things to do. Many provide advice, referral, life skills training and a range of direct and indirect linkages with other services, including health and substance dependency practitioners, who may provide input to the centre. Day-centres are usually direct access services, although some have closed sessions for specific client groups, for example women.

Direct access hostels

Direct access hostels offer same-day access to basic institutional accommodation, and increasingly prioritize people who are sleeping rough at the point of referral. There were about 2700 such bed spaces in London in 1998, representing a reduction of about 75% over two decades.[9] They are staffed 24-hours a day, and generally provide a comparable range of support services to day-centres. People are no longer encouraged to live in direct access hostels for long periods, and resettlement into longer-term accommodation has become a critical function.

Street outreach services

Street outreach teams make contact with homeless people in the places they are known to frequent, particularly the areas where people sleep out. This demands specialist engagement skills and techniques,[10] as well as careful attention to safety, and to the rights of the individuals who are approached.[4] Outreach in the form of 'CAT teams' (contact and assessment teams) is integral to the current government policy of targeting homelessness services at rough sleepers.[11]

SPECIALIST MENTAL HEALTH SERVICES

The main way PMH nursing is made available to single homeless people within specialist programmes, is through multidisciplinary teams targeting this client group. Although some services are based in a fixed site (e.g. a clinic), contact with clients is generally made through 'secondary outreach',[12] i.e. by engaging with the existing clients of voluntary sector services within the venues provided by those services.

Most teams work across multiple venues (i.e. within several host homelessness services inside a city or Health Authority patch). Contact is available through discrete sessions and by appointment. Referrals are made either directly by the client or a peer, by staff in the voluntary sector service, or people are referred on to the specialist team by gatekeepers in mainstream mental health services.

The composition of each team is the product of varied funding regimes, joint working arrangements and local priorities. Mental health professionals may work alongside GPs, nurse practitioners, dentists, chiropodists, drug and alcohol workers, social workers, trainers, housing workers, health development workers and 'link workers'.[13] There is a focus on primary care provision, although some teams, for example START in South London, have a mental health focus.[14]

Some homelessness services have semi-formal, local relationships with mental health care providers, through access to a PMH nurse,[15] or to fast-track assessment for individual clients. Others directly employ nurses to work with their clients. In Spitalfields, London, an exceptional nurse-led primary health care centre for homeless people is being piloted.[16]

Table 47.1 shows how mainstream mental health and homelessness services are largely complementary and interdependent, even if the terminology and foci for intervention differ. This chapter will consider how PMH nurses work across these two sectors.

Extending nursing into homelessness services: the case management model

The broadly defined concept of 'case management' best encompasses the range of roles required of PMH nurses working within specialist homeless services, in particular in its emphasis upon engagement, advocacy and service linkage. In the US this approach has formed the 'cornerstone of efforts to serve people who are homeless' for two decades, and is the only method supported by something like an evidence base.[6] The approach is gradually gaining recognition in the UK.[7]

The PMH nurse rarely manages a defined caseload of homeless people. Collaborative working practices and ways of recruiting staff from other services are, therefore, threaded through what follows. We would also stress that implementing these approaches is never a linear process. Homeless people often have far more

TABLE 47.1 Crisis support and rehabilitative functions of mental health and homelessness services

Short-term (crisis) functions		
	Mental health services	Single homelessness services
Definition of crisis	Psychotic breakdown, acute distress, risk to others, risk to self	Sleeping rough, homeless, unable to manage/at risk of losing accommodation
Crisis response (supportive intervention)	Intensive therapeutic contact, assertive outreach, crisis team or home treatment team contact, carer support	For homeless people: food, clothes, practical help, support, assessment, referral For those threatened with homelessness: advocacy, housing advice, liaison
Crisis response (substitutive intervention)	Hospital accommodation, treatment, care, containment, safety measures, medication, therapy	Hostel or shelter accommodation, food, warmth, support, cleaning facilities, health referral
Long-term (rehabilitative) functions		
	Mental health services	Single homelessness services
Intended outcome (behavioural/lifestyle change)	Living with maximum independence Rehabilitation Relapse prevention Community integration Symptom management	Living with maximum independence Resettlement Tenancy sustainment 'Meaningful occupation' Self-management of drug/alcohol problem
Interventions to achieve outcome	Community mental health team contact Medication Day hospital Cognitive-behavioural therapy Occupational therapy	Resettlement/floating support team contact Generic support services Day-centre Advocacy Life-skills training

pressing needs to fulfil than adherence to a support programme, and single consultations will need to encompass multiple interventions across the spectrum of case management roles.

Table 47.2 identifies the key roles of professionals working with homeless people.[6,17]

THERAPEUTIC FUNCTIONS

Client identification, outreach and engagement

Engagement requires a complicated set of skills and attitudes. It includes being able to establish and develop trusting and caring relationships, responding quickly to client need priorities, being dependable but flexible, and being adept at covertly assessing a client's often changing needs for intensive services or personal space.[6]

Many homeless people associate the PMH nurse role with the stigma of being perceived as 'mad', or with custodial or policing functions. An attitude of humility and willingness to learn from both the clients and the staff of the host service will ensure that such prejudices and fears are reduced.

Our experience suggests that the following practices are effective in nurturing engagement with homeless people.

❑ **Be known as available for a range of supports.** Few people will approach you for a 'mental health consultation'. Try to address people's perceived needs, which will often relate to day-to-day survival. Do not force the pace or introduce service objectives too quickly. An ability and willingness to sort out benefit problems, advocate across a wide range of services, and successfully take on a variety of instrumental roles for people is essential.

❑ **Offer regular contact opportunities.** Establish fixed times when you can be approached, ideally covering periods of morning, afternoon and early evening, with a flexible provision for unstructured participation in the project's activities. Modes of working should encompass one-to-one consultations on an as-required and appointment basis, and casework support consultations with homelessness service staff.

❑ **Assimilate.** Ensure that you fit into the host service by dressing appropriately and reinforcing the rules.

TABLE 47.2 Functions of case management for homeless people

THERAPEUTIC FUNCTIONS

1 **Client identification and outreach:** to attempt to enrol clients not using normal services
2 **Assessment:** to determine a person's current and potential strengths, weaknesses and needs
3 **Planning:** to develop a specific, comprehensive, individualised treatment and service plan
4 **Client advocacy:** to intercede on behalf of a specific client or a class of clients to ensure equity and appropriate services
5 **Linkage:** to refer or transfer clients to necessary services and treatments and informal support systems
6 **Monitoring:** to conduct ongoing evaluation of client progress and needs
7 **Crisis intervention:** assisting clients in crisis to stabilize through direct interventions and mobilizing needed supports and services
8 **Direct service:** provision of clinical services directly to the client

SYSTEMIC FUNCTIONS

9 **System advocacy:** intervening with organizations or larger systems of care in order to promote more effective, equitable, and accountable services to a target client group
10 **Resource development:** attempting to create additional services or resources to address the needs of clients

The homelessness service staff should be partners in every component of the case management process. Participation in homelessness service team meetings will cement your position as a resource, as well as yielding insights into staff perceptions of the mental health needs of individual clients.

❏ **Work off-site.** For example, accompany people to appointments, or to the shops or to a café. This can be a powerful catalyst for the engagement process. It demonstrates that you are honoured, not ashamed, to be in their company. Some clients will only be accessible away from service locations[10] – many regard day-centres and hostels as dangerous.

Assessment

Outcome-focused assessment is probably the single most powerful tool available to the PMH nurse attempting to materially improve the lives of single homeless people. This meshes assessment with advocacy and service linkage functions. Appropriate assessment can open doors to a range of benefits: social security payments, housing placements, probation (as opposed to custodial sentencing), care management, mental health service treatment, and access to crisis services.

A key problem for clinicians is that, often, only frag-

ments of people's histories and careers of service usage are available.[4] Family and long-standing friends often are inaccessible. The client will probably not have a GP with any breadth of knowledge of their mental health. Assessment information may thus be overly weighted by the immediate perceptions of the person's needs (in particular their crisis needs) by staff in the homelessness service, and clients.

To augment core assessment skills, consider the following:

❏ **Be opportunistic.** The PMH nurse needs to be able to assess for multiple needs in single episodes of client contact – there is no guarantee the person will return at a time convenient to you. Such episodes may be fleeting and initiated in busy places, and the most pressing issue may be obscured by a superficially mundane request for help.

❏ **Tailor assessment content and format to mesh with other services.** In homelessness work, assessments are multifunctional, not solely the foundation of nursing or MDT interventions. You may be the only specialist a service user is willing or able to see. You will be asked to corroborate a range of needs and special circumstances. This means building a understanding of the operational criteria of the different services dealing with these needs.

❏ **Incorporate information from staff from homelessness services.** Provide clear guidelines as to what behaviours staff should be particularly aware of, and how to record information (e.g. exact quotations or descriptions of behaviour rather than judgements like 'He is acting paranoid').

❏ **Ensure that gatekeepers to secondary mental health services are informed.** This particularly includes professionals assessing people for compulsory hospital admission, or responding to reports or presentations of crisis. Homeless people are often routinely perceived as so far removed from the norm that judgements as to whether they are in actual crisis, or in 'normal chaos' are very difficult to make. The crisis admission route is particularly important for homeless people.

Planning

It cannot be over-emphasized that the planning task needs to be carried out in the spirit of mutual collaboration with the client and that the client's expressed needs drive the whole process.[7]

Colleagues from the homelessness service will undertake some of the key interventions that will follow assessment. Also, ongoing contact between you and the client cannot always be taken for granted, and you may move into a planning stage before completing an assessment.

These issues shape the task of planning interventions in the following ways:

- **Commence planning on initial contact.** Planning should be concurrent with engagement and assessment, and should ensure attention to every applicable case management task. Staff need to *know* they are responsible for tasks, particularly when planning occurs across agencies.
- **Collaborate.** Plans will often need to be incremental and linked to gains as perceived by the client. Goals involving motivation or behavioural change will often need a long, planned lead-in of sustained supportive contact from specific team members. A frank discussion of potential resources will ensure that reasons for not wanting particular services (e.g. negative experiences of associated services in the past) are understood and addressed.

Case study 47.1 Planning

Donette is a PMH nurse providing two four-hourly sessions a week to the residents and staff of a direct access hostel. About a quarter of the people she sees every week are new to the service. Her case notes consist of a weekly summary of what she and the team have learnt about a person, followed by a plan consisting of a list of actions to be completed by herself and the hostel staff over the following week or fortnight. Her colleague, Kate, is the hostel keyworker for Gareth, a 23-year-old man who is new to the area, vague about his history and involved in crack cocaine use. He presents as shy and elusive to staff, but there have been instances of verbal hostility, particularly towards people he is not familiar with. He has also expressed persecutory ideas. He says he has used inpatient mental health services in the past. He has started to confide in a team member and express the fear that he will be 'dead before too long'. The initial plan was as follows.

1   Register Gareth with the Broadway Practice (who employ a drug dependency worker) and offer to accompany him to initial appointments (Kate/hostel team).

2   Encourage Gareth to talk one-to-one to a trusted staff member as often as possible. Allow him to set the pace and discuss his fears. What has brought him here? What has helped, what has not? What has kept him going? (Kate/hostel team).

3   Attempt, with his permission, to locate and contact his previous service provider(s) for more specific information about his history (e.g. Why did he leave his accommodation? What was the discharge summary from his last period in

hospital?) (Kate will contact housing providers. Donette will contact mental health services).

4   Record examples of the speech and behaviour that are of concern to staff and other residents. Include the context (time of day, people present, level of intoxication if any, anything else that seems important) (Kate and Team).

5   Reinforce Donette's availability to Gareth in drop-ins, or by appointment at a time which suits him. If he is comfortable, discuss his use of drugs, his perceptions of his habit and past use of drug and mental health services (Donette, Kate and Team).

6   Complete initial risk assessment and crisis plan (Donette).

Client advocacy

In an ideal world, 'pure' advocacy services, distinct from support providers, would be available to homeless people. There is evidence that such services are needed and effective, particularly when they employ formerly homeless people.[1,18] In reality, providers must adopt advocacy functions if the referral stage of linkage to benefits and services is to happen.

The interface between specialist mental health services for homeless people and mainstream mental health services will usually be a contested area. Good joint working arrangements do not compensate for limited resources and mainstream services ill-suited for homeless people's use. In this context, advocacy should encompass the following:

- **Use assertive referral methods.** Referrals of homeless people 'upstream' – to mainstream services – will often need to be sustained, educational about homelessness issues, documented, explicit about the outcome desired, and referenced to that service's criteria. Accompanying clients to assessments is supportive, and demonstrates your scrutiny of the process to the assessor.
- **Assist colleagues in homelessness services in advocacy and referral work.** Encourage staff to adopt the focus and methods outlined above, discourage vagueness and a sense that mainstream services will always be able to 'sort it out'. Educate colleagues about how to access the decision-making structures within mental health care services.

Linkage

We need to identify homeless and mentally ill people as important resources rather than as individual problems to be tackled.[19]

Convincing a client that making a referral could bring a benefit, and the target service that the referral is appropriate, are integral to the planning and implementation processes. The critical component of this linkage process is the bridging role of the support worker. This role involves building a therapeutic alliance based on hopefulness and an appreciation of the proven strengths and resources of the client. The US experience is that such 'low-demand' engagement may extend for *many years* before lifestyle change occurs, particularly where substance dependency occurs alongside mental illness.[20]

Important components of bridging work are as follows:

❑ **Share 'process information'[21] with clients.** Referral systems often reinforce client passivity and disregard the security of personal information. Informing the person in detail about what they might expect from a referral *process*, as well as possible service *outcomes* (including potentially negative experiences), is an essential part of a rights-based approach.

❑ **Maintain an awareness of a wide range of resources.** This includes mainstream and independent sector support services (dealing with mental health and drug and alcohol issues) and therapy services. Also self-help and mutual help groups accessible to homeless people; education and training resources; opportunities for creative expression (e.g. writing, acting, the arts); and online initiatives in all of those areas.[22]

❑ **'Critical time interventions',[23]** i.e. workers based in homelessness services providing long-term (at least 9 months) focused support during major transitions in clients' lives (e.g. transfer to a lower support environment), in likely areas for difficulties (e.g. money management, medication).

Case study 47.2: The bridging role

Tony is a 37-year-old man who has spent considerable time in institutions: children's homes, borstals and prison. He had been asking for a lot of one-to-one time with his keyworker following a serious assault in which he was left for dead. He presented with a mixture of anger, sadness, despair, desperation and fear. Sessions always involved tears, sometimes shouting and statements of great violence towards third parties. He also described periods of complete numbness and depersonalization.

Underlying this disclosure and discharge of emotion was a hunger to understand why history kept repeating itself. In his struggle to maintain relationships he asked, 'is it too late to change?' After a series of sessions with his support worker and the PMH nurse it was agreed to refer Tony for psychotherapy. He was accompanied to two assessments, both of

which resulted in the therapy service declining to work with him. One assessor suggested 'residential rehabilitation with anger management', the other that he needed hospitalization. This was crushing for him.

Tony agreed that the nurse could write a brief assessment and offer this to potential therapists for pre-assessment. A therapist was eventually recommended by another client, and he agreed to talk to Tony based on the written assessment. He came to the hostel and saw him with his support worker. Despite many ups and downs, three years later they are still in regular contact. The therapist and his support worker have helped Tony explore his honesty, courage and determination for history not to repeat itself, and he has moved forward in his life.

Monitoring

Outcomes linked to sustained 'resettlement' and 'meaningful occupation' are the gold standards for homelessness services.[24] We propose outcome measures that complement these without compromising the distinctive therapeutic role of the PMH nurse.

The evaluation of nursing interventions must include an understanding that changes in lifestyle and behaviour, which contribute to improved *health* (in every sense of the word), are difficult for anyone. For homeless people – with restricted access to resources – the obstacles are far greater. Any of the outcomes listed in Table 47.3 may result from the efforts of a range of disciplines, in conjunction with clients' own tenacity.

Direct service provision and crisis intervention

A primary therapeutic role of the PMH nurse is to plan for and manage crisis collaboratively. The advanced prac-

TABLE 47.3 Some outcomes in work with homeless people

- Retaining the person in the service for longer periods (as opposed to their returning to the streets or being excluded)
- Engagement with primary health care service (in-house)
- Benefit income is increased, also ability to manage cash
- Reduced use of hospital
- Safer use of alcohol and/or drugs, safer sexual practices
- Engagement with support/resettlement programme
- Engagement with mental health practitioner/s
- Participation in occupational activities* for homeless or rehoused people
- Participation in service decision-making/management activities (e.g selecting staff)
- Participation in mainstream occupational activities*

*Training, education, leisure, sport, artistic, employment

TABLE 47.4 The feelings of homeless people about health care services, from McCabe et al.[27]

Theme	Attributes of the theme
Committed care	Providers do not give up on people (even if non-compliant), able to appraise for a variety of health problems (not just expressed needs at the time); thorough care; sticking with the person; non-punitive (e.g. if appointments are missed).
Respectful engagement	Perceptions of support, of care, empathy, acceptance and respect from provider. Not feeling rushed, being addressed by name, feeling good about self as a result of being respected.
Trust	Belief, faith and confidence in health care providers. Trust allows for sharing sensitive information without fear of it being used against them. Also refers to credibility attached to provider's recommendations.
Assumption free	Treatment not tainted by negative pre-judgement or prejudice against homeless people, e.g. homeless people are transient, non-compliant, unreliable and mendacious.
Inclusionary care practices	Being able to access needed care, included in decisions, allowed to reject decisions without penalty to further care. Minimal paperwork, awareness and accommodation of homeless people's lifestyle issues, respect for homeless people's ability to prioritize health care choices.

titioner in this field should also develop additional expertise, particularly in substance dependency work.

- **Groupwork.** These sessions may have a range of emphases: health promotion, for example medication or first aid;[25] user involvement and participation[26]; support and resettlement;[14] or promote artistic, sporting or therapeutic activity.
- **Joint working.** Jointly case managing with homelessness agency staff, clients presenting with frequent crises, hostile behaviour or safety needs, is a pragmatic and enabling extension of the nursing function. This demands careful negotiation and a thorough mastery of communication systems in the homelessness agency. Roles may be shared, or separately delineated. There are opportunities for mutual role modelling and learning and the PMH nurse may also offer clinical supervision.

Finally in this section, we would emphasize that little positive work can be undertaken with homeless people without close attention to and awareness of their lived experience of support services. Table 47.4 summarizes the results of an elegant US study exploring service users' feelings about the provision of health care services in a range of homelessness services.[27]

Systemic interventions

> Inadequate housing, homelessness, and family poverty are structural issues but are no less amenable to intervention than the health conditions they engender. The way they differ is in the type of intervention they require ... Advocacy is structural therapeutics.'[28]

The current UK policy emphasis upon 'joined up' public services provides increased opportunities for PMH nurses in the homelessness sector to take lead roles in developing services and promoting inclusive ways of working. Homelessness services can be innovative development partners, although the tension between business needs and clients' needs is often more palpable than in other areas of mental health care.

Maureen Crane, through her work with older homeless people (street outreach work, creating and evaluating a service, researching and writing about problems and solutions),[14] is an exemplar of the PMH nurse as practitioner of what Roberts calls 'structural therapeutics'[28] which links the domains of individual and public health. It restores clinicians' historical role, which has been to develop and publicize the organizational and environmental improvements that enhance people's health, particularly the health and safety of those experiencing extremes of deprivation.

Systemic interventions include the provision of training to housing and homelessness service staff. This is a form of structural advocacy that is integral to the work of many specialist health and homelessness teams. Training health service staff about homelessness issues is, sadly, less widespread. We have included in Table 47.5 some typical examples of questions asked of PMH nurses by homelessness service staff. These illustrate the bewilderment many experience when dealing with mental health services. All the issues raised in these queries make ideal subjects for training, and a case study approach, setting the issues in context, is often appropriate.

QUESTIONS ASKED BY STAFF IN HOMELESSNESS SERVICES

Service operational issues

- Why are personality disorder diagnoses barriers to mental health provision?

- Why can't mental health services and substance misuse services co-ordinate better?
- Why has this client been kept in hospital for a long time/summarily discharged?
- How can I get involved in joint care planning with this person and mental health services?
- Why won't the crisis team attend the hostel during crises?

Safety issues

- What can we do about this person's self-harming?
- This person says they want to kill themselves. What shall we do?

Technical knowledge issues

- What does this section of the Mental Health Act mean?
- What happens if this person starts or stops taking this drug?
- What happens if this person mixes this drug with alcohol or street drugs?
- How can we help this person manage their physical illness?

CONCLUSION

A recent NHS proposal to establish a career pathway for nurses working with homeless people, and establish 'social exclusion nursing' as an area for consultant-level nursing practice, was disappointing in its neglect of PMH nursing.[13] We believe that PMH nurses' ability to move between therapeutic, health promotion and all-round 'fixer' roles is particularly valued by homeless people.

We would wish to see a skill base encompassing the philosophy of 'social exclusion nursing' embedded in nursing curricula, as opposed to becoming a specialism. Most mental health service users would benefit from the case management approaches we have highlighted. We have found that there are many more opportunities to develop innovative services *out* of the traditional clinical area than in it, and would commend this way of working to any PMH nurse interested in the challenges we have outlined.

REFERENCES

1. Brandon D, Morris L. Towards social inclusion: peer advocacy with homeless people. In: Ramon S (ed.) *A stakeholder's approach to innovations in mental health services*. Brighton: Pavilion, 2000.
2. Bines W. The health of single homeless people. In: Burrows R, Pleace N, Quilgars D (eds). *Homelessness and social policy*. London: Routledge, 1997.
3. Pleace N, Quilgars D. Health, homelessness and access to health care services in London. In: Burrows R, Pleace N, Quilgars D (eds). *Homelessness and social policy*. London: Routledge, 1997.
4. Timms P, Borrell T. Doing the right thing – ethical and practical dilemmas in working with homeless mentally ill people. *Journal of Mental Health* 2001; **10**: 419–26.
5. Barker P J, Keady J, Croom S, Stevenson C, Adams T, Reynolds W. The concept of serious mental illness: modern myths and grim realities. *Journal of Psychiatric and Mental Health Nursing* 1998; 5: 247–54.
6. Morse G. A review of case management for people who are homeless: implications for practice, policy and research. In: Fosburg L, Dennis DL (eds). *The 1998 national symposium on homelessness research*. U.S. Department of Housing and Urban Development and the U.S. Department of Health and Human Services [online] 1999 [cited 2002 Jan 12]. Available from: URL: http://aspe.hhs.gov/progsys/homeless/symposium/toc.htm
7. Gournay K. Case management. In: Sandford T, Gournay K (eds). *Perspectives in mental health nursing*. London: Baillière Tindall and RCN, 1996: 31–52.
8. Llewellin S, Murdoch A. *Saving the day: the importance of day centres for homeless people*. London: CHAR, 1996.
9. Social Exclusion Unit. *Rough sleeping*. London: Cabinet Office, 1998.
10. Erickson S, Page J. To dance with grace: outreach and engagement to persons on the street. In: Fosburg L, Dennis DL (eds). *The 1998 national symposium on homelessness research*. U.S. Department of Housing and Urban Development and the U.S. Department of Health and Human Services [online] 1999 [cited 2002 Jan 12]. Available from: URL: http://aspe.hhs.gov/progsys/homeless/symposium/toc.htm
11. Rough Sleepers Unit. *Coming in from the cold, progress report on the government's strategy on rough sleeping*. London: Department for Transport, Local Government and the Regions, 2001.
12. Timms P. Management aspects of care for the homeless mentally ill. *Advances in Psychiatric Treatment* 1996; **2**: 158–65.
13. London Standing Conference for Nurses, Midwives and Health Visitors Nursing and Homelessness Group. *Nursing and homelessness*. London: NHS, 2001.
14. Warnes A, Crane M. *Meeting homeless people's needs, service development and practice for the older excluded*. London: King's Fund, 2000.
15. Wood A, Sclare P, Love J. Service innovations: a service for the homeless with mental illness in Aberdeen. *Psychiatric Bulletin* 2001; **25**: 137–40.

16. Rennells B. *Spitalfields PMS pilot, first wave nurse-led PMS pilot.* Proceedings of King's Fund Seminar, 29 November 2001, London, UK.

17. Willenbring ML, Ridgely MS, Stinchfield R, Rose M. *Application of case management in alcohol and drug dependence: matching techniques and populations.* Rockville, MD: National Institute on Alcohol Abuse and Alcoholism, 1991.

18. Fleischmann P, Wigmore J. *Nowhere else to go: increasing choice and participation for the users of supported housing.* London: Single Homeless Project, 2000.

19. Brandon D. Homeless in Cambridge? *Journal of Mental Health* 1998; **7**: 325–9.

20. Oakley D, Dennis D. Responding to the needs of homeless people with alcohol, drug, and/or mental disorders. In: Baumohl J (ed.) *Homelessness in America.* Phoenix Arizona: Oryx, 1996: 179–86.

21. Park G, Barrington L. Loose connections, bringing together agencies working with single homeless people. London: King's Fund, 2001.

22. For example ABC Tales (URL: http://www.abc-tales.com) and Groundswell (URL: http://www.oneworld.groundswell.org.uk).

23. Susser E, Valencia E, Conover S, Felix A, Tsai W, Wyatt RJ. Preventing recurrent homelessness among mentally ill men: a critical time intervention after discharge from a shelter. *American Journal of Public Health* 1997; **87**: 256–62.

24. Rough Sleepers Unit. *Preventing tomorrow's rough sleepers, a good practice handbook.* London: Department for Transport, Local Government and the Regions, 2001.

25. Hinton T, Evans N, Jacobs K. *Healthy hostels – a guide to promoting health and well being among homeless people.* London: CRISIS, 2001.

26. Glasser N. Giving voice to homeless people in policy, practice and research. In: Fosburg L, Dennis DL (eds). *The 1998 national symposium on homelessness research.* U.S. Department of Housing and Urban Development and the U.S. Department of Health and Human Services [online] 1999 [cited 2002 Jan 12]. Available from: URL: http://aspe.hhs.gov/progsys/homeless/symposium/toc.htm

27. McCabe S, Macnee CL, Anderson MK. Homeless patients' experience of satisfaction with care. *Archives of Psychiatric Nursing* 2001; 15: 78–85.

28. Roberts I. Deaths of children in house fires. *Br Med J* 1995; **311**: 1381–2.

Chapter 48

SERVICES FOR PEOPLE REQUIRING SECURE FORMS OF CARE

Colin Holmes*

HISTORICAL CONTEXT

The beginnings of secure provision

In the early 19th century, when institutional care for 'lunatics' started to become widespread across Europe, North America and the British colonies, almost all facilities were 'secure'. Wards or blocks were locked, patients were monitored and escorted at all times, the whole complex was surrounded by high walls, and entry and exit were through a single imposing 'main gate' controlled by the gatekeeper. The asylum therefore typically constituted an appropriate destination for people who had committed minor offences and were found to be insane. From the very beginning, most asylums had a number of 'criminal lunatics', and acquired special facilities to accommodate patients detained under criminal or lunacy legislation.

Special verdicts and/or sentencing arrangements had long existed in Europe, and evidence that courts recognized the diminished responsibility of some people with mental disorders appears in the earliest Greek literature and the works of Aristotle and Plato. Legislation in respect of lunatics appeared in Britain in 1800, when *The Criminal Lunatics Act* enabled courts to detain 'at His Majesty's Pleasure' persons found to be 'insane on arraignment', that is at the time they appear in court. The courtroom was an important, highly public site for testing and legitimating the emerging psychiatric expertise, and not surprisingly, the Medical Superintendents of European and North American asylums led the groundbreaking debates about the legal implications of insanity.[1–2] Their views often met with strong criticism, since the excuses afforded by the new 'mental science' were widely thought to be at odds with common-sense notions of justice. Indeed, it was Queen Victoria who, after several attempts on her life, complained that to describe the perpetrators as 'Not Guilty by Reason of Insanity', whether or not they were subsequently confined 'at Her Majesty's Pleasure', was at odds with the facts, a view taken by many who regarded them as guilty even though they were insane. It was not until 1883 that Her Majesty's preference was reflected in law, when *The Trial of Lunatics Act* enabled courts to return a verdict of 'Guilty But Insane', and subsequent legislation reinstated the 'not guilty' element. The ground-breaking case which set the standard for determinations of insanity in homicide cases was that of Daniel MacNaughtan (there is much dispute over the correct spelling of this name). MacNaughtan attempted to shoot the British Prime Minister Robert Peel in 1843, his shot missed and killed Peel's Secretary. He was found to be insane, and out of his trial came a principle, 'the M'Naughten Rules', based on the ability to distinguish right from wrong. MacNaughtan's case has been explored in great depth by Moran.[3]

*Colin Holmes is Adjunct Professor at James Cook University in Townsville, Australia. Previously he was Professor of Mental Health Nursing at Nepean, Sydney.

In Scotland, 'diminished responsibility' because of mental disorder, was established as a defence to murder since at least the 18th century, reaffirmed in the case of *R. v Dingwall* in 1867, and upheld ever since. It was not until the *Homicide Act* of 1957 that it was introduced into English law, which nevertheless continued to resist the notion of a defence based on 'irresistible impulse', long accepted in most other European countries. In the United States, a strict application of the M'Naghten Rules has tended to prevail in most states, despite the formulation of modern alternatives, notably the 'Durham Rules' of 1954. Detailed histories of the insanity defence and its evolution are given by Fingarette,[4] Robinson,[5] and Boland.[6]

Alongside the development of the legal basis for special consideration of mentally disordered offenders there has been a corresponding development of options for disposal, and of associated services. The first asylums catering primarily for criminal lunatics were those built in Australia, which was settled as a penal colony for the United Kingdom's most undesirable and dangerous offenders. There is some evidence that transportation to Australia was more likely if the offender exhibited signs of 'degeneracy', such as madness, drunkenness, or sexual perversion but, in any case, the deprivations of the journey to Australia undermined the mental and physical health of even the fittest transportees. There was, therefore, a high level of lunacy among the convicts arriving in the colony, and initially most of the patients of Australia's asylums were convicts. They were subject to harsh and neglectful treatment, since they were considered to be especially dangerous. Australia's first psychiatric facility, Castle Hill Asylum in Sydney, New South Wales, opened in 1811 for 30 patients, with medical services provided by Dr William Bland, who was himself serving a sentence for causing death by duelling. Much of the direct care was provided by the most troublesome convicts as a form of punishment, a practice not officially abandoned until late in the century. Castle Hill was closed in 1826, and by this time a terrible and punitive facility for women, called a 'factory prison', had opened at Parramatta, near Sydney. It was gloomy, ill-ventilated and dilapidated, and housed insane convicts as well as the 'criminal insane', i.e. those found to be insane at the time of their offence. In Tasmania, the site of Australia's second penal colony, facilities likewise initially catered for the convict population, with New Norfolk Asylum taking its first lunatic convict patient in 1829. Interestingly, the Medical Officer at New Norfolk at this time was Dr John Meyer, who later became Medical Superintendent at Broadmoor Criminal Lunatic Asylum in England. By the 1850s, New Norfolk was notorious for its use of electric shocks, blistering, cold showers and emetics, both to treat and punish its

patients: it was Tasmania's last institutional psychiatric facility, closing in February 2001.

Thus, although not the first to provide separate facilities, Australian asylums were among the first in the world to cater primarily for mentally ill offenders, and as the proportion of colonists increased in relation to convicts, it became important to distinguish between the criminal insane, insane convicts and the general insane, and to resolve questions as to where they should be cared for and under whose authority. This prompted the establishment of some designated facilities for criminal and convict lunatics, but these distinctions and the need for separate facilities remain contentious to this day.[7–8]

The first separate facility for criminal lunatics anywhere in the world appears to have been Dundrum Criminal Lunatic Asylum, near Dublin, Ireland, which opened in 1850 at the urging of Lord Chancellor Sugden. It was built to house 80 male and 40 female patients, and, rather surprisingly, was reported to be a bright and cheerful place, although patients wore grey and black striped clothes in the style of the prisoners of the day. Today, Dundrum offers a national forensic service to the Republic of Eire. Its more famous English equivalent, Broadmoor Criminal Lunatic Asylum, was not opened until 1863, but was much larger and by 1882 had some 500 patients. It remained under the jurisdiction of the Home Office, which administers Britain's prisons, until 1949 when it became part of the National Health Service. In Scotland, both male and female criminal lunatics were housed in a special wing of Perth Prison from 1865, and no other special facilities appear to have been developed until the opening of Carstairs State Hospital in 1957, when patients were transferred from Perth Gaol.[9]

In Canada, Rookwood Asylum in Kingston, Ontario, was built by convicts and opened specifically for criminal lunatics in 1856. It was an impressive four storey bluestone building with room for 180 patients, and remained part of the penitentiary system until 1877, when its name was changed to Kingston Asylum for the Insane. The first American facility specifically for the criminal insane appears to have been the New York State Asylum for Insane Convicts at Auburn, New York, which opened in 1859, initially for 80 patients. In 1891 it moved to new, larger premises, known as the Matteawan State Hospital, but this also became overcrowded and in 1900 another facility was opened, the Dannemora State Hospital. It should be noted that while the history of psychiatry is a massive scholarly industry, little attention has been paid to the history of forensic psychiatry,[10] and there are almost no published resources devoted specifically to the history of day-to-day care.

The lessons and legacy of history

The origins of secure services for mentally ill people in the English-speaking world are emblematic of a time when secure services were the norm. Although 'secure services' or 'forensic services', are today reserved for a very special and challenging group of patients, they continue to reflect these origins, and many of the issues and dilemmas faced in the 19th century still face us today. The early Australian lunacy services, for example, immediately faced the question as to whether separate provision should be made for the criminal insane and the convict insane, that is those who are found to be insane prior to sentencing, and those who become insane while serving a sentence, and whether this provision should, in turn, be separate from that for the civil insane. This entailed the question as to who should have responsibility for these various services, and where they should be located. Many colonial authorities felt that the convict insane should remain the responsibility of the prison department and cared for in prison, while the criminal insane should be the responsibility of the health department and cared for in asylums. The less popular view was that all insane persons, of whatever origin or status, should be cared for in the health system. This view was championed by many who worked in the prison system and saw psychologically disturbed prisoners as disruptive, dangerous or vulnerable, and a negative influence on other prisoners and the smooth running of the prison. An outspoken supporter of this approach was William Neitenstein, the head of the New South Wales prison department at the turn of the century, who argued as early as the 1880s that sex offenders should be located in asylums rather than in prisons, so that they could receive appropriate treatment. In practice, services in Australia, and most countries, developed in an 'ad hoc' fashion, subject to the preferences and interests of successive political, medical and other authorities, and was a victim of their generally negative and neglectful approach to both offenders and the mentally ill. As a result, some services have remained prison-based, some are exclusively based in the health system, and yet others are located within prison facilities but serviced by health system personnel. In Britain, the question of who provides what health services to prisoners, was carefully reconsidered in 2000–2001, in the light of scandalous conditions and unacceptable standards, and there are strong calls for them to be handed over in their entirety to the Department of Health.[11] This recently happened in Tasmania, Australia, for similar reasons.

Associated with these questions about the location of, and responsibility for, services for mentally ill offenders, have been difficulties with legislation, which has generally failed to keep track of advances in the understanding and treatment of people with mental illnesses, with increased understanding of offender behaviour, and with developments in penological thinking and practice. Today's criminal legislation has changed very little since the precedents established in the early 19th century by which an offender was judged to have been insane and therefore legally excusable. Inadequate and outdated criminal and civil legislation, often interpreted according to outdated precedents, has inhibited the development of the most appropriate systems of care, and underwritten an administrative complexity which has tended to make the operation of services cumbersome and acted against the interests of the patient. Historically, transfers between service systems and facilities, for example, were extremely difficult to arrange and long delays were frequent. Such difficulties continue to plague forensic psychiatric services, and now involve the added problem of how legislation can facilitate rather than inhibit continuity of care in the community, and enable professionals to operate effectively in and across services which are never actually 'seamless', despite the aspirations of policy makers.

Another group of questions that arose in the early days of the asylum system concerned the appropriate level of security for different types of patient, and how the special precautions necessary for dangerous criminal and convict patients could be reconciled to the therapeutic aspirations of the asylum and to the comparatively less intrusive security needs of other patients. In recent times, the relationship between therapy and security, or care and custody, persists as a practical and psychological problem facing those who plan, manage and provide care, and has been debated almost *ad nauseam*.[12] The issue of varying levels of security is also raised today in response to the expectation that each patient will receive individualized care appropriate to their particular needs, and the requirement, expressed in a number of health standards, human rights statements, and laws, that each be cared for in the least restrictive environment possible. This can only be achieved if security is seen as an element in an individual care plan,[13] rather than as a characteristic of a facility. Only recently have the practical issues of establishing, maintaining and reviewing security in forensic settings been the subject of publication.[14]

The historical record is also directly relevant because early lay and professional discussions concerning this group of patients uses evaluative language expressive of attitudes which would today be widely considered discriminatory, demeaning and in all respects politically incorrect, but which was entirely acceptable in its day. This highlights several continuing but neglected problems. Firstly, it blatantly testifies to the fact that the patients concerned are, indeed, sometimes extremely obnoxious or morally repulsive, and that relating to them therapeutically, might be problematic. Secondly, it raises the problem as to the relationship between madness and badness, how these are conceived, and how society should respond when they are met in the same individual, a problem with which we are still struggling.[15] Thirdly, it illustrates the problem of public and political negativity toward mentally ill offenders, who are still liable to be seen principally as criminals, for whom punitive, prison-like conditions are appropriate; most obviously, this means that care is expected to be delivered in facilities built a century or more ago, when such attitudes were the norm, and this has an impact on efforts to create therapeutic environments with graduated levels of security, and on efforts to reintegrate patients back into the community. These problems, in turn, raise the question of how to reconcile increased resourcing for such services with the fact that resources are limited and the needs of mentally ill offenders must be weighed against those of other, apparently more deserving, people.

Finally, the early history is important because it rehearsed the difficult question as to the extent to which criminal behaviours are, of themselves, legitimate targets of professional psychiatric intervention, and Neitenstein's call for the removal of sex offenders to asylums is a case in point. During the early part of the 19th century, protracted disputes occurred concerning the extent to which evidence presented by psychiatrists, or 'alienists', regarding a person's actions should be taken into account in determining questions of guilt and sentencing. In fact, the courts tended to prefer 'common-sense' explanations of defendants' behaviour, and of their level of culpability, and it took many years for medicine to establish authority in presenting such evidence. These disputes also revealed the ways in which the discourses of law and medicine interact in the highly charged context of the courtroom, exposing the limitations of psychiatric explanation and evoking fears that it seeks to undermine the pursuit of justice. Precisely these phenomena still operate today whenever psychiatry is transported into the courtroom, and its authority continues to be challenged from a range of public and professional sources.[16–19]

TERMINOLOGY

A simple strategy to help medicine establish its authority in relation to lunacy during the early 19th century, particularly in the courtroom, was to develop a technical discourse, with a plethora of obscure terms, the aim being to give the appearance of precision and certainty as to the nature of the problem, and to exclude and confuse those outside the profession. This discourse was initially chaotic and haphazard, with each 'alienist' preferring his own particular descriptive terms, but the level

of standardization gradually increased, even though competing theories and diagnostic systems persisted, and today forensic psychiatry mostly employs the terminology of the *Diagnostic and Statistical Manual of the American Psychiatric Association* ('DSM-IV-R'). It also uses many terms and phrases that are rarely encountered elsewhere, or which have unclear or special meanings. For their part, nurses need to understand terminology that has developed in three contexts – organizational, clinical and legal – and it is important to be clear about the basic terms.

- ❑ *Forensic* – has its origins in the Latin word meaning 'forum', that is a court or debating chamber; except in classical studies, where it is still used to refer to such forums, it means 'relating to courts of law'.
- ❑ *Forensic psychiatry* – that form of psychiatry relating to courts of law. Since law has civil and criminal aspects, the term can be used to refer to involvement in civil cases, such as the provision of expert opinion in divorce and child custody proceedings, insurance and damages cases, employment law, challenges to wills, and the regulation of professions: this usage is common in the United States. In other countries it is generally reserved for psychiatry applied to criminal cases. Nevertheless, it is rare in practice for forensic psychiatric services to be reserved exclusively for people who have appeared in a court of law. Most services assume a much wider range of responsibilities, notably in assessing, advising on, and sometimes managing, patients who present with especially challenging or dangerous behaviours, either transiently or chronically; and, the policies of many forensic units allow for such individuals to be admitted as local needs dictate.
- ❑ *Forensic psychiatrist* refers to a psychiatrist who works in forensic settings, although it entails no specialist qualifications and its use is a matter of custom and practice. Specialist training is available to psychiatrists in some countries, but is not mandatory.
- ❑ *Forensic psychologist* refers to a psychologist who works in forensic settings. Specialist training is widely available at postgraduate level and the term is increasingly protected by professional organizations which, in Australia and the United States, have significant forensic sections.
- ❑ *Forensic nursing* should be used to refer to all forms of nursing provided as part of forensic services, although job descriptions do not generally include the word 'forensic' and its use almost exclusively characterizes the setting in which the nurse works, rather than upon their qualifications, these having become available only in the last few years. In the United States, a major role for forensic nurses is the care of victims of crime, especially victims of sexual

assault, and these nurses are increasingly being given special titles. Elsewhere, the offender is the focus of forensic nursing, and engagement with victims, or even offenders' significant others, is unusual.

❑ *Forensic mental health nursing*, or *forensic psychiatric nursing*, should be reserved for the forensic branch of mental health or psychiatric nursing, but again it does not appear in job descriptions, and is based on the setting in which the psychiatric nurse works rather than upon their qualifications. It is widely thought to be important to make a distinction between forensic and non-forensic roles, and to identify the distinctive skills and expectations of those working in forensic settings.[20–23] The study of nursing in secure environments conducted by the Faculty of Health, University of Central Lancashire, on behalf of the United Kingdom Central Council for Nursing, Midwifery and Health Care represents the most extensive study and review of the role of the forensic nurse conducted thus far, and is an extremely valuable resource for anyone interested in forensic mental health care.[24] It is the Council's most requested publication, and is available free of charge via their website. The Scottish National Board has produced extensive documents on the enhancement of the forensic mental health nursing role, likewise available free of charge via the Board's website.[25] Opinion is divided as to whether a distinction between forensic and non-forensic nursing roles can be sustained,[26] and as to the future identity of forensic nurses,[27,28] but the case for a separate identity appears to be at least as strong as that for distinguishing any other specialty within nursing (see Robinson and Kettles[29] for an international consideration). Most obviously, the client group served comprises primarily forensic patients and, whether in an institutional or community setting, the problems being managed are significantly linked to criminal offending, unlike those normally faced by non-forensic mental health nurses.

❑ *Corrections nursing* is a term used in the United States and Australasia to refer to all forms of nursing provided within the prison system. Such services may be the responsibility of the health system, the penal system, or a mixture of both. *Prison nursing* is the equivalent term in the UK, Ireland and Canada. However, since correctional services are increasingly extending care to settings other than prison facilities, including a variety of periodic detention centres, and the community, the value of the term 'prison nursing' is debatable.

❑ *Forensic patient* is widely used to distinguish patients coming under the jurisdiction of forensic services from other service users. The term should be used with caution because not all facilities providing forensic services restrict their clientele to individuals who have come into conflict with the law or are subject to the jurisdiction of a court. Similarly, not all forensic patients are cared for by services designated as forensic, especially when they are in transitional accommodation prior to discharge or are living in the community and may be absorbed into the caseloads of non-forensic services. The State of New South Wales, Australia, is perhaps unique in defining the term in law.

❑ *Mentally ill offender*, although most obviously referring to a mentally ill person convicted of an offence, is sometimes defined in criminal legislation, each statute wording the definition in slightly different ways. In some contexts, it refers to those people once called 'criminal lunatics', that is people found to be mentally ill prior to sentencing, but in others it includes the 'convict insane', that is those found to be mentally ill while serving a custodial sentence. 'Mental illness' for these purposes is usually taken to be as defined in civil legislation, notably Mental Health Acts, though not all such Acts refer to 'mental illness', preferring other terminology. The phrase is problematized by the *Diagnostic and Statistical Manual of the American Psychiatric Association*, since this abandons the term 'mental illness' completely, in favour of 'mental disorder'. In any case, it should not be used to describe all people who use forensic services, because many of these people are not convicted offenders, but have perhaps been remanded for pre-trial assessment. Furthermore, forensic services frequently include services to people who have just been taken into custody and are being assessed at a police station, prior to any court appearance; and, in some places, the clientele includes non-forensic patients for whom appropriate secure provision is otherwise unavailable.

❑ *Mentally disordered offenders* is a term used in some jurisdictions where the distinction between 'mental illness' and 'mental disorder' is incorporated into civil or criminal legislation. It often includes people who have a psychological problem not amounting to a mental illness, such as may arise as a result of post-traumatic brain damage, intellectual disability, or transient drug-induced organic states. In some countries, such as Britain, forensic psychiatric services for those suffering from personality disorder, or a sexual abnormality, are made available through the health system, while in others, such as Australia, they are provided, if at all, exclusively within the penal system.

❑ *Criminally insane* is an adjective or noun, largely historical, referring to those whose criminal acts were attributed to their insanity.

❑ *Convict insane* is likewise historical, referring to those who become insane while serving a custodial sentence.

❑ *Court Liaison Nurse/Officer (Mental Health Court Support Worker)* refers to a nurse who conducts psychiatric assessments of defendants, presents their findings in court, and makes recommendations as to the appropriate disposal of defendants.[30,31]

Forensic terminology is developing as services expand, new roles emerge, and the language of professionals become more precise, and the short descriptions given above should be regarded only as a starting point.

CORE PRINCIPLES OF A QUALITY FORENSIC SERVICE

The equivalence principle

Nurses working in forensic settings must accept that mentally ill offenders are entitled to receive care of the same standard as they could reasonably expect were they not offenders. Although it is not beyond question, this simple principle – sometimes called 'the equivalence principle' – provides a legally and ethically secure basis for clinicians of all disciplines, upon which services for mentally ill offenders should be organized and delivered. It means that all the standards and conditions of care, all the ethical and professional codes, practice guidelines, accreditation criteria, quality assurance expectations, legal safeguards, and so forth, which apply in non-forensic settings must apply in forensic ones; and, that care must be provided in accordance with local, national and international covenants, conventions and laws. The overwhelming majority of the literature champions the equivalence principle, but it might be useful here to consider the problems that it might present to nurses and other clinicians.

Firstly, in accordance with the equivalence principle, people with mental disorders should receive mental health services appropriate to their needs, irrespective of their history of criminal offending. This is in the public interest since the individual will present less risk of further offending if their illness is effectively treated. Importantly, this unequivocally ties forensic care into risk assessment and reduction, which is often cited as an area of expertise distinguishing forensic and non-forensic roles in nursing. However, it raises many questions about the extent to which psychiatry is concerned with offending behaviour *per se*, since not all such behaviour is obviously the result of or even related to the individual's mental disorder. This links to the concept of 'dangerousness', which can be regarded as a reflection of the risk of re-offending and the seriousness of the offence

anticipated. Some authorities have argued that the risk of further offending should not be a matter for psychiatry, and forensic psychiatry appears to be divided as to whether it should be involved in assessing dangerousness.[32–35]

A second problem with the equivalence principle is that nurses in particular may find it difficult to meet patients when they know that their offending behaviour has been particularly unpleasant or horrendous. In some cases, nurses simply find it psychologically difficult, while in others they may find it morally repugnant and may consciously challenge the principle that all people should receive the same level of care. This issue has received almost no acknowledgement in the literature, and yet some resolution is necessary if nurses are to avoid consequences harmful to all parties concerned.[36]

Finally, an obvious distinguishing feature of much forensic care is that it is delivered in secure settings, and this may undermine or even be at odds with the equivalence principle. A widely accepted standard is that treatment and care will be provided in the 'least restrictive environment' compatible with the legitimate right of the community to be protected from unacceptable levels of danger, and the protection of the individual patient from unacceptable risks of serious damage to self or serious deterioration.[37] Deciding what constitutes the most appropriate level of security in individual cases is a difficult task. An important contribution can be made by a well-founded and continuous risk assessment process, which directly influences treatment and management decisions.

Similarly, applying the equivalence principle means that confidentiality of all patient information will be respected, regardless of whether the person is serving a prison sentence. This can be especially problematic, however, since information about escape plans, for example, or about a patient's murderous thoughts in relation to a specific staff member, or about risky sexual or drug behaviours in the facility, can not remain confidential, and a judgement must be made as to which information should be passed on to prison authorities in order to avoid possible harm to others. Where care is delivered within a prison system, confidentiality may be almost impossible.

In addition to these practical problems, there are a number of moral objections to the equivalence principle, which ought to be considered by nurses. The commonest concern:

❑ The claim that in a context of resource shortage, a judgement has to be made as to which groups are most deserving; it is difficult, according to this view, to argue for increased funding of services for mentally ill offenders when set alongside the needs of sick children.

❏ The claim that since offenders have broken the social contract they can no longer claim rights equal to those of law-abiding citizens.

❏ Some offenders are amoral beings, in the sense that they have no respect for the normal moral conventions, and effectively live outside the community of moral beings; they are therefore not owed the moral respect that membership of that community entails.

Individuals who provide health care in forensic settings must ponder these and similar issues and come to a reconciliation or understanding which allows them to maintain their professional and therapeutic roles.

Standards for a quality forensic service

Assuming, then, that mentally ill offenders are entitled to a quality service, we might ask exactly what such a service would be like. Firstly, it would reflect international and national covenants establishing standards of services for mentally ill people. In Britain, this would include the seven evidence-based standards listed in the *National Service Framework for Mental Health* (September 1999),[38] which fleshes out the policies announced in the paper *Modernizing Mental Health Services* (1998).[39] The Framework notes the commitment of the British Government to work toward the elimination of mixed sex accommodation in all National Health Service facilities; although little progress had been made in this regard by the end of 2001, it makes clear the nature of future forensic services. Local service providers are required to translate these national expectations and standards into a workable care delivery programme. In the case of forensic services, however, this suggests a level of cross-systems cooperation that is only just beginning to materialize.

In Australia, standards are laid down as part of the National Mental Health Strategy, comprising the *Mental Health Statement of Rights and Responsibilities*, the *National Mental Health Policy*, and the Australian Health Ministers' *Second National Mental Health Plan*.[40–42] The latter document explicitly states that it 'is relevant for the whole system of mental health service delivery' (p. 6), and thus includes forensic services. The Plan identifies 'forensic populations' as one of several 'target groups for whom improved service access and better service responses are essential'. In addition, the Health Departments of some Australian states have begun to develop standards and sets of expectations for mental health services. The New South Wales Health Department framework for the development of mental health care, for example, gives a clear statement as to the level of services that users can expect. In Canada, there

are a number of statements establishing standards of service for mentally ill offenders, notably the *Standards for Health Care* published in 1994.[43] In New Zealand, a detailed framework for forensic mental health services appeared in March 2001, with a strong emphasis on the integration of community and institutional care.[44] It reports the results of a national survey, and highlights a host of issues that need to be addressed, but says disappointly little about the standard of service that clients can expect in the future. Indeed, even its two-page statement of the underlying philosophy of care is presented as a list of questions.

There are many examples of excellence in forensic care. The Reaside Clinic in the West Midlands of England opened in 1987 as a 'state of the art' forensic psychiatric service, and has articulated very clearly the features of a quality forensic service in its leaflet *The Philosophy of the Reaside Clinic* (1998).[45] This states that patients should be cared for:

❏ with regard to the quality of care and with proper attention to the needs of individuals;

❏ as far as possible in the community, rather than in institutional settings;

❏ under conditions of no greater security than is justified by the degree of danger they present to themselves or to others;

❏ in such a way as to maximize rehabilitation and their chances of sustaining an independent life;

❏ as near as possible to their own home; and

❏ with respect for their rights as citizens.

The high security State Hospital at Carstairs in Scotland offers another example, articulating more specific clinically oriented targets. The hospital reconsidered its approach to patient care in light of numerous reports about poor conditions, and in response to recent NHS reports and practice statements. The outcome is that it is implementing the *Carstairs Hospital Health Improvement Programme* (1998)[46] which lists the following improvements:

❏ developing a systematic and comprehensive approach to the assessment of dangerousness and offending behaviour;

❏ developing a treatment approach to the management of anger;

❏ developing a range of specialist treatment interventions covering sexual and other behaviour problems such as fire raising;

❏ developing structured treatment and education programmes in drug and alcohol abuse;

❏ developing a more co-ordinated approach to women's services;

❏ reviewing the clinical, environmental and social configuration of every ward;

- developing more scientific risk assessment and risk management;
- promoting best practice to ensure clinical effectiveness through the development of research and audit, and clinical guidelines;
- developing and implementing a health promotion strategy;
- introducing an independent arm to advocacy;
- improving external collaboration to encourage the development of a nationally integrated framework of forensic psychiatric and social services;
- reviewing the needs of patient's relatives and friends, with a view to providing them with better support and information;
- implementing quality human resources, information and estate strategies to support all of the above; and
- ensuring the above developments represent sound value for money for the public purse.

This gives an interesting indication of the issues that major forensic institutions are currently addressing, and of the changing roles of nurses and other clinicians.

In addition to these kinds of statements about standards expected of forensic services and the clinical services they should offer, a few authorities have issued ethical or professional codes regulating the conduct of clinicians in forensic settings. These obviously supplement those which already regulate the profession at local and national level. In New South Wales, for example, the booklet *Corrections Health Service Professional and Ethical Guidelines*[47] is now in its third edition and deals with some of the key ethical issues faced by staff. It lists some of the differences between personal and professional relationships and explains ways in which professional boundaries may be especially susceptible in forensic settings. It covers issues such as promises, confidentiality, sexual behaviour and staff-inmate relationships, and professional and unprofessional behaviour generally. These *Guidelines* could be regarded as a useful starting point for any service wishing to develop policies and educational programmes addressing professional conduct in forensic settings, and in the USA, the National Council of State Boards of Nursing's document *Professional Boundaries* deals with very similar issues.[48]

Services 'appropriate to need'

In accordance with the equivalence principle, statements about the quality of services for mentally ill people repeatedly affirm that they must be 'appropriate to their needs', and when this is applied to mentally ill offenders we are confronted by some important challenges. Most obviously, it is not easy to work toward such a service

when so little research has been conducted to establish precisely what those needs are and when the literature is mostly limited to specific settings.[49–51] Researchers at the University of Birmingham have published a substantial review of the health care needs of prisoners in England and Wales, which includes a section on mental health needs,[52] but the only discussion exclusively forensic is that by Cohen and Eastman,[53] who conclude by questioning whose needs will be met by the services being envisioned in current British policy and planning.

When it comes to the special needs of specific groups, although we have already noted the British policy of working toward separate facilities for men and women, the particular problems confronting women who need forensic psychiatric care have only recently become the subject of research and discussion.[54–57] The most substantial publication currently available, *Women and Secure Psychiatric Services: A Literature Review*, was prepared by the School of Policy Studies at Bristol University and submitted to the NHS Centre for Reviews and Disseminations in June 1998.[58] The report offers conclusions in the areas of policy, research and practice and is a valuable resource.

The special needs of young people in forensic care have also only recently started to attract attention,[59–64] and there appears to be almost nothing which addresses the nursing care of this group. There is also only a small literature addressing the needs of members of ethnic and cultural minorities,[65–67] some of which are seriously over-represented in forensic settings, not least in Australia.

Recognizing vulnerability and responding to abuses

A quality forensic service should acknowledge that its clientele will include many who should be regarded as vulnerable individuals. It should have a strategy for recognizing, and dealing quickly and effectively with, suspected cases of abuse, as well as strategies for minimizing, monitoring and learning from cases of abuse. There must be clear and accessible procedures for staff and patients indicating how to respond to abuse or suspected abuse, including appropriate lines of communication. Abuse or exploitation may constitute a criminal offence, and/or professional misconduct and/or breach of contractual conditions, and so there must also be clear, accessible statements about options relating to disciplinary or criminal proceedings. Most importantly, it should be recognized that mentally ill offenders enjoy the same legal protections and resources as any other person, and this must be scrupulously observed: they should have unhindered access to legal advice, for example, and be able to institute appropriate inquiries and proceedings. There must be policies and procedures, which minimize the risk that patients will be abused, but which also protect staff and others from wrongful accusations. Nurses should be fully aware of these procedures and adopt an advocacy role in relation to their use by patients and colleagues. Adopting such a role is sometimes not easy and there must also be a system in place for the protection of any person, staff or patient, who could be considered a 'whistleblower' and therefore at risk. It is significant that because of the seriousness of this risk, formal procedures for the protection of whistleblowers are a legal requirement for health services in many countries.

In forensic settings, it is possible that if information relating to a patient were to become openly known, that person would become vulnerable, in that it might make them a target for harassment or assault, or otherwise put them at risk of exploitation, by other inmates or patients. Clear and carefully observed policies relating to patient confidentiality are therefore highly relevant to the issue of protecting potentially vulnerable patients. Lastly, the vulnerability of any particular patient must feature in assessments of risk, and be taken into account in treatment programmes, in day-to-day management and in discharge planning. Needless to say, the nurse is a key player in the conduct of these processes, and in the protection of vulnerable individuals.

Risk assessment and management

This in turn relates to the nurses' role in risk management. 'Risk' here covers risk to one's own safety, health, and quality of life – material, cultural and spiritual – as well as risk to others. It may apply to further offending, accidental or deliberate self-harm, suicide, homicide and violence to others, vulnerability to sexual abuse, stalking and harassment, material exploitation, property damage, public nuisance, neglect or abuse of dependants, intimidation and threats to others, and reckless behaviour such as dangerous driving, and multiple drug abuse with consequent exacerbation of mental disorder and offending risk. Forensic psychiatric services worldwide are attempting to place clinical and management decision-making on a sound evidence-based footing, and this includes assessments of the risks posed by mentally ill offenders to themselves and the community. In a quality forensic service, risk assessment procedures are formally developed and conducted, and based on a subtle blend of multidisciplinary clinical judgement, research evidence, and standardized tests, for which staff are appropriately trained. For this reason, a massive literature has appeared around the topic of risk in recent years, and there is a growing literature on nurses' use of violence prediction tools (e.g. Almvik and Woods[68]). There are

still too few publications, however, dealing with the role of nurses in risk assessment generally, although those available are excellent starting points.[69–71] The New Zealand Ministry of Health's *Guidelines for Clinical Risk Assessment and Management in Mental Health Services*,[72] is typical of many system-wide statements, and likewise represents an excellent starting point for developing an understanding of how a service responds to the challenge of risk management.

PROBLEMS, CURRENT DEVELOPMENTS AND PROSPECTS

Many aspects of forensic care continue to pose challenges and are evoking novel responses. First, there are politico-organizational problems: the historical legacy of poor facilities and poor practice, of bad reputations fuelled by continuing scandals and of a lack of interest among politicians competing for resources; definitional problems and consequent disputes over authority and legitimacy in the face of medical domination, the need to create a professional identity, and related problems in the recruitment and retention of high quality staff; not least, it might be argued that services continue to be organized around bureaucratic convenience rather than patient need, and that a radical rethink is probably required in most jurisdictions. In addition, the proliferation of private prisons and the gradual emergence of private forensic services, requires that they be subject to appropriate regulatory mechanisms, and that effective working relationships with public sector services be established.

Second, there are many new, as well as long-standing, clinical problems, such as:

- ❏ how far forensic services, and especially clinicians such as nurses, should be concerned with understanding, assessing and managing risk and dangerousness, especially when that danger is not directly related to an individual's mental illness;
- ❏ matching patients to the appropriate level of security;
- ❏ determining the role of the patient in clinical decision-making;
- ❏ how to overcome the counter-therapeutic attitudes and practices encountered among some prison/corrections staff and police officers.

Practical strategies for dealing with these problems are being sought, but progress is sometimes undermined by the vested interests of existing agencies in maintaining the status quo.

On a more positive note, forensic services worldwide are burgeoning, and with increased funding comes increased accountability and service innovation, which are now contributing to radical improvements in quality. Current developments include the adoption of the 'clinical governance' approach,[73,74] discussed elsewhere in this text, which is being actively pursued in a number of forensic services, notably those in South Australia. One of the key features is an emphasis on clinical supervision and evidence-based practice, both of which are now becoming accepted as aspirations for forensic settings.[75] In addition, debates about the restrictive nature of traditional health-system divisions of labour, based on the orthodox 'disciplines', are beginning to take place. Forensic mental health appears to be a prime example of an area of practice in which effective and efficient service delivery calls for a postdisciplinary approach.[76]

However, the most obvious and encouraging development in recent years has been the explosion of forensic research and publication. Among the pioneering texts on forensic mental health care, many primarily address nursing issues, express a nursing perspective or are written for nurses.[28,79–81] There are a number of important articles and book chapters elucidating forensic mental health nursing,[82,83] as well as texts dealing with broader issues include.[84,85] These are all well-written and important texts, often breaking new ground and setting a high standard for the future. They are testimony to the sophisticated new breed of forensic mental health professionals who combine intellectual acumen with clinical experience in order to promote high quality, evidence-based practice. Such individuals are vital to overcoming the numerous problems facing forensic services, and augur well for the prospects of a quality service which benefits mentally ill offenders and the community.

REFERENCES

1. Ray I. *A treatise on the medical jurisprudence of insanity.* Boston: Little Brown, 1838.

2. Prichard JC. *On the different forms of insanity in relation to jurisprudence.* London: Baillière, 1842.

3. Moran R. *Knowing right from wrong: the insanity defence of Daniel MacNaughtan.* New York: Free Press, 1981.

4. Fingarette H. *The meaning of criminal insanity.* Berkeley: University of California Press, 1972.

5. Robinson D. *Wild beasts and idle humours: the insanity defence from antiquity to the present.* Cambridge, MA: Harvard University Press, 1996.

6. Boland F. *Anglo-American insanity defence reform: the war between law and psychiatry.* Aldershot: Dartmouth Publishing, 1999.

7. Barclay W. *Discussion paper: a study of corrections mental health services in New South Wales.* Sydney: Corrections Health Service, 1997.

8. Bluglass R. *Review of forensic mental health services, New South Wales.* Matraville, NSW: Corrections Health Service, 1997.

9. McComish AG. The development of forensic services in Scotland 1800–1960. *Psychiatric Care* 1996; **3**(4): 153–8.

10. Forshaw D, Rollin H. The history of forensic psychiatry in England. In: Bluglass R, Bowden P (eds). *Principles and practice of forensic psychiatry.* Edinburgh: Churchill Livingstone, 1990: 61–102.

11. HM Prison Service Working Group. *Nursing in prisons: report by the working group considering the development of prison nursing, with particular reference to health care officers.* HM Prison, the NHS Executive and the National Assembly for Wales; undated. Available at: http://www.doh.gov.uk/prisonhealth/nursinginprisons.pdf Accessed 20 April, 2002.

12. Burrow S. Therapy versus security: reconciling healing and damnation. In: Mason T, Mercer D (eds). *Critical perspectives in forensic care: inside out.* London: Macmillan, 1998: 171–87.

13. Tarbuck P. The therapeutic use of security: a model for forensic nursing. In: Thompson T, Mathias P (eds). *Lyttle's mental health and disorder*, 2nd edn. London: Baillière Tindall, 1994: 552–70.

14. Dale C, Gardner J. Security in forensic environments: strategic and operational issues. In: Dale C, Thompson T, Woods P (eds). *Forensic mental health: issues in practice.* Edinburgh: Baillière Tindall and The Royal College of Nursing, 2001: 251–73.

15. Feinberg J. Sickness and wickedness: new conceptions and new paradoxes. *J Am Acad Psychiatry Law* 1998; **26**(3): 475–85.

16. Barton WE, Sanborn CJ (eds). *Law and the mental health professions: friction at the interface.* New York: International Universities Press, 1978.

17. Dershowitz AM. *The abuse excuse: and other cop-outs, sob stories, and evasions of responsibility.* Boston: Little Brown and Company, 1994.

18. Arrigo BA. *The contours of psychiatry: a postmodern critique of mental illness, criminal insanity, and the law.* New York: Garland, 1996.

19. Buchanan A. *Psychiatric aspects of justification, excuse and mitigation: the jurisprudence of mental abnormality in Anglo-American criminal law.* London: Jessica Kingsley, 2000.

20. Burrow S. An outline of the forensic nursing role. *British Journal of Nursing* 1993; **2**: 899–904.

21. Burrow S. The role conflict of the forensic nurse. *Senior Nurse* 1993; **13**(5): 20–5.

22. Royal College of Nursing. *Buying forensic mental health nursing: an RCN guide for purchasers.* London: Royal College of Nursing, 1997.

23. McCourt M. Five concepts for the expanded role of the forensic mental health nurse. In: Tarbuck P, Burnard

P, Topping-Morris B (eds). *Forensic mental health nursing: policy, strategy and implementation*. London: Whurr, 1999: 149–61.

24. Faculty of Health, University of Central Lancashire. Nursing in secure environments: a scoping study conducted on behalf of the United Kingdom Central Council for Nursing, Midwifery and Health Visiting. London: UKCC, 1999. Available at: http://www.fnrh.freeserve.co.uk/ Accessed 20 April, 2002.

25. National Board for Nursing, Midwifery and Health Visiting for Scotland, 2000. Continuing professional development portfolio: a route to enhanced competence in forensic mental health nursing. Available at: http://www.nbs.org.uk Accessed 27 March, 2002.

26. Evans A, Wells D. An exploration of the role of the Australian forensic nurse. Research report to Royal College of Nursing Australia. Canberra: RCNA, 1999.

27. Mercer D, Mason T, Richman J. Professional convergence in forensic practice. *Australian and New Zealand Journal of Mental Health Nursing 2001*; **10**: 105–15.

28. Sekula K, Holmes D, Zoucha R, DeSantis J, Olshansky E. Forensic psychiatric nursing: discursive practices and the emergence of a specialty. *Journal of Psychosocial Nursing 2001*; **39**(9): 51ff.

29. Robinson D, Kettles A (eds). *Forensic nursing and multidisciplinary care of the mentally disordered offender*. (Forensic Focus 14). London: Jessica Kingsley, 1999.

30. Hillis G. Diverting people with mental health problems from the criminal justice system. In: Tarbuck P, Burnard P, Topping-Morris B (eds). *Forensic mental health nursing: policy, strategy and implementation*. London: Whurr, 1999: 36–50.

31. New South Wales Law Society. Justice and mental health systems cheer new court liaison program. *Law Society Journal* 1999; **37**(8): 12.

32. Mullen PE. Forensic mental health. *British Journal of Psychiatry* 2000; 176: 307–11.

33. Petrunik M. *Models of dangerousness: a cross jurisdictional review of dangerousness legislation and practice*. Report prepared for the Policy Branch, Ministry of the Solicitor General of Canada, 1994. Available at: http://www.sgc.gc.ca/epub/ Accessed 27 March, 2002.

34. Rose N. Governing risky individuals: the role of psychiatry in new regimes of control. *Psychiatry, Psychology and Law* 1998; **5**(2): 177–95.

35. Prins H. Will they do it again? *Risk assessment and management of criminal justice and psychiatry*. London: Routledge, 1999.

36. Holmes CA. *Caring and not caring: the case of mentally ill offenders*. Royal College of Nursing Australia Conference: Health Ethics Futures. Hamilton Island, Queensland, Australia, July 25–28, 2001.

37. Forensicare. *Forensicare – Victoria's forensic mental health service*. Melbourne: Victorian Institute of Forensic Mental Health, 1999. Available via: http://www.forensicare.vic.gov.au/ Accessed 20 April, 2002.

38. Department of Health (UK). *National service framework for mental health* 1999. Available at: http://www.doh.gov.uk/pub/docs/doh/mhmain.pdf Accessed 20 April, 2002.

39. Department of Health (UK). *Modernising mental health services: safe sound, supportive* 1998. Available at http://www.doh.gov.uk/nsf/mentalh.htm Accessed 20 April, 2002.

40. Australian Health Ministers. *Mental health statement of rights and responsibilities*. Canberra: AGPS, 1991. Available at: http://www.health.gov.au/hsdd/mentalhe/mhinfo/standards/nsrr.htm Accessed 20 April, 2002.

41. Australian Health Ministers. *National mental health strategy*. Mental Health Branch, Commonwealth Department of Health and Family Services. Canberra: AGPS, 1992. Available via: http://www.health.gov.au/hsdd/mentalhe/mhinfo/nmhs/index.htm Accessed 20 April, 2002.

42. Australian Health Ministers. *Second national mental health plan*. Mental Health Branch, Commonwealth Department of Health and Family Services. Canberra: AGPS, 1998. Available at: http://www.health.gov.au/hsdd/mentalhe/mhinfo/nmhs/plan2.htm Accessed 20 April, 2002.

43. Correctional Service of Canada. *Standards for Health Care Correctional Service of Canada* 1994. Available via: http://www.csc-scc.gc.ca/ Accessed 20 April, 2002.

44. Ministry of Health (New Zealand). *Services for people with mental illness in the justice system: framework for forensic mental health services* 2001. Available at: http://www.moh.govt.nz Accessed 27 March, 2002.

45. Leaflet. The philosophy of the Reaside Clinic, Reaside Clinic, Great Park, Birmingham.

46. The Carstairs Hospital Health Improvement Programme (1998) has now been implemented. Their new Health Improvement Plan 2002–2005. Available at: http://www.show.scot.nhs.uk/tsh/

47. NSW Corrections Health Service. *Professional and ethical guidelines for corrections health service nurses* 3rd edn. Sydney: Corrections Health Service, 1998.

48. National Council of State Boards of Nursing (USA). *Professional boundaries: a nurse's guide to the importance of appropriate professional boundaries* 1996. Available at: http://www.ncsbn.org Accessed 27 March, 2002.

49. Taylor PJ, Butwell M, Dacey R, Kaye C. *Within maximum security hospitals: a survey of need*. London: SHSA, 1991.

50. Maden A, Curle C, Meaux C, Burrows S, Gunn J.

Treatment and security needs of special hospital patients. London: Whurr, 1995.

51. Pierzchniak P, Farnham F, De Taranti N, *et al.* Assessing the needs of patient in secure settings: a multi-disciplinary approach. *Journal of Forensic Psychiatry* 1999; **10**(2): 343–54.

52. Marshall T, Simpson S, Stevens A. *Health care in prisons: a health care needs assessment*, 2000. Department of Public Health and Epidemiology, University of Birmingham. Available at http://www.pub lichealth.bham.ac.uk/department Accessed 27 March, 2002.

53. Cohen A, Eastman N. *Assessing forensic mental health needs: policy, theory and research.* London: Gaskell, 2000.

54. Hemingway C (ed.) *Special women? The experience of women in the special hospital system.* Aldershot: Avebury, 1996.

55. Veysey BM. Specific needs of women diagnosed with mental illness in US jails. In: Levin BL, Blanch AK (eds). *Women's mental health services: a public health perspective.* Thousand Oaks, CA: Sage, 1998: 368–89.

56. Kenney-Herbert J. Health care of women prisoners in England and Wales: a literature review. *Howard Journal of Criminal Justice* 1999; **38**(1): 54–66.

57. Storey L, Murdock D. Women in secure care. In: Dale C, Thompson T, Woods P (eds). *Forensic mental health: issues in practice.* London: Baillière Tindall and The Royal College of Nursing, 2001: 179–88.

58. Lart R, Payne S, Beaumont B, Macdonald G, Mistry T. *Women and secure psychiatric services: a literature review.* Bristol: School for Policy Studies, Bristol University; 1998. Summary available at: http://www. york.ac.uk/inst/crd/report14.htm Accessed 20 April, 2002.

59. Cocozza J (ed.) *Responding to the mental health needs of youth in their juvenile justice system.* Seattle: National Coalition for the Mentally Ill in the Criminal Justice System, 1992.

60. Bailey S, Dolan M. *Adolescent forensic psychiatry.* London: Butterworth-Heinemann, 1999.

61. Kurtz Z, Thornes R, Bailey S. Children in the criminal justice system and secure care systems: how their mental health needs are met. *Journal of Adolescence* 1998; **21**(5): 543–53.

62. Loeber R, Farrington DP (eds). *Serious and violent juvenile offenders.* Thousand Oaks, CA: Sage, 1998.

63. Grisso T. Juvenile offenders and mental illness. *Psychiatry, Psychology and Law* 1999; **6**(2): 143–51.

64. Nicol R, Stretch D, Whitney I, et al. Mental health needs and services for severely troubled and troubling young people including young offenders in an NSH region. *Journal of Adolescence* 2000; **23**: 243–61.

65. Fernando S, Ndegwa D, Wilson M. *Forensic psychiatry, race and culture.* London: Routledge, 1998.

66. Kaye C, Lingiah T (eds). *Race, culture and ethnicity in psychiatric practice: working with difference.* London: Jessica Kingsley, 1999.

67. McKeown M, Stowell-Smith M. Language, race and forensic psychiatry: some dilemmas for anti-discriminatory practice. In: Mason T, Mercer D (eds). *Critical perspectives in forensic care: inside out.* London: Macmillan, 1998: 188–208.

68. Almvik R, Woods P. Predicting in-patient violence using the Broset violence checklist (BVC). *International Journal of Psychiatric Nursing Research*, 1999; **4**(3): 498–505.

69. Woods P. How nurses make assessments of patient dangerousness. *Mental Health Nursing* 1996; 16(4):20–22.

70. Woods P. Risk assessment and management. In: Dale C, Thompson T, Woods P (eds). *Forensic mental health: issues in practice.* Edinburgh: Baillière Tindall and The Royal College of Nursing, 2001: 85–97.

71. Raven J. Managing the unmanageable: risk assessment and risk management in contemporary professional practice. *Journal of Nursing Management* 1999; **7**: 201–6.

72. Ministry of Health (New Zealand). Guidelines for clinical risk assessment and management in mental health services. Wellington: Ministry of Health in partnership with the Health Funding Authority, 1998. Available via: http://www.moh.govt.nz/moh.nsf Accessed 20 April, 2002.

73. Lees N, Withington J. Involving service users. In: Dale C, Thompson T, Woods P (eds). *Forensic mental health: issues in practice.* Edinburgh: Baillière Tindall and The Royal College of Nursing, 2001: 109–26.

74. HM Prison Service Working Group. *Clinical governance in prison health care: a discussion document.* HM Prison, and the Department of Health, 2001. Available at: http://www.doh.gov.uk/prisonhealth/clingov.pdf Accessed 20 April, 2002.

75. Duffy D. Clinical governance: a framework for quality in forensic mental health care. In: Dale C, Thompson T, Woods P (eds). *Forensic mental health: issues in practice.* Edinburgh: Baillière Tindall and The Royal College of Nursing, 2001: 53–60.

76. Rogers P, Gournay K, Topping-Morris B. Clinical supervision for forensic mental health nurses: the experience of one medium secure unit. In: Tarbuck P, Burnard P, Topping-Morris B (eds). *Forensic mental health nursing: policy strategy and implementation.* London: Whurr, 1999: 171–89.

77. Holmes CA. *Postdisciplinarity in mental health care: an Australian viewpoint.* Nursing Inquirer 2001; 8(4): 230–39.

78. Mason T, Mercer D (eds). *Critical perspectives in forensic care: inside out.* London: Macmillan, 1998.

79. Tarbuck P, Burnard P, Topping-Morris B (eds).

Forensic mental health nursing: policy, strategy and implementation. London: Whurr, 1999.

80. Dale C, Thompson T, Woods P (eds). *Forensic mental health: issues in practice.* Edinburgh: Baillière Tindall and The Royal College of Nursing, 2001.

81. Kettles A, Woods P, Collins M. *Therapeutic interventions for forensic mental health nurses.* London: Jessica Kingsley, 2001.

82. Kirby SD, Maguire N. Forensic psychiatric nursing. In: Thomas B, Hardy S, Cutting P (eds). *Stuart and Sundeen's mental health nursing: principles and practice,* UK edn. St Louis: Mosby, 1997: 395–409.

83. Mason T, Mercer D. Forensic psychiatric nursing. In: Clinton M, Nelson S (eds). *Advanced practice in mental health nursing.* Oxford: Blackwell Science, 1999. 236–59.

84. Kaye C, Franey A (eds). *Managing high security psychiatric care.* Rosebery, NSW: MacLennan and Petty: 1998.

85. Chaloner C, Coffey M (eds). *Forensic mental health nursing: current approaches.* Oxford: Blackwell, 1999.

IMPORTANT WEBSITES

Australian Institute of Criminology. Available at: http://www.aic.gov.au/
Includes downloadable copies of relevant reports, publications information, research reports, and news items.

Correctional Service of Canada. Available at: http://www.csc-scc.gc.ca/
Offers many research reports in summary and in full text; newsletters, and links.

Dave Sheppard Associates. Available at: http://www.davesheppard.co.uk/
British site containing a massive database of mental health legislation, government reports, year-by-year catalogues of significant events, including offences in which mental health played a part, absconding and 'untoward events' inquiry reports, and links to other useful sites.

National Criminal Justice (NCJRS). Available at: http://www.ncjrs.org/
National Institute of Justice (NIJ). Available at: http://www.ojp.usdoj.gov/nij/
US sites giving access to searchable databases of references, abstracts and full-text materials on all aspects of forensic mental health, criminology and crime.

Phil Wood's Forensic Nursing Resource Site. Available at: http://www.fnrh.freeserve.co.uk/
This is currently the most comprehensive and up-to-date forensic mental health nursing site on the Internet, with scores of useful links, lists of publications, references, full-text articles, research reports, and international news on all forensic issues.

Chapter 49

THE PSYCHIATRIC INTENSIVE CARE UNIT

Cheryl Waters* and Andrew Cashin**

INTRODUCTION

Psychiatric intensive care exists to maximize safety and support while promoting independence for people who are an acute risk to themselves or others. The whole province of psychiatric intensive care is beleaguered by therapeutic conundrums and quandaries. To illustrate:

❑ How is a balance struck between the caring and controlling functions of nursing?
❑ Is psychiatric intensive care about treatment or containment?
❑ How does one satisfy the competing needs for safety and privacy?
❑ How is the central tenet of least restriction practiced in an environment where safety and risk management are crucial?

These are only a few of the questions that need to be considered when nursing patients in a *psychiatric intensive care unit* (PICU). Furthermore, in no area of practice, more so than in the PICU, is the ability to evaluate one's own motives and desires more important for the nurse.

In this chapter some of these issues and challenges will be examined alongside a discussion about the nature, goals, purposes and methods of nursing care in a PICU. We will explore how one might negotiate some of these impasses and the intentions behind nursing actions and attitudes when caring for the acutely mentally ill in need of intensive treatment.

DESIGN

The designs of PICUs vary greatly. Invariably designed to meet local needs, there is no consensus on design.[1] However, although there are general design principles, there are large variations in how these principles are operationalized. PICUs tend to be small wards, often with between eight and 10 beds. They are usually locked and have higher staff to patient ratios than in other units.[2] They are also carefully furnished and attention is given for example to covering possible points for the connection of ligatures, which may be used to cause self-harm. The individual's need for privacy is balanced against the need to be able to see what patients are doing in order to maximize safety as well

*Cheryl Waters is a Senior Lecturer at the University of Technology, Sydney, Australia, where she is responsible for post-graduate research degree education.
**Andrew Cashin is a family counsellor with the Autism Association of New South Wales. He has a Diploma of Applied Science, Bachelor of Health Science and Master's of Nursing by thesis in which he explored the efficacy of seclusion as a psychiatric emergency intervention. Presently he is a doctoral student at the University of Technology Sydney, School of Nursing, Midwifery and Health.

as prevent elopement.[3] The design of the unit should allow for clear observation of patients at all times, even as it provides the semblance of privacy and an environment in which they can feel safe and supported. To make this possible the units are often structured so that patient areas surround and are visible to a central nursing area. Further, a balance is sought between a high stimulus environment that can be the result of having a number of highly acute people in the same small area, and the need for a relaxed, healing environment. Watkins[4] reports the evidence from the Sainsbury centre survey of 1988 that noted that collectively the design of PICUs in the UK needs improvement to meet treatment needs and maintain a therapeutic atmosphere conducive to recovery.

FOCUS OF CARE

Although the physical environment of the PICU is central to the achievement of its goals perhaps what is more important to consider are the aims and objectives of nursing care in the PICU and how these are best achieved.

By definition the focus of care in the PICU is the intensive care of patients with acute mental illness: patients who are an acute risk to themselves or others because of suicidal, homicidal or assaultive behaviour. This means that as a rule the patients in PICUs are sectioned under the local mental health act: they are usually there involuntarily, as anyone who could agree to admission and hospitalization would usually be cared for on a more open unit. The purpose of PICUs is to provide short-term or brief treatment[5,6] with a focus on risk assessment and management. In other words, the PICU is like any intensive care unit in that the patients are acutely in need of intensive care.[7] The patients have the benefit of a somewhat controlled environment until they improve and move on, to a less acute unit or to the community. The spirit of all mental health acts at this time is to treat in the least restrictive environment.[8,9] Therefore, the type of person who might be admitted is further limited to someone who cannot be treated in a less restrictive environment.

It is important to bear in mind that the treatment and time in PICU is only one part of an overall treatment plan and process. The PICU is not merely about containment, nor is it a punishment block that can be used to coerce patients into compliance with treatment programmes on other units.[3] The PICU is the setting for treatment during one phase of the illness experience. In a study by Gentle[10] nursing staff characterized their perceptions of the patients in PICU as 'the unwanted' (by other parts of the service) and the goal of the PICU as 'keeping everyone in'. Perhaps of even more concern was

the description that the therapeutic environment was 'a vague goal'. The outlook expressed by these nurses is a concern if it reflects a socially constructed view of PICU shared by nurses, carers, other mental health professionals, and the community at large.

Views such as these will have an impact on the outcomes of care because they will influence all concerned. Staff may experience lower morale and patients a sense of hopelessness. As a result of these beliefs it could be difficult to conceive of admission to the PICU as merely a step in the recovery process or ebb in the tide of the person's illness experience.[11] If nurses are to feel valued and to value the care they give in these settings, and to achieve their therapeutic ambition of helping the person integrate this chapter in their life, PICU has to be believed to be more than a 'dumping ground' for unwanted patients, and nursing care more than just 'baby-sitting'. The sense of hopelessness embodied in the beliefs expressed above would infect carers and patients alike to the extent that the time in PICU would be perceived as a waste. Admission to the PICU should not remove patients from the path to achieving their therapeutic goals. Therefore, the goals for the stay in PICU need to be clear and, to the extent that it is possible, agreed upon. Clear goals make achievements obvious. Even small gains can be noticed and celebrated. The potential effect on morale and hopefulness is obvious.

Clear goals for the admission are a necessary prerequisite for effective care. The actual assessment of the patient has to be fully undertaken before admission, and that assessment needs to take place with regard to a well-defined set of objectives, and a clear, recovery focused philosophy for the unit. It is necessary to be clear about why someone is being admitted, in order to know what must occur for him or her to have achieved the goals of the admission and not stay on any longer than required. Severimuttu[12] showed that out of 33 admissions, all of which had clear goals established prior to admission, only two admissions resulted in stays in the unit in excess of 12 days. Unfortunately, in this age of reactive clinical planning, unless clear goals and desirable outcomes are established beforehand, there is the risk that the main drive for discharge will be when the bed is required for another client with ill defined needs.[12] This has the further effect of reinforcing negative perceptions about both PICU nursing and admission to these units.

OBSERVATION AND ENGAGEMENT

There has been much recent (2000–2001) debate about the relationship between observation and therapeutic engagement. This debate has taken place on the

Psychiatric Nursing List (a UK bulletin board for mental health nurses and others. The discussions are available if you search the archives for the list at the website www.jiscmail.ac.uk/lists/psychiatric-nursing.html). The upshot from such discussion cautions that the distinction between close observation and therapeutic engagement could be a false one. Especially in the PICU as the close contact and higher staff-to-patient ratios mean that patients are engaged with staff when they need them, and that because of the higher presence and visibility there does not need to be a specially designated attentiveness.

In keeping with the characteristics of those patients who would benefit from PICU, their condition is uncertain and unstable. The nurse in the PICU needs to develop an ongoing awareness of the potential for harm. Observation is perhaps one of the fundamentals of skilled nursing and it is a difficult intervention to carry out in a manner that is both non-intrusive and effective. As the civil rights of the person admitted to the PICU have been suspended it logically follows that she or he has the right to be kept safe. The premise underlying involuntary containment in a PICU is that the patient is not in the position to take responsibility for his or her actions. The legal burden for the patients' actions consequently largely falls on the hospital while they remain an involuntary patient in the PICU. Patients who are assessed as at risk in acute psychiatric wards may be placed under close observation in order to maintain intensified and prolonged assessment.[13] 'Close' refers to the ongoing state of attentiveness cultivated as one of the core attributes of PICU nursing. This attentiveness includes a continuous process of risk assessment.[3] A much debated matter in acute care and PICU nursing is this activity of close observation, how the patient might interpret it and what it signifies in terms of the relationship between the nurse and those in their care.

When you know what to look for, you will be struck by the craft displayed by adept and accomplished nurses when they are 'observing' patients. The fact that they always seem to be available to patients when most needed, and that when outbursts occur they have anticipated it and offer a calm and stable presence. Early in your career you might interpret the masterful ability to be present to the environment and those in it, as apparently doing nothing, hanging about, and socializing with the patients and enjoying a game of pool (although, disappointingly, this may in fact have been true on occasion). Years of attentive experience allow an automatic processing of the gestalt of the PICU environment and the unconscious sifting of the relevant cues from the irrelevant in an ongoing process of observation, which has become so refined, it appears virtually effortless. This is an accomplishment that is at the core of mental health nursing craft, and which cannot be taught, but only

learned by attentive and curious involvement in the milieu.[14] From this it can be seen how, in the hands of an expert nurse, close observation and engagement are inexorably linked.

No event or situation is by itself a stressor. What shapes our reaction to any situation is our interpretation of it, what it means for us. There is no separable reality out there as such, only events and situations that are perceived in a meaningful way peculiar to the individual. The challenge of nursing in the PICU is to develop an alliance where we can have access to this meaning through shared dialogue. It is only through the creation of this unique and privileged conversational space that we have the opportunity to assist the patient to reframe their experience and put a new perspective on it. A large part of the therapeutic work in the PICU is creating this shared space. This could be called therapeutic engagement.

Therapeutic in this sense broadly means any interaction that opens up a conversational space to examine the person's life-story. The person who has become the patient in the PICU has a view of what is happening to them, why they are in the position of patient, why they are reluctantly in a hospital, and what is going to happen to them. The illness experience, in the initial stages of admission at least, may contribute strongly to the meanings constructed by the patient. Someone who is experiencing acute psychotic illness, by definition, will construct his or her world from this frame of reference and interpret his or her experiences in care correspondingly.

Perception of admission to the PICU

1 John believes that his family and workmates are trying to put him in a government experimental programme where his organs will be replaced with mechanical devices. When the police picked him up and he was admitted under the act to the local PICU, he became very distressed. Anyone who comes near him is warned not to accept any injections, food or drink, because it contains an anaesthetic.

2 Anne, who is very depressed, believes she has been locked away with these strangers because she has not appreciated or been thankful for her family. She has been sent there to languish from the incurable illness, the knowledge of which they are withholding from her.

MULTI-STORIES LIVES

Once a dialogue is opened, or a conversational space has been created, then the business at hand is to work with the person's story. The space that is created makes room for the evolution of a new chapter in the narrative of his/her life. One function for the nurse in the PICU is to listen in an active way to this story. The nurse's focus is on recovery – not from the medical disease as such but from the consequences of the illness and the distress and dis-ease it creates in the person's life. One way to access this and to help rewrite this impact is through respectful attention to the stories patients tell us.

The work of Michael White and his colleagues[16,17] from the Dulwich Centre in Adelaide, South Australia, offers some insights into the role of story and narrative in the shaping of people's lives and the restructuring of peoples experiences. From this work we can appreciate that the lives of people and patients are shaped by the stories they engage with to give their lives meaning: shaped in order to remain true to these internalized stories. The undertaking for the attentively listening nurse is to help deconstruct the meaning to highlight the difference between the reality of the world in which their way of being is problematic, and these internalized stories.

It is now important that we consider the point of involvement in the patient's narrative in PICU and how it might be different to the goals of such an involvement in other contexts.

1   One way of thinking about *narrative* is to consider how we all use it to make sense of things. The stories we tell about our life are the expression of our experiences of a life as it is lived and how we interpret it. We can use patients' narratives to engage with them and to demonstrate respect for their experiences and interpretations. As a result we learn more about the consequences of the illness in their life and are better situated to be involved in their recovery. Without this connection we risk having inadequate comprehension for effective intervention. So patients' stories also provide us with 'frames of intelligibility' with which to make sense of their beliefs and behaviours.

2   Another reason that narrative is important relates to the idea of reality orientation. The concept of reality orientation is widely evident in mental health literature. Keltner and colleagues[2] refer to the process as acknowledging the affective component, but not the content, of delusional ideas. The concept centres on the premise of avoiding the reinforcement of delusions. In a practical sense reality is what the person perceives it to be. The PICU nurse's goal is to orientate this reality to that which is required to allow the person to progress towards a less restrictive environment. In the long term the goal is to help the patient ultimately recreate a self-identity based on a preferred storyline. In the short term there needs to be movement towards a better storyline – one that is more consistent with the best explanation nurses have for culturally and historically accumulated insights about acceptable and health promoting behaviours. In this the nurse is the mediator for sense making. Therefore we as nurses need to listen and help people re-author their stories by inserting some well-placed questions and comments that lead the person to reflection on the utility of some of their beliefs and behaviours. Both the patients and our insights can be bought to bear in the search for more fitting ways of being. At the very simplest level this could be called reality orientation and is one of the goals for engagement through narrative approaches.

Given that the stay in the PICU is usually short-term, goal-directed work on a whole life-story is definitely not achievable. The issues that need immediate attention are what lead up to the admission and what needs to happen here and now in terms of behavioural change and risk reduction that will allow the person to regain control of their life and move to a less restrictive environment.

3   Transitions: Longer-term *re-authoring* is ongoing. The narrative of a person's life is constantly evolving. The preferred story is the basis for longer-term goals and the material to work on in the next setting. Taking this material into the next setting provides continuity in the person's treatment in different settings. The open ward, or step-down setting may not provide enough opportunity to complete the work of re-authoring the life-story and this work will need to continue into the community. The ongoing process of re-authoring and editing the narrative can form the basis of a community treatment programme and provide further continuity and connection as the person moves through the service. If she or he needs readmission, there is some predictability that may lead to a shorter admission. If part of each admission is not about making sense of, and integrating the experience, then subsequent admissions may be as scary and unpredictable as the first admission.

Out of the telling and retelling of the story, and the reorientation to a reality that is plausible and congruent with the expectations of society, comes the possibility of the return of control and movement to a different treatment setting. The decision to legally return control is often medical. However, it is nurses who have the most contact with patients in the PICU and have the greatest opportunity to engage the patient and do the work at hand of eliciting and editing the story.

POWER AND CONTROL

In the PICU a fundamental purpose of the nurse's involvement and engagement is to negotiate the timely and appropriate return of control to the patient. One of the challenges of PICU nursing is the delicate balance necessary in the separation of the controlling and therapeutic functions. Nursing negotiates this continuum continually in PICU and the balance will change depending on the patient's ability to exercise self-control and establish achievable goals for themselves.

Medication can be a challenge to the process of engagement, particularly if administered against the person's wishes. The nurse in the PICU has a role in administering prescribed medication. This includes routine and emergency medication. The administration of medication can involve forced interaction between the person in the role of nurse and the person who has been assigned the role of patient. This can become a ritual of testing the limits and asserting the right to choice. Aggressive incidents may occur with increased frequency at this time, as the nurse must force contact. Contact is forced, as the nurse must attempt to connect even in the face of clear and overt messages from the patient that it is not their wish for contact at this time.

The nurse can only negotiate with and for the patient within the limits defined by the law and the overall treatment plan. The challenge for the nurse is to maintain the goal of engagement and build a therapeutic alliance in the situation of having to exert coercive influence over the patient. It is the nurse who assumes these interactions: not other health professionals. These types of interactions are difficult to comprehend for reluctant patients and may have the effect of confirming their suspicions.

The bottom line may be that as in any ICU the patient may need to take medication to stabilize and subsequently regain control of their life. If the person is an involuntary patient the right to consent has been withdrawn. The bottom line may well involve the forced administration of medication, be it via intramuscular or intravenous route. (The new short-acting depot antipsychotic medications are marketed on the basis of the need for less frequent administration. Hence, there could be less need for interactions of this sort.) Choices will need to be made about how to negotiate forced interactions around medication, and possibly food and fluid. The nurse needs to reflect on his or her investment in this power struggle, and whether decisions are based on their perceived investment. It can be difficult in the face of such interactions to maintain clear boundaries and separate out our reactions: to be sure that what is being done is a response to the patient's clinical need and not in response to fear and uncertainty. Neilson and Brennan[18] note that the 'nurses' therapeutic skills may be tested to the limit by patients' challenging behaviours, and nursing skills in observation and therapeutic engagement contribute directly to the maintenance of a safe environment and the ongoing process of risk assessment' (p. 154). Patients in PICU are rarely grateful for admission and what they perceive as forced treatment. Consequently, it is important to have put some serious time, both individually and as a treatment team, into thinking about how to align oneself with and for the resistive patient: how to develop and be part of a therapeutic alliance that may be barely friendly or even civil. Social norms for behaviour and interaction cannot be used to judge the reasonableness of a patient's comportment. Before these interactions begin the goals for care need to be clear, as do the limits within which to operate. This can only occur if there is good support and communication between all members of the treatment team and if adequate opportunities exist for the development of self-knowledge and clinical practice skills. This will be touched on again before the end of the chapter.

DOCUMENTING THE JOURNEY

The nurse has a responsibility in the documentation of the patient's journey through the PICU by writing progress notes and revising the care plan or individual service plan. What is documented is the progress on the goals chosen for the patient, by the patient if possible. It is not necessarily a reflection of the progress with medical goals, or organizational goals. There are other forums for these. The notes will become a living record of the patient's personal journey during their stay in the PICU. Documentation will allow progress in line with the predetermined goals to be monitored in a consequential way. It allows others on the treatment team to continue the work in a meaningful and consistent way and it provides the history and description that is used to acknowledge that the time has come to leave the PICU. During a review of the patient's time in PICU and when approaching the termination of the relationship with the primary care nurse, documentation allows an appreciation of the magnitude of the person's journey so far. This is an occasion to affirm the progress made[15] to this point. It also allows for work towards a shared understanding of what the time in the PICU has meant for the patient to help integrate this into the overall health care experience and their personal journey.

CHALLENGES AND OPPORTUNITIES

Working in a PICU by definition involves intensive contact with acutely ill patients. These people are often the very reluctant and hostile recipients of care. Nurses deal most frequently and most intensely with patients and they are also responsible for the overall milieu. Violence is common.[3,19] The setting poses challenges to personal resources on many levels. One of the challenges may come when we are caused to re-evaluate the source of the affirmation of our nursing worth: of the meaningfulness of our labour. As nurses, whether appropriate or not, we frequently rely on patients, or their significant others, to validate the worth of our efforts. Grateful patients and relatives often seem to make the job worthwhile. There are a number of reasons why this validation is not forthcoming in the PICU. Firstly, when caring for reluctant patients this validation may not come at all, or if it does, it is often with hindsight on the part of the patient, and a long time after the fact.

Secondly, it is not always easy to understand our own motivations in caring for patients and in wanting acknowledgement and appreciation. Without adequate preparation and support it is possible that the nurse will seek to get their own needs met through their patients. This is inevitably destructive for the relationship and for the well-being of the patient. The therapeutic relationship is not a relationship of equals:[20] it exists to serve the patient.

In order to support nurses to plot a course through the perils of the PICU, access to clinical supervision of nursing practice is imperative. Not only can good supervision provide the essential support necessary to restoring emotional and psychological balance, but it will also provide the essential learning context focused on challenging clinical issues.[21] Without support the PICU nurse is prone to burnout, followed shortly after by 'move out'. This support comes from being part of a functional team[3] and from participating in appropriate learning and restorative activities.

The PICU can cause family or friends to feel conflicted. Having a friend or family member in a PICU may not offer the same confirmation of the severity and legitimacy of illness that a medical or surgical intensive care unit may. When discussing a physically sick friend or relative the information that they are in, or were in, intensive care is used as a benchmark of the seriousness of the illness. Furthermore, in these settings it is taken for granted that the patient values the efforts made on his or her behalf to help a return to wellness. As noted earlier patients are often reluctant to receive care in the PICU.[1] Significant others are also confronted with issues of stigma and questions about cause and fault in regard to mental illness. The person in care may be detained against their will, and they are certainly conscious and verbal: they often express the belief that they should be allowed to leave or not be forced to go to hospital. Significant others are often torn between their long-term commitment to these people and their view of the ben-

efits of hospitalization: they are often blamed for alerting mental health teams. The patient may express a very deep sense of betrayal. The responses of significant people to admission to the PICU will influence how the patient perceives of it both now and at future encounters. Accordingly the PICU nurse has an important part to play in working with carers when they have contact with the unit.

Gratitude

It is not uncommon to meet a person some years after they have spent time with you as a patient, and to have them share with you a particular episode of care, an interaction that validated their worth as people, that meant something to them in a deep and meaningful way. At the time nothing is said as the person struggles with the acuity of their illness and the labour of finding meaning in the experience.

CONCLUSION

The intensity signified in psychiatric intensive care is complex. At the most basic level the acuity of illness requires a care that is intense. There is a high staff-patient ratio. This is no different to any other intensive care environments in which nurses practise. A further level of intensity is manifested in the nurse–patient relationship. In many ways this differs from other intensive care environments in which technological care is of equal importance. The only machines that go 'ding' in the PICU are the personal alarms worn by nursing personnel. The primary instrument for the nurse in the PICU is the self and the self needs to be healthy and resilient to serve both patients and the nurse's needs well. In order to be able to participate in the nurse–patient relationship in a therapeutic manner, issues of power and control must be worked through, else the only one having their needs met may be the nurse. The privilege for nurses in the PICU is the access it enables to people in life crises who are vulnerable but who are also confronted by possibilities and opportunities. The danger is that the person may remain overwhelmed by the experience of their illness. The opportunity lies in their potential to consider their life and revise both the current and future chapters to incorporate new and more adaptive ways of being. This work of editing and rewriting is the basis of the work to continue in other settings and may underpin continuity of care.

REFERENCES

1. Clinton C, Pereira S, Mullins B. Training needs of psychiatric intensive care staff. *Nursing Standard* 2001; **15**(4): 33–6.

2. Keltner NL, Schwecke L, Bostrom C. *Psychiatric nursing*, 3rd edn. St Louis: Mosby, 1995.

3. Brown K, Wellman N. Psychiatric intensive care: a developing speciality. *Nursing Standard* 1998; **12**(29): 45–7.

4. Watkins P. *Mental health nursing: the art of compassionate care*. London: Read Educational and Professional, 2001.

5. Lehane M. Intensive care for acute mental illness. *Nursing Standard* 1995; **9**(36): 32–4.

6. Severimuttu A. National association of psychiatric intensive care units. *Nursing Standard* 1999; **13**(31): 31.

7. Kidd P, Wagner K. *High acuity nursing*, 2nd edn. Stanford, CA: Appleton and Lange, 1997.

8. McCoy SM, Garritson S. Seclusion the process of intervening. *Journal of Psychiatric Nursing and Mental Health Services* 1983; **21**(8): 8–15.

9. Garritson SH, Davis AJ. Least restrictive alternative: ethical considerations. *Journal of Psychiatric Nursing and Mental Health Services* 1983; **21**(12): 17.

10. Gentle J. Mental health intensive care: The nurses' experience and perceptions of a new unit. *Journal of Advanced Nursing* 1996; **24**(6): 1194–200.

11. Barker P. The Tidal Model: developing an empowering, person-centred approach to recovery within psychiatric and mental health nursing. *Journal of Psychiatric and Mental Health Nursing* 2001; **8**(3): 233–40.

12. Severimuttu A. Starting from scratch. *Nursing Standard* 1996; **10**(34): 26–7.

13. Neilson P. A secure philosophy. *Nursing Times* 1992; **88**(8): 31–3.

14. Benner P. *From novice to expert*. California: Addison Wesley, 1984.

15. Epston D, White M. Termination as a rite of passage: Questioning strategies for a therapy of inclusion. In: Neimeyer RA, Mahoney MJ (eds). *Constructivism in psychotherapy*. Washington, DC: American Psychological Association, 1995: 339–54.

16. White H. *The content of form: narrative discourse and historical representation*. Baltimore: Johns Hopkins University Press, 1987.

17. White M. Narrative therapy outline. In: *Dulwich Centre Conference on Narrative*. Adelaide, 1999.

18. Neilson P, Brennan W. The use of special observation: an audit within a psychiatric unit. *Journal of Psychiatric and Mental Health Nursing* 2001; **8**:147–55.

19. Severimuttu A, Lowe T. Aggressive incidents on a psychiatric intensive care unit. *Nursing Standard* 2000; **14**(35): 33–6.

20. Fishwick M, Tait B, O'Brien AJ. Unearthing the conflicts between carer and custodian: Implications of participation in Section 16 hearings under the Mental Health (Compulsory Assessment and Treatment) Act (1992). *Australian and New Zealand Journal of Mental Health* 2001; **10**(3): 187–96.

21. Butterworth T, Carson J, Jeacock J, White E, Clements A. Stress, coping, burnout and job satisfaction in British nurses: findings from the Clinical Supervision Evaluation Project. *Stress Medicine* 1999; **15**(1): 27–33.

Chapter 50

EARLY INTERVENTION IN PSYCHOSIS

Paul French*

INTRODUCTION

The term 'early intervention' is currently used to describe a range of strategies that have been developed for working with people with psychosis.[1] These various approaches have attracted a great deal of attention from clinicians, researchers and policy makers. In support of these developments, The National Health Service in England has recently committed itself to the development of 50 teams to provide early intervention for people with psychosis.[2] It appears that these teams will be focusing upon those people with first episode psychosis in an attempt to identify them early and thereby affecting the duration of untreated psychosis (DUP). The hope would be that teams could work with individuals and families to quickly bring symptoms under control, minimize residual symptoms and reduce subsequent episodes of relapse, sometimes called the critical period hypothesis.[3] However, there are other early intervention strategies which require discussion in order to understand fully the range of interventions available. Relapse prevention work has also been included in the early intervention paradigm as the aim of this strategy is to identify early signs of relapse and then offer interventions that are geared towards preventing relapse. Finally, the last strand of this paradigm, which is also generally considered to be a more radical approach, is the detection of people at high risk of developing psychosis. This may allow the development of a primary preventative intervention for psychosis. These various strategies will now be discussed in more detail indicating the theory behind them and their application to practice.

RELAPSE PREVENTION

Relapse prevention is utilized with people who have an existing psychotic disorder with the aim of minimizing further episodes of relapse. Relapse is defined by 'the emergence or exacerbation of positive symptoms which tends to be preceded by subtle changes in mental functioning up to 4 weeks prior to the event'.[4] Relapse prevention, therefore, offers a way in which these subtle changes can be identified, monitored and acted upon as soon as possible in order to prevent a relapse from occurring.

Theoretical background

The period prior to relapse is known as the prodromal period and is normally characterized by changes in the

*Paul French qualified as an RMN in 1989, and since then has worked in inpatient and community settings and also as a lecturer practitioner. His main interest is in the development of cognitive models and interventions for individuals at high-risk of developing psychosis in an attempt to develop primary preventative interventions.

person's mood, behaviour and thoughts, which appear 2–6 weeks prior to relapse. In numerous illnesses there can be evidence of the onset of that illness prior to the emergence of full-blown symptoms. This is very often through the emergence of subclinical symptoms and a range of other indicators heralding the onset of the illness. Prodromes in psychosis appear to be typified by, for example, tension, eating problems, concentration problems, sleeping difficulties, depression, social withdrawal, anxiety, dysphoria and irritability and may also include pre-psychotic signs such as suspiciousness and mild feelings of paranoia.[5] The first studies that attempted to identify common signs of a prodromal phase in psychosis used a retrospective design and found that the majority of patients and their carers reported particular changes in thoughts, feelings and behaviours prior to episodes.[6–8] Patients have expressed a strong interest in learning about early warning signs of the illness and relapse and rated it second most important out of an agenda of over 40 topics.[9] It has also been found that patients tend to monitor their own symptoms and also initiate responses to changes in symptoms[7] (e.g. engaging in diversionary activities, seeking professional help, resuming or increasing medication) and this is despite a lack of guidance from services. If these early signs and symptoms can be identified then they may present an opportunity to act quickly in order to offer treatments aimed at minimizing symptoms and the possibility of preventing subsequent relapse. Interventions in relapse prevention have generally been aimed at medication and support. However, a recent trial of cognitive therapy aimed at relapse demonstrated that psychological interventions could be utilized to minimize relapse.[10] Significantly the most frequent thoughts reported by patients are fears of hospitalization and the consequences of this. It is hypothesized that these thoughts trigger strong emotions, which, in turn fuel the cognitions, and the whole process may then spiral out of control.

Practical application

The process of undertaking relapse prevention entails detailed questioning about certain crises in order to understand the process of relapse as experienced by the individual. There are a number of questionnaires available to guide this process, and the Early Signs Monitoring System[8] has been extensively utilized and has useful probes to elicit information. Once this process is complete (and this can include interviewing family members) an action plan can be devised in collaboration with the person, significant family members and those in the care team. This should include strategies of monitoring, assessment, intervention, and further assessment. The interventions can be derived from psychological intervention previously undertaken. Increased support with practical issues and targeted medication to assist in the management of symptoms can be helpful. A relapse plan can be initiated at any point in a person's care. There is no requirement that it is undertaken by community staff; indeed, ward based staff may be ideally situated to initiate this intervention. By the time the patient is discharged from hospital the details of the process of relapse may be forgotten. It is also conceivable that once the recovery process has begun then some people may want to forget about the episode and not wish to discuss the details associated with relapse, what McGlashan calls the 'sealing over' process.[11] To capitalize on this window of opportunity the timing of interventions is crucial and implementation in inpatient units is therefore indicated. Finally, other psychological interventions such as family interventions have been most successfully implemented when introduced during periods of admission and this could well be the case with relapse prevention.

FIRST EPISODE CARE

The emphasis in this stage is to work with people who have recently experienced a diagnosis of schizophrenia. This approach to early intervention draws upon literature that has challenged the prevailing Kraeplinian view of schizophrenia as being an illness that is characterized by progressive deterioration throughout its course. For many years this view has driven our concepts and treatment protocols of schizophrenia and has potentially added to the stigma associated with this illness. However, there is evidence that points to an alternative conceptualization, which is the critical period hypothesis.[12] Birchwood has argued that during the first five years of diagnosis, interventions should be maximized in an effort to minimize any symptomatology while retaining any skills, contacts and positive aspects of the person's life. This approach attempts to alter what has previously been felt to be a biological determinate of prognosis and is the thrust behind this aspect of the early intervention paradigm.

Theoretical background

The length of time between the onset of psychosis and the subsequent delay in treatment has been termed the duration of untreated psychosis (DUP). The average length of DUP has been found to be approximately one year.[13,14] A number of studies have found that a longer DUP is associated with poorer prognosis,[15] and one study found it to be the most important predictor of treatment response in a large group of first admission patients.[16] Therefore, a strategy to reduce DUP would be of great importance clinically. Once an illness has been diagnosed, there is evidence that it does not necessarily follow a deteriorating course. We know that one third to one half of people receiving a diagnosis of schizophrenia will experience a single episode or multiple episodes with no residual symptoms in between episodes, the remainder experiencing multiple episodes with residual symptoms.[17] Generally speaking, mental health services do not come into contact with the former group of people. They focus upon the latter group and this can shape conceptualization of the illness by clinicians. In the early stages of the illness there is no obvious way of identifying what course the illness will run and what the prognosis will be. This has meant that a watch and wait approach has been taken; however an alternative view is that if interventions were maximized then perhaps this could influence the course of the illness.

Practical application

It appears that the sooner someone has access to treatment then potentially the better the prognosis. Services need to be able to identify cases early and have access to a range of treatment options. However, many services have finite resources and are frequently over-burdened. Their focus is predominantly working with what has been termed the 'seriously mentally ill' (SMI) population as driven in the UK by the care programme approach (CPA). The concept of SMI in this context is not a particularly useful one, if it prevents some patients in the very early stages of a psychotic episode from accessing services when they most need it.

New cases of psychosis are fairly rare. Rates of psychosis in the general population are 3:100, but this is a lifetime prevalence rate. One strategy to boost the chances of early detection could be the development of educational and awareness materials for the general public and those professionals who would be most likely to come into prodromal cases such as GPs, primary care teams, university counsellors and voluntary organizations that deal with young people in distress. Research to test the efficacy of this design has been undertaken in Norway through the TIPS project,[18] which uses educational material in newspapers, radio, cinema, television and leaflets sent to houses for the general public. At the same time those people who are likely to come into contact with prodromal cases such as schools and primary care teams are provided with videos, lectures and educational material in an effort to raise awareness of psychosis and tackle stigma associated with schizophrenia.

Once prospective new cases are identified at an early stage then it becomes a priority to engage with the individual and also their family or carers. Engagement has been recognized as a vital component of many aspects of psychiatric care including case management, and there is a wealth of literature on engagement strategies. These will not be discussed in detail here. People working within community mental health teams (CMHTs) generally have excellent engagement skills and have experience of working with clients with existing mental illness, although they need to be aware of the specifics of working with people with early onset psychosis. The person may not wish to discuss matters associated with their illness, adopting a sealing over recovery strategy.[11] This may well affect the way in which the person engages with all aspects of their treatment from psychological interventions to medication. An ability to recognize different recovery styles and work within these styles can be useful. Typically the most effective way of engaging people is to work on problems they themselves identify and not on a service-based agenda of needs.

Treatment should have its emphasis within community settings, attempting to minimize hospital admissions, as this whole process can be associated with trauma.[19] Managing episodes through home treatment teams may minimize this trauma. Community treatment teams should be well-educated, motivated and positive about outcomes and potential ways to impact upon prognosis. Ideally these teams should be distinct from other services, with members focusing their efforts towards first episode care. In the early stages diagnosis is frequently uncertain and a symptom-orientated approach to management may prove more fruitful. In terms of medical treatment, the newer atypical drugs, which have minimal side-effect (compared to typical anti-psychotic drugs), should be utilized; however side-effects such as weight gain and sexual dysfunction are still present in the preparations. Pharmacists can be valuable members of the team and can offer expert advice, although they are not frequently utilized. Alongside pharmacological management of symptoms, comprehensive psychological management should take place. Cognitive-behavioural therapy (CBT) has been the most widely researched psychological intervention for psychosis, with significant evidence indicating the efficacy of this form of intervention. There is a range of potential CBT interventions that could be employed at this point. Also family interventions should be offered and not just to high expressed emotion (EE) families but also to low EE families as well.

PRIMARY PREVENTION

This overall approach can be viewed as potentially one of the most exciting developments in psychosis research and intervention. For many years people have been attempting to identify what factors contribute towards the development of psychosis. The aetiology of schizophrenia and related psychotic disorders is at present unknown, but there is a general consensus amongst researchers and clinicians that a stress vulnerability model best accounts for the available evidence.[20–23] These models suggest that there is a biological vulnerability to the disorder, but that transition to psychotic illness is mediated by exposure to environmental stressors.

Theoretical background

The biological vulnerabilities associated with psychosis have attracted a great deal of attention. For example, vulnerability has been attributed to genetic predisposition[24] and to events that might subtly damage the developing nervous system, such as foetal exposure to the influenza virus.[25] Theories of this sort aim to explain why some individuals appear to be at greater risk of developing psychotic symptoms compared with others. Up till now the most effective method of identifying groups vulnerable to schizophrenia, has been to identify children whose parents had a diagnosis of schizophrenia and follow up their children, thus identifying an at-risk population. However, the major flaw associated with it is that the majority of people who develop psychosis have no family history. Therefore, large numbers of individuals will be missed if this is used as an identification strategy.

A development on this approach has been to incorporate lessons learnt from the relapse intervention work where prodromal experiences were utilized. As mentioned previously, relapse prodromes have been used in relapse prevention work. There has been increased interest in the initial prodrome since a study in Australia identified people in the initial prodrome and found that 40% of their population made the transition to psychosis.[26] This indicates that the identification of high-risk individuals is a possibility and further work is being undertaken to improve the ability to predict who will develop psychosis.[27]

Accurate identification of clients in the initial prodromal phase of psychosis may indicate that an intervention aimed at this population could result in primary prevention of psychosis, as Falloon[28] has demonstrated. There is a range of treatment options available for schizophrenia and these have been extensively reviewed.[29] By far the most common and generally accessible treatment for psychosis is medication. However, the drugs used to treat psychosis have a range of side-effects; even the atypical anti-psychotics while showing fewer side-effects such as movement disorders, still have a number of unpleasant side-effects associated with them. Therefore, to use medication as a treatment option for this high-risk group would mean exposing the majority to side-effects of neuroleptic medication when they may never go on to develop psychosis. This clearly has ethical considerations[30] and little or no justification.[31] A solution would be to employ a treatment strategy with no physical side-effects and one that targets the problems that are causing concern. A psychological intervention would, therefore, be indicated. Cognitive-behavioural therapy (CBT) for psychosis has been around for almost 50 years, starting with a single case study.[32] The accumulating body of evidence to support this treatment option has now reached the point where randomized controlled trials have demonstrated its efficacy.[33–36] CBT would appear the most appropriate treatment strategy to be offered during the initial prodrome in an effort to minimize symptoms and possibly prevent the transition to psychosis. Cognitive models to describe the onset of psychosis have been described.[37–39] These models draw upon the extensive work of others who have developed established models to understand specific symptoms of psychosis.[40,41]

There is now good evidence to suggest that identification of high-risk groups is possible.[26,42] However, there is little evidence to suggest that CBT will be able to prevent the onset of psychosis. A randomized controlled trial is currently being undertaken[42] and there are case studies[37] and case series suggesting the possibility of this kind of intervention. This form of intervention would generally require a radical change in clinician's view of the concept of psychosis. There exists a strong belief in the medical model of psychosis. However, there is also a range of evidence suggesting that psychological processes have a large part to play in the development and maintenance of symptoms. Hallucinations are not specific to psychosis; they can be found in a wide range of presentations. In fact in certain circumstances they are considered absolutely normal. For example let us consider for a moment the death of an elderly man who has been married for 50 years to the love of his life (his childhood sweetheart). When his wife tells us that she frequently hears him calling her name and she has seen him sat in his favourite chair, we do not immediately consider the prescription of neuroleptic medication. Rather we spend time normalizing this experience. For a number of years we have been exposed to normalizing information regarding psychotic symptoms associated with schizophrenia and this approach is a well-established intervention. However, to fully embrace the concept of normalization we should believe that psychotic symptoms can indeed be understandable.

Formulation-driven approaches, which promote the understanding of symptoms, should apply.

Practical application

It is important to consider what can be offered, if anything, to this at-risk group. Will it be the identification of at-risk cases? Is it identification and monitoring? Is it identification and treatment? What criteria will be used to classify a case as high risk? What will treatment consist of? If psychological treatments are going to be used are there sufficiently skilled clinicians to deliver these interventions? What services and treatments are available if someone makes the transition to psychosis? These questions should all be considered when developing a strategy for at-risk populations.

Teams should take stock of their existing resources, links and networks and should build upon existing links with primary care in the initial stages. However, it is important to remember that identification of existing cases can be hard enough, and identifying at-risk groups can be even harder. The primary care teams who are likely to come into contact with this group can be helped by providing easily understood and an over inclusive referral criteria. It should then be up to the specialist team to undertake an assessment of the individual in order to come to a decision whether they fit into a high-risk criteria or not, which may require more than one assessment session. If the person is not suitable, the client should be told about which other options are available to them. If suitable, the person should be monitored as a minimum in order to observe if they make the transition to psychosis. If they do, treatment should begin as discussed in the section above. If treatment is going to be offered to people in the high-risk group prior to transition to psychosis this should not include antipsychotic medication, as this would be unethical. If pharmacological treatments are going to be considered they should target the symptoms for which the person is help seeking such as anxiety, depression, sleep disturbance. The treatment of choice at this stage should be cognitive therapy designed specifically for this group. This treatment is structured, time limited, problem and goal-orientated and has proven efficacy in treating psychotic and non-psychotic symptoms. It requires the therapist to have a wide-ranging knowledge of cognitive models and their application, but also access to clinical supervision to assist with difficult aspects of the cases. Psychological interventions with this client group are especially challenging, not only in terms of necessary skills but also in terms of changing our perceptions of psychosis as being a medical condition that requires medical intervention, to an understandable process amenable to psychological intervention.

Case study 50.1

A 17-year-old man, John is referred to psychiatric services from his GP due to concerns from his family that his behaviour is becoming increasingly 'odd'. He finally agreed to be seen by his GP and appeared sullen, withdrawn and preoccupied although denied any present concerns. His family stated that he is spending increased amounts of time isolated in his room in the family home and they can occasionally hear him talking to himself while alone. They also report that he is eating very little and tends to sleep during the day rather than at night. John admits to smoking cannabis frequently in the past, but denies any current use. No other drug or alcohol use. Up until recently he had a girlfriend and used to go out with her and his friends, although since his break-up with his girlfriend he hardly goes out and does not see his friends. They are tending to ring him less and less as time passes.

John is sent an appointment to attend an outpatient appointment at his local mental health unit and on receipt of this becomes angry and increasingly withdrawn from his family. John does not attend this appointment, which causes further tension in the family. Another appointment is arranged and his family takes him to the appointment. He is finally assessed and it is felt that he may be depressed with some paranoid ideas, which are related to his drug use. He is given a prescription for anti-depressants, a follow-up appointment and the number of a local voluntary organization that works with young people.

John does not contact the voluntary organization or take medication and he does not attend his follow-up appointment. Things become steadily worse within the family home as John's behaviour deteriorates to the point where he assaults one of his elderly neighbours and the police are involved. They take him to a local casualty department where he is felt to be experiencing a psychotic episode, and he is formally admitted. Unfortunately the local unit has no beds and he is sent to another unit some distance away, which makes it difficult for his family to visit. These factors impact upon how John and his family view the services and they feel as though they have been let down.

DISCUSSION

Case 50.1 describes some of the difficulties associated with the onset and development of psychosis. In the initial stages it can be hard to define the difference between adolescent behaviour, drug-induced symptoms and the onset of psychosis. Frequently clinicians do not consider the development of psychosis for many reasons, such as not being willing to stigmatize individuals. However, offering non-stigmatizing services, which target people's problems and engage them and their family with services can overcome this. John does display some signs indicating potential risk and engaging with John and his family at this stage could be extremely beneficial. If services can be geared towards a wait and see approach with more emphasis placed on engagement of potential at-risk individuals, offering flexible appointments, this may affect how services are perceived and subsequent engagement. Unfortunately many services are geared towards crisis provision as opposed to prevention, due to limited resources. Unfortunately this process may not only affect how people engage with services, but also the efficacy of the treatments on offer whether pharmacological or psychological.

CONCLUSION

This chapter has discussed a range of interventions available for people with psychosis under the umbrella of early interventions. However, these treatment options clearly operate at different points in the person's illness. It is important that clinicians and managers are aware of the different forms of early intervention in order that they can tailor services to deliver these forms of intervention. Clients deserve access to these interventions and clinicians should strive to develop skills to deliver them. Some aspects of these interventions are extremely challenging to the conceptualization of psychosis; however, the rewards for professionals and their clients could be immense.

REFERENCES

1. French P, Walford L. Psychological approaches to early intervention for psychosis: what it is and what it can achieve. *Mental Health Care* 2001; **4**: 158–61.

2. Department of Health. *The NHS Plan, a plan for investment, a plan for reform.* London: The Stationery Office, 2000.

3. Birchwood M. The critical period for early intervention. In: Birchwood M, Fowler D, Jackson C (eds). *Early intervention in psychosis: A guide to concepts, evidence and interventions.* Chichester: John Wiley, 2000.

4. American Psychiatric Association. *Diagnostic and statistical manual of mental disorders (DSM)*, 4th edn. Washington DC: APA, 1994.

5. Birchwood M. Early intervention in psychotic relapse. In: Haddock G, Slade P (eds). *Cognitive-behavioural interventions with psychotic disorders.* London, New York: Routledge, 1996.

6. Herz M, Melville C. Relapse in schizophrenia. *American Journal of Psychiatry* 1980; **137**: 801–12.

7. McCandless-Glincher L, Mcknight S, Hamera E, Smith BL, Peterson K, Plumlee AA. Use of symptoms by schizophrenics to monitor and regulate their illness. *Hospital and Community Psychiatry* 1986; **37**: 929–33.

8. Birchwood M, Smith J, Macmillan F, Hogg B, Prasad R, Harvey C, Bering S. Predicting relapse in schizophrenia: the development and implementation of an early signs monitoring system using patients and families as observers. *Psychological Medicine* 1989; **19**: 649–56.

9. Mueser KT, Bellack AS, Wade JH, Sayers SL, Rosenthal CK. An assessment of the educational needs of chronic psychiatric patients and their relatives. *British Journal of Psychiatry* 1992; **160**: 674–80.

10. Gumley AI, Power KG. Is targeting cognitive therapy during relapse in psychosis feasible. *Behavioural and Cognitive Psychotherapy* 2000; **28**: 161–74.

11. McGlashen TH. Recovery style from mental illness and long-term outcome. *Journal of Nervous and Mental Disease* 1987; **175**: 681–5.

12. Birchwood M. The critical period for early intervention. In: Birchwood M, Fowler D, Jackson C (eds). *Early intervention in psychosis: a guide to concepts, evidence and interventions.* Chichester: Wiley, 2000.

13. Loebel AD, Lieberman JA, Alvir JMJ, Mayerhoff DI, Geisler SH, Szymanski SR. Duration of psychosis and outcome in first episode schizophrenia. *American Journal of Psychiatry* 1992; **149**: 1183–8.

14. Barne TRE, Hutton SB, Chapman MJ, Mutsatsa S, Puri BK, Joyce EM. West London first episode study of schizophrenia: clinical correlates of duration of untreated psychosis. *The British Journal of Psychiatry* 2000; **177**: 207–11.

15. Crow TJ, Macmillan JF, Johnson AL, Johnstone E. The Northwick Park study of first episodes of schizophrenia: II. A randomised controlled trial of prophylactic neuroleptic treatment. *British Journal of Psychiatry* 1986; **148**: 120–27.

16. Drake RJ, Haley CJ, Akhtar S, Lewis SW. Causes of duration of untreated psychosis in schizophrenia. *The British Journal of Psychiatry* 2000; **177**: 511–15.

17. Hegarty JD, Baldessarini RJ, Tohen M, Waternaux C, Oepen G. One hundred years of schizophrenia: A meta-analysis of the outcome literature. *American Journal of Psychiatry* 1994; **151**(10): 1409–16.

18. Larsen TK, Johanessen JO, McGlashen T, Horneland M, Mardal S, Vaglum P. Can duration of untreated psychosis be reduced. In: Birchwood M, Fowler D, Jackson C (eds). *Early intervention in psychosis: a guide to concepts, evidence and interventions.* Chichester: Wiley, 2000.

19. Meyer H, Taiminen T, Vuori T, *et al.* Post-traumatic stress disorder symptoms related to psychosis and acute involuntary hospitalisation in schizophrenic and delusional patients. *The Journal of Nervous and Mental Disease* 1999; **187**: 343–52.

20. Gottesman II. *Schizophrenia genesis: the origins of madness.* San Francisco: Freeman, 1991.

21. Gottesman II, Shields J. *Schizophrenia: the epigenetic puzzle.* Cambridge: Cambridge University Press, 1982.

22. Neuchterlein KH, Dawson M. A heuristic vulner-

ability stress model of schizophrenic episodes. *Schizophrenia Bulletin* 1984; **10**: 300–312.

23. Zubin J, Spring B. Vulnerability: a new view of schizophrenia. *Journal of Abnormal Psychology* 1977; **86**: 103–26.

24. Murray RM, McGuffin P. Genetic aspects of psychiatric disorders. In: Kendell RE, Zealley AK (eds). *Companion to psychiatric studies*. Edinburgh: Churchill Livingstone, 1993.

25. McGrath J, Murray R. Risk factors for schizophrenia: from conception to birth. In: Hirsch SR, Weinberger DR (eds). *Schizophrenia*. Oxford: Blackwell Science, 1995: 187–205.

26. Yung A, Phillips LJ, McGorry PD, *et al*. A step towards indicated prevention of schizophrenia. *British Journal of Psychiatry* 1998; **172** (Suppl. 33): 14–20.

27. Miller TJ, McGlashan TH. Early identification and intervention in psychotic illness. *American Journal of Psychiatry* 2000; **157**(7): 1041–50.

28. Falloon IRH. Early intervention for first episodes of schizophrenia: a preliminary exploration. *Psychiatry* 1992; **55**: 4–15.

29. Lehman AF, Steinwachs DM, Dixon LB, *et al*. Translating research into practice: the schizophrenia Patient Outcome Outcomes Research Team (PORT) treatment recommendations. *Schizophrenia Bulletin* 1998; **24**(1): 1–10.

30. Yung A, McGorry PD. The prodromal phase of first episode psychosis: past and current conceptualisations. *Schizophrenia Bulletin* 1996; **22**: 353–70.

31. Bebbington P. Early intervention in psychosis: pharmacotherapeutic strategies. In: Birchwood M, Fowler D, Jackson C (eds). *Early intervention in psychosis: a guide to concepts, evidence and interventions*. Chichester: Wiley, 2000.

32. Beck AT. Successful outpatient psychotherapy of a chronic schizophrenic with a delusion based on borrowed guilt. *Psychiatry* 1952; **15**: 305–12.

33. Drury V, Birchwood M, Cochrane R, Macmillan F. Cognitive therapy and recovery from acute psychosis: a controlled trial. I. Impact on psychotic symptoms. *British Journal of Psychiatry* 1996; **169**: 593–601.

34. Kuipers E, Garety P, Fowler D, Dunn G, Bebbington P, Freeman D, Hadley C. London–East Anglia randomised controlled trial of cognitive-behavioural therapy for psychosis. I. Effects of the treatment phase. *British Journal of Psychiatry* 1997; **171**: 319–27.

35. Tarrier N, Yusupoff L, Kinney C, McCarthy E, Gledhill A, Haddock G, Morris J. Randomised controlled trial of intensive cognitive behaviour therapy for patients with chronic schizophrenia. *British Medical Journal* 1998; **317**: 303–7.

36. Sensky T, Turkington D, Kingdon D, *et al*. A randomized controlled trial of cognitive-behavioral therapy for persistent symptoms in schizophrenia resistant to medication. *Archives of General Psychiatry* 2000; **57**(2): 165–72

37. French P, Morrison AP, Walford L, Knight A, Bentall RP. Cognitive therapy for preventing transition to psychosis in high-risk individuals: a single case study. In: Morrison AP (ed.) *A case book of cognitive therapy for psychosis*. Brunner–Routledge, London, 2002.

38. Garety PA, *et al*. A cognitive model of the positive symptoms of psychosis. *Psychological Medicine* 2001; **31**: 189–95.

39. Morrison AP. The interpretation of intrusions in psychosis: an integrative cognitive approach to hallucinations and delusions. *Behavioural and Cognitive Psychotherapy* 2001; **29**: 257–76.

40. Bentall RP, Kinderman P, Kaney S. The self, attributional processes and abnormal beliefs: towards a model of persecutory delusions. *Behaviour Research and Therapy* 1994; **32**: 331–41.

41. Morrison AP. A cognitive analysis of the maintenance of auditory hallucinations: are voices to schizophrenia what bodily sensations are to panic? *Behavioural and Cognitive Psychotherapy* 1998; **26**: 289–302.

42. Morrison AP, Bentall RP, French P, *et al*. A randomised controlled trial of early detection and cognitive therapy for preventing transition to psychosis in high risk individuals: study design and interim analysis of transition rate and psychological risk factors. *British Journal of Psychiatry* 181 (Supplement **43**: 78–84).

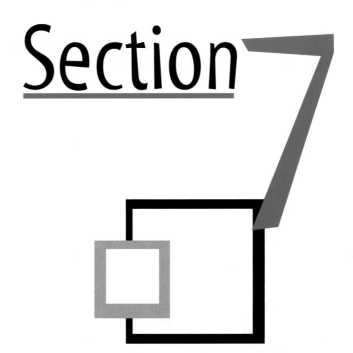

Section 7

Some standardized processes of nursing practice

Preface to Section 7

As members of the multidisciplinary team, nurses have discrete responsibilities. In earlier sections, some of the broad principles and the value base of nursing practice were illustrated. In this section we consider how nurses might fulfil more specific roles in the development or delivery of specific *aspects* of mental health service provision.

The section begins with the process of admission to hospital and ends with the changing role of nurses in the administration and prescription of medication. These two chapters illustrate both the tradition of care and treatment – hospitalization and medication – but also how practice is changing, as a result of political, economic and philosophical factors, all of which impinge on our appreciation of the quality of care.

We have chosen here to illustrate some of the standardized processes that form the bedrock of nursing practice: how nurses assess the risk of suicide or self-harm; engage with people deemed to be at risk; keep appropriate and adequate records of care and prepare for the discharge process; enable the delivery of special treatments, like ECT; and help to promote mental health.

This section encompasses, therefore, many of the dimensions of the role of the psychiatric-mental health nurse: from the specifically *psychiatric* dimensions of keeping suicidal people safe, to the more *developmental* aspects of care associated with mental health promotion.

Chapter 51

ADMISSION TO A PSYCHIATRIC UNIT

Angela Simpson* and Jerome Wright**

THE CRISIS AND OPPORTUNITY OF HOSPITAL ADMISSION

The person on the brink of admission to an acute inpatient unit is invariably frightened. This fear is commonly compounded by the growing realization of the need for admission to inpatient psychiatric care. For the person in crisis the scale of personal change can seem overwhelming. It is not uncommon for the person to feel as if a breaking point has been reached, destabilizing the 'self' and the person's perception of him/herself in the future. Following such a breakdown, people commonly find themselves in a situation in which they need to redefine themselves and their relationships, and begin to question the direction of their lives.

Nurses working in acute inpatient settings are in close contact with people in distress. As a result, they can find the experience of working *with* people in crisis, unnerving. People in crisis respond in different ways to distress, so the ward environment is often characterized by uncertainty and unpredictability. In these conditions, nurses may begin to question their ability to respond effectively and may even doubt their skill in supporting people in crisis. A gap between what the person in crisis

needs and what nurses *feel* able to provide, can lead nurses to question their purpose, role and potential usefulness. A reaction to this occupational stress may lead nurses to seek to *control* the environment, leading to criticism that acute admission wards provide custodial rather than therapeutic care.[1–3]

Failing to recognize acute admission wards as highly complex and innately 'fear-full' places is a fundamental error when seeking to create and sustain a caring and therapeutic environment. Fear has positive as well as negative effects. It frees us from complacency, stimulates action and above all, brings us face to face with our shared humanity or common human experience. From this starting point acute admission wards might be freed from the presence of overwhelming fear and control, and the development of fundamentally humanizing, and caring, environments may be realized.

THE FUNCTION OF ACUTE ADMISSION WARDS

The overall numbers of people admitted to acute admission units is rising.[2] Demographic, economic and societal

*Angela Simpson is a Lecturer in Mental Health Nursing at the University of York, England. She was the team leader of the acute psychiatric Nursing Development Unit at Cedar Ward in Harrogate and currently is a doctoral student at the University of Newcastle.

**Jerome Wright is a Lecturer in Nursing at the University of York, England. He has a strong clinical nursing background in a variety of care specialties including acute mental health care, Community Psychiatric Nursing and as a Clinical Nurse Specialist in Liaison Psychiatry. Jerome has a particular interest in the care of people in acute distress and for those with concurrent physical health problems and has written and published on HIV and mental health nursing and mental health in primary care.

changes, and the widening gap between the rich and poor, all have a major impact upon people's mental health. The nature and organization of existing mental health services – including rapid closure and inadequate replacement provision – also has adversely affected the way that acute admission wards function.

However, seeing hospital as the hub of mental health services, portrays a hospital-centric view of mental health care; one in which the community is seen as a resource for the hospital rather than the other way around. This requires a fundamental repositioning of mental health services from the traditional service-led function to a 'service-user-centric' model. Such a move encapsulates the shift from 'what services offer' to 'what people need'. From such a perspective, support is offered through respect, and active engagement, helping people to interpret and make sense of their own experiences, offering choice, information and a continuity of care.[4–7] Incorporating these human conditions into the milieu of acute inpatient care shifts the focus away from the ward as a repository for the most troubled and vulnerable to a place of healing and recovery where caring relationships can be established.

NURSING ALONGSIDE THE PERSON IN ACUTE DISTRESS

Mental health nurses should be 'natural allies' of people in emotional crisis.[8] The close proximity of the nurse to the person in crisis affords an opportunity to develop close alliances with people in care, establishing relationships that foster hope and growth, while also providing practical and emotional support. Two core nursing values: *empowerment* and *curiosity* allow nurses to develop such close rapport.

The nurse who seeks to actively empower the person in crisis acknowledges the person as 'an expert of the self', and as such identifies strongly with the need to place the person at the centre of decision-making. To empower the person, nurses demonstrate an awareness of the persons' needs, the need to promote personal choice, to provide information, to allow time to complete tasks and to discuss future care options.[9]

Maintaining a fundamental sense of curiosity about the person and their experience is also necessary. Peplau[10] spoke of a 'gentle curiosity'; a willingness to relate and a concern to provide people with the support they need to free themselves from their distress. This is more than a fleeting attention, offered only when the person's speech or actions demand it, but is an active engagement and dialogue; seeing the task of the person in crisis as developing an understanding of themselves. For people in acute distress this can be challenging and traumatic 'work in progress'. Recovery from psychologi-

cal or emotional distress is not a tidy process and it does not necessarily involve the absence of symptoms,[11] since the person might resolve to live with or work through distress. Thus, individual caring relationships that are established in crisis, might best instil the prospect of limitless possibilities within the person.

The first 72 hours of any person's admission to an acute inpatient ward are pivotal to the establishment of the helping relationship and are likely to have a significant impact on the person's experience of crisis and their view of the prospect for recovery. Here, a case illustration follows Jon and his family through the first three days following admission to an acute psychiatric unit.

Case study 51.1

Jon is 17 years old. He has recently returned to live in the family home after spending a year living in a shared house with fellow students. He has dropped out of his studies and spends his time isolated in his bedroom. Contacts with his friends have deteriorated. There is growing tension between Jon and his brother. Unlike Jon, Andy has graduated from college, has found himself a job which he enjoys and has a wide circle of friends. This growing tension resulted in an incident where Jon threatened and physically assaulted his brother. Jon's family is becoming increasingly concerned about him, especially his irritability and growing emotional distance. They seek advice from their GP. Jon admits to the family doctor that he has been hearing voices since he left home and that these are scary because they are critical and derogatory. The situation between Jon and his brother continues to deteriorate and the family is at breaking point. The GP arranges for a psychiatrist to visit and it is recommended that Jon be admitted to hospital for further assessment.

MEETING THE PERSON IN CRISIS

The decision to admit Jon to an inpatient admission unit is medically led, but is made in collaboration with Jon, his family and the nursing team. In preparing to meet Jon, the nurse takes the opportunity to discuss what is already known about him, seeking the views of the medical team regarding the purpose of the hospital admission. In Jon's case the family situation is vital so, where possible, the nurse takes the opportunity to discuss the wider social situation, with the team, which has been involved recently. This background information gives the nurse some idea of what to expect from Jon and his family on admission. More especially, the nurse develops early insight into Jon's own view of his admission to hospital, helping the nurse to gauge if Jon is likely to be a willing, or reluctant, participant.

Medical colleagues are likely to have already begun to form a 'working hypothesis' regarding an early diagnosis of Jon's condition, which will be reflected in conversations with the nursing team and records relating to the admission. While taking into account the views of medical colleagues, it is important that nurses remain open-minded. The nursing focus will place considerable emphasis on attempting to understand Jon's *experience* of distress, identifying strongly with Jon's interpretation of his own experience.[12]

Although acute inpatient units offer a responsive crisis service, there is usually always a time interval between the ward receiving notification of the need for admission to hospital and the person arriving on the ward. This time is put to good use by nurses who, in preparing to meet Jon:

❑ Collate all available information about Jon and his family, liaising with other members of the multiprofessional team who have already established contact – such as medical and primary care colleagues.
❑ Make appropriate preparations on the ward, creating a comfortable bed space for him.

Prior to admission, the nursing team should identify the nurse who is best placed to be Jon's key nurse. This will involve:

❑ Providing a consistent source of contact for Jon and his family.
❑ Working closely with Jon, providing the conditions in which a constructive, helping relationship might be developed.
❑ Accepting responsibility for co-ordinating Jon's care.
❑ Liaising with the nursing team and wider multiprofessional team to co-ordinate Jon's care while he is in hospital.

Prior to admission nurses concern themselves with creating the conditions in which Jon might experience a strong sense of 'togetherness' or 'attachment'. The nursing team should be aware that Jon is likely to identify closely with the nurse undertaking the admission interview,[13] so in most cases this nurse becomes best placed to further develop the key-nurse relationship.

Arrival at the unit

People react in different ways to the experience of hospital admission. Typical responses can include a sense of hopelessness questioning 'What good is this going to do?' Others sometimes feel rejected by family or those close to them. Some people, especially those compulsorily admitted, feel angry or irritated by the prospect. Whatever the view of the person about their admission, the nurse must accept the person as they are within the crisis, and allow this to be the starting point of constructive helping.

Taking an interest in how the person presents on arrival to the ward will inform the key nurse about the level of the person's discomfort and distress. This distress should be acknowledged by the key nurse who:

❑ Introduces her/himself to Jon, explaining that (s)he is a nurse on the ward who has special responsibility to work closely with him.
❑ Empathizes with Jon's situation.
❑ Seeks guidance from Jon about what can be done now to make him more comfortable.
❑ Recognizes the social discomfort experienced by Jon, who is clearly outside of his usual environment

The key nurse is well aware that the experience of being admitted to hospital, or having a family member/close associate admitted to hospital, is stressful. As such, the key nurse communicates interest in Jon, his family and friends and his situation and is careful to demonstrate respect. Although the situation is far from 'normal', commonly nurses are able to break this difficult 'social ice' by gently normalizing the situation. Nurses do this by remaining relaxed (although quietly confident) and paying immediate attention to the comfort needs of Jon and his family who need:

❑ Private space on the ward to talk with each other, and the nurse.
❑ Refreshments.
❑ A place in which it is possible to smoke (if required).
❑ To know where Jon's bedroom is located.
❑ To be shown where the bathroom/toilets are located.
❑ To identify with the key nurse as a consistent and helpful presence.

Orientating the person to his new surroundings helps Jon to feel at ease on the ward. These early attempts to ease the distress of the admission process can be likened to friendship building. The person in distress expects nurses to function as both friend and professional.[14] Admitting Jon to hospital allows the nurse the opportunity to extend simple kindness, in a genuine attempt to develop a personable relationship characterized by mutual understanding and warmth. Jon and his family might find some comfort in the fact that although the situation is an unusual one for them, it is not unusual for the key nurse.

The ward as a safe haven

Jon needs to be reassured that the ward is safe. The nurse communicates this in two ways. Firstly, interpersonal safety and trust are nurtured through the beginnings of the helping relationship. Here the nurse develops a personable relationship with Jon and his family and provides information in an easy and relaxed manner, but is also competent and responds to situations requiring professional knowledge and expertise. Secondly, the nurse communicates issues of wider personal safety directly to the person on admission. Jon's attention is drawn to some basic ground rules that maintain the safety of everyone, whether residing, visiting or working within the unit. These usually include:

❑ The need to store all medications in a clinical room.
❑ The need for every person to hand in sharp objects.
❑ No alcohol to be drunk or stored on the ward.
❑ No illicit substances to be used or stored on the ward.
❑ The need for everyone to treat each other with courtesy and respect.

While these ground rules help to instil confidence that the ward is safe, the nurse should also discuss with Jon the team's expectations that everyone will treat one another, and the environment, with respect. Although people will experience episodes of distress from time to time, the nursing team should clearly articulate the importance and expectation that everyone concerned will attempt to support each other through extending concern and respect. When distressed, the person is expected to extend the same degree of concern for others, they would expect for themselves, while also being respectful of the environment. These are the conditions that will help the person to best support himself and support others, while allowing nurses to provide support to Jon and other people admitted to the ward.

Preparing for the admission interview

The nurse begins, tentatively, to develop an understanding of Jon and his wider, family situation. However, it is important to note that these impressions remain 'impressions' until they are carefully explored with Jon. The nurse uses the admission interview to explore Jon's perceptions of his experience. The timing of the admission interview itself is important. Although most people admitted to hospital like Jon are willing and able to talk through their situation in more detail, on admission some are initially unwilling or unable to engage in this process. It is important to recognize that the quality of the interview and the opportunity within it for constructive engagement, is pivotal to therapeutic helping. The

admission interview is best undertaken as a collaborative process, so the nurse seeks to create the conditions in which Jon might become a willing and active participant in the process.

The nurse takes the time to discuss with Jon what he might expect from the admission interview, gauging his willingness and potential ability to collaborate. At this early stage (s)he needs to demonstrate a willingness to work with Jon as a person, responding to his individual needs. This means allowing time and space to make decisions, but more especially, allowing personal choice whenever it is possible to do so. These conditions help to reduce fear. As Jon retains control and independence, autonomy is promoted and respected. This also means, however, that in some respects the nurse is following the lead of the person in care.

While the process of conducting the admission interview necessarily involves the nurse asking questions and recording supporting information it is important that the interview doesn't descend into a remote, impersonal 'tick box' exercise. The nurse is challenged to overcome the organizational need to collate specific information, and the nursing aim of striving to meet with the person, developing an increased understanding of Jon the 'person' and his experience of crisis. Creating the condition in which such human contact can occur, requires a degree of preparation. Jon needs to understand why the admission interview is necessary, and also must be informed that information collected and written down will be shared with other members of the multiprofessional team. To prepare Jon for the admission interview and win collaborative support for the process, the nurse:

❑ Explains the interview process.
❑ Gives Jon copies of the paperwork to be completed.
❑ Encourages him to ask questions.
❑ Counters concerns that it is a lengthy process by reassuring him that it can be completed at his pace, allowing time for a break if necessary.
❑ Understands that Jon might not be able to complete the interview in one attempt. Where this occurs it is the nurse's responsibility to continue to attempt to create the conditions in which Jon might settle to this collaborative task.

THE ADMISSION INTERVIEW: THE PERSON AS A PERSON

The admission interview provides the nurse with a valuable opportunity to make human contact with Jon. This is *the* forum in which the skilful nurse begins to sow the seeds of a constructive helping relationship. At the admission interview the nurse listens carefully to Jon's account of his *experience* of distress and investigates with him how this affects his ability to live everyday life.[12] Adopting this approach allows the nurse to demonstrate early concern and understanding for Jon as a person. It also helps to instil early confidence in Jon that his perceptions and concerns might best be addressed within a constructive and supportive relationship as opposed to facing this alone.

The admission interview is not a routine chore and is best approached by nurses who possess a keen interest and an open mind. According to Barker[12, p.43] the admission interview serves the nurse with opportunity to:

❑ Develop a relationship with the person.
❑ Establish trust.
❑ Promote professional closeness and collaboration.
❑ Start to identify problematic patterns in the person's actions.
❑ Identify how the person's personal resources might help the person to overcome distress.

The admission interview achieves its optimum potential when both parties experience it as a 'human to human' activity. For nurses this might mean accepting the need to leave their 'professional' status to one side, choosing instead to give something of themselves, placing emphasis on attempting to understand Jon's 'human crisis' in a 'human way'. In developing this line of enquiry the nurse will explore:

❑ Jon's perception of the circumstances that have resulted in the hospital admission.
❑ How Jon views himself now within the crisis.
❑ How it feels to *be* Jon.
❑ How things have changed for Jon and how he feels about this.
❑ Jon's view on the family crisis.

In finding out more about Jon and his situation, the nurse is likely to begin to gauge the extent of his personal distress. Assessing the extent to which the person might be a risk to themselves or other people is an important feature of the admission interview. The nurse will have developed an awareness of how Jon's experience and situation are effecting his ability to live and will also have developed some understanding of the extent to which Jon feels his situation to be inside or outside of his own control. During the admission interview, the nurse will develop a sense of how Jon sees himself in the future. The extent to which he feels optimism or hopelessness are important elements of this process. Felt hopelessness is strongly associated with personal risk.[15] The admitting nurse therefore needs to question Jon sensitively with regard to the issue of personal safety, discussing how Jon and the ward team can work together to maintain and maximize meaningful interpersonal engagement while seeking also to maximize personal safety.

Recording the interview collaboratively

During the interview the nurse begins to formulate an understanding of Jon, his condition, and situation. Having listened carefully and made observations, the nurse checks his/her perceptions and understandings with Jon, to clarify their accuracy and to avoid making assumptions. Striving to achieve this degree of accuracy helps to convey genuine concern and respect. At some point, the observations made by the nurse and Jon will need to be recorded. Progressive nursing teams will recognize the value of offering Jon the opportunity to write down his own experience in his own words.[15] If Jon doesn't feel able to do this, the nurse agrees the language to be used within the documentation and writes this down on his behalf. The nurse might choose to use direct quotes made by Jon, as his language is likely to closely reflect his experience. Undertaken in this way, the admission interview has the potential to be fundamentally empowering, as the person in care is involved in a transparent documentary process, which is inherently collaborative. More especially, by completing the admission assessment with Jon, he retains a degree of control within the process.

Negotiating care

Jon needs to maintain a sense of purpose regarding the hospital admission. This is achieved when a plan of care for the next 72 hours is developed collaboratively. The nurse discusses with Jon what he might expect to happen over the next few hours and days. Jon needs to be informed of the degree of individual contact he can expect from his key nurse and also any structured group activity he might be expected to attend. Jon needs to understand that these opportunities exist so that he might learn through his own experience, but also through the wider experience of others. It is not uncommon for people in distress to feel as though they are not worthy of help themselves, but they can invariably be persuaded to offer support to others. This is a highly constructive starting point for people who are reluctant to share their experiences with others.

Beyond this, Jon also needs to know how to access nursing support quickly should he begin to feel a growing sense of unease and distress. The nurse must also ensure that Jon receives support without needing to ask for it. Jon needs to develop an awareness at this early stage that the primary purpose of the admission to hospital is for him to find the words to articulate his distress. Jon needs to get to know and understand his distress while being supported in a safe and purposeful care environment.

As the admission interview draws to its natural conclusion, the nurse takes the opportunity to thank Jon for working through the process and acknowledges that the task may well have been a difficult one for Jon to undertake. The nurse remains optimistic indicating a willingness to continue to work constructively with Jon.

Key points

The nurse conducting the admission interview:

❑ Views the admission process as a unique opportunity to make 'human contact' with Jon. This is not a routine, menial or paper based task. Rather it provides the nurse with the opportunity to develop awareness of Jon's experience of distress and how this affects the way he lives.

❑ Allows the nurse to provide simple, practical support to enable Jon to become comfortable within the ward surroundings.

❑ Is quietly, but authoritatively, supportive, mixing informal friendly support with practical expertise.

❑ Looks beyond diagnostic labels, developing a keen interest in Jon's view of what is happening for him.

❑ Is keenly attentive, listening to Jon, allowing him time to identify with his experience and feelings, while remaining watchful.

❑ Recognizes that helping relationships are developed over time in small steps. The developing sense of 'togetherness' helps to create the conditions in which Jon might begin to feel safe and emotionally supported.

❑ Avoids making assumptions, about Jon's experience. Rather, demonstrates interest and respect by carefully checking Jon's interpretation of his experience.

The nurse conducting the interview will have obtained a large amount of information about Jon, his experience of distress and his view of his current situation. This will be communicated to other nurses and the wider multiprofessional team. Shared awareness of Jon and his situation helps the team to plan purposeful and constructive care for the next few days.

CHANGING PRESENTATION OF THE PERSON IN CRISIS

Although the nurses will have worked carefully with Jon collecting further information regarding his situation and condition, they need to recognize that this assessment represents a snap-shot of Jon's experience and is subject to continual change. Jon's changing needs are illustrated as his story of distress continues to unfold.

> During the night Jon again experiences some scary voices, which he said were telling him that his life is worthless. He briefly talks to the nursing staff on duty about this but is not willing to talk at length. The following day Jon is observed packing his belongings and says that he is leaving. He seems distracted and single-minded.

Working with the person in acute distress involves responding constructively and purposefully to meet the person's needs. Such help is best constructed when the nurse accepts the person where they are emotionally seeking to expand their knowledge of the person's unique experience of distress.

The primary focus of nursing involves attempting to understand the experience of the person in crisis as opposed to attempting to *explain* it.[12] This is an important distinction. Here, the nurse who seeks to explain Jon's experience is likely to focus on Jon's recent voice hearing and view this in a restricted way, regarding this as a feature of his illness, which might best be managed through increased observation and perhaps medication. This limits Jon's involvement in the potential solution and restricts his ability to learn through his experience of distress. It also re-enforces the view that Jon is *ill* and therefore in need of medical attention.

The nurse who seeks to understand Jon and his experience, and views this as the primary (although not exclusive) focus of nursing, will avoid applying diagnostic criteria to Jon's experience of distress, but instead will focus attention on:

❑ Recognizing Jon's increasing distress as a human response to crisis.

❑ Providing Jon with a safe space to articulate his experience.

❑ Accepting his experience of distress, without judging him.

❑ Seeking further clarification about what is happening now.

❑ Allowing Jon to talk through his distress, exploring what is happening for him.

❑ Exploring all of the options available, discussing the likely consequences of proposed actions.

❑ Identifying Jon's strengths that might help him manage this crisis.

In seeking to understand the person's experience, the crisis, and the situation, nursing employs a shift in emphasis away from the medicalization of the life problems. This involves caring *with* the person, within which the experience of distress is openly shared and available strengths and opportunities are explored and utilized. There may be a need for medical treatment within this situation, but equally there may not. To gauge this need with compassion and understanding of Jon's human needs, nurses must retain their caring focus, viewing nursing as unique and valued in its own right. By seeking to understand Jon's human experience, the nurse creates the opportunity for Jon to discuss his distress. This involves the person in identifying with a range of opportunities that exist within the crisis and seeks to support the person through the process. The range of opportunities available to the person in crisis is expanded rather than restricted and wherever possible the nurse maximizes opportunities for the person to make their own choices. More especially the person in crisis begins to acknowledge that the solution to the crisis and the problems of living rests within him/herself. Thus, caring retains an empowering and optimistic focus and the person in crisis is supported throughout the experience of distress. The nurse shares the journey toward recovery with the person in crisis.

Key points

- ❏ The nurse works *with* the person in crisis, empathically and pragmatically. The nurse avoids over-reacting to the crisis situation, seeking instead to develop her understanding of the person and their situation through constructive dialogue.
- ❏ The nurse approaches crisis situations with openness and curiosity.
- ❏ The nurse does not jump to early conclusions, keeps calm allowing the person to articulate their distress.
- ❏ Where possible, the nurse promotes choice.
- ❏ The nurse gently points out possible limitations within the person's own thinking.
- ❏ The nurse seeks to de-escalate the situation while minimizing whenever possible the need for the use of control.

REFERENCES

1. Sainsbury Centre for Mental Health. *Acute problems: A survey of the quality of care in acute psychiatric wards*. London: Sainsbury Centre for Mental Health, 1998.
2. Muijen M. Acute hospital care: ineffective, inefficient and poorly organised. *Psychiatric Bulletin* 1999; **23**: 257–9.
3. Barker S. *Environmentally unfriendly: patients' views of conditions on psychiatric wards*. London: Mind, 2000.
4. Lewis SE. A search for meaning: making sense of depression. *Journal of Mental Health* 1995; **4**: 369–82.
5. Deegan P. Recovery as a journey of the heart. *Psychiatric Rehabilitation Journal* 1996; **19**: 91–7.
6. Read J. What do we want from mental health services? In: Read J, Reynolds J (eds). *Speaking our minds*. Milton Keynes: Open University Press, 1996.
7. Faulkner A. Evidence of what? *Mental Health Nursing* 2000; **20**(6): 3.
8. Repper J. Adjusting the focus of mental health nursing; incorporating service users' experiences of recovery. *Journal of Mental Health* 2000; **9**(6): 575–87.
9. Faulkner M. Empowerment and disempowerment; models of staff/patient interaction. *Nursing Times Research* 2001; **6**(6): 936–48.
10. Peplau H. *Interpersonal relationships in nursing*. New York: Putnam, 1952.
11. Anthony WA. Recovery from mental illness: the guiding vision of the mental health service system in the 1990s. *Psycho-social Rehabilitation Journal* 1993; **12**: 55–81.
12. Barker PJ. *Assessment in psychiatric and mental health nursing*. Cheltenham: Stanley Thornes, 1997.
13. Altschul AT. *Patient–nurse interaction*. Edinburgh: Churchill Livingstone, 1972.
14. Jackson S, Stevenson C. What do people need psychiatric and mental health nurses for? *Journal of Advanced Nursing* 2000; **31**(2): 378–88.
15. Barker P. The Tidal Model: developing an empowering, person-centred approach to recovery within psychiatric and mental health nursing. *Journal of Psychiatric and Mental Health Nursing* 2001; **8**(3): 233–40.

Chapter 52

ASSESSING RISK OF SUICIDE AND SELF-HARM

John R Cutcliffe*

INTRODUCTION

Some people with mental health problems may be at risk of committing suicide or otherwise harming themselves seriously. Consequently, the assessment of such possibilities is a vital part of nursing practice. Although nurses are encouraged to think about how they might *prevent* the occurrence of suicide and self-harm, the possibility of prevention lies in the usefulness of assessment and the careful use of the results of such an assessment.

Assessing risk is a complex and imperfect science. This chapter outlines some ways of approaching the development of a standardized approach to the nursing assessment of suicide and self-harm.

Definitions

Distinctions between forms of *self-harm* (sometimes called parasuicide) and *suicide* are problematic, not least because of the practical difficulties in determining the person's intent.[1] Consequently, a precise definition, which differentiates between self-harm/parasuicide and

suicide is difficult. However, suicide has been defined in Webster's Thesaurus as:

> the act or instance of taking one's own life voluntarily and intentionally.

Whereas self-harm/parasuicide has been defined as:

> any non-fatal act in which an individual deliberately causes self-injury or ingests a substance in excess of any prescribed or generally recognized therapeutic dose.[2]

It has been argued[1] that this definition is too non-specific. Perhaps this next definition is more concise.[3]

> Self-harm is commonly defined as an individual's intentional damage to a part of his or her body, without a conscious intent to die, although the result might be fatal.

Historically, many definitions of suicide, parasuicide and self-harm, overlap and even conflict. However, parasuicide and self-harm are distinguished from suicidal intent or ideation. Indeed, it has been pointed out[3] that the confusion surrounding these terms is heightened by

*John Cutcliffe is chair of Nursing at the University of Northern British Columbia, Canada. He has been involved in Mental Health nursing since 1987. His clinical work has concentrated on the areas of 'challenging behaviour' and 'humanistic therapy'. His substantive areas of research/teaching are hope/hopeless, care of the suicidal person and clinical supervision. He has over 100 publications in peer reviewed and professional journals, eight book chapters and five books.

the inclusion of 'suicide' in the word parasuicide. Since suicide implies a death wish, this is misleading. Here *self-harm* will be used.

There appears to be a significant difference between the act of suicide and the act of self-harm, and not only a difference in the outcome. Furthermore, while self-harm questions have been included in some suicide risk assessments,[4] this can be misleading, not only for the person but also for the interpretation of the results. Therefore, I acknowledge the differences between self-harm and suicide and address them separately. Also, I need to add a caveat. In differentiating between suicide and self-harm, I am not suggesting that the issues are not linked, and that anyone who self-harms is, by the nature of the differences, not at risk of suicide. As pointed out,[3] some people who self-harm do go on to take their own life. However, there is evidence that shows that over 95% of people who self-harm do not go on to take their own lives.[3,5]

ASSESSING RISK OF SELF-HARM

Several variables appear to be linked to increased risk of self-harm.[6] These include:

❏ being single or divorced;
❏ being unemployed;
❏ having a recent change in living situation;
❏ having a mental disorder;
❏ having a previous self-harm incident.

While acknowledging the limitations of this study,[6] the most important risk factors identified were: younger age and being female. In a related study,[7] the risk factors identified were:

❏ high incidence of psychiatric illness (affective disorders in particular);
❏ psychiatric co-morbidity;
❏ family distress; history of sexual and/or physical abuse.

These studies help us to assess the presence of 'conventional risk factors'. However, there is a growing recognition that such assessments may have significant limitations. As highlighted above, one conventional risk factor is that of young women having higher rates of self-harming than young men. Nevertheless, rates of self-harm in populations are not static; patterns of self-harming behaviour change. For example, a contemporary study of attendance for self-harm injuries at a West Midlands hospital[1] indicated that the rates are rising in young men far quicker than in young women. Similar findings are reported in additional, related studies.[8,9] These findings led the authors to state that:

if the rate continues to rise faster in men, the traditional excess of self-harm presentations in women will be eroded.[1]

Thus, risk assessment tools based solely on these conventional risk factors could be misleading and potentially, inaccurate.

Other studies have considered additional risk factors. A study that explored the specificity of risk assessment for self-harm found that the most potent short term predictor of self-harm repetition was a high score on the Beck Hopelessness scale, whereas in the longer term the number of previous self-harm incidents was the major predictor.[10] Another study[11] concluded that patient characteristics alone are an insufficient explanation of the risk of self-harm and that alternative considerations are available. Anderson[12] agreed, offering a case for consideration of the internal and external factors and their interactions in the person's life, in that they allow shape and depth to be added to the assessment.

Self-injurious acts have a symbolic meaning. The form of self-harm should not be regarded as a random act. As a general rule, self-injurious behaviour, particularly in people who have been given the diagnostic label of 'multiple personality disorder' or 'borderline personality disorder' is *communication*-orientated rather than death-orientated.[3] Although it would be unwise to adopt a '*cavalier*' attitude towards suicide attempts, typically such clients have offered a range of reasons for self-harming behaviour. Thus, risk assessment for self-harm should consider the following dynamics:

❏ self-harming as a means to release intrapersonal tension;
❏ self-harming as an expression of 'letting the badness flow out';
❏ self-harming to assuage a sense of guilt;
❏ self-harming to harm the rejecting object (e.g. the abuser) by harming what is dear to them, i.e. the self-harmer;
❏ self-harming as a way to interrupt the person's feelings of 'internal deadness';
❏ self-harming as a metaphor for 'blood letting'.

Each of these dynamics is thus associated with a history of previous incidents of self-harming. Indeed, previous incidents of self-harm are perhaps the clearest indicator of current risk of self-harm.[10,11,14] A history of childhood sexual abuse appears to be the clearest indicator of increased risk of self-harm, particularly if the duration of the abuse is long, if the perpetrator is known to the victim and if force/penetration are used.[3] However, although these high-risk indicators are important, checking for their presence should form only one part of a more thorough assessment. Given the overlap and parallels with suicide, we should now consider the assessment of suicide.

ASSESSING SUICIDE RISK

Since suicide is a multi-faceted, complex phenomenon, it clearly needs a pluralistic, multi-dimensional and multi-professional response.[15] This complexity and multifactorial nature is mirrored in the assessment of suicide risk, where precise assessment of the extent of risk is extremely difficult to achieve. This is particularly the case when practitioners use simplistic and 'isolated' assessment tools in the hope that these provide enough accurate information to gauge suicidal risk. According to Morgan,[16] traditionally, at least in clinical psychiatry, this simplistic and 'isolated' approach was concerned with matching the 'patient' with a set of risk factors, each of which had a statistically positive correlation with increased suicide risk. Considering the complexity of the dynamics and social processes of suicide, and the often highly individual nature of each person involved, it is unsurprising that, in isolation, this approach had many limitations. While such tools can be accurate over the long term, they can be very unspecific and insensitive over the short term;[16] creating a large number of false-positives (people regarded to be at high risk of suicide when they are not), and false-negatives (people regarded to be at low risk of suicide when they are actually at high risk).

As a 'golden rule', the fundamental basis of risk assessment must be a full and thorough clinical evaluation of each individual.[16] While I support this position, I would add the following reservations:

1   Full and thorough clinical evaluations require a degree of 'clinical judgement'. If they are to develop this clinical acumen, inexperienced members of staff need time and 'first hand' experience of clients deemed to be a high risk of suicide.

2   The current emphasis on 'evidence based practice' would suggest that full and thorough clinical evaluations are best served when they are underpinned with evidence.

Although Morgan recognized the limitations of risk assessment tools[16] he acknowledged that they could provide useful checklists, helping guard against complacency and over confidence. In keeping with Morgan's argument, and considering the two-stage caveat above, the rest of this chapter focuses on the Nurses' Global Assessment of Suicide Risk.

THE NURSES' GLOBAL ASSESSMENT OF SUICIDE RISK (NGASR)[a]

Several studies have shown[17,18] that within practice, the detection of suicide risk, in a population of psychiatric inpatients, poses many problems. However, mental health care staff recognized the need for a system that would not inhibit the development of the staff's judgement while simultaneously supporting their assessment of suicide risk with an evidence-based tool. Importantly, given their clinical judgement, based on years of experience,[19] the tool was intended to augment rather than replace the experienced clinician's judgement. As Motto et al.[20] pointed out:

> A scale can only be a supplement to clinical judgement and should not, on its own, override contradicting information.

On its own, risk assessment does not necessarily constitute evidence-based practice. However, as noted specific variables are associated with increased risk of suicide.[21,22] However, current research suggests that it is unlikely that there is one specific predictor which indicates high suicide risk.[15-17] Nevertheless, a risk assessment tool that enabled clinicians to assess for the presence and influence of these predictor variables, would mean that, at least, part of the clinician's assessment becomes evidence based. Crucially, this has the additional influence of raising the nurses' awareness of the problem of suicide and factors associated with risk, helping them become more vigilant.

A crucial problem in developing a suicide risk assessment tool is that high-risk issues for one individual cannot be generalized for a larger population. Similarly, high-risk factors for large populations do not necessarily translate and apply to the individual.[20] However, even an imperfect instrument can serve a useful purpose, especially for those who are less confident or experienced: especially if the instrument could then be rated (and validated) in practice.

The NGASR involves a simple scale with 15 items. The tool was designed so that all the information necessary to score each of the predictor variables could be able to be extracted during the admission interview. By highlighting the predictor variables that may be pertinent to the client, and summarizing the respective scores, a total score is possible. This score correlates with an (estimated) indication of the level of potential suicide risk. Additionally, subsequent risk assessment ratings, aided by the use of the tool, mean that all the formal and informal collection of data to (e.g. observations of the client's mood and behaviour, records of interactions with nurses, other clients and additional health care staff) may be 'summarized' and repeated on a regular basis, providing an indication of changes in apparent suicide risk.

The NGASR was based on a review of the relevant empirical literature, which indicated that the presence

[a] For a more comprehensive explanation of the background and development of the risk assessment tool see Cutcliffe JR, Bassett C. Introducing change in nursing: the case of research. *The Journal of Nursing Management* 1997; **5**: 241–7.

(and influence) of some variables appeared to suggest a higher degree of risk than others. Thus, not all indicators of suicidal risk, were given the same 'weighting' or score. The most potent indicators in the NGASR – those with a higher statistical correlation with suicide – are weighted with a score of three, the remainder being allocated a score of one.[17,20,21,23–26]

An additional difficulty in designing risk assessment tools involves determining the demarcations between degrees of risk. As noted already, suicide is complex and models that suggest that one is either 'at risk' or 'not at risk' are simplistic. After reviewing case notes, and talking to the families of 'completed' suicides, I identified four discrete levels of suicidal risk. Two distinct categories of risk exist – namely: extremely high risk and very low risk. Extremely high risk refers to that state of being that might be likened to a state of 'psychiatric emergency'. The person is extremely vulnerable; requires the highest degree of engagement and input from the mental health nurse and would present with a number of high-risk factors (variables) and maybe some other risk factors too. Since it would not be prudent for mental health nurses to claim that a client presents with no risk of suicide, the author described the category that represents the least risk as, low risk of suicide. These individuals would thus score low and present with few (if any) of the risk factors. A further two categories were

TABLE 52.1 The Nurses' Global Assessment of Suicide Risk

Predictor variable	Value
Presence/influence of hopelessness	3
Recent stressful life-event	1
e.g. job loss, financial worries, pending court action	
Evidence of persecutory voices/beliefs	1
Evidence of depression/loss of interest or loss of pleasure	3
Evidence of withdrawal	1
Warning of suicidal intent	1
Evidence of a plan to commit suicide	3
Family history of serious psychiatric problems or suicide	1
Recent bereavement or relationship breakdown	3
History of psychosis	1
Widow/widower	1
Prior suicide attempt	3
History of socioeconomic deprivation	1
History of alcohol and/or alcohol misuse	1
Presence of terminal illness	1
Total =	25

added; intermediate and high risk. Again, given the complexity of suicide and the multiple factors that can be involved in predicting risk, a single third category was felt to be rather simplistic and didn't allow enough for the interplay of risk factors and the cumulative degree of risk that multiple factors combined indicated.

RATIONALE FOR THE 15 KEY INDICATORS[b]

1 There is considerable evidence that feelings of hopelessness are highly correlated with suicide risk.[21,22,25] Recent studies suggest that hopelessness, often associated with a depressive state, is a greater indicator of risk than the depressive state itself. Furthermore, hopelessness is not unique to depressive states; people with recurrent forms of mental and/or physical distress, personal or social problems can develop a sense of pervasive hopelessness. Various scales estimate a person's level of hope. Thus, if the nurse wishes to assess this area in more detail, to verify his/her initial assessment, he/she might draw upon one of these tools.

2 Holmes and Rahe[27] produced a list of life-events, which appeared to 'carry' a certain degree of associated stress. In certain circumstances, and particularly if there are cumulative stressful life-events, these can lead the person to think about suicide as a 'way out'. Details of these events can be determined during the admission interview and/or from any existing professional reports, e.g. social work reports.

3 Although not associated exclusively with mental illness,[28] the experience of hearing voices or 'delusional' beliefs can be disturbing. When such 'voices' take on a persecutory tone or content, this can contribute to the person's sense of hopelessness. Furthermore, some voices/beliefs may contain more explicit messages of self-harm or destruction. Although suicidal acts as a result of such 'messages' is not overly common[15] they can nevertheless encourage a person towards suicide.

4 A relationship exists between depression and suicide.[29] When depression is manifest in the form of loss of interest or pleasure, then this can be regarded as further indication of potential suicidal risk.[21] This does not apply only in people with a formal diagnosis of depression, but may also be evident in people with other severe forms of mental or physical distress.

---

[b] Due to space and word limitations, references for each of these risk factors have been restricted. For a more comprehensive explanation of the supporting literature see Cutcliffe JR, Barker P. Developing an instrument to help mental health nurses assess the risk of suicide: the Nurses' Global Assessment of Suicide Risk (NGASR). *Journal of Psychiatric and Mental Health Nursing* (in press).

5 Some studies into predictive risk factors in suicide have indicated that a withdrawal from interpersonal and social interactions is associated with increased risk.[30] Such withdrawal can be one of the first warning signs that the person is experiencing difficulty in maintaining the pattern of everyday living. That is not to suggest that anyone who spends time alone should automatically be considered to be at risk of suicide. It is more a matter of changes in patterns of interpersonal and social interaction; a change in the balance of time spent alone against time spent with others.

6 Although the expression of suicidal intent is not always conclusive evidence of genuine intent,[16] such warnings should not be ignored, and may be genuine indications of increased thoughts about suicide. Some studies have indicated that some 'cries for help' have passed by unnoticed.[18] Yet, such warnings can also be evidence of clients 'reaching out' for help.

7 Any evidence of a specific plan to commit suicide represents a major risk factor, especially if the person attempted to keep the plan secret.[20] Such plans may be uncovered by accidental discovery of physical evidence, or perhaps by way of something(s) that the person says which either allude to such a plan, or reveal part of it.

8 A further predictor that needs to be considered is that of a family history of serious psychiatric problems or suicide.[26] Such a history can compound the person's sense of hopelessness and inevitability. When significant family members have committed suicide, this can, inadvertently, serve as a model for the person's hopelessness.

9 A recent bereavement or relationship breakdown should be considered as another significant risk factor.[20,21,26] Loss and bereavement affect the person in many different ways, yet one frequently reported commonality of unresolved bereavements appears to be loss of hope.[31] Consequently, the person may be left feeling like ending his/her life in response to the loss and these feelings can be compounded by the concomitant loss of hope. This may particularly be the case when the bereaved was the person's primary source of human, interpersonal support.

10 Where the person has a history of psychosis, then the risk of suicide appears to be slightly increased.[26,29] Although it is accepted as an axiom that not all people who suffer from and live with a psychosis also experience suicidal thoughts, the person's process of reasoning can be impaired/altered.

11 Previous empirical studies have shown that when the person is a widow/widower, then the risk is slightly increased.[20] This is particularly the case if the person has not reached any 'resolution' to their bereavement or has not 'adapted' to their loss. It is important to remember that in contemporary society, this predictive variable also includes the loss of 'common law' spouse and the loss of a same-sex life partner.

12 Any indication or evidence of a prior suicide attempt is a significant indicator of current/future suicidal risk.[32]

13 Suicide is a multifactorial event that does not happen in isolation from the world in which the person lives in. Thus, it can be precipitated by both internal phenomenon and external events, in addition to external circumstances. For example, a history of socioeconomic deprivation (e.g. poor housing, unemployment, low quality of life) appears to be associated with increased risk of suicide.[32]

14 Further studies have supported the findings of Barraclough et al.[29] and continue to suggest that a history of alcohol and/or substance misuse is associated with a higher risk of suicide.[15] This may particularly be the case when the concept of 'spontaneous act' suicides and people using alcohol/drugs in order to gain the courage to go through with the suicidal act, is taken into account.

15 Finally, some people who are suffering from a terminal illness consider suicide.[15] Either as a means of dealing with physical pain, or as a means of taking an element of control/dignity, or as a way of dealing with the prospect of further holistic deterioration and loss (euthanasia).

DEVELOPING AN EVIDENCE BASE FOR SUICIDE RISK ASSESSMENT

Formal assessment tools for estimating suicide risk constitute only a part of the assessment process. Nevertheless, they are a useful part of the 'bigger picture' and perhaps have particular value for less experienced staff. In addition to formal risk assessment tools, a full clinical assessment may include some (or all) of the following.

❑ The clinical judgement of all practitioners involved. Particular value may be attached to the judgement of a practitioner who has established a strong relationship with the client; or someone who has spent long periods of time in the company of the client.

❑ Ongoing assessments evaluations (whether based on a risk assessment tool or not) that piece together to

TABLE 52.2 NGASR and corresponding levels of risk and suggested engagement

Score of 5 or less = low level of risk estimated.
Suggested level of engagement:
Level four

Score between 6 and 8 = intermediate level of risk.
Suggested level of engagement:
Level three

Score between 9 and 11 = high level of risk.
Suggested level of engagement:
Level two

Score 12 or more = very high level of risk.
Suggested level of engagement:
Level one

form a cumulative 'picture' of the person's potential risk.

❑ Data/information gained during the initial admission interview and subsequent interviews with the client, family and/or significant others.

Having identified that formal interviews (admission interviews and subsequent assessment interviews) can also play a key part in more accurate assessments of a person's risk of suicide, it is necessary to consider some of the questions that might be asked in such interviews. Each interview needs to be conducted with extreme sensitivity and empathy, and should conclude with an emphatic declaration of support, care and concern for the individual. Also, each interview is likely to be unique, since it will involve the unique situation, personality and presenting needs of the particular client. Therefore, the questions included in box two should be regarded as guidelines and not 'check lists' of questions that the nurse follows unthinkingly.

CONCLUSION

It is important to be realistic and to recognize the limitations of self-harm and suicide prevention.[15] According to Alvarez,[34] suicide has existed throughout history and the complete eradication of suicide is highly unlikely. Nevertheless, there remains a great deal that mental health nurses can do to minimize the risk of self-harm and suicide. Inextricably linked to minimizing this risk is accurate assessment of self-harm or suicidal risk. While acknowledging that risk assessment tools are only one aspect of a more thorough assessment of risk, the NGASR provides nurses with a standardized instrument, which might assist them with this challenging process, and may be of particular worth to less experienced (and student) nurses.

TABLE 52.3 Suggested questions for suicidal risk assessment interview

When you think about your current situation and difficulty, do you think that it can improve, that things can turn out well?

How much pleasure do you gain from your life; from those activities and relationships that used to give you pleasure?

How hopeful do you feel, do you feel that you still have hope on a day-to-day basis?

At the start of the day, how do you feel about the day to come and how you will be able to cope?

Does your current situation make you question the point or purpose of it all; of your situation or even your life/existence?

Would you describe yourself as feeling desperate or experiencing a sense of despair?

How does the thought of having to face another day make you feel?

Have you ever felt or believed that you are a burden, and if so, could you say in what way; a burden to whom?

Have you ever thought about or wished that it would all end?

Have you ever thought that death would be a relief; that death would present a way out; or wished that you were dead?

Have you ever thought of ending your life? How often do you have these thoughts? How compelling are they?

Have these thoughts ever led you to attempt to take your own life?

If you experience such thoughts, how able are you to resist them? What do you do to resist them? How can we help you when you experience such thoughts?

How serious do you think you are about wishing to harm yourself, and if you were in my position, would you be concerned about your safety?

Are you able to give me any reassurance about your safety or do you feel the need for extra interpersonal support and security right now?

What, if anything, could make you feel more at risk of harming yourself?

How easy for you is it to ask for help, particularly when you are feeling particularly vulnerable of harming yourself?

What do you need right now?

How can I help you right now?

What degree of interpersonal support and security do you feel you need right now?

Adapted from refs 16 and 34.

REFERENCES

1. Kinmond KS, Bent M. Attendance for self-harm in a west midlands A&E department. *British Journal of Nursing* 2000; **9**: 215–20.
2. Krietman N. *Parasuicide*. Chichester: Wiley, 1977.

3. Santa Mina EE, Gallop R. Childhood sexual and physical abuse and adult self-harm and suicidal behaviour: a literature review. *Canadian Journal of Psychiatry* 1998; **43**(8): 793–800.

4. Stuart G. Self-protective responses and suicidal behaviour. In: Stuart G, Laraia MT (eds). *Principles and practices of psychiatric nursing*, 7th edn. New York: Mosby, 2001: 381–400.

5. Anderson R. Assessing the risk of self-harm in adolescents: a psychoanalytic perspective. *Psychoanalytic Psychotherapy* 2000; **14**(1): 9–21.

6. Welch SS. A review of the literature on the epidemiology of parasuicide in the general population. *Psychiatric Services* 2001; **52**(3): 368–75.

7. Read GFH. Trends in adolescent and young adult parasuicide population presenting at a psychiatric emergency unit: a descriptive study. *International Journal of Adolescent Medicine and Health* 1997; **9**(4): 249–69.

8. Hawton K. Attempted suicide. In: Clarke DM, Fairburn CG (eds). *Science and practice of cognitive-behavioural therapy*. Oxford: Oxford University Press, 1997: 285–312.

9. McLoone P, Crombie IK. Hospitalisation for deliberate self-poisoning in Scotland from 1981–1993: trends in rates and types of drugs used. *British Journal of Psychiatry* 1996; **169**: 816.

10. Sidley GL, Calam R, Wells A, *et al*. The prediction of parasuicide repetition in a high-risk group. *British Journal of Clinical Psychology* 1999; **38**(4): 375–86.

11. Burrow S. The deliberate self-harming behaviour of patients within a British special hospital. *Journal of Advanced Nursing* 1992; **17**: 138–48.

12. Anderson M. Waiting for harm: deliberate self-harm and suicide in young people – a review of the literature. *Journal of Psychiatric and Mental Health Nursing* 1999; **6**: 91–100.

13. Marmer SS, Fink D. Rethinking the comparison of borderline personality disorder and multiple personality disorder. *Psychiatric Clinics of North America* 1994; **17**: 743–71.

14. Kreitman N, Casey P. Repetition of parasuicide: an epidemiological and clinical study. *British Journal of Psychiatry* 1988; **153**: 792–800.

15. Hawton K. Causes and opportunities for prevention. In: Jenkins R, Griffiths S, Wylie I, *et al.* (eds). *The prevention of suicide.* London: Department of Health/HMSO, 1994: 34–45.

16. Morgan G Assessment of risk. In: Jenkins R, Griffiths S, Wylie S (eds). *The Prevention of Suicide.* London: Department of Health/HMSO, 1994: 46–52.

17. Goldstein RB, Black DW, Nasrallah A, Winokur G. The prediction of suicide: sensitivity, specificity and predictive value of a multivariative model applied to suicide among 1906 patients with an affective disorder. *Archives of General Psychiatry* 1991; **48**: 418–22.

18. Morgan HG, Priest P. Suicide and other unexpected deaths among psychiatric in-patients. The Bristol confidential inquiry. *British Journal of Psychiatry* 1991; **158**: 368–74.

19. Menghella E, Benson A. developing reflective practice in mental health nursing through critical incident analysis. *Journal of Advanced Nursing* 1995; **21**: 205–13.

20. Motto JA, Heilbron DC, Juster RP. Development of a clinical instrument to estimate suicide risk. *American Journal of Psychiatry* 1985; **142**: 680–86.

21. Fawcett J, Scheftner W, Clark D, Hedeker D, Gibbons R, Coryell W. Clinical predictors of suicide in patients with major affective disorders: a controlled prospective study. *American Journal of Psychiatry* 1987; **144**: 35–40.

22. Weisharr ME, Beck AT. Hopelessness and suicide. *International Review of Psychiatry* 1992; **4**: 177–84.

23. Beck AT, Weissman M, Lester D, Trexler L. The measurement of pessimism: the hopelessness scale. *Journal of Consulting and Clinical Psychology* 1974; **42**: 861–5.

24. Pokorny AD. Prediction of suicide in psychiatric patients: report of a prospective study. *Archives of General Psychiatry* 1983; **40**: 249–57.

25. Young MA, Fogg LF, Schefter WA, Fawcett JA. Interactions of risk factors in predicting suicide. *American Journal of Psychiatry* 1994; **151**: 434–5.

26. Powell J, Geddes J, Hawton K. Suicide in psychiatric hospital in-patients. *The British Journal of Psychiatry* 2000; **176**(3): 266–72.

27. Holmes TH, Rahe RH. The social readjustment rating scale. *Journal of Psychosomatic Research* 1968; **11**: 213–18.

28. Romme M, Hoing A, Noorthoorn E, Escher A. Coping with hearing voices: an emancipatory approach. *British Journal of Psychiatry* 1992; **161**: 99–103.

29. Barraclough B, Bunch J, Nelson P, Sainsbury P. A hundred cases of suicide: clinical aspects. *British Journal of Psychiatry* 1974; **125**: 355–73.

30. Charlton J, Kelly S, Dunnell K, Evans B, Jenkins R. Trends in suicide deaths in England and Wales. *Population Trends* 1992; **69**: 6–10.

31. Cutcliffe JR. Hope, counselling and complicated bereavement reactions. *Journal of Advanced Nursing* 1998; **28**(4): 754–61.

32. Gunnell D, Frankel S. Prevention of suicide: aspirations and evidence. *British Medical Journal* 1994; **308**: 1227–33.

33. Barker P. *Developing the security plan: guidance notes.* Newcastle: Newcastle City Health Trust, 1999.

34. Alvarez A. *The savage God: a study of suicide.* New York: WW Norton, 1974.

Chapter 53

ENGAGEMENT AND OBSERVATION OF PEOPLE AT RISK

John Cutcliffe*

Suicide is a form of behaviour as old as man himself but the phenomenon has been described in differing ways according to the attitudes prevalent within society at various times in history.[1]

THE POLICY CONTEXT

While suicide cannot be considered to be a recent phenomenon,[1,2] attention to the problem has increased during recent years. In the UK, over a decade ago, the 'Health of the Nation'[3] identified suicide as a major cause of death among specific groups. One group identified was those people who suffer from mental illness, and one of the health care targets highlighted was to reduce the number of people with mental illness who commit suicide by 33%.

More recently, 'Modernizing Mental Health Services: safe, sound and supportive'[4] observed that suicide was the second most common cause of death in those aged under 35 years. Although it was acknowledged that the rate has begun to decline, there are still over 4000 deaths annually in England, with people with severe mental illness representing one of the highest at-risk subgroups.

Latterly, in the long awaited 'National Service Framework for Mental Health',[5] it was proposed that local health and social care communities should prevent suicides, but suggested only (again) the need for 'safe hospital accommodation' and 'ensuring that staff are competent to assess the risk of suicide'. Thus, it can be seen that the problem of suicide has received greater attention and, for the mental health nurse, such attention may be timely.

Mental health nurses (MHNs) working in inpatient settings have 24-hour responsibility for caring for people at risk of suicide.[6] Thus MHNs have, potentially, a major input into the everyday lives of suicidal inpatients. Furthermore, they can draw upon a well-established literature, which has highlighted the link between suicide and a number of factorsa. However, within this literature, one finding is consistent, and that is the need for pluralistic, interactive theoretical models of suicide, and suicide response, especially within mental health nursing practice.[7] Despite the MHNs vital responsibility for safeguarding people at risk of harm, and the potential to offer therapeutic intervention, exactly how they should go about providing this care is not well understood. Furthermore, although the phenomenon of suicide is well documented, relatively little attention has been paid to examining the explicit nursing role, or how the clients perceive the care provided, and its relative merits and limitations. Nevertheless, the MHN should be familiar with this literature, such as it is, when considering the care of the suicidal client. Therefore, it is

*John Cutcliffe is chair of Nursing at the University of Northern British Columbia, Canada. He has been involved in Mental Health nursing since 1987. His clinical work has concentrated on the areas of 'challenging behaviour' and 'humanistic therapy'. His substantive areas of research/teaching are hope/hopeless, care of the suicidal person and clinical supervision. He has over 100 publications in peer reviewed and professional journals, eight book chapters and five books.

appropriate to consider to the two most common approaches to providing care for suicidal clients.

OBSERVATION AND ENGAGEMENT

Despite the recognition that suicide is a complex, multi-faceted phenomenon, requiring sophisticated and integrated approaches to care, many texts appear to emphasize the need to 'treat' the underlying affective mood disorder.[8] A similar emphasis is espoused by Rawlins[9] who suggested that a suicidal client needs to be:

> given anti-depressant medication to elevate his mood and make him more amenable to treatment. Electroconvulsive treatment (ECT) is an additional treatment that has proved effective.

Similarly, authors such as Pritchard[8] offer some generic suggestions for the care of the suicidal client (e.g. input from a variety of clinicians, improved socioeconomic conditions, social skills training). These broad, and perhaps long-term interventions (lithium therapy, anti-depressant therapy and ECT) have been shown to be effective in the management of depression. However, crucially, Gunnell and Frankel[10] point out that several retrospective reviews of the treatments received by psychiatric patients provided no consistent evidence that these therapies reduce the likelihood of suicide. Furthermore, ignoring their questionable efficacy with respect to 'treating' the suicidal client, it is fair to say that they do not appear to say much about the more acute problems facing nurses when they attempt to engage with suicidal clients.

Some texts appear to advocate an even more '*masculine*' approach to caring for suicidal clients, when they suggest further 'interventions' include removing harmful items (such as belts, socks!) and placing the client on 24 hours a day observations on a one-to-one basis.[9] Rawlins[9] is by no means the only author to suggest 'close' or 'special' or 'one-to-one' observations as the primary intervention for care of the suicidal client. As a result, for people who are deemed to be 'at risk' of suicide, 'observation' has increasingly become the prime focus of care. Furthermore, these levels of observation are most often 'set' by psychiatrists perhaps with little regard to the demands this might make on nursing staff, emotionally and logistically. In his insightful study of special observations of suicidal psychiatric inpatients, Duffy[11] reported similar findings. Duffy noted that, in each case studied, special observation was formally prescribed by a doctor, usually a junior. Perhaps more importantly, despite the fact that special observations are *prescribed*, they are invariably carried out by nurses. As a result, special observation had become, specifically,

a nursing activity. Duffy[11] also noted nurses' discomfort with being identified (by some disciplines) as custodians rather than therapeutic practitioners.

The MHN needs to be aware that 'close' or 'special observations', are currently common practices in the 'care' of the suicidal client. Any text that claims to be addressing the care of the suicidal client needs to include some examination of the practice. Furthermore, knowledge of the nuances of such practice, including its limitations, should stand the aspirant MHN in good stead. While individual units, wards and/or NHS Trusts may well have their own policy on 'close or special observation', these share key commonalities. One such example is provided in Table 53.1.

Observation: safe and effective?

Despite the continued emphasis on 'observation' as the *modus operandi* for the care of the suicidal person, it is increasingly being called into question and as a result alternative models of care are being considered. Although nurses' use of observation and 'specialling' has been in evidence for almost 25 years, the therapeutic value of such approaches to care have long been questioned. The practice of observation was developed as a means to inform medical staff of the status of the patient. It served the function of assuring the 'absent' doctor of the physical safety of the patient. Yet as statistics for suicide in inpatient settings (and my own research experience of attending over 90 suicide or open verdict inquests) illustrate, observation as a caring practice is a woefully weak intervention. For up to one third of the suicides committed while inpatients, many of these were 'under' levels of observation. Where observation policies exist, there is a great deal of inconsistency in the interpretation of the policies and yet further problems with actioning or carrying out these observations. The Standing Nursing and Midwifery[12] report, and work arising from it, may well address some of these problems. However, additional problems remain.

Service users' experiences of close observation is critical to any consideration of its utility. In the UK, evidence from Newcastle[13] and York[14] indicates that while being 'under observation', users felt neither safe nor supported. One user summed up the experience succinctly when he stated:

> some do closes (observation) nicely. They talk to the patient like a friend and still carry on with their other duties. But others are like robots. When the patient moves they follow like zombies.

Alternatively, a service user in Fletcher's[14] study noted:

> They didn't actually ask me if I was feeling suicidal. Just went everywhere with me and a member of staff stated:

'I would be happy to say to somebody, "Don't try anything because I am going to be with you all the time and I don't want that responsibility on me"'.

More recent evidence from Oxford[15] and Bradford[16] further supports this position. Jones *et al.*[15] found that most of the research subjects in their study did not like the experience of being observed, found it intrusive and that some nurses didn't talk to the users at all during the observation period. This was found to be a particularly negative experience. Similarly, in Dodds and Bowles[16] attempt to dismantle observation and move towards a more 'care' orientated system, the following findings were established:

❑ incidents of deliberate self-harm reduced by two thirds;

❑ violence and aggression reduced by over a third;
❑ staff sickness fell by two thirds;
❑ absconding declined by half; and
❑ there was no increase of suicides during the corresponding period (18 months).

Importantly, they stated:

the effect on patient care has been striking: patients are more engaged with their named nurses, better informed and more involved with their care.

It comes as no surprise that the therapeutic value of observation is being questioned.

The operation of observation

Inextricably linked to the alleged value (or otherwise) of observations is the matter of who carries them out. Extensive shortages of RMNs across the UK has led to a reliance on Bank or agency staff. In Gournay *et al.*'s[17] study, they found that bank nurses provided between 23.6 and 36.3% of the staff compliment. Quite rightly, they condemned this as unacceptable. While such figures vary across the UK, this pattern is by no means exclusive to London.[16] Compounding this situation, in many (most) parts of the country, observation is carried out in the main by support staff, bank/agency staff and students.[18] Consequently, observation is invariably regarded as a low skill activity, often carried out by staff who, by their junior or transient nature, have only limited knowledge of the person. According to Dodds and Bowles[16] this is 'counterproductive', and contributes little in the way of assessment and treatment, or to the development of new approaches to acute inpatient care. This situation leaves nurses in reactionary, custodial roles and despite the rhetoric of 'supportive observation', the nurse is often construed as a custodian, if not a doorman.

As a means of intervention for people who are suicidal, observation is:

❑ A system designed originally to inform doctors and now, at least in part, is concerned with meeting the needs of the organization.
❑ Fails up to one third of those people it aims to protect. These numbers are even more alarming when the number of people who go on to harm themselves once the 'observation' restrictions have been lifted, are considered.
❑ A crude, 'custodial' form of intervention, given the highly complex, convoluted and sophisticated care needs of this client group.
❑ Implemented, mainly, by transient (bank/agency) staff or support staff with minimal training.

TABLE 53.1 'Close observation' policy

1. The level of observation should be determined by risk assessment, be a constituent part of the plan of care and be recorded in medical/multidisciplinary notes.
2. Observation levels are prescribed by the responsible medical officer.
3. A nurse may increase the level of observation following a risk assessment (but must inform the RMO and the multidisciplinary team as soon as possible).
4. The planned delivery of the close observations will be organized by the nurse in charge of the shift; and recorded on an observation rota. This rota will identify the member of staff delegated to undertake observations for a specific time-span.
5. All staff must be clear of their specific responsibilities and sign to confirm that they have completed the span of observation.
6. Close observations should not be carried out by the same nurse for a duration of longer than 2 hours.
7. When passing on the responsibility for close observations to another nurse, the following must be discussed; the level of observation, the nature of the risk, restrictions of patient's movement, any special consideration, any relevant information concerning the patient's mood or behaviour, and ensure that the level of observation is understood.
8. Every effort should be made to promote a therapeutic relationship with the patient; minimizing the distress caused by the process.
9. The patient should be informed of the level of observations.
10. Significant others, where confidentiality allows, should be informed of the level of observations.
11. The allocation of staff to close observations should take into account aspects of the individual's needs, e.g. gender, ethnicity.

From the Standing Nursing and Midwifery Committee.[12]

❏ Does little (if anything) to address the genesis or route of the person's problems, which led him/her to feel suicidal in the first place.

❏ Is highly stressful for the nurses who participate.

ENGAGEMENT – INSPIRING HOPE

The complexity of people at risk of suicide or self-harm is axiomatic. Such people need highly specific, and sophisticated, forms of care. There is a growing recognition that the nursing care of people who are at risk of suicide or self-harm needs to re-focus on a more manifest form of care and support, rather than upon tightening up the *policing* strategy of observation. Given the complex and sophisticated nature of the problem of suicide, it is maybe of no surprise that there is no 'singular' treatment or intervention that appears to address the problem. However, there is a growing body of evidence that indicates that there are two linked, basic interpersonal processes that appear to be key for mental health nurses in providing care for the suicidal client: *engagement* and *inspiring hope*.

Engagement comprises several processes: forming a relationship – a human/human connection, conveying acceptance and tolerance and hearing and understanding. Any other interpersonal intervention provided to help people address their suicidal feelings needs to be grounded in such a relationship. This serves as the grounding for other interventions, but also is a powerful intervention in itself. The relationship conveys the message that the nurse 'cares about' the client, and that his/her life has value. Providing nursing care for the suicidal client is more focused on ways of *being* as opposed to *doing*. The value and importance of this fundamental interpersonal process is referred to throughout the limited research into care of the suicidal client. For example, studies have indicated the following:

❏ the value of compassion and emotional identification when caring for the suicidal client, in addition to the trust that is built through regular contact between client/nurse;[19,20]

❏ the need to consider one's own attitudes towards suicide in order that the nurse can ensure they do not distance themselves from the client;[21]

❏ the importance of relating to suicidal clients;[21]

❏ the value of engaging in twice weekly counselling sessions with some suicidal clients;[22]

❏ and the value of nurses initiating contact with suicidal clients, and attending to clients' basic needs (including the value of physical contact with suicidal clients).[23]

Bound up with this process of engagement is the unconditional acceptance and tolerance of the suicidal client. Caring practice for the suicidal client is concerned with unconditional acceptance and tolerance, removing any sense of coercion of psychological pressure. The presence of these qualities, alone, in the nurse would not be enough. They also have to be conveyed or demonstrated in a 'genuine' manner. All too frequently unfortunately, clients who have attempted to take their own life, encounter disapproving attitudes.[21-22] Attitudes range from contempt – believing that the client is taking up valuable space and time that could be used for someone who has 'a real problem' – to ignorance, lacking any understanding of why anyone would wish to take their own life. Condemnation, criticism or contempt can only exacerbate the client's feelings of worthlessness and hopelessness, which led to their suicidal behaviour. Consequently, the potential therapeutic value of conveying a sense of complete acceptance and tolerance becomes clear.

Studies have shown how nurses caring for suicidal clients confirmed, rather than criticized their emotions and feelings;[20] Given that suicidal clients are highly vulnerable,[21] nurses' offer of unconditional positive regard and empathy, is valuable if not essential.[24,25] Similarly, nurses must accept suicidal clients' feelings, be open and have time for the person.[23]

The third component of engagement is concerned with listening, hearing and understanding. This may appear obvious but creating and providing the environment where the client can begin to explore, discuss and resolve his/her thoughts and feelings, is crucial in addressing the client's desire to harm himself. This hearing and understanding need not be regarded as a form of sophisticated counselling, but is more a matter of attending to the client, encouraging him/her to explore his thoughts and feelings, and providing the opportunity for the client to express painful emotions without being judged or condemned. Studies have illustrated that: nurses caring for suicidal clients emphasized listening to clients;[20] the value in hearing the clients when they are ready to talk;[23] the therapeutic value of hearing and empathizing with the suicidal client[24,25] and the value of listening without prejudice.[21]

INSPIRING HOPE

There is an abundance of evidence that identifies hopelessness as a key element in determining whether or not someone will commit suicide rather than merely considering it.[26] It is clear that suicidal people need hope, and MHNs are ideally placed to be one such source of hope. However, recognition of the importance of hope in MH nursing is a relatively recent phenomenon. Only now is it gaining recognition as being central to the therapeutic potential of the nurse–patient relationship, and to the quality of the person's life. Despite this pivotal position, the indications are that the inspiration of hope is low on the clinical agenda, and consequently it should be noted that, at this moment in time, there is no specific theory or research that informs nurses of how to inspire hope in suicidal clients. Nevertheless, there is growing evidence, which suggests that hope inspiration appears to be a subtle, unobtrusive, implicit process.[28] Hope inspiration appears to be bound up with the necessary and sufficient human qualities in the nurse and the projection of these into the environment (and client).

Although hope appears to have an important influence on some people's lives, the processes of hope inspiration needs to remain subtle and implicit rather than overt. According to Frankl,[27] one cannot be forced to hope; hope cannot be commanded or ordered. Such a view clearly resonates with inspiring hope in suicidal clients, where such clients cannot be 'forced' to feel less suicidal. Therefore, theories which suggest that the inspiration of hope appears to be bound up with the presence of certain 'human qualities', and the interpersonal (spiritual) connection between clients and MHNs appears to have resonance with Frankl's[27] views.

A significant component of hope inspiration appears to be the relationship between hope and caring. Hope is inherent in caring practices. Research into the inspiration of hope, in a variety of disparate client groups, highlights that the presence of another human being, who demonstrates unconditional acceptance, tolerance and understanding, as (s)he enters into the caring practice, simultaneously inspires hope.[28] Three of the processes involved in engaging with suicidal clients have been identified: forming a relationship, conveying acceptance and tolerance, and hearing and understanding. Each of these shares a great deal of similarity with the subtle processes of hope inspiration. Consequently, we can theorize that hope inspiration for suicidal client, may well also be bound up with demonstrating unconditional acceptance, tolerance and understanding, as the MHN engages in 'caring' practice.

Vaillot[29] made similar remarks when she described the link between caring and hope inspiration when she said:

> There is no simple, possibly no satisfactory answer to the question, how does one inspire hope in patients? Knowledge, techniques, good planning and sound assessment of nursing care are necessary and indispensable, but they are the tools one has in order to nurse.

However, the attitude of caring does go some way to answering this question. As Vaillot[29] added:

> the nurse inspires hope by what she is more than what

she does … it is a salutary effect on the patient from the fact that it is an expression of the nurse's caring.

Where people at risk of suicide are concerned, the caring relationship must be developed as a 'hope-inspiring' form of engagement. Effective nursing is predicated on effective engagement with the person. Only through engaging with the person, will the nurse come to understand the nature of the person's needs, and what might need to be offered to address them. The nurse's engagement with the suicidal person must be dedicated to understanding the nature of that hopelessness, and to developing the means to re-instill hope. The value of this hope-inspiring form of engagement is illustrated in the following case studies.

Illustrations

Each of these case studies is based on real care situations. In the interests of confidentiality, names and any personal details have been changed.

Case study 53.1: Walter

History and context

Walter was a 24-year-old man with a history of cutting and self-mutilation. He had experienced over 10 previous admissions. Walter has been diagnosed as suffering from 'multiple personality disorder', schizophrenia, a sociopathic personality disorder and demon possession! He expressed some difficulty with close inter-personal relationships and described himself as homosexual. He has had several previous 'suicide attempts', although on each occasion, he was always 'found in time'.

Overview of care

At the beginning of Walter's care episode, the nursing staff carried out an assessment of his suicide risk using the NGASR (see Chapter 52) and determined that he presented with a low risk of suicide. However, this potential risk was identified as a need, and together with Walter, a care package was negotiated. A range of interventions/practices, all of which were based on the 'Engagement: hope inspiration' approach for care of the suicidal client, were implemented:

❏ 'One-to-one' sessions with Walter and his nurse were arranged. These occurred three times a week, in a quiet room. This formal structured, undisturbed time provided Walter with the chance to experience the undivided attention of someone who was willing to work with him. Walter would use this time however he wanted; he would set the 'agenda', but most commonly he would turn to talking about his particular outlook on the world.

- On every day, one of the nurses involved in Walter's care would discuss with him how Walter intended to use the day, what (if any) activities Walter would like to participate in. Additionally, they would explore how the nursing team could assist him with those activities (e.g. share a meal together, attend and participate in any ward based groups).
- When Walter was feeling vulnerable, it was negotiated that a nurse would make a purposeful contact with Walter every hour. Frequently, this purposeful contact was subsumed within some larger interpersonal contact, e.g. we would often go for long walks, enjoy a cup of coffee together.

Case study 53.2: Johnny

History and context

Johnny was a 62-year-old man, who has been married to the same woman for nearly 40 years. He has two grown up children and three grandchildren. Over the past two years he has been experiencing what he describes as 'funny turns'. His appetite appears to be good but he often wakes up very early in the morning and cannot get back to sleep. He runs a local gymnasium which he says he does enjoy, but it also causes him a lot of pressure and stress. He has recently started taking antidepressant medication, prescribed by his GP. When things are bad, sometimes he says, 'sometimes I feel like ending it all' but he is looking forward to his retirement. On admission, he says he feels 'hopeless' at the moment and that his thoughts about 'ending it all' are more frequent and pervasive.

Overview of the care

Johnny's care began with an assessment of his suicide risk using the NGASR, which determined that he presented with a high risk of suicide. For the first few days of his care, we negotiated a 'package' of care with him and agreed that we would review this after three days. As with Walter, a range of interventions/practices, all based on the 'Engagement: hope–inspiration' approach, were implemented:

- We agreed, that due to our concern for Johnny's well being, he would not be left alone during this three-day period. We felt he needed a high level of engagement; thus there would always be a nurse very close to him (physically close). We explained to Johnny that this physical closeness was a gesture of our concern for him, not a custodial intervention. Furthermore, this physical closeness would provide a range of opportunities for Johnny and his nurse to engage in dialogue or activities.
- This high level of engagement was used purposefully to encourage Johnny to talk about his thoughts and feelings; to enable him to vent his painful emotions, for the nurse to listen to him, and provide unconditional acceptance and support.

- Each day his level of suicidal risk was assessed using the same assessment tool, and due to the high level of engagement and the relationship established, this was felt to be highly accurate.
- Occasionally, we would sit quietly together.
- We would read together or play board games.
- Latterly, we would look at his choices and options, beginning to challenge, subtly, some of his more 'hopeless' or 'negative' constructs.

After several days of this high level of engagement, his risk assessment showed that his level of suicidal risk was declining, and therefore his care was re-negotiated accordingly.

CONCLUSION

Suicide represents a growing problem, particularly for the mental health nurse. MHNs need to familiarize themselves with interventions that they might use when caring for, with and about suicidal people. Although there are similarities between the use of observation and the use of engagement, to care for suicidal clients, the difference lies in the emphasis. Engagement is concerned with inspiring hope, and with exploring and attempting to understand the nature of the person's problems that led them to feel suicidal. Engagement is concerned primarily with addressing the person's need for emotional and physical security, rather than serving the needs of the organization. When one considers the benefits of engagement[25] and the failings of the current 'observation' focused approach, the need to abandon observation in favour of engagement becomes clear.

REFERENCES

1. Rosen G. History in the study of suicide. *Psychological Medicine* 1971; **1**: 267–85.
2. Aldridge D. *Suicide: the tragedy of hopelessness.* London: Jessica Kingsley Publishers, 1998.
3. Department of Health. *Health of the nation.* London: HMSO, 1990.
4. Department of Health. *Modernising mental health services: safe, sound and supportive.* London: HMSO, 1998.
5. Department of Health. *National service framework for mental health.* London: HMSO, 1999.
6. Higgins R, Wistow G, Hurst K. *Psychiatric nursing revisited. The care provided for acute psychiatric patients.* London: Whurr, 1998.
7. Rickelman BL, Houfek JF. Toward an interactional model of suicidal behaviors: cognitive rigidity, attributional stylem stress, hopelessness and depression. *Archives of Psychiatric Nursing* 1995; **9**: 158–68.

8. Pritchard C. Psychosocioeconomic factors in suicide. In: Thompson T, Mathias P (eds). *Lyttle's mental health and disorder*, 2nd edn. London: Baillière Tindall, 1998: 276–95.

9. Rawlins RP. Hope–hopelessness. In: Rawlins RP, Beck AT (eds). *Mental health nursing – a holistic life cycle approach*, 3rd edn. St Louis: Mosby, 1993: 257–84.

10. Gunnell DJ, Frankel S. Prevention of suicide: aspirations and evidence. *British Medical Journal* 1994; **308**: 1227–33.

11. Duffy D. Out of the shadows: a study of the special observation of suicidal psychiatric in-patients. *Journal of Advanced Nursing* 1995; **21**: 944–50.

12. Standing Nursing and Midwifery Advisory Committee. *Practice guidance: safe and supportive observation of patients at risk: mental health nursing – addressing acute concerns.* London: Department of Health, 1999.

13. Barker P, Walker L. *A survey of care practices in acute admission wards.* Reports submitted to the Northern and Yorkshire Regional Research and Development Committee. Newcastle: University of Newcastle, 1999.

14. Fletcher RF. The process of constant observation: perspectives of staff and suicidal patients. *Journal of Psychiatric and Mental Health Nursing* 1999; **6**: 9–14.

15. Jones J, Ward M, Wellman N, Hall J, Lowe T. Psychiatric inpatients' experiences of nursing observation: a United Kingdom perspective. *Journal of Psychosocial Nursing* 2000; **38**: 10–19.

16. Dodds P, Bowles N. Dismantling formal observation and refocusing nursing activity in acute inpatient psychiatry: a case study. *Journal of Psychiatric and Mental Health Nursing* 2001; **8**: 173–88.

17. Gournay K, Ward M, *et al.* Crisis in the capital: inpatient care in inner London. *Mental Health Practice* 1998; **1**: 10–18.

18. Barker P, Cutcliffe JR. Clinical risk: a need for engagement not observation. *Mental Health Care* 1999; **2**(8): 8–12.

19. Sainsbury Centre for Mental Health. *Acute problems: a survey of the quality of care in acute psychiatric admission wards.* London: Sainsbury Centre for Mental Health, 1998.

20. Talseth AG, Lindseth A, Jacobson L, Norberg A. Nurses' narrations about suicidal psychiatric inpatients. *Nordic Journal of Psychiatry* 1997; **51**: 359–64.

21. Davidhizar R, Vance A. The management of the suicidal patient in a critical care unit. *Journal of Nursing Management* 1993; **1**: 95–102.

22. Rogers P. Assessment and treatment of a suicidal patient. *Nursing Times* 1993; **90**: 37–9.

23. Talseth AG, Lindseth A, Jacobson L, Norberg A. The meaning of suicidal in-patients' experiences of being cared for by mental health nurses. *Journal of Advanced Nursing* 1999; **29**(5): 1034–41.

24. Long A, Reid W. An exploration of nurses' attitudes to the nursing care of the suicidal patient in an acute psychiatric ward. *Journal of Psychiatric and Mental Health Nursing* 1996; **3**: 29–37.

25. Long A, Long A, Smyth A. Suicide: a statement of suffering. *Nursing Ethics* 1998; **5**(1): 3–15.

26. Weisharr ME, Beck AT. Hopelessness and suicide. *International Review of Psychiatry* 1992; **4**: 177–84.

27. Frankl V. *Man's search for meaning: an introduction to logotherapy.* New York: Harper and Row, 1959.

28. Cutcliffe JR, Grant G. What are the principles and processes of inspiring hope in cognitively impaired older adults within a continuing care environment? *Journal of Psychiatric and Mental Health Nursing* 2001; **8**: 427–36.

29. Vailot M. Hope: the restoration of being. *American Journal of Nursing* 1970; **70**: 268–73.

Chapter 54

RECORD KEEPING

Martin F Ward*

INTRODUCTION

Many nurses turning to this chapter will probably think, 'Well I don't need to read this because I know all about record keeping'. On the face of it they may be right. My guess is that they would be wrong. By assuming that we already know something we probably end up knowing a lot less than we think we do. Such a position is out of step with both the philosophical stance of contemporary multidisciplinary practice and the professional development expectations of individual nurses.

The reality may be more problematic. Most nurses are exposed to good record keeping principles as students and receive no more instruction, coaching or guidance for the rest of their careers, unless a crisis occurs, precipitating a management-led insistence that they review local policies or seek the guidance of national standards. Considerable evidence suggests that most practising nurses find it difficult to reconcile their professional ideals with the way that they regularly record information concerning patient progress. When questioned closely, research participants regularly express doubts about the efficacy of their written communications, frustration with the systems they have to use and the limitations of the infrastructures they see as inhibiting this vital aspect of their work. Audits, both local and national, and public inquiries continue to highlight record keeping as a major factor in the escalation of serious and untoward incidents into tragedies.

THE FUNDAMENTALS OF GOOD RECORD KEEPING

Among other things, records should be clear, concise and legible. However, such principles are not enough because the written record of one professional – as a source of information for another – involves more than having a clean and legal document. Such simplicity confuses the differing needs for a *complex* 'professional record' with the more straightforward requirements of a 'legal document'.

Records have to serve a purpose. In health care that purpose may involve more than just a communication about the state of a person's well-being. By first identifying the *purpose* of record keeping we can describe what needs to be done to make it effective, while at the same time disentangling the *legal* from the *professional* requirements. This will also help us identify the different forms of records required to meet our different purposes. In doing so, this raises the status of record keeping from a mundane activity to one of sophistication, requiring high levels of professional skill.

*Martin Ward has been a psychiatric nurse, tutor and researcher for over 30 years. He was the Director of the Royal College of Nursing's Mental Health Nursing Programme at Oxford and presently is an Independent Consultant in Mental Health.

Record purpose and integration of care

If a nurse records information quickly, merely as an end product to some other activity, then record keeping risks becoming a secondary process, with no great significance. As a first principle, record keeping should be:

> Integral to the overall process of care; carrying equal status to any other component; needing to be considered with the same attention to detail as the intervention itself.

The reason for this is quite clear. Records are part of the intervention. Nurse–patient contact time needs to be planned if it is to be effective. It has to fit an operational process that builds up into a picture of care. Each contact has to be evaluated and its impact measured. Finally, it has to be recorded, not just because protocol dictates that it should, but as part of this overall picture. Change or progress cannot be measured without baselines, from which comparisons can be made. If we do not record details of what has taken place, historically, in our various contacts with the patient, how else can we know when we need to revise our interventions? How can continuity between practitioners be maintained unless everyone has access to details of what happened in their absence? How can the memory of one observation endure, clearly, over weeks or even months? How can patients make a real contribution to their own care if there is no record that will help them to see themselves as others do? Finally, how can care be truly evaluated if there are important gaps in the chain of recorded events, or if lack of precision blurs all events into a single story of everyday routine?

Seeing the recording process as secondary to – or divorced from the care process – devalues nursing and dilutes the impact of concerted teamwork. None of the above outcomes from the recording process can be achieved successfully without the attention to detail demanded by good record keeping. Recognizing that recording and care are on the same continuum enables the practitioner to appreciate the importance of identifying the purpose of the recording.

A clinical illustration

Janine, a nurse on a busy in-patient acute unit, receives a telephone call from a patient who has gone home to collect some personal belongings. Archie tells the nurse that his home has been burgled. He is distraught and abusive on the phone. He resists her first attempts to calm down and threatens to hurt himself unless something is done to help him, *immediately*. As his primary nurse, Mike, is off duty, Janine has no direct responsibility for Archie. As no-one else is available Janine must handle the situation herself. Archie is becoming increasingly agitated and starts shouting down the

phone. Janine asks him to describe what has happened in his home and, while he is talking she opens his care record. Carefully documented records of care plan outcomes highlight that Archie responds well to active listening. Further reading gives two examples of previous incidents. However, the primary nurse has underlined a section that tells that analysis of previous conversations indicates that Archie does not like to be given the option of making difficult decisions. Janine manages to diffuse the situation by prompting more controlled discussion and by offering to phone the police once Archie has returned to the unit where he can give an interview.

In the clinical illustration, previous care records highlighted key and significant information that could be used as a way of ensuring that others could work for the patient's benefit. Primary concerns about the patient's response to perceived threats were the primary purpose of the written record and, as a result, were integral to care itself.

It could be argued that an experienced nurse would have the skills to work all this out for herself while on the phone with Archie. But, why should she have to experiment and risk prolonging or exacerbating Archie's difficulties? The recorded information helped Janine to resolve the situation quickly and Archie was calm enough to return to the unit safe in the knowledge that someone understood and cared enough to help. More importantly, Archie received care that reduced his distress, reducing the possibility of the situation escalating into a real emergency. The continuity between responses of his primary nursing team and this 'outsider' would only reinforce his confidence in his care programme.

Good record keeping has to be seen as having a specific purpose and integrated with the process of care delivery. The production of appropriate records is, therefore, a state of mind and is as philosophically bound as any model of care. This mindset has been referred to as a 'symbol of professionalism'.[1] However, as such it can cause conflict and tension when set against organizational requirements. In his ethnographic research Allen described nurses on a surgical ward having difficulty reconciling their professional ideals about the quality of their records with the way that they were viewed by their employing organization, the time available to complete them, and the credibility with which they were viewed by other members of the clinical team. In the USA, tension between nurse driven documentation and the perceptions of that work by other disciplines, was seen – in one case – as a cause for a breakdown in support between different working groups, to the detriment of patients.[2] In that study, the nurses were advanced psychiatric practitioners and the problems were resolved by increasing the amount of significance that their records had to the process of care. Further examples of this way of thinking can be found in Japan,[3] Sweden[4] and Norway[5] as well as the UK.[6,7]

Professional development

In the same way that individual practitioners need to update themselves in relation to changes in health care attitudes and techniques, so too it is important that they regularly review how they record information generated by those changes. If we accept the link between recording and care delivery we also accept that development in each area are interdependent. Research has shown that not only does an ongoing programme of reviewing personal record keeping improve the efficiency of this activity but it also raises awareness of the necessity to view such work as central to clinical effectiveness.[8] This pilot scheme included six-monthly updates and evaluations of nurses' adherence to a documentation system, linked to their care delivery process, and demonstrated the benefits of attributing continued importance to the recording process. Another project exploring the effects of a 30-week multidisciplinary mental health education programme carried out in the UK, identified communication as part of the core skills of mental health workers. However, it was concluded that programme participants tended to overestimate their skills in the two key areas of care planning and record keeping.[9]

Practice-based research from both the UK and North America clearly identifies the links between the application of research within a clinical environment and the absolute necessity to modify the supporting recording activities.[10–13] However, the two processes in these studies, *care delivery* and *record keeping*, were not separate entities, but part of the same process, with one equally informing the other. Similarly, in a large study to identify the cognitive impairment of 3954 elderly primary care patients effective documentation was seen as the key to improving diagnostic evaluations.[14] In all these studies the need for educational development within record keeping was identified as a prerequisite for change.

Formal education programmes can only account for a small proportion of the professional development of any practitioner during the course of their career. Conversely, record keeping is a daily event. Likewise, the growth in understanding of a way of doing something, or the increase in personal technology, is a cumulative process with each day building on the last. Formal education can usually only address primary issues relevant to a group or section of the working community, identified by stage of training, exposure to specific working methods or seniority, etc. In effect, these educational programmes aggregate knowledge to create standardized development. While the ability to generate summative improvements in care quality is important, it is not designed to meet the needs of individual practitioners. Record keeping itself is not a static thing and improvements in computer technology, for example, have created a whole new generation of documentation possibilities, with software packages enabling multilayered record keeping to follow a patient throughout the whole of their care.[15]

Ongoing professional development can benefit from an exploration of individual records in a far more dynamic way. Cutcliffe[16] outlined the need to record information from clinical supervision sessions. If one takes his discussion to its logical conclusion it also shows the importance of using written records as a method of supervision itself. Reviewing evidence of actual clinical work through the written record of the supervisee, then jointly developing strategies for understanding both the clinical work and its subsequent recording would seem to have benefits for both activities. Discussions about what a nurse did in given circumstances or how they did or did not resolve conflict can easily be shrouded by poor memory or preconceived ideas about their own effectiveness. The written record can be used as an *aide memoir* for reflective discussion. Exploring the ways information was recorded would be the first step in improving the performance of the nurse. It would also show the importance of matching recording purpose to those of clinical intention. Significantly, it would also highlight the loop within which these two elements exist; the quality of one being interdependent upon the quality of the other. Matching a recording process to fit the requirements of clinical actions calls for different forms of recording. The more skilled nurses become at recognizing this, the more sophisticated and effective they become at responding appropriately to the changing needs of individual patients.

This need to identify different forms of record keeping for different purposes has far reaching implications. One failing of the current hierarchy within psychiatric-mental health nursing (at least in the UK) is the accepted convention that junior nurses act as key workers or primary nurses, while more senior clinical staff act as managers or consultants. Consequently, documents supporting the work of a clinical team are often the products of the junior staff. Additionally, senior staff may provide clinical supervision, but this is not standard practice. Unless junior staff seek advice and/or regular supervision, their own record keeping becomes the benchmark or 'standard' and they have limited opportunities to develop this important professional skill. Record keeping is only as good as the person who makes the record. If there are no quality goals, or the quality remains static, the value of those records will gradually diminish. Clearly, senior practitioners need to contribute regularly to the recording process, even if this requires a change in the infrastructure within which the nurses work.

To this situation one must also add the problems associated with the implementation of certain models or ways of delivering nursing. If the philosophical basis of care centres on a high degree of patient autonomy, the recording process for contact with that patient needs to reflect this. Fowler offered a good example,[17] in relation to the application of Peplau's theory of interpersonal relations, about interpersonal working with patients and the difficulty of recording these interactions. In Fowler's view, the holistic nature of Peplau's work did not easily fit with a record keeping system. While acknowledging this fact, the author recommended that nurses develop a recording style, in the form of a commentary, that best suited the approach, i.e. the clinical contact being reflected in the recording purpose.

LEGAL REQUIREMENTS AND GOOD PRACTICE

Practitioners need to recognize the difference between professional and legal accountability. In countries where there is specific mental health legislation (such as the UK, Canada, Australia and New Zealand), the process of care delivery is provided within a framework that sets parameters for the circumstances under which that care can be delivered.[18,19] For example, determining when they can be treated against their wishes, the period of their hospitalization, and their access to appeal, protects patient rights. Other medico-legislation combines with this to ensure confidentiality and access to patient records. Increasingly, legislation demands that care should be:

❏ appropriate to the needs of the individual;
❏ of the highest quality; and
❏ complies with new ideas and technology.

In effect such legislation sets the scene for care delivery but does not prescribe the nature of the care to be delivered. It leaves clinical decision-making to the clinician.[20] Professional accountability, therefore, is very much a personal choice, albeit guided by standards of professional conduct.[21]

Conversely, the nature of medically related record keeping is determined by strict rules that have to be complied with to ensure not only confidentiality, but also the maintenance of standards.[22,23] Although, decisions concerning these issues should not be left to individual choice, evidence from service reviews suggest that this is not always the case.[24,25] While nurses have choice over the care that may be offered, and therefore

determine the purpose of the associated record keeping, they do not have choice about the framework of the records themselves, nor the standards that have to be met to make them an accepted legal document. Separating the legal from the professional requirements of good record keeping enables the nurse to identify clearly the framework upon which they base the choice element of the work. Only once nurses are aware of what has to be done to comply with legal standards, can the construction and design of the records, which fit the purpose of care, proceed.

The following is a summary of the key points governing legally acceptable records and standards of good practice. All recorded entries *must* be:

❏ **Legible** – i.e. written in the national language and readable.
❏ **Written in blue or black ink** – both for necessary copying purposes and to make the text bold.
❏ **Signed and dated by the recorder** – initials are only acceptable where a code is provided to enable auditors to clearly identify the recorder.
❏ **Deletions must also be signed and dated** – mistakes or crossings out within the text have to be sanctioned by the recorder.
❏ **Originals** – photocopies of documents fade or discolour over time and can seriously hamper the reader's ability to decipher what is written. Entries must be made on original documents. Where it is necessary for a copy of notes to be made this fact must be clearly stated on the file itself.
❏ **Abbreviations avoided** – abbreviations can mean different things to different readers, and nothing at all to others; may cause confusion and are generally the result of sloppy unidisciplinary professionalism.
❏ **Stored in a locked cabinet or safe place** – access must be only to those who have direct patient responsibility or who need to have information about the patient for legal or professional reasons i.e. multi-disciplinary team members in clinical decision-making roles.
❏ **Available to those who have legal access to them** – where appropriate this will include the patient's legal representatives with permission given by the patient representatives of the Mental Health Act Commission or similar bodies and authorized auditors.

Entries *should*:

❏ **Involve patients** – where possible patients should be involved in documenting the impact of the care they receive, as well as designing and evaluating it.
❏ **Be relevant to the patient in whose file they are being made** – complicated observations about the interactions between different patients should be divided

into sections and placed in each patient's records thus ensuring that all the patients involved have a record of the event and not just one patient.

❑ **Be concise** – accurate and to the point. More words do not necessarily mean more information and health professionals need to know the facts as quickly as possible. If the facts are hidden in rhetoric they are likely to be missed or the record itself ignored.

❑ **Record progress** – repeat entries of 'slept well' and 'no change' are pointless. It should be assumed that if no entry is made in a progress record there is no change from the previous entry. Only things that are different need to be reported.

❑ **Be information sensitive** – key or significant information that influences care decisions should be highlighted or placed on a separate data sheet for ready access.

❑ **Be systematic** – all entries for a particular patient should follow a pattern as determined by the purpose of the recording.

❑ **Be sequential** – if entries have to be made in retrospect they should be clearly marked accordingly.

❑ **Be recorded on the appropriate document** – most case files contain any number of different documents and entries need to be in the right place.

❑ **Be coded** – in a way that enables a reader to see which pieces of the total record fits with other entries.

❑ **Not be repeated** – if it is necessary to place the same entry on different document either use an accepted coding system to refer the reader to the original entry as with care plans and evaluation records or review the use of the documents themselves to avoid over-reporting.

❑ **Be multidisciplinary** – although this may not always be possible, systems that encourage different disciplines to use their own records have been shown to be poor communicators of relevant health care information and key factors in the event of complex care failing to support individual patients.

PROBLEMS ASSOCIATED WITH GOOD RECORD KEEPING

Patient involvement

While most practitioners accept the principle of patient involvement in the design, delivery and evaluation of their care as a fundamental part of contemporary psychiatric care, for many it remains unclear as to how such ideals can be operationalized. When considering the possibility of patients helping to construct their own care record alarm bells often go off because such records

are seen to be the domain of practitioners. However, this can only be the case if sensitive information is to be withheld from the patient or if they are too disturbed to be able to make either a genuine contribution or appreciate what is being asked of them. Of course, there are more sinister reasons, that the entries themselves are derogatory to the patient as a person, badly written or patently incorrect.[26]

With the growth in discreet computer software that enables different aspects of the patients file to be displayed at any given time[27] it is possible to restrict the amount of access that a patient has. Even with traditional paper records access should not be a problem. The patient should already have access to their own care plan, indeed should have been encouraged to help construct it, why then should they not have access to the reporting data charting the impact and progress of that care plan? If individual practitioners are having difficulty finding ways of reducing the tokenism of patient involvement, sharing the responsibility for completing some of the patient's records with patients themselves may be a good place to start.

Multidisciplinary record keeping

Multidisciplinary or joint record keeping has been the focus of much debate over the past decade. Despite evidence to suggest that it *reduces* duplication, *increases* both practitioner reporting effectiveness, *enhances* transfer of data across teams, *raises awareness* of the contributions of individual team members, and provides a clearer picture of care overall,[28] the approach is still resisted by many. Several factors may be involved, not least the possible poor quality of individual disciplines' record keeping. However, as Rigby *et al.* reported, modern technology and new ways of recording dictate that all members of a care team use similar recording mechanisms.[29] Yet, other members of the team may need to be convinced of the effectiveness of such a radical move. One way of achieving this is for nurses to tailor their recording so that it fits with both the purpose of the care offered and is written in such a way as it becomes accessible to other disciplines. Adherence to the recording principles described within this chapter would also improve the overall quality of nursing records and thus make their inclusion in joint records a valuable asset.

'Organizational straightjackets' – the documents themselves

In this era of quality improvement, clinical governance, audit and cost effectiveness many organizations have demonstrated their desire to improve efficiency by developing standardized recording documentation.[30–33] While there are obvious benefits for an organization to implement such schedules within a psychiatric setting say for audit and quality assurance purposes, they tend to ignore the nature and purpose of some of the more interpersonal and reflective aspects of mental health care. Some authors[34,35] argue that the recording purpose has to dictate the record, not the other way around. Liberto and colleagues posed the question as to what happens to the anecdotal information gathered during a conversation, an observation or an incident? They suggested that individual practitioners adapted their recording style to fit with that of the organization but that they included more subjective and anecdotal data within a commentary. This would then be accessed readily by others, but not confused with factual reporting. What takes place between patients and nurses is not always clear. Standardized recording demands answers and requires the recorder to make quick decisions about

what is experienced or observed. This challenges much conventional wisdom in contemporary psychiatric-mental health nursing and, as a result, more open reporting styles need to be developed. Such a style of reporting may get 'messy' from an audit perspective, but reducing complex patient information into checklists is clinically counterproductive.

Consider a clinical environment where all disciplines use the same recording device, patients are encouraged to write in their own records, record keeping is regarded as a part of the care process and is, therefore, commiserate with care actions and nurses are encouraged to explore more personalized approaches to documentation. The record for the event described at the beginning of this chapter might read like the illustration in Figure 54.1.

This example offers only a snap-shot of what is possible. There is no 'rocket-science' here, just good sense and clear recording. What is important is that the record

Entry 45, 18th April 2002 15:30hrs	Archie phoned the unit in an agitated state shouting that his flat had been burgled. I found it difficult to calm him down and he threatened to harm himself if I did not do something to help him. He was genuinely upset, and for obvious reasons. Referred to Entry nos. 27 and 31 for some idea how to deal with this. Mike's notes enabled me to ask Archie to come back to the unit and I would phone the police for him. He agreed and is on his way. Janine Wilson, Staff Nurse (Janine Wilson)
Entry 46, 18th April 2002 16:20hrs	Archie has returned (refer Entry 45). Still upset but calmer and no longer shouting. Contacted police on 01865 123456 and spoken with PC Wilson – they will send someone to interview Archie this evening. Will talk to Archie to see if anything else can be done. Janine Wilson, Staff Nurse. (Janine Wilson)
Entry 47, 18th April 2002 17:00hrs	Thank you Janine, I feel a lot better now. Can someone sit with me when the police come? Archie Raymond
Entry 48, 18th April 2002 17:30hrs	Can Janine, Archie and Mike meet with me tomorrow, 19th April at about 11:00 to see if we can alter Archie's support programme please (refer Entry 45). Alan Bennett, Senior Reg Alan Bennett
Entry 49, 18th April 2002 18:20hrs	Meeting arranged (refer Entry 48). Janine Wilson, Staff Nurse (Janine Wilson)
Entry 50, 18th April 2002 20:15hrs	Archie Raymond interviewed Re: break-in. Malcolm Wilson (M. Wilson PC 234)
Entry 51, 18th April 2002 21:00hrs	I want to talk tomorrow about how I can deal better with these situations (refer Entry 45). I was very frightened when I got home and if it had not been for Janine would have done something stupid. Janine says there are several ways we can approach this so I will be better prepared in the future. The meeting should be good. Janine Wilson, Staff Nurse (Janine Wilson) and Archie Raymond

FIGURE 54.1 Example of record keeping

itself is part of what actually happened, not an after-thought.

CONCLUSION

Record keeping is a complex and dynamic process and cannot be relegated to the status of an 'also-ran'. If care is to be regularly tested against outcomes, measured for its effectiveness, modified or even totally changed to reflect new ideas and technology, ideology or philosophy, it has to be supported by a recording process which is both fit for the purpose and as robust as the clinical intervention itself.

The written records of any professional group testify to the working activities of that group. There will always be problems associated with maintaining high quality, informative and practical records, within a work environment that may be stressful, complex and time consuming. Nonetheless, if the nurses' contribution to this process is disjointed, lacks depth and is poorly prepared it will diminish the contribution that nurses make to the delivery of care. In effect, this will devalue the contribution of nursing generally within the mental health care team. While nursing will no doubt attempt to find other ways of preserving its reputation the real losers in this situation are the patients. Failure to see the importance of good nurse record keeping, targeted to purpose and intrinsically linked to care delivery, is a failure to see the importance of nursing in the relief of suffering for those with mental health problems.

REFERENCES

1. Allen D. Record-keeping and routine nursing practice: the view from the wards. *Journal of Advanced Nursing* 1988; **27**: 1223–30.

2. Glair-Gajewski C, Trigoboff E. Formulation of a systematic method of documentation for nurse-led mental health groups. *Journal of New York State Nurses Association* 1993; **24**: 16–18.

3. Kataoka K. Evaluation of mental health, psychiatric care, and welfare planning at a public hospital. *Seishin Shinkeigaku Zasshi* 1996; **98**: 865–9.

4. Andersen T, Johansson BM, Lindberg M, Stenwall R. New documentation routines in psychiatry in Vasterbotten: unified structure for better quality of care. *Lakartidningen* 1999; **96**: 2102–6.

5. Am T, Riaunet A. Integrated psychiatric care planning. *Tidsskrift for Den Norske Laegeforening* 1997; **117**: 1759–62.

6. Briggs M, Dean KL. A qualitative analysis of the nursing documentation of post-operative pain management. *Journal of Clinical Nursing* 1998; **7**: 155–63.

7. Moloney R, Maggs C. A systematic review of the relationships between written manual nursing care planning, record keeping and patient outcomes. *Journal of Advanced Nursing* 1999; **30**: 51–7.

8. Bernick L, Richards P. Nursing documentation: a program to promote and sustain improvement. *Journal of Continuing Education in Nursing* 1995; **25**: 203–8.

9. Parsons S, Barker P. The Phil Hearne course: an evaluation of a multidisciplinary mental health education programme for clinical practitioners. *Journal of Psychiatric Mental Health Nursing* 2000; **7**: 101–8.

10. Schubert DS, Billowitz A, Gabinet L, Friedson W. Effect of liaison psychiatry on attitudes toward psychiatry, rate of consultation, and psycho-social documentation. *General Hospital Psychiatry* 1989; **11**: 77–87.

11. Talashek ML, Gerace LM, Miller AG, Lindsey M. Family nurse practitioner clinical competencies in alcohol and substance use. *Journal of American Academy of Nurse Practitioners* 1995; **7**: 57–63.

12. Russell L. The importance of wound documentation and classification. *British Journal of Nursing* 1999; **8**: 1342–3, 1346, 1348 passim.

13. Dowding D. Examining the effects that manipulating information given in the change of shift report has on nurses' care planning ability. *Journal of Advanced Nursing* 2001; **33**: 836–46.

14. Callahan CM, Hendrie HC, Tierney WM. Documentation and evaluation of cognitive impairment in elderly primary care patients. *Annals of Internal Medicine* 1995; **122**: 422–9.

15. Bingham RM. Increasing the effectiveness and efficiency of academic advising through computerization. *Computers in Nursing* 1997; **15**: 137–40.

16. Cutcliffe JR. To record or not to record: documentation in clinical supervision. *British Journal of Nursing* 2000; **9**: 350–5.

17. Fowler J. Taking theory into practice: using Peplau's model in the care of a patient. *Professional Nurse* 1995; **10**: 226–30.

18. Ta A. Supervision of psychiatric patients. *Canadian Nurse* 1997; **93**: 47–8.

19. Foster B. Ethical practice and legal responsibility for duly authorized officers: achieving a balance. *Australian and New Zealand Journal of Mental Health Nursing* 1998; **7**: 41–5.

20. Wallace M. The legal framework for mental health nursing. *Collegian* 1996; **3**: 11–20.

21. NMC Code of professional conduct. London. Nursing and Midwifery Council. 2002.

22. NHSE. *Keeping the record straight.* London, NHS Executive, 1993.

23. UKCC. *Standards of records and record keeping.* London, United Kingdom Central Council for Nurses, Midwives and Health Visitors, 1998.

24. Sainsbury Centre for Mental Health. *Acute problems: a survey of the quality of care in acute psychiatric wards.* London, Sainsbury Centre for Mental Health, 1998.

25. Sainsbury Centre for Mental Health. *National Visit 2: A visit by the Mental Health Act Commission to 104 mental health and learning disability units in England and Wales: Improving care for detained patients from black and minority ethnic communities.* London, Sainsbury Centre for Mental Health, 2000.

26. Keefe RH, Hall ML. Private practitioners' documentation of outpatient psychiatric treatment: questioning managed care. *Journal of Behavioural Health Service Research* 1994; **26**: 151–70.

27. Milholland DK. Privacy and confidentiality of patient information. Challenges for nursing. *Journal of Nursing Administration* 1994; **24**: 19–24.

28. Walsh C. Patient records improve with unified case notes. *Nursing Times* 1998; **94**: 52–3.

29. Rigby MJ, Roberts R, Williams JG. Objectives and prerequisites to success for integrated patient records. *Computer Methods and Programs in Biomedicine* 1995; **48**: 121–5.

30. Corben V. The Buckinghamshire nursing record audit tool: a unique approach to documentation. *Journal of Nursing Management* 1997; **5**: 289–93.

31. Mongiardi F. Language of care. Record keeping needs a common framework. *Nursing Standard* 1998; **12**: 20.

32. Baker JG, Shanfield SB, Schnee S. Using quality improvement teams to improve documentation in records at a community mental health center. *Psychiatric Services* 2000; **51**: 239–42.

33. Kallert TW, Schutzwohl M, Leisse M, Becker T, Kluge H, Kilian R, Angermeyer MC, Bach O. Standardized documentation system for the complementary sector of psychiatric care. Development and trial in Saxony. *Psychiatrische Praxis* 2000; **27**: 86–91.

34. Barbiasz JE, Hunt V, Lowenstein A. Nursing documentation: a format not a form. *Journal of Nursing Administration* 1981; **11**: 22–6.

35. Liberto T, Roncher M, Shellenbarger T. Anecdotal notes. Effective clinical evaluation and record keeping. *Nurse Education* 1991; **24**: 15–18.

Chapter 55

DISCHARGE PLANNING

Martin F Ward*

INTRODUCTION

Imagine that you board a plane, sit in your seat for hours, being offered an endless supply of refreshments and indigestible meals, yet have no idea where you are going nor how long it would take. Then, when you land, you are not told where you are but are herded from the aircraft and left in the terminal building.

Imagine that you had been admitted to a psychiatric unit and that the same level of information had been offered you. The analogy may seem like a strange one, but whereas few of us have ever been admitted to a psychiatric unit, most of us have flown. Even on short flights we crave information about where we are, how long before we land and what the weather is like at the destination. We have some sort of travel arrangements and our destination is usually something we can visualize and, as a consequence, feel comfortable with. It has a purpose and we feel safe. Conversely, the patient in the psychiatric unit, given none of the relevant information, finds it difficult to make sense of the journey (the admission) and probably feels very insecure about the destination (the discharge)!

If we would not accept the consequences of a meaningless and blind journey why do we so often accept for our patients the clinical limitations imposed by unplanned discharge?[1] The point of a journey is to arrive. Equally, the purpose of a hospital admission is to be discharged in a state of health that enables the person to sustain him/herself as independently as possible. One is part of the other. Both constituting the reason and both being part of the outcome. To divorce one from the other risks leaving nurses incapable of delivering appropriate interventions during the admission period that will lead, eventually, to discharge.

However, as Breeze points out,[2] in contemporary psychiatric practice throughout most of the world, the emphasis placed upon risk and its assessment has created something of a paradox for nursing. On the one hand nurses accept that, theoretically, the purpose of admission is successful discharge. Yet, on the other they are confronted with the constraining influences of insufficient inpatient facilities that are prone to generating unplanned discharge for certain patients, supervised discharges that require significant and, often incomplete, community resources, the requirement of a seemingly endless supply of suitably trained key workers and for many patients the absence of any meaningful lifestyle once discharged.[3] Is it any wonder, therefore, that many nurses find it difficult to rationalize harsh reality with high professional expectations.[4] To fully understand the complexity of discharge process as the rubric for clinical efficacy it is necessary to explore both the nature of different care continuums and the roles and values of those involved.

---

*Martin Ward has been a psychiatric nurse, tutor and researcher for over 30 years. He was the Director of the Royal College of Nursing's Mental Health Nursing Programme at Oxford and presently is an Independent Consultant in Mental Health.

DISCHARGE GOALS

There are four basic forms of discharge from an inpatient mental health unit:

1 **Short stay or acute**. Anything from a few days to a few weeks, possibly repeated several times within a care sequence but always with the purpose of reducing dependence upon care staff before it takes place.

2 **Rehabilitation or long stay**. Often referred to as continuing care but this does not fully do it justice for the discharge itself is based around reversing a long-term trend of dependence upon staff and producing independence of them. The goal here is not so much the maintenance of a level of self-sufficiency but more the re-acquisition of lost skills and the confidence to use them.

3 **The so-called 'revolving door'**, often a combination of the above two. Goals will vary according to patient needs but will nearly always involve programmes to enable patients to achieve a level of concordance with community treatment and the implementation of skills for self-determination.

4 **Against medical advice**. Always clinically unplanned and often caused because of patient dissatisfaction with treatment or conditions of care, whether warranted or not. The patient goal is usually based upon frustration with progress, a sense of infringement upon personal space or conflict with treatment targets. For those requiring care there is usually a very poor outcome from such a discharge.[5]

5 **Completion of treatment**. Although the concept of cure has little or no meaning within mental health care, patients do achieve levels of self-determination, decision-making and absence of symptoms that demand absolute discharge. They are recognition of personal success and their goal is simply to allow people to lead their own lives.

With the exception of last type the goals of these discharges are predicated upon the assumption that professional support will be needed over-time after inpatient care. In other words, the inpatient process is only part of the over-all package of care. However, there is another form of discharge, with a different goal, that usually only occurs from a community source.

Some authors describe generic goals for discharging patients who fall into the categories listed above.[6] Gibson identifies the goals of a rehabilitation service as being linked specifically to those of patients, and particularly those suffering the effects of severe and enduring mental health problems such as schizophrenia. Producing measurable gain in functioning, promoting independence and self direction and implementing care designed to help the patient live a meaningful life in the least restrictive environment are the central goals upon which discharge is based. Gibson, along with most other authors and researchers, also suggests that treatment concordance within the community reduces recidivism and therefore includes work that promotes this as part of the discharge goal.

These goals would seem to be consistent with the outcomes of planned discharge as can be seen when considered against outcome research carried out to explore the lives of patients currently living in the community. A longitudinal comparative study carried out in Berlin[7] demonstrated that the main gain for patients who had worked through a planned discharge programme designed to meet their individual needs was in the area of social functioning. Significantly, the presence of psychiatric symptoms was the same for both the inpatient control group and those in the community. The main goals for discharge for these long-term patients had been to mobilize community resources in the areas of accommodation, employment and social interaction, described in other German research as 'vocational rehabilitation'.[8] The results of the Hoffmann study were also supported by work carried out to explore the impact of mental health case managers on social functioning[9–11] as well as that undertaken enabling patients to evaluate the effectiveness of their own care in the community.[12]

What is important about these studies is that they show how linking inpatient therapeutic processes to rehabilitation activities designed to meet discharge goals, then resourcing the ongoing support of these goals once discharged, has a better chance of bringing about a successful conclusion to the care package. They also demonstrate that planned discharge does not occur by accident but by design and the Canadian study pointed out unplanned discharges more often result in re-admission.[1] In Australia Owen *et al.* showed that the re-admission rate to an inpatient acute unit within six months of discharge was as high as 38% even when the community resource was well financed and integrated between health and social care agencies.[13] The major determining factor for re-admission was not so much the quantity of the community resource, but the quality of the planning prior to discharge in mobilizing resources that would most successfully meet the needs of the individual patient. A failure on the part of inpatient care staff to use discharge goals as determinants for treatment packages will inevitably result in disjointed movement between the two parts of the service.

ADMISSION TO DISCHARGE – THE CARE CONTINUUM

Re-admission rates for psychiatry are important indicators because they provide us with some clues as to the effectiveness of the original discharge. However, reliance upon them alone may actually weaken the case for improving the planning that goes into a discharge. For those requiring intensive support and hospitalization being discharged does not mean that they are well, it simply means that a new stage in the care process has been reached. People have to return to hospital, in all walks of medicine and for all sorts of reasons. For the same reasons that people move from inpatient care to community care they may well need to move back again. The problem is not so much the re-admission but the inference that the care, or indeed the patient, has in some way failed within the community. Statistics detailing re-admission rates tell us only that X% of patients had to return to hospital, they do not provide information about why, nor do they tell us anything about the discharge planning during the preceding admission. Predicting re-admission[14,15] seems a rather futile exercise unless the work is designed to establish what needs to be done to improve the rates, or better still, explain them.[16]

Consider the following example:

Case study 55.1

A young male patient, diagnosed as suffering the effects of schizophrenia, is admitted to his local acute inpatient unit for the third time in 12 months. Staff on the ward refer back to his case records for information about previous admissions and discharge activities. Having read the research that shows historical knowledge about prior re-admissions is a main indicator for predicting future re-admission they conclude that the patient will more than likely return to hospital following this admission. They construct a care package in-line with that which he received during previous admissions because whilst in hospital he responded well to it. After three weeks he is deemed well enough to return to the care of the community team and is discharged. Two months later he is re-admitted and the staff show no surprise at his reappearance.

Question: 'Who failed in this situation?'
Answer: 'It's not that simple!'

Why? Well for a start the patient may well have received the correct care whilst in hospital and the discharge package may well have been appropriate for his needs. Secondly, as a young man he may have encountered new threats to his personal integrity that could not have been predicted within any care package and thirdly, spending small amounts of time being hospitalized may have been the right way to help him through this phase of his illness. On the other side of the coin, no-one checked to see what the contextual problems associated with the requirement for re-admission were; secondly, no subsequent alterations were made to either the treatment or

discharge patterns in the absence of key community data and finally, the staff simply assumed he would return and his re-admission affirmed their clinical judgement. No-one actually failed, but no-one actually succeeded either. Unfortunately, staff decision-making was reinforced and consequently beliefs about the patient's ability to sustain himself within the community diminished. If the balance of failure shifts further towards the patient from the care staff so their desire to individualize his care will begin to fade.

Consider again the work of Owen *et al.* in 1997. They concluded that re-admission was necessitated as a result of poor fit between patient needs and aftercare facilities. However, the project was undertaken against the backdrop of a large hospital closure programme with established health and social aftercare facilities. What is not explicit within this work is how the patients were prepared prior to discharge nor how the aftercare quality was evaluated in relation to the requirements of individual patients. Discharge begins with admission and ends, if and when, the patient has to be re-admitted when the cycle begins once again. What the predictive qualities of psychiatric re-admission tell us are several things: (i) many patients may need re-admission; (ii) the preparation for discharge has to fit their individual requirements; (iii) community resources have to fit the goals of discharge; (iv) much can be learnt from exploring the effectiveness of previous inpatient episodes and associated discharges; and (v) care and discharge for each subsequent admission has to be tailored to fit individual requirements at that time, not those of previous admissions.

Admission, for a community team will mean something different to that of an inpatient team, yet the same principles apply to both groups. The real difference is that the point of care contact is altered, thus admission means being supported by a community nurse, discharge albeit temporary means transferring to the inpatient facility. In both cases links between the care teams and the patient should remain intact especially if re-admission is anticipated, maybe even planned for in the case of the community team.

Viewed from this perspective it is easier to understand the concept of discharge being the starting point for admission. When a patient begins the supportive period attributed to community care the community nurse should already have been party to developing the discharge programme. They may be identified as a key worker or case manager and their responsibilities for that patient will have begun during the inpatient stay. The unplanned inpatient discharge produces severe problems for community staff, but so too does the planned discharge that did not have involvement from staff having to implement it. Similarly, patients who are re-admitted to inpatient facilities should return with careful records of progress from the community team, enabling a thorough analysis of the circumstances that brought about the event.

However, this does not fully explain the situation experienced by staff receiving a new admission, to all intents and purposes, an unknown entity. In this case the whole purpose of admission will be to resolve immediate problems and return the individual back to their own life, with as little negative impact on that life as possible. The nurse has to develop a picture of what that life looks like and discharge has to be considered in the light of that information. Thus, care delivered to that patient has to be delivered with one eye on what, for them, is considered to be normal. As we will see later, probably the main source of this information is the patient him/herself but for now suffice to say that the goal of discharge has to fit what the patient thinks they need to be able to return to their own home. Though objectives of care set within the nursing process may well be small and immediate, there has to be a wider view of the reasons for those objectives. Remembering that much of the rehabilitation process is geared towards sociological as well as psychological functioning the provision of clinical therapies or therapeutic activities has to be made in order to operationalize those areas. Certainly symptoms have to be addressed, especially those that produce fear and misery, insecurity and the will to live, but they need not necessarily be the sole determinants for discharge. Indeed, many ex-users of mental health services lead relatively successful lives, yet still experience psychiatric symptoms that would confound the majority of society. It is the patients' ability to deal with these symptoms that is important and very often this requires very sophisticated personal strategies on their part. Ironically, often the successful support required by these individuals is far less sophisticated, being simply an understanding person who appreciates what they are doing and is there for them on a regular basis or when they need them.[17–19] One Danish study shows that although discharged patients' general level of life satisfaction tends to be lower than that of the general population one factor that increases this level is the close relationship that develops between themselves and a health care professional who genuinely appears to care about them.[20] This is confirmed by similar studies in the UK,[4,21] the USA,[22,23] Japan,[24,25] Sweden,[26] India[27] and the Netherlands.[28]

PATIENT INVOLVEMENT

As already mentioned the key source of information about expectation of care is the patients themselves. Yet, it would minimize the involvement of patients if we only view their role within care as providing information alone. The construction, delivery and evaluation of that care all fall within their remit. In the context of this chapter their commitment to the construction of a dedicated plan of their own discharge would seem to be an ideal way of achieving this. A study carried out in four Nordic countries considered the problems associated with what they described as 'discharge lags'.[29] These were situations where discharge was delayed because of a lack of community resources. However, the authors also discussed several factors that increased the continuity between inpatient and community and one of these was the involvement of the patient in planning their own discharge. There are other issues to consider.

For many years data concerning patients who absconded from inpatient care was regarded as proof simply that some patients would leave against medical advice. However, Bowers et al.[30] undertook a series of 52 interviews in the East End of London with patients who returned following absconding. The reasons given for leaving were both rational and in the main contextual to the care process. Within the clinical area they described being bored, frightened by other patients and feeling trapped and confined, whilst extraneous factors included feeling cut off from relatives and friends, having household responsibilities or being worried about the security of their home or property. Psychiatric symptoms, though mentioned, were not usually the primary cause for leaving. Of course, some patients left impulsively often following bad news about anticipated leave or discharge. Collectively these described causes provide us with a clue to the admission activities of these patients. It is unlikely that they were actively involved in the development and delivery of their own care because had they been so much of this absconding may have been averted. For example:

Case study 55.2

Tony is becoming agitated because he needs to get home to sort out bills that he tells his primary nurse are accumulating on his door mat. Having been an inpatient on the unit for nearly two weeks he has had no opportunity to check this fact but logic tells him that life is going on outside and he has responsibilities that have to be met. The primary nurse tells him that she will get Tony's social worker to go to his house and sort things out. Tony is happy with this. Two days later, having had no feedback and becoming increasingly concerned, he asks again for news of the social worker's visit only to be told that the nurse has not been able to contact him yet but will try again later. Twenty minutes later Tony goes missing.

Question: 'Who failed in this situation?'
Answer: 'The system.'

The 'system' here is the organizational structure that excluded Tony from his own care activities and the bureaucratic processes that gave personal responsibility to others that should have been his. Had the nurse and Tony been working together the nurse would have appreciated the importance of the home situation on Tony's ability to concentrate on his mental health problems, and indeed may even have concluded that they were one and the same thing. One of the key recommendations of the Bowers et al. work was that serious consideration be given to the patient's meaning of an admission.[30] If it could be argued that effective return to the community was the main objective then it is clear that the work of the care team is to deliver care that is designed to promote this. If Tony has no say in this aspect of the care package, when exactly does he have involvement? If he is in a position to be accompanied to his home, either by his primary nurse or a community nurse working in an inreach capacity the immediacy of such action would reduce the anxiety he feels and working with the nurse would enable him to resolve the problems created by the bills.

However, the 'system' has to be designed so that it places the patient at the heart of the care team, and not the care staff. To paraphrase Bowers et al., serious consideration has to be given to the patient's meaning of being *discharged* from hospital and the only person who can tell you that is the patient. If the discharge begins with admission then surely the patient has to be actively participating in clinical decision-making from the very beginning, not at the point of discharge when all the decisions about him have already been made.

Similarly, when the patient has returned to the community as part of a planned package of care and is now working with community staff the issue of involvement remains paramount. For a discharge package to work it has to be agreed by all parties. Compromise may be required from both parties but this is all part of individualizing care. Much work has been carried out showing that some patients are either re-admitted or commit suicide following discharge from an inpatient facility.[31–33] This research showed that lack of patient involvement in discharge planning was a major contributing factor to these events. Recidivism has been shown to be reduced when the patient is able to see the necessity to continue with treatment regimes following discharge.[34–36] Yet, to do so the patient has to see the importance of the treatment long before they return home. The process of discharge begins with the admission, or at the start of their rehabilitation programme.

MULTIDISCIPLINARY WORKING

Joint patient-care staff planning using carefully described rehabilitative goals can only truly be said to function properly when the care staff themselves are working as an integrated team. It is not the purpose of this chapter to address the issues of multidisciplinary or multi-agency working in its widest sense but careful examination of the literature reveals that one aspect of the discharge process can be heavily influenced by effective teamworking, that of risk consideration. Undoubtedly the decision for a patient to leave the protective confines of an inpatient facility to re-establish themselves in the community can be a period of high risk within their overall care package. Research exploring the nature of suicide following discharge,[33] violence after discharge,[37] the complex problems associated with dual diagnosis[38] and even patient experiences of their own discharge[39] are testament to this. Christ et al. (1994) identified that risk screening on admission not only speeded up discharge but targeted potential difficulties long before discharge was reached, thus reducing the necessity for possible re-admission. However, such screening required input not just from the inpatient team but also multi-agency staff working in the community. The 'system' in this situation needed to have cooperation and co-ordination consistent with one organization, not the polemicism associated with traditional arguments about inpatient vs. community. It also required staff to work together with the patient irrespective of professional boundaries.

When all of these factors are put together an example of a planned discharge might look like this:

Case study 55.3

Christine was re-admitted to an acute inpatient unit accompanied by both her daughter and Mike the community psychiatric nurse (CPN) having had a relapse in her ability to cope with daily living activities at home. There was a substantial increase in expressed clinical symptoms that had, in part, been brought about by deterioration in the relationship between herself and her husband. Mike had been working with Christine over a four-month period and had been in regular contact with both social care staff helping with accommodation and finance issues, as well as Christine's psychiatrist at the outpatient clinic. Mike was able to feedback to the inpatient primary nurse relevant information concerning Christine's changing need pattern and a review of the multidisciplinary records provided a picture of the progress of care to date. Christine had previously been discharged with a minimum supervision package under the terms of the care programme approach (CPA) meaning that

---

Mike had acted as her key worker both prior to discharge as well as afterwards. Mike's original inreach work had enabled him to work with Christine on developing discharge goals but the relationship between patient and spouse had not been targeted at that time.

Within the first few days a discharge plan was developed based on Christine's own perception of what she felt she needed to achieve and she was screened for risk factors that might impede her once back in the community. These included self-harm after arguments with her husband and wandering off on her own when she could not contact her daughter. Christine set cognitive targets for herself that included personal strategies and seeking help. When met these would indicate that she had both overcome the risk factors and reached a point at which she felt she was ready for discharge. Over a hospitalization period of five weeks the immediate problem of expressed symptoms was dealt with, enabling Christine to concentrate on her relationship difficulties. She worked with her primary nurse and the psychologist to construct and practice strategies for dealing with her identified relationship problems and both the daughter and husband were invited to take part in this work where appropriate. In the meantime Mike met with the social worker and these family members and discussed ways of working together with professional support once Christine was discharged.

Finally, a discharge letter was faxed through to Christine's GP as the primary care team would later play a crucial role in monitoring the impact of her care package. Following a series of team meetings, which Christine attended, the decision was made for her to have a trial period at home on leave to see how her new strategies and the overall support package functioned. Additionally, the social worker had secured more suitable rented accommodation for the family. At the end of a controlled discharge period Christine was discharged, with Mike providing regular weekly feedback both to the community mental health team and the inpatient primary nurse. Christine was re-admitted 18 months later following the complete breakdown of her marriage.

Question: 'Who failed in this situation?'
Answer: 'No one! And certainly not Christine.'

CONCLUSION

Effective discharge has to be considered the optimum for all admissions whether they be inpatient or community. The process of discharge has to be targeted to a goal or series of goals with individual patients determining the specific nature of these goals. The patient's involvement with the rest of the multidisciplinary team is a major determinant for the success of both the admission and its discharge and re-admission need not necess-

arily be seen as a failure of care if the work that went into the original discharge was appropriate and patient-centred. How these criteria are operationalized within any given service will ultimately depend upon the skill of the practitioners and the motivation of the patients. However, some things are clear.

Nurses have a key role to play in the provision of appropriate discharge and aftercare. Their unique position as the main point of professional contact for patients places the burden of care firmly on their shoulders and in the 21st century one of their key roles will be the co-ordination of aftercare.[40] They have the skills, and with the right resources should also have the opportunity, to affect the implementation of evidence to support their work.[41] Similarly, medical staff need to realize that the presence or absence of clinical symptoms is only one factor within a patient's discharge profile, and not necessarily a primary one.[42] Patients themselves place far more emphasis on the quality of their life and its social orientation than do health care professionals.[17]

All sorts of factors will come into play in determining whether a patient is equipped for discharge, many of them beyond the control of care staff and not least of them whether s/he should have been in hospital in the first place[43–45] and finally, just because community aftercare is provided it does not necessarily mean that it is appropriate, or that patients take advantage of it. Herein lies a note of caution. A UK study[46] reported that 77% of their patient sample received aftercare but 56% had no identified key worker and most lacked any long-term forward planning linking inpatient care to community living. Thus the point made earlier in this chapter returns to remind us that irrespective of the organization, the resources and the 'system' in place, if nurses and care staff generally do not have a mindset that sees discharge planning as integral to the total package of care they provide patients will continue to suffer the effects of poor professional insight.

REFERENCES

1. Gillis K, Russell VR, Busby K. Factors associated with unplanned discharge from psychiatric day treatment programs. A multicenter study. *General Hospital Psychiatry* 1997; **19**: 355–61.
2. Breeze J. Can paternalism be justified in mental health care? *Journal Advanced Nursing* 1998; **28**: 260–5.
3. Moore C. Discharge from an acute psychiatric ward. *Nursing Times* 1998; **94**: 56–9.
4. Ward MF, Cutcliffe J, Gournay K. *The nursing, midwifery and health visiting contribution to the continuing care of people with mental health problems: a review and UKCC action plan*. London: United Kingdom Central

Council for Nursing, Midwifery and Health Visiting, 2000.

5. Pages KP, Russo JE, Wingerson DK, Ries RK, Roy-Byrne PP, Cowley DS. Predictors and outcome of discharge against medical advice from the psychiatric units of a general hospital. *Psychiatric Services* 1998; **49**: 1187–92.

6. Gibson DM. Reduced rehospitalizations and reintegration of persons with mental illness into community living: a holistic approach. *Journal of Psycho-social Nursing and Mental Health Services* 1999; **37**: 20–5.

7. Hoffmann K, Kaiser W, Isermann M, Priebe S. How does the quality of life of long-term hospitalized psychiatric patients change after their discharge into the community? *Gesundheitswesen* 1998; **60**: 232–8.

8. Kallert TW, Leisse M. Rehabilitation concepts of schizophrenic patients treated in community psychiatry. *Rehabilitation (Stuttgart)* 2000; **39**: 268–75.

9. Ford J, Rigby P. Aftercare under supervision: implications for CMHNs. *British Journal of Nursing* 1996; **5**: 1312–16.

10. Carter AM. Case management in psychiatric inpatient recapture. *Military Medicine* 1997; **162**: 44–50.

11. Ward MF, Armstrong C, Lelliott P, Davies M. Training, skills and caseloads of community mental health support workers involved in case management: evaluation from the initial UK demonstration sites. *Journal of Psychiatric and Mental Health Nursing* 1999; **6**: 187–97.

12. Lelliott P, Beevor A, Hogman G, Hislop J, Lathlean J, Ward MF. 'Carers' and users' expectation of services – user version CUES-U, a new instrument to measure the experience of users of mental health services. *British Medical Journal* 2001; **179**: 67–72.

13. Owen C, Rutherford V, Jones M, Tennant C, Smallman A. Psychiatric rehospitalization following hospital discharge. *Community Mental Health Journal* 1997; **33**: 13–24.

14. Walker R, Minor-Schork D, Bloch R, Esinhart J. High risk factors for rehospitalization within six months. *Psychiatric Quarterly* 1996; **67**: 235–43.

15. Masaki N, Fujita T, Kai S, Zaitsu Y, Hira Y, Kondoh K, Yamashita K, Hatada K. Readmission among discharged psychiatric patients and its correlates. *Nion Koshu Eisei Zasshi* 1997; **44**: 372–83.

16. Thornicroft G, Gooch C, Dayson D. The TAPS project. 17: Readmission to hospital for long term psychiatric patients after discharge to the community. *British Medical Journal* 1992; **305**: 996–8.

17. Gerber GJ, Coleman GE, Johnston L, Lafave HG. Quality of life of people with psychiatric disabilities 1 and 3 years after discharge from hospital. *Quality of Life Research* 1994; **3**: 379–83.

18. Montgomery P, Johnson B. Chronically mentally ill individuals re-entering the community after hospitaliza-

tion. *Journal of Psychiatric and Mental Health Nursing* 1998; **5**: 497–503.

19. Martin DP, Diehr P, Conrad DA, Davis JH, Leickly R, Perrin EB. Randomized trial of a patient-centered hospital unit. *Patient Education and Counseling* 1998; **34**: 125–33.

20. Folker H, Jensen BM. Study of selected methods of self-assessment of health, quality of life and satisfaction with treatment. Use among patients four weeks after discharge from a psychiatric ward. *Ugeskr Laeger* 2001; **163**: 3347–52.

21. Bruce J, Watson D, van Teijlingen ER, Lawton K, Watson MS, Palin AN. Dedicated psychiatric care within general practice: health outcome and service providers' views. *Journal of Advanced Nursing* 1999; **29**: 1060–7.

22. Bostelman S, Callan M, Rolincik LC, *et al*. A community project to encourage compliance with mental health treatment aftercare. *Public Health Report* 1994; **109**: 153–7.

23. Goodwin R, Lyons JS. An emergency housing program as an alternative to inpatient treatment for persons with severe mental illness. *Psychiatric Services* 2001; **52**: 92–5.

24. Ito H, Shingai N, Yamazumi S, Sawa Y, Iwasaki S. Patient perceptions and satisfaction of psychiatric services at their discharge. *Seishin Shinkeigaku Zasshi* 1999; **101**: 138–47.

25. Ito H, Shingai N, Yamazumi S, Sawa Y, Iwasaki S. Characteristics of nonresponders to a patient satisfaction survey at discharge from psychiatric hospitals. *Psychiatric Services* 1999; **50**: 410–12.

26. Kjellin L. Compulsory psychiatric care in Sweden 1979–1993. Prevalence of committed patients, discharge rates and area variation. *Social Psychiatry and Psychiatric Epidemiology* 1997; **32**: 90–6.

27. Mahato C. Schizophrenia patients: duration of hospital care and returning to the self care ability. *Nursing Journal of India* 2000; **91**: 11–12.

28. Monden MA, Duindam JM. Conditional discharge of three committed psychiatric patients, the ambulatory practice. *Nederlands Tijdschrift voor Geneeskunde* 2000; **144**: 1548–51.

29. Saarento O, Oiesvold T, Sytema S, *et al*. The Nordic Comparative Study on Sectorized Psychiatry: continuity of care related to characteristics of the psychiatric services and the patients. *Social Psychiatry and Psychiatric Epidemiology* 1998; **33**: 521–7.

30. Bowers L, Jarrett M, Clark N, Kiyimba F, McFarlane L. Absconding: why patients leave. *Journal of Psychiatric Mental Health Nursing* 1999; **6**: 199–205.

31. Goldacre M, Seagroatt V, Hawton K. Suicide after discharge from psychiatric inpatient care. *Lancet* 1993; **342**: 283–6.

32. Geddes JR, Juszczak E. Period trends in rate of suicide in first 28 days after discharge from psychiatric hos-

pital in Scotland, 1968–92. *British Medical Journal* 1995; **311**: 357–60.

33. Aleby L, Shaw J, Amos T, *et al.* Suicide within 12 months of contact with mental health services: national clinical survey. *British Medical Journal* 1999; **318**: 1235–9.

34. Collins-Colon T. Do it yourself. Medication management for community based clients. *Journal of Psychosocial Nursing and Mental Health Services* 1990; **28**: 25–9.

35. Christ WR, Clarkin JF, Hull JW. A high-risk screen for psychiatric discharge planning. *Health and Social Work* 1994; **19**: 261–70.

36. Lloyd A, Horan W, Borgaro SR, Stokes JM, Pogge DL, Harvey PD. Predictors of medication compliance after hospital discharge in adolescent psychiatric patients. *Journal of Child and Adolescent Psychopharmacology* 1998; **8**: 133–41.

37. Tardiff K, Marzuk PM, Leon AC, Portera L. A prospective study of violence by psychiatric patients after hospital discharge. *Psychiatric Services* 1997; **48**: 678–81.

38. Flynn PM, McCann JT, Fairbank JA. Issues in the assessment of personality disorder and substance abuse using the Millon Clinical Multiaxial Inventory MCMI-II. *Journal of Clinical Psychology* 1995; **51**: 415–21.

39. Armitage S, Kavanagh K. Hospital nurses' percep-tions of discharge planning for medical patients. *Australian Journal of Advanced Nursing* 1996; **14**: 16–23.

40. McGihon NN. Psychiatric nursing for the 21st century. The PACED model. *Journal of Psycho-social Nursing and Mental Health Service* 1999; **37**: 22–7.

41. el-Guebaly N, Hodgins DC, Armstrong S, Addington J. Methodological and clinical challenges in evaluating treatment outcome of substance-related disorders and comorbidity. *Canadian Journal of Psychiatry* 1999; **44**: 264–70.

42. Carmin CN, Ownby RL. The relationship between discharge readiness inventory scales and the brief psychiatric rating scale. *Hospital and Community Psychiatry* 1994; **45**: 248–52.

43. Hall MJ, Kozak LJ. Long-stay patients in short-stay hospitals. *Advanced Data* 1993; **1**: 16.

44. Gantt AB, Cohen NL, Sainz A. Impediments to the discharge planning effort for psychiatric inpatients. *Social and Work Health Care* 1999; **29**: 1–14.

45. McDonagh MS, Smith DH, Goddard M. Measuring appropriate use of acute beds. A systematic review of methods and results. *Health Policy* 2000; **53**: 157–84.

46. Hall AD, Puri BK, Meehan K, Read JH. An investigation into the practice and benefits of statutory aftercare in an inner city psychiatric service. *International Journal of Clinical Practice* 1997; **51**: 355–8.

Chapter 56

THE NURSE'S ROLE IN THE ADMINISTRATION OF ECT

Joy Bray*

INTRODUCTION

The prescribing and administration of electroconvulsive therapy (ECT) remains one of the most controversial areas in psychiatry. To have an understanding of the nurse's role it is important to consider the arguments about ECT, relating these to the patient's wishes and the available evidence base.

> I know ECT works well for me when I am seriously depressed and unable to do anything for myself. I have a right to choose to have it. It is the only way I have of regaining myself and my life quickly when I am seriously depressed. If I don't have it I am unable to do anything for around 6 months – with ECT it is over in a few weeks. Without ECT I would have lost my job and most of the things I value in life.
>
> Woman – ECT in last 2 years

> The ECT affected my memory long term, has slowed down my thinking process and has damaged my ability to associate words and ideas. Because of this my speech is sometimes not as fluent as it was before I had ECT. I cannot recognize some of the faces of people I have

known for some time. My confidence and self-esteem are very low and the ECT treatment has contributed to this.
>
> Woman – ECT in last 2 years

These directly opposing statements are taken from a MIND survey of experiences of having ECT.[1] Some find it a life saving procedure and are grateful to be offered it, others find it degrading and distressing, leaving them with permanent side-effects, usually memory loss. Mental health professionals should be able to discuss the benefits and difficulties of any treatment with the person involved and their relatives or carers. However, ECT is a treatment which can be prescribed as an emergency in most countries, and administered *without* patient consent (at the time of writing, in the UK this is framed by the Mental Health Act [1983]). This can make the administration an ethically and emotionally difficult process.

This chapter will focus on the patient's experience and associated distress, rather than enter into the debate about ECT. The evidence base underpinning the administration of ECT will be considered, alongside contraindications and alternative treatments, and the key

---

*Joy Bray is Senior Lecturer at Homerton College, Cambridge, England. She has had past training in CBT, psychotherapy and groupwork and is clinically involved working with individuals in distress from psychosis. She works closely with an inpatient unit considering how to make the environment and experience positive for all involved.

issues around consent, and the procedure itself, will be discussed using available UK guidelines.

ECT AS TREATMENT

The Department of Health[2] has defined ECT as:

> ... a treatment involving the passage of an electric current across the brain. The treatment is only administered to an anaesthetized patient who has also been administered a muscle relaxant. The electric current induces seizure activity in the brain which is necessary for the therapeutic effect of treatment.

ECT is particularly indicated in very severe depression. Depression is probably best viewed as a syndrome rather than a single pathological entity. ECT is of specific value in the treatment of patients who display psychomotor retardation and/or depressive delusions or hallucinations. Those who are this severely depressed may refuse, or be unable, to eat and drink, with a consequent high risk of mortality; it may also be considered that the individual is at risk of committing suicide though they will be unable to act on this feeling when this depressed. ECT also has a limited use in the treatment of other disorders such as catatonia (where the person will be withdrawn and may seem to be in a stupor) and mania. It can be used when drug treatments have proved ineffective or are inadvisable (for example with depressed individuals who have a cardiac condition; in neuroleptic malignant syndrome and schizophrenia specifically where there are predominantly negative symptoms).[3]

Although one of the commonest reasons given for administering ECT is that it prevents suicide, this assumption can be challenged. On reviewing the literature, Challiner and Griffiths[4] were unable to definitively endorse this assumption and presented evidence to the contrary, that ECT does not necessarily prevent suicide in those with severe depression.[a]

An impression of the incidence of the treatment can be found in the Department of Health survey, January 1999 to March 1999, where 2800 patients received ECT treatment. Of these 900 were male and 1900 female, 44% of male patients and 36% of female patients receiving the treatment were 65 years and over. It should be noted that there is a preponderance of female patients prescribed ECT and those over 65 years of age.

Some patients will always choose ECT as a first-line treatment, citing that it has decreased a fear of having depression again and that it worked.[5] There is evidence, however, that up to one third of individuals experiencing ECT find it deeply and lastingly traumatic. It may exacerbate feelings of shame, failure and badness, which are already features of their depression. Many such people might wish to avoid the treatment if offered again. An apparently successful outcome may simply be indicative of compliance and powerlessness, allied to a fear of confiding one's true feelings to the staff.[6]

ECT: THE EVIDENCE BASE

Given its controversial status, patients need to be offered the opportunity to discuss their treatment with an informed nurse.

1   Patients must be given information on the nature and purpose of the treatment and any serious side-effects, though this need not be an exhaustive list of every possible risk.

2   They must be able to understand the nature and purpose of the treatment.

3   Their consent must be given without undue force, persuasion, or influence being bought to bear on them.[7, p.196]

A study found that nurses with a more positive response to ECT had a greater knowledge base in that area. It was also noted that knowledge of ECT in nurses is not adequate and needs some improvement.[8]

There are three areas of evidence to consider:

❑   The experience of individuals having ECT.
❑   The evidence suggesting the efficacy of ECT.
❑   Known side-effects.

MIND[9] and UKAN[10] (United Kingdom Advocacy Network) both published surveys of people's experience of receiving ECT. While the respondents' comments make difficult reading as individuals have found it emotionally and psychologically damaging, it must be noted that the research method (a distributed questionnaire) is more likely to access people who were either very satisfied or unsatisfied with treatment; these groups will have retained stronger memories and feelings, and therefore be more likely to respond to a questionnaire. Both positive and negative comments were accessed; however they were predominantly negative. These surveys showed that:

❑   Out of 418 respondents, depression was the most common diagnosis for recipients of ECT.
❑   34% of those given ECT most recently were not aware that they could refuse consent for treatment.
❑   15% had the opportunity to consult an independent advocate before making a decision.

---

[a] For a critical presentation of evidence arguing against ECT see Johnstone L. *Users and abusers of psychiatry*, 2nd edn. London: Routledge, 2001.

❑ 60.5% of those given ECT most recently were not (as far as they can remember) given any information about side-effects.

❑ 84% of respondents said they had experienced unwanted side-effects as a result of having ECT.

❑ In the short term 36% found the treatment helpful or very helpful and 27% unhelpful or damaging.

This highlights the need for better provision of information, the need to involve advocacy services, and to monitor side-effects more systematically. However the small numbers in the sample must be noted and the fact that elderly people were under-represented. This is important as the Department of Health has noted that elderly people (in particular women) are the most frequent recipients of ECT; this means that their experiences are not accessed and included.

When anticipating, or during the course of ECT, 32.5% felt hopeful that it would help them recover, but 45.5% recipients felt anxious. Without wishing to minimize the anxiety felt, it also needs to be recognized that anxiety is a normal feeling prior to anaesthesia where there is a lack of control and fear of the unknown. The attitude in ECT nursing care is moving towards that of general nursing, where it is recognized that information prior to anaesthesia is important and reduces anxiety.[11] In a review of the literature related to a fear of and objection to ECT it was noted that despite modifications in technique and education (there was no comment on the quality of this education) anxiety had not reduced over the years. The authors suggest that some patients gradually develop a pathological fear of ECT over the course of treatment, and this creates a significant obstacle to compliance. This clinical phenomenon was first described in the 1950s, but is still often unrecognized today.[12] This may lead the clinical team to underestimate the level of fear involved and therefore not work to minimize it or offer alternative treatments.[b]

The effectiveness of ECT

It has frequently been argued that there is little quality research on the benefits of ECT, specifically improvement in mental state. Many of the early studies, which 'proved' the efficacy of ECT, were methodologically flawed. Where ECT was compared to simulated ECT, double blind procedures were not employed. This meant that the patient assessor knew who *had*, and who *had not* received ECT, thus allowing for potential bias in assessment of recovery.

The frequently cited claim that ECT can reduce sui-

cide, was tested in a longitudinal study. The authors concluded that there was no evidence to support the belief that ECT prevents suicide in those with severe depression.[13] ECT does produce short-term improvements on depression rating scales for some people, but this is not sustained beyond 4 weeks.[14] However there is evidence indicating that depressed patients, who have not responded to anti-depressant treatment, recover if treated subsequently with ECT.[15] A fixed number of treatments should not be prescribed, as it is clear that patients can respond after only a few treatments. Instead, there should be a regular psychiatric assessment to monitor improvement.[16] The frequency of administration of ECT needs consideration. In a well-controlled trial the rate of response was significantly more rapid with ECT administered three times weekly, but was associated with more severe memory impairment. There has been a continued debate around the efficacy of unilateral (where electrodes are placed on one side of the head only) versus bilateral (placed on both sides). During the 1980s bilateral was strongly advocated as being more effective, and as having comparable resulting side-effects when compared to unilateral ECT; previously it was thought that unilateral minimized side-effects. However the Royal College of Psychiatrists have noted the variation in the ability of those administering ECT and in the machinery used. They now advise that the decision to use unilateral or bilateral electrode placement should be based on the appraisal of advantages and disadvantages for each patient. If unilateral ECT is given, the electrodes should be widely separated. Because the therapeutic equivalent of unilateral and bilateral depends on a high standard of administration, bilateral ECT is recommended where the expertise of those administering is in doubt. Twice weekly is an optimum schedule for bilateral ECT, unless clinical indications require the more rapid anti-depressant effect of three times weekly.[17]

Continuation of anti-depressant drug treatment is essential after successful ECT because nearly half the depressed patients who recover with ECT will relapse within 12 weeks without drug treatment. For all patients, the four months following treatment is the critical time for relapse.[18]

HOW ECT MIGHT WORK

Differing theoretical perspectives afford differing views of ECT.

❑ From a sociological perspective, mental illness is

[b] The Department of Health is currently funding a project to discover consumer perspectives on ECT, SURE (Service User Research Enterprise) is carrying out the work, and the researchers have all been users of mental health services. One of the aims of the work is to contribute to information being provided for patients in the future.

viewed as a social phenomenon, rather than biologically determined, and ECT is seen as effectively silencing people, thereby legitimizing the lack of attention paid to our malfunctioning society.[19]

❑ Social learning theory characterizes ECT acts as a *negative reinforcer* resembling early theories of punishment. Although this view is now largely discarded, some people obviously feel *as if* they are being punished or threatened.

❑ Although the therapeutic effect of ECT remains unclear – *how* it works – the seizure stimulated, is fundamental to the process. The apparent efficacy of chemically induced seizures suggests that electricity itself is not essential.[20]

It is suggested that the therapeutic action derives from the induction of a generalized seizure of adequate quality and duration. Short generalized, missed, focal or unilateral seizures have little or no therapeutic effect. If an ECT-induced seizure is to have a therapeutic effect, the stimulus given must induce seizure activity throughout the whole brain, which is a generalized seizure. These are associated with a variety of alterations in brain function for example, alterations in cerebral blood flow and metabolism, protein and other biosynthetic processes membrane and neurotransmitter function.[21]

Four weeks is the usual duration of the artificial euphoria that usually follows a closed-head injury. This may explain the therapeutic effect of ECT, though this also means recognizing that some brain damage is a consequence of ECT.[22] While it is generally accepted that ECT causes a certain amount of brain damage, the amount and severity is continuously debated. However the *definitive* therapeutic action of ECT remains unknown at present.

ECT: UNWANTED SIDE-EFFECTS

The severity and longevity of unwanted side-effects of ECT remains a contentious issue. A series of side-effects may occur immediately after treatment including headache, muscular aches, nausea, drowsiness, weakness and anorexia. In the first week, memory problems and headaches are the most prominent side-effects.[22] While there is continued professional debate around long-term memory loss, the current professional consensus is that there is no *irrefutable* evidence for long-term memory loss; it is considered that the valid and reliable scientific evidence is not there. However there are a multitude of patient narratives which evidence this but these do not have their base in scientific rigor and so it is difficult for some professional groups to consider these as credible evidence. Memory loss is not routinely tested for following the administration of ECT, and until this happens long-term memory loss will not be considered proven beyond doubt. However the evidence for short-term memory loss is recognized and acknowledged.[23]

Another expert opinion supports the view that ECT causes brain damage and that it irrefutably interferes with long-term memory. It has been argued that the degree of damage varies between individuals and that the key manifestation is memory loss. This is disturbing enough but there are probably other losses, such as the ability to think clearly or to learn new facts. There may also be cumulative memory loss. This may well not be more clearly identified since it is not routinely tested for by psychiatrists, before and after the administration of ECT.[24]

Patients have commented on and written about the effect of ECT on their long-term memory, making both sad and powerful reading. However their impact on the prescribing of ECT is unknown. The most commonly reported side-effects are headaches, drowsiness, confusion and loss of past memories. The most commonly reported permanent side-effects are memory loss and difficulty in concentrating. The following excerpts are chosen to demonstrate that as far as is known geographical location, gender and ethnicity have no bearing on the experience of side-effects.[25]

> I can remember very little of this year, after having ECT in September. I found once I came home I would meet people while out, knew them but could not place them or remember their names.
>
> Woman – Wales

> I found myself unable to play the guitar and sing songs and tunes I had been playing for 25 years.
>
> Man – Yorkshire

> Creativity, reading and things that I enjoyed and was patient in doing went down sharply.
>
> Pakistani woman – London

> I have long and short-term memory impairment, I have serious cognitive damage. I cannot do any work with figures, numbers mean nothing to me. I have great difficulty reading. I was a taxi driver for 20 years. Now I can only find my way if I have my carer present to give directions. I do not know my left from my right.
>
> Woman – Yorkshire

These extracts[25] do not provide a definitive argument against ECT, since the same publication includes many statements of support for the use of ECT. However, this does provide evidence that side-effects are a real, and very distressing problem for a proportion of patients. The persistent memory loss, which some individuals experience, has been related to the patient having chronic depressive symptoms, which can include impaired memory. While this is relevant it still disregards much of the evidence from patients and ensures the patient's experience is regularly undermined.

Mortality associated with ECT is thought to be similar to that of general anaesthesia in minor surgical procedures (approximately two deaths per 100,000 treatments). Despite the use of ECT for people with physical illnesses (which render them unsuitable for anti-depressant treatment) and the prevalence of use with elderly patients it is believed by many clinicians to carry a lower mortality rate than the use of anti-depressant drugs.[26] Johnstone argues against this and suggests that mortality is consistently under-reported.[27]

ALTERNATIVE TREATMENT

ECT is unsuitable for some patients because of an underlying medical condition. Others object to the treatment and so alternatives need to be considered. Cognitive behaviour therapy is rarely offered to older people, yet there is evidence that CBT in the physically healthy older adult is effective in decreasing depression, and treatment gains are maintained at follow-up.[28] The importance of psychological therapies, medication and bereavement counselling is acknowledged by the UK ECT Forum. Indeed they advocate the use of adjunct therapies stating that the positive effects of ECT are short-lived.[29]

Transcranial magnetic stimulation (TMS) is a relatively new treatment, involving the focal application of magnetic energy to the cerebral cortex, thus inducing small electrical currents. Subconvulsive repetitive TMS does not involve loss of consciousness, loss of memory or seizure and so avoids the difficulties around administering ECT and the available evidence suggests that the therapeutic effect is comparable.[30]

Finally there is considerable evidence showing that exposure to family and social disadvantage (particularly multiple) during childhood can predispose individuals to major depression in adulthood.[31] This is not to suggest that ECT is always inappropriate, but rather to consider the need for preventative methods which could enable this vulnerable population to live a more healthy life.

INFORMED CONSENT: THE ETHICAL DIMENSIONS OF ECT ADMINISTRATION

The legal framework of the relevant state or country frames the concept of informed consent. Professional guidelines exist for use in conjunction with the relevant mental health legislation, to enable best practice from clinicians.[32,33]

In the UK there are three routes by which a person may receive ECT:

1 **With their consent**. Consent implies that a person has been given the information about the proposed treatment necessary to make an informed decision. Even among patients with severe mental disorder, who may be considered most likely to benefit from ECT, the majority can make valid decisions about receiving it. Consent must be freely given and based on an adequate understanding, of the *purpose*, *nature* and *likely effects* and *risks* of treatment. This should include an indication of success rates and available alternatives. Consent should be for a specified number of treatments given during a stated period of time.[34] *Consent may, however, be withdrawn at any time.*

2 **Without consent under the Mental Health Act 1983**. In the period January to March 1999 in England 2800 patients received ECT treatment. 700 of these patients were formally detained while receiving the treatment, and of these 59% did not consent to treatment.[35] Where a patient cannot consent to ECT the proper course of action is to use the Mental Health Act 1983, Sections 2 and 3. Administration of ECT is covered by Part IV of the Mental Health Act, Section 58 ('treatments requiring the patient's consent or a second opinion') and 62 ('urgent treatment'). Consent to ECT should always be sought by the *Responsible Medical Officer* (usually the patient's medical consultant) and the patient may withdraw consent at any time. If the patient refuses or withdraws consent, a second medical opinion is sought, appointed by the Mental Health Act Commission, who will interview and assess the patient. In emergencies compulsory ECT may be given (under Section 62) without the second opinion safeguard if it is necessary either to save the patient's life, because their physical condition is so fragile, or prevent deterioration of such. In this case the Commission should be informed so that a second opinion may be provided as soon as possible.[36]

3 **Without consent under the Common law**. Where a person lacks the capacity to consent to treatment but is not detained under the Mental Health Act and has not refused treatment (for example a confused and depressed elderly person), ECT may be given without consent. In this situation doctors have the right to treat the person 'in their best interests' under common law. However, a second opinion from a consultant colleague is recommended, and the situation should be discussed with relatives.[37]

However, these safeguards appear, at times, to be disregarded. Some of the survey respondents noted above said that they had consented 'under duress' or had felt 'coerced'. A number said they had been threatened with the use of the Mental Health Act if they did not comply. Consequently, they felt pressured and lost the second opinion safeguard.[38] However, in a study comparing the views and outcomes of consenting and non-consenting patients receiving ECT, the outcomes in non-consenting patients were equivalent to those seen in consenting patients; more than 80% believed they had benefited from treatment. This does, of course, leave 20% believing they had not benefited.[39] The ECT survivors network (*ECT Anonymous*) suggests that informed consent isn't worth the paper its written on, unless the person can say no and still avoid the application of a 'section'.[40] The Mental Health Act aims to protect civil rights, yet it also gives almost total power, regarding decisions about treatment, to the medical profession, at the expense of the patient's autonomy. The Act operates within a medical model framework, giving precedence to the medical treatment of symptoms.[41] Alternatively, some individuals believe that they benefit from ECT, but are afraid to speak out as they fear negative reactions from other users and professionals who are vociferous opponents of ECT.[42] The role of advocates and advanced directives are central to the future resolution of this issue.

NURSES' DILEMMAS OVER ECT

As noted, ECT remains controversial. In some US states the treatment is banned. One of the most important ethical aspects of ECT is whether the therapeutic benefits outweigh the risks. Given that there is no conclusive evidence to identify ECT as the treatment of choice in major depression, each case needs individual assessment in the light of the most recent studies. This means that nurses have a responsibility to care for and support the patient during the whole process of deliberation and treatment. It can be argued that there are suitable alternatives to the prescribing of ECT; these include intensive nursing care, cognitive behaviour therapy and psychotherapy, which seem to be rarely considered. This is presumably because of the extra cost which would be incurred and also because the patient group most frequently prescribed ECT are elderly women who do not have a strong political voice. When the patient has had full information and freely consents to the treatment I would suggest that there is no dilemma, as we acquiesce to the patient's wishes. However if, having provided full information and having discussed any dilemmas with the patient and the family/carers, the patient still refuses consent, I would suggest that this wish be respected and the multidisciplinary team consider alternative treatment.

THE NURSING ROLE AND FUNCTIONS

The nurse's role in ECT involves three distinct but related areas:

- ❑ Preparation of the patient.
- ❑ Care during the procedure.
- ❑ Care following the procedure.

Although general principles may be outlined for each area, there is a need to individualize care through carrying out a comprehensive assessment,[43] using standardized assessment tools where relevant, within a nursing framework, such as the Tidal Model.[44]

An account of a patient's experience of ECT sets the scene for the overview of the procedure.

Case study 56.1: Richard's story

Richard is a man in his thirties who was given a diagnosis of schizophrenia 5½ years ago. He is a striking, vibrant man with an appealing, arresting voice and an obvious sense of humour.

When Richard was first prescribed clozapine this coincided with the beginning of a severe autoimmune illness. Richard had always had a depressive element to his schizophrenia. However he was prescribed ECT partly because the medical opinion was that continued administration of atypical antipsychotic medication constituted an unwarranted physical danger. His ECT was administered on an outpatient basis and he had two treatments out of the ten prescribed. When asked, 'What helped?' Richard said: 'The ECT nurse had been there for years, she was called Electric Annie. She was a real nurse, very caring but appropriately so. She was calming and reassuring, you felt you were the most important thing. This was important because the process itself is very scary. She had a generally friendly and reassuring manner, she said things like "Don't worry you won't know anything about it". But she was honest, and that was the most important thing. She said I'd have a stinking headache after and would feel quite unpleasant. And I did! Afterwards I got the king of all migraines. She made sure I got a cup of tea after (a hot one would have been nice) and later I got two paracetamol, which didn't touch the headache.

The worst thing was being wheeled on a trolley through the hospital. This hadn't been explained to me, and the anaesthetist was late and couldn't find the veins. But I don't remember a great deal. The nurse was very good with my mum as well. She came with me and the nurse calmed her down, as she was very apprehensive. My mum came because Caroline [long-term partner] wouldn't come. She was against me having it [ECT]. It's not good to do it without the consent of the nearest and dearest, it was so damaging for us. Caroline hasn't participated in any of my treatment since, which has been awful for me. It had a real impact'.

The treatment was stopped after two sessions because of the partner's fears and a different atypical anti-psychotic was commenced.

Key principles of the nurse's role in ECT

1 Ensuring that the psychological needs of patients and statutory requirements are met.

2 Monitoring the patient's physical well-being.

3 Assisting and supporting medical staff in the use of equipment.

4 Supporting and educating patients' relatives and significant others.

5 Supporting, guiding and educating all grades of nursing staff so as to facilitate improvements in ECT practice.[45, p.114]

Each mental health service should possess relevant practice and procedure guidelines, framed within state/national directives from relevant professional bodies. ECT should take place in a purpose built clinic within a hospital, with a waiting area, treatment clinic and *separate* lying recovery, and sitting recovery, areas. The *ECT Nurses Forum* states that good practice requires that the patient escort should always be a qualified nurse, who is known to the patient and is responsible for the person's follow-up care for up to four hours after treatment. ECT is an area of specialist practice and every ECT suite should have a specialist nurse co-ordinator who sees patients before treatment as well as in clinic. This nurse should carry out pre and post-treatment nursing assessments, monitor the patients progress and feed this back to the relevant clinical team.[46] Regrettably, clinical guidelines have, in the recent past, often been poorly implemented for whatever reason.[47]

Patient preparation

Psychological preparation

❑ Education of, and discussion with, patient and family/carer. This should be repeated as often as requested. Video and written information should be offered that might be viewed or read afterwards. Time should be made available to answer queries following this (fact sheets are available from e.g. RCP and RANZACP)[c]. The patient's anxiety can be overwhelming and will need to be understood within the context of a potentially threatening procedure. Best practice suggests that preparation be carried out by the patient's primary nurse.

❑ Many clinics offer educational and orientation visits to relatives/carers prior to treatment.

❑ Memory diaries can be employed as a way of helping the individual re-orientate themselves following treatment; these contain information which the patient finds meaningful and can contain current or old material. Developing the diary is work that the primary nurse can carry out as a collaborative effort.

Physical preparation

❑ Tests need to be done to ensure physical fitness prior to a general anaesthetic; chest X-ray; electrocardiogram (ECG); baseline electroencephalogram (EEG), blood count and erythrocyte sedimentation rate (ESR). (Cardiovascular complications are the major cause of death associated with ECT. Blood tests assess current health and consider any other relevant pathology.)

❑ Ensure the patient understands that they need to fast for 6 hours before the general anaesthetic (to prevent regurgitation and inhalation of undigested food during the anaesthesia). A low-fat meal is advised the evening before.

❑ Patients prescribed cardiac and antihypertensive drugs may take these with sips of water only.

Day of treatment

❑ Ensure that the patient has fasted.

❑ Property should be deposited for safe keeping (e.g. rings, necklaces).

❑ Loose, comfortable clothes should be worn, which can be readily opened at the front for monitoring equipment to be positioned (e.g. ECG leads).

❑ Spectacles may be worn, but not contact lenses.

❑ Hair must be clean and dry for optimal electrode contact, and hair ornaments removed to prevent contact with the electrodes.

❑ Nail varnish and make up should be removed, to allow monitoring of changes in colour, which may indicate cardiovascular functioning.

❑ Measure the patient's temperature, pulse, respiration rate and blood pressure to provide a baseline measure.

❑ Immediately prior to treatment ask the patient to visit the toilet to empty their bladder.

Outpatient preparation

❑ Patients should be encouraged to report to day surgery or the ECT clinic well before treatment commences, to ensure adequate psychological and physical preparation.

---

[c] Royal College of Psychiatrists. *The ECT handbook*. London: RCP. 'A factsheet for you and your family', page 103. The Royal Australian and New Zealand College of Psychiatrists. *New Public Information Statement – Electroconculsive Therapy Explained*. http://www.ranzcp.org/statements/other/ect.htm

- ❏ Patients are advised how long they will be in clinic and are asked to be accompanied by a relative/friend and not to return to an empty house.
- ❏ Patients advised to avoid alcohol or driving for the rest of the day.
- ❏ If the patient is unaccompanied the clinic manager is to ensure that he/she does not leave the clinic until fully recovered and does not drive home.

The escort nurse may use a checklist to ensure preparation is complete. The key role is to act as the patient's advocate, offering support and reassurance, ensuring that the patient's privacy and dignity are maintained and relaying the patient's anxieties, if expressed, to the core team. Some patients benefit from being accompanied by a relative/friend throughout treatment. If clinic staff consider that the patient will benefit, they may remain present throughout all treatment stages. The patient may request information at any time, and this is provided to reduce anxiety. The patient may withdraw consent at any time before anaesthesia commences.

Care during the procedure

1. The patient is accompanied from the waiting area into the ECT suite and introduced to the members of the ECT team, and their roles explained if needed.
2. The patient removes footwear and any aids (false teeth, spectacles, hearing aid etc.).
3. The treatment nurse may place cardiac monitoring leads on the patient's chest. EEG leads may be positioned – some clinics routinely use EEG tracings to monitor the seizure this is good practice as it ensures that a generalized seizure has occurred and allows accurate timing of the seizure. A pulse oximeter is clipped to the patient's finger to monitor oxygen saturation. Blood pressure is monitored via an automatic cuff.
4. Patients are encouraged to lie on their back with the friend/carer or primary nurse within easy reach.
5. The clinic nurse assists the anaesthetist and psychiatrist and the primary nurse attends to support the patient.
6. The anaesthetist inserts a peripheral venus line to deliver the muscle relaxant (usually suxmethonium chloride) and the intravenous anaesthetic (usually propofol or thiopentone sodium). The drug is titrated to the patient's age, weight and physical condition.
7. As the muscle relaxant takes effect the anaesthetist provides oxygen (as the muscles assisting respiration are temporarily paralysed) by mask using positive pressure ventilation.
8. A bite block may be inserted as the patients jaw muscles are directly stimulated in ECT and may clench.[48]
9. The treating psychiatrist is responsible for the electrical stimulation and seizure monitoring. The electrical stimulation causes a brief generalized seizure, twitching of the fingers and toes may be observed. Limbs will need supporting only if the seizure is exceptionally brisk. A seizure lasting 30–60 seconds is generally considered adequate. Characteristic EEG changes will be observed and monitored by the treating clinician. A seizure longer than 120 seconds should be terminated using a benzodiazepine.
10. Anaesthetic staff will continuously ventilate the patient with pure oxygen until he/she is able to breathe spontaneously.
11. Vital signs should be monitored after the treatment and compared to baseline.

Care after the procedure

Responsibility for this phase is with a nurse competent in recovery techniques.

- ❏ The patient is placed in the three quarter prone recovery position and a clear airway maintained.
- ❏ A nurse remains with the patient throughout the recovery stage. TPR and B/P are monitored every 15 minutes.
- ❏ People take differing times to recover and should not be rushed. The nurse should provide frequent reassurance and reorientation, repeating the information until the patient can remember. The relative or friend may wish to take this role. Confusion may be an unwanted effect. The primary nurse may be able to use material from the memory diary to help orientation. It is important to document the presence of confusion.
- ❏ Patients who are fully conscious and responsive to verbal commands and willing to move should be accompanied to a quiet area in the ECT suite and given refreshment, an important consideration for comfort and rehydration.
- ❏ The patient should be asked if there are any unwanted effects such as headache or nausea (the patient may not always say so, spontaneously). Prescribed medication should be administered and checked for efficacy.
- ❏ Accompany an inpatient back to their ward where

they may well want to rest. The primary nurse will be responsible for monitoring their condition for a reasonable interval (usually 4 hours) following their return.

- ❑ Night staff will continue to observe the patient the night following treatment.
- ❑ The patient may well want to discuss their experience of treatment, issues, which were disturbing, and also what was helpful, this information can usefully be integrated into the care plan.
- ❑ Continued monitoring and discussion of side-effects is important and may indicate a need to alter prescribed treatment, e.g. increased dosage of analgesia.
- ❑ An assessment of mental state between treatments is essential to monitor improvement or otherwise, standardized assessment tools are used such as the Beck Depression Inventory.

CONCLUSION

The administration of ECT continues to be a controversial and emotionally difficult area of nursing care, although if the underpinning philosophy of care ensures a collaborative approach to the individual and their relatives/carers the principal is sound and has the potential to aid effective care. However ECT does not exert a therapeutic effect for all patients, therefore the prescribing of ECT and its administration warrants careful consideration and monitoring. Poor practice in the area of administration has been evident in systematic audits carried out in the UK; it is important that nurses involved in the administration of ECT have a specific training and are professionally accountable for their actions. An aspect of care, which seems to be poorly performed, is that of providing the person and family/carer with information, about both the procedure and possible side-effects. It is vital that any nurse involved with the administration of ECT is well-educated in all aspects of the treatment. By involving independent advocates throughout the process, any felt lack of information can be rectified and the individual will be able to give a true informed consent. Working collaboratively means that individuals who choose, and may request ECT, should be enabled throughout the process. It seems an anachronism that in the 21st century we are relying on an individual to almost choose their treatment rather than making the judgement from a recognized empirical evidence base. However it can be argued that offering a person an informed choice for treatment with ECT, alongside the notion that alternative effective treatments are equally available and offered in an unbiased way, is a reasonable basis for care.

REFERENCES

1. Pedler M. *Shock treatment, a survey of people's experiences of electro-convulsive therapy.* London: MIND, March 2001.
2. Department of Health. *Statistical Bulletin. Electroconvulsive therapy: survey covering the period from January 1999 to March 1999, England.* London: Department of Health, 1999.
3. Royal College of Psychiatrists. *The ECT handbook.* London: Royal College of Psychiatrists, 1995. [New edition published February 2002.]
4. Challiner V, Griffiths L. Electroconvulsive therapy; a review of the literature. *Journal of Psychiatric and Mental Health Nursing* 2000; **7**: 191–8.
5. Perkins R. My three psychiatric careers. In: Barker P, Campbell P, Davidson B (eds). *From the ashes of experience.* London: Whurr Publishers, 1999.
6. Johnstone L. Adverse psychological effects of ECT. *Journal of Mental Health* 1999; **8**(1): 69–85.
7. Johnstone L. *Users and abusers of psychiatry*, 2nd edn. London: Routledge.
8. Gass JP. The knowledge and attitudes of mental health nurses to electro-convulsive therapy. *Journal of Advanced Nursing* 1998: **27**: 83–90.
9. Pedler *op. cit.* (2001).
10. United Kingdom Advocacy Network. Ukan's national user survey. *Openmind* 78 Dec 1995/Jan 1996.
11. Heide Baldwin. Personal communication, July 2001. Chair of the ECT Nurses' Forum, UK.
12. Fox HA. Patients' fear of and objection to electroconvulsive therapy. *Hospital and Community Psychiatry* 1993; **44**(4): 357–60.
13. Milstein V, Small JG, Small IF, Green GE. Does ECT prevent suicide? *Convulsive Therapy* 1986; **2**: 3–6.
14. Brandon S, Cowley P, McDonald C, Neville P, Palmer R, Wellstood-Eason S. Electroconvulsive therapy: results in depressive illness from the Leicestershire trial. *British Medical Journal* 1985; **288**: 22–5.
15. Prudic J, Sackeim H, Devanand DP. Medication resistance and clinical response to electroconvulsive therapy. *Psychiatry Research* 1990; **31**: 287–96.
16. Rodger CR, Scott AIF, Whalley LJ. Is there a delay in the onset of the anti-depressant effect of electroconvulsive therapy? *British Journal of Psychiatry* 1994; **164**: 106–9.
17. Shapira B, Tubi N, Drexler H, Lidsky D, Calev A, Lerer B. Cost and benefit in the choice of ECT schedule. *British Journal of Psychiatry* 1998; **172**: 44–8.
18. Royal College of Psychiatrists *op. cit.*, 1995.
19. Wallcraft J. ECT: effective, but for whom? *Openmind* 1993; **62**: 14.
20. Fitzsimmons LM, Mayer R. Soaring beyond the

cuckoo's nest: health care reform and ECT. *Journal of Psycho-social Nursing* 1995; **33**: 10–13.

21. Royal College of Psychiatrists *op. cit.*, 1995.

22. Breggin P. *Brain disabling treatments in psychiatry.* New York: Springer, 1997.

23. Calev A, Gaudino E, Squires N, Zervas I, Fink M. ECT and non-memory cognition: a review. *British Journal of Clinical Psychology* 1995; **34**: 505–15.

24. Sterling P. *Written testimony to the New York State Assembly.* May 31st 2001. ukan@can-online.org.uk

25. Pedler *op. cit.*, March 2001.

26. Royal College of Psychiatrists *op. cit.*, 1995.

27. Johnstone L. *op. cit.*, 2001.

28. Heffern WA. Psychopharmacological and electro-convulsive treatment of anxiety and depression in the elderly. *Journal of Psychiatric and Mental health Nursing* 2000; **7**: 199–204.

29. Baldwin H. Personnel communication *op. cit.*, 2001.

30. The Royal Australian and New Zealand College of Psychiatrists. *College Statement – Electroconvulsive Therapy Explained.* August 2001 – www.ranzcp.org/statements/ps/ps40.htm

31. Sadowski H, Ugarte B, Kolvin I, Kaplan C, Barnes J. Early life family disadvantages and major depression in adulthood. *British Journal of Psychiatry* 1999; **174**: 112–20.

32. The Royal Australian and New Zealand College of Psychiatrists *op. cit.*, 2001.

33. Royal College of Psychiatrists *op. cit.*, 1995.

34. Pippard J, Taylor P. ECT, the law and consent to treatment. In: Freeman CP (ed.) *The ECT handbook.* London: Royal College of Psychiatrists, 1995.

35. Department of Health *op. cit.*, 1999.

36. Department of Health and the Welsh Office. *Code of Practice Mental Health Act 1983.* London: HMSO, 1993.

37. Pippard J, Taylor P. *op. cit.*, 1995.

38. Pedler *op. cit.*, 2001.

39. Wheeldon TJ, Robertson C, Eagles JM, Reid IC. The views and outcomes of consenting and non-consenting patients receiving ECT. *Psychological Medicine* 1999; **29**(1): 221–3.

40. Openmind. UKAN's national user survey. Openmind 78. Dec 1995–Jan 1996.

41. McCarthy J. Electro-convulsive therapy: can compulsory treatment ever be ethical? *Mental Health Care* May 1999; **2**(9): 308–9.

42. Mahony C. Sparks still fly. *Nursing Times* 2000; **96**(5).

43. Barker PJ. *Assessment in psychiatric and mental health nursing.* Cheltenham: Stanley Thornes, 1997.

44. Barker PJ. *The Tidal Model.* University of Newcastle, 2000.

45. Halsall SM, Lock T, Atkinson A. Nursing guidelines for ECT. In: Freeman (ed.) *The ECT Handbook.* London: Royal College of Psychiatrists, 1995.

46. Baldwin H. Personal communication *op. cit.*, 2001.

47. Duffett R, Lelliot P. Auditing electroconvulsive therapy: the third cycle. *British Journal of Psychiatry* 1998; **172**: 401–5.

48. Stuart GW, Laraia M. *Stuart and Sundeen's principals and practice of psychiatric nursing,* 6th edn. Missouri: Mosby.

Chapter 57

MENTAL HEALTH PROMOTION

Judy Boxer*

All health and social policy is significant in the realm of mental health promotion. Health promotion is a synergy between health education and healthy public policy. The prevention of mental illness and the promotion of mental health are only possible if environmental, fiscal, economic and social policies are in place to support the basic foundations for health. Whether they relate to jobs, training, accommodation or equal opportunities, they are all vital parts of a mentally healthy society. They influence the foundations for health and ultimately its promotion.[1]

RATIONALE

At the start of this new millennium some of the ideas and vision I have held for so long do now seem to have materialized into reality, namely into a coherent strategy defined by the current government and a clearer plan and timetable to work toward.[2] How students learn about mental health promotion is vital if this approach is to maintain the profile it deserves in mental health training. Here I intend to identify why this is and what has been achieved to date. There are general themes that need to be considered and are essential for practitioners to address. These should form the core of a mental health worker's competence and be clearly identified in each stage of the process of care by all mental health staff.

KEY THEMES AND DEFINITIONS

- ❑ What constitutes 'good' mental health or well-being?
- ❑ What is the International/European and National perspective on mental health promotion?
- ❑ What are the costs and benefits of mental health promotion for practitioners?
- ❑ How best can practitioners be included in evaluating strategic approaches and incorporate them in to service delivery?

*Judy Boxer is a Senior Lecturer in the School of Health and Social Care, Sheffield Hallam University, England

- How does a vision of mental health promotion survive the journey from policy to practice?
- What are the resource implications?
- How can service-users be more involved in mental health promotion?
- Whose responsibility is it to co-ordinate action planning for mental health promotion at Trust or local authority level?
- How do educationalists support students in identifying the relevance of theory to practice?
- Does mental health promotion require both generic and specialist skills and are these skills being developed in both higher education and the range of practice settings?

Key definitions

Several definitions of mental health promotion exist, underpinned by theoretical analysis and debate and evidence from practice.[3] Although some are identified here, readers need to bear in mind that however helpful definitions are as a starting point for understanding they are also 'value loaded'.[4] They reflect the philosophy and practice of prevention, education and health promotion; similarly, the choice of a mental health promotion definition will reflect the focus of personal, professional style and influence the choice of intervention (see Fig. 57.1).

Mental health promotion aims to enable people to manage life events, both predictable and unpredictable, by increasing self-esteem and a sense of well-being. To achieve this through working with individuals, groups and communities to improve life skills and quality of life as well as trying to influence the social, economic and environmental factors that can have an impact on mental health[5]

Mental health promotion involves any action to enhance the mental well-being of individuals, families, organizations or communities[2]

Mental health promotion is developing positive mental health both for, and with, the community in general and individuals who may have mental health problems. It includes self-help, service provision and organizational skills. The concept of mental health promotion recognizes that an individual's mental health is inextricably linked to their relationship with others, their lifestyle, environmental factors and the degree of power they can exert over their lives[1]

FIGURE 57.1

HISTORICAL OVERVIEW

The historical development of mental health promotion has over the years been piecemeal and limited in any clear national strategy of what constitutes mental health and how to maintain it in a society that places innumerable pressures on individuals in all aspect of our lives. Mental health promotion has clear links with public health concerns, such as the environment we live in, with poverty, inequality and all those pressures that are both seen and felt by all of us throughout the life cycle. The experience of oppression we know dampens the spirit and psyche and can lead to major mental health problems at any stage of life. There are a number of examples of 'good practice' in adult, older adult and children's mental health services as to how mental health promotion can challenge and empower service users in addressing the link to oppression and mental illness.[6]

The problem has been how to synthesize some very complex and abstract ideas and at the same time remain practical. In the past mental health students have been disadvantaged by a lack of knowledge of the subject by both educationalists and practitioners. It must be remembered that mental health promotion is also one aspect of general health promotion and prevention.[7,8] In the UK the Health of the Nation[9] first identified the need to tackle major public health issues like coronary heart disease and accidents as well as mental illness, through health promotion. The emphasis on 'solving' the problems of mental illness has led to a range of public health approaches, which can be identified, from the late 19th century to the present day (Table 57.1).

From the days of the earliest public health movements, the prevention of ill-health and the promotion of

TABLE 57.1

ACTIVITY	FOCUS
Late 19th century Public Health Acts and Medical Officers of Health	Environmental issues
Early 20th century Immunization and family planning	Personal preventive medicine
World War II Hospital and treatment services	Medical and drug intervention
Present day Social and economic determinants of health	Healthy public policy

positive health was realized by social and environmental policy changes not simply medical advances or interventions. Inter-agency working is a core aspect of mental health practice and those interested in mental health promoting activities need to acquire knowledge and understanding of key government initiatives that tackle health and social inequality, such as Health Action Zones and New Deal for Communities. The requirements of individual practice will be summarized later. Historically the problem with agreeing a comprehensive definition of health has been widely discussed. As mental and physical health is inter-related, we need to examine these concepts further. Approaches to health education and health promotion have discrete features, which Naidoo and Wills[10] identified as:

❑ medical or preventive;
❑ involving behaviour change;
❑ educational;
❑ empowerment; and
❑ social change.

EXISTING MODELS OF HEALTH PROMOTION

The following diagrams (Figs 57.2, 57.3 and Table 57.2) illustrate models of health promotion that represent stepping-stones to clearly identifying a useful approach to promoting mental health.

These illustrate ways that individuals and countries, have tried to develop an understanding of the context of mental health in different parts of the world, and to be proactive in the information people can access about the

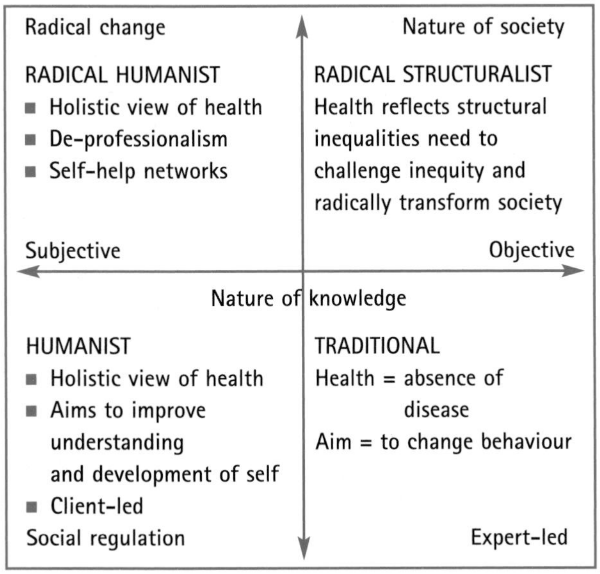

subject. The balance between a medical and social paradigm is a desired outcome as to how different countries tackle mental health problems as part of a wider framework of health and social care delivery.[11]

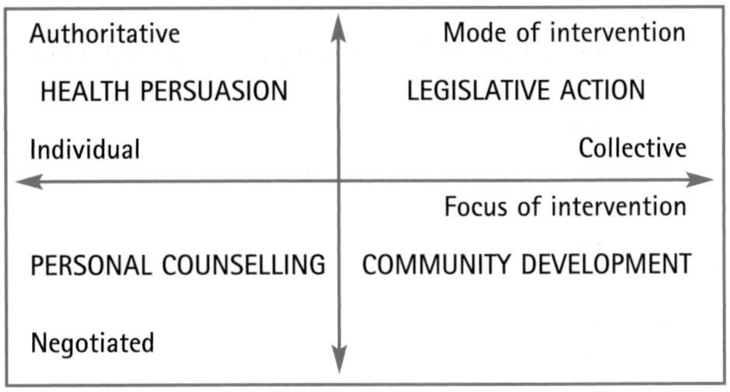

FIGURE 57.3

TABLE 57.2

DISEASE MANAGEMENT
■ Curative services
■ Management services
■ Caring services

DISEASE PREVENTION
■ Preventive services
■ Medical services
■ Behaviour change

HEALTH EDUCATION
■ Agenda setting
■ Empowering and support
■ Information flow

POLITICS OF HEALTH
■ Social actions
■ Policy development
■ Economic and fiscal policy

WORLD HEALTH APPROACHES TO MENTAL HEALTH PROMOTION

Because good health depends on so many different factors, many sectors need to be involved in health promotion. The World Health Organization WHO[12] identified five objectives, which form the basis for improving mental and physical health:

❑ Build healthy public policy.
❑ Create supportive environments.
❑ Strengthen community action.
❑ Develop personal skills.
❑ Re-orient health services.

To achieve these objectives and effectively improve the health of the population many organizations need to work together. While health and social services have an

FIGURE 57.2 Four paradigms of health promotion. (adapted from Caplan and Holland, 1990[30])

important role to play, their work is most effective when complemented by other sectors such as education, recreation, and environment, central and local government, commerce, industry and the non-statutory and voluntary sectors. Social integration and support are also important, so the involvement of community organizations and individual members of local communities is vital. Health is understood in a holistic sense, as defined by the World Health Organization in 1948:

'Health is a state of complete physical, social and mental well-being, and not merely the absence of disease or infirmity. Within the context of health promotion, health has been considered less as an abstract state and more as a means to an end that can be expressed in functional terms; as a resource which permits people to lead an individually, socially and economically productive life. Health is a resource for everyday life, not the object of living. It is a positive concept emphasizing social and personal resources as well as physical capabilities'.[10]

A UK report on mental health[9] identified more comprehensively how the 'community' is a resource that might stimulate change and deliver public health policy. The WHO places great importance on the community as an important resource and setting for tackling the causes and effects of mental health problems. This ranges from self-help and mutual aid, through lobbying for changes in mental health care and resources, carrying out educational activities, and participating in the monitoring and evaluation of care, to advocacy to change attitudes and reduce stigma. Consumer groups have emerged as a powerful, vocal and active force, often dissatisfied with the established provision of care and treatment. These groups have been instrumental in reforming mental health.[10]

The WHO places mental health in as much a social as a medical context and recognizes that successful health and mental health promotion generally involves change at a number of levels. This includes individuals and the family, organizations, communities and society. This should be translated at the macrogovernmental level to policy and action designed to actively support the right of all citizens to good health. More recently, health promoters have come to perceive health in socioecological terms, recognizing the fundamental link between health and conditions in economic, physical, social and cultural environments. Policy makers are beginning to look beyond the traditional health care illness oriented system to improve population health, in recognition that in addition to biological factors, health is also determined by external factors such as poverty, housing, environment and social support.

Given the social context of mental health it is useful to examine the range of new social regeneration initiatives currently being implemented. These can contribute significantly to mental health promotion. They also offer

practitioners new cross discipline resources, models and methodologies and as part of this a whole new partnership approach with local people and mental health service users. This new 'regeneration' context will be explored further.

MENTAL HEALTH PROMOTION POLICY OVERVIEW

> Mental health policy is dominated by a value system torn between individual consumerism and social structural change. This is borne out in the tensions of mental health policy that is based on degrees of social control while at the same time advocating policy for independence and empowerment.[1]

Policy developments of mental health have largely been dominated by a medical paradigm. The relationship between mental illness and social problems such as deprivation has not fully been acknowledged and a lack of vision has all too often fostered a divide between inpatient and community provision in its widest sense. However, the inclusion of mental health service users is at the heart of key policy initiatives and is clearly identified in the UK's National Service Framework for Mental Health,[14] Older Adults[15] and Making it Happen.[2] Figure 57.4 highlights the criteria for health promotion and provides an example relevant to mental health.

STRATEGY AND MENTAL HEALTH PROMOTION

Any successful strategy requires the necessary building blocks. A strategic approach concerns itself with purpose, and intentions to act, as well as being the plan itself. Such an evolving process may have very broad aims, as identified in the NHS Plan[14] or be locally determined by a campaign at local neighbourhood level. From a mental health perspective, identified themes act as a blueprint for action.[16] The example in Table 57.3 takes into account recent UK Government strategic thinking.

Here I offer a brief overview of supporting documents related specifically to mental health promotion, which show the transition from government approaches such as Key Area Handbook: Mental Illness[17] to the latest document, Making it Happen.[2]

The aim of the Key Area Handbook – Mental Illness, was to identify strategic objectives at individual, group and agency level by:

❑ Reducing the incidence of mental illness and suicide by the ability to cope in stressful situations.

Approach	Aims	Methods	Worker/client relationship
Medical	To identify those at risk from disease	Primary health care (detection of depression)	Tends to be expert led with more passive, conforming client
Behaviour change	To encourage individuals to take responsibility for their own health	Persuasion through one to one advice Information, e.g. medication and compliance	Expert led Dependent client Maybe victim-blaming culture
Educational	Increase knowledge and skills about healthy lifestyles	Information Explanation of attitudes through small groupwork Development of skills, e.g. post-natal depression group	May also be expert led May also involve client in negotiation or partnership
Empowerment	To work with clients or communities to meet perceived needs	Advocacy Negotiation/Networking Facilitation – service-user led initiative, e.g. User-focused monitoring	Health promoter as facilitator Service-user empowerment
Social change	To address inequalities in health based on factors such as race, gender, class and geography	Development of organizational policy, e.g. PALS Legislation, e.g. financial entitlement for user involvement activities	Entails social regulation and requires top down as well as bottom up approaches

FIGURE 57.4 Relevance to mental health promotion. (adapted from McCulloch and Boxer[13])

❏ Countering fear, ignorance and stigma about mental illness and creating a more positive social climate in which it becomes more acceptable to talk about feelings, emotions and problems. It is also to seek help without fear of labelling or feeling a failure.

❏ Preventing the deterioration of an existing mental illness.

❏ Improving the quality of life of people with long-standing, recurrent or acute mental health problems. This includes family and friends.

❏ Maintaining and improving social functioning.

The main thrust of the policy placed a great onus on both practitioners and service users to identify medium to long-term strategies that focused on vulnerable people at risk of social isolation or exclusion, emphasizing groups with mental illness. Given the relative neglect of the mental health of the population as a whole, other measures were necessary. Tackling the problem of mental illness as a public health issue was recognized more clearly in another Department of Health publication[18] and made clear a range of interventions that could form an action plan for mental health promotion as a public issue rather than a private one (Table 57.4).

TABLE 57.3 Mental health themes that help determine strategy

- **A rationale:** Background information giving the reasons for producing a mental health strategy, e.g. Health improvement

- **An analysis of needs:** Can be both quantitative and qualitative with an increased emphasis required on the felt experience of service users, e.g. National Service Framework for Mental Health

- **Stocktaking:** The context in which current services, support and activity in the mental health field takes place. This involves quality assurance mechanisms such as clinical audit and governance, e.g. Making it Happen

- **Philosophy and principles:** The values and principles upon which the strategy is based

- **Aims:** What is it that those producing the strategy are trying to do?

- **Actions, activities and methods:** How the aims can be achieved, e.g. Problem Tree, Making it Happen

- **Measurements and targets:** Monitoring and evaluation on achieving aims

- **Dissemination and implementation:** Gaining agreement, ownership, and responding to views and comments of individuals, groups and organizations. An implementation process for a strategy may also include a costed operational plan for funding or re-allocating funding to achieve the strategy's aim

TABLE 57.4

- Community participation
- Health information
- Community transport
- Welfare benefit provision within health settings
- Social support
- Use of media
- Service specifications for inter-agency work by health promotion units
- Targeting of health promotion in settings
- Multiple settings community-based health promotion

REGENERATION AND MENTAL HEALTH PROMOTION

Health and mental health policy

Repper[19] offered a comprehensive summary of mental health policy development from the 1950s to the present in an analysis of social inclusion and mental health. She defines a pattern of deinstitutionalization in the 1960s to the current 'plethora of policy and recommendations' in response to the community care agenda of the 1970s and 1980s.

In the last decade health policy has shifted from experimentation with market forces back to a rediscovery of inequalities and poverty. The previous Conservative administration set up a contractual framework of purchasers and providers to secure health improvement. With it came a national health strategy, 'Our Healthier Nation' with long-term targets for key illness areas including mental health.[20] The new Labour administration has reaffirmed the principles of the NHS seeking to increase investment and structural change. Recognizing that the root causes of ill health are multifactorial they have seen health service provision as one of many services and interventions for public health improvement. This has culminated in a range of regeneration and urban renewal policy relevant to mental health.

Over the last several years the Government has launched a range of area-based initiatives to help tackle social exclusion and reduce inequalities. Each initiative has specific objectives relating to education, health, employment, crime prevention, urban regeneration and wider social well-being. They also contain other common characteristics. These include: a focus on areas and communities where there is a need for priority action; support for innovative approaches; strong local involvement; new partnerships; flexibility and responsiveness in public programmes.

For example, the three main regeneration policies using an Action Zone approach – focusing on a specific geographical area – aim to intervene at several levels. At the individual level in terms of employment Action Zones, at the community or organization level for Health Action Zones, at a service or strategic level for Health Action Zones. The New Deal for Communities Initiative includes many of the aims of the specific action zones to deliver improvements at a neighbourhood level. This is directly comparable with a mental health promotion strategy that aims to promote public mental health at all levels in society.

Public health: mental health

> The opportunity now exists to make the structural changes that will sustain the momentum for the new public health initiative ... Yet all this laudable activity still assumes that 'public health' is essentially a professional activity, doing things to people's health. But in the new information age it is the public themselves who will drive the agenda. The one thing that will sustain the momentum is providing open access to individuals to comparative information about their own health, environment, and health care.[2]

MAKING IT HAPPEN: A GUIDE TO DELIVERING MENTAL HEALTH PROMOTION (DOH, 2001)

The definition of mental health promotion in this document can only be used as a base line for the requirements of mental health promotion. This key document outlines the main ways that people can be supported, who are trying to promote mental health as well as providing guidelines for the implementation of the National Service Framework for Mental Health: Standard One (NSF). There are case studies and practice objectives to support initiatives in all parts of the country and some of these will be identified later. The NSF requires effective working between health and social services and there is a clear aim and process to meeting Standard One (Table 57.5).

The shift in emphasis back to public mental health is being identified in a much more comprehensive way and comes at a time when other policy documents outline key strategic approaches to this problem.[21] In 'Making it Happen' a model has been used,[22] (Table 57.6) previously identified by Whitehead.[3]

These four levels have now been condensed to three (see Table 57.7) and each one is relevant to individuals at risk, vulnerable groups in society, people with mental health problems and the whole population. The Commonwealth Department of Health and Aged Care identify five key areas to consider in terms of these key targets: individual factors; family factors; school context; life-events and situations; and community and cultural factors. There is a need to identify expected outcomes and what the benefits of mental health promotion are at a macro level (Table 57.8)[2].

⌨ TABLE 57.5 Standard One NSF[14]

Aim

To ensure health and social services promote mental health and reduce the discrimination and social exclusion associated with mental health problems.

Health and social service should:

- Promote health for all, working with individuals and communities.
- Combat discrimination against individuals and groups with mental health problems, and promote their social inclusion.

Meeting Standard One will require action across whole populations, as well as programmes for individuals at risk.

Performance will be assessed nationally by improvements in the psychological health of the population, measured by the National Psychiatric Morbidity Survey and by a reduction in suicide rates. At local level health improvement programmes (HimPs) should include evidence of action to:

- Combat discrimination against the social exclusion of people with mental health problems.
- Promote mental health in schools, workplaces and neighbourhoods; for individuals at risk; and for groups who are most vulnerable.

⌨ TABLE 57.6

- Strengthening individuals
- Strengthening communities
- Improving access to essential facilities and services
- Encouraging macroeconomic and cultural change

⌨ TABLE 57.7

- **Strengthening individuals:** or increasing emotional resilience through interventions designed to promote self-esteem, life and coping skills, e.g. communicating, negotiating and parenting skills.
- **Strengthening communities:** this involves increasing social inclusion and participation, improving neighbourhood environments, developing health and social services which support mental health, anti-bullying strategies at school, workplace health, community safety, childcare and self-help networks.
- **Reducing structural barriers to mental health:** through initiatives to reduce discrimination and inequalities and to promote access to education, meaningful employment, housing and services and support for those who are vulnerable.

⌨ TABLE 57.8

STRATEGY

- Agreeing a vision and setting aims and objective

What does the strategy hope to achieve?

- Mapping existing initiative

Identifying gaps and duplication

- Identifying key settings and target group

Local needs assessment to agree key settings and target groups

- Making the links with policy initiatives with supporting goals

For example, National strategy for neighbourhood renewal, health and safety Executive's securing health together, mental health information strategy, Sure Start, Lifelong Learning

- Identifying key stakeholders

Whose commitment will be essential to the delivery of the strategy?

How will key stakeholders be involved/consulted?

What steps will be taken to involve users, carers and local communities?

- Selecting interventions

What are the chosen interventions, who are they targeting, in which settings?

- Finding the evidence to support the approach taken

What strength of evidence is available to support the interventions selected?

- Establishing indicators of progress

What kind of indicators will demonstrate progress?

- Building in evaluation

How will the interventions/different components be evaluated?

How will the overall strategy be evaluated?

- Identifying staffing and resource implications

Does the present workforce (across all sectors) have the capacity to deliver the strategy?

Have any skills/training/capacity development needs been identified?

How will the workforce/skills gaps be addressed?

Implementing policy: whose responsibility?

Key elements of 'Making it Happen' provide practical advice but something more is needed to make sure that at local level information is co-ordinated and easily available to all. The Mental Health Promotion Project is one of a number of projects linked to the Mental Health Task force with a key objective being to help support the implementation of the NSF and the NHS Plan. By early 2002 Trusts and local authorities were required to develop and agree evidence-based mental health promotion strategy based on local need. Local Implementation Teams have to have in place a self-assessment framework with criteria that can be used to judge whether services have met targets and outcomes. An example of this is shown in Table 57.9.

TABLE 57.9

- Be based on an assessment of local needs to identify key settings and target groups
- Demonstrate a clear rationale for selected interventions which are based on the evidence or which, through their implementation, can add to the evidence base
- Include action to reduce discrimination against people with mental health problems
- Show evidence of links to mainstream community development initiatives to promote social inclusion, such as neighbourhood renewal, education action zones, etc.

Developing your competence and skills in mental health promotion

The following myths have been identified by people working in the field and former students who have, until recently been limited in the availability of material on the subject. The responses show positive ways in which practice could be enhanced. The Internet is a focal point for resources about mental health and illness. However, it can be difficult to know how to access the information about mental health promotion specifically. The section on recommended reading gives some of the most useful documents and websites. The need to engage in dialogue with people working in this way is paramount and should be an essential part of the supervision process (see Fig. 57.6).

Myth 1: 'It's too large a subject'
This myth has its roots in the assumption that because the factors influencing mental health are so numerous and complex that the task is best left alone or it is something that someone else does.

Myth 2: 'We do it anyway'
This myth is the 'mental health promotion by default' argument. Good practice should equate to a health promoting practitioner but however good professionals intentions are or their practice, oppression and inequality disempower individuals because of the power imbalance in being a user of statutory mental health services.

Myth 3: 'There is little that can be achieved immediately'
Good communication skills and listening and acting within a public health perspective are deemed essential for health and social care professionals in light of the current policy initiatives and service development plans. How practice is implemented, as well as what is practised is important. A leaflet or a small scale project will not radically alter perceptions or society. Yet if the small scale is planned and evaluated or audited and then championed, it can start to sway and influence organizations and the public they serve. One clear example of this is the development of Mental Health User Focused Monitoring[24]

Myth 4: 'Our focus is on those with severe and enduring mental illness'
Fear of a practice drift towards people with less disabling mental illness or problems is a concern. People with severe and enduring mental illness have as much right for their mental health to be promoted as any citizen. It still holds true that the philosophy and principles of mental health promotion are based upon the need for the foundations for health to be in place. Recent initiatives to tackle the problem of acute in-patient care provide an example of an attempt to do this.[26] Ensuring access to treatment and care by being able to offer choice and services that are culturally and ethnically sensitive, working in partnership with dignity and respect for service users problems are all practical steps toward promoting the mental health of those diagnosed with mental illness.

Myth 5: 'We don't have the skills'
Mental health is seen as a technical activity requiring resources and training beyond the realm of ordinary practice or as rooted in community and social models of health, far removed from professional practice until more recently. There are considerable attitudinal shifts that can and should be incorporated into educational and training strategies for all health and social care professionals. We are all potential users of mental health services and we all operate in the social sphere. As such we have understanding and misunderstanding to formulate emotionally health-enhancing practice. By being exposed and prepared to learn from community work, primary care and the mental health service-user movement, we can all become more sophisticated practitioners of mental health promotion.

FIGURE 57.6 Some common myths. (adapted from McCulloch and Boxer[1])

Developing practice

A range of skills is required to be effective in promoting mental health. Many of these are considered as core competencies for mental health practice, such as identified in The Capable Practitioner.[26] The additional skills required for community work and neighbourhood participation will depend very much on role and function.

An important area for skill development is in terms of understanding the mental health service-user movement and how users and carers are actively engaged at various levels of strategic planning, service development, advocacy, e.g. PALs, User Voice, care and treatment and monitoring processes.[23]

Case study

I work as an external co-ordinator for a user focused monitoring project funded by Derbyshire Mental Health Services Trust in England. The project has been running for two years and was supported because of the requirements of the NSF and a commitment by this Trust to take the needs and opinions of service users at the heart of the service. The Sainsbury Centre for Mental Health had taken a clear role in clarifying a process of qualitative analysis that was service user led and implemented and had a key objective in identifying a recommendation the Trust could act on in the light of the findings.[25]

Using the problem tree approach outlined in Making it Happen, the framework for the project is outlined under the headings provided to show the key elements required for professionals and service users to work in partnership (see Tables 57.10–57.14).

Further developments in user-focused approaches can be found in the suggested reading lists. Other

TABLE 57.10

THE PROBLEM: DEVELOPING A USER FOCUSED MONITORING PROJECT FOR A LOCAL MENTAL HEALTH TRUST

The CAUSES of this problem are:
- No clear policy guidelines on service user involvement in the monitoring of treatment and services
- Finding sustainable funding sources for the project
- Feeling isolated as it is hard to access information about what is going on in other parts of the country
- Continued dissatisfaction with current mental health services, especially in-patient wards
- Lack of appropriate skills for service users wanting to get involved in the project, such as interviewing, communication and questionnaire design
- Too little value placed on service user experience and understanding of mental health problems and how to best resolve them.

TABLE 57.11

The EFFECTS on mental health service users are:
- The continuation of oppressive practices, discrimination and a lack of comprehensive and integrated services having a negative impact on treatment outcomes and emotional well-being
- Lack of potential and purpose being realized
- Not being able to access an empowering approach to mental health problems (read J's account)
- Missing out on the opportunity to engage with staff and other service users in a different and more egalitarian way

TABLE 57.12

A SOLUTION to this problem is:
- To develop a service user focused monitoring project as part of an overall strategy for service user involvement that is supported and encouraged by people working at executive, ward, community and voluntary levels.

TABLE 57.13

The OBJECTIVE would be achieved by:
- Setting up a user focused monitoring steering group
- Providing a proposal to the Trust Board
- Advertising for service users who would like to be involved in interviewing other service users and undertake a process of selection
- Plan and deliver a training programme in communication and interviewing skills for service users
- Identify key areas to be monitored twice yearly
- Design and use a semi-structured interview schedule
- Analyse the findings Take forward recommendations for change at key levels of Trust organization, e.g. clear link with clinical governance

TABLE 57.14

The RESULTS of these actions are:
- Published reports of the findings of each monitoring process
- Providing evidence of the problems and how they have been tackled and solutions found.
- Better communication between people at all levels of the Trust
- Resolution of mental health problems by being involved with the project even if people experience a relapse of symptoms
- Link to a National network of service user led projects

examples of good practice are in Appendix Four of Making it Happen.[2] The following diagram identifies the key areas of service user involvement in mental health services in Derbyshire (see Fig. 57.7). It provides an example of the necessary integration of the work of strategic development, clinical governance and the link to the divisional management teams. Service users need to be at the heart of service planning and by addressing these developments as mental health promoting the requirements of the NSF: Standard One, for Mental Health and Making it Happen are being met.

MENTAL HEALTH SERVICE USER ACCOUNT OF USER-FOCUSED MONITORING PROJECT

J's story

Being involved in the UFM project has been the most positive experience I have had since first becoming ill 12 years ago. From the very outset it was both challenging and exciting. Even the advert, which appeared in the local press, seemed to leap up from the page and, quite literally, I was on the phone applying before I had finished reading it. The advert was for people who had experience of the mental health services, to come forward to be trained to interview other service-users to allow them a 'voice'. Implicit in the advert was the recognition that, as users of mental health services, we could make a unique contribution to this project, that we are capable of reasoned intelligent thought and hold valid opinions worth listening to. In fact, we had a role to play in the modification of services and their delivery.

This attitude was diametrically opposed to the one I came across when first ill so I was being given the chance to turn a deeply traumatic experience into a uniquely qualifying attribute ... an opportunity too valuable to miss. Things got better still, we had five days of training, which included constructing the questionnaire and being trained to use it. The fact that we were paid for this training gave additional credibility to the project as it emphasized that we were valued and considered worth the investment. This was reinforced by the calibre and status of those who trained us. We are a diverse group but those five days united us and we became a mutually supportive group. We interviewed many different people in a variety of situations. Almost without exception people had thought deeply about the issues and their answers were considered fair and reasonable. They were lavish with praise when it was appropriate and some even indicated that they refrained from overburdening key-workers they recognized as being stretched. Negative comments were backed up with relevant examples. The majority of the people I met seemed to agree to the interview because they had something important to say which they felt would improve outcomes for others as well as themselves. Before we actually started the interviewing 'for real', I was slightly concerned that talking in depth with people who might be extremely distressed or ill just might bring me down and affect my own mental health. In practice this did not happen. Most interviews took place with two interviewers so there was immediate support but the most helpful thing was that once you started interviewing you realized that the interviewee was entrusting you with a message that had to be carried forward. That is not to say that some interviews were not distressing, they were, especially those with people who self-harm, who casually recounted the punitive attitudes of those who have contact with them and there were others who lived in awful conditions. Of course I would come away upset and sometimes angry but at the same time I knew the whole project was designed to improve things

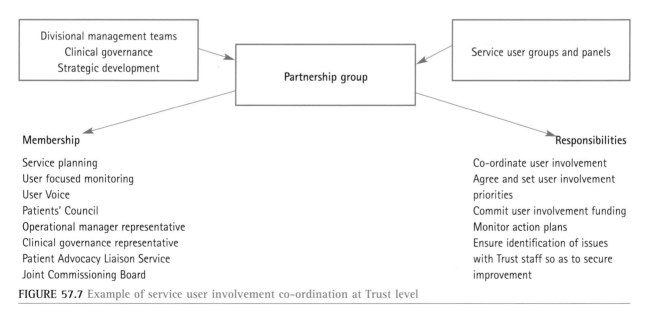

FIGURE 57.7 Example of service user involvement co-ordination at Trust level

Partnership group

Divisional management teams
Clinical governance
Strategic development

Service user groups and panels

Membership

Service planning
User focused monitoring
User Voice
Patients' Council
Operational manager representative
Clinical governance representative
Patient Advocacy Liaison Service
Joint Commissioning Board

Responsibilities

Co-ordinate user involvement
Agree and set user involvement priorities
Commit user involvement funding
Monitor action plans
Ensure identification of issues with Trust staff so as to secure improvement

for these people and that knowledge was extremely empowering. When I applied to this project it was because I wanted the user's voice to be heard by the service providers and I believe that is being accomplished. What I did not expect and what for me personally has been the greatest benefit, is that at last I have managed to achieve closure on my own negative experiences of so many years.[25]

DEVELOPING SKILLS AND COMPETENCE IN MENTAL HEALTH PROMOTION

The core of mental health practice skills in mental health promotion are increasingly based on an ability to be adaptable as opposed to the more prescriptive or traditional necessity of nursing practice. Interestingly, education and training in social work defines and identifies the core values that lend themselves to being 'health promoting' but are still not an integrated part of nursing curricula. Fundamental to this is the necessity of being able to relate to and appreciate the effects of oppression and how this manifests in vulnerable people. There is an inextricable link between mental illness and racism for example, that still has not been understood clearly enough or has reached all of mainstream practice in how people from black and minority ethnic groups are treated in mental health settings.[27] As identified, there is a framework for mental health promotion to help guide practice and there is also a framework for anti-oppressive practice which needs to be considered as equally important in our role as mental health workers. Dalrymple and Burke[28] offer these key elements to practice:

- ❏ Personal self-knowledge.
- ❏ Knowledge and an understanding of the majority social systems.
- ❏ Knowledge and understanding of different groups and cultures.
- ❏ Knowledge of how to challenge and confront issues on a personal and structural level.
- ❏ Awareness of the need to be 'research minded'.
- ❏ Commitment to action and change.

For students to be able to learn effectively about mental health promotion the key elements for both theory and practice are:

- ❏ Anti-oppressive practice.
- ❏ Ethical practice.
- ❏ Empowerment of self and others.
- ❏ Self-awareness and reflection at the level of the personal and professional commitment given to the above.
- ❏ Holistic interpretation.
- ❏ Co-operative/social practice.

- ❏ Therapeutic and culturally sensitive.
- ❏ Awareness of feminist theory and practice.
- ❏ Experiential and action-based learning.
- ❏ Refining knowledge and experience.

SUMMARY

Hopefully it has become clear that mental health promotion is a core aspect of our practice as mental health workers. As a strategic approach it has the support of World Health Organizations and Governments. It is a necessity not a luxury. Our mental stability as described in this chapter has consequences at macro and micro levels and it is clear that it is important to build on core skills that extend the boundaries of partnership with agencies other than health and social services. I have identified the main initiatives that currently exist but it is up to each of us as to how much we see our role as linked to community and neighbourhood regeneration approaches. The need to understand strategic thinking is important to be able to develop practice that is health promoting. This hopefully mirrors the developments in mental health practice as envisaged in the Capable Practitioner[26]. I have identified the importance of practice being anti-oppressive and culturally sensitive and this is vital in terms of working in areas with diverse ethnic populations and the clear link that mental health issues have to religious and cultural beliefs. There is a growing body of knowledge and evidence about mental health promotion and the websites addresses provided are an essential resource in networking and making links with others trying to initiate projects within the requirements of mental health policy. The key points addressed in this chapter are listed below.

Summary points

Having identified the key elements of mental health promotion you should have a clearer idea of:

- ❏ What mental health promotion is.
- ❏ What are the main policy themes and strategic framework for its effective implementation.
- ❏ What your part is in helping to implement the requirements of these policies and practice initiatives.
- ❏ Be able to access examples of good practice.
- ❏ See mental health promotion as a core activity of mental health nursing and practice.
- ❏ Be able to participate as a citizen in promoting health and acting as a role model for others.
- ❏ Identify your own mental health needs and use this a basis for reflective and critical theoretical analysis and skill development.

❏ Identify how you are developing partnerships with service users in promoting health across primary, secondary and tertiary services.

WEBSITE INFORMATION ABOUT MENTAL HEALTH PROMOTION

❏ Mentality: www.mentality.org.uk
❏ Department of Health, mental health related topics: www.doh.gov.uk/mentalhealth
❏ Mind out for mental health: www.mindout.net
❏ Mental health foundation: www.mentalhealth.org.uk
❏ Sainsbury Centre for Mental Health: www.scmh.org.uk
❏ Mental health media: www.mhmedia.com
❏ Mental health promotion updates: www.doh.gov.uk/mental
❏ Mental health promotion project group: www.doh.gov.uk/mental
❏ Kings Fund: www.kingsfund.org.uk
❏ World Health Organization: www.who.int
❏ World Federation for Mental Health: www.wfmh.org
❏ Clifford Beers Foundation: www.charity.demon.co.uk
❏ New Deal for Communities: www.regeneration.uk.com

REFERENCES

1. McCulloch G, Boxer J. *Mental health promotion: policy, practice and partnerships.* London: Baillière Tindall, 1997: 30.
2. Department of Health. *Making it Happen: a guide to delivering mental health promotion.* London: HMSO, 2001 p 27.
3. Whitehead M. Tackling inequalities: a review of policy initiatives. In: Benzeval M, Judge K, Whitehead M (eds). *Tackling inequalities of health: an agenda for action.* London: King's Fund, 1998.
4. Tudor K. *Mental health promotion.* London: Routledge, 1996.
5. Macdonald G. *Promoting mental health: a report for the health education department.* London: HEA, 1994.
6. McCulloch G, Boxer J. *Mental health promotion: policy, practice and partnerships.* London: Baillière Tindall, 1997: 9.
7. Health Education Authority. *Community action for mental health.* London: HEA, 1998.
8. Department of Health. *Mental health promotion update.* London, Issue 3: Feb 2002. http://doh.gov.uk/mental
9. Department of Health. *The Health of the Nation: a strategy for health in England.* London: HMSO, 1992.
10. Naidoo J, Wills J. *Health promotion: foundations for practice.* London: Baillière Tindall, 1994.
11. World Health Organization. *Mental health: new understanding, new hope.* World Health Report. Geneva: WHO, 2001.
12. World Health Organization. *Ottowa Charter: the first international conference on health promotion.* Geneva: WHO, 1986.
13. McCulloch G, Boxer J. *Mental health promotion: policy, practice and partnerships.* London: Baillière Tindall, 1997: 34.
14. Department of Health. *National service framework for mental health – modern standards and service models.* London: DOH, 1999.
15. Department of Health. *National service framework for older adults – modern standards and service models.* London: DOH, 2001.
16. McCulloch G, Boxer J. Mental health promotion. In: Thompson T, Mathias P (eds). *Lyttle's mental disorder,* 3rd edn. London: Baillière Tindall, 2000.
17. Department of Health. *The NHS Plan.* London: DOH, 2000. Department of Health. *The Health of the Nation – key area handbook: mental illness.* London: DOH, 1994.
18. Department of Health. *Variations in health.* London: DOH, 1995.
19. Repper J. Interventions in mental health practice. In: Thompson T, Mathias P (eds). *Lyttle's mental disorder,* 3rd edn. London: Baillière Tindall, 2000.
20. Department of Health. *Saving lives: our healthier nation.* London: DOH, 1999.
21. Palmer S. Editorial. From public health to the health of the public. *British Medical Journal* 1998; **317**: 550–51.
22. Department of Health. *Making it Happen: a guide to delivering mental health promotion.* London: HMSO, 2001: 22.
23. Rose D. *Users' voices.* London: The Sainsbury Centre for Mental Health, 2000.
24. Boxer J. *UFM audit of CPA Springboard Project Derby:* Southern Derbyshire Mental Health Services, 2000.
25. The Sainsbury Centre for Mental Health. *Acute Solutions.* London: SCMH, 2999.
26. The Sainsbury Centre for Mental Health. *The capable practitioner: a framework and list of the practitioner capabilities required to implement the national service framework.* London: SCMH, 2001.
27. Alexander Z. *Study of black and ethnic minority issues.* London: Department of Health, 1999.
28. Dalrymple J. Burke D. *Anti-oppressive practice: social care and the law.* Buckingham: Open University Press, 1995.
29. Caplan R, Holland R. Rethinking Health Education Theory. *Health Education Journal* 19990; **49**(1): 10–12.

Chapter 58

MEDICATION IN NURSING PRACTICE: THE PSYCHIATRIC NURSE AND PRESCRIBING AUTHORITY

Nancy M Daniels* and Gail B Williams**

INTRODUCTION

Hildegard Peplau founded the first Graduate Programme in Psychiatric-mental Health Nursing at Rutgers University in New Jersey, USA, 1952. The focus of this programme was on teaching nurses the role of the psychotherapist along with fostering the role of the clinical nurse specialist.[1] In Peplau's view, given nurses' close contact with patients, the role of the nurse as psychotherapist or counselor was predominant. 'In the ensuing decades, other graduate programmes in psychiatric nursing followed this innovative model'.[1]

Since then, the influence of Peplau's thinking about psychiatric nursing and, in particular interpersonal relations, has spread worldwide, influencing the development of nursing curricula in most Western countries. Arguably, the public in all such countries, but especially in the USA, has benefited from psychiatric-mental health nurses' willingness to seek higher levels of education and to assume ever-increasing levels of responsibility.[2]

The scope of practice within psychiatric-mental health nursing in the USA has made remarkable progress despite its relatively short history. In addition to developing the nurse–patient relationship along more formal therapeutic, educative or counselling lines, psychiatric-mental health nurses began to develop roles as autonomous providers of psychotherapy following the establishment of educational programmes based upon Peplau's leadership.[1] As changes in the health care needs of the United States evolved, the demand for high quality health care professionals also increased and the emergent developments in nursing role functions in the USA have become models for practice development in many Western countries, but especially in the UK.

Psychiatric-mental health nurses began to seek and obtain prescriptive authority in many states of the USA in the 1980s and 1990s. Today approximately 48 of the 50 US states offer prescriptive authority to advanced practice nurses. Increasingly, this North American initiative is becoming a model, worldwide, but especially in the UK, Australia and New Zealand, where legislation is likely to be passed soon, approving prescribing privileges for psychiatric-mental health nurses who have acquired the appropriate level of postgraduate education.

*Nancy Daniels MN APRN BC is a clinical nurse specialist in private practice at the Alamo Mental Health Group in San Antonio, Texas. She provides psychotherapy and prescription medication management for patients ages 18–101.

**Gail Williams PhD, RN is currently Associate Professor and Co-Director of the Center for Violence Prevention at The University of Texas Health Science Center at San Antonio School of Nursing in San Antonio, Texas. The Center for Violence Prevention is dedicated to the development and nurturance of multidisciplinary collaboration in research, education and clinical practice that advances the knowledge on violence related health needs of citizens and communities within South Texas.

During the past three decades these authors have witnessed a remarkable growth in nurses' professional self-confidence and in public confidence in nursing. A major influence on the role of the psychiatric-mental health nurses has involved a paradigm shift in psychiatric- and mental health nursing practice. Psychiatric-mental health nursing has moved from the largely psychodynamic perspective portrayed by Peplau, to a more comprehensive biopsychosocial model of practice.[1] Indeed, nursing as a whole has undergone a paradigm shift, in which there have been efforts to replace the traditional cure model with the *care* model. Caring has long been considered by many as an essential concept of nursing and so too with psychiatric-mental health nurses. Indeed, caring has been described as the essence of nursing practice.[3] However, caring has often been depicted as a moral ideal rather than a task-oriented behaviour, with the focus on the caring moment experienced between the nurse and patient.[3,4] Along with this paradigmatic shift psychiatric-mental health nursing has embraced 'caring' as the core of therapeutic interactions.[5]

> Caring as an interpersonal relationship focuses specifically on the nurse–patient relationship and the self-actualizing and healing effect the caring relationship can beget.[6]

As psychiatric-mental health nursing evolves, research will be needed to continually contribute to the unified body of knowledge necessary for the discipline and to accommodate the ever-changing need of patients.

The evolution of autonomous practice

In this chapter, the evolution of an autonomous practice in nursing is presented. Guidelines for competency in prescribing medications will be addressed along with a discussion of nursing's *legal authority* regarding prescriptive authority. Practical examples cases illustrating the blend of prescriptive authority and psychotherapy will be presented to highlight the evolving role of the psychiatric-mental health nurse. Finally implications for the role of the psychiatric-mental health nurse in the 21st century will be considered. Although the issues and examples described derive from experience of nursing in the USA, it is assumed that similar issues either have emerged, or will undoubtedly emerge, in other countries. Given that the development of prescribing authority within the broader role of the psychiatric-mental health nurse was first developed in the USA, it is appropriate that the 'American experience' be used as an exemplar.

REQUIREMENTS FOR COMPETENCY IN PRESCRIBING MEDICATIONS

With a broad knowledge base in assessment, diagnosis, treatment and prevention, psychiatric-mental health nurses can provide patients with access to high quality *holistic* nursing care. In today's psychiatric setting this holism has taken on added meaning. Originally holism in psychiatric-mental health nursing meant an integrated approach to the patient, respecting the inseparable nature of mind and body. In the last decade psychiatric-mental health nursing – at least within most Westernized countries – had to address the philosophical nature of this holism.[7] To practice holistically the psychiatric-mental health nurse had: ' … to acquire and maintain a grasp of biology of emotional experience in the same way that nurses had traditionally used psycho-social or psychodynamic viewpoints to understand the experience of those receiving psychiatric-mental health nursing care'.[7] Stuart contended that: 'psychiatric nurses thus entered the 1990s with the challenge of integrating the expanding bases of neuroscience into the holistic biopsycho-social practice of psychiatric nursing'.[8] The advances made in understanding the brain have posed both opportunities and challenges for psychiatric nurses.[8] McCabe cautioned that psychiatric-mental health nursing can no longer be content with an aging paradigm rooted in older knowledge and beliefs but must acknowledge the new paradigm, in which the brain is the central focus of psychiatric nursing.[9]

A new paradigm of nursing

According to Kuhn, a paradigm includes the beliefs and values shared by a given community and as such paradigms are significant for a discipline.[10] Psychiatric-mental health nursing as a community is challenged to create a new paradigm. From a historical perspective nursing and psychiatric nursing has been cognizant that nursing is a process.[9] It has been suggested that psychiatric-mental health nursing's new paradigm be ' … contextually situated within the process and notion of relationship'.[9] Nursing's endeavour to expand the definition of holism can be viewed as an attempt to make this paradigmatic shift.[7]

Holism can be viewed as an emphasis on the importance of the whole and the interdependence of the parts. Today with the advent of psychobiologic knowledge, holism has been redefined to include 'prescriptive privileges' for advanced practice nurses, which are commonplace in the United States of America.[7] 'The public has acknowledged the integrated knowledge of advanced practice psychiatric-mental health nursing and through legislated changes has imbued the practice arena with new responsibilities'.[7] By combining psychotherapy with the prescription of medication, advanced practitioners have the opportunity to provide a truly holistic level of psychiatric care. Also, the patient's access to health care providers and health care is greatly improved.

Competency standards

The *American Psychiatric Nursing Association* published a position statement in 1994,[11] setting standards of competency for nurses in the USA that included the following:

- ❏ Licensure as a registered nurse (or Advanced Practice Registered Nurse) by a State Board of Nursing.
- ❏ Master's degree in nursing.
- ❏ Certification as a specialist by the American Nurses Credentialing Center.
- ❏ Demonstrated competence in physical assessment, neuroscience and clinical psycho-pharmacology.

The authors presume that when other countries begin to explore the practical reality of nurse prescribing, similar competency standards to those outlined above will be a necessary part of such a development.

The Advanced Practice Registered Nurse

Legislation in the United States has allowed advanced practice registered nurses *APRNs* to prescribe medications. APRNs are defined as licensed registered nurses with a Master's degree and a depth of knowledge of psychiatric-mental health nursing theory. Additionally they must have supervised clinical practice and competence in advanced psychiatric-mental health nursing skills.[12] In the USA, nursing practice is regulated at the state level. This means that all 50 states have different sets of nursing laws. While there is similarity among states with regard to the laws permitting registered nurses to practice, at the advanced practice level the laws are widely different. Maintaining professional cohesiveness in this environment is a compelling challenge for the nurses and the nursing profession.

To maintain professional integrity, practitioners must be competent for the roles they assume. The prescribing of medications has become an integral component of the advanced practice role. If advanced nursing practice in psychiatric mental health nursing is to be holistic, nurses must, at the same time, continue to practice as psychotherapists. We cannot forget that medications influence, and are influenced by, the psychodynamics of the therapeutic relationship. To provide holistic care there needs to be an integration of care for *mind* and *body* that

incorporates medication management through prescriptive privileges. This approach has been proposed as a means to capitalize on the unique expertise of the advanced practice registered *nurse*, while simultaneously increasing patient access to quality and cost-effective health care.[12]

Advanced practice registered nurses with prescriptive privileges may prescribe pharmacologic agents to manage symptoms, and improve the functional status of patients with psychiatric disorders. Such *medication management* involves knowledge and clinical experience and is not without challenges. The following factors must be taken into consideration when prescribing any pharmacologic agent:

1. There are no medications prescribed for the treatment of mental disorders and stress-related dysfunctional behaviours whose actions are *limited* to the central nervous system (CNS).

2. Many patients may be receiving other prescribed and non-prescribed medications or using substances such as *alcohol, caffeine, nicotine* or *illicit drugs of abuse* (e.g. cocaine) that have actions in the CNS.

3. Many medications and other substances may effect the body's ability to *absorb*, the liver's ability to *metabolize*, and the kidney and liver's abilities to eliminate medications targeted at the CNS.

Because of these factors, any advanced practice registered nurse, authorized to prescribe medications, needs extensive *knowledge* of basic and clinical pharmacology.

Prescriptive authority

Prescriptive authority was granted to nurses in the USA as a result of a statute enacted by a state legislature. After the statute was enacted, rules of practice were produced, usually by the regulatory boards for nursing and medicine. There are two general types of prescriptive authority: *substitutive* and *complementary.*[13]

- ❏ **Complementary prescriptive authority** provides that the nurse must have a written practice protocol *and* provide prescriptions under the supervision of a licensed physician. In some states there is a requirement for a practice protocol for each diagnostic category the nurse intends to treat. In Texas, for example, the protocol is more general and covers scope of practice and lines of authority for supervision.[14] The majority of states that offer prescriptive authority to psychiatric-mental health nurses do so under complementary authority.
- ❏ **Substitutive prescriptive authority** is more autonomous. In this arrangement, the nurse is an

independent practitioner. There is *no* requirement for physician supervision.

In addition to restrictions on practice autonomy, some states limit the nurse's ability to prescribe controlled substances. Others require the use of a formulary system in which drugs that can be prescribed must be listed.

Along with this variation in laws regulating nursing practice, there is the additional challenge in deciding what to call these nurses with advanced skills and prescriptive authority. Traditionally, in the USA the term 'Nurse Practitioner' has been used to refer to the nurse who is able to provide primary care to children and adults. Psychiatric-mental health nurses have preferred the term 'Clinical Specialist' because of a desire to retain the professional identity with the role of psychotherapist. But with the psychotherapist who is able to perform a physical examination and prescribe medication, the term 'Psychiatric-mental Health Nurse Practitioner' may be more descriptive. The challenge before the profession is to develop a title that meets the needs of the profession and is acceptable to the public.

Advanced practice nursing titles

Current titles for advanced practice nurses also vary considerably. In some states these nurses are called *Advanced Practice Nurses* (APN) while in others they are titled *Advanced Practice Psychiatric-Mental Health nurses* (APPN). In still others they are *Advanced Registered Nurse Practitioners* (ARNP) or *Advanced Practice Registered Nurses* (APRN). The American Nurses Association and the American Psychiatric Nurses Association are endeavouring to address this titling issue.

The demands of the advanced-practice nursing role are bringing about curriculum changes in graduate nursing programmes. Whereas the emphasis has previously been on training in psychotherapy, there is now interest in developing clinicians and or practitioners who are able to provide biological therapy as well as psychotherapy. Both aspects of care require a considerable body of knowledge and it is important for educational institutions to do justice to both.[15–17] To prescribe medications in either a complementary or substitutive authority arrangement, specialty-focused graduation education is essential.

It seems likely that the differing limitations on practice autonomy, and the presence of differing titles given to nurses with prescribing authority, will be repeated – and perhaps added to – when other countries follow the US example. The UK, for example, has employed the title of 'clinical nurse specialist' for many years and more recently has introduced the concept of the 'nurse consultant'. However, it remains unclear whether or not these *particular* groups of nurses, with their particular educational profiles, will be the nurses who will assume the responsibilities of prescribing authority.

THE ROLE OF PRESCRIBER AND PSYCHOTHERAPIST

Holistic psychiatric care requires that nurses understand the patients' biological, psychological, social and spiritual needs. Nursing education serves as a framework for a lifetime growth process in which nurses continually seek to learn and acquire clinical skills and wisdom. As nursing continues to evolve, the scope and depth of skills required for practice will also evolve. Some of the finest (and toughest) teachers for nurses are the patients to whom they provide care.

To illustrate the evolving role of the psychiatric-mental health nurse in practice, we offer three case studies, which depict this role. While drawn from our personal clinical practice, in no way do these cases reflect the range of patients seen in the contemporary psychiatric-mental health nursing. They do, however, provide an example of how the psychiatric-mental health nurse, within this new evolving role, may combine the various aspects of care. [*All three patients gave consent to present their cases and all names are fictitious, to preserve anonymity.*]

Case study 58.1: June

June is a 35-year-old married mother of two school age children. She was referred for treatment by her primary care physician due to 'mood swings'.

On initial interview she was tearful and frustrated. She complained of extreme irritability and negative thoughts. She had intrusive recollections of verbal abuse by her strict father and conflict with her mother. She was unable to sleep well and unable to concentrate.

Her symptoms had a particular pattern that she had identified for herself. During and after her menstrual period she was cheerful and could cope with her children, her job and her husband. Her unhappy childhood was a distant memory and did not concern her on a daily basis. Around the middle of her menstrual cycle, she noticed increasing fatigue, hypersomnolence and difficulty concentrating. This began around the time of ovulation and worsened for the next week. The following week she experienced increased energy associated with insomnia and irritability. She was concerned at her tendency to lose control and shout at her husband and children. She had experienced panic attacks that had taken her to an emergency room fearing she was having a heart attack. Her work performance was impaired and at times she could not go to work. Academic performance also became very difficult.

These symptoms would resolve the day after the beginning of menstrual bleeding. Then she would again experience two

---

weeks of normal mood, subjective happiness, good coping skills, good quality sleep and good concentration.

June met criteria for premenstrual dysphoric disorder (PMDD). This occurs in 3–5% of menstruating women.[18] The severity of the symptoms can have a substantial impact on various aspects of a woman's life such as interpersonal relationships and work performance. In women who experience this, they suffer repetition of the symptoms approximately 430 times in their lives.

The mood symptoms of PMDD are thought to be caused by sensitivity to the effects of progesterone. While higher levels of oestrogen which are present in the earlier phase of the menstrual cycle can lift the mood, progesterone can lower the mood. It is thought that progesterone activates the monoamine oxidase system and thus lowers levels of serotonin and norepinephrine in the central nervous system. This process is the reverse of the effect of monoamine oxidase inhibitors that have the effect of increasing levels of serotonin and norepinephrine.

June was intelligent and insightful. She had kept a record of her own symptoms and patterns of occurrence. We agreed on a trial of sertraline beginning with 25 mg per day. She noticed improvement immediately, but the improvement was not sustained. Over the next few weeks we adjusted the dose to 100 mg per day as she began to tolerate the medication. She achieved complete remission of symptoms.

Case study 58.2: Robert

Robert was a 78-year-old man who lived alone. He had been divorced for many years and had estranged himself from his adult daughter. He had been considered irascible and eccentric for a number of years. He was socially withdrawn, had poor personal hygiene and poor quality diet. His daughter made efforts to care for him, but he was somewhat uncooperative. He would allow her to give him prepared meals and would occasionally let her take him to a physician.

In September 1997, his daughter noticed that he was, alternately, laughing and crying. At times he did not respond to his name and appeared to be having visual hallucinations. His daughter brought him to our crisis clinic for evaluation.

It was not possible to conduct a complete interview. Robert was silly and unco-operative. A Folstein Mini Mental Status[19] exam was attempted with little success. His daughter could give some history, but this was sketchy since she did not see him frequently. There was no evidence that he drank alcohol.

Robert's blood pressure was 90/60 and his pulse was 120. He had facial oedema and oedema of his hands. His legs were very oedematous and the right leg had infected stasis ulcers with purulent drainage. In addition, Robert had suffered dementia for some time. Superimposed on this was acute delirium resulting from congestive heart failure and sepsis.

Robert was transferred to the Emergency Department immediately. His diagnosis was septic shock due to cellulitis of the right leg and right side heart failure. Robert died two days later.

It is not uncommon for physical illnesses to present with psychological symptoms or for psychological illnesses to present with physical symptoms. The astute clinician is obliged make an accurate diagnosis.

Case study 58.3: Hector

Hector was a 58-year-old man who suffered from chronic back pain. He was referred by a psychiatrist for hypnotherapy and medication management.

Hector's back pain had begun after a work related injury ten years before. He had slipped and fallen on a wet floor. He sustained a fractured vertebra and a herniated disc. Two back surgeries seemed to have worsened the pain. He had become disabled and could no longer work as a meat cutter. He became depressed and withdrawn. He felt hopeless and thought of suicide to end his misery. The surgeon offered another attempt at surgical correction, but could not assure this would help.

On interview, Hector made little eye contact. He was stoical about his pain. His entire life was focused on coping with pain, from moment to moment. He was unable to enjoy contact with his friends or family. He was requiring large doses of narcotic analgesics but receiving little benefit.

His diagnosis was major depression due to chronic pain. In patients who experience pain for more that six months, almost 100% become depressed. Anti-depressants are not only helpful for the depression, but also reduce the patient's sensitivity to pain.

Treatment options were discussed with Hector and he agreed to a trial of venlafaxine. This drug has the ability to affect serotonin, norepinephrine and dopamine systems. Drugs that effect norepinephrine are often beneficial adjuncts in the treatment of pain.[20] Hector was prescribed the extended release preparation and the dose was increased over three weeks time to 150 mg twice daily. Venlafaxine can cause hypertension in some patients, so his blood pressure was checked at each office visit. His mood improved steadily.

Over the next several weeks tramadol was added, which is a serotonin drug that is used for pain not depression. The dosage was increased to 100 mg three times daily. After beginning this drug, it was possible to taper and discontinue narcotic analgesics.

Along with the pharmacotherapy for pain, hypnosis for Hector's pain was employed. He was a good candidate for hypnosis. While he was not a psychologically minded person, he had a strong sense of aesthetics. He enjoyed making things look nice and loved to talk about beautiful places he had seen. All hypnosis is self-hypnosis; this treatment works well for the patient who desires it.[21,22] Over the course of a year, Hector improved steadily. While he still has pain, he says it now bothers him less. He is able to enjoy his family and friends. He goes to family gatherings and to church. He has even become involved in local politics. He is raising a small herd of goats and is able to make extra money for himself. He employs self-hypnosis when he feels the need.

INTO THE FUTURE

The nursing profession faces many challenges in all countries in the 21st century. The importance of standardization of the titling and education of advanced practice nurses, in particular, has been emphasized. However, as noted, apart from specific states within the USA, there are few examples of how such standardization might become a part of mainstream practice. However such standardization will be necessary if nursing is to be viewed as a credible authority, by other professions and by the public. At present advanced practice nurses are required to have specific skills and credentials.[23] According to Gilliss, the advanced practice nurse is required to have a basic nursing education, basic licensure, graduate degree in nursing and experience in the area of specialization.[23] In addition advanced practice nurses are expected to possess comprehensive assessment skills, diagnostic expertise, ability to manage health and illness problems, and the proficiency to assess and intervene with complex systems.[23] The skill base of advanced practice nurses also includes ability to analyze research findings.[23] The ability to provide leadership, cooperation and collaboration and exercise autonomy is integral to the advanced practice role.[23] Education of advanced practice nurses has made strides in the last decade and will continue to evolve to meet the health care demands of the future. According to Andrews, the advanced practice nurse has the distinct advantage of '… bringing knowledge and expertise from the unique perspective of nursing to the advanced practice arena'.[24] As such the advanced practice nurse is not a physician extender or physician substitute.[24] While physician and nurses will collect and utilize similar data, the difference lies in what they do with the data.

The profession of nursing, as a whole, will need to continue to pay attention to financial compensation for all nurses if it is to continue to attract and retain the brightest and the best. While these challenges, at times, seem nearly insurmountable; the benefit to health care consumers is increased access to care on a global basis.

CONCLUSION

It has long been recognized that nurses have often recommended suitable medications to physicians for their patients. Assuming the responsibility for prescription of medication, combining this with the delivery of psychotherapy, is a part of the natural evolution of psychiatric-mental health nursing in the USA and looks set to become a model for similar developments in many other countries. It has been shown that nurses with advanced educational preparation are able to assume this autonomy in practice and meet the challenges of the public in a way that is both holistic and caring. This represents a development of nursing practice to meet the changing needs of health care provision in the 21st century.

REFERENCES

1. Shea C. Careers in advanced practice nursing. In: Shea C, Pelletier L, Poster E, Stuart G, Verhey M (eds). *Advanced practice nursing in psychiatric and mental health care*. St Louis: Mosby, 1999: 1–34.

2. Moller M. The business of psychiatric-mental health nursing: cents and sensibility. *Journal of the American Psychiatric-Mental Health Nurses Association* 1999; **5**: 54–61.

3. Watson J. Nursing: *Human science and human care – a theory of nursing*. New York: National League for Nursing Press, 1985.

4. McCance K, McKenna H, Boore J. Caring: theoretical perspectives of relevance to nursing. *Journal of Advanced Nursing* 1999; **30**: 1388–95.

5. Fishel A. Psycho-social and behavioral health care. In: Shea C, Pelletier L, Poster E, Stuart G, Verhey M (eds). *Advanced practice nursing in psychiatric and mental health care*. St Louis: Mosby, 1999: 185–219.

6. Kiser-Larson N. The concepts of caring and story viewed from three nursing paradigms. *International Journal for Human Caring* 2000; **4**: 26–32.

7. McEnany G. Psychobiologic influences: chronobiology. In: Shea C, Pelletier L, Poster E, Stuart G, Verhey M (eds). *Advanced practice nursing in psychiatric and mental health care*. St Louis: Mosby, 1999: 221–42.

8. Stuart G. Roles and functions of psychiatric nurses: competent caring. In: Stuart G, Laraia M (eds). *Principles and practice of psychiatric nursing*. St Louis: Mosby, 2001: 2–13.

9. McCabe S. The nature of psychiatric nursing: the intersection of paradigm, evolution, and history. *Archives of Psychiatric Nursing* 2002; **2**: 51–60.

10. Kuhn T. *The structure of scientific revolutions*. Chicago: University of Chicago Press,1962.

11. American Nurses Association. *A statement on psychiatric mental health. Clinical nursing practice and standards of psychiatric-mental health clinical nursing practice*. Washington, DC: American Nurses Publishing, 1994.

12. Laraia M. Psychopharmacology. In: Stuart G, Laraia M (eds). *Principles and practice of psychiatric-mental health nursing*. St Louis: Mosby, 2001: 572–607.

13. Talley S, Brooke P. Prescriptive authority for psychiatric clinical specialists: framing the issues. *Archives of Psychiatric-mental Health Nursing* 1992; **6**: 71–82.

14. The Texas APN. *The resource guide for practice*. Texas Nurses Association, 1997. Web site: http://www.texas nurses.org

15. Delaney J, Chisholm M, Clement J, Merwin E. Trends in psychiatric mental health nursing education. *Archives of Psychiatric-mental Health Nursing* 1999; **12**: 67–73.

16. Naegle M. Prescription drugs and nursing education: knowledge gaps and implications for role performance. *Journal of Law, Medicine and Ethics* 1994; **22**: 257–61.

17. Johnson B. The 5 R's of becoming a psychiatric-mental health nurse practitioner: rationale, readying, roles, rules and reality. *Journal of Psycho-social Nursing* 1998; **36**: 20–24.

18. Yonkers KA, Halbreich U, Freeman E, *et al.* Symptomatic improvement of premenstrual dysphoric disorder with sertraline treatment. *Journal of the American Medical Association* 1997; **278**: 983–8.

19. Folstein M, Folstein S, McHugh P. Mini-mental state: a practical method for grading the cognitive state of patients for the clinician. *Journal of Psychiatric Research* 1975; **12**: 189.

20. Virani A, Mailis A, Shapiro L, Shear N. Drug interactions in human neuropathic pain pharmacotherapy, Pain 73. *Toronto: International Association for the Study of Pain: Elsevier Science B.V.,* 1997.

21. Zahourek R. *Clinical hypnosis and therapeutic suggestion in nursing.* Orlando: Grune and Stratton, Harcourt Brace Jovanovich, 1985.

22. Barber J, Adrian C. Psychological approaches to the management of pain. *New York: Bruner Mazel,* 1982.

23. Gilliss C. Education for advanced practice nursing. In: Hickey J, Ouimette R, Venegoni S (eds). *Advanced practice nursing: changing roles and clinical applications.* Philadelphia: Lippincott, 2000, 34–45.

24. Andrews J. Roles of the advanced practice nurse. In: Robinson D, Kish C (eds). *Core concepts in advanced practice nursing.* St Louis: Mosby, 2001: 261–8.

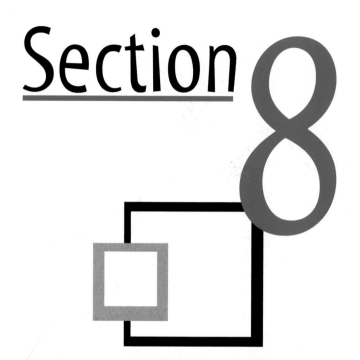

Section 8

Legal, ethical and moral issues

Preface to Section 8

The field of mental health has long been the focus of controversy and debate. The problems of living, which represent the material substance of psychiatric diagnoses, are deeply embedded in society and culture, and are framed by both professional and lay understandings of what it means to 'be human'.

In this section we consider mental health across some wider contexts.

To what extent does mental health legislation differ across different countries and cultures?

What are the core ethical challenges presented to nurses in the course of their working lives, and where do these ethical and moral dilemmas come from?

People who become psychiatric patients are men and women, with differing or changing sexual preferences. To what extent is their sexuality and gender relevant to their status as patients or clients or people in care?

Psychiatry is a powerful institution and people in care often feel the effects of that power on an acutely personal level. In a 'free' society, how do we begin to understand the concepts of freedom and consent, as they might apply in mental health care?

Finally, we return to our roots, metaphorically, and consider how mental health care might be delivered in a culturally meaningful way. In an increasingly multicultural society, what are the important considerations for the development of culturally appropriate care?

Chapter 59

PSYCHIATRIC LEGISLATION: AN INTERNATIONAL PERSPECTIVE

Shaun Parsons*

This chapter examines the role of the Law in mental health from an international perspective, focusing on the overall use and meaning of the Law, and assumptions of mental illness underpinning these legal interpretations.

THE DOMINANCE OF THE WESTERN MODEL

In this chapter I shall try to discuss the use of mental health legislation from an international perspective. However, it is apparent that the form of mental health legislation used in the Western democracies is applied, almost universally, across the world. There are procedural differences between the application of Mental Health Law in different countries, and also differences in the administration and review of the law. However, the essence of the law in every country is almost universal.[1,2] This state of affairs presides even when the culture, from which the legislation is derived, has a different philosophical basis to Western society, for example countries of the Far East.[3] Due to the hegemony of Western approaches to psychiatry and the law, the Western system will be examined here in depth, paying particular emphasis to the assumptions underpinning Western approaches to psychiatric legislation. However, some of the key procedural differences between jurisdictions

using Mental Health Law will also be explored, particularly the checks and balances that aim to ensure that the law is not abused. The role of the nurse in mental health legislation will also be considered.

The Western viewpoint

In Western societies, mental illness is broadly seen as a form of social deviancy. In many ways the Law surrounding mental illness is structured similarly to the other main form of social deviancy focused on by Western law – criminal acts. In both criminal law and mental health legislation the person deviating from a societal norm can be removed from society. The person who steals may be arrested, tried and if convicted, imprisoned – thus being removed from society. The individual with mental health problems can be detained, usually under specific mental health legislation. In most jurisdictions they are detained in a place of safety until assessed by a psychiatrist. If the person is found to have a mental health problem, and crucially if found to be a danger to themselves or others, then they can be detained and treated against their will.

In the cases of people who have broken the law, and those who are deemed to have psychiatric symptoms

*Shaun Parsons is a Lecturer in Clinical Psychology at the University of Newcastle and he practises as a Forensic Psychologist in NHS. His research interests include the monitoring and treatment of sex offenders in community and prison settings and the interaction between the police and people with mental health problems.

that lead to detention, there is a perceived need to protect the individual *and* society from their actions or potential actions. In both cases society has formulated a view of *normalcy* within the bounds of which members of society are expected to operate. In both cases these laws are based upon assumptions of what is normal or abnormal behaviour. Thus stealing, trespassing or murder are neither expected nor tolerated in Western society; such acts are seen as a form of social deviancy. In the case of mental health the boundaries are less clear, but it is considered generally unacceptable to threaten to take your own life, seem to have significant thought disorder or act in a variety of disinhibited ways in public. From this viewpoint social deviancy is dealt with by removal from society. This is recognized by society by its investiture of the power of forcible restraint in only two groups of people, the police and the mental health professionals, particularly the psychiatrist. Both groups have the power to take the individual expressing social deviancy into custody and hold them against their will until experts determine their disposal. It is at this point that the comparison between the two approaches appears to diverge. In the case of people who break the criminal law, society punishes them by either imposing a fiscal penalty or detaining them in prison for a period determined by a Magistrate or a Judge, until they are released. In English law, only in the more severe crimes – such as murder – is a sentence open-ended, and criminals held until they are no longer considered a danger to society. For those detained under Mental Health Law in most Western systems, there are no such boundaries to their detention. This is because the detainee is not being punished, but *treated*, and therefore does not receive a sentence, but rather, is detained until judged to no longer be a danger to themselves or to others. Again, most Western systems allow for a review of the detention, which is usually an independent assessment of the detainee's mental state, or an appeal against the detention.

Given the similarities between the operation of the criminal justice and mental health detention laws and their common foundation of social deviancy, it is unsurprising that both systems overlap considerably. Almost 70% of prisoners held in prison in England and Wales have mental illness[4] and in most Western countries there is a ready exchange, almost a revolving door, between the two systems. In England and Wales, as provision for mental health services has declined, the number of people with mental health problems in the criminal justice system has increased. Further evidence of commonality between the two systems is the sharing of powers between mental health professionals and Law Enforcement officers. In most Western systems there is provision to remove people from the criminal justice systems with mental health problems and to transfer

their detention to hospital. Also the police usually have the power to detain someone showing social deviancy in a pattern that may indicate that mental illness is present. In some jurisdictions this power is formalized. For example, in England and Wales, the police can detain someone under the Mental Health Act of 1983 using Section 136. Therefore, a non-psychiatric professional has the power to detain under *Mental Health* legislation. In other jurisdictions the power of the police is less formal. For example in Oregon, in the United States, the police may arrest someone and take them for assessment, but they are using public *order* laws not public *health* laws.

Key assumptions

There are several key assumptions upon which the Western system is based and these will be briefly discussed.

The Western system is based upon two principles:

1 The view that psychiatric systems are best conceptualized as an *illness* and, as such, the illness is treatable and perhaps even curable. This viewpoint has both proponents and opponents. However, the debate will not be discussed here. Interested readers should consult the chapter on Psychiatric Classification (Chapter 14) or Boyle[4,5] and Parsons and Armstrong.[6]

2 The view that society has a moral right, and indeed a duty, to protect the majority from the minority and also to protect those whom it judges to be incapable of protecting themselves.

This second point is essentially the balance of personal freedom and right of expression against the right of society to protection from some of its members. In Western systems the state judges that it has the prerogative and duty to exercise its right. However, the state also sees it as its duty to operate these powers at the minimal level possible so as not to impinge upon personal freedom, human rights or freedom of expression. In democracies, this power is seen as bestowed by the people and operated in the name of the people. It is argued that if people wish to change either the criminal or Mental Health Laws, then they would vote for political parties who supported the changes that they wished and then would enact them once in office. The same philosophy argues that in England and Wales the police enforce the law by consent. Again this point will not be explored or justified here. For a more detailed argument see Szasz[7] and Parsons and Armstrong.[6]

Within the Western democracies no other system

of mental health legislation is in operation. Some jurisdictions allow more extensive powers, such as the UK, while others have a more liberal interpretation of their duties towards those with mental health problems, such as Italy and in some states in the USA. In all jurisdictions the use of mental health legislation is criticized by some as an erosion of the rights of the mentally ill or even the criminalization of mental illness. In nearly all the Western democracies there are calls for tighter, and more prescriptive, legislation, even in jurisdictions that already possess considerable legislation, such as the UK. For example, following a number of high profile cases in which members of the public have been assaulted and/or killed by people with mental health problems, and also when individuals known to have personality disorders have sexually assaulted and killed members of the public, there has been considerable public pressure to increase restrictive legislation. The UK government has been urged to increase powers of compulsion and detention under a new Mental Health Act, and to extend the power of detention to those with dangerous and severe personality disorder. There also have been calls to extend the power of detention for those with mental health problems in community as well as hospital situations, with people in the natural community being compelled to take medication and undergo community treatment for their mental health problems.

DIFFERENCES BETWEEN JURISDICTIONS

There are very few differences between jurisdictions in their use of psychiatric law, however, the issue of Judicial as opposed to psychiatric power, and the role of nurses in enforcing psychiatric legislation, will be briefly examined.

Judicial vs. psychiatric powers

The degree of power invested in mental health professionals, particularly psychiatrists, varies between jurisdictions. In some jurisdictions, such as many states in the USA, the psychiatrist has the sole power to detain an individual with mental health problems. However, it is rare that a review process, as discussed above, does not temper this power. For example, in England and Wales the power to detain is shared between two doctors and also a social worker with specific mental health training. Any person detained may also lodge an appeal to a mental health tribunal, to overturn the detention. However in these examples the power remains medical, as there is no involvement of the Judiciary. In other jurisdictions the role of the medical profession is advisory,

and the actual power to detain and the decision to detain rests with a local judge or magistrate. The psychiatrist can advise that a person is detained but ultimately the decision is a non-medical one, although based upon medical advice. Belgium is an example of a country where the decision to detain is made by a justice of the peace and the role of the medical profession is purely advisory. Appeals against the detention are also made through the civil courts.[1] In theory, the involvement of the judiciary should protect an individual's rights and allow for a non-medical, non-specialist opinion to be heard. However, there is no evidence to suggest that this difference is significant for the patient, and the process remains a medical one.

The role of the psychiatric mental health nurse

In very few jurisdictions does the nurse have the power to detain an individual against their will, under mental health legislation that differs from the powers of civil arrest granted to most citizens of Western democracies. Certainly the nurse does not share the psychiatrist's ability to recommend detention of someone not currently detained. In most jurisdictions the nurse has the power to restrain and hold an individual already detained, if they attempt to leave the unit in which they are being treated. In some cases this power is formalized within mental health legislation, such as the nurses holding power in Section 47 of the Mental Health Act in England and Wales, while in others the power to detain is covered by existing law. For example, in Belgium a nurse or doctor may detain someone under Belgium's laws which regard the refusal to 'help someone in need' as a criminal act.[1] In this case a detained individual attempting to leave would be identified as a person in need and those caring for them would be obliged to act.

OTHER CULTURAL DEFINITIONS OF MENTAL ILLNESS

Before discussing other systems again, the hegemony of the Western model should be highlighted. There is hardly a country in the world, whatever its location and culture, which does not have a version of Western mental health legislation on its statute books. The dominance of the Western view of psychiatric systems as an illness that needs to be treated cannot be overstated. Nevertheless the viewpoints of the societies upon which this viewpoint has been imposed often reflect fundamental differences from the Western view of illness generally, and psychiatric systems in particular.

Although most states have a form of Western psychiatric legislation the application and use of this legislation varies considerably. Leff[8] for example argued that in Southern African society people who hear voices or have visual hallucinations may be described as mentally ill if they go to see a psychiatrist and a Western system of detention is in operation,[9] but within their own community such an experience was seen as something of a status symbol. Thus it would be unlikely that such individuals would come to the attention of psychiatric services as they would be tolerated, and perhaps even revered, by the society and community around them.

A similar situation can be seen in the religious views of hallucinatory phenomena. Throughout the history of Christianity many people have reported visions of Christ or the Virgin Mary, or have heard the voices of these figures. Far from being thought of as mentally ill these people have been seen as blessed, for example, the case of Bernadette Soubirous of Lourdes. Bernadette was a young woman who lived in the town of Lourdes in the South of France in 1858. One day, when gathering firewood, she saw and heard what she believed to be the Virgin Mary, the mother of Christ, who told her to ask the priests to build a shrine to her in a small grotto and to visit again. Bernadette told others of her visit and she returned a number of times to the grotto with an increasing audience. Each time she could see the apparition but others could not. On one occasion in front of 400 people the apparition told her to drink from a stream, which was apparently invisible, and represented by a pool of muddy water. Bernadette scraped the ground where the water was and from the hole a spring of water began to flow. Bernadette told others of her vision, which only she could see, and also explained that those who believed and who were ill might be cured if they bathed in the water. Since then Lourdes has become a Holy place to Roman Catholics and a number of apparently inexplicable cures have been recorded.

However, from the viewpoint of Western psychiatry and Western science, many of these events could be explained using a rational approach. Bernadette was of an age at which early symptoms of psychosis often develop. Caves and grottos are often associated with water courses, which run close to the cave floor and digging into a cave floor might well release a flow of water, especially as there was already water there. Finally in the normal statistical distribution of the outcomes of any illness, outliers at the extreme bounds of probability must occur if enough cases are examined. Therefore, in any apparently terminal illness we would expect a small number of people to spontaneously recover, an apparently miraculous cure. In a site attracting very ill people it is unsurprising that these rare, unusual, but nevertheless expected resolutions of illness should become

associated with Lourdes. If 100,000 individuals with cancer visit Lourdes, then it is reasonable to assume that at least two or three may appear to spontaneously go into remission.

Depending on the viewpoint adopted, both explanations are rational and acceptable. To a believer who already accepts the supernatural presence of God, the religious explanation is acceptable and rational. To a non-believing scientist, the story consists of few coincidences and the psychotic symptoms of a young woman. In the 19th century south of France, a deeply Catholic and religious area, the religious explanation was accepted and Bernadette was ultimately Canonized as a saint. In the technological France of the 21st century, it would be interesting to see the response to Bernadette now. Canonization and belief in Bernadette's story would be unlikely, and a detention under France's Mental Health Laws and enforced treatment with antipsychotic medication would be the more probable outcome.

This illustrates that psychiatry cannot be seen in isolation from the culture in which it develops. Even if Western psychiatric laws are on the statute books, they may not be applied, or may be applied in very different ways from apparently identical laws in Western democracies.

MENTAL HEALTH LAW AND POLITICAL CONTROL

The use of Mental Health Law to control political dissent is an extreme form of the Western view of psychiatric illness as social deviance. In generally totalitarian regimes, for example, as existed in the late Union of Soviet Socialist Republics, it was common to label political dissent as mental illness. This may be carried out overtly or covertly. When exercised overtly, the State's position is that the society is so perfect, rational and beneficent that no sane person would dissent or criticize it. Carrying out such dissent must, therefore, be prima-facie evidence of mental illness. Individuals who do dissent are then treated under existing Mental Health Laws. Such a standpoint can be hard to justify especially in a modern technologically advanced society, so totalitarian regimes have resorted to a more covert use of mental health legislation. In these situations a dissenter is detained and treated for a mental illness and symptoms of the mental illness may well be induced using drugs or other techniques. In both cases the psychiatric institution is at best a prison and at worst an institution or a tool of state aggression. Regrettably there are still examples of regimes that commit these violations of human rights around the world.

ENACTING MENTAL HEALTH LAW IN WESTERN COUNTRIES

In this section the way in which mental health legislation is enacted and applied in the Western democracies is examined by using the example of the law as written and applied in England and Wales. The mental health legislation in force at the time of writing this chapter was the Mental Health Act (1983),[10] however, a new mental health act, with extended powers, was in the process of being formulated. This is not intended as a comprehensive guide to the MHA, but is used to illustrate how a jurisdiction enacts Mental Health Law.

Three phases of compulsory admission under the MHA will be discussed:

❏ Assessment.
❏ Treatment.
❏ The appeal/review process.

The parts of the MHA which deal with people with serious mental health problems who have broken the law, will then be examined. The MHA 1983 states in Section 1 that the scope of the act is to deal with the reception, care and treatment of mentally disordered patients, the management of their property and other related matters. This is an extremely wide-ranging statement, essentially saying that the MHA has the power to control and intervene in every aspect of a mentally disordered person's life.

A further important point about Section 1 of the MHA is that it then attempts to define the types of mental health problems within the scope of the act from a legal, as opposed to a psychiatric/medical, perspective. Therefore the definition of mental disorders is split into four types:

1 **Severe mental impairment**: this means a state of arrested or incomplete development of mind, which includes severe impairment of intelligence and social functioning and is associated with abnormally aggressive or seriously irresponsible conduct on the part of the person concerned.

2 **Mental impairment**: this means a state of arrested or incomplete development of mind (not amounting to severe mental impairment), which includes *significant* impairment of intelligence and social functioning and is associated with abnormally aggressive or seriously irresponsible conduct on the part of the person concerned

Severe mental impairment and mental impairment are generally used to apply to those with learning difficulties, who exhibit abnormally aggressive or seriously irresponsible behaviour. It is therefore important to note that simply having a full scale intelligence quotient in the learning disability range does not allow the individual to be sectioned.

3 **Psychopathic disorder**: this means a persistent disorder or disability of mind (whether or not including significant impairment of intelligence) which results in abnormally aggressive or seriously irresponsible conduct on the part of the person concerned

When compared to other mental disorders treatment of psychopathy is difficult. Psychopathy in the MHA is a legal definition and there are several different definitions of psychopathy used by psychiatrists and psychologists. Therefore the legal definition of psychopathy encompasses a heterogeneous population, which makes targeting any treatment problematic. In addition, many psychiatrists have questioned the treatability of those identified with having psychopathy and therefore argue that they should not be detained under the MHA.

4 **Mental illness**: this category is not defined and is therefore left open to interpretation. This is, however, established through common practice and case law (previous legal cases involving the act which have set precedents) as meaning the opinion of psychiatrists backed up by the official classifications of mental illness.

Compulsory admission to hospital for assessment

In the MHA 1983 the provision to detain for psychiatric assessment is provided by Section 2 which provides the authority for someone to be detained in hospital for assessment for a period of 28 days on the recommendation of two medical practitioners. The section cannot be renewed after the 28 days have passed and although the letter of the law would allow a new Section 2 to be imposed in reality this would be seen as an inappropriate use of the act. If an admission is seen as being urgent then the person can be admitted under Section 4 of the MHA which allows a single medical practitioner to detain someone for up to 72 hours, during this time once a second medical opinion is obtained the Section 4 can be converted into a Section 2.

Finally an individual who is already a patient in a psychiatric unit on a voluntary basis may be sectioned under Section 2 or Section 3 if their medical condition is judged to demand it. If a doctor feels that a person should be detained under the MHA but the person tries to leave a Section 5.2, doctor's holding power, may be used to detain the individual for up to 72 hours while a Section 2 or Section 3 is obtained. Nurses have a similar power if they feel that the person is suffering a mental disorder and that for either the patient's or others protection they should be prevented from leaving until a doctor can impose a Section 5.2. A Section 5.4 can only be used to restrain an individual for 6 hours and cannot be extended and should only be used when a doctor cannot attend to place a Section 5.2.

Compulsory treatment

Compulsory treatment under the MHA (1983) is provided under Section 3. Section 3 provides the authority for someone to be detained in hospital for treatment and again it requires agreement by two medical practitioners. The person detained must be judged to have a diagnosis of mental illness, severe mental impairment, psychopathic disorder or mental impairment. Section 3 can be for 6 months and it may be renewed for a further 6 months and then can be renewed again for periods of a year. Those applying for the section must also make the case that the treatment cannot be provided unless the person is detained under Section 3. A key point is that in the case of psychopathic disorder or mental impairment any treatment undertaken under Section 3 must be likely to alleviate or prevent a deterioration of his condition and the treatment must be necessary for the health or safety of the person being restrained or for the protection of others.

Appeals and scrutiny of detention

Appeals against detention under the MHA are not judicial but rather are made to a specially convened body under the Act, the Mental Health Review Tribunal (MHRT). The MHRT is convened by the hospital/unit responsible for the detention and is made up of 'hospital managers' these are not managers of the unit but are people asked to represent the hospital or unit on the MHRT. The members of the committee are medical, legal and lay people with the latter usually having expertise in some aspect of social care. Individuals are usually represented by lawyers and the committee is operated on formal quasi judicial lines. The MHRT has the power to reverse, confirm or modify the detention. In the case of Section 2 appeal can be made in the first 14 days of detention and in the case of Section 3 during the first six months and at subsequent renewals.

A further level of scrutiny and guidance is given by the Mental Health Commission which is a special health authority and has the power to appoint doctors to give second opinions, receiving treatment plans, drawing up a code of practice and preparing guidance notes.

In theory under the MHA (1983) there is a substantial independent, fair and impartial reviewing system, however, in practice the Act has been criticized for not convening MHRTs quickly and for being an intimidating and remote review procedure. However, it can also be argued that a quasi judicial system established locally is more approachable and less intimidating and less prone to delays than a judicial system of review and appeal.

CONCLUSION

As noted at the beginning, when this chapter was commissioned I was asked to produce a review of mental health legislation around the world. However, I quickly found that at least on the surface the dominance and hegemony of Western society was complete and that apart from relatively minor technical difference in the application of Mental Health Laws, these laws were broadly similar in all jurisdictions. What did differ were the extent to which the Laws were used and applied and the extent to which they effected local beliefs. Many non-Western societies have a different worldview of mental health problems and systems. Even disorders such as schizophrenia, which can be shown to have a markedly similar presentation and course around the world, are perceived differently in non-Western cultures.

It can be seen from the example of the MHA (1983) that mental health legislation is an extremely powerful instrument of control over the citizen's freedom. However, it can also be seen that the spirit of the Act is that of an instrument designed to assist people and to protect them and society and that there is a formidable and comprehensive set of safeguards in place to prevent abuse of the Act. If psychiatric disorders are accepted, and there is compelling evidence that such diagnoses, while by no means being perfect, do represent real illness and are associated with significant distress, then some form of mental health legislation becomes a moral imperative.[6] Therefore the challenge for the 21st century in Mental Health Law is to create compassionate and user friendly laws that also respect local culture. Those enforcing such legislation, and exercising powers given to them by the state, have a duty to Act compassionately and in the best interests of the individual. The role of the nurse here is crucial, as the individual being detained has a right to expect that those who carry out most of their daily care should be their guide and advocate through the potentially frightening and complex mental health legislation.

REFERENCES

1. Van Lysebetteb T, Igodt P. Compulsory psychiatric admission: a comparison of English and Belgian legislation. *Psychiatric Bulletin* 2000; **24**: 66–8.

2. Dosa A. New legislation on civil commitment in Hungary. *Medicine and Law* 1995; **14**: 581–7.

3. Kitamura F, *et al.* Method for assessment of competency to consent in the mentally ill. *International Journal of Law and Psychiatry* 1998; **21**: 223–44.

4. Singleton N, Meltzer H, Gatward R, *et al. Psychiatric morbidity among prisoners in England and Wales.* Office for National Statistics, 1998.

5. Boyle M. *Schizophrenia a scientific delusion.* London: Routledge, 1990.

6. Parsons S, Armstrong A. Psychiatric power and authority: a scientific and moral defence. In: Barker P, Stevenson C. *The construction of power and authority in psychiatry.* Oxford: Butterworth Heinemann, 1999.

7. Szasz T. The case against psychiatric power. In: Barker P, Stevenson C. *The construction of power and authority in psychiatry.* Oxford: Butterworth Heinemann, 1999.

8. Leff J. *Psychiatry around the globe. A transcultural view.* New York and Basel: Marcel Dekker, 1981.

9. Oosthuizen H, Fick G, Els C. Legal status of the mentally disordered person in South African law. *Medicine and Law* 1995; **14**: 601–9.

10. Department of Health and the Welsh Office. *The Mental Health Act (1983).* London: The Stationery Office, 1983.

Chapter 60

ETHICAL ISSUES IN PSYCHIATRIC AND MENTAL HEALTH NURSING

Richard Lakeman*

INTRODUCTION

Interpersonal relationships lie at the heart of psychiatric and mental health nursing. The nurse and person are part of a web of relationships encompassing family, friends, colleagues, organizations, communities and wider society. These groups have an interest in, and expectations about, the nature of the relationship between the nurse and person. The person often finds themselves in a relationship with nurses at a time of extreme powerlessness, distress, vulnerability and estrangement from others, compounded by the stigmatizing effects of being labelled and treated as mentally ill. How nurses use their personal and professional power, in relation to the person, and how they balance the expectations and wishes of all interested parties, has profound ethical implications.

Ethics is about human action, what one ought to do, and forms of belief about right and wrong human conduct.[1] Ethics may also be viewed as the basis for choosing the kind of professional life we believe we should lead, so that we need not look back with regret in the future.[2] The practical purpose of ethics should be to provide guidance to the nurse on the 'right' course of action in a given situation. Nurses are involved in ethical inquiry whenever they spend time considering what they should do in relation to others and may be said to

be practising ethically when they choose to do the 'right thing' and can provide an ethical justification for their actions. In psychiatric and mental health nursing, uncertainty about the right course of action and ethical problems are encountered on a day-to-day basis. Consequently, nurses need highly developed skills in ethical reasoning and ethical problem-solving.

ETHICAL THEORY

An ethical problem may be said to arise when moral principles conflict in a given situation. An **ethical dilemma** may be likened to an **avoidance–avoidance conflict** in which there may be several alternative courses of action but each one of them is negative or in some way punishing. Examination of conflicting principles can alert one to a problematic ethical situation. However, the solution to the problem may not be readily apparent. Seedhouse[3] suggests that a willingness by health workers 'to do the right thing' or 'to be moral' is insufficient to ensure ethical practice. People need tools in the form of an understanding of ethical theory and philosophy to guide and justify their actions. It is, however, beyond the scope of this chapter to provide more than a sketch of some of the key features of a few ethical theories.

*At the time of publication Richard Lakeman is the Clinical Nurse Consultant of the Mobile Intensive Treatment Team in Townsville, North Queensland. He has previously worked in teaching and other psychiatric inpatient and community settings. To find out more about Richard please visit: http://www.geocities.com/HotSprings/8517/

Deontological theories

Deontological theories are concerned with 'duty' and beg the question 'What is my duty in a given situation?'. Many people believe it their moral duty to obey God. However, this can be problematic as there are irreconcilable differences between people regarding what the will of God is. Others also deny the existence of any 'divine' voice of authority. An influential alternative to theological ethics was proposed by Kant, who suggested a universal law, which demands '… that we should only act in accord with a given principle or set of principles if we can, at the same time, reasonably will that it should be binding on all others through space and time'.[4] In many instances Kant's 'categorical imperative' prescribes a very clear duty to act. For example, it would be unconscionable to lie to anyone regardless of the consequences, because of the chaos and damage caused if all people were permitted to lie in all circumstances. The ability to reason is central to Kantian notions of morality. Without the capacity to reason, one cannot enjoy full status as a moral citizen.

Consequentialist (teleological) theories

A broad range of theories hold that actions may be judged good or bad depending on the consequences they produce. Contention exists over what counts as good consequences (e.g. material gain, happiness, freedom, dignity, etc.) and whose good should be promoted (e.g. self, the in-group, the profession, society, or all people equally). Utilitarianism is a theory that proposes that an act may be judged good or bad depending on whether it promotes the greatest balance of good *over* bad, happiness *over* unhappiness, and pleasure *over* pain. The world tends to be viewed in terms of peoples' collective and overall interests. When considering where to invest scarce health resources a utilitarian perspective would require an investment to ensure the *greatest good* for the *greatest number*. While at face value this appears appealing, it may also serve as a justification to discriminate and alienate minority groups, or minority points of view.

Moral principles

When people make statements such as 'it isn't fair' or 'do no harm' they are perhaps unwittingly appealing to moral principles. While, there may be disagreement about which principle might carry the most weight in a given situation, or how principles might be used, there is general agreement that the principles of autonomy, non-maleficence, beneficence and justice underpin ethical behaviour in health care.

Autonomy is a principle that implies that people ought to be free to choose and act any way they wish, providing that their actions don't violate or impinge on the moral interests of others. Autonomy means having respect for the self-determination or decision-making of others. Maintaining or promoting people's autonomy and some form of equitable partnership poses one of the greatest ethical problem for psychiatric nurses in their relationships with people in distress.[5–8] In psychiatric and mental health nursing autonomy is frequently overridden in the interest of promoting the principle of **beneficence** or 'doing good'. Unfortunately, what counts as good and who should be the arbiter of what is good are contentious questions. For example some people argue that suppression of symptoms through medication is a hindrance to real recovery and that the adverse effects of psychotropic drugs are often worse than experiencing the illness itself.[9] Forcibly administering medication against a person's will is a clear breach of a person's autonomy, yet may be justified by the health professional as being in the person's best interests. Such actions are always ethically problematic and require a legal mandate to act.

'Madness', more recently called 'mental illness', has long been recognized as a class of experience, which may profoundly affect the capacity of people to make free, and rationale choices. Plato is credited with saying that, 'a man … either in a state of madness, or when affected by disease, or under the influence of old age, or in a fit of childish wantonness, himself no better than a child …' could not be held accountable for his crimes.[10] The Kantian notion of morality is focused on the rational being[11] and someone who is unable to reason from this point of view does not possess free moral agency and cannot be held to account for their actions. However, people's reasoning is seldom totally impaired.

Mental health professionals are often called upon to make judgements about a person's **capacity** to make autonomous choices for official purposes (e.g. to determine if a person requires civil commitment under a Mental Health Act) and during their everyday encounters with people. Even when people are deemed to be severely mentally ill, with some degree of impaired judgement, they are likely to continue to possess intact decision-making capacity in at least some areas. Health professionals, therefore, require skill in recognizing the person's current strengths or 'ablement' to protect and promote the person's autonomy.

Non-maleficence means to do no harm and has long been claimed as 'the first' principle of ethical health care. The meaning of harm is open to interpretation but certainly extends to psychological, social, or spiritual harm or suffering. The principle of non-maleficence would provide justification to condemn any act, which might cause another avoidable suffering. The principle of non-maleficence requires nurses to take heed of the experience of patients and to recognize the potential suffering that illness and treatment may cause. For many people the experience of treatment and hospitalization is fraught with traumatic and harmful experiences as illustrated by an extract from Susie's story:[12]

> Nothing compared with the horror of this psychiatric unit. It was the most traumatic experience I have ever had ... It was just total madness, twenty-four hours a day, no privacy, all my personal belongings were stolen. I was sexually abused by another patient. I was assaulted. I had no safe space. They were trying to de-stim (sic) me in a very unsafe environment ... using punishment.

As well as considering Susie's story in terms of non-maleficence, one may also consider that she had been treated unjustly and did not deserve to be exposed to abuse in any circumstances. **Justice** is a term that may be considered in several ways. For example justice may be considered as fairness, or revenge (retributive justice), or an equal distribution of benefits (distributive justice) or as equality. Justice in its various forms is a core ethical concept, and is used as a justification for action, or breached, in a myriad of ways in relation to people with mental illness.

The various conceptions of justice can come into play in any given situation. Often this is a recipe for conflict, as illustrated here:

Case study 60.1

John went without treatment for a psychotic disorder because he lived in a rural area where services were not available. He shot and killed a family member when psychotic, believing him to be possessed by a devil. He was found not guilty of murder because of insanity and was remanded in a psychiatric forensic unit for treatment. He responded quickly to treatment but was not released for some years, because of the public reaction to a 'murderer' not serving a reasonable sentence. On discharge he was unable to find reasonable accommodation because of the publicity surrounding the case and was unable to find employment because of his history of mental illness.

That John went without early recognition, treatment or care is an issue of distributive justice. Despite responding to treatment, and presumably posing no great risk to others if adequately supported, his continuing incarceration became an issue of retributive justice (or punishment). This in itself was unfair as he was found 'not guilty' because of insanity. Neither was his experience of discrimination 'fair' when he was discharged. The principles of *retributive justice* and *justice as fairness* conflicted in John's situation and no doubt impeded his recovery.

Sometimes the ethical principles at stake in a given situation may be vague, but may be refined further into **moral rules**. For example, the rule 'tell the truth' (**veracity**) arises from the principle of autonomy, which recognizes that rational people ought to be free to choose. Telling a lie therefore would deprive a person of the information needed to make a rational choice. Consequently, nurses are obliged to be truthful towards people in their care. While telling a blatant lie may be ethically indefensible in many situations, telling the 'whole truth' can sometimes be destructive. Lawler[13] coined the term '**minifism**' to describe '... verbal and/or behavioural techniques which assist in the management of potentially problematic situations by minimizing the size, significance, or severity of an event involving a patient'. 'Good' health professionals are likely to modify their 'gut responses' or manage their self-presentation in their interactions with people, to minimize the harmful impact of revealing their responses. For example, a nurse may be disgusted by a person's incontinence or body odour. However, being brutally honest about their feelings may shame the person or otherwise cause a loss of dignity. To prevent such harm, the nurse may sensitively prompt or assist the person to attend to self-care. The person may ask 'This must be really disgusting?' or state 'I'm disgusting' but the sensitive nurse will modify their response to minimize the incident in an effort to maintain the person's dignity.

Reflection

❑ Which ethical principles do you value the most and why?
❑ When considering an ethical course of action do you primarily consider the consequences of the action or the action itself?
❑ What ethical theory do you identify with and why?

Virtues

A virtues approach to ethics emphasizes the moral character of the person through the question: 'What sort of person should I be?' In practice the resolution of ethical problems begins with a recognition that situations are ethically problematic[14] or that the person is vulnerable.[15] In the example outlined above, the nurse may be said to have acted compassionately by minimizing his or her response to the person's incontinence. Virtues provide the disposition that enables a person to reason well and to act according to the right reasons.[16,17] Virtues may also provide an intuitive choosing of the right course of action when moral principles conflict.

The virtues that nurses need depend on the roles they choose or are required to assume.[18] Early nurse education stressed obedience, and loyalty to the doctor. However contemporary nurses require other virtues such as courage, to realize roles such as advocate. Some virtues which are useful for psychiatric nursing include:[17,19]

❏ **Compassion** – the capacity to share another person's suffering and to appreciate their humanity and vulnerability.
❏ **Humility** – remembering that we do not possess all the answers, which inclines us towards listening and learning from others.
❏ **Fidelity** – which provides a commitment to help other people and reminds us that clients have a claim on us that endures even when they refuse the treatment we offer.
❏ **Justice and courage** – provide not only an inclination to do what is right and fair, but also provide a motivation to act to protect others interests even at some personal cost.

Virtues may not be learned in the same way as principle based theories of ethics. They are necessary, but insufficient, to ensure ethical behaviour. However, virtues like clinical knowledge and skill may be developed through such practices as reflection, good mentorship and supervision.

Reflection

Consider someone you work with whom you consider to be a virtuous person. How does he or she demonstrate virtue?

Criticism of traditional approaches to ethics

Traditional Western philosophical ethics has failed to provide an account of, or prescribe a unifying morality, which has utility in all situations. The impartiality and detachment associated with traditional ethical decision-making is also at odds with the lived experience of psychiatric nurses, which is characterized by involvement and value laden clinical judgement. Spreen Parker[20] suggests that dialogue between people concerning their individual needs, desires and values is seen to threaten the impartiality required to make principle based decisions and, '… moral reasoning is confined to an abstract monologue, rather than a relational, embodied dialogue between human beings struggling to make sense of deeply perplexing situations'. At least some nurses have suggested that traditional approaches to ethical problems are antithetical to the practice of nursing founded on an ethos of care, which stresses involvement and the highly contextualized nature of human relations.[21,22]

Further criticisms of traditional approaches to ethics centre on their failure to address the systematic and systemic oppression of whole peoples, cultures and groups such as the mentally ill. Johnstone[23] suggests that mainstream bioethics is ethnocentric and sexist in nature and has '… only limited practical value and application in the realms of clinical practice in the health care arena'. An evolving ethic of care[24] and feminist approaches to ethics[25] offer different lenses to examine the nature of ethical problems, and prescribe factors other than principles – for example relationships and institutionalized oppressive structures – that require consideration in ethical enquiry.

THE MANY ETHICAL DIMENSIONS OF PSYCHIATRIC NURSING

Culture and moral pluralism

Globalization facilitated by communication technologies, ease of travel, and news media have made it increasingly obvious that people can and do have vastly different worldviews including conceptions of what is good or proper conduct. All people exist within and are inextricably part of a culture, which colours the way they see, make sense of, and interact with the world. Culture – among other things – consists of the values or abstract ideals held by the members of a given group, and the norms or definite rules and principles people are expected to follow.[26] Culture exists prior to ethics not the other way round.[4] A cursory review of cultural differences reveals a moral pluralism, which must be explored and negotiated if nurses are to claim ethical sensitivity or practice. It is not enough to rely on tradition, appeal to authority, adherence to the law, or to simply follow instructions to ensure ethical practice. To act ethically requires as a starting point an awareness of factors, which colour and shape our view of the world.

The traditions and practice of Western psychiatry and psychiatric nursing arise largely from Western values and views of health and wellness. These views are value laden. They are embedded in institutional processes and are often taken for granted by health professionals. For example, most health professionals would accept the 'holistic' notion of people being biological, psychological, social and spiritual beings. In practice however, Western psychiatry and psychiatric institutions tend to view the origins of mental distress as biological, which might in turn manifest as psychological, or social symptoms. Treatment is primarily biological (i.e. drug treatments) with adjunctive psychological (e.g. psychotherapy) or social (e.g. family education or therapy) interventions. In contrast (as illustrated in Fig. 60.1), people from traditional indigenous cultures such as Australian Aboriginal, or New Zealand Maori are likely to conceive of distress quite differently, viewing the root cause of distress as being of spiritual or social origin,

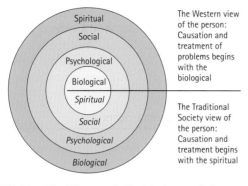

FIGURE 60.1 The Western 'holistic' view and the traditional 'cultural' view of the person.

giving rise to psychological or biological symptoms. The problem itself may be located in the family group or community rather than the individual.

In traditional cultures when a person manifests with what may appear to be symptoms of psychosis or depression, the problem may be viewed as arising from some spiritual or social transgression, possibly of a family member or an ancestor. Treatment may involve prayers or rites, or 'making good' the perceived wrongdoing. In such circumstances a biological deterministic view and treatment of the person may not merely reflect a difference of opinion or a benign approach to care but may cause irreparable damage to the person through removing hope of recovery or estrangement from those that might best be able to help.

The importance of respect for cultural difference and culture as fundamental to understanding and the promotion of health, is slowly being recognized (see the ICN Code of Ethics[27]). Respect for cultural difference requires, as a starting point, an examination of one's own values, as well as the 'taken for granted values and assumptions' that guide everyday behaviour. Culture permeates every facet of human understanding, and provides the threads of the moral fabric upon which are woven the many relationships which psychiatric and mental health nurses enjoy.

Reflection

- What do you value?
- What is your personal understanding of the term mental health?
- Contrast your values and ideas about mental health with someone from a different cultural background.

Power and discourse

It has already been suggested that people experiencing mental illness often engage in relationships with psychiatric nurses when they have diminished power. A practical purpose of ethics is to guide the use of power by health professionals. This power is often made invisible, or legitimized through the use of language, and often reflects the worldview of the dominant culture. Foucalt[28] described the formulation of communicative processes on the basis of power, as 'discourse'. The world of clinical practice has its own language and logic, which is self-sustaining, in that it serves as a justification for action.[29]

The particular worldview – or 'ideology' – to which clinicians are aligned in practice, is founded on assumptions about what it means to be a person, what it means to be distressed, and what it means to nurse the distressed person. These assumptions are never value-neutral. Almost invariably they are bound by culture and often serve to subjugate or take away the power of others. The psychiatric discourse shapes people's stories, which are invariably stories of dysfunction and pathology. This is not to say that psychiatric discourse is bad *per se*. However, it is wrong to assume that psychiatry has the only story to tell in relation to people that are distressed. Indeed 'narrative therapy' acknowledges that the stories that communities of persons negotiate and engage in, give meaning to their experience. Narrative therapy aims to assist people to tell alternative stories, or 're-author' their lives according to preferred stories of strength and courage.[30] In considering the moral lives of psychiatric nurses in relation to communities, groups, and individuals the nurse must be mindful of the power of language, attuned to the various discourses that shape reality, and open to alternatives.

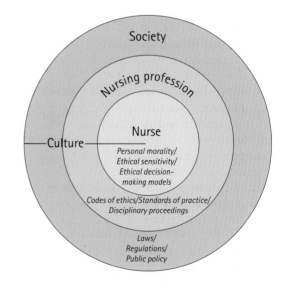

FIGURE 60.2 The moral lives of psychiatric nurses.

Psychiatric nurses and society

It may be useful to think of the moral lives of psychiatric nurses as having many dimensions and encompassing a number of key relationships (see Fig. 60.2). At the 'macro' level nursing is part of society and reflects, maintains and promotes certain societal interests. Governments are concerned with the best way to tackle societal problems and dictate what is considered proper conduct towards others through the passing of laws and regulations.

The mentally ill have been, and continue to be, poorly served by societies and have often experienced abuse, infringement of **human rights** and discrimination. Most Western countries have now adopted the United Nations resolution on the protection of persons with mental illness and the improvement of mental health care.[31] This is an international agreement, which requires member countries to ensure that people with mental illness are able to exercise all the civil, political, economic, social and cultural rights enjoyed by others. It also sets out standards for care and treatment and articulates the right for people to be treated in the **least restrictive environment**.

In contemporary Western societies the criminal justice and mental health systems have a mandate for **social control**, i.e. legally mandated and defined roles to contain, control or modify certain types of behaviour deemed undesirable. The threshold for interfering or restricting a person's liberty in order to assess or treat mental illness involuntarily has typically been raised to diminished rationality, lack of insight and imminent and serious risk of harm to oneself or others.[5] Nevertheless, even if involuntary assessment is legally mandated, people continue to be entitled to claim other **rights**. Some rights claims require a clear legal and ethical duty of the nurse (e.g. the right to information requires that people be told of their legal status). However, in some instances it may be uncertain where the nurse's duty lies in relation to rights claims. For example people may claim a right to legal advice or an alternative medical opinion. The nurse has a clear duty not to impede the person from seeking such advice but they may not be bound to facilitate it. The right to be treated with **respect** appears to be fundamental but like notions of beneficence it is open to interpretation.

In the best possible world one might safely rely on the laws of society as the framework required to behave ethically. Unfortunately, blindly following the law is perhaps the lowest level of moral comportment. Nurses who colluded in the extermination of the mentally ill in Nazi Germany, and the labelling as mentally ill and forced medication of political dissidents in the Soviet Union, might claim that they were acting lawfully. However few (at least from a position of detachment) would conclude that they were acting ethically. At best the law can provide only a crude guide to ethical behaviour in the nurse–person relationship through providing negative sanctions for extreme forms of immoral behaviour, e.g. physically abusing a patient, and defining the circumstances under which certain rights may be breached in the provision of treatment.

Reflection

- Make a list of rights.
- For each right identified, consider what duty a nurse may have in relation to those rights.

The nursing profession

Nurses are part of a profession, which implies a body of knowledge and set of values held by its members. Professions only exist in the context of society and reflect many of the values of that society. Codes of ethics and standards of practice reflect the publicly declared values of professions. Theories, while less publicly accessible, provide the professional with some framework to understand and guide their work. Watson[32] has described nursing as a 'moral ideal'. Certainly 'grand' nursing theories paint an ideal picture of the nurse's work. No 'grand' nursing theory adequately deals with the problem or the role of nursing in compulsory treatment. Nevertheless, nurses can look to their profession for more specific guidance on how to be and behave in relation to other people.

Reflection

- Review the ICN Code of Ethics[27] and study the standards under each element of the Code.
- Reflect on what each standard means to you. Think about how you can apply the standard in your nursing practice.
- Use a specific example from experience to identify ethical dilemmas and standards of conduct as outlined in the Code. Identify how you would resolve the dilemma.

The nursing profession, through regulatory bodies, is able to **censure** members for behaving in an unprofessional (viz unethical) manner, or acting beyond the **boundaries** of professional conduct. At a less formal level nurses may regulate their own conduct through discourse about professional boundaries. A boundary marks out territory, or the margins of an entity. A boundary violation in relation to nursing practice implies that someone is not behaving, as a nurse should, and that they are being something else. Boundary discourse appeals to elements of principle, rule-based and virtue ethics as well as etiquette. There are a number of potential areas of boundary violation:

- ❏ **Competency** – Practising beyond one's competency or training.
- ❏ **Roles** – Practising outside of institutional roles.
- ❏ **Physical contact** – Inappropriate touching, or sexual contact.

- ❑ **Space and place** – Undertaking therapeutic interventions outside of usual hours of work or in an inappropriate geographic space (e.g. in someone's bedroom).
- ❑ **Remuneration** – Receiving or soliciting gifts or favours for work done.
- ❑ **Dress and appearance** – Dressing provocatively or in an intimidating manner.
- ❑ **Communication** – Using inappropriate, derogatory, or overfamiliar language.
- ❑ **Intimacy** – Becoming 'too close' to clients; disclosing too much about oneself.

Some boundary violations reflect an unequivocal wrongdoing. For example, most professional bodies take a dim view of practitioners having sexual relationships with clients, in part because the client is always the more vulnerable party. However, the margins of professional boundaries are often blurred. Nurses experience an ongoing tension between the need to maintain distance from clients with the desire to establish therapeutic relationships.[5] Distance may play a role in maintaining a sense of safety but a degree of intimacy is almost always needed to develop trust and identification with the helper. Physical contact may be an important communicative device that can convey compassion and at times institutional roles may be unhelpful and confining. Nevertheless, consideration of professional boundaries is an everyday issue for most nurses.

Reflection

Consider each of the boundary areas described above and for each identify behaviour which is:

- ■ outside of the boundaries of professional nursing practice;
- ■ safely within the boundaries of practice;
- ■ on the margins.

Nurse and patient

The nurse is in the centre of the circle and must perform activities that are instrumental to the profession of nursing and wider society, and at the same time are in the direct interests of the person in care. This causes problems when the interests and demands of different parties conflict. The language of 'patient rights' has come to permeate discourse in psychiatric services.[4] Such rights and remedies are enshrined in legislation. However, such developments do not ameliorate the ethical problems of practice. For example, nurses are challenged to consider 'how' they might promote and protect rights (for example, choice and autonomy) at a time when society also demands that rights are subjugated, under the umbrella of protecting itself from the perceived threat of those with mental illness. Many of the ethical problems that arise within the psychiatric nurse–person relationship are a reflection of the tension, which comes when the demands of society and of medicine conflict with the ideals of nursing.

As has already been discussed, a frequently encountered problem in psychiatric practice is balancing the principles of personal autonomy with beneficence. Another concept to consider is that of **paternalism**. Beauchamp and Childress[18] define paternalism as 'the intentional overriding of one person's known preference or actions by another person, where the person who overrides justifies the action by the goal of benefiting or avoiding harm to the person whose will is overridden'. Compulsory treatment is a dramatically paternalistic practice. However, a far more frequent and subtle paternalistic practice is 'rationing' a person's cigarettes, refusing someone permission to go for a walk, or attempting to bend the will of another through coercive methods.

The method by which others try and influence or directly control another's behaviour may vary in terms of the gravity of the ethical problems that arise. MacKlin[11] described a continuum of interpersonal behaviour control methods:

- ❑ **Coercion** – involving a threat of force or bodily harm.
- ❑ **Manipulation** – involving deception to change behaviour; a lesser threat or covert threat.
- ❑ **Seduction/temptation** – involving the offer of enticements; playing to the 'weak will' of another.
- ❑ **Persuasion** – involving reason and argument.
- ❑ **Indoctrination/education** – involving the provision of education or activity (for example role modelling).

The use of or threat of force is considerably more ethically problematic than weaker methods of influence, but all attempt to override a person's free will and interfere with their autonomy. Lützén[33] described 'subtle coercion' as a common practice, which may be conceptualized as an interpersonal and dynamic activity, involving one person (or several) exerting his or her will on another. This requires a judgement of the patient's competency, acting strategically, modifying the meaning of autonomy, justifying coercive strategies and ethical reflection. The following incidents create conflicts in decision-making and require the nurse to assess the person's capacity for autonomy and sometimes engage in subtle coercion:

- ❑ patient's refusal of treatment, food or self-care;
- ❑ searching through and keeping patient's belongings;
- ❑ patients wanting to leave hospital;
- ❑ self-destructive behaviour; and
- ❑ patients being unable to communicate their own needs.

Whenever coercive methods are used there is a potential breach of ethics, in that the person's autonomy is compromised. Sometimes people are controlled in covert and subtle ways: for example a person is admitted voluntarily to an inpatient psychiatric unit but comes to appreciate that if they choose to leave that they will be prevented by nurses from doing so. In other instances nurses may use force (for example physically restraining a person), or otherwise more profoundly limiting their autonomy through the use of **seclusion** (preventing a person from interacting with others). The use of **physical restraint** and seclusion may be legally sanctioned within some psychiatric hospitals, to prevent harm to the person or others. However, people often experience these practices as coercive, frightening, punishing and harmful.[34,35] In response to behaviour from patients that engenders fear in others, nurses are often constrained by a lack of knowledge about non-coercive alternatives to restraints or seclusion.[35] The ongoing development of intrapersonal skills to deal with one's own fear and anxiety, as well as the development of interpersonal skills to defuse the anxiety and allay the fear of others, is an ethical imperative for nurses.

Reflection

- How do you respond to fear and anxiety?
- How might your responses affect the care that you provide?
- What might you do to allay the fear of others?

A further area of ethical tension, arising from balancing autonomy with beneficence, is the maintenance of **privacy**. The two areas of privacy related to mental health care include access to personal information and access to personal space. Privacy allows one to express characteristics and desires that one would not wish to reveal to others, *and* the freedom to control one's self-presentation.[36] People within acute psychiatric inpatient services are frequently under close observation or video surveillance and have severely limited opportunities to control self-presentation. People under the care of assertive outreach teams or receiving intensive psychiatric follow-up in their homes also experience an invasion of privacy. This can engender a sense of shame, embarrassment and violation, and can affect a person's identity. Surveillance can cause harm and nurses must balance the potential harm of close monitoring and breaching an individual's privacy, with the potential harm that may arise if the person's privacy is maintained.

Reflection

- Imagine how it might feel to have your behaviour constantly observed by others.
- If you have the opportunity, request colleagues or tutors to place you in a seclusion room or in physical restraints for an undisclosed period of time. Discuss the experience with others.

ETHICAL DECISION-MAKING

In practice, people rarely employ a formal ethical reasoning process when choosing how to act in relation to others. Benner[37] proposes that an ethic of care must be learned through experience, because it is dependent on recognition of '… salient ethical comportment in specific situations located in concrete specific communities and practices, and habits'. However there will be dilemmas and problems, which emerge in everyday practice, that are perplexing or require nurses to highlight, negotiate and justify to others, solutions to ethical problems. In such circumstances a problem-solving process may be usefully employed. It is beyond the scope of this chapter to provide a detailed account of any one ethical decision-making process (for further study, see Refs 3 and 4). All nurses, however, will be familiar with a basic problem-solving process, which involves assessment, diagnosing, planning, implementing and evaluating. Assessment involves identifying and describing the relevant ethical elements in a situation. The following questions may be useful to consider in assessment:

- What is the situation (provide a rich description)?
- Who has an interest in the outcome of the decision and what are their views on the right course of action?
- What are the choices available?
- What may be the possible consequences of each choice?
- What resources are required for each course of action?
- How might each choice impact on relationships with others?
- What principles or values stand to be compromised by each choice?
- What principle or value should take precedence in this situation?
- What are the rights of the parties involved?
- What duties arise from these rights?
- What are the legal requirements in the situation?
- Who ought to be involved in decision-making?

After careful examination of a situation it may be found that there is no ethical problem at all, but rather there is a problem of communication, law or policy that can be resolved through means other than ethical reasoning. If it appears that a dilemma or ethical problem remains, goals need to be set and a plan of action made. The plan may involve compromise, negotiation, further consultation, education or mediation. Lastly, the plan needs to be carried out and evaluated. Teams or groups may undertake this process. Indeed when faced with a dilemma it is generally better not to carry the burden alone, but to seek advice or supervision from others.

Limited moral agency of nurses

Even if nurses possess exceptional skills in ethical reasoning this does not necessarily confer the freedom to undertake the ethical course of action. Nurses are frequently constrained from exercising free moral agency.[38] In part this is because of the instrumental nature of nursing to medicine and the status of nursing within the health care system.[39,40] Quite simply nurses are often legally required to do the bidding of medicine, 'the team' or others. Profoundly ethical decisions relating to a person's rationality, insight, competency, or risk are couched as 'diagnostic' decisions or 'clinical judgements' which, according to psychiatric discourse and frequently the law, are the purview and territory of medicine. Nurses are often legally required to carry out 'doctors orders' to administer drugs, contain people under court orders, restrain, seclude otherwise restrict people's liberty. Nurses are often required to be the enforcers of compulsory treatment orders and contain the responses of people to being treated against their will. Yet, nurses are usually ancillary to 'clinical' and treatment decisions, or when decisions are made in 'teams' psychiatric discourse tends to dominate.

In a recent study, Lützén and Shreiber[41] found that the '… nature and resolution of ethical decisions about patient care were contingent on whether or not the cultural or management milieu of the workplace was supportive of nursing practice, that is, a place in which personal and professional growth was encouraged or not'. They suggest that nurses working in some contexts have limited choices because they work in a system that does not provide opportunities to challenge assumptions and work towards changing non-therapeutic environments, without risking personal sanctions. Nursing ethics must contend with the problem of many nurses having little, if any, say in ethical decision-making, and the problems of negotiating ethically problematic situations where the contributions and concerns of nursing are rendered invisible.[39,42]

Exposure to the ethical problems of practice can and ought to cause some **moral distress**. However, the power of discourse, the security of tradition and deference to psychiatric authority can lull the nurse into **moral complacency**, or the discarding of once cherished values. Moral discomfort may be functional if channelled into solving the problems of institutionalized oppression, and hegemonic discourse which inhibit nurses from acting freely and creating a truly collaborative health care ethic.[40] Barker[43] suggests that '… we face a major ethical dilemma in choosing between our faith in biomedical explanations of ill-health, on the one hand, and listening to, and learning from, the people in our care … on the other'. It may be that a greater challenge is accommodating and valuing different points of view, multiple realities and above all not abandoning those people who find themselves in situations that provoke our own moral distress or discomfort.

A pressing and ongoing ethical problem that psychiatric nurses face is realizing the purpose of nursing in relation to people that are distressed or suffering. It is easy and at times enticing to reduce nursing to a set of discrete roles or tasks such as 'managing risk', assessment, or administering treatments. However, while helpful, such tasks do not necessarily address what the person most needs, which may be to find meaning in suffering. As Frankl observed,[44] 'Suffering ceases to be suffering in some way at the moment it finds a meaning'. Assisting people to grow, find meaning in experience, connect with others and reconnect with self, reflect elements of true caring which are constantly threatened by competing discourses and human nature which compels one to flee from suffering. A fruitful starting point for ethical practice regardless of the context is for nurses to reflect on and refine their own philosophical basis of nursing care.

Psychiatric and mental health nursing is an ethical undertaking. The psychiatric nurse is often involved in complex messy situations, involving real people who hold differing accounts of a situation and have different and conflicting interests. Above all, psychiatric nursing practice involves a relationship with people who experience suffering. Ethical practice is more likely when the nurses has knowledge of ethical theory, the possession of clinical knowledge, skill, and virtues such as compassion, an awareness of one's own values and the values of others, and an awareness of the ethical dimensions of everyday psychiatric discourse.

REFERENCES

1. Beauchamp TL. *Philosophical ethics: an introduction to moral philosophy*, 2nd edn. New York: McGraw-Hill, 1991.

2. Barker P. Where care meets treatment: common ethical conflicts in psychiatric care. In: Barker P (ed.) *The philosophy and practice of psychiatric nursing*. Edinburgh: Churchill Livingstone, 1999: 199–212.

3. Seedhouse D. *Ethics: the heart of health care*. Chichester: John Wiley, 1988.

4. Johnstone M-J. *Bioethics: a nursing perspective*, 3rd edn. Sydney: Harcourt Saunders, 1999.

5. Fisher A. The ethical problems encountered in psychiatric nursing practice with dangerously mentally ill persons. *Scholarly Inquiry for Nursing Practice* 1995; **9**(2): 193–208.

6. Forchuk C. Ethical problems encountered by mental health nurses. *Issues in Mental Health Nursing* 1991; **12**(4): 375–83.

7. Garritson SH. Ethical decision making patterns. *Journal of Psycho-social Nursing* 1988; **26**(4): 22–9.

8. Lützén K, Nordin C. Benevolence, a central moral concept derived from a grounded theory study of nursing decision making in psychiatric settings. *Journal of Advanced Nursing* 1993; **18**: 1106–11.

9. Coleman R. *Recovery an alien concept*. Gloucester: Handsell Publishing, 1999.

10. Conrad P, Schneider JW. *Deviance and medicalization: from badness to sickness*. St Louis: C.V. Mosby, 1980.

11. MacKlin R. *Man, mind and morality: the ethics of behavior control*. Englewood Cliffs: Prentice-Hall, 1982.

12. Crooks S. *Susie's story*. In: Leibrich J (ed.) *A gift of stories*. Dunedin, NZ: University of Otago Press, 1999: 9–15.

13. Lawler J. *Behind the screens: nursing, somology, and the problem of the body*. Melbourne: Churchill Livingstone, 1991.

14. Lakeman R. Commentary on 'Where care meets treatment: common ethical conflicts in psychiatric nursing'. In: Barker P (ed.) *The philosophy and practice of psychiatric nursing*. Edinburgh: Churchill Livingstone, 1999: 213–16.

15. Lützén K, Evertzon M, Nordin C. Moral sensitivity in psychiatric practice. *Nursing Ethics* 1997; **4**(6): 472–82.

16. Armstrong AE, Parsons S, Barker PJ. An inquiry into moral virtues, especially compassion, in psychiatric nurses: findings from a Delphi study. *Journal of Psychiatric and Mental Health Nursing* 2000; **7**: 297–306.

17. Lützén K, Barbarosa da Silva A. The role of virtue ethics in psychiatric nursing. *Nursing Ethics* 1996; **3**(3): 202–11.

18. Beauchamp T, Childress J. *Principles of biomedical ethics*, 4th edn. New York: Oxford University Press, 1994.

19. Christensen RC. The ethics of treating the 'untreatable' (editorial). *Psychiatric Services* 1995; **46**(12): 1217.

20. Spreen Parker R. Nurses' stories: the search for a relational ethic of care. *Advances in Nursing Science* 1990; **13**(1): 31–40.

21. Kurtz RJ, Wang J. The caring ethic: more than kindness, the core of nursing science. *Nursing Forum* 1991; **26**(1): 4–8.

22. van Hooft S. Acting from the virtue of caring in nursing. *Nursing Ethics* 1999; **6**(3): 190–201.

23. Johnstone M. Keynote address. In: *Health care ethics: opening up the debate, 1995*. Massey University, Palmerston North, NZ: Unpublished, 1995, pp. transcript 1–18.

24. Simms LM, Lindberg JB. *The nurse person: developing perspectives for contemporary nursing*. New York: Harper and Row, 1978.

25. Sherwin S. *No longer patient: feminist ethics and health care*. Philadelphia: Temple University Press, 1993.

26. Giddens A. *Sociology*, 2nd edn. Oxford: Polity Press, 1993.

27. International Council of Nurses. *The ICN Code of Ethics for Nurses*. ICN, 2000.

28. Foucalt M. *The birth of the clinic: an archaeology of medical perception*. New York: Pantheon, 1973.

29. Goffman E. *Asylums: essays on the social situation of mental patients and other inmates*. Harmondsworth: Pelican Books, 1961.

30. Lobovits D, Epston D, Freeman J. narrativeapproaches.com./narrative%20papers%20folders/sax.htm Finding Common Ground between Human Service Seekers, Providers and Planners: A Reauthoring Conversations Approach.

31. United Nations. *The protection of persons with mental illness and the improvement of mental health care*. United Nations, 1991.

32. Watson JK. *A handbook for nurses*, 6th edn. London: The Scientific Press, 1921.

33. Lützén K. Subtle coercion in psychiatric practice. *Journal of Psychiatric and Mental Health Nursing* 1998; **5**: 101–7.

34. Johnson ME. Being restrained: a study of power and powerlessness. *Issues in Mental Health Nursing* 1998; **19**(3): 191–206.

35. Mohr WK, Mahon MM, Noone MJ. A restraint on restraints: the need to reconsider the use of restrictive interventions. *Archives of Psychiatric Nursing* 1998; **12**(2): 95–106.

36. Olsen DP. Ethical considerations of video monitoring psychiatric patients in seclusion and restraint. *Archives of Psychiatric Nursing* 1998; **12**(2): 90–94.

37. Benner P. The role of experience, narrative and community in skilled ethical comportment. *Advances in Nursing Science* 1991; **14**(2): 1–21.

38. Yarling RR, McElmurry BJ. The moral foundation of nursing. *Advances in Nursing Science* 1986; **8**(2): 63–73.

39. Liaschenko J. Ethics and the geography of the nurse–patient relationship: spatial vulnerabilities and gendered space. *Scholarly Inquiry for Nursing Practice* 1997; **11**(1): 45–59.

40. Lakeman R. Nurses are more than tools: instrumentality and implications for nursing ethics. In: King J (ed.) *Mental health nurses for a changing world: not just surviving*, 3–7 September 2000. Broadbeach, Queensland: Australian and New Zealand College of Mental Health Nurses, 2000: 204–12.

41. Lützén K, Shreiber R. Moral survival in a nontherapeutic environment. *Issues in Mental Health Nursing* 1998; **19**(4): 303–15.

42. Liaschenko J. The shift from the closed to the open body – ramifications for nursing testimony. In: Edwards SD (ed.) *Philosophical issues in nursing*. London: Macmillan Press, 1998: 11–30.

43. Barker P. Patient participation and the multiple realities of empowerment. In: Barker P (ed.) *The philosophy*

and practice of psychiatric nursing. Edinburgh: Churchill Livingstone, 1999: 99–116.

44. Frankl V. *Man's search for meaning: an introduction to logotherapy.* New York: Pocket Books, 1963.

Chapter 61

SEXUALITY AND GENDER

Alec Grant*

A male nurse got my address from my notes and decided to visit me at home while I was on leave. I was still pretty unwell and very drugged up and so I stupidly let him into my house. You can probably guess the rest ...

Diane, User and freelance Mental Health Consultant[1],[†]

One gay man said that he and his partner were generally made to feel awkward by (mental health) workers ... One lesbian said that staff made inappropriate comments; another ... reported being generally made to feel awkward; and one bisexual woman was told not to have any physical contact with her same-sex partner ... (some) reported incidents of physical and sexual violence in what are supposed to be therapeutic environments. One incident involved sexual assault and rape on a woman by a male nurse.

Golding[2],[††]

We have several long-term adult patients struggling to deal with sexual impulses. The staff avoid discussing this topic with the patients and are at a loss when trying to intervene. We have no classes or educational material on appropriate expression of sexuality. Our hospital prohibits any kind of touching – including hugs, holding hands and kissing. Specifically, what do you say to someone (who will likely be locked up for a long time) who wants to have a normal physical relationship with another human being? Does anyone out there currently have information on this topic or have you found some interventions that are helpful with your patients?

Lori Hutchison, Nurse[1],[†]

INTRODUCTION

When I began writing this chapter in the summer of 2001, the United Kingdom's *Royal College of Nursing* (RCN) bulletin announced that nurses would play a bigger role in promoting sexual health,[3] as part of the English Department of Health's Sexual Health Strategy. The *RCN Equality Network* also reported that it had organized a stand, for the first time, at the recent London Lesbian and Gay Mardi Gras.[4]

In contrast to what Goffman might have described as 'front-stage corporate impression management',[5] the lived experience for many service users – and for some psychiatric-mental health nurses – may not rest comfortably with these up-beat messages from the nursing establishment. Lori Hutchison's Internet posting at the

---

*Alec Grant is a Principal Lecturer at the University of Brighton, UK. His key interests are in clinical supervision, cognitive behaviour therapy and the impact of organizational issues on practice.

[†]All citations from the Psychiatric Nursing discussion list[1] are personal communications. The Internet address for the list appears in the references at the end of this chapter.

[††] Brackets added by author.

beginning of this chapter suggests that service users, in some clinical settings, will find it difficult to express important aspects of their sexuality because of organizational and cultural factors, and that at least some nurses feel unhappy about this. The quote from Golding's mental health awareness research on lesbian, gay and bisexual issues tells us that psychiatric-mental health nursing still needs to confront institutional homophobia. Finally, Diane's experiences, as a woman service user, illustrate the current power imbalances between female (users) and male (nurses), and the vulnerability of women receiving community care. To give adequate context to a further exploration of these issues, we need to outline the key terms and assumptions and clarify their meanings.

TERMINOLOGY

Gender will refer, here, to the *social* aspects of sexuality, in terms of the subjective individual and social experience/s of *'femaleness'* or *'maleness'*, and related behaviours. *Sexuality* can be considered as both a broad and narrow concept. In broad terms it may be thought of as:

> ... encompassing the most intimate feelings and deepest longings of the heart to find meaningful relationships ... the totality of being human ... Sexuality reflects our human character not solely our genital nature ...[6]

This broad definition encapsulates the noblest aspects of human growth and development. I return to this in the conclusion, when speculating on future possibilities for psychiatric-mental health nursing. The focus of the chapter is, however, mainly on sexuality in the narrow terms of its 'genital nature'. This is to counter the trend towards the inadequate representation of genital-sexuality in psychiatric-mental health nursing literature, and practice settings.

You never see a nipple in the Daily Express

This trend can be explained, partly, by inter-related cultural and organizational factors. Nursing – both in academic writing and practice – may suffer from a variant of the phenomenon described by John Cooper Clarke in his poem *'you never see a nipple in the Daily Express'*.[7] Nursing, at least in Britain, seems to be characterized by sexual asepsis – purged and sanitized, it is spared the discomfort that attends discussions of genital sexuality and its relation to the darker side of nursing practice and work settings. A good example is the occasional article in the *Nursing Times*, which reminds readers of the 'inappropriateness' of overtly genitally-sexualized talk or behaviour among (usually inpatient) service users.[8]

Equally, in the quality nursing research journals (in contrast to published research from the broader world of social science), qualitative accounts are rarely convincing in human terms – sexually-charged swear words are consistently absent from quoted dialogue.

In organizational terms, several factors operate to 'airbrush' the genital-sexual needs, lives, behaviour and abuse from the picture. Medical hegemony continues to define the reality and experiences of service users, through talk of 'illness' or 'disease' rather than in fully human terms.[9] Fineman[10] reminds us that the bureaucratic organizational settings, within which nurses and patients interact for extended periods of time, are subject to – often tacit and unseen – rules around displays of emotion. Genital-sexual behaviour and talk is thus frequently likely to be regarded as a 'backstage', private activity,[5,11] inappropriate for the public world of day-to-day psychiatric business as usual.

Unfortunately – at least for some individuals – the failure to acknowledge and respond in fully human terms to the fact that all of us, nurses and users, have genital-sexual dimensions to our lives, is likely to lead to various forms of clandestine 'backstage' activity, including sexual abuse. Ironically, in a circular way, such activity is tacitly sanctioned by the failure of organizations – service and education – to confront issues of gender and genital-sexuality, and by the potential for abuse, sexual and otherwise, inscribed within the process of *institutionalization*.[12] This will be touched on again later.

OVERVIEW

The overall aim of this chapter is to put gendered, genital sexuality back into the psychiatric-mental health nursing dialogue, in specific and selected ways. A brief exploration of the emergence of the concepts in psychiatric-mental health nursing will clarify their importance for service users and nurses. Following this, the theme of power imbalance and abuse will be addressed, using a variety of sources of evidence related to accounts of abusive practice, none being viewed as necessarily 'the best', 'most reliable' or 'objective'. The implications for good nursing practice will be suggested, along with an important current example and, finally, I will consider what are, in my view, some of the most important future issues for psychiatric-mental health nurses concerning sexuality and gender.

SEXUALITY AND GENDER

Emergence of the concepts

Dexter[13] described sexuality as first appearing as a curricular topic for psychiatric nurses in the 1982 training syllabus. Despite this, a decade later, perhaps reflecting the cultural unwillingness to deal openly with the subject, in the newly-designated 'mental health nursing' Nolan's *History of Mental Health Nursing*[14] contained no gendered and sexualized accounts, characters, issues or problems.

Thankfully, there are several more fully human historical studies, which contrast with this sanitized perspective. Gittins[15] sensitively used the memories of women and men – inpatients and nurses – who lived and worked in Severalls Psychiatric Hospital in England between 1913 and 1997, to construct a fascinating picture of the various forms of sex and gender-related experiences and practices, tolerated within this total institution.

Chatterton[16] traced the development, historically, of psychiatric-mental health nursing during the 20th century, asserting substantial differences from general nursing, including specific forms of gendered divisions of labour between men and women in mental health nursing. Chatterton's work can be read as tacitly emphasizing the patriarchal nature of bureaucratic organizational life in psychiatric institutions, which allowed for the possibility of various forms of gendered abuse of power.[17] These include the difficulties of men and women occupying the same space, and the prejudice and maltreatment that has traditionally been the experience of many lesbian and gay service users.

Various authors[18–20] have addressed the tendency for women to have experienced sexual abuse at the hands of mental health professionals, and the problems that women with such experiences may have in mixed sex wards. Thilbert[21] explored mental health ideology and care in relation to gender and sexuality. She dealt specifically with her difficulties as a lesbian developing empowering groups for women users in a community mental health centre, and the impact this had on the group.

From the perspective of lesbian, gay and bisexual service user experience, Golding[2] and McFarlane[22] highlighted the ways in which mental health services have reflected societal prejudices, in directly oppressing and pathologizing homosexual and bisexual people through systematic mistreatment over time. In Golding's view people fail to reveal their sexuality to staff for fear of discrimination or abuse. Many are concerned that their right to confidentiality will not be respected, and fear prejudice from health care workers. Such fears have justification in the face of reports of prejudice and abuse that some nurses and other mental health workers and users exhibit towards non-heterosexual users.[2,22]

Implications for users and nurses

The failure of some psychiatric-mental health nursing historical literature to acknowledge and address issues around gender and sexuality adequately, seems to reflect the broader cultural and organizational tendencies in nursing scholarship and practice. Despite this, a sizeable body of research and strategic literature alerts us to the fact that, both historically and currently, psychiatric-mental health nursing takes place in gendered, genitally-sexualized practice settings. Consequently, the overt and covert behaviour of mental health staff – reflective of broader societal prejudices and gendered attitudes – may disadvantage vulnerable service users. Let us elaborate on some of the abuse trends outlined above.

Women users in inpatient settings

Newton[18] defined mixed male and female acute wards (currently being reversed in Britain[20]) as potentially problematic for women. Given the evidence that 'a disproportionate number of women who come into contact with mental health professionals have at some time suffered physical and sexual abuse', these women are highly vulnerable.[20] Similarly, Glenister cited the findings of The Mental Health Act Commission in 1993,[23] where in mixed-gender acute wards:

> Women feel very frightened to sleep in dormitories or single rooms leading from corridors that are easily accessible to male patients ... a woman suffering from puerperal depression was admitted informally with her baby ... said she was nervous of venturing away from her room ... she spent long periods standing as a sentry at her door.

Barton[12] has also helped us to understand how the nature of psychiatric institutions lend themselves to the perpetration of abuse generally and, potentially, sexual abuse specifically, because of the power imbalance inscribed within the process of *institutionalization*:

> Brutality, browbeating, rough handling, harshness, teasing and general ill-treatment always lie latent in institutions, smouldering and ready to burst into flames at any time ... The presumption that such things do not or cannot happen has been shown again and again to be naïve and fatuous.

Glenister noted that managerial supervision in and of itself is insufficient to combat abusive institutionalized practice.[19] In the early days of my research on the impact of organizational factors on clinical supervision, an inpatient nurse (man) from the same organization was prosecuted for coercing a depressed woman inpatient into a sado-masochistic sexual relationship. After his conviction and imprisonment, the then Director of Mental Health noted in the local press that this kind of thing shouldn't happen again as there were 'systems of in-house supervision in place'.

This view rests on the rather naïve assumption that nurses feel safe enough, or are willing enough, to openly disclose their own abusive acts,[24] or that they, or their community colleagues,[25] feel and act *professional* enough to embrace the scrutiny that supervision – managerial or clinical – would bring, as an audit check on their own potential for abuse. Goffman described the 'face-saving' and 'impression management'[5] common to interpersonal relations. In many settings, especially inpatients, clinical supervision fails to take account of these factors.[24] Additonally, at least some groups of community psychiatric-mental health nurses may have more of an investment in concealment, than openness to professional scrutiny.[25] This is a frightening phenomenon when the vulnerability of female service users living alone in the community is considered.

Vulnerability at home – intimidation on the wards

I once witnessed a nurse grab hold of a patient in a blatantly sexual way. I was horrified and asked what the nurse was doing. I did complain at this, but my complaint was never taken forward. Instead three male nurses came up to me and asked me what I was doing, was I trying to get so-and-so the sack. Very intimidating … I am in no way suggesting that all sexual abuse in the inpatient setting comes from staff, but I am not alone in having had nurses making inappropriate contact with patients in their own homes.

Diane, User and freelance Mental Health Consultant[1]

Diane's experiences suggest obvious implications for psychiatric-mental health nursing practice. The nurse misused his power in sexually abusing her, in the safety (for him) of her own home. Diane, as a first time inpatient was both under-informed and under-confident of her rights as a service and as a human being. When she complained about the sexual abuse she had witnessed, institutional, cultural and organizational forces conspired against her in the intimidating response she received.[12,19]

Of course, not only women users are vulnerable in mental health care settings. A community psychiatric nurse researcher noted:

Although it is largely women who are likely to be sexually abused/attacked within psychiatric/therapeutic situations, men are also subject to unwanted attentions sometimes, including by staff. I have worked with two male clients who were visited at home by male inpatient nurses shortly after discharge. Both of those clients also reported sexual advances by a male nurse or assistant when an inpatient.[1]

Lesbian, gay and bisexual experiences

The overall conclusion from Golding's research, was that at least some lesbians, gay men and bisexuals who use mental health services do not feel safe enough to come out to both staff and users within them. Many of Golding's participants feared:

prejudicial attitudes and discriminatory treatment, physical and verbal abuse, isolation, rejection, and the pathologization of their sexualities as mental disorders.[2]

Such concerns are not unjustified, as McFarlane's later study showed.[22] A 'climate of fear' can exist for many lesbians, gay men and bisexuals, which is of course detrimental to their mental health. Many of Golding's participants reported experience of prejudice, discrimination, harassment, and occasional sexual violence and rape.[2]

The de-classification of homosexuality as a mental disorder by the American Psychiatric Association in 1973 and the World Health Organization in 1992 may not have deterred some mental health professionals who – according to both Golfing and McFarlane – continue to view homosexuality as a mental disorder (and, perhaps, find it morally abhorrent). Half of Golding's research participants reported that they had been told they might have fewer problems if they 'hid' or tried to 'change' their sexuality. Some reported that their partners had not been treated on an equal par with the partners of heterosexual users. Similarly, some staff had used the excuse that partners were not 'legally' next-of-kin or 'nearest relative', thus denying equal rights to lesbian, gay and bisexual partners.

Further, Golding argued that the majority of mainstream mental health services do not have information resources that are of any use to lesbian, gay and bisexual people, thus further isolating them. One option is to 'come-out', which is by no means a risk-free thing to do.

EMERGING IMPLICATIONS FOR GOOD PRACTICE

Psychiatric-mental health nurses need to reflect, constantly, on the *therapeutic interpersonal boundaries* between user and nurse. In particular, we need to ask: what are the distinct characteristics of a helping relationship in mental health care? How does this compare and contrast with other 'relationships': for example, those based on friendship, romance, or outright sexual exploitation?

In maintaining appropriate boundaries, nurses need to understand the relationship between 'fantasy lives' and 'lived relationships'. Without fantasies, including sexual images and thoughts, we would fail to thrive and develop as humans. However, each of us needs to distinguish between fantasy and reality. Vulnerable individuals – users and nurses – can often become confused about this distinction and risk acting upon fantasy, as if it were reality. This is especially the case if we have no supportive facility to help us express, and work through, our confusion. For nurses, this takes the form of clinical supervision. For users it involves similarly facilitative relationship with mental health workers.

The safety needs of service users are of crucial importance. Nurses need to recognize and challenge any practice that undermines the safety of users. This includes a focus on the environmental and organizational conditions that give rise to the potential for abuse. These include the problems inherent in many mixed-sex wards; the vulnerability of clients both in inpatient and community settings; and the heterosexist bias in the organization and provision of mental health care.

Clinical supervision represents one possible mechanism for good practice in the area of sexuality and gender. This might 'protect patients from nurses and nurses from themselves'.[26] Nurses should, however, be mindful of the relative lack of adequate clinical supervision in psychiatric-mental health nursing. This is, in turn, related to cultural and organizational problems including a lack of ownership of, and resistance to, its provision.[24]

In the broader context, today's students of psychiatric-mental health nursing may be more willing than their forebears to explore issues around gender and genital-sexuality in non-defensive ways. They may question, challenge and begin to make sense of the widespread embargo on discussing and dealing with these issues, whether in work-settings, in the literature or in nursing academe.

Lesbian, gay and bisexual users

In addition to the general issues raised above, more specific concerns arise around the needs of lesbian, gay and bisexual users. Golding and McFarlane[2,22] have suggested the need for uniform training for mental health staff in meeting the needs of these groups, to help them access appropriate services. McFarlane argued that raising the visibility of lesbians, gay men and bisexuals, including helping supporting workers to 'come out', would be helpful in the process of acknowledging and accepting *all* sexual orientations. In turn, this might minimize the potential for non-heterosexual behaviour to be pathologized.

Good practice in the expression of sexuality in institutional settings

A provincial hospital in British Columbia, Canada may well be unusual in having privacy suites – locations within the hospital. These offer patients a private and dignified setting for emotional or sexual intimacy. All suites contain reminders to practice safe sex, condoms, and a panic alarm, and have a degree of supervision by staff. To quote a little from Riverview's policy:[27]

> The desire for sexual intimacy is natural and the expression of this desire by consenting adults enhances the quality of life of many individuals. Education regarding sexuality is important for healthy sexual relationships. Patients at Riverview Hospital have a right to sexual intimacy in a private and dignified setting where they are as safe from harm as is reasonably possible. Sexually active patients are safer from harm when sexual activity occurs in a privacy suite within the Hospital than when it occurs elsewhere in the Hospital or grounds.

It may be instructive for readers of this chapter to speculate on how well or badly their own health care organizations measure up to the Riverview example. The Riverview provision, although appealing at first glance, may also raise some interesting questions. For example, by what means do staff ensure that the 'degree of supervision provided' is conducted sensitively as opposed to voyeuristically?

THE FUTURE

It is assumed that people need to strive towards personal growth and more fully human relationships.[28,29] This applies, whether they are users or providers of mental health services. However, this cannot be done in a vacuum. The environmental and organizational context of mental health activity – such as the effects on gender and sexual (broad and narrow) experience and behaviour characteristic of different care environments – need to be taken into account.

Nurses who engage in continual reflective practice, around the positive and negative impact of gender and sexuality, and their environmental and organizational contexts, are more likely to be helpful in facilitating human relating. In practice, a key question for future psychiatric-mental health nursing practice is: considering our definitions of sexuality (both broad and narrow) how might psychiatric-mental health nursing have a more positive impact on the nurse–user relationship?

Sexuality as human relatedness

Thematically complementing sexuality in its broad sense, Barker[28] (supported by Wilkin[30]) has argued eloquently for a unique philosophy of psychiatric-mental health nursing, which re-conceptualizes mental health difficulties as human problems in living. This focus, encapsulated in Barker's 'Tidal Model',[31] assumes that the proper role of the nurse is to assist, or co-facilitate individuals with such problems in the process of their resolution. It is further assumed that users:

> ... know what are their needs, or can be helped to recognize or acknowledge these, and from this minimally 'empowered' position, may be helped to meet these needs, in the *short*, rather than in the medium or longer-term.[32]

From a different, but potentially complementary perspective, Clarke[33] urges nurses to practice 'ordinary decency', in the spirit of according service users the respect that they would like themselves, were they on the receiving end of care delivery.

In and of themselves, these views are laudable, absolutely relevant to the voiced needs of many contemporary services users,[33,34] and should be pursued in the spirit of respecting the potential for human-ness and human growth that proceeds from a broad notion of sexuality. However, to realize this, students of psychiatric-mental health nursing will need to balance these models and philosophies with the following broader contextual issues. Attention should be paid to how the process of institutionalization[12] insidiously shapes abusive practices. Also worthy of consideration are the ways in which the management of emotional life in bureaucratic organizations[10] tends to relegate sexual activity as 'inappropriate', thus forcing it underground. The effects of visibility on what Wilkin describes as master – as opposed to second rate – craftsmanship,[30] arguably allows for potentially more abuse by nurses working in the community,[1] while some ward nurses may have institutional support for bad practice.[12,19] Finally, the impact of heterosexism in shaping services[2,22] must also be challenged.

Meanwhile, in cyberspace

On the psychiatric nursing discussion list,[1] debate continues to ebb and flow, regarding the potential for sexual abuse created by certain types of environment. In a discussion occurring in May 2001, opinions varied between those who were against mixed-sex wards because of the potential for abuse, and those who thought that wards should mirror society. Some of the latter considered that an important aim of the inpatient experience was to maintain elements of social reality and promote appropriate living skills, including the ability to live with members of the opposite sex. Ironically, Bowers (the list manager) in his posting on this strand dated the 25th May 2001 wrote:

> I was struck again by the importance of the issue when I read Thomas *et al.* (*Psychiatric Bulletin* 1995;**19**: 600–604)[35] this morning. One third of female inpatients report some form of sexual harassment, most of which was not reported to staff because the women excused the perpetrators because of their mental illness. In a small number of cases, the perpetrators were staff. Only 57% of female patients felt safe on the wards ... Thought provoking, isn't it?[1]

REFERENCES

1. Psychiatric nursing list homepage: http://www.city.ac.uk/barts/psychiatric-nursing

2. Golding J. *Without prejudice: mind lesbian, gay and bisexual mental health awareness research*. London: Mind Publications, 1997 (tel: 0181 519 2122).

3. Royal College of Nursing. Greater role for nurses in sexual health. *RCN Bulletin* 2001; **32**: 1.

4. Royal College of Nursing. RCN joins in the fun at Mardi Gras. *RCN Bulletin* 2001; **32**: 7.

5. Goffman E. *The presentation of self in everyday life*. London: Penguin (Pelican) Books, 1971.

6. Webb C. *Sexuality, nursing and health*. Chichester: John Wiley, 1985.

7. Clarke JC. *You never see a nipple in the Daily Express*. http://www.cyberspike.com/clarke/nipple.html

8. Nazarko L, Aylott J, Andrews A. How should nurses respond to patient's sexual needs? *Nursing Times* 2000; **96**(5): 3–9.

9. Barker P, Stevenson C (eds). *The construction of power and authority in psychiatry*. Oxford: Butterworth Heinemann, 2000.

10. Fineman S (ed.) *Emotion in organizations*. London: SAGE Publications, 1996.

11. Lemert C, Branaman A. *The Goffman reader*. Oxford: Blackwell,1997.

12. Barton R. *Institutional neurosis*, 3rd edn. Bristol: Wright, 1976.

13. Dexter G. *Psychiatric nursing skills: a patient-centred approach*, 2nd edn. Chltenham: Stanley Thornes, 1997.

14. Nolan P. *A history of mental health nursing*. London: Chapman and Hall, 1993.

15. Gittens D. *Madness in its place: narratives of Severalls Hospital: 1913–1997*. London: Routledge, 1998.

16. Chatterton C. Women in mental health nursing: angels or custodians? *International History of Nursing Journal* 2000; **5**(2): 11–19.

17. Parkin W. The public and the private: gender, sexuality and emotion. In Fineman S (ed.) *Emotion in organizations*. London: SAGE, 1996.

18. Newton S-A. Women and mental health nursing. In: Sandford T, Gournay K (eds). *Perspectives in mental*

health nursing. London: Baillière Tindall, published in association with the RCN, 1996.

19. Glenister D. Coercion, control and mental health nursing. In: Tilley S (ed.) *The mental health nurse: views of practice and education.* Bodmin, Cornwall: Blackwell Science, 1997.

20. NHS Executive. *Safety, privacy and dignity in mental health units: Guidance on mixed sex accommodation for mental health services, 2000.* Available at website: http://www.doh.gov.uk/pdfs/mhmixedsexaccom.pdf .

21. Thilbert D. Working with women. In: Barker P, Davidson B. *Psychiatric nursing: ethical strife.* London: Arnold, 1998.

22. McFarlane L. *Diagnosis homophobic: the experiences of lesbians, gay men and bisexuals in mental health services.* London: PACE (the Project for Advice, Counselling and Education), 1998 (email: pace@dircon.co.uk; tel: 0171 700 1323).

23. The Mental Health Act Commission: Fifth Biennial Report 1991–1993. In: Glenister D. Coercion, control and mental health nursing. In: Tilley S (ed.) *The mental health nurse: views of practice and education.* Oxford: Blackwell Science, 1997.

24. Duncan-Grant A. *Clinical supervision activity among mental health nurses: a critical organizational ethnography.* Portsmouth: Nursing Praxis International, 2001.

25. Morrall P. *Psychiatric-mental health nursing and social control.* London: Whurr, 1999.

26. Barker P. Psychiatric nursing. In: Butterworth T. and Faugier J. (eds). *Clinical supervision and mentorship in nursing.* London: Chapman and Hall, 1992.

27. Riverview Hospital. *Policy and procedure manual: patient sexuality: responsibility and support.* July 31, 1998. Website: http://www.bcmhs.bc.ca/

28. Barker P. *The philosophy and practice of psychiatric nursing.* Churchill Livingstone: London, 1999.

29. Barker P, Davidson B (eds). *Psychiatric nursing: ethical strife.* London: Arnold, 1998.

30. Wilkin P. The craft of psychiatric and mental health nursing practice, chapter 4. In: Barker P (ed). *Psychiatric and mental health nursing: the craft of care.* London: Arnold, 2002.

31. Barker P. The Tidal Model: developing and empowering, person-centred approach to recovery within psychiatric and mental health nursing. *Journal of Psychiatric and Mental Health Nursing* 2001; 8(3): 233–40.

32. Barker P. Doing what needs to be done: a respectful response to Burnard and Grant. *Journal of Psychiatric and Mental Health Nursing*, Commentary section. 2002; 9(2): 232–6

33. Clarke L. *Challenging ideas in psychiatric nursing.* London: Routledge, 1999.

34. Campbell P. Listening to clients. In: Barker P, Davidson B. *Psychiatric nursing: ethical strife.* London: Arnold, 1998.

35. Thomas C, Bartlett A, Mezey GC. The extent and effects of violence among psychiatric in-patients. *Psychiatric Bulletin* 1995; **19**(10): 600–604.

It may be timely for psychiatric-mental health nursing to challenge the cosy overemphasis of caring enshrined in person-centred curricular approaches and give more attention to considering what they need to do to avoid fulfilling their future institutional capacity to engage in 'violence, coercion and control'.[1] The notion of the self-actualizing user also seems fatuous in the light of environmental and organizational problems in inpatient[10] and community mental health care.[14] These serve to disadvantage users and will be addressed more specifically later.

Soft cop or nurse?

Consider the view of Simpson,[55] a community psychiatric-mental health nurse researcher, with recent clinical experience of assertive outreach work targeted at homeless mental health clients. He described a bleak and invidious picture of today's British community psychiatric-mental health nurse trapped between two worlds:

> ... (despite the sense of the need to maintain a therapeutic role) the supervision register brought in alongside CPA (Care Programme Approach) increased the sense of the CPN (Community Psychiatric-mental health nurse) as soft cop ... the soft police control role is experienced by many nurses as shifting the emphasis towards monitoring people – making sure you keep in contact with people ... this results in a blame culture ... organizational blame and avoiding risk. All emphasis is in maintaining contact and being seen to do that. If someone commits suicide or kills someone then the finger of blame points at the CPN.
>
> The supervision register didn't work and has been scrapped in line with refinements to the CPA...CPNs are taking on the care coordinator role ... having to do more case management and overseeing, with less time to have hands on care with the client ... some would say that's okay ... employing more community support workers ... that respond to a clients' need for a far more accessible, more practical, less talking in jargon worker. The argument against is that to be effective as a CPN you have to have a close relationship with a client.
>
> There's a lot of good stuff in the NSF (National Service Frameworks for Mental Health) ... plans for very positive stuff for when things go wrong. However, alongside of that are proposals for the new law (new Mental Health Act) with the emphasis on risk ... with more involvement in sectioning. The argument for: good relationship means a better person to section. The argument against: that this is relationship destroying.

Misery without tears

A question emerging for nurses from the above discussion is 'to what extent do existing constructions of service users enhance or inhibit empowerment?' For a broader and more detailed response to this question, readers of this chapter may wish to consult the excellent work of both Parker and his colleagues[56] and Barker and Stevenson.[57] For the moment it is useful to give a specific example of how user-freedom and consent may in reality be enhanced or undermined by assumptions prevalent in the research literature. The 'compliance therapy' research of Gray et al.[58] illustrated the tendency of some British nurse researchers to make (arguably) morally unacceptable, absolutist 'truth claims' from the results of their quantitative paradigm research.[59] Gray and Gournay have been charged with ignoring the issues of social control implicit in their work, where some patients may not have the choice of opting out of a medico-social structure and where:

> Power is built into the social fabric of mental illness of which we are all a part. It is difficult to compete with the power of money and the new-found knowledge that money can generate.[60]

Long,[60] with support from major qualitative researchers,[59] argued that it behoves quantitative psychiatric-mental health nursing researchers to abandon the fallacy of considering their approach the most *superior* and *only* window in the world worth looking through, and of being above consideration of the ethical and philosophical implications of their methods. Similarly Gergen[61] highlighted the 'cultural imperialist' position taken by those who fail to attend to the power-imbued, socially constructed nature, of what passes for 'neutral' science, where statistical outcomes portray 'human beings with the tears wiped off'.

In contrast, user-focused research may offer an additional empirical approach to enable individuals with mental health problems to articulate their needs in ways less distorted and influenced by what many regard as a thinly disguised social control and economic agenda. Users, from the so-called severe and enduring end of the mental health spectrum were recently trained to conduct research among others with the same severity of problem.[13] Emerging conclusions were that users are perfectly capable of making balanced judgements on the services they receive, and indeed are more likely to open out to researchers who have been through similar experiences.

To conclude this section, it seems apparent that, to accord users adequate respect, psychiatric-mental health nurses need to grapple with the problems around user freedom and consent, in the context of *both* user and nurse identity construction *and* the rhetoric of empowerment.

I will now discuss ways in which acute inpatient and community cultures and environments undermine user freedom. More attention will be paid to problems in acute inpatient environments, because of the overwhelming evidence – at least in Britain – of their intrinsically abusive nature. My aims are to focus the reader's critical awareness of some problem areas and highlight possible solutions emerging from contemporary research.

ACUTE PSYCHIATRIC WARDS

> ... acute wards resemble jails and by extension, the nurses jailors.[62] I have been discounted both as an agent in my own life ... recently, I was told 'Just remember who you are. You're only a patient'.[10]

A reduction over the years in long stay facilities, and the failure to provide adequate community services, has led to increased pressures on the use of acute-psychiatric services. The general picture of acute inpatient wards in England is bleak: while costly in accounting for two-thirds of mental health budgets,[63] there is little evidence that inpatient stays are clinically effective[64] or cost-effective interventions across the range of mental health crises,[65] providing little more than custodial care.[66]

Patients admitted on a voluntary basis often experience the admission as coercive, with many subsequently attempting to leave, only to be compulsory admitted to prevent them from doing so.[67] Patients may want to leave because psychiatric inpatient units are, generally speaking, unpleasant environments. There seems to be a consensus across the user, carer and professional literature that acute inpatients often feel deprived of therapeutic activity and sufficient contact with nurses, and at times feel unsafe and at risk of physical and sexual assault.[1,28,68,69] Patients on acute wards also report boredom because of the limited recreational activity available. They have limited participation in, and information about, their care which may often be poorly planned and co-ordinated.[70] Further research, which seems to have established reasonably well that high emotion is a significant factor in worsening the experience of false beliefs and voice hearing[71] suggested, somewhat paradoxically, that acute inpatient environments may often be likely to provoke a worsening of the symptoms they purport to manage and reduce.

A frequent reason given for trained nursing staff being unable to use their psychotherapeutic skills in acute settings is that they are overworked, spending a disproportionate amount of time on administrative and co-ordination duties, and managing time-limited crises, at the expense of ongoing, in-depth patient care.[72,73] Nurses have reported decreasing work satisfaction and poor morale, with recruitment, retention and staff sickness as associated problems.[73] Consequently, agency nurses staff many wards. Given the above, it is unsurprising that the nursing of service users in inpatient settings emerges as a site of struggle over client freedom.[10]

Alternatives to acute care are few however, and acute inpatient nurses in Britain today are, in the main, set up for failure. The introduction of clinical governance[74] into the National Health Service aims to increase clinical accountability within trusts and improve on the delivery of patient-centred evidence-based practice. Jarring with this expectation, and in keeping with the general picture of problems in acute inpatient care described above, Flanagan's[75] small scale qualitative research of acute inpatient psychiatric-mental health nursing suggested that nurse-patient contact was both limited and usually informal. Over-stretched nurses focused most of their energies on a minority of more difficult to manage clients at the expense of less troublesome ones. These nurses were unable to identify specific interventions drawn from research or underpinned by a clear theoretical rationale. Only a small percentage felt that they had sufficient and appropriate training to prepare them for working with psychotic individuals and, equally, few admitted to reading about or discussing recent research or developments in practice.

SECLUSION, RESTRAINT AND SPECIAL OBSERVATION

Without suggesting that it is acceptable practice, it is understandable from the above picture that seclusion and restraint are much used interventions. A systematic review carried out for the Cochrane Library[76] on the empirical status of seclusion and restraint for people deemed as suffering from serious mental illnesses concluded that there are no controlled studies in existence that evaluate the usefulness of seclusion or restraint among those people. Indeed, in support of Sallah,[77] there are potentially serious adverse effects for the use of these techniques, described in the qualitative studies included in the review. The review concludes with the recommendation that alternative ways of dealing with unwanted or harmful behaviours need to be developed.

One method of controlling and containing the most disturbed patients, considered imminently at risk of harming themselves or others is through observation. Observation has however recently been described as a 'woefully weak intervention whose limited effectiveness can be judged by the one-third of people who commit suicide while inpatients'.[78] Bowers and Park[79] in their review of the literature on special observation (SO), while conceding that the procedure is based on clinical pragmatism and traditional custom and practice rather than evaluative research, take a more balanced view. They argue that there is little agreement between health care areas about what nurses should do during SO, but report that under certain circumstances the practice can be therapeutic. Conversely, they summarize evidence to suggest that in other circumstances nurses find it stressful and patients dislike it.

Nurses who find the process stressful do so because, among other reasons given, it is frequently regarded as a low status activity, thus delegated to junior or untrained staff, and because the paternalistic process tends to influence styles of nurse–patient interactions which infantilize the patient receiving SO. Perhaps a more fundamental reason for nurses finding the procedure difficult is the problem of SO placing nurses in a position where patients' rights to privacy and human dignity are temporarily suspended for safety reasons.

From the perspective of the service user, the evidence is equivocal. Inpatients may either feel isolated, degraded, policed, coerced and lacking in interaction with their observer, or understood and accepted.[79] Jones et al.[80] reported the findings of a pilot study from the perspective of the patient, where the experience was predominantly described by most clients as negative. What made observation more palatable was the observing nurse interacting more with the client and providing information about the observation process.

Bowers and Park soberly conclude that SO may be effective for some types of patients and not others, and that different levels of SO may have differing efficacy in different circumstances.[79] For example, a highly intrusive level of SO might be an effective strategy in preventing the suicide, in the short term, of users with severe depression, but completely counterproductive with the violent, paranoid patient. The degree of efficacy might also depend upon what the observer does during SO, and how skilled or otherwise they are.

Re-focusing

Partly triggering a vigorous psychiatric nursing list dialogue entitled 'engagement versus obs' in the Spring of 2001,[34] Dodds and Bowles[62] provided an alternative to 'formal observation' in re-focused nurse activity. This work builds on the research of Barker and Cutcliffe who argued that clinical risk in acute psychiatric-mental health inpatient nursing merited engagement rather than observation strategies.[81] In a case study of radical changes to the management of inpatients in an acute English inner city male admission ward, Dodds and Bowles took the view that, arising from a culture of acute psychiatry characterized by medical dominance, formal observation undermines and violates patients' rights and inhibits the development of satisfying supportive relationships between nurses and inpatients.

The objective of their 're-focusing' project was to reclaim nursing control over care in order to reduce

formal observations, replacing 'control' oriented with 'care' interventions, progressing from an individual to a group basis over time. The incidence of formal observation was gradually reduced over a six-month period, with nurses spending increasingly more time with patients in one-to-one settings, 'enabling alternative nursing interventions to be collaboratively developed with the patients'. Eighteen months into the project, one-to-one observations were totally discontinued, a change which:

> ... has released a significant amount of nursing time. Within the first year of the project, nurses began to provide a weekly programme of activities for patients that continues presently; a programme is published which informs patients what to expect in the coming week ... community meetings introduced with an agenda determined by patients and staff.

The authors also reported, among other improvements in the general area of client freedom, reductions in inpatient suicide rates, in deliberate self-harm, in absence without leave, in violent incidents on the ward and in staff sickness. They described a major change in the characteristics of patient care, with:

> ... patients ... more engaged with their named nurses, better informed and more involved in their care. All patients now hold their own copies of care plans and discuss them before and after their review with medical staff, on a minimum of a weekly basis.

The most important benefit for clients arising from this project was described as the 'gift of time', which the authors argue is one of the key elements of psychiatric-mental health nursing, valued more highly than any other intervention experienced whilst in hospital.[82]

In summary, acute inpatient environments present considerable challenges to over-stretched psychiatric-mental health nurses keen to enhance client freedom in, and consent for, the inpatient experience. Building on earlier research,[81] the promising work of Dodds and Bowles does however suggest a radical, successful and empirically supported alternative to more traditional custodial responses.

THE COMMUNITY EXPERIENCE

The care programme approach (CPA)[83] governs the psychiatric management of people with mental health problems living in the community. However, Rose[13] found that the majority of users in her study didn't know what the CPA was for; were clearly not, as advocated, involved in drawing up their care plan; didn't know that they had a plan; who their CPA contacts were, or who to contact in a crisis. Mental health professionals were found to assess service users according to their needs, often interpreted as 'problems'. Rose argued that most users in her study felt that their strengths and abilities had not been considered, and reported that what was missing from their care was a 'sympathetic ear and the chance to talk about ordinary things'. This report indicates that, despite the rhetoric of empowerment, and despite locating users in the community at the centre of their care, at least some may not feel meaningfully involved in making collaborative decisions at any level or stage of the process.

Skulduggery

With Rose's findings in mind it is useful at this point to turn to the work of Morrall,[14] who studied the professional context and practice among community psychiatric-mental health nurses (CMHNs). Athough his work was local and qualitative, thus by no means generalize able to all community settings, it speaks to the overall problem of user freedom and consent. It suggests the probability that at least some groups of CMHNs contribute to practice conditions which may undermine the expressed and actual needs of service users around empowerment.

Morrall found that CMHNs in his study organized their caseloads on an arbitrary basis, while being unable to clearly articulate their role. Moreover, they did not in the main receive or accept guidance on the form of intervention appropriate for their clients. Clients were often discharged without an adequate objective evaluation of how ready they were for this.

Supporting previous observations of the behavioural strategies CMHNs use in managing their caseloads, Morrall argued that the group he studied would not in the main openly disagree with the unwelcome control exerted upon them by consultant psychiatrists. Instead, they used in his words 'skulduggerous contrivances' to combat this:

> One CPN stated that when given an 'inappropriate' referral by the psychiatrist, one or two visits are made to the client before she or he is discharged, rather than simply refusing to accept the client in the first place.

Morral reported the trend of CMHNs either resisting or not having clinical supervision, and adopting sometimes covert techniques to manipulate caseload size. They also exhibited a reluctance to discuss clients on a regular basis with referring agents, including the basis and rationale for their decisions to discharge clients.

The work of Rose and Morrall may help readers of this chapter to consider the extent to which local community psychiatric-mental health nursing practice resembles or deviates from the authors' findings. It

might also help preparation of a more acceptable future ethical identity. The key issue is the extent to which aspects of user freedom and consent is undermined by professionals who actively conceal their practices, and employ covert tactics to avoid engaging with some clients. The major challenge for readers attracted to community psychiatric-mental health nursing as their chosen field is for them to manage their future professional and ethical identities in such a way as to avoid being socialized into skulduggerous practice.

My own experience of teaching on BSc courses in community psychiatric nursing at the University of Brighton does suggest that CMHN students are, in the main, unaccustomed to regular, effective and meaningful clinical supervision. Indeed most seem resistant to, and defended against, the concept. This trend must be considered in the broader phenomenon of the relative failure of clinical supervision to impact significantly on the work of psychiatric-psychiatric-mental health nurses. In large part, this can be at least partly explained in terms of resistance among psychiatric-mental health nurses, their managers, and writers on clinical supervision in nursing to consider the impact of, or seriously engage with, crucial organizational factors.[84]

THE FUTURE

> It is clear that mental health workers and mental health service users are talking and listening together more. What is open to question is both the quality of discussion and the boundaries of debate.[10]

All professions constituting the future mental health service workforce will need to be trained to respond to the needs of service users more effectively.[13] It follows that students must receive adequate and appropriate education and training to do so.[10] A major challenge for lecturers, users, carers and psychiatric-mental health nursing students in the future, is to prepare for this while striving to retain and – in the interests of users and carers – ethically enhance a nursing identity.[10,21] The dialogue must become more open, and less characterized by professional and institutional forms of denial. Educators must therefore abandon an anachronistic *over-investment* in humanistic assumptions and principles and take on board strategies for helping nurses respond helpfully to the multiple identities and needs of 21st century mental health users. This process must include some attention in curricula to the ways in which organizational factors in mental health care settings reduce the likelihood of classroom learning producing effective organizational change and practice.[1,15,85,86]

Nurse educators must also recognize that both clinical and educational areas will probably continue to function for the foreseeable future as blame cultures.[87] Such cultures are, theoretically at any rate, likely to work against liberating professional education agendas. For the foreseeable future, many psychiatric-mental health nurses, like their teachers, will continue to be socialized into an agenda of avoiding creative risk taking, and are likely to fall back on the kind of established custom and practice, ultimately undermining of client freedom and consent, favoured in many acute and community settings.[21,85,86]

To balance the above problems, the future will also hopefully see the burgeoning of an already established community of multi-identity psychiatric-mental health nurses and service users.[20,21,34] There are ongoing dialogic possibilities for solving ethical issues around freedom and consent by participation in the psychiatric nursing list, to some degree fulfilling the need expressed by the user movement in Britain to improve on the 'quality of discussion and the boundaries of debate' between users and psychiatric-psychiatric-mental health nurses.[10]

CONCLUSION

In this chapter I have tried to broaden the dialogue on the problems of freedom and consent for psychiatric-mental health nurses and service users, moving away from a myopic focus on legal issues only. With an eye to the future, I hope to have helped readers develop their conceptual, theoretical and empirical vocabulary to begin to meaningfully combat professional and institutional denial and selective attention around important aspects of user freedom and consent. The overarching challenge for the psychiatric-mental health nurse of the future is to give much more attention than has hitherto generally been the case to listening to, and taking seriously, the experiences and concerns of the people they purport to empower.[10] In this regard, the last word must go to Dunn[11] who has recently reminded us that:

> ... wherever the mentally ill and their loved ones ... try and make their voices heard, there is such an overwhelming catalogue of misery reported that I do not have the slightest doubt that there is very considerable cause for concern about their treatment. If I had to sum it up in one brief sentence, I would say that the overwhelming complaint made by the mentally ill and their families is that of not being listened to or not being taken seriously.

REFERENCES

1. Glenister D. Coercion, control and mental health nursing. In: Tilley S (ed.) *The mental health nurse: views of practice and education*. Bodmin, Cornwall: Blackwell Science, 1997.

2. Department of Health and Welsh Office. *Code of Practice Mental Health Act 1983*. London: The Stationery Office, 1999.

3. Mind: The Mental Health Charity. *Mind the law: capacity*. London: Mind, May 2000.

4. Applebaum PS, Griiso T. The MacArthur treatment competence study: 1. Mental illness and competence to consent to treatment. *Law and Human Behaviour* 1995; **19**: 105–26.

5. Department of Health. *Reference guide to consent for examination or treatment*. London: Department of Health, March 2001 (copies available free from: Department of health, PO Box 777, London SE1 6XH, or from NHS Response Line 0541 555 455, or from the Department of Health website on: www.doh.gov.uk/consent.

6. Department of Health. 12 key points on consent: the law in England. http://www.doh.gov.uk/consent/twelvekeypts.htm , March 2001.

7. Green C. When is a patient capable of consent? *Nursing Times* 1999; **95**(7): 50–51.

8. Grisso T, Appelbaum PS. *Assessing competence to consent to treatment: a guide for physicians and other health professionals*. New York: Oxford University Press, 1998.

9. Lord Chancellor. *Making decisions: The Government's proposals for making decisions on behalf of mental incapacitated adults*. London: HMSO, 1999.

10. Campbell P. Listening to clients. In: Barker P, Davidson B. *Psychiatric nursing: ethical strife*. London: Arnold, 1998.

11. Dunn C. *Ethical issues in mental illness*. Aldershot: Ashgate, 2000.

12. English National Board. *Regulations and guidelines for the approval of institutions and programmes*. London: ENB, 1996.

13. Rose D. *Users' Voices: The perspectives of mental health service users on community and hospital care*. London: The Sainsbury Centre for Mental Health, 2001.

14. Morrall P. *Mental health nursing and social control*. London: Whurr, 1999.

15. Morrall P. Clinical sociology and empowerment. In: Barker P, Davidson B (eds). *Psychiatric nursing: ethical strife*. London: Arnold, 1998.

16. Barker P, Davidson B (eds). *Psychiatric nursing: ethical strife*. London: Arnold, 1998.

17. Newell R, Gournay K (eds). *Mental health nursing: an evidence-based approach*. London: Churchill Livingstone, 2000.

18. Clarke L. *Challenging ideas in psychiatric nursing*. London: Routledge, 1999.

19. Barker P. *The philosophy and practice of psychiatric nursing*. Churchill Livingstone: London, 1999.

20. Grant A. Psychiatric nursing and organizational

power: rescuing the hidden dynamic. *Journal of Psychiatric and Mental Health Nursing* 2001; **8**: 173–88.

21. Grant A. Knowing me knowing you: towards a new relational politics in 21st century mental health nursing. *Journal of Psychiatric and Mental Health Nursing* 2001; **8**: 269–75.

22. The Sainsbury Centre for Mental Health in collaboration with the University of Central Lancashire, Health and Ethnicity Unit. National Visit 2. A visit by the Mental Health Act Commission to 104 Mental Health and Learning Disability Units in England and Wales. *Improving care for detained patients from black and minority ethnic communities.* London: The Sainsbury Centre for Mental Health, 2000.

23. Jennings S. *Creating solutions: developing alternatives in black mental health.* London: King's Fund Publishing, 1997.

24. Warner L, Nicholas S, Patel K, Harris J, Ford R. National Visit 2. A visit by the Mental Health Act Commission to 104 mental health and learning disabilities units in England and Wales. *Improving care for detained patients from black and minority ethnic communities. Preliminary report.* London: The Sainsbury Centre for mental Health in association with The University of Central Lancashire, 2000.

25. Copsey N. *The provision of community mental health services within a multi-faith context.* London: The Sainsbury Centre for Mental Health, 1997.

26. Newton S-A. Women and mental health nursing. In: Tilley S (ed.) *The mental health nurse: views of practice and education.* Bodmin, Cornwall: Blackwell Science, 1997.

27. Thilbert D. Working with women. In: Barker P, Davidson B (eds). *Psychiatric nursing: ethical strife.* London: Arnold, 1998.

28. NHS Executive. *Safety, privacy and dignity in mental health units: guidance on mixed sex accommodation for mental health services.* London: NHS Executive, 2000.

29. Orme J. *Gender and community care: social work and social care perspectives.* New York: Palgrave, 2001.

30. Kohen D (ed.) *Women and mental health.* London: Routledge, 2000.

31. Golding J. *Without prejudice: MIND lesbian, gay and bisexual mental health awareness research.* London: MIND Publications, 1997.

32. McFarlane L. *Diagnosis: homophobic: the experiences of lesbians, gay men and bisexuals in mental health services.* London: PACE (the Project for Advice, Counselling and Education), 1998 (email: pace@dircon.co.uk).

33. Coleman R. The politics of the illness. In: Barker P, Stevenson C (eds). *The construction of power and authority in psychiatry.* Oxford: Butterworth Heinemann, 2000.

34. Psychiatric Nursing List homepage: http://www.city.ac.uk/barts/psychiatric–nursing

35. Lakeman R. Psychiatric nursing. The Internet: facilitating an international culture for psychiatric nurses. *Computers in Nursing* 1996; **16**(2): 87–9.

36. Bowers L. Constructing international professional identity: what psychiatric nurses talk about on the Internet. *International Journal of Nursing Studies* 1997; **34**(3): 208–12.

37. Clarke L. Nursing in search of a science: the rise and rise of the new nurse brutalism. *Mental Health Care* 1999; **21**: 270–72.

38. Cannon B, Coulter E, Gamble C, Jackson A, Jones J, Sandford T, Sharkey S, Ward M, West L. Personality bashing. *Mental Health Care* 1999; **21**: 319.

39. Ritter S. Insulting distortion. *Mental Health Care* 1999; **21**: 319.

40. Rogers P. Persecution complex. *Mental Health Care* 1999; **21**: 319.

41. Barker P. Arrested development. *Mental Health Care* 1999; **21**: 393.

42. Stevenson C. Power and control. *Mental Health Care* 1999; **21**: 393.

43. Duncan-Grant A. Misrepresentation, stereotyping, and acknowledging bias in science: responses to Liam Clarke. *Mental Health Care* 1999; **21**: 336–7.

44. Gournay K. What to do with nursing models. *Journal of Psychiatric and Mental Health Nursing* 1996; **2**(5): 325–7.

45. Barker PJ, Reynolds B. Rediscovering the proper focus of nursing: a critique of Gournay's position on nursing theory and models. *Journal of Psychiatric and Mental Health Nursing* 1995; **3**(1): 75–80.

46. Repper J. Adjusting the focus of mental health nursing: Incorporating service users' experiences of recovery. *Journal of Mental Health* 2000; **9**(6): 575–87.

47. Dallard D. What does counselling do? A critical re-examination of Rogers' core conditions. *Mental Health Care* 1999; **21**: 383–5.

48. Rotter JB. Generalized expectancies for internal versus external control of reinforcement. *Psychological Monographs* 1966; **80**.

49. Diclemente CC, McCounnaughy EA, Norcross JC, Prochaska JO. Integrative dimensions for psychotherapy. *International Journal of Eclectic Psychotherapy* 1986; **5**(3): 256–73.

50. Fennell M. *Overcoming low self-esteem: a self-help guide using cognitive-behavioural techniques.* London: Robinson, 1999.

51. Snyder CR, Ilardi SS, Cheavens J, Michael ST, Yamhure L, Sympson S. The role of hope in cognitive behaviour therapies. *Cognitive Therapy and Research* 2000; **24**(6): 747–62.

52. Bandura A. *Social learning theory.* London: Prentice-Hall, 1977.

53. Rogers CR. *On becoming a person: a therapist's view of psychotherapy*. London: Constable, 1988.

54. Wetherell M, Maybin J. The distributed self: a social constructionist perspective. In: Stevens R (ed.) *Understanding the self*. London: Sage, in association with The Open University, 1997.

55. Simpson A. Personal communication, 2001.

56. Parker I, Georgaca G, Harper D, McLaughlin T, Stowell-Smith M. *Deconstructing psychopathology*. London: Sage, 1999.

57. Barker P, Stevenson C (eds). *The construction of power and authority in psychiatry*.Oxford: Butterworth-Heinemann, 2000.

58. Gray R, Gournay K, Taylor D. New drug treatments for schizophrenia: implications for mental health nursing. *Mental Health Practice* 1997; **1**: 20–23.

59. Denzin NK, Lincoln YS (eds). *Handbook of qualitative research*, 2nd edn. Thousand Oaks, California: Sage, 2000.

60. Long A. Have we the right to deny people their right to embrace their emotional pain? *Journal of Psychiatric and Mental Health Nursing*; 2001; **8**: 85–92.

61. Gergen KG. *An invitation to social construction*. London: Sage Publications, 1999.

62. Dodds P, Bowles N. Dismantling formal observation and refocusing nursing activity in acute inpatient psychiatry: a case study. *Journal of Psychiatric and Mental Health Nursing* 2001; **8**: 183–8.

63. Kennedy P. Mental health: implementing the national service framework (Editorial). *Health Policy Matters* 2000; **1**: 1.

64. The Sainsbury Centre for Mental Health. *Acute problems: a survey of the quality of care in acute psychiatric wards*. London: The Sainsbury Centre for Mental Health, 1998.

65. Minghella E, Ford R, Freeman T, Hoult J, McGlynn P, O'Halloran P. *Open all hours: 24-hour response for people with mental health emergencies*. London: The Sainsbury Centre for Mental Health, 1998.

66. Mental Health Act Commission and the Sainsbury Centre for Mental Health.*The national visit: a one-day visit to 309 acute psychiatric admission wards by the MHAC in collaboration with the Sainsbury Centre for Mental Health*. London: Sainsbury Centre for Mental Health, 1997.

67. Fanham FR, James DV. Patients' attitudes to psychiatric hospital admission. *The Lancet* 2000; **335**: 594.

68. The Sainsbury Centre for Mental Health. *Acute problems: a survey of the quality of care in acute psychiatric wards*. London: The Sainsbury Centre for Mental Health, 1998.

69. Department of Health. *Modernising Mental Health Services*. London: HMSO, 1998.

70. Moore C. Acute psychiatric wards: what do patients get? *Mental Health Practice* 1998; **1**: 12–13.

71. The British Psychological Society. *Understanding mental illness: recent advances in understanding mental illness and psychotic experiences*. A report by the British Psychological Society Division of Clinical Psychology. Leicester: The British Psychological Society, 2000.

72. Gijbels H. Mental health nursing skills in an acute admission environment: perceptions of mental health nurses and other mental health professionals. *Journal of Advanced Nursing* 1995; **21**: 460–65.

73. Higgins R, Hurst K, Wistow G. Nursing acute psychiatric patients: a quantitative and qualitative study. *Journal of Advanced Nursing* 1999; **29**: 52–63.

74. Department of Health. *The new NHS*. HMSO: London, 1997.

75. Flanagan T. Mental health nursing in the acute inpatient setting: unravelling the chaos. Research paper presented at: *Developing evidence to enhance practice, 6th Annual INAM Research Conference*. University of Brighton, 2001.

76. Sailas E, Fenton M. Seclusion and restraint for people with serious mental illnesses. The Cochrane Library (Oxford) 2001. Issue 2. Website: http://www.update–software.com/abstracts/ab001163.htm

77. Sallah D. Alternatives to seclusion. In: Tilley S (ed.) *The mental health nurse: views of practice and education*. Bodmin, Cornwall: Blackwell Science, 1997.

78. Barker P, Cutcliffe J. Hoping against hope. *Open Mind 101* January/February 2000; 18–19.

79. Bowers L, Park A. Special observation in the care of psychiatric inpatients: a literature review. *Issues in Mental Health Nursing* 2001; **22**: 769–86.

80. Jones J, Lowe T, Ward M. Inpatients' experiences of nursing observation on an acute psychiatric unit: a pilot study. *Mental Health and Learning Disabilities Care* 2000; **4**(4): 125–9.

81. Barker P, Cutcliffe J. Clinical risk: a need for engagement not observation. *Mental Health Practice* 1999; **2**(8): 8–12.

82. Jackson S, Stevenson C. The gift of time from the friendly professional. *Nursing Standard* 1998; **12**: 31–3.

83. Department of Health. National Health Service and Community Care Act. London: HMSO, 1990.

84. Grant A. *Clinical supervision among mental health nurses: a critical organizational ethnography*. Portsmouth: Nursing Praxis International, 2001.

85. Morgan G. *Images of organization*. Thousand Oaks, California: Sage, 1997.

86. Grant A, Mills J. The great going nowhere show: structural power and mental health nurses. *Mental Health Practice* 2000; **4**: 6–7.

87. Department of Health. *An organisation with a memory: report of an expert group on learning from adverse events in the NHS Chaired by the Chief Medical Officer*, 2000. http://www.doh.gov.uk/orgmemreport/index.htm

Chapter 63

PROVIDING CULTURALLY SAFE CARE

Anthony J O'Brien* and Erina Morrison-Ngatai**

INTRODUCTION

The encounter between a nurse and a service user may involve an interaction between two people from very different backgrounds. For both the nurse and the service user, a wide range of beliefs, experiences, norms and values will influence perceptions of mental health, mental health care, and treatment. Many of these have their origin in cultural identity. The therapeutic relationship is influenced by two sets of cultural beliefs and values – those of the nurse and those of the service user. The role of the nurse is to develop a relationship, which recognizes and respects the service user's culture, and the influence of cultural identity on the therapeutic encounter.

Here, we shall discuss the issue of *culture* as it relates to mental health nursing. We aim to provide a basis for mental health nurses to reflect on their own cultural identity and that of the people they care for. We shall not provide prescribed responses for engaging with people whose cultural identities are different from one's own. Rather, we shall suggest a process of reflection on cultural identity, and on the impact of cultural difference on interactions between nurse and service user. Although the term 'culture' is most frequently used to

refer to ethnic culture, it can usefully be applied to a range of differences, including those of gender, sexuality, physical ability, age and religion. Here, 'culture' refers only to ethnic culture, although it is recognized that the discussion may also have relevance to various forms of group *belonging*.

Research and theory on the 'need for nursing'[1,2] provides a theme, which integrates this chapter with other sections of this book. Embedded in the three levels of need identified by this body of work is the need for cultural respect and affirmation. As with other human needs, cultural needs do not necessarily show themselves to the nurse, and should not be identified independently by the nurse. Instead the service user should be engaged in identifying those needs. The need for engagement as a basis for providing culturally safe care recognizes the relationship between nurse and service user as central to the process of providing appropriate care. Without a relationship of empathy and trust service users are not likely to identify cultural needs, and so will not be able to avail themselves of opportunities for support in meeting those needs.

We draw on New Zealand experiences in the development of the concept of cultural safety. Consistent

*Tony O'Brien is a general and a psychiatric nurse, presently working as senior lecturer in mental health nursing at the University of Auckland, New Zealand. He is interested in social issues in mental health nursing and in ways of reducing coercion in mental health care. He is a fifth generation pakeha New Zealander of Irish and Scots ancestry.
**Erina Morrison-Ngatai is of Te Arawa–Ngati Whakaue, Kahungungu–Rakaipaaka, and Tainui–Ngati Maru descent. Currently she lectures in mental health nursing, provides leadership in cultural safety and Maori health within the undergraduate and postgraduate programmes at Massey University. Active professional service includes vice president of the ANZCMHNInc., NZ Councillor and Maori Caucus member. Current research activities focus on Maori mental health nurses, and clinical indicators for standards of practice.

with the view that reflection on cultural identity is the basis for providing culturally safe care to others, the chapter should be seen in light of the authors' cultural identities and context. The first author (AO) is a pakeha[a] male academic and the second author (EMN) is a Maori[b] female academic. We work in a postcolonial New Zealand society that is meeting the challenges of restoration and redress for past events, and of the neo-colonization process of globalization. A range of research and literature provides an international perspective. While the model of cultural safety we outline is considered to be applicable beyond New Zealand, like models of nursing and mental health care, it needs interpretation in local contexts if it is to fully acknowledge the realities of individual nurses and service users.

RACE, ETHNICITY AND CULTURAL IDENTITY

The concept of race has its origins in anthropologists' attempts to classify human beings based on observable differences in physical attributes. Many early writings on race, including those of prominent theorists of psychiatry, reflect views of the innate superiority of white people over other races.[3,4] Because of these associations the term 'race' is less used currently.[4] The term refers to human groupings based on biologically determined racial characteristics. In the health sciences it is now more common to speak of 'ethnicity', a term that implies a sense of group belonging, which is self-claimed and not imposed on the basis of observable physical attributes.[5] However the concept of ethnicity recognizes the biological basis of physical characteristics of ethnic groups. The terms 'race' and 'ethnicity' are sometimes used interchangeably.

Culture can be defined as a set of traditions, beliefs, values and practices shared by members of a social group.[5] While it is commonly thought that culture and ethnicity are synonymous, the concepts are not identical. A person is born with particular characteristics, some of which are attributable to ethnicity, in the biological sense discussed above. Frequently, individuals are influenced by characteristics of more than one ethnic group. For instance a person may have Indian, Chinese and Caucasian ancestry, resulting in a blend of physical characteristics. However if we wish to understand that person's beliefs, values and behaviour, we will need to know about the self chosen group affiliations of that person, or their culture.

Members of a single ethnic group will have different experiences of what it means to be a member of that group. However the language used to describe ethnicity reflects the tendency to make generalizations, which have the potential to become stereotypes. The term 'Asian American' covers people from 40 different ethnic groups, who speak 30 different languages.[6] To make sound clinical decisions about the mental health needs of members of this group it is necessary to recognize its diversity.[7] Also, as Pilgrim and Rogers[4] note, within different cultures there are differences in the experience of mental distress, for example those based on gender. These examples illustrate the need to be aware that general categories such as 'Asian', 'Polynesian' or 'African' provide, at best, a partial picture of an individual's cultural identity.

Nurses need to recognize that identification of 'culture' can be a form of imposition, in which a nurse classifies a service user, based on the nurse's beliefs or expectations about that person's cultural preferences. This is especially so if the nurse's classification is based solely on observed characteristics such as skin colour or facial features, rather than on the person's expressed cultural preferences.

CULTURAL DIFFERENCES IN CLINICAL PRACTICE

Consideration of the impact of culture on clinical practice begins with a review of the culturally determined nature of Western psychiatry. The illness model of mental distress is a construct developed by Western psychiatry, but one which contrasts sharply with traditional ways of thinking, for example those of Indian, African, and Asian cultures,[4] and with traditional Maori cultural beliefs.[8] Also, Western models of mental health care are based on the ideal of disengagement of the self, so that the search for mental health becomes a search for an ideal individual self. This is reflected in models of psychotherapy and treatment, which assume a universal self, free of the influences of culture.[9] This approach does not recognize paradigms of traditional cultures, for example Maori cultural beliefs of good mental health, as an outcome of harmony with oneself, one's family, community, ancestors, creator and the environment.[10] Within Western models of mental health, culture is considered to provide the content (thoughts, perceptions, feelings) associated with mental illness, while the form (depressed mood, psychosis) is considered to be culture free. Leff[11] presents evidence from studies in a wide range of countries, which suggests that functional psychosis is a universal human experience. However he cautions that this conclusion should be interpreted carefully, as the instruments used in the studies 'were

---

[a] The term 'pakeha' is used in New Zealand to refer to people of Anglo, Celtic or Caucasian ancestry.
[b] Maori people are the indigenous people of Aotearoa/New Zealand.

constructed in the West and may have imposed a cultural stereotype on the patient populations examined' (p. 42).

Whatever the influence of culture on the content or form of mental illness, when people come into contact with mental health services, culture has a significant role to play. A significant body of evidence suggests that ethnicity influences presentation to services, assessment, and decisions about care and treatment.[12] Ethnicity has also been found to influence pathways to care, diagnosis, prescribing patterns and use of ECT.[4] While there are many factors that may mediate the influence of ethnicity (such as age, social isolation, gender, socioeconomic status, severity of illness), it seems that ethnicity is a significant factor in service users' involvement in mental health care. Working at the 'care face'[13] of mental health brings nurses into close contact with service users, in situations where ethnic difference may play a crucial role in shaping relationships.

One area of nursing practice that has been influenced by ethnicity is nurses' perceptions of dangerousness. When behaviour is perceived to be dangerous there are a number of responses available to nurses. These range from 'one-to-one' intervention and supported time out, through to coercive measures such as seclusion and restraint. Nurses' responses to acts of violence may be influenced by the ethnicity of the service user. In a study of violence in inpatient units there was no difference, based on ethnicity, in rates of compulsory detention.[14] However, the same study reported that non-violent black[c] patients were four times more likely than non-violent whites to be admitted to a locked unit. Another study found that restraint was almost four times more likely to be used following violence by black than white service users,[15] suggesting that nurses may have a lower tolerance of violence by blacks than by whites.

While there is clear evidence that rates of diagnosis and decisions about treatment and care are influenced by clinicians' perceptions of ethnicity, there is also concern that insufficient attention may be given to the influence of biological differences between different ethnic groups. Metabolism of psychoactive medications, development of side-effects and adverse effects, and thresholds of effectiveness have all been shown to have some variability related to ethnicity.[16] The effects of these differences may be further compounded by cultural differences in help-seeking, expression of symptoms, and patterns of communication.[16] Nurses need to be familiar with the specific effects of psychoactive medications on different ethnic groups, and of cultural differences in patterns of response.

Although a person's experience of mental distress and illness is influenced by culture, it is important to

In a recent audit of case notes in 11 out of 22 mental health services in New Zealand[17] it was found that in 65% of cases, service users were not given the opportunity to identify their cultural needs. In addition, 28% of service users were not offered support for those cultural issues they did identify. Encouragingly, in 65% of cases Maori cultural advisors were consulted regarding the care of Maori service users. However only 23% of Maori service users were offered cultural assessment, in accordance with the requirement of the New Zealand Mental Health Standard.[18] For the purposes of this study, identification of ethnicity by the nurse was not considered to represent an opportunity to identify cultural needs. Assessment is a key aspect of nursing care, and is crucial to planning appropriate care. Without an opportunity to identify cultural needs, service users are not able to access cultural support, and this is likely to adversely affect their engagement with and response to care. Providing an opportunity to identify cultural needs is dependent on the establishment of rapport, and should be negotiated with the service user.

FIGURE 63.1 Identification of cultural needs.

note the diversity within contemporary cultures. Nurses should not assume that all members of a particular culture subscribe to a particular view of that culture. Cultures are dynamic, adaptive and changing, and an individual's behaviour cannot be predicted solely on the basis of their ethnicity. Also, identification with one culture does not preclude beliefs and practices that are consistent with another. A person who is ethnically Japanese may have experience of other Asian cultures, which may have influenced their cultural identity. They may live and work within a Western society, and yet feel strongly committed to traditional Japanese cultural practices at the time of a death or other culturally significant event. The idea that culture equates to ethnicity can lead to unhelpful stereotypes that, in health care, may prevent individuals from making their needs known and seeking appropriate support. Figure 63.1 summarizes the results of New Zealand research documenting clinical nursing practice in the area of identification of cultural needs.

Developing effective responses to cultural difference

Nurses learn, through therapeutic relationships, to respond effectively to the emotional distress of service users. Part of this process involves reflection on the experiences, assumptions and skills the nurse brings to

---

[c] While 'black' does not refer to a particular ethnicity, it is a term used to refer to non-white minorities, particularly in Britain.

Stage One: Dualism	Clinical example
At this stage of development nurses rely on authority to provide answers to questions of cultural difference. They typically look to literature and the opinions of experts to guide their thinking although their own beliefs are strongly held. A statement characteristic of this stage is 'Culture doesn't matter to me. I treat everyone the same regardless of their culture'. The nurse at this stage is not aware that she cannot step outside her own culture, and that her interactions are, in part, culturally determined.	The nurse conducts an assessment interview and records the service user's ethnicity after asking the patient to select ethnicity from a list provided on the assessment form. There is no discussion of whether the categories available reflect the person's cultural identity. The nurse believes that while it is important to acknowledge cultural identity, this can be achieved on the basis of ethnicity. There may be an assumption that the person will make any special needs known, and so no inquiry about special cultural needs is undertaken. Any requests regarding cultural needs are responded to on the basis of the same treatment to all patients regardless of particular cultural needs.
Stage Two: Relativism	Clinical example
This stage involves awareness of the diversity of cultural perspectives, but the nurse may feel that all views have equal validity. Authorities, including cultural authorities, are simply one more opinion. There appears to be no basis for action that is better than another. A nurse might say: 'We all have our own views, but none of us can claim to be right. Even members of the same culture might have different views. We should try to respect them all'. This statement recognizes diversity both between and within cultures, but that diversity is seen as invalidating actions that are committed to a particular cultural perspective.	As part of the assessment interview the service user is asked to identify their ethnicity, but also asked if the available categories accurately reflect their cultural identity. Additional comments or issues are recorded after discussion with the service user. The nurse is aware that ethnicity does not determine cultural beliefs, and asks if there are any particular cultural needs. Specific needs will be addressed if the resources for doing this are immediately available. If there are no resources immediately available this is simply recognized as a limitation of the system.
Stage Three: Evolving commitment	Clinical example
The nurse at this stage is able to both recognize diversity of cultural perspectives, and commit themselves to a course of action. The action is informed by the realities of the nurse's culture, his place in the power relationships of health care, and the realities of the culture of the service user. Commitment is demonstrated in the statement: 'People don't always feel safe to identify their cultural needs. We need to create a safe environment in which needs can be expressed, and provide the right supports so that those needs can be met'. The nurse making this statement is aware that factors outside the individual nurse–patient relationship influence the health care encounter, and consciously uses the power of her position to benefit the patient.	The nurse creates a safe environment for the assessment interview, perhaps by involving members of the service user's family, with consent of the service user. The service user self identifies his ethnicity, and is given an opportunity to identify any specific needs or concerns. When specific needs are identified by the service user the nurse talks to colleagues and members of the service user's cultural group to establish ways of providing appropriate cultural support. Support is provided only in consultation with the service user. The nurse reflects on the impact of social processes on the health care encounter and uses the experience to further his own knowledge of resources and supports available, and to make that knowledge available to other nurses in the service.

FIGURE 63.2 Developing cultural safety in the process of assessment. Adapted from Woods PJ, Schwass M 1993, Cultural safety: a framework for changing attitudes. *Nursing Praxis in New Zealand* 1993; 8(1): 4–15.

the therapeutic relationship. The increasing ethnic diversity of countries in which mental health nursing is practised suggests a need for reflection on cultural identity as part of the process of development of nursing skills. Power differences in the nurse–patient relationship place the onus for recognizing and responding to cultural difference with the nurse, rather than the service user.[19]

The diverse cultural needs of users of health services require that nurses develop approaches to care that recognize and respect the culture of service users.

❑ **Cultural sensitivity** involves awareness of cultural difference and knowledge of some of the culturally specific beliefs and practices that may influence service users' engagement with care.

❑ **Cultural competence**, is defined as 'respect for, and understanding of, diverse ethnic and cultural groups, their histories, traditions, beliefs and value systems'.[7] This recognizes the need for nurses to be sensitive to the culture of service users, and to respond to cultural diversity within the service user group. Wells has identified the need for cultural competence to extend beyond the individual, and embrace institutional change.[20]

- ❑ **Cultural proficiency** begins with examination of cultural biases, those 'cultural values and beliefs that are internalized through the socialisation process',[20, p.193] and includes organizational change within the educational institutions and health services.
- ❑ **The concept of cultural safety** meets Wells' criteria for cultural proficiency, but also requires reflection on the particular history of the society in which health care is provided.

CULTURALLY SAFE CARE

Cultural safety differs from cultural sensitivity, cultural competence and cultural proficiency by envisaging a process of change from sensitivity, through awareness, to safety. Consistent with other Western countries, the early response of New Zealand nursing to cultural difference was to promote cultural sensitivity. However by 1988 Maori nurses suggested that sensitivity to cultural difference was not sufficient to address differences in the health status of different ethnicities and the concept of cultural safety was developed.[21] Cultural safety developed as a means of addressing ethnic differences in health status between Maori and non-Maori New Zealanders. Mental health remains one of the main areas of concern for Maori health.[8] Although it originated in New Zealand, cultural safety, has applicability in other social contexts.[22,23]

Cultural safety has been defined as:

> The effective nursing of a person/family from another culture by a nurse who has undertaken a process of reflection on her/his own cultural identity and recognizes the impact of the nurses's culture on his/her own nursing practice.[24]

Although cultural safety was originally developed as a response to the disproportionate health problems of Maori, the concept is considered to be applicable to all cultures.[25] Any people who differ from a dominant culture are potentially at risk and can benefit from culturally safe care. This is particularly so for immigrant groups, for example Pacific Island people in New Zealand, Vietnamese in Australia, West Indians in the UK or North African immigrants to European countries.

Cultural safety begins with analysis of the historical relationships between the different groups that make up a society. The focus of cultural safety is on the social positions of these groups rather than solely on their distinctive cultural beliefs or practices as a basis for developing culturally safe relationships with service users.[25] From this basis, health is placed in a political and historical context. Cultural safety focuses on the social, economic, political and historical influences on health.[23] Because the political and historical context of each society is unique, cultural safety needs to be given specific meaning within local contexts. The principle of recognition of the histories of different cultures within different societies, the historical relationships between different cultures, and in particular, issues of power differences between cultures is a significant extension of concepts such as cultural sensitivity and cultural competence.

Nurses learning to be culturally safe practitioners begin with reflection on their own cultural identity and history, and move, through guided education, to commitment to personal and political change. Woods and Schwass[22] depict this process of change as occurring in three stages: *dualism*, *relativism* and *evolving commitment*. The model of change is outlined in Figure 63.2, with an example of development of cultural safety in the process of assessment.

Cultural safety and collaborative care

The process of psychiatric and mental health nursing involves establishing collaborative therapeutic relationships with service users on the basis of their need for nursing care.[1] Barker's *Tidal Model* of mental health nursing stresses the need for the person's experience of mental distress or illness to be understood by the nurse. It also emphasizes provision of 'support and services a person might need to live an ordinary life' (p. 234). However, development of understanding between nurses and service users is influenced by differences that must be negotiated by the nurse.[19] In cross-cultural encounters the paradoxical nature of nursing is apparent. After researching nurses' experiences of cross-cultural caring Spence concluded that: 'Trying to be oneself in a way that enables others to be themselves, under circumstances that are intrinsically never fully knowable, is unlikely to be free of tension'.[26]

The nurse who is focused on establishing a therapeutic relationship will consider both her own cultural identity and that of the service user in her assessment and plan of care. Making sense of the experience of mental distress or illness requires understanding of the influence of culture on that experience. Because of the sheer diversity of service users' cultural identities in relation to that of the nurse, it will not be possible for nurses to understand all the possible cultural influences the nurse and service user bring to the therapeutic relationship. As a minimum, the nurse should reflect on her own cultural identity and how that may influence her engagement with service users.

Collaborative care relies on therapeutic communication, which reflects the cultural backgrounds of nurses and service users. Communication patterns are influenced by culture, with many communication patterns being culture-bound. In a study of Chinese service users' communications patterns with nurses, unique cultural influences were identified.[27] While the nurses were aware that Chinese culture had a significant effect on therapeutic communication, their communication strategies tended to reflect the Western models of their nursing education. The authors concluded that 'to be therapeutic with clients from diverse backgrounds, nurses need to understand the intricacies of different cultures'.[27] The researchers recommended that Chinese service users would benefit from nurses' improved understanding of culturally bound communication strategies. We would add that understanding the culture of others does not involve becoming an expert or authority on those cultures.

In the New Zealand context Morrison-Ngatai[10] has discussed a Maori model of communication, which, while consistent with principles of therapeutic communication, respects the cultural identity of Maori service users. The *Te Niho-Mako* model 'fosters the inherent need for Maori, of connecting, linking and bonding'.[10] The three concepts, which form the model are *tata*, *kupu*, and *tika*. Their nearest equivalents in pakeha terms are attending, listening, and etiquette. While the first two concepts are familiar, the third refers to rightness of the situation: feelings and thoughts are expressed in ways that are sometimes verbal, sometimes physical. Within the *Te Niho-Mako* model spontaneity, rather than reserve, is valued. The model is recommended to nurses caring for Maori service users, although is regarded as of particular value in situations where Maori care for Maori (*see the discussion below on culturally specific services*).

The dominant interpersonal model of mental health nursing is a Western construct, having been developed within a North American cultural context and then adopted in other Western and non-Western countries. However the practice of mental health nursing needs to be responsive to the realities of the diverse cultures in which it takes place, in order to provide care that service users experience as culturally safe.

Service user involvement

It can be useful to consider issues of culture in the context of moves to involve users of services in planning, provision and evaluation of mental health services. Mental health services have traditionally been organized around the needs of service providers, rather than service users[28,29] and have reflected the cultural values of the provider group. However users of services are disproportionately members of minority cultures, whose values are not always recognized in the services provided.

Involvement of service users has meant that nurses have had to consider how their practice best meets the needs of the people they care for.[28,29] One way of meeting the needs of culturally diverse groups is to involve those groups in the provision of services. Service users can be involved in direct care roles or in advisory roles aimed at promoting the cultural safety of the service. Nurses can expect to work alongside service users and can learn from both the service experience and cultural experience this group has to offer.

Involvement in services can extend to managing service provision. Pierre[30] describes the role of a company formed by service users to provide services to ethnic minority service users in Liverpool. In providing services the company seeks to create a non-racist environment which challenges institutional processes encountered by ethnic minorities in mainstream services. Pierre concludes that 'user involvement is not an impossible dream, but a necessary possibility and a desirable antidote to the uncaring, unhelpful and unwanted image of psychiatry currently portrayed among black users'.[30]

The cultural safety model calls for changes at an institutional level in order that mental health services are safe for members of all cultures. It also draws attention to issues of power in the provision of mental health services. Service users from over-represented ethnic groups can be involved in the provision of mainstream services (those which are available to all members of the community), or in the development of culturally specific services to members of their own communities.

Culturally specific services

Another response to the over-representation of service users from minority cultures is the development of services provided by members of those cultures for service users of their own culture. Culturally specific services aim to overcome the problem of cultural domination often experienced in mainstream services, and to meet the needs of service users in ways that are consistent with their cultural beliefs. In New Zealand there are now over thirty culturally specific mental health services for Maori service users.[8] While the same range of treatment options available in mainstream services is available in Maori services, the staff are all Maori, and committed to observing Maori protocol in providing services.

Staff of culturally specific services may be nurses or other health professionals, or they may be employed especially for their cultural knowledge and skills. This will include traditional and contemporary cultural knowledge. Culturally skilled staff work alongside clinical staff, providing treatment programmes that are likely to include cultural activities and incorporate cultural protocols within standard forms of treatment.

While culturally specific services may be useful for members of over-represented minorities, caution needs to be exercised in offering service users choice in participating in culturally specific services. We have already discussed the important issues of choice in cultural identity, and the same caution needs to be exercised in offering culturally specific care. If clinicians ascribe culture on the basis of ethnicity, then there may be misunderstandings in offering culturally specific care.

Culturally specific services have the potential to offer a real alternative to service users, which challenges the dominant Western values of mental health services. Nurses from over-represented ethnicities need educational opportunities aimed at developing the unique combination of cultural and clinical skills necessary to provide culturally specific care. They need to recognize that culturally safe care requires structural change supported by allocation of resources in order to address the effects of historical processes.

FUTURE DEVELOPMENTS

It is likely that, in the future, mental health services will need to respond to increasing ethnic diversity amongst service users. This is particularly so in light of continuing population movements occurring throughout the 21st century. This will place demands on individual nurses to reflect on the nature of their own cultural identity and the implications of cultural differences for their encounters with service users. Nurses will also need to develop a broad range of cultural skills and knowledge, although they cannot be expected to become experts in the cultures of service users. Services will need to consider how to recruit and retain nurses from over-represented ethnic groups, and may need to provide culturally specific services for some populations. Individual, institutional and social change is necessary to meet the challenges of cultural diversity.

While much of the responsibility for addressing issues of providing culturally safe care rests with service managers and funders, individual nurses can also take action to improve their responsiveness to service users from cultures different to their own. *Clinical supervision* offers an opportunity for reflection on cultural issues, including cultural identity, power and the nurse's ability to respond to cultural needs. Supervision with nurses from different cultures is one way of facilitating this, either as supervisors or as participants in group supervision.

Opportunities to develop cultural knowledge and skills may also present themselves in the form of service development and education, liaison with cultural services and discussion with colleagues and service users. Nurses need to focus on development of cultural awareness and skills as part of their professional development, and as part of their commitment to meeting the full range of needs of service users.

The continued relevance of interpersonal models of mental health nursing will depend on their capacity to respond to the demands of increasing cultural diversity. The nursing relationship has been described as frequently 'one way traffic'.[2] Concepts such as collaborative care mark nursing's commitment to know and respond to the other, recognizing that the capacity to know another person is limited by the nurses' perceptions of 'otherness'. For nurses to more fully offer themselves to service users, the cultural dimension of the nursing relationship needs to be acknowledged and explored.

REFERENCES

1. Barker P. The Tidal Model: developing an empowering, person-centred approach to recovery within psychiatric and mental health nursing. *Journal of Psychiatric and Mental Health Nursing* 2001; **8**: 233–40.

2. Barker P, Jackson S, Stevenson C. The need for psychiatric nursing: towards a multidimensional theory of caring. *Nursing Inquiry* 1999; **6**: 103–11.

3. Fernando S. 'Race', criminality and forensic psychiatry. A historical perspective. In: Kaye C, Lingiah T (eds). *Race, culture and ethnicity in secure psychiatric practice. Working with difference*. London: Jessica Kingley, 2000: 49–54.

4. Pilgrim D, Rogers A. *A sociology of mental health and illness*, 2nd edn. Buckingham: Open University Press, 1999.

5. Fernando S. *Race, culture and psychiatry*. London: Tavistock/Routledge, 1988.

6. Oakley LD. Sociocultural context of psychiatric nursing care. In: Stuart G, Laraia M. *Stuart and Sundeen's principles and practice of psychiatric nursing*, 7th edn. St Louis: Mosby, 2000: 135–46.

7. Bush CT. Cultural competence: implications of the Surgeon General's report on mental health. *Journal of Child and Adolescent Psychiatric Nursing* 2000; **13**: 177–8.

8. Durie M. Mental health and Maori development. *Australian and New Zealand Journal of Psychiatry* 2000; **33**: 5–12.

9. Carnevale FA. Towards a cultural conception of the self. *Journal of Psycho-social Nursing* 1999; **37**(8): 26–31.

10. Morrison-Ngatai L. Communication in practice. An insight into the dynamics of communication for Maori. Implications for mental health nurses. *Paper presented at 23rd Annual Conference of the Australian and New Zealand College of Mental Health Nurses*, Adelaide, South Australia, October 20–23, 1997.

11. Leff J. *Psychiatry around the globe. A transcultural view*. London: Gaskell, 1988.

12. Spector R. Is there racial bias in clinicians' perceptions of the dangerousness of psychiatric patients? *Journal of Mental Health* 2001; **10**: 5–15.

13. Barker P, Whitehill I. The craft of care: towards collaborative caring in psychiatric nursing. In: Tilley S (ed.) *The mental health nurse. Views of education and practice.* Oxford: Blackwell, 1997: 15–27.

14. Noble P, Rogers S. Violence by psychiatric inpatients. *British Journal of Psychiatry* 1989; **155**: 384–90.

15. Bond CF, DiCandia CG, McKinnon JR. Responses to violence in a psychiatric setting: the role of patients' race. *Personality and Social Psychology Bulletin* 1988; **14**: 448–58.

16. Mohr W. Cross-ethnic variations in the care of psychiatric patients. A review of contributing factors and practice considerations. *Journal of Psycho-social Nursing* 1998; **36**(3): 16–21.

17. O'Brien TP, O'Brien AJ, Morrison-Ngatai L, McNulty N, Skews G, Ryan T. *Clinical indicators for mental health nursing standards of practice.* Report to Health Research Council of New Zealand, 2002.

18. Standards New Zealand. *National Mental Health Sector Standard.* Wellington: Standards New Zealand, 2001.

19. Walsh C. Negotiating difference in mental health nursing in New Zealand. In: Tilley S (ed.) *The mental health nurse. Views of education and practice.* Oxford: Blackwell, 1997: 172–85.

20. Wells MI. Beyond cultural competence: a model for individual and institutional cultural development. *Journal of Community Health Nursing* 2000; **17**: 189–99.

21. Ellison-Loschman L. Giving a voice to health consumers. *Kai Tiaki. Nursing New Zealand* 2001; **7**(1): 12–13.

22. Woods PJ, Schwass Cultural safety: a framework for changing attitudes. *Nursing Praxis in New Zealand* 1993; **8**(1): 4–15.

23. Brown AJ, Fiske J-A. First Nations women's encounters with mainstream healthcare services. *Western Journal of Nursing Research* 2001; **23**: 126–47.

24. Nursing Council of New Zealand. *Guidelines for cultural safety in nursing and midwifery education.* Wellington: Nursing Council of New Zealand, 1996.

25. Polaschek NR. Cultural safety: a new concept in nursing people of different ethnicities. *Journal of Advanced Nursing* 1998; **27**: 452–7.

26. Spence DG. Hermeneutic notions illuminate cross-cultural nursing experiences. *Journal of Advanced Nursing* 2001; **35**: 624–30.

27. Arthur D, Chan HK, Fung WY, Wong KY, Yeung KW. Therapeutic communication strategies used by Hong Kong clients with their Chinese clients. *Journal of Psychiatric and Mental Health Nursing* 1999; **6**: 29–36.

28. Epstein M, Orr AM. An introduction to consumer politics. In: Clinton M, Redmond S (eds). *Advanced practice in mental health nursing.* Oxford: Blackwell, 1999: 1–16.

29. Repper J. Adjusting the focus of mental health nursing: Incorporating service users' perspective of recovery. *Journal of Mental Health* 2000; **9**: 575–87.

30. Pierre SA. Psychiatry and citizenship: the Liverpool black mental health users' perspective. *Journal of Psychiatric and Mental Health Nursing* 2000; **7**: 249–57.

Section 9

The development of mental health nursing

Preface to Section 9

Where nurses once were content to call themselves 'psychiatric nurses', in many countries they now choose to describe themselves as 'mental health nurses'. The assumption is clear – there is some distinction between the two titles: each must connote a specific kind of practice.

In this section we consider how mental health nursing might develop, and what it might entail, which would distinguish it from the 'old order' of psychiatric nursing.

We begin with a consideration of the importance of clinical supervision, which serves as the medium for growing the kind of 'reflective practitioner' who might both understand nursing practice and be sensitive to the personal foibles and defences of the *person* who is the nurse.

The concept of *mental health* nursing is less than 20 years old and in many countries is only emerging as a way of speaking about nursing, rather than practising it. What might distinguish this alternative form of nursing practice from its psychiatric elder? How might nurses know when psychiatric nursing was indicated or when the more developmental form of mental health nursing should be the focus of practice?

Collaboration has been a feature of many of the chapters in earlier Sections of this book. In this penultimate section, we consider how the contemporary concept of collaboration might be no more than an echo of Nightingale's principles for nursing practice. How might a 21st century nurse learn to 'go with the Flo' in developing genuinely collaborative care?

Finally, we consider the responsibility that nurses have to base their practice on the best available evidence. Nursing care is rarely free at the point of delivery, although in many economies the costs are largely hidden. However, nurses have a responsibility to deliver their service wisely, shaping this from the best research guidance available. How do nurses find this important source of intelligence and how might they distinguish the good advice from the trivial?

Chapter 64

CLINICAL SUPERVISION

Peter Wilkin*

> I am a part of all that I have met;
> Yet all experience is an arch wherethro'
> Gleams that untravell'd world, whose margin fades
> For ever and for ever when I move.
>
> Alfred, Lord Tennyson, *Ulysses*

INTRODUCTION

Psychiatric-mental health nurses (PMH nurses) spend their working lives sailing in an ocean of emotions. As they strive to build alliances with distressed and inaccessible people, affective riptides constantly threaten their own sense of emotional balance. In the space of one shift, they can encounter the abject despair of deep depression, witness the confusion and chaos of psychosis, or share in the hallelujah of someone's recovery. Shaken by the turbulence of madness, they are not always sure if the disturbance springs from without or within.

As in all human relationships, there is no exact science to inform our craft and we rely heavily on experience to navigate us through each and every psychiatric situation. Yet, as Coleridge[1] declares, 'the light which experience gives is a lantern on the stern, which shines only on the waves behind us!' In the absence of any absolute truths, it makes good sense to extract the oils from our nursing experiences to fuel the lamps that light up our future practice. Clinical supervision offers the PMH nurse a 'lamp of lightning'[2] to 'that untravell'd world', where her raw and unedited nursing experiences can be survived and understood[3] and where she will come to know both herself and the patient in a deeper, more intrinsic way. Through the process of clinical supervision, the raptures and heartaches of her clinical experiences will slowly ripen into experiences of learning.

CLINICAL SUPERVISION – WHAT DOES IT REALLY MEAN?

As the nursing literature on clinical supervision steadily grows, most authors present a definition similar to but always different from the last one. Rather than adding to the confusion, I shall offer you two, brief interpretations that already exist, both of them from PMH nurses. The first example is provided by Tania Yegdich,[4] who believes that 'the nature of clinical supervision, has as its narrative, the patient's human suffering. What is examined in supervision is the effect of the patient's suffering

*Peter Wilkin is the Primary Mental Health Service Leader in Rochdale and Clinical Supervision Module Leader at Manchester Metropolitan University. His professional priorities are the welfare and development of his colleagues and the personal growth of psychiatric service users. His therapeutic approach is conversational, combining pragmatism with unconditional regard.

on the nurse's ability to respond, interact and to *think* (author's italics)'. Here, Yegdich takes us straight back to that sea of emotion that is the PMH nurse–patient encounter. She sees supervision as a place that contains the anxieties that spill out of the clinical episode, allowing the PMH nurse time and space to 'think'. This is a scary business, as it inevitably involves recognition of our mistakes and second-class craftings. Yet, as every clinical supervisor worth her salt knows, the history encapsulated within our past clinical encounters contains the knowing best suited to inform all our future practice. In its crude form it lies dormant within us, like a book unread gathering dust on a shelf. It is only when we open the covers of such an experience that the full story is revealed. Then, and only then, can we analyse and assimilate this information into our belief systems.

The second example is provided by Phil Barker,[5] who believes that 'supervision in psychiatric nursing has two main aims: to protect people in care from nurses and to protect nurses from themselves'. The irony in Barker's statement delivers his concerns like a head on a plate. Like Yegdich, he can see how the PMH nurse is hooked by the patient's distress. Driven by the anxiety this causes within her, the PMH nurse reacts against the patient's anguish in a desperate attempt to eradicate it. Despite her conscious healing intentions, the nurse's agenda is borne from within herself. It is an act of separation, which serves only to negate the experience of the patient. Barker's recognition of just how much PMH nurses give of themselves is reflected in the latter part of his statement. Without a reliable network of support, constant caring can lead to emotional exhaustion and eventual burn-out.[a] While clinical supervision in itself is no guarantee against this happening, it surely reduces the potential.[6]

So, for theoretical purposes, we can break down clinical supervision into its major components. On the one hand, it provides regular space for PMH nurses to sit down, drop their shoulders and share with their supervisor any clinical material that is affecting how they are feeling. On the other hand, clinical supervision offers a forum for the PMH nurse to present any piece of her clinical work for exploration and discussion. The supervisor will structure the discussion in a way that will enable the PMH nurse to revisit her clinical moments and feel them happening once more. This revisiting process allows the nurse to construct a deeper and more colourful picture of her chosen clinical incidents. She can ask questions of herself in relation to the patient. She can wonder *why* she was *how* she was, said *what* she said, *did* what she did. She can begin to understand why

she behaved in a certain way and how the patient might have interpreted it. She can come to know herself from the inside and slowly own her own prejudices and defences. Ultimately, she can begin to adjust her beliefs and attitudes and, through the supervisory process, come to know the patient. Emotionally liberated and with lucent thought, the PMH nurse can return to the practice field, her new-found freedom more likely to kindle a similar process in the patient.

Brigid Proctor's supervisory tasks

While I have chosen to break down clinical supervision into two primary functions of support and development, other authors have created their own preferred ways of presenting the subject. There are now numerous models of supervision being employed, usually designed to meet the needs of a specific discipline (e.g. PMH nurses, health visitors) or therapeutic persuasion (e.g. person-centred counselling, psychodynamic psychotherapy). Despite the existence of so many approaches, it feels prudent to highlight just one which, besides having been adopted by many in its unabridged form, seems to have become the foundation for many other subsequent models. Brigid Proctor's[7] 'Supervision Alliance Model' promotes a non-hierarchical, relationship-based approach to supervision, which puts the process of nursing at 'the heart of the matter'.

Within Proctor's model lie the three tasks of supervision, which drive it along. The restorative task, Proctor believes, needs to 'come first', in that it provides vital support on which to pitch the other two tasks. The formative task describes the reflective process that enables the nurse to learn from her clinical experiences. Finally, the normative task is probably the one which nurses have struggled with the most. It is the task that addresses our professional accountability and, as such, carries with it a mandate to confront and challenge any nursing practice that seems either unethical or unsafe.

Taken at face value, such a task seems not only acceptable but also quite reassuring from every perspective. Unfortunately, there have been widespread examples of 'supervision' being introduced into PMH nursing teams as something much more scrutinizing and directive.[8] The boundary stones between clinical supervision and managerial supervision have not always been acknowledged and some PMH nurses have been subjected to managerial monitoring and even appraisal under the guise of clinical supervision.[9] Other supervisory systems have been imposed on nurses with no prior

---

[a] Freudenberger (1980, p. 2) describes 'burn-out' as 'a demon born of the society and times we live in' and defines a sufferer of the phenomenon as 'someone in a state of fatigue or frustration brought about by devotion to a cause, way of life, or relationship that failed to produce the expected reward' (p. 13). Since Freudenberger introduced the term in 1980, it has been adopted by the nursing profession to represent the debilitative effects of accumulated work-related stress which, if left untreated, results in stagnation and, ultimately, can result in emotional collapse. (Freudenberger HJ. *Burn-out*. USA: Doubleday, 1980.)

discussion and little or no training for either the supervisors or the supervisees.[10] The horror stories that such experiences generate travel quickly, causing other PMH nurses to resist clinical supervision, seeing it as a form of managerial inspection and control.[11] This is so sad as, contrary to becoming a form of surveillance, clinical supervision was always intended to be an exploratory and emancipating experience.

While Proctor[12] has chosen to divide supervision into three separate components, it is nigh on impossible to identify such lines of demarcation in practice. As the supervision flows, these three tasks become transposed and often fused together. There is a necessary fluidity within the supervision session that enables the supervisor to respond to the constantly shifting needs of the PMH nurse.

THE SUPERVISORY RELATIONSHIP

Knowing how and when to respond to the supervisee shares many similarities with the craft of caring. The supervisor must always take her direction from the PMH nurse. He is the customer and he must be allowed to decide what piece of clinical practice to present in the session.[13] Despite the carried implications of 'giver' and 'receiver', all individual responsibilities are embraced by the supervisory relationship. There must be mutual trust, respect and honesty: enough 'togetherness' to guarantee that the supervisory journey is a shared undertaking with clear boundaries agreed beforehand.

This is not to say that the supervisory relationship should be cosy and without conflict. The clinical material presented by the PMH nurse will, at times, contain nursing errors and highlight a lack of experience and knowing. This is completely acceptable. It merely confirms what we already accept: that PMH nursing is a difficult craft and, irrespective of the nurse's grade and training, we spend much of our clinical time crafting in the dark. However, there will be an inevitable tension as the supervisor gradually lights up the bits that, as they dawn, the PMH nurse would rather push back into the shadows again. Such moments are pivotal to the productiveness of clinical supervision. The supervisor must feel confident enough to address these issues; the PMH nurse must be willing to join her in exploring them. The destination is always a mystery until the PMH nurse suddenly realizes he is 'there': back where he started, yet knowing the place for the first time.[14]

Clinical supervision and transference relationships

PMH nursing is a relationship-based activity. It involves human beings meeting and interacting and renders both the patient and the PMH nurse susceptible to being shanghai'd by their emotions.[15] Why do we suddenly find ourselves drawn to a particular patient, and then embark upon a fairly reckless mission to 'rescue' him – oblivious to the opinions and contributions of others? And why do we actively avoid Mrs X, who keeps herself to herself and spends most of her time lying on her bed? Or why do we feel so angry towards the young man who has just been admitted again following yet another overdose of tablets? Well, often we do not even ask ourselves such questions, much less discover the answers. Consequently, our emotionally charged nursing reactions fail to provide the 'good enough'[b] nursing care that every patient is entitled to.

Freud[16] referred to all such subconsciously driven behaviour as counter-transference reactions: automatic and impulsive rejoinders by the therapist to the similarly subliminal transference reactions of the patient. He believed that patients, who had been emotionally wounded in their early childhood, unconsciously treated the therapist as though he was the original perpetrator of the trauma (e.g. an abandoning father, an indifferent mother, or an abusive teacher). Freud named this unconscious behaviour a transference reaction. Predictably, if the therapist failed to identify the transference and, as a consequence, reacted back, this was seen as a counter-transference reaction. It is, of course, quite possible for the initial transference reaction to come from the therapist, prompting a counter-transference reaction from the patient.

Case example

Danny is a young man who had been admitted to an acute psychiatric ward after taking a huge overdose of tablets. His childhood could only be described as horrendous. His father left home when he was still an infant and his stepfather used to beat him and his older sister. When he was nine years old, his mother killed herself: he found her hanging in the cellar. He was separated from his sister and placed with several foster parents, all who said they could not cope with Danny. At the age of eighteen, he had moved in with his sister and her boyfriend, who introduced him to heroin. Danny became very depressed and this is his third hospital admission following an overdose. Lou, a PMH nurse on the

---

[b] It was the psychoanalyst, Donald Winnicott, who introduced the concept of the 'good-enough' mother into psychoanalytic theory. I have used the term, with some licence, to represent the clinical supervisor who is able to survive the PMH nurse's fears and frustrations (carried with him from the PMH nurse–patient encounter) by emotionally containing him and encouraging him to charter his own course through these difficulties. (Winnicott DW. *Playing and reality*. London: Routledge, 1971.)

ward, is 38 years of age. She is Danny's care co-ordinator. She is a very caring nurse and has tried hard to engage Danny. He has rejected all her attempts to care in a very aggressive way. He verbally abuses her and accuses her of not genuinely caring at all.

Curiously, the nurse often introduces aspects of the PMH nurse–patient relationship, unconsciously, into the supervision session. It is as if a parallel process[18] is being played out, as the PMH nurse unconsciously casts himself as the patient, and his supervisor as himself. While an in-depth understanding of such phenomena is not necessary for the PMH nurse/supervisee – an awareness of the existence of such complex processes may serve to illustrate that the role of clinical supervisor should never be taken on without preparation and training. To do so would be irresponsible, resulting in a second-class service to both the supervisee and the patient.

Analysis

Danny's reactions to Lou's attempts to care are inappropriate. It is a transference reaction, unconsciously fuelled by his childhood traumas. He is equating Lou with his mother, who he has never forgiven for not protecting him and for abandoning him in such a horrific way. He is projecting all his unresolved feelings onto Lou in an attempt to punish her. He is determined to make her suffer. When she 'gives up on him', as he suspects she eventually will, this will also confirm to him that he is worthless and unlovable.

While we have the benefit of the above analysis, Lou does not. If she is able to work out what is going on with Danny, then she is much less likely to take it personally and fall into a counter-transference reaction. However, even the most experienced nurse has her 'blind spots' and unconsciously 'reacts back' at times. All our interactions are a scandal to theory. They arise out of the chaos of our personalities and we are never completely sure what we are going to say until after we have said it. Nor are we always aware why we choose to 'be' with someone in a particular fashion. In situations such as these, clinical supervision is 'like hearing a welcome voice when lost in the dark'.[17] Powered by kind concern, the supervisor splashes the PMH nurse with enough light to bring the unfamiliar slowly into focus.

Having acknowledged the correlation between the PMH nurse–patient relationship and the supervisory relationship, we can now take a look at the actual mechanics of the supervisory process. How does clinical supervision lead the PMH nurse beyond his threshold of knowing to become a more informed and holistic practitioner?

TURNING 'LIVED EXPERIENCE' INTO 'LEARNING EXPERIENCE'

When the PMH nurse steps into the supervision session, he will already know all he needs to know! Why, then, should he need to come along to supervision in the first place? Because, although the knowing is within him, much of it will be the 'unthought known'[c].[19] The PMH nurse 'knows enough' to be able to make sense of any piece of clinical practice. He has the capacity to understand himself and to understand the patient. He carries with him a wealth of knowing: enough to provide him with the basic equation from which to understand and to learn from his most reliable guide – the patient. What he does not have are the internal eyes with which to recognize and utilize such knowing. The role of the clinical supervisor is to guide the PMH nurse's thoughts to the clinical incidents that need to be unfolded. Wrapped within those moments of practice are the unthought knowns that need to be accessed for clarification, insight and illumination.

Rather than leading the PMH nurse down a particular reflective road – which would imply that an ideal route exists – the supervisor offers signposts that point in many directions.[20] These indicators take the form of Socratic questions[d] about the PMH nurse's casework:[21]

> 'I wonder if you realize what you've just said?'
> 'Perhaps you could have responded differently?'
> 'I sense a shift in your mood?'

The supervisor is there to provide the PMH nurse with options, not answers.[22] Whichever way the PMH nurse chooses to go, he will navigate his own exploratory course. He will struggle through the anxieties of not-knowing until all the fragments of insight slowly fit together. He will come upon a knowing that really means something to him; a knowing full of new potential for both him and the patient. He has turned his lived experience of clinical practice into a learning experience.

---

[c] Tania Yegdich must be afforded the credit for introducing Christopher Bollas's concept of the 'unthought known' into the supervisory arena.[4] I have introduced the 'unthought known' to describe the supervisee's 'knowing' (in relation to his encounter with the patient) that has not yet surfaced into consciousness. Through her communication with the supervisee, the supervisor is able to 'be' with him and, simultaneously, feel the 'being' of the patient. It is from this connective state that the supervisee's unthought known gradually emerges from emotional storage to become consciously knowable. (Bollas C. *The shadow of the object: psychoanalysis of the unthought known.* London: Free Association Books, 1987.)

[d] Socratic questioning is an approach which encourages the supervisee to actively explore a problem and unearth his own 'knowing' (as opposed to having the answers given to him). It is often employed to guide the reflective process in the form of structured prompts (e.g. 'what were you feeling at that point?', 'what would you really like to say to that patient?', 'how could you do that differently?').

Reflection

Clinical supervision is and has to be a collaborative experience.[23] Both the supervisor and the PMH nurse need to identify a template of action that slots into each supervision session: a frame that offers reassuring familiarity but, also, stimulates the journeywork necessary to turn lived experience into learning experience. Many models of supervision employ a form of guided reflection as the wheelwork that drives the session.[24,25] It is relationship based and structured with cues that turn the reflective journey in a progressive manner.[26]

With the nurse–patient relationship at the very heart of it, reflective practice has become an effective medium in the PMH nurse's growth and development. It offers an experiential learning cycle that takes the 'wealth of untapped knowledge embedded in the (nurse's) practices' and converts it into learning.[27] The cyclical nature of reflective practice ensures an open-ended final stage that always connects up to the starting point. It is a seamless process that employs reflexivity as a means to reinterpreting the clinical encounter in order to inform future practice.[28]

The organization as a stakeholder

Hopefully, I have presented clinical supervision for what it is meant to be: regular, structured 'time out' for PMH nurses, offering them a safe space to reflect upon their contact with patients and to learn and know more by doing so. Yet, despite its obvious potential and the steady flow of literature promoting clinical supervision, it has not been adopted – certainly not in the way it is advocated – as a cornerstone of clinical practice.[29] Although high-profile clinicians,[30] academics,[31] professional bodies[32] and the Department of Health[33] have campaigned for its introduction into nursing, the commitment within the nursing profession in general has not been there.[34]

While an educated guess suggests that supervision is more prevalent in PMH Nursing than in any other branch of nursing, research shows that, even within this specialist field, working examples of bona fide clinical supervision are sparse.[35] There are a number of reasons for this. Generally speaking, clinical practice – together with the administrative tasks that it generates – is seen as the main priority of nurses. This is certainly the case as far as most psychiatric services managers are concerned. Their priorities are the availability of enough nurses to staff the wards and minimize the risk of violence, suicide, self-harm and absconding. There is also a cost implication here,[36] in that providing supervision and providing cover for nurses to leave the clinical area needs paying for. Again, service managers seem reluctant to allocate a portion of their budget to fund non-clinical activities.

Surprisingly, some PMH nurses seem to collude with their managers by choosing to prioritize hands-on nursing,[37] even at the expense of their own emotional wellness. While a historical and cultural work ethic drives certain nurses to stay clinically available throughout the length of their shifts, emotional burn-out renders the busy clinical area a less-threatening option for others. Sadly, the former will doubtlessly join the ranks of the latter at some stage of their working lives if they are allowed to continue emotionally (and often physically) flogging themselves without being suitably looked after. While clinical supervision is by no means a panacea for all the difficulties encountered by PMH nurses,[38] it is designed to acknowledge them and to 'help turn down the heat' of the clinical encounter.[39] Withholding clinical supervision, whatever the reason, is both counterproductive and unacceptable. PMH nurses are precious individuals who deserve to be treated as such.

Although PMH nurses are the most visible beneficiaries of any clinical supervision that they share in, they are, of course, not the only ones. If the clinical supervision is 'good enough' then it is hard to argue against the patient and his carers also reaping rewards in terms of better, more informed clinical interventions. The supervisor, too, should gain from every supervisory encounter, enriched by her own discoveries that spring from the supervisory relationship. Managers – stretching upwards as far as chief executives – could enjoy the harvest of a more settled workforce, happier to be in a more nurturing environment. The list goes on. If clinical supervision is celebrated and its positive effects broadcast loudly, people will be more likely to appreciate its impact and more willing to support its implementation.

How is clinical supervision delivered?

Every system of clinical supervision needs the stability of an organizational mandate – official permission to 'act' – to ensure its implementation and survival. With no organizational guy ropes to hold it down, it could be swept away at any time.[40] If clinical supervision is established within your team, you may or may not have a say in how you access it. Bearing these realities in mind, let us look at what should be available to every practising PMH nurse, from the moment he joins the team until the day he leaves it.

Firstly, the PMH nurse should be able to choose his own supervisor:[41] preferably a supervised clinician whom he knows and trusts and with whom he feels safe enough to share his clinical practice. This person should be an experienced supervisor herself and preferably someone who has undergone preparatory training before taking on the role.[42] If the PMH nurse has any special supervisory needs, these should be welcomed and addressed. Hawkins and Shohet[43] highlight the need to provide culturally sensitive supervision for those who work with people from ethnic minority groups. Similarly, PMH nurses who constantly work in 'subcultures' (e.g. gender specific work) may have different supervisory needs.

The debate as to whether or not line managers should provide clinical supervision continues to rattle on. The argument swings both ways. Some would say that line managers are best placed to understand the nurse's clinical dilemmas.[44] Others believe that the hierarchical component would influence the manager's agenda.[45] And would the PMH nurse feel comfortable enough to share his practice and his inevitable mistakes with his manager? There are other variables to be considered, particularly the manager's non-clinical role (if that is so) and, of course, the availability of good enough supervisors. While freedom of choice would eradicate most of these dilemmas, it may not be an option if supervisors are scarce.

Once the supervisor has been identified (or allocated), a contract needs to be negotiated between PMH nurse and supervisor. The contract should outline all the elements that are needed to ensure the provision of safe, regular clinical supervision.[46] The frequency, duration, time and place, provision for cancellations, agreed methods of recording, review date, and a shared understanding of the confidentiality boundaries, all need to be included. Role boundaries, issues of accountability, presentation frameworks, individual and joint responsibilities and expectations are also essential ingredients in the contracting stage of supervision. The more detailed the contract, the safer the foundation that supports the supervisory relationship.

While not necessarily a contractual issue, the mode of delivery does need to be addressed at the contracting stage. What will be the format of the clinical supervision? Will it be provided on a one-to-one basis, or will it be group supervision?[47] Predictably, there are advantages and disadvantages with both formats,[48] although it may well be resource driven and a fait accompli as to which is provided.

If clinical supervision has either not been offered to you at all or falls short of the standards laid out in this text, you have justified cause for complaint. As a practising PMH nurse you need and deserve good enough clinical supervision. If your complaints fall on stony ground, consider other avenues of appeal. Try not to be afraid of lobbying senior managers or Trust executives. If possible, take your protest forward with like-minded others. Or perhaps you could look outside your immediate team for clinical supervision? Never give up – clinical supervision is vital to your survival and development.

WORKING EXAMPLES OF CLINICAL SUPERVISION

With the rudiments of clinical supervision now outlined, the following synopses provide some genuine case illustrations from the field of PMH nursing.

Synopsis 1

Helen, a community PMH nurse, came into supervision feeling 'stuck', 'guilty' and 'rejected'. Despite her desire to work with Charles in a person-centred way, the Organization's overriding medical approach had intruded into her nursing care. She wanted to provide Charles with information about his prescribed drugs so that he could make an informed choice about taking them. He had misinterpreted her best intentions as an attempt to cajole him into taking medication. She had subsequently become the victim of a rather vigorous negative transference reaction from Charles. Not having realized what was going on, she had unconsciously reacted back by becoming a medical messenger of the organization. She had adopted a defensive position, focusing on the possible consequences if Charles decided not to take his medication. She now felt 'a failure', unable to work out how to respond to Charles if he 'was still cross' with her when she next visited him.

The supervision session provided Helen with time and space to reflect on her clinical incident. She had felt 'hurt' when Charles had verbally attacked her. 'I only really wanted what was best for him', she complained. It gradually dawned on her that she had fallen into the role of 'injured parent'. This had prevented her from hearing what Charles had to say and responding to his distress. Through re-experiencing her own hurt from the nurse–patient encounter, she had come to know that Charles, too, was suffering. Freed from her own despair, she could revisit Charles with enough room inside her to carry and survive his anger. Helen left the session feeling 'free' and ready to accept Charles just as she finds him. She would sit with him and respond to however he needed to be.

Synopsis 2

Michelle, a community PMH nurse, had turned up to our supervision session five minutes late. She seemed unsettled and reluctant to start and confessed to having 'nothing to discuss'. Some gentle searching on my behalf uncovered Michelle's busy schedule and, in particular, a patient who had dominated most of her morning. She now found herself falling behind and desperately needing to 'catch up'. Supervision, she felt, was impeding her from doing so. She was desperate to make her escape and respond to the 'neediness' of patients once more.

It took a huge effort from Michelle to reflect on her urge to dash off and rescue people. As we focused on the patient whom she had been with all morning, I sensed a shift in Michelle's 'being'. She became passive and quite childlike, I thought. I found myself working hard, having to lead her much more than usual. She seemed reluctant to contribute and, when she did, she was introducing obstacles and blocking off potential therapeutic pathways. Michelle had become that 'needy' patient. She was thwarting my attempts to help her and, simultaneously, demonstrating her 'helplessness'. It was now my turn to feel the frustration of being strung along and having to work extra hard.

When I shared this parallel process with Michelle she shook her head in amazement. Now she could see that, by reacting to the patient's 'needy' behaviour, she was both perpetuating it and avoiding having to explore just why the patient was so regressed. This keyed into some much wider issues for Michelle, particularly her reluctance to ask for help when she needed it from her colleagues (although she was quick to provide it for others). It was a theme that Michelle would reflect on at length in future clinical supervision sessions, resulting in a huge stride forward in both her personal and professional development.

Synopsis 3

Diane, a PMH nurse, presented Albert, aged 77 years, in supervision. He had made a serious suicide attempt ten weeks ago and had eventually been admitted to the psychiatric ward from the Surgical Intensive Care Unit. Yesterday, he had been discharged home and Diane had said 'a final goodbye to him'. Albert's wife had died just over 12 months ago and he could see no reason whatsoever for living out his own life. Diane had developed a very deep therapeutic relationship with Albert and this, together with a truly, multidisciplinary team approach and the love of his children, had generated hope within him. Diane cried huge tears in our session: tears that carried her joy at witnessing Albert's recovery, tears that expressed her sadness at having to 'let go' of him, and tears that released all the emotions that she had carried over the past eight weeks.

Diane had needed the clinical supervision session to sort out her feelings and cry away some of the emotional overload that she had been carrying. It had also provided me with a golden opportunity to celebrate with Diane the 'healing power' of her caring.[49]

CONCLUSION

Clinical supervision should be a genuine clinical interlude, taken with the organization's blessing. It is time out – for you, the PMH nurse – to recall your clinical encounters and to share those experiences through a dialogue with someone you consider to be a good enough supervisor. As you sit down ready to engage in clinical supervision, you might just feel the butterflies fluttering around in the pit of your stomach. This is a good sign. It is the anxiety borne from the emotional distress of the patient. It is anxiety loaded with conundrums: will the patient survive my caring? Will I survive my caring? Am I helping or hindering? What am I carrying that belongs to the patient? And what is the patient carrying that I need to take back as mine?

Although you already know the answers to all these questions, your knowing is, as yet, unthought. Yet the real learning that is spawned within the supervision session is no intellectual exercise. It does not come from books or papers; and it is certainly not given in the form of solutions by the supervisor. It is a learning that germinates in the in-betweenness of supervisor and PMH nurse. By speaking a shared language of feelings, they can experience the immediacy of the PMH nurse's clinical material and savour its discovered yield. Having cast aside the moonshine of intellectual speculation, the PMH nurse comes to know through an 'education of the heart'.[e]

Engaging in clinical supervision enables the PMH nurse to develop a deeper understanding of his clinical experiences. He can 'revise the way in which the past is understood and the future anticipated'.[50] However, the experienced PMH nurse knows that his 'experience is never limited, and it is never complete'.[51] In the gloaming of the nurse–patient encounter, he is beholden to remake himself at every given opportunity. Clinical supervision is the agency specifically created for him to be able to do so.

REFERENCES

1. Coleridge ST. Aids to reflection: moral and religious aphorisms XXV. In: Beer J (ed.) *The collected works of Samuel Taylor Coleridge: Vol. 9, Aids to reflection, 1831.* New Jersey: Princeton University Press, 1993.

2. Wilkin P. Clinical supervision and community psychiatric nursing. In: Butterworth T, Faugier J, Burnard P (eds). *Clinical supervision and mentorship in nursing,* 2nd edn. Cheltenham: Stanley Thornes, 1998: 189.

3. Wilkin P. Supportive supervision as a means of

---

[e]'We shall never learn to feel and respect our real calling and destiny, unless we have taught ourselves to consider every thing as moonshine, compared with the education of the heart', Scott, W. – letter to J.G. Lockhart, August 1825, quoted in: Lockhart, JG. *Life of Sir Walter Scott*, Vol.6, Chapter 2, Edinburgh: Cadell, 1837.

enabling self-awareness. *Nursing Times Learning Curve* 1998; **3**(3): 10–11.

4. Yegdich, T. *Borne to be free: enduring the unthought known in supervision and therapy.* Conference paper presented at the Rozelle Annual Winter Symposium, July, Sydney, Australia, 1996: 95–102.

5. Barker, P. Psychiatric nursing In: Butterworth T, Faugier J, Burnard P (eds). *Clinical supervision and mentorship in nursing,* 2nd edn. Cheltenham: Stanley Thornes, 1998: 67.

6. Yegdich T. An Australian perspective on clinical supervision. In: Cutcliffe JR, Butterworth T, Proctor B (eds). *Fundamental themes in clinical supervision.* London: Routledge, 2001: 271.

7. Proctor, B. Training for the supervision alliance attitude, skills and intention. In: Cutcliffe JR, Butterworth T, Proctor B (eds). *Fundamental themes in clinical supervision.* London: Routledge, 2001: 25–46.

8. Power S. *Nursing supervision: a guide for clinical practice.* London: Sage, 1999: 12–13.

9. Yegdich T. Clinical supervision and managerial supervision: some historical and conceptual considerations. *Journal of Advanced Nursing* 1999; **30**(5): 1195–204.

10. Scanlon C, Weir WS. Learning from practice? Mental health nurses' perceptions and experiences of clinical supervision. *Journal of Advanced Nursing* 1997; **26**: 295–303.

11. Northcott N. Clinical supervision – professional development or management control? In: Spouse J, Redfern L (eds). *Successful supervision in health care practice: promoting professional development.* Oxford: Blackwell Science, 2000: 10–29.

12. Proctor B. Training for the supervision alliance attitude, skills and intention. In: Cutcliffe JR, Butterworth T, Proctor B (eds). *Fundamental themes in clinical supervision.* London: Routledge, 2001: 25–46.

13. Page S, Wosket V. *Supervising the counsellor: a cyclical model.* London: Routledge, 1994: 68–71.

14. Eliot TS. Little Gidding. In: *T.S. Eliot, collected poems, 1909–1962.* London: Faber and Faber, 1942.

15. Hughes L, Pengelly P. *Staff supervision in a turbulent environment: managing process and task in front-line services.* London: Jessica Kingsley Publishers, 1997: 79–98.

16. Freud S. *The dynamics of transference,* standard edition, Vol. 12. London: Hogarth Press, 1912: 97–108.

17. Barker P. Psychiatric nursing. In: Butterworth T, Faugier J, Burnard P (eds). *Clinical supervision and mentorship in nursing,* 2nd edn. Cheltenham: Stanley Thornes, 1998: 78.

18. van Ooijen E. *Clinical supervision: a practical guide.* London: Churchill Livingstone, 2000: 169–70.

19. Yegdich T. *Borne to be free: enduring the unthought known in supervision and therapy.* Conference paper presented at the Rozelle Annual Winter Symposium, July, Sydney, Australia, 1996: 95–102.

20. Wilkin P. Clinical supervision: helping to make it work. *Mental Health Nursing* 1999; **19**(2): 18–22.

21. Overholser JC. The Socratic method as a technique in psychotherapy supervision. *Professional Psychology: Research and Practice* 1991; **22**(1): 68–74.

22. Jacobs D, David P, Meyer DJ. The supervisory encounter: a guide for teachers of psychodynamic psychotherapy and psychoanalysis. New Haven: Yale University Press, 1995: 186.

23. Anderson H. *Supervision as a collaborative learning community,* 4 pages, 2000. Supervision, Internet, 11th February, 2002, available: http://www.harlene.org/Pages/supervisionbulletin.htm

24. Driscoll J. *Practising clinical supervision: a reflective approach.* London: Baillière Tindall, in association with the Royal College of Nursing, 2000: 17–32.

25. Lillyman S, Ghaye T. *Effective clinical supervision: the role of reflection.* Dinton: Quay Books, 2000.

26. Johns, C. *Becoming a reflective practitioner: a reflective and holistic approach to clinical nursing, practice development and clinical supervision.* Oxford: Blackwell, 2000.

27. Benner, P. *From novice to expert: excellence and power in nursing practice.* California: Addison-Wesley, 1984: 11.

28. Johns, C. *Becoming a reflective practitioner: a reflective and holistic approach to clinical nursing, practice development and clinical supervision.* Oxford: Blackwell, 2000: 61–71.

29. Wilkin P, Bowers L, Monk J. Clinical supervision: managing the resistance. *Nursing Times* 1997; **93**(8): 48–9.

30. Barker P. *The philosophy and practice of psychiatric nursing.* London: Churchill Livingstone, 1999: 183–95.

31. Butterworth T. Clinical supervision as an emerging idea in nursing. In: Butterworth T, Faugier J, Burnard P (eds). *Clinical supervision and mentorship in nursing,* 2nd edn. Cheltenham: Stanley Thornes, 1998: 1–18.

32. United Kingdom Central Council. *Position statement on clinical supervision for nursing and health visiting.* London: UKCC, 1996.

33. Department of Health. *Clinical supervision for the nursing and health visiting profession.* CNO Letter (94) 5. London: HMSO, 1994.

34. Cutcliffe JR. An alternative training approach in clinical supervision. In: Cutcliffe JR, Butterworth T, Proctor B (eds). *Fundamental themes in clinical supervision.* London: Routledge, 2001: 47–63.

35. Grant A. Clinical supervision and organisational power: a qualitative study. *Mental Health Care* 2000; **31**(12): 398–401.

36. Department of Health. *Clinical supervision: a report of the Trust Nurse Executives' workshops.* London: HMSO, 1994.

37. Cottrell S, Smith G. *Suspicion, resistance, tokenism and mutiny: problematic dynamics relevant to the implementation of clinical supervision,* 8 pages, 2000. The development of clinical supervision in nursing, Internet, 11th February, 2002, available: http://www.clinical-supervision.com/article.htm

38. Carson J, Butterworth T, Booth K. Clinical supervision, stress management and social support. In: Butterworth T, Faugier J, Burnard P (eds). *Clinical supervision and mentorship in nursing.* Cheltenham: Stanley Thornes, 1998: 62.

39. Barker P. Psychiatric nursing. In: Butterworth T, Faugier J, Burnard P (eds). *Clinical supervision and mentorship in nursing,* 2nd edn. Cheltenham: Stanley Thornes, 1998: 78.

40. Wilkin P. Clinical supervision and community psychiatric nursing. In: Butterworth T, Faugier J, Burnard P (eds). *Clinical supervision and mentorship in nursing.* Cheltenham: Stanley Thornes, 1998: 200.

41. Bond M, Holland S. *Skills of clinical supervision for nurses: a practical guide for supervisees, clinical supervisors and managers.* Buckingham: Open University Press, 1998: 79.

42. Hawkins P, Shohet R. *Supervision in the helping professions,* 2nd edn. Buckingham: Open University Press, 2000: 106–24.

43. Hawkins P, Shohet R. *Supervision in the helping professions,* 2nd edn. Buckingham: Open University Press, 2000: 88–105.

44. Johns C. *Becoming a reflective practitioner: a reflective and holistic approach to clinical nursing, practice development and clinical supervision.* Oxford: Blackwell Science, 2000: 56.

45. Bond M, Holland S. *Skills of clinical supervision for nurses: a practical guide for supervisees, clinical supervisors and managers.* Buckingham: Open University Press, 1998: 18–19.

46. Power S. *Nursing supervision: a guide for clinical practice.* London: Sage, 1999: 116–30.

47. Milne D, Oliver V. Flexible formats of clinical supervision: description, evaluation and implementation. *Journal of Mental Health* 2000; 9(3): 291–304.

48. van Ooijen E. *Clinical supervision: a practical guide.* London: Churchill Livingstone, 2000: 31–4.

49. Benner P. *From novice to expert: excellence and power in nursing practice.* California: Addison-Wesley, 1984: 220.

50. Warnke G. *Gadamer: hermeneutics, tradition and reason.* Cambridge: Polity Press, 1987: 29.

51. James H (1884). *The art of fiction.* Temecula: Reprint Services Corporation, 1992.

Chapter 65

THE POSSIBILITY OF GENUINE MENTAL HEALTH NURSING

Gary Rolfe* and Lyn Gardner**

A ROSE BY ANY OTHER NAME ...

Anyone involved in nursing during the past two decades will have noticed some sweeping and far-reaching changes in the profession. One of the most obvious, but one which has been largely uncontested, is the change in title that occurred in the UK in the early 1990s, from *psychiatric nurse* to *mental health nurse*. For many nurses, this change has probably been seen as largely insignificant in comparison to other major innovations, such as the move from the institution and into the community, the development of the multidisciplinary team, and the introduction of a *National Service Framework* (NSF) for mental health.[1] Furthermore, those nurses entering the profession more recently have only ever seen themselves as mental health nurses. And in any case, the more poetic reader might conclude: 'What is in a name? A rose by any other name would still smell as sweet.' Here, I shall argue that there is a great deal in a name; that the words we use to describe ourselves and what we do have a real and sometimes profound influence on our thoughts and actions. Seen in this way, the change of name not only *reflects* wider changes occurring in the profession, but also to some extent *initiates* them.

This relationship between language and the world it seeks to describe is well-recognized by many in the profession, and is reflected in the seemingly continual changes in the terminology used to describe those on the receiving end of nursing care, from the 'wild lunatics shouting insults in the streets'[2] of the 16th century to the more respectful 'service user' of today. Both the labelled and the labellers recognize that certain terms have stigma attached to them, and the regular changes in terminology over the years reflect the observation that, however 'pure' and unsullied any new terminology starts out, the stigma of the old labels quickly attaches itself to the new.

But labels do not simply describe the way that the world currently is, they also shape the way that it might develop. Thus, the ongoing debate over the past twenty years about whether the people we nurse should be referred to as *patients*, *clients*, *consumers* or *service users* (along with several more esoteric terms) is far more than simply a choice between different forms of address, since each label has different connotations about what the user might expect from the service and vice versa.

The term 'patient' was originally introduced to shift the focus from the 'lunatic' who had no control over her

---

*Gary Rolfe is a psychiatric nurse and Reader in Practice Development at the University of Portsmouth. His main interest is in practitioner knowledge and helping health care professionals to explore their own practice through action research.

**Lyn Gardner is a lecturer in mental health studies at the University of Southampton. Her main interest lies in the exploration of women's experiences of mental distress/illness, and she is currently researching women who self-mutilate/self-harm.

actions and therefore required only custodial care, to the idea of an illness which was amenable to treatment and therefore offered hope of a return to normal life. While the label 'patient' connotes an illness no different from physical conditions (indeed, it suggests that mental illness *is* a physical condition), it can also lead to a medical relationship in which the patient plays a largely passive role and expects to be 'cured' of her 'disease' through the administration of physical treatments such as medication and ECT. Mental illness is therefore something that the patient 'has' and that doctors and nurses attempt to remove.

The term 'client', introduced in the 1980s, suggests a more active and business-like relationship between a professional and a lay-person, similar to that encountered in other professions such as law. This term was soon replaced by 'consumer' to reflect the market economy prevalent in the UK at the end of the last century, and suggests the provision of a paid service and the possibility of 'shopping around' for the best deal, with the balance of power shifted somewhat away from the professional. Similarly, 'service user' retains the element of choice but without the cost implication. However, each of these alternative terms suggest that the user approaches the service provider with a problem that she wishes to be resolved, whereas the real-life situation is frequently rather different, since it often involves a degree of coercion, if not outright compulsion. As one 'consumer' remarked, 'Survivors of the mental health system are no more consumers of mental health services than cockroaches are consumers of Rentokil'.[3]

For this reason, many nurses have reverted to the term 'patient' as a more honest (if not entirely accurate) description of the role of the service user, while some users prefer to see themselves as 'survivors' of the mental health system. We can see, then, that while the terminology employed by the service to describe itself, the services it offers, and the recipients of those services, might *reflect* the times, it also *proactively* determines the way in which those services are perceived and might therefore influence their future development.

FROM PSYCHIATRIC TO MENTAL HEALTH NURSING

The change in terminology from 'psychiatric nursing' to 'mental health nursing' might therefore have more than merely a symbolic significance; rather, it might be seen as a deliberate attempt to influence the way in which the profession conducts itself and what it expects from the practitioners and users of the services it provides. In particular, it might be seen as an indication of the intent to shift the focus of the service from psychiatric *illness* to mental *health*, and from treatment to prevention.

This shift in focus is illustrated, in England, by Standard One of the *NSF* where it states that health and social services should work to 'promote mental health for all' and attempt to 'combat discrimination against individuals and groups with mental health problems, and promote their social inclusion'.[4] The move was applauded by the *Sainsbury Centre for Mental Health*, in their review of the NSF, where they highlighted the links between 'adverse life conditions' and poor mental health.[5] This implies a broader role for mental health nurses, yet it is not clear what form that role may take, and as Tudor[6] has pointed out, there is considerable confusion and 'conceptual ignorance' about the term mental health promotion. A person with a diagnosed mental illness may still achieve a sense of 'wellness', and thus mental health nurses already perform a health promotion role in enabling the individual to achieve that end. Yet a broader mental illness prevention role, as set out in the NSF, is perhaps a new departure.

The change in terminology has been gradual, and probably originated in the USA. Stuart and Sundeen[7] traced the origins of American psychiatric nursing back to 1873, but it was not until a century later that we see the term 'mental health nursing' employed. Initially, both the old and the new terms were used together, for example, in the American Nurses Association's certification of psychiatric mental health nurse generalists and in the publication of *Standards of Psychiatric-Mental Health Nursing Practice*.[8] Interestingly, while Stuart and Sundeen record this gradual shift in terminology, they make no explicit comment on it, and perhaps significantly retain the term 'psychiatric nurse' in the title of their influential textbook.

As with most innovations in nursing, there appears to be a ten-year lag between the USA and the UK, with the term 'mental health nursing' being introduced into the UK along with the *Project 2000* curriculum in the mid 1980s. Thus, the 'Course Development Guidelines' published in 1989 by the English National Board for Nursing, Midwifery and Health Visiting (ENB) introduced the new branch programme by pointing out that:

> This branch is entitled 'Mental Health' in recognition of the fact in all aspects of work the nurse will be promoting optimum mental health of both a **restorative** and **preventative** nature.[9]

Thus, the previous qualification of Registered Mental Nurse, with its focus on the illness model of psychiatry, was replaced in 1989 with the qualification of Registered Nurse (Mental Health) with a focus on 'optimum mental health'.

It is perhaps worth exploring further these changes in terminology introduced by the ENB in the late 1980s. The wording of the titles of the new branch programmes was the subject of some discussion at the time, and several mental health nurses pointed out that the adult and child branches were named after groups of people, while the remaining two branches were named after conditions. Thus, adult nursing entailed working with *all* adults and child nursing entailed working with *all* children, whereas mental health nursing included only a particular subgroup of adults and children. This, it was claimed, reflected the inferior position of mental health and learning disabilities nursing, which could be seen merely as specialities or subdisciplines of adult and child nursing. Furthermore, it is interesting to note that the Learning Disabilities branch was originally entitled 'The Branch Programme in Mental Handicap Nursing', and included a whole page of justification for retaining the old label, beginning:

> In common with other groups who attempt to develop a working language to convey meaning, difficulty is experienced when we use the term 'mental handicap'. It is recognized that in many respects the term is confusing, uncomplimentary and unsatisfactory. It is employed because it is still used as a general statement.[10]

We can see in this statement at least a tacit recognition of the power of labels to influence attitudes. However, whereas learning disability nurses fought for a change in terminology, the move from psychiatric nursing to mental health nursing was accepted, in general, uncritically. Indeed, the shift in focus to health education and illness prevention was seen by many as a positive move, and has been reinforced in policy documents throughout the 1990s from 'Health of the Nation',[11] with its emphasis on suicide prevention, to the 'National Service Framework for Mental Health', which addressed 'the *mental health needs* of working age adults',[12] and whose first standard specifically aimed to 'promote mental health for all'.

THE PROMISE OF MENTAL HEALTH NURSING

One of the first textbooks in the UK to embrace the new terminology was Reynolds and Cormack's *Psychiatric and Mental Health Nursing* in 1990, and we can see in this title a reflection of the American strategy of initially retaining both terms. Interestingly, however, Reynolds and Cormack did not use them interchangeably, but rather distinguished between 'clients with a psychiatric diagnosis' and 'those who have mental health problems but who do not necessarily have such a diagnosis'.[13] Clearly, if such a distinction was invoked on a national scale, then the new mental health nurse would have a rather limited clientele, and not one that is in line with the current policy focus on serious and enduring mental illness.

However, by the time that Wright and Giddey's textbook *Mental Health Nursing* was published three years later, Burnard, writing in the Foreword, noted that:

> The term 'mental health' has largely replaced 'psychiatry' and this reflects the move towards prevention of mental illness and the promotion of positive health …[14]

This switch in terminology is also reflected in the 1997 rewrite for a UK readership of Stuart and Sundeen's *Principles and Practice of Psychiatric Nursing*. While Stuart and Sundeen retained the term 'psychiatric nursing' from initial publication in 1979 through all subsequent editions, the UK version of the book was entitled *Mental Health Nursing: Principles and Practice*. In the UK edition, the now outdated term 'psychiatric nurse' is defined as:

> the nurse whose main focus is within the institutional setting of a hospital. The term also implies the close connection that nursing had with the medicalization of madness and mental illness.[15]

In contrast, mental health nurse is a more contemporary term that has derived from the shift of emphasis from illness to health and the changes made to service delivery. The term suggests more positive attitudes towards mental health problems through strategies of prevention and intervention.[16]

The authors identify *mental health* nursing with the role of the community psychiatric nurse (CPN) which began to emerge in the 1970s. These CPNs 'believed in early intervention and health promotion as the key principles in mental health',[17] whereas 'the skills base of nurses who worked for many years in large traditional hospitals may not be appropriate for today's acute admission or community work'.[18]

We can see in this simple and cursory analysis of the terminology that the title 'mental health nurse' implies a number of changes from the earlier 'psychiatric nurse'. First and foremost, it suggests a focus on illness prevention and health promotion delivered mainly in community settings, but also a move away from a medical model approach to treating mental illness to a more socially oriented view. But as a number of writers have pointed out, this change of focus to some extent conflicts with the policy drive in the UK towards working with people with serious mental illness as outlined in the documents *Working in Partnership*[19] and *Building Bridges*.[20] Rogers and Pilgrim, for example, argue that the term 'mental health services' is a misnomer, since 'most of what are called mental health services actually respond to people with a diagnosis of mental illness'.[21] In a similar vein, Barker adds that:

> Increasingly, psychiatric services are described as *mental health* services, despite maintaining their focus on

dealing with manifest illness, using traditional forms of psychiatric intervention.[22]

To resolve this apparent conflict, we need to look more closely at some of the implications of the change in emphasis from illness to health.

MENTAL HEALTH NURSING AND THE PREVENTION OF ILLNESS

One of the problems with this shift of focus is that whereas mental illness is well defined and categorized in terms of signs, symptoms and diagnoses, there appears to be no generally accepted definition of mental health. As Torkington points out, there are no precise formulae, criteria or measurable objectives, and mental health has different meanings for different individuals and demographic groups.[23] Health is widely recognized as a social construct that varies according to age, gender, race, culture and social class. Furthermore, some definitions view health as merely an absence of illness, whereas others see it as the presence of various attributes such as individuality, creativity and fulfilment of potential. Perhaps because of these difficulties in defining and setting objectives for health, Rogers and Pilgrim note that government policy in the UK has focused largely on mental illness *prevention* rather than mental health *promotion*.

Health educationalists usually classify illness prevention into three types (see Table 65.1).

Primary mental illness prevention

Primary mental illness prevention could theoretically involve the entire population. However, in practice the strategies are mostly restricted to those at greatest risk of mental illness, usually identified through social and demographic indicators such as poverty and poor housing. Rogers and Pilgrim point out that whereas the USA has focused specifically on primary prevention, the UK has in the past had no such policy. Newton[24] has identified four possible reasons for this lack of emphasis on

TABLE 65.1 (adapted from Rogers and Pilgrim 1996)

Primary prevention	Anticipation and pre-emption of mental illness
Secondary prevention	Intervention at an early stage in the causation and occurrence of mental illness
Tertiary prevention	Minimization of the effects associated with existing mental illness, such as prevention of relapse or symptom management

primary prevention. Firstly, she argues that there is a conceptual vagueness surrounding the concepts both of mental illness and illness prevention, which makes it difficult successfully to plan services. Secondly, the knowledge gained from research about effective interventions is not, for whatever reason, being put into practice. Thirdly, she claims that most service planning is short-term and *ad hoc* and there is little incentive to invest in long-term prevention strategies that might not show results for decades. And fourthly, prevention has social and cultural implications that extend far beyond the scope and remit of the health services, making full implementation extremely difficult. Furthermore, evidence from the USA suggests that even when wide-ranging social reforms are initiated as the main thrust of a primary prevention strategy, it is likely to have little impact on the incidence of mental health problems.[25] Perhaps for these reasons, strategy in the UK has in the past focused mainly on secondary and tertiary prevention. It remains to be seen how the goals of primary mental health promotion as set out in Standard One of the NSF will be achieved.

Secondary mental illness prevention

Secondary mental illness prevention focuses on early intervention, perhaps even before the patient is being troubled by the condition. The onus of secondary prevention has traditionally fallen largely on general practitioners and other primary health care services, and has centred on a strategy of screening for various symptoms and psychiatric conditions. Yet developments in early intervention with people experiencing psychotic disorders[26] have provided opportunities for mental health nurses to take an active role in secondary prevention work.[27]

Risk assessment is often thought to be enhanced by the use of rating scales,[28] which identify patients who fall into high risk categories. For example, a rating scale for suicide risk might include psychiatric and socioeconomic factors that are often associated with suicide attempts. However, Kelly,[29] has pointed out that these scales are at best merely an adjunct to clinical judgement. As a Department of Health training manual noted:

All these factors are well-known statistical correlates of suicide and must not be ignored. They do, however, present problems in the day-to-day clinical situation. Many individuals will possess these characteristics yet not commit suicide, and suicide can occur in people of very different characteristics.[30]

It continued:

Suicide risk in any individual can only be assessed effectively by full clinical evaluation consisting of a thorough review of the history and present illness, assessment of mental state and then a diagnostic formulation.[31]

Secondary mental illness prevention is perhaps not as simple and straightforward as its proponents might claim it to be, and can involve a great deal of investment in time and money for perhaps a limited outcome.

In addition, secondary intervention makes the twin assumptions that patients are unhappy with their symptoms (indeed, that they are even *seen* as symptoms by the patient) and that they wish to receive treatment at this early stage of their illness. If, as we claimed above, health and illness are social constructs that are defined differently by different groups and individuals, then illness prevention can be seen as the imposition of a norm or ideal onto the patient with which she may disagree. An extreme example might be the construct of suicide, which is seen by the nurse as a sign of a mental illness but which could be seen by the patient as a rational solution to an intractable problem, or even as a fundamental human right. A different example might be deliberate (*sic*) self-harm, which might be construed by the individual as a lifestyle statement (think, for example, of body piercing),[32] or even as a physical treatment to reduce tension and anxiety.[33] Similarly, auditory hallucinations, usually considered to be a symptom of psychotic illness, might be construed by the person experiencing them as anything from a religious experience to merely an aspect of normal everyday life.[34] There is a real danger, then, that secondary mental illness prevention can involve an unwelcome and unasked for incursion into the life of the patient, who might find herself with a psychiatric label (and, in extreme cases, with psychiatric treatment) for something that she regards as normal, or at least as outside the remit of psychiatry. Furthermore, victim blaming is always a danger in a culture that emphasizes the importance of participation by the patient in the maintenance of her own mental health. For example, it is tempting to blame the non-compliant patient or the patient who leads what is seen by the nurse as an unhealthy lifestyle for the situation she finds herself in, much as smokers are sometimes blamed for their physical health problems.

Tertiary mental illness prevention

Tertiary prevention focuses on individuals who already have a diagnosis of mental illness, and aims to prevent relapse and minimize existing symptoms. As in the case of secondary prevention, however, patients do not always welcome tertiary mental illness prevention. Indeed, some patients are simply not interested in treatments of any kind, whether primary, secondary or tertiary. For some, it might be the patient's friends or family

who initiate treatment when she does not consider herself to be ill. Some might regard certain symptoms as pleasurable rather than distressing, for example, the manic episodes of bipolar disorder. Others might consider the treatment or its side-effects to be less desirable than the symptoms it is designed to reduce. Yet others wish for something other than illness prevention or symptom management; as one service user put it, what she required was refuge, 'a non-medical place run by people who understand what I'm going through, where I could go for respite when my life is impossible'.[35]

THE POSSIBILITY OF GENUINE MENTAL HEALTH NURSING

There is, perhaps, a certain irony in the current situation. At least in the UK, the switch from psychiatric nursing to mental health nursing occurred at a time when the profession, driven (in England) by the 1982 mental nursing syllabus, was already in transition from a medically dominated to a socially oriented discipline. The irony is that, by adopting an illness prevention model of mental health nursing rather than focusing on health promotion, psychiatric nursing was sucked back into the medical model. As Rogers and Pilgrim argue:

> A mental illness prevention approach has a narrow focus. It derives from the natural sciences – in particular, medicine. Also, it has been located in the institutions of public health/welfare, at a particular historical time and place in the development of the welfare state. In other words, an emphasis on illness will inevitably tie prevention to the knowledge base, practices, and institutional forms of a single profession – medicine.[36]

The promise of mental health nursing of a move away from the medical model might therefore be seen to have had the opposite effect. Furthermore, by continuing to pursue this medical model approach, the unique role of the nurse is becoming increasingly threatened. There is very little that the mental health nurse is now expected to do that cannot be done equally well either by a practitioner from a different profession or else by a non-professional who has been specifically trained in one particular aspect of the role of the mental health nurse.

This brings us to the question posed by Barker: 'what exactly has *psychiatric* nursing to do with *mental health* nursing?'[37] For Barker, the answer is both simple and profound: mental health is defined not merely as the absence of illness, but as a positive state in its own right. Citing Freud, Barker equates mental health with the capacity to love and work, and particularly to *love*. The promotion of mental health is therefore concerned as much with the spiritual as with the physical and the mental; as much with the soul or spirit as with the body and the mind. As he continues:

> The failure to acknowledge the spiritual distress of mental illness is the most damning indictment of our current 'mental health services'. All too often we discover that we have successfully treated the illness but have either damaged or lost the person in the process.[38]

Mental health nursing is therefore not concerned merely with illness prevention, but neither is it concerned with health education. For Barker, the job of the mental health nurse is not to tell patients about their illness, but to allow them to tell *us* about it:

> I am often asked, is it not important for me to be able to tell patients and their families what they are suffering from? The answer is, for me, a clear 'No'. People tell me what they are 'suffering' from! My responsibility is to be able to help them express themselves to the best of their abilities.[39]

For Barker, the true focus of mental health nursing is the building of what is sometimes referred to as a therapeutic relationship, a relationship that enables the patient to tell her story and thereby to begin her *own* recovery and growth. Barker refers to this as an 'alliance' whereby 'nurses can join with people in their distress, metaphorically accompanying them ... on that "search for truth"'.[40] It is a 'caring with' rather than a 'caring for'.

Perhaps we might be permitted a musical analogy. The mental health nurse plays the piano accompaniment while the patient sings the song; and it is the singing of the song, the telling of the story, that is also the therapy. Mental health nursing is therefore a 'being with' the patient, accompanying her while she finds *herself*. This might seem simple, even trivial, and yet the 'not knowing' required of the mental health nurse goes against all the expectations placed on her by the service, her colleagues and her patients. The perceived role of the nurse is to provide answers, and yet Barker tells us that we do not know, we *cannot* know, the answers for each of our individual patients. He adds that:

> When I joined the field almost 30 years ago, if it wasn't psychoanalytic, in one form or another, it wasn't worth the candle. Today if it isn't cognitive – or, increasingly, cognitive-behavioural – many believe that it is not state-of-the-art. Long ago I realized that 'not knowing' was a respectable position.[41]

This observation about the perceived importance of cognitive-behavioural interventions is reinforced at the highest level. Professor Sir David Goldberg of the Institute of Psychiatry in London writes in the Preface to Newell and Gournay's textbook '*Mental Health Nursing: an evidence-based approach*' that:

> The arrival of nurse therapists ... has transformed the role of the psychiatric nurse from mainly custodial and supportive to being the purveyor of active – and often highly effective – interventions. The cognitive-behavioural approach is referred to repeatedly and is likely to set mental health nursing on a new course in the next century.[42]

There is no denying the relevance and importance to psychiatry of cognitive-behavioural therapy, and even of analytic psychotherapy. However, to refer to it as mental *health* nursing is perhaps stretching the point, if by health we mean a positive *process* of growth rather than simply the absence of illness. It might at best be referred to as *psychiatric* nursing, and at worst as something other than nursing entirely, since clearly not all cognitive-behavioural therapists are nurses. There is, of course, a place for this psychiatric nurse, who 'responds to people's distress by helping to contain it, delimit it, or otherwise "fix" it',[43] but this approach to nursing is rooted firmly in the medical 'illness prevention' model of 'caring for', and is at best a static holding strategy; it might prevent a deterioration in the patient's condition, but it does little to promote the growth that is necessary for a true state of health.

TWO ROSES, TWO NAMES ...

And so, back to terminology, to the words we use to describe who we are and what we do. We started this chapter by charting a shift in terminology from 'psychiatric nurse' to 'mental health nurse', and the past decade has seen a battle for ownership of this new label. The two principal sides in this battle have been what we might call the technological and the humanist, or what one commentator has personalized as 'Gournayism versus Barkerism'.[44]

However, battles are usually fought over disputed territory, in this case over ownership of the term 'mental health nursing' and all that it implies. We have argued in this chapter that Gournay's body- and mind-oriented technical interventions such as CBT are better described as 'psychiatric nursing', reflecting their grounding in illness prevention and the medical model. Similarly, Barker's spirit- or soul-oriented humanistic (non)interventions better meet the criteria of 'mental health nursing', reflecting their grounding in human growth and development. Seen in this way, Gournayism *versus* Barkerism becomes Gournayism *and* Barkerism; there is not one but two territories, and there is no reason why the nurse should not travel back and forth between them, or even stand on the border with one foot in either camp. *This* is the possibility of a genuine mental health nursing.

REFERENCES

1. Department of Health. *National service framework for mental health.* London: HMSO, 1999.

2. François Colletet. Cited in Foucault M. *Madness and civilization.* London: Routledge, 2001: 33.

3. Cited by Barker I, Peck E. *Power in strange places: user empowerment in mental health services.* London: Good Practices in Mental Health, 1987.

4. DOH, *op. cit.*

5. Sainsbury Centre for Mental Health. *The national service framework for mental health: an executive briefing.* London: Sainsbury Centre for Mental Health, 1999.

6. Tudor K. *Mental health promotion: paradigms and practice.* London: Routledge, 1996.

7. Stuart GW, Sundeen SJ. *Principles and practice of psychiatric nursing,* 3rd edn. St Louis: C.V. Mosby, 1987.

8. Ibid., p. 7.

9. English National Board for Nursing, Midwifery and Health Visiting. *Project 2000 – A new preparation for practice: guidelines for course development.* London: ENB, 1989: 30, their emphasis.

10. Ibid., p. 20.

11. Department of Health. *The Health of the Nation: a strategy for health in England.* London: HMSO, 1992.

12. DOH, *op. cit.* (Executive summary, p. 3, our emphasis).

13. Reynolds W, Cormack D. *Psychiatric and mental health nursing: theory and practice.* London: Chapman and Hall, 1990: ix.

14. Wright H, Giddey M. *Mental health nursing: from first principles to professional practice.* London: Chapman and Hall, 1993: xii.

15. Thomas B, Hardy S, Cutting P. *Stuart and Sundeen's mental health nursing.* Chicago: Mosby, 1997: 3.

16. Ibid., p. 3.

17. Ibid., p. 7.

18. Ibid., p. 8.

19. Department of Health. *Working in partnership: a collaborative approach to care.* London: HMSO, 1994.

20. Department of Health. *Building bridges.* London: HMSO, 1995.

21. Rogers A, Pilgrim D. *Mental health policy in Britain.* Basingstoke: Macmillan, 1996: 142.

22. Barker P. *The philosophy and practice of psychiatric nursing.* Edinburgh: Churchill Livingstone, 1999: 83.

23. Torkington, S. Perspectives in mental health. In: Martin P (ed.) *Psychiatric nursing.* London: Scutari Press, 1995: 1–19.

24. Newton J. *Preventing mental illness.* London: Routledge, 1988.

25. Rogers and Pilgrim, *op. cit.*

26. Birchwood M, Smith J, Macmillan J, Hogg B, Prasad R, Harvey C, Bering S. Predicting relapse in schizophrenia: the development and implementation of an early signs monitoring system using patients and families as observers. *Psychological Medicine* 1989; **19**: 649–56.

27. Lancashire S, Haddock G, Tarrier N, Baguley I, Butterworth AC, Brooker C. Effects of training in psycho-social interventions for community psychiatric nurses in England. *Psychiatric Services* 1997; **48**(1): 39–41.

28. Maphosa W, Slade M, Thornicroft G. Principles of assessment. In: Newell R, Gournay K (eds). *Mental health nursing: an evidence-based approach.* Edinburgh: Churchill Livingstone, 2000: 103–20.

29. Kelly S. Suicide and self harm. Ibid., 2000: 187–206.

30. Department of Health. *Suicide prevention: the challenge confronted.* London, HMSO: 1994: 19.

31. Ibid.

32. Steele V. *Fetish: fashion, sex and power.* Oxford: Oxford University Press, 1996.

33. Babiker G, Arnold L. *The language of injury: comprehending self-mutilation.* Leicester: The British Psychological Society, 1997.

34. Romme M, Escher S. *Accepting voices.* London: Mind, 1993.

35. Lindow V. A service user's view. In: Wright H, Giddey M, *op. cit.,* p. 27.

36. Rogers and Pilgrim, *op. cit.,* p. 146.

37. Barker, *op. cit.,* p. 79.

38. Ibid., p. 90.

39. Ibid., p. 85.

40. Ibid., p. 89.

41. Ibid., p. 59.

42. Newell and Gournay, *op. cit.,* pp. ix–x.

43. Barker, *op. cit.,* p. 89.

44. Grant A. Knowing me knowing you: towards a new relational politics in 21st century mental health nursing. *Journal of Psychiatric and Mental Health Nursing* 2001; **8**: 269–80.

Chapter 66

NURSE–CONSUMER COLLABORATION: GO WITH THE FLO!

Cynthia Stuhlmiller*

INTRODUCTION

The idea of forming collaborative relationships with consumers of mental health nursing can be seen as nothing more than commonsense. However, it requires the 'right attitude' and can be challenging, given the restrictive bureaucratic systems within which nurses operate. Nonetheless, the idea of nurses working collaboratively with consumers[a] is not new. Arguably, the historical foundation for the nursing profession rests on the notions of collaboration, participation and empowerment outlined by Florence Nightingale in 1859 in her 'Notes on Nursing'. Admittedly she was not directly addressing issues related to people with a mental illness. However, her theme of advocating for human rights of patients and families is clear and strong. Hildegard Peplau – considered the grandmother of psychiatric nursing – also believed that nursing is informed by participation, involvement, and collaboration with the patient and their support network.

To this day, the most enduring concept central to the discipline of nursing remains the value and importance of the *nurse–patient relationship* and its inherent characteristics that influence the experience of illness and recovery. The interpersonal aspects of relating enable the nurse and person to understand each other more fully – including the distress, suffering, strengths, and possibilities of the consumer and the nurse's abilities and limitations to help in the realization of health.

If mental health nursing is founded on the concept of relating and collaborating, why then is there an escalation of dissatisfaction in health care relationships[1]? Could it be that care based on the meaningful human-to-human connection of mutual respect and trust has eroded? Furthermore, why does every mental health care reform agenda have as a priority 'consumer and carer participation in planning, implementation and evaluation of mental health service delivery'? Does this preoccupation signal that the basic principles of collaboration continue to be largely ignored or discounted? What has kept nurses from embracing the fundamental principles of their profession to become strong leaders in the field of mental health care?

Some of these questions will be explored here, by revisiting the basics of good nursing as they apply to mental health collaboration. '*Go with the Flo*' is a call for nurses to re-examine and act on the principles set down

*Cynthia Stuhlmiller, Professor of Nursing (mental health) Flinders University, Adelaide Australia, has enjoyed an exciting and varied career in nursing. Cutting across all of her experiences remains a commitment of promoting human connection as she maintains that it is among the most fundamental and important determinants of health and wellness.

[a] Consumer is the term currently in vogue. However, I agree with Barker and prefer the term person, person nursed or person-in-care. These terms, including patient and client will be used interchangeably.

by Florence Nightingale. Her views are contemporary and timeless. Her plea for restoration of basic values, commitment, and informed moral action that leads to social and political reform transcends time and is particularly prophetic for the 21st century. Perhaps her voice has finally come of age.

An overview of ideologies and tensions in mental health care is offered, followed by models and principles of collaboration, concluding with some illustrations of collaboration. I urge you to consider how everyday mental health nursing is about being proud, confident, and outspoken about the importance of working collaboratively with consumers or doing good nursing.

HISTORICAL IDEOLOGIES AND TENSIONS

The evolution of treatment for people with a mental illness provides an understanding from which current day issues concerning collaboration with consumers have emerged. Until the 16th century it was thought that devils or evil spirits possessed people who displayed unusual or deviant behaviour. Such people were left, by and large, to fend for themselves. In the 17th and 18th century the mentally ill were provided with food and shelter along with criminals and poor people. In the 19th century asylums were built to house the increasing number of people considered insane and medical doctors were put in charge to treat them under the auspices of medical science as madness came to be understood as mental illness (see Chapter 2 for a fuller discussion).

In the 20th century the work of Freud, Bleuler and Kraepelin, significantly advanced the worldview of mental illness as theories about the science of the mind began to proliferate.[2] Ironically the practice of treating people through objective clinical study was a breakthrough from the previous system of accusing 'mad persons' of demonic possession.[3] By the 1950s, the introduction and success of psychotropic drugs in controlling people reinforced the scientific notion that mental illness is a result of neurological dysfunction and biochemical imbalances. In the 1960s, the civil rights movement in the United States drew attention to the status of blacks, women, and other disenfranchised groups. Activists began to consider that the inhumane conditions found in custodial mental hospitals might be contributing to mental illness. Along with a faith in psychotropic drugs, deinstitutalization and establishment of community mental health centres in the United States began.[4] Other Western nations followed.

Anti-psychiatry and the consumer movement

At the same time, the established paternalistic professional attitude towards mental patients, who used science to claim to know what was best for the person, was challenged as the era of anti-psychiatry unfolded. Assertions by powerful critics such as Laing,[5] Goffman[6] and Szasz[7] that mental illness might be a myth questioned the legitimacy of the psychiatry and highlighted its exploitative, social control, practices. Efforts to overthrow the medical model and to challenge the enormous power of the mental health system, saw professionals and 'ex-mental patients' exploring together alternatives to psychiatric treatment.[3] This political force, first dominated by professionals, evolved in the 1970s under the direction of groups such as the Mental Patients' Liberation Movement.

Despite these efforts, psychiatry survived by acting defensively and asserting its medical identity – although suspicion of credibility remained.[8] In the past 30 years, the consumer movement has advanced as public education levels have increased, awareness of the power differential has grown, the dangers of medical technology have become amplified, and a general distrust of experts become apparent.[9] With an emphasis on individual rights to full participation in decision-making about care, the public is no longer blind to the coercive dimension of psychiatry. Yet, this has not eased the stigma of mental illness, nor has consumer participation become widespread.

As we enter the age of *post-psychiatry*, the limits of psychiatry and anti-psychiatry will be clarified and the voices of consumers and carers will take centre stage.[8] Less optimistic views assert that the priority for cost containment, expressed through managed care in the United States, threatens progress and is destroying both the medical and mental health care system. Speaking for the *National Coalition of Mental Health Professionals and Consumers*, Karen Shore stated:

> Managed care deprives citizens of three basic rights: the right to choice, the right to privacy, and the right to make their own treatment decisions. Clinicians and hospitals are chosen and retained if they make a profit for the managed care company, not because of their skill, training, or ethics.[10]

Where do mental health nurses stand in this climate? I believe that the basic tenets of nursing will take on increasing importance as health care becomes even more focused on 'magic bullets' and quick fix solutions. As caring practices are replaced by business solutions, the cry for humanistic connection becomes louder. The way forward in mental health nursing will require joining forces with consumers to embrace in a new way, a genuine way, the true spirit of collaboration that our profession has been founded on.

I agree with Shanley[11] who pointed out that both consumers and mental health nurses have much in common in terms of their powerlessness and sense of being undervalued. This commonality creates an opportunity for building collaborative links to influence delivery of care. He warned that both mental health nurses and consumers need to take risks – individually and collectively – to deal with entrenched views and to give up the safety and security of the medical model. While the call for political activism is vital in Shanley's view, my aim is slightly less ambitious. A revitalization of old nursing ideals taken up with courage, conviction, and pride will go a long way toward fuelling the bigger agenda. If a stated goal of nursing is to enable people to recover and make their own choices, then let's do it. Let's relinquish the paradigm of control and dominance that, in theory, has never belonged to nursing. Let's go with the Flo!

THE PRINCIPLES OF COLLABORATION

Models of collaborative mental health nursing based on equity and empowerment have proliferated over the years. As Peplau claimed, the nurse–patient relationship was the crux of psychiatric nursing and led to mutual growth promotion.[12] Kendell's nursing system embraced the need for emancipatory nursing strategies, to improve health through liberation from oppression, and to increase empowerment.[13] She argued that nursing was an arm of oppression with its purpose to maintain the current system of inequity. She believed that nurses should help oppressed people fight back against social systems and political groups that keep them down. The nursing care partnership model[14] also challenged the dominance of psychiatry and presupposed that a reciprocal and chosen partnership would increase the quality and safety of life. The nurse client alliance model[15] emphasized that it is critical that the nurse move between closeness and keeping distance, giving support and presenting challenges. Empowerment as a goal was a means to lessen the powerlessness, helplessness, subordination, and loss of control of clients.[16]

Indeed these models point to the inextricable linkage of empowerment, as facilitated through partnership, collaboration, participation, the nurse–patient relationship and alliance, to health. Empowerment refers to both a process of being in charge of one's own life and a goal of gaining authenticity and autonomy. This occurs by recognizing and promoting the potential, abilities, and competencies of the person to meet their own needs, solve problems, and mobilize resources to control their own lives. Or, as Barker and Ritter[17] suggest, the word enabling [people to do for themselves] can replace empowerment as more practical concept

Yet the goal of empowerment, involving equity and autonomy, is somewhat contradictory in the mainstream mental health system where one person holds power over the other – and is paid to do so. As consumers point out, 'The very unequal power relationships between the two groups [consumers and staff], the history of paternalism; the 'reserve powers' which our society gives to professionals to withhold liberty, to forcibly inject; etc. all militate against the development of relationships which can truly be described as *partnership*'.[18]

Regardless of current health care arrangements, bureaucratic restrictions, hierarchical structures, or dominance of the medical model, there is much that a nurse can do in his or her everyday practice to work collaboratively within consumers toward improving relationships and outcomes. However, the conditions for promoting empowerment are reliant on the nurses' attitude toward the person.

ENGAGEMENT AND POSITIVE CONNECTEDNESS

The quality of the relationship between nurse and consumer – and their support – network influences the success of collaboration. The nurse who listens, observes, investigates and conveys interest, concern, and understanding, will maximize the likelihood that the consumer will engage collaboratively. Nightingale tells us that it is only through engagement that ways to maintain or bring back health for the person can be discovered:

> Pathology teaches the harm that disease has done. But it teaches nothing more. We know nothing of the principle of health ... except from observation and experience [of the person].[19]

Engagement on the part of the nurse means giving full attention:

> All hurry of bustle is peculiarly painful to the sick ...
> Always sit down when a sick person is talking business to you, show no signs of hurry, give complete attention and full consideration if your advice is wanted.[19]

Obstacles to engagement include failure to find a common ground or connection. This could include unwillingness – of either the nurse or consumer – to open up, explore, identify, and pursue a shared goal. Even if the person is severely compromised and unable to participate in their care, the nurse, through a sense of shared humanity, will always find a way to connect even if it is through a smile, gentle touch, or an attempt to provide comfort.

Connectedness is about shared humanity. Although

we may all be different, we are more alike than unlike. Nightingale talks about this as an empathetic understanding of the patient as drawn from the nurses own experience. Putting yourself in the place of the other is an ethical demand of nursing. Consider, as Nightingale says, 'what it must be like for patients to see the same walls, ceiling, and surroundings during confinement'[19] or to a person with a mental illness what it might be like to be frightened, disoriented, or misunderstood. 'Find out the fancies of patients', says Nightingale, 'they are the most valuable indications of what is necessary for their recovery'.[19]

Positive connectivity develops progressively, beginning with the patient, or even the nurse, expressing vulnerability. The nurse might say: 'I am not sure how to help, perhaps you can tell me'. Or, 'I too was frightened by that, what can we learn about it?' As an aside, too many incidences of aggression and violence go unexplored collaboratively. It is unacceptable to merely remove the nurse and medicate the patient – which often is the response. At some point the opportunity arises to learn from each other about what has happened, and how each responded, such as: 'you said, I felt, you did, I became scared, you reacted'. This helps to build mutual understanding and competency.

When the nurse addresses the person as a fellow human, further disclosure is encouraged. Despite the literature that cautions against disclosure, emphasizing the need to avoid burdening the person being cared for, certain types of disclosure can help to create a meaningful bond that fosters collaboration. Providing opportunities for the consumer to be involved and take responsibility results in a mutual investment with mutual risk-taking and trust. The more each person in the relationship feels valued the more each person will invest in collaboration.

Reciprocity and trust

Nightingale acknowledged the importance of reciprocity when she said:

> I do not say don't tell them of your anxieties – I believe it is good for him and good for you too. But if you tell him what is anxious, surely you can remember to tell him what is pleasant too. A sick person does enjoy hearing good news.[19]

This statement highlights the reciprocal nature of nursing that can benefit all involved. Nightingale went on to explain that genuineness and truth go hand in hand:

> I would appeal to all attendants of the sick to leave off this practice of attempting to cheer up the sick by making light of their danger and by exaggerating their probabilities of recovery. No mockery in the world is so hollow as the advice showered upon the sick.[19]

Realistic, authentic, communication fosters trust and enhances collaboration. Nightingale pointed out the consequences when not being trustworthy:

> Always tell a patient and tell him beforehand when you are going out and when you will be back, whether it be for a day, an hour or ten minutes … If you go without his knowing it, and he finds it out, he will never feel secure again that the things that depend upon you will be done when you're away, and in 9 out of 10 cases he will be right. If you go without telling him when you will be back, he can take no measures nor precautions as to the things which concern you both, or which you do for him.

Well over a century later, studies continue to reaffirm Flo's observations. For example, Repper, Ford and Cooke[20] found that four strategies applied by community nurses contributed to trust building in order to engage patients in their own care. They are:

1 realism;
2 taking the long-term perspective;
3 client-centred flexibility; and
4 positive empathetic understanding of the client.

Thorne and Robinson[1] argue that reciprocal trust is a necessary component of satisfying effective health care relationships. From the consumer's perspective, reciprocal trust has a significant impact on the experience of receiving health care and on the development of competency to deal with illness. Being trusted by one's health care professional is described as an affirming and validating phenomenon; one which promotes self-esteem and fortifies the health care relationship.

Consumers outline ways that they attempt to reduce the status differential between themselves and their health care professional. They report using gift-giving, inquiring about the professional's health and family life, joking, expressing concern for the professional's work conditions, and rationalizing errors as strategies aimed at humanizing their health care encounters.[1]

Professionals however do not always understand nor care about the patient perspective. Instead, they often base their decisions upon a set of values distinct from and contradictory to the patient's own.[1] Resistance to building reciprocal trust with patients may be found in the balance of power. Social distance between patients and providers has serviced as a mechanism for preserving authority. Reciprocity therefore poses a threat to the power afforded professionals who gain their identity and self-esteem through their position.[1] This may be particularly true for nurses who already feel powerlessness to have the edge on a group with even less power. In addition, reciprocity engenders fear that familiarity might breed excessive demands on the part of consumers.[21] Thus, the notion of reciprocal relationships in mental health challenge the accepted social order by magnifying the insecurity of health care professionals who feel that the need for their service is greater than anything that they are capable of providing.[1]

Advocacy and joining forces

The nurse as an advocate has arisen from the need for people in states of compromised health or vulnerability to be protected, not only from the experience of illness, but more significantly from the conditions and institutional processes that claim to care and cure.[22] Advocacy was the main agenda of Nightingale in her outspoken views that patients had 'The right to sewage, clean air and water'. Peplau too[23] claimed that the primary responsibility of nurses is advocacy for patients, consideration of their needs, and an interest in the person as having dignity and worth. When the nurse works collaboratively with the consumer, he or she will take notice and be solicited to respond when both the obvious and less obvious violations to the person and their care plan are being undermined. Horsfall[24] specified further that the nurse is obliged to prevent human rights abuse or neglect and support consumers' access to the least restrictive environment. Advocacy occurs on both an individual and collective level.

On the individual level every mental health nurse is responsible, regardless of the setting, for ensuring that consumers are informed about their rights, diagnosis, medications, treatment options. They need to understand the information and be supported in their choices.

On a broader level mental health nurses have advocacy responsibilities that include: developing, implementing and evaluating policies to prevent consumer right infringements; monitoring mental health settings vis-à-vis consumer rights neglect or abuse; speaking out to maintain safe work conditions;[24] and questioning service providers who use stereotypes or diagnostic labels rather than individual assessments to refer to people.[25] While some of these responsibilities require additional personal confidence and support, it is clear that there is a range of advocacy issues that will only be accomplished through the collective collaboration to influence the political will.

The following issues identified by consumers require retraining and restructuring of attitudes and systems:[24]

❑ access to 24 hour crisis care;
❑ escape from stigma by professionals, lawyers, and the public;
❑ good quality community services;
❑ choice of case manager;
❑ access to advocacy resources in all settings including complaint procedures;

❑ real support and treatment options to choose from;
❑ feedback opportunities regarding service policies;
❑ access and choice of affordable housing;
❑ vocational rehabilitation choices and employment opportunities.

As Horsfall pointed out, these issues can only be accomplished through collaboration with consumers, other health professionals, community development organizations, social justice groups, health policy makers and administrators. This is a wider political agenda yet, as Champ[24] suggested, understanding the concerns of consumer activists can provide nurses with valuable insights and questions about the social, cultural, and political contexts in which nurses practise. In return, consumer activists can become strong allies for nurses, supporting their own concerns about ensuring quality services, equity of access, and adequate funding.

Here I shall describe several collaborative initiatives with which I have been involved and found rewarding. I end with a summary of practical suggestions and tips for collaboration.

THERAPEUTIC COLLABORATION

I have long been influenced by an early experience in therapeutic collaboration. The idea of 'being with' not 'doing to' was concretized during my volunteer work at *Soteria House*, a residential treatment programme for people experiencing psychosis of schizophrenia in San Jose, California. The growth model of anti-psychiatry and the therapeutic community guided the philosophy of care.[26] Treatment consisted entirely of person-to-person interaction based on acceptance, respect, tolerance, commitment, and a positive expectation of recovery. No medications were used or hierarchical structures imposed. I learned a great deal from the residents. They taught me how human touch, involvement, concern, hope, comfort and understanding had a powerful impact on their experience of health and healing. I witnessed many occasions of improvement and recovery.

More specifically, collaborative involvement at Soteria required a redefinition of disease, roles, and expectations. The degenerative incurable illness of schizophrenia was redefined as a development crisis. Staff were non-professional helpers. Therapists were not therapists or expert fixers, but also helpers. No-one possessed any specific power or authority over others. Helpers communicated to the residents that much could be learned from one's experience of psychosis. Thus the labelling, invalidating, hiding away from the community, expectations that pills could mask pain and suffering, and 'doing to' people was all eliminated.[26] An egalitarian, fraternal, and communal residence was developed, where helper tasks were principally defined by the needs of the residents themselves. Helpers had lots of time and used it to aid residents in identifying, experiencing, and dealing with life problems. The motto 'just don't do something, stand there' captures the type of collaboration I learned about.

Interestingly during my time at Soteria, one resident, Bob, was transferred from the Veterans' Hospital where I also worked. After a period of regression – likely caused by the absence of the structure and institutional rules, he began to make some dramatic changes. At Soteria I was no longer his nurse but a helping friend. As he improved we set out for a goal of going to a jazz club on a date, as he hadn't been well enough to be in public in over 8 years. I will never forget the evening. We interacted like long lost pals going out for food and music. He saddled up to the bar, drank coke and entered conversations with others about his military experiences. I had never heard these stories as he had been in a medicated stupor for years. Reminiscent of Oliver Sacks book, *Awakenings*, the funding for the Soteria project was cut, Bob went back to the Veterans' Hospital and to this day he remains locked in a secure ward, gesturing and mumbling under a cloud of anti-psychotic drugs.

This experience changed me forever. The idea that patients possess personal wisdom that if listened to or noticed teaches us how to guide their care has been a driving force of my practice. In my pioneering (late 1970s) work with Vietnam Veterans suffering the effects of war stress, it was the Veterans themselves who taught us how to develop ways to be helpful so that they might reintegrate their experiences in meaningful ways.

Mental health nursing is about being respectful, taking notice, and not rushing in with a set of pre-determined protocols. This approach guards against iatrogenic outcomes, such as those that can be witnessed from current day psychological debriefing practices. The widespread assumption that traumatic events lead to persistent long-term negative psychological consequences can create a self-fulfilling prophecy and undermine people's natural restorative processes. To suggest that people will be worse off as a result of trauma is to shortchange them from the possible strengths, capacities, and growth that can be discovered. A mental health nursing approach based on salutogenesis (that which fosters health and wellness) rather than the pathogenic (that which fosters disease or pathology) is firmly derived from this paradigm of nursing.

RESEARCH COLLABORATION

Many years ago a consumer approached me to help conduct a training course for other consumers to become research interviewers of their peers. As I dug through my resources in preparation, I came across a basic text on communication and interviewing skills for beginning nurses. That became our starting point. What evolved over the course of seminars and workshops was a most thrilling experience. Having taught nursing for many years, my seasoned class of consumers knew much about nursing and possessed the most superb interviewing skills already. Of course, they had experienced more interviews than most people in a lifetime. As it turned out, I had very little to offer. Their astute sensitivity, timing of questions, reflective interest, wisdom about the hierarchical politics that unfold in interviews and overall knowledge of pitfalls and safety nets in interview situations was stunning. The data uncovered by the consumers in the actual project revealed much more than had been previously obtained in any other project. My respect and humility became intensified.

EDUCATIONAL COLLABORATION

My belief that some of the best teachers of nurses are those who have been nursed[24] is the focus of my current work in undergraduate education. I have developed a programme aimed to enable students to learn from consumers about mental health and illness through adventure-based outdoor activities. The project uses a collaborative education model that underpins the teaching and learning approach. A pilot of the project occurred in 2001. Forty mental health consumers and 80 third-year undergraduate nursing students participated in a two-day outdoor educational camp entitled: '*Inside Out: Adventures in Mental Health Nursing*'. Together they explored issues of mental health and illness through experiential and perceived high-risk challenges. The following outcomes were reported:

❑ Reduction of stigma as consumers and students came to know, trust, and count on each other in order to succeed in the adventure challenges.
❑ Increased self-esteem, self-efficacy, and overall sense of well-being as consumers and students confronted and worked through personal and professional mental health issues.
❑ A shift in student beliefs and attitudes toward people with mental health problems as evidenced by subsequent student clinical work and the resultant 200% increase in the number of students selecting to enter mental health nursing.
❑ Increased confidence and competency of consumers as active participants and teachers of nurses as evidenced by subsequent personal and work choices.

These statements capture the common responses:

Nurses: 'I discovered that underneath all mental illness, we are all human … strip away the illnesses, find a common theme, anything that you may share as interest with a client, then communication will be easy'.

'My views about mental illness definitely changed, I was surprised at just how 'normal' the consumers were. This experience definitely broke down the stereotypes of mental health and the negative feelings I had about mental health. I learned something about myself too'.

'I can't believe the trust that people developed in a one hour activity, the openness of consumers and what people can achieve with support and how much encouragement helps.'

Consumers: 'I gained extra confidence in myself and through gaining the ability and confidence to open up and talk to others'.

'The mental and physical challenges made me feel more positive about my own life and I realized just how influential stress and negative thoughts, words, actions can effect well-being'. 'It was great to have the shoe on the other foot. Here I was teaching the same kinds of people who used to put me in seclusion.'

Many consumers have subsequently organized camping trips, other socializing events, and have expressed interest in further involvement in teaching students. The students who participated spread the word to those who did not attend. The result is that a great number of the students have selected to enter mental health nursing. This is an unprecedented result as previously, mental health nursing was rarely considered to be an attractive career option for nurses.

These results could not have been achieved as quickly or powerfully in clinical or academic settings. The naturalistic environment removed institutional barriers and expectations by creating a novel and level playing field. The experiential approach challenged all participants equally, enabling mutual recognition and commonality. The activities were geared for challenge, success, and fun thereby promoting teamwork, trust-building, problem-solving, competency, and well-being. In combination, these conditions created a powerful learning experience that had immediate, longer-term, and possibly sustaining effects. The components essential to the success of the programme included the collaborative education model and the adventure approach.

In 2002, the expanded programme will include an overnight stay. In addition, consumers who participated in the inaugural camp will team up with educators to provide spot lectures and targeted activities. Besides the two full day adventure camp, one full day and two half days have been reserved at the University for a consumer driven seminar series. For example, a lecturer will give one half of a presentation, with theoretical information about mental illness or psychotropic medications. The other half will be given by a consumer who will bring the material to life by providing an inside story. I am certain that undergraduate nurses will long remember this seminar series with practical understanding.

TIPS FOR DEVELOPING 'COLLABORATION'

Various principles, issues and examples of specific collaborative initiatives were illustrated above. By now you may be wondering how you can make the rewards of collaboration part of your everyday practice. The following outline recaps things that have already been discussed and offers additional ways and means as suggested by consumers.

❑ Pay attention to the interpersonal aspects of relating that foster collaboration (engagement, connectedness, trust, reciprocity, respect, advocacy).
❑ Take care of your own personal baggage that might interfere with collaboration.
❑ Take care of your work stress and pick up your attitude.
❑ Get feedback – consumers will tell you in what ways you are helpful and not so helpful.
❑ Empower yourself – claim your practice, be confident, clear and proud of what you do.
❑ Create situations that increase contact between staff and patients.
❑ Engage in fun activities – sing, dance, play music, tell jokes etc.
❑ Use experiential metaphors to highlight therapeutic issues – go through an obstacle course and think of how it reminds you of life's challenges.
❑ Consider together how a mental health nurse can be likened to a tour guide.[27]
❑ Read books and/or watch movies together and critique.
❑ Write letters 'to the editor' together, respond to nursing journal articles.
❑ Create your own support network.
❑ Assert some control over your working environment – pick flowers together and beautify the environment.
❑ Engage in political activity.
❑ Maintain an emphasis on empowering the environments and structures where individuals can grow.
❑ Hold community meetings and identify collaborative projects, i.e. plant a garden.
❑ Create opportunities for clients to become more involved in self-help initiatives.

- ❑ Surf the net together to find information and support resources.
- ❑ Create a resource file or index card with local resources, hotline numbers.
- ❑ Create your own web page together.
- ❑ Providing support and training for consumer participation.[28]
- ❑ Allow patients to contribute to the clinical records – have them provide documentation regarding their progress.
- ❑ Have consumers generate criteria for employment opportunities.
- ❑ Invite consumers to participate in employment interview panels.
- ❑ Involve consumers in staff performance management reviews.[28]
- ❑ Invite consumers to provide inservices on medications, illness experiences etc.
- ❑ Include consumers to participate in staff education sessions – for example while teaching staff about cognitive-behavioural therapy conduct the sessions on the ward with the patients – *in vivo* presentations.
- ❑ Facilitate consumer friendly meetings.[28]
- ❑ Participate in a research project together such as count how many cups of coffee are consumed each day, replace standard coffee with decaffeinated, observe the results.
- ❑ Attend consumer meetings together.
- ❑ Become a consumer advocate by serving on a board of directors for a consumer group.
- ❑ Put the shoe on the other foot, participate in a role reversal session with a consumer.
- ❑ Play the Lemon Looning game with consumers – a board game like monopoly where each station on the board invites participants to experience the life of a consumer, i.e. lose your weekend pass, get extra medications, get detained.

Ideas for collaboration are limitless. Working together can make your work and the consumer's work less stressful, more exciting, and more rewarding. Be creative and most of all, have fun. The future of mental health may well rest on the nature and quality of forming successful collaborative relationships with consumers.

As Champ said:

> Increasingly nurses will find themselves working along side consumer representatives, advocates, and consultants on committees and boards of government Health regions and services are now encouraged to budget for consumer participation and involvement. In some services consumer workers coordinate consumer issues and initiatives, ensuring that consumers' perspectives are included in all aspects of the functioning of the service. This includes everything from including budgetary concerns to ensuring consumer satisfaction with outcomes.[24]

Mental health nursing today requires strong voices, being in the world courageously and convincingly and conveying a new proclamation for reform in the personal, public, political, and social spheres.[29] Calls for health care and system reform are just as worldwide today as they were in Nightingale's time. These are calls for you to recapture the foundational principles of our profession to deal with social, political, and even scientific injustice. These are calls to counterbalance scientific know-how and quick fixes with informed comfort and care measures. As Nightingale emphasized, be concerned with the quality of life. Attend to the aesthetics of your surroundings – light, colour, air, space, and nature. Create healing environments where the patient is an active and reactive participant in his or her own care rather than as a passive recipient. Be concerned with relationships and unity and wholeness. Jean Watson[29] echoed Nightingale, the contexts for all of these approaches are basic public health issues that are humanitarian as well as scientific and political. Nightingale's thinking calls for collaboration between nurses and consumers as a mandate for health.

REFERENCES

1. Thorne SE, Robinson CA. Reciprocal trust in health care relationships. *Journal of Advanced Nursing* 1988; **13**: 782–9.

2. Keltner N, Schwecke L, Bostrom C. *Psychiatric nursing: a psychotherapeutic management approach.* St Louis: Mosby, 1991.

3. Frank KP. *The anti-psychiatry bibliography and resource guide.* Vancouver: Press Gang, 1979.

4. Shrives L. *Basic concepts of psychiatric-mental health nursing*, 4th edn. Philadelphia: Lippincott, 1998.

5. Laing R. *The divided self: an existential study in sanity and madness.* Baltimore: Penguin Books, 1965.

6. Goffman E. *Asylums: essays on the social situation of mental patients.* New York: Double Day/Anchor, 1961.

7. Szasz T. *The myth of mental illness.* New York: Harper and Row, 1961.

8. Bracen P, Thomas P. Postpsychiatry: a new direction. *British Medical Journal* 2001; **322**: 724–7.

9. Pellergrino E, Thomasma D. *For the patients' good.* New York: Oxford University Press, 1988.

10. Shore K. The issues facing ethical mental health care. Address at the Nurses' March on Washington Capitol Building. *The National Coalition of Mental Health Professionals and Consumers*, http:www.the nationalcoalition.org/march.html 1996.

11. Shanley E. Common experiences of mental health

nurses and consumers: ingredients of a symbiotic relationship? *Australian and New Zealand Journal of Mental Health Nursing* 2001; **10**(4): 243–52.

12. Peplau H. In: O'Toole A, Welt S (eds). *Interpersonal theory in nursing practice. Selected works of Hildegard Peplau*. New York: Springer, 1989.

13. Kendell J. Fighting back: promoting emancipatory nursing actions. *Advances in Nursing Science* 1992; **15**(2): 1–15.

14. Schroeder C, Maeve M. Nursing care partnerships at the Denver nursing project in human caring: an application and extension of caring theory in practice. *Advances in Nursing Science* 1992; **15**(2): 25–8.

15. Hummelvoll JK. The nurse–client alliance model. *Perspectives in Psychiatric Care* 1996; **32**(4): 12–20.

16. Jones P, Meleis A. Health is empowerment. *Advances in Nursing Science* 1993; **15**(3): 1–14.

17. Barker P, Ritter S. Commentary. *Journal of Psychiatric and Mental Health Nursing* 1996; **3**: 141–4.

18. Victorian Mental Illness Awareness Council. *Developing effective consumer participation in mental health services: The report of the lemon tree learning project.* 1997: 5–6.

19. Nightingale F. *Notes on nursing: what it is, and what it is not.* Commemorative edition. Philadelphia: JB Lippincott, 1992.

20. Repper J, Ford R, Cooke A. How can nurses build trusting relationships with people who have severe and long-term mental health problems? Experience of case managers and their clients. *Journal of Advanced Nursing* 1994; **19**: 1096–101.

21. Lazare A, Eisenthal S, Frank A, Stoeckle JD. Studies on a negotiated approach to patienthood. In: Gallagher EB (ed.) *The doctor–patient relationship in the changing health care scene.* Washington DC: United States Department of Health, Education and Welfare, 1976: 119–39.

22. Curtin LL. The nurse as an advocate: a philosophical foundation for nursing. *Advances in Nursing Science* 1979; **1**(3): 1–10.

23. Peplau H. Another look at schizophrenia from a nursing standpoint. In: Anderson C (ed.) *Psychiatric nursing 1974–1994: a report on the state of the art.* St Louis: Mosby, 1995.

24. Horsfall J, Stuhlmiller C, with Champ S. *Interpersonal nursing for mental health.* Sydney: MacLennan and Petty, 2001.

25. Keglovits J, Meder M. Advocacy, clients rights, and legal issues. In: Wilson H, Kneisl C (eds). *Psychiatric nursing*, 5th edn. Menlo Park: Addison-Wesley, 1996: 208.

26. Mosher LR, Menn A. Community residential treatment for schizophrenia: two-year follow-up. *Hospital and Community Psychiatry* 1978; **29**(11): 715–23.

27. McAllister M. Conquistadors and ruins: metaphors for a post positivist world. *The Australian Electronic Journal of Nursing Education* 2000; **5**(2): 1–17.

28. Connor H. Collaboration or chaos: a consumer perspective. *Australian and New Zealand Journal of Mental Health Nursing* 1999; **8**(3): 79–86.

29. Watson J. Notes on nursing: guidelines for then and now. In: Nightingale F. *Notes on nursing.* Commemorative edition. Philadelphia: J.B. Lippincott, 1992: 80–5.

Chapter 67

BUILDING PRACTICE FROM RESEARCH

Mark Fenton*

> So far as the laws of mathematics refer to reality, they are not certain. And so far as they are certain, they do not refer to reality.
>
> Albert Einstein, *Geometry and Experience*[1]

INTRODUCTION

This chapter skims the surface of how research can help inform practice. There are obvious gaps in the areas it covers, the main one being the omission of use of qualitative research to inform clinical practice. While I acknowledge this gap from the beginning, I also add a caveat: the problems I outline in using quantitative research to inform practice, also exist for the use of qualitative research. However, there is one other, important, reason for focusing on the quantitative dimension of health care research: this is a key contributor to the development of evidence-based health care and, as such, raises critical issues concerning the evidence-base that might be necessary for the future development of psychiatric-mental health nursing. The kind of research – and its attendant problems – that is addressed here, is the kind of research that has the most direct application to the development of the 'evidence base' of mental health care.

The process of inquiry

Research provides information that we cannot get from other sources; such as personal and technical experience; the opinion of respected peers, or well-designed guidelines. Some interventions we make as mental health nurses may not need research; situations that fall under national legislation, like mental health laws to detain or treat people against their will; or when the evidence is so overwhelming that research is unnecessary, like being the other side of a solid door when someone is prone to hitting out at the nearest person to them. However, there are times when we do not know what would be the best way to help somebody, or the research is conflicting.

Imagine that you are a recently qualified nurse, working on an acute admissions ward, based in the grounds of the local District General Hospital, which provides an out of hours assessment service for people following a self harm attempt. As you become more experienced, you will eventually be asked to go across and assess someone. Knowing that you will be faced with this very real problem of assessing someone who has recently survived a self-harm attempt, you decide to do some preparation in learning how *best* to treat someone, to prevent reoccurrence or repetition of self-harm. The responsibility lies with you to provide a thorough assess-

---

*Mark Fenton trained as a psychiatric nurse in Salford, UK, and after working in various parts of the country, eventually undertook a psychodynamic training. After family changes necessitated further moves, he has ended up working in the epidemiology of research into the care of those with schizophrenia.

ment, a plan of treatment and to deliver and evaluate that care. You vaguely remember from a lecture that the use of a cognitive-behavioural approach was effective in reducing repetition in attempts at self-harm, so you look in your notes from your lecture and take out the book that was recommended reading.[2] The chapter recommends using cognitive-behavioural therapy as a means to prevent repetition.

Being the diligent practitioner you are though, you also look around for further information and search the Cochrane Library for a systematic review and come across one which includes one of the authors of the chapter in the book.[2,3] In the systematic review, the author's conclusion is:

> There still remains considerable uncertainty about which forms of psycho-social and physical treatments of self-harm patients are most effective, inclusion of insufficient numbers of patients in trials being the main limiting factor. There is a need for larger trials of treatments associated with trends towards reduced rates of repetition of deliberate self-harm. The results of small single trials which have been associated with statistically significant reductions in repetition must be interpreted with caution and it is desirable that such trials are also replicated.[3]

Now, you experience the classic 'conflict of information' for which research is famous. One source says to use cognitive-behavioural therapy, while the more recent report says that there is considerable uncertainty and more research is needed. How do you make sense of this?

Here, I shall outline how you might appraise research to inform your clinical practice, looking specifically at factors that might reassure you that the results are reliable.

RESEARCH

Research comes in many different forms and flavours, with two main groupings based on qualitative and quantitative research methodologies. This chapter will focus mainly upon the use of quantitative research, but all the problems identified are applicable to using qualitative research.

The main difference between qualitative and quantitative research is the end result, with quantitative research having a numerical answer (how many people got better using Therapy A versus Therapy B), and qualitative research giving a synthesis of observations of the topic, for example, behaviour. However, this is only a general rule. The qualitative researcher may also have used quantitative methods to arrive at their outcome, and as is more increasingly common, quantitative research also gives a description of observed behaviours or outlines a belief system. To engage in a polemical argument about not being able to reduce people to num-

bers, and not being able to come to any conclusion about the outcome in qualitative research is to misunderstand that they are both quite different tools used to do different jobs. For example, to answer the question 'What are my chances of getting rid of the voices taking drug A versus no drug or drug B?' needs research using quantitative methods, whereas to answer the question of what it is like to live with a chronic disease such as schizophrenia, or how to make the best choice when choosing which long-term care home to place a relative needs research using qualitative methods.

Types of quantitative research

Fundamental to quantitative research is comparison between groups or individuals. Three common methods used are cohort studies, case controlled studies or intervention studies, such as the randomized controlled trial (RCT). While the end result will be a numerical one, each methodology serves a very different purpose.

When we use a case–control study to investigate the association between an exposure and an outcome, we start by identifying individuals with the outcome of interest (cases), and compare them to individuals without this outcome (controls). We obtain information about one or more previous exposures from cases and controls, and compare the two groups to see if each exposure is significantly more (or less) frequent in cases than in controls.

The case–control method (in particular, the method of analysis) was developed in the early 1950s as an approach to the problem of investigating risk factors for diseases with long latent periods, where cohort studies are impractical.

An early example of a case–control study was one examining the association between cigarette smoking and lung cancer, published in 1950[4] by Doll and Hill. That study was an example of the use of case–control design to investigate risk factors for a rare disease.[4] Case–control studies are also used to investigate causes of a new disease.

Cohort studies start by measuring exposure to a risk factor of interest. Individuals are classified by their exposure status, and then followed over a period of time to see whether they develop one or more outcomes. Cohort studies are particularly useful for studying rare exposures; studying multiple outcomes, or defining the natural history of disease and the sequence of events.

Intervention studies are similar to cohort studies. In a cohort study, the starting point is the exposure. In an intervention study, however, rather than observing the presence or absence of a 'naturally occurring' exposure, the investigator allocates the exposure (or intervention) to one group within the study population.

The remainder of the subjects, who do not receive the intervention, act as a control group.

This simple outline of three types of methods used in quantitative research highlights the need for comparison, which is fundamental if any claim is made about cause of an outcome, for example A causes C while B does not, or A is better than B. Because comparison has been made with another appropriate group, the comparison demonstrates the outcome is greater or less than a group in similar circumstances.

SYSTEMATIC REVIEWS

There is a fourth type of numerical study that is becoming more frequently used, which is meta-analysis. Meta-analysis occurs when more than one study is found on the same subject and the results combined to give a summative overview. These are often presented in a systematic review.

In 1979, Archie Cochrane, a British epidemiologist, was asked by the Department of Health to look at the quality of practice with the UK National Health Service. He said of medicine:

> ... it is surely a great criticism of the profession that we have not organized a critical summary, by speciality or subspecialty, adapted periodically, of all relevant randomized controlled trials.[5]

Why do we need reviews of treatments?

As mentioned above, the sheer volume of information available and limited time to read makes it impossible to even contemplate keeping up to date with all current research. So it is not unusual to depend on reviews. These may be reviews supplied in a textbook, via a colleague's opinion, a lecture, a review article in a journal, a consensus statement, or a guideline. Reviews often use the results of trials and try and summarize their results in order to provide a time-efficient way of gaining an overview of a particular subject area. Most reviews however are subjective.

Why systematic reviews?

Those who have designed randomized trials have tried to be objective and scientific. If a trial were presented to an academic journal without a 'methods' section the chance of it being taken seriously would be small. Medicine and nursing, however, operate a double standard. On one hand the trial has to be undertaken with scientific rigour, while on the other, the reviews of those trials are often no more than opinion.

Traditional reviews of treatments within health care are often not verifiable and consensus of what constitutes good practice is often based, not on the best, objectively appraised evidence, but on unscientific reviews.[6] These traditional reviews frequently have no methods section whatsoever and do not attempt to describe how data was identified and assimilated. The means by which the conclusions in most reviews were drawn are frequently unclear, subjective and unscientific. In 1987, Mulrow showed that 86% of reviews in major North American general medical journals were opinion, rather than evidence-based.[7]

Traditional reviews of treatment may have results radically different from what the best available, systematically summarized evidence would say. There is no reason why mental health nursing should be any different from any other discipline. By employing basic survey methodology, similar to that described above for evaluating trials, the reviewing process can become more systematic, quantitative and therefore open to interpretation and valid criticism.

What are systematic reviews?

A systematic review has explicit criteria by which relevant data are identified. Often these data are in the form of randomized controlled trials (RCTs). Reviewers would pre-state what participant group was of interest (for example, those with schizophrenia), what intervention was to be the focus of the review (i.e. family intervention vs. standard care) and what outcomes were of interest (e.g. relapse, family burden and cost). There would be a crystal-clear search strategy for these studies so anyone could replicate the findings. Reviewers would explain, before even seeing the trials, how they were to be selected, data extracted and, where possible, summated in a meta-analysis.[9]

As if the need for scientific rigour is not enough there are other advantages to trying to summate data. Most of the time penicillin is a very powerful intervention for uncomplicated bacterial infections and it would not need a large controlled trial to show its clear advantage over placebo. Most of the treatments undertaken by metal health nurses are likely to be less potent, with more subtle effects that need the 'magnifying glass' of a large trial to clarify. Much trial research is underpowered and cannot make any reasonable recommendations about the effectiveness or harm that an intervention may cause.[9] Summating trials where the participants, interventions and outcomes have been similar (meta-analysis) attempts to increase the power of the reviewer to clarify exactly what the effects of treatments are.

Pooling several studies may also allow greater generalizability of results. For example, a mental health nurse may be asked to work within a community mental health team (CMHT) that serves a middle-class rural area. This nurse is unclear as to the efficacy of this type of care and uses CINAHL to identify relevant studies. They find eight citations, none of efficacy, and a systematic review.[11] The other seven citations focus on patterns of referral, the use of zoning, the pressures and rewards of working in a CMHT, the effects of sharing letters with clients, two citations on managing CMHTs and one on a community mental handicap team. The systematic review, however, identifies four studies. One from Australia, Canada, and two from London pooling results from all over the world, many different care cultures and situations. As the individual trial findings were not substantially different from each other, she should feel more reassured as to generalizability of their findings.

As with all research, systematic reviews, with or without meta-analysis, can be poorly undertaken and not pay due attention to the inclusion of biases. Meta-analysis may be undertaken on limited subsets of data and therefore still lack power that would have been available if all trials were combined.[12] Even if all relevant published material is summated, if there is strong publication-bias (where studies with more positive results have a greater chance of being published), the adding up of a one-sided data set can be misleading.[13] Systematic reviews of treatment trials cannot be read uncritically. They may often be the best available evidence of what helps or harms but they should not be a means of scientific tyranny. Their methods and results must be carefully scrutinized, passed through the filter of common sense and clinical experience and then applied.

USING RESEARCH TO INFORM PRACTICE

Can I use single reports of research to inform my practice?

While the simple answer to this question is 'yes', there are some things the reader needs to do at various stages of reading a paper. Research using any methodology is prone to leaving the reader uncertain as to what they should do in response to the research. Often researchers write for other researchers rather than clinicians; using outcomes such as a rating scale that will never see the light of day in a clinical area. There are some quick and easy ways of assessing a paper though to see whether a paper set out to answer a question that is relevant to the reader, using the questions in Tables 67.1–67.5 taken from the Critical Appraisal Skills Programme.[14] However, once deciding that a report is worth reading, the skills to judge whether the results can be viewed as reliable are also required.

The busy clinician does not have available much time to read copious amounts of research to answer a clinical question. Surveys of medical staff find that the time available is less than one hour per week,[8] and there is no reason to think other disciplines have more time than that available to them. There are also over 20,000 biomedical journals published worldwide each year. Given the huge scale of even trying to keep up to date, it becomes obvious that no one person could do so. So having reliable stepping off points, where the reader decides to not continue reading a paper, makes sense.

TABLE 67.1 Questions to ask of a review

- Were the questions and methods clearly stated?
- Were the methods used to find studies comprehensive?
- Were explicit methods used to determine which studies were included?
- Was the methodological quality of the studies assessed?
- Was the selection of studies reproducible and free from bias?
- Were differences in study results adequately explained?
- Were results combined appropriately?
- Were the conclusions supported by the data cited?

Sacket 2000[8]

TABLE 67.2 Are the results of the trial valid?

Screening questions
- Did the trial address a clearly focused issue?
- Is a trial (RCT) an appropriate method to answer this issue?

The two screening questions in Table 67.2 are filters that allow the reader to decide if this study is relevant to answering a question of effectiveness. If the reader cannot answer yes to the above questions, then the research is unable to answer a question about whether an intervention will work. Surveys of research into the care of those with schizophrenia[15] show that much of the research is insufficient to answer most questions about the effectiveness of many interventions. The World Health Organization has also declared that the randomized controlled trial is the gold standard to answer questions of effectiveness in mental health care.[16]

After deciding that the paper might answer a question of effectiveness, the reader should then decide whether the results are valid or not.

Table 67.3 gives five questions the reader should answer to decide if again they can continue to use this study to inform their practice. Chalmers[17] showed that in studies where the assignment of participants can be manipulated, the results of those studies over-estimate positive results by a magnitude of nearly 20%. When the same interventions are assessed in studies with no control, the over-estimation of effect is by approximately 50%.

In a survey of 2000 studies into the care of those with schizophrenia,[15] it is shown that in recent drugs trials, up to 60% of those who began the study left before its completion six weeks later. Do you lose nearly 60% of those you care for in six weeks? An inference which can be drawn from such losses to follow-up is that either these participants bear no resemblance to the people you come into contact with, or the research is doing something so toxic, that what is happening to the study participants is very different to what happens clinically. The potential for results being biased increases when those that leave a study are not accounted for at the end of the trial, as the potential for those that do leave being systematically different to those that stay are high.

It seems logical that we should expect all participants to be treated equally within a study; however, it is not always the case that this is so. For example, Chouinard[18] completed a study into the use of risperidone versus haloperidol. In this study, the risperidone was given at 2, 6, 10 and 16 mg a day, while all those on haloperidol were given a fixed dose of 20 mg of haloperidol. In the conclusions, it is said that risperidone causes less extrapyramidal side-effects than haloperidol, when 30 of the 92 taking risperidone, and 14 of the 21 taking haloperidol experienced these types of side-effects. It is clear

TABLE 67.3 Questions assessing validity of research using randomized controlled methodology

- How were patients assigned to treatment groups?
- Were participants, staff and study personnel 'blind' to treatment?
- Were all of the participants who entered the trial properly accounted for at its conclusion?
- Aside from the experimental intervention were the groups treated in the same way?
- Did the study have enough participants to minimize the play of chance?

TABLE 67.4 What are the results?

- How are the results presented?
- What is the main result?
- How precise are these results?

TABLE 67.5 Will the results help locally?

- Can the results be applied to the local population?
- Were all important outcomes considered?
- Should policy or practice change as a result of the evidence contained in this trial?

though that the dose of haloperidol is much higher than one would expect to see in use in the UK, with no flexibility of dose of the comparator, a drug known to be fairly toxic and a cause of these types of side-effects, especially at high dose. This example also illustrates the question of blinding within studies. A double blind study is where both the person receiving the treatment and the person giving the treatment are blind to which intervention is being given. In the study,[18] the people receiving haloperidol are likely to have received this drug previously, therefore recognizing the side-effects they were experiencing were likely to be caused by the 'old' treatment, thus invalidating the blinding process. It is also likely that the person supervising the participants could take an educated guess as to what treatment the person was being given from the reports of side-effects. What does seem to be important regarding blindness is the independence, or blindness of the person undertaking the evaluation. It may not actually be possible to have any blinding in a study, and is probably impossible when undertaking studies of social interventions.

Prior to undertaking a study, researchers are required to state the hypotheses of their intended study, and identify how they will consider someone to have improved. Using a power calculation derived from the expected effect on those taking an experimental treatment as opposed to its comparator, it is possible to work out how many people need to be included in each arm to demonstrate a statistically significant effect, which would not be expected to be caused by chance alone.

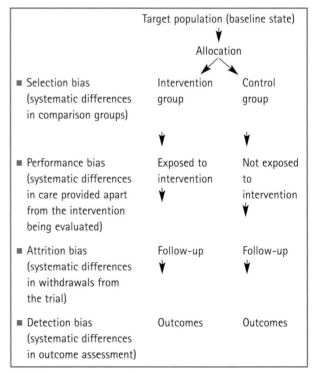

FIGURE 67.1 Sources of bias.

The survey undertaken by Thornley and Adams[15] shows that the average study size undertaken into the care of those with schizophrenia was of 60 people, exactly the same size groups as what is considered the first RCT. This study in 1948 was undertaken to assess the effectiveness of streptomycin, where the outcome was of changes in chest X-ray appearances and mortality in the two groups.[19] It seems we may have dutifully followed the early model of undertaking RCTs, without taking into account the methods may need to change with different outcomes. For example, to demonstrate a difference of 10% between two groups (intervention group vs. control group), using one of the most commonly used rating scales in mental health trials, the Brief Psychiatric Rating Scale[20] that can be said to be statistically significant, and not down to chance alone, needs 150 people in each arm of the study (300 total).

Figure 67.1 summarizes the potential areas of concern when assessing whether the results of a study are valid or may be biased. Bias refers to any error in the design or conduct of a study that results in a conclusion, which is different from the truth. There are many potential sources of error in research, often referred to as bias. The main areas where bias can creep in are: selection, performance, attrition and detection bias. A biased study is one that does not give a true representation of the situation we want to describe or the association we want to analyse.

As mentioned above, a common outcome in trials into the care of those with schizophrenia is the BPRS. As the reader of those trials, how would you expect to see the results presented?

When you see two graphs, what do you think when you see a line steadily increasing or decreasing to the right? Many times when reading a study, it is not uncommon to find that is exactly the result. A graph with no meaningful data attached to it (i.e. numbers of people who experienced either a good or bad event), and a line increasing or decreasing, depending on the outcome, with the graph increasing for good outcomes, and decreasing for bad.

This is a useful result if you want to know how to get a line to go up or down, but fairly meaningless when faced with a person who wants to know if the treatment you are initiating or recommending is going to help them. You may read something, which says in the abstract, it works. In fact, in very few studies I have read do they say anything other than 'it works'. So much so, that you would think everything works, yet clinically, we realize there is a gap between what people say works and what does work in practice.

Not everyone gets better. The use of rating scales to evaluate an outcome is more common than seeing an outcome such as getting on with daily activities or not getting into trouble in close relationships. A way to answer the question of 'what is the main result?' is to identify what has been measured. If it's mental state using a rating scale, it is unlikely to be useful in telling you anything clinically.

We then need to ask how precise these results are. In doing so, the reader needs to know that the researchers took every care in avoiding either hidden or overt bias of detection. Marshall[21] undertook a study into the use of unpublished rating scales, and found that researchers who use a scale that has never been published find positive results, which do not seem replicated after the rating scale is published and peer reviewed. The only thing being different is the scale is published. You the reader have to decide whether a result is useful for informing your practice.

As the majority of us do not use rating scales in our clinical practice, it can be argued that they do little to inform the reader of the ability of an intervention to make a difference.

In asking can results be applied locally, the reader needs to know that the participants in the study are similar to those they are working with. In a meta-meta review of the use of depot medication,[22] which reported on nine systematic reviews into all drugs licensed in the UK for the use as maintenance depot medication for those with schizophrenia, a conclusion the authors came to was that the research had not been undertaken in people who are unwilling or unable to take medication on a regular basis, but on people who seemed to be stable in their illnesses, and compliant with treatment, and willing to undertake research.

So for all the research undertaken into the use of depot medication, it does not say whether it is a useful tool in people who are unable or unwilling to take medication, the very people it will be used for.

Tollefson[23] reports the largest recent study undertaken in people with schizophrenia, using a drug called olanzapine. A total of 1996 people started the study. For a side-effect to be reported in the study report,[23] at least 10% of those entering the study had to experience the side-effect. Using this method of reporting, rare but important side-effects potentially do not get reported.

It is important also to consider that the trialists consider all possible confounders. For example, if you were to look at research into the number of coffee drinkers who also experience cancer, you could find a positive association. If, however, the researchers failed to ask if the coffee drinker was also a smoker, an important confounder would be missed (lots of coffee drinkers are also smokers). This was the case when early research was undertaken into the possible causes of HIV infection in males. Early on, the association was made between the use of amyl-nitrates, or poppers, and HIV infection. The use of poppers was a confounder in this instance, as the amyl-nitrate was used by males to relax the anal sphincter in anticipation of sexual intercourse, among other things.

When asking should policy or practice change, it is useful to remember the difference between statistical, and clinical significance:

> … Researchers and readers of research often focus excessively on whether a result is statistically significant (i.e. not likely the result of chance). However, just because a test shows a treatment effect to be statistically significant, it does not mean the result is *clinically* important. For example, if a study is very large (and therefore has a small standard error), it is easier to find small and clinically unimportant treatment effects to be statistically significant. A large randomized controlled trial compared rehospitalizations in patients receiving a new heart drug with patients receiving usual care. A 1% reduction in rehospitalizations was reported in the treatment group (49% rehospitalizations vs. 50% in the usual care group). This was highly statistically significant ($P<0.0001$) mainly because this is a large trial. However, it is unlikely that clinical practice would be changed on the basis of such a small reduction in hospitalization.[24]

CONCLUSION

This chapter has shown that although research can provide answers, there are certain limitations within the methodologies of the research process, which may lead to bias in the conclusions drawn, or which may limit the applicability of research findings and what answers can be given. I have also shown that some research may not be clear in its focus, or designed to answer the question it set out to. I have emphasized the 'quantitative' end of the research spectrum. However, similar problems can and do emerge in qualitative forms of inquiry, albeit influenced by different factors. (For a consideration of the parameters, and problems, of qualitative forms of research, see Leininger,[25] Morse and Field,[26] Holloway and Wheeler,[27] and Stevenson[28].) It is worth remembering, however, that despite its perceived importance, research is just but one of the tools we have at our disposal, when it comes to developing practice.

For example, Thompson and Dowding[29] found that an influential factor upon our practice is the recommendations of respected peers. Others have found that our practice doesn't change much from that we were taught in our training, while others have found that our practice is dictated by what the patient will accept, or the hospital will pay for. This may be all we need.

However, when a detailed look has been undertaken of practices within medicine, many interventions have been found to be ineffective, harmful or in rare circumstances, the cause of death. Is there any reason to suspect that the interventions we undertake in mental health are

any the more effective, less harmful, and on the odd occasion, not killing the people we set out to treat?

You may not be able to answer some questions from research, as the methods used are limited or not designed to answer the question it set out to. However, you still need to navigate your way through the mass of information available. Hopefully, this chapter will give you some guidance in what is going to be helpful, and perhaps more importantly, what is not. Only you can answer the question about how happy you are with the reasons that you undertake certain interventions in a particular way at a particular time. However, on the occasions that you need to reach for the research to inform you, you will find that it is tarnished and as prone to bias as advice from the locals in my pub. There is very little as powerful as something having worked once. Yet it is the tool we have.

REFERENCES

1. Einstein A. *Sidelights on relativity*. London: Methuen, 1922.
2. Hawton K. In: Clark DM, Fairburn CG, Gelder MG. *Science and practice of cognitive behaviour therapy*, Chapter 12. Oxford: Oxford University Press, 1997: 285–313.
3. Hawton K, Townsend E, Arensman E, Gunnell D, Hazell P, House A, van Heeringen K. *Psycho-social and pharmacological treatments for deliberate self harm* (Cochrane Review). The Cochrane Library, Issue 4, 2001. Oxford: Update Software.
4. Doll R, Hill AB. Smoking and carcinoma of the lung: preliminary report. *British Medical Journal* 1950; ii: 739–48.
5. Cochrane AL. 1931–1971: A critical review, with particular reference to the medical profession. In: *Medicines for the year 2000*. London: Office of Health Economics, 1979.
6. Antman EM, Lau J, Kupelnick B, Mosteller F, Chalmers TC. A comparison of results of meta-analysis of randomized controlled trials and recommendations of clinical experts. Treatment for myocardial infarction. *Journal of the American Medical Association* 1992; **268**: 240–8.
7. Mulrow CD. The medical review article: state of the science. *Annals of Internal Medicine* 1987; **106**: 485–8.
8. Sackett DL. Surveys of self-reported reading times of consultants in Oxford, Birmingham, Milton-Keynes, Bristol, Leicester, and Glasgow, 1995. In: Rosenberg WMC, Richardson WS, Haynes RB, Sackett DL. *Evidence-based medicine*. London: Churchill-Livingstone, 2000.

9. Pharoah FM, Mari JJ, Streiner D. *Family intervention for schizophrenia* (Cochrane Review). The Cochrane Library, Issue 4, 2001. Oxford: Update Software.

10. Systematic overview of controlled trials helps clarify treatment effects. *Drug and Therapeutics Bulletin* 1992; **30**: 25–7.

11. Tyrer P, Coid J, Simmonds S, Joseph P, Marriott S. *Community mental health teams (CMHTs) for people with severe mental illnesses and disordered personality* (Cochrane Review). The Cochrane Library, Issue 2, 2002. Oxford: Update Software.

12. Yusuf S, Wittes J, Probstfield J, Tyroler HA. Analysis and interpretation of treatment effects in subgroups of patients in randomized clinical trials. *JAMA* 1991; **266**: 93–8.

13. Hughes MD. The impact of stopping rules on heterogeneity of results in overviews of clinical trials. *Biometrics* 1992; **48**: 41–53.

14. Critical Appraisal Skills Programme http://www.phru.org.uk/~casp/resources/index.htm.

15. Thornley B, Adams CE. Content and quality of 2000 controlled trials in schizophrenia over 50 years. *British Medical Journal* 1998; **317**(7167): 1181–4.

16. WHO Scientific Group on Treatment of Psychiatric Disorders. *Evaluation of methods for the treatment of mental disorders.* WHO: Geneva, 1991.

17. Chalmers I, Hetherington J, Newdick M, *et al.* The Oxford Register of Perinatal Trials: Developing a register of published reports of controlled trials. *Controlled Clinical Trials* 1986; **7**: 306–24.

18. Chouinard G, Jones B, Remington G, *et al.* A Canadian multicenter placebo controlled study of fixed doses of risperidone and haloperidol in the treatment of chronic schizophrenic patients. *Journal of Clinical Psychopharmacology* 1993; **13**: 25–40.

19. Hill AB. The clinical trial. *British Medical Bulletin* 1951; **7**: 278–82.

20. Overall J, Gorham D. The Brief Psychiatric Rating Scale. *Psychological Reports* 1962; **10**: 799–812.

21. Marshall M, Lockwood A, Bradley C, Adams C, Joy C, Fenton M. Unpublished rating scales: a major source of bias in randomised controlled trials of treatments for schizophrenia. *British Journal of Psychiatry* 2000; **176**: 249–52.

22. Adams CE, Fenton MKP, Quraishi S, David AS. A systematic review of depot neuroleptic drugs for people with schizophrenia. *British Journal of Psychiatry* 2001; **179**: 290–9.

23. Tollefson GD, Beasley CM, Tran PV, *et al.* Olanzapine versus haloperidol in the treatment of schizophrenia and schizoaffective and schizophreniform disorders: results of an international collaborative trial. *American Journal of Psychiatry* 1997; **154**: 457–65.

24. Sheldon TA. Estimating treatment effects: real or the result of chance? [Editorial]. *Evidence-Based Nursing* 2000; **3**: 36–9.

25. Leininger MM. *Qualitative research methods in nursing.* London: Grune and Stratton, 1985.

26. More JM, Field PA. *Nursing research: the application of qualitative approaches.* London: Chapman and Hall, 1996.

27. Holloway I, Wheeler S. *Qualitative research for nurses.* Oxford, Blackwell Science, 1996.

28. Stevenson C. Taking the pith out of reality: A reflexive methodology for psychiatric nursing research. *Journal of Psychiatric and Mental Health Nursing* 1996; **3**(2): 103–10.

29. Thompson C, Dowding D. *Clinical decision making and judgment in nursing.* Edinburgh: Baillière Tindall, 2001.

Section 10

The future of psychiatric-mental health nursing in context

Preface to Section 10

Psychiatric and mental health nursing has, traditionally, been a vocation, based on traditional notions of human service. More recently it has aspired to be a profession, with its standards and regulatory bodies for the control and monitoring of 'good practice'. Now it seeks to become a discipline, with its own knowledge base, which although unique might complement and enable the work of other members of the multidisciplinary mental health team.

In this concluding section I invited some colleagues to prepare some forecasts: where did they think nursing would be in the years ahead and what did they think might be important influences on the development of the profession, or the emergence of the discipline.

Needless to say, very different answers emerged to these questions, which may have been a function of the authors themselves or the context within which the authors were viewing the future. All of the forecasts are, however, helpful. They suggest the possible direction of nursing practice but appreciate that forecasts can often be wrong.

Europe, Japan, the USA and Australia and New Zealand were chosen as the settings for these forecasts for the simple reason that each represents a significant social and or cultural base for the development of mental health practice. As the reader will find, although there exists some common human ground, what is deemed to be important for the immediate future of mental health nursing is changeable when crossing continents.

In drawing the book to a close I make an effort to link with the historical introduction in Section 1, with a reflection on the virtue of caring. Of necessity this includes a consideration of how society and the institution of psychiatry, thinks about mental health and ill health, and how the culture of nursing might continue its own unique framing of the *experience* of health and ill health.

Chapter 68

THE EUROPEAN CONTEXT

Seamus Cowman*

INTRODUCTION

In health care Ministries across Europe, the realization is dawning that European Union (EU) law has profound consequences for the organization of health care systems. In some countries there are public and private partnerships and across many countries there are serious concerns being expressed about the availability and level of publicly funded health care systems. Duncan[1] suggests that there is a paradox in European terms in that for years there was pressure from many interest groups for the EU to be 'doing something' about health. Yet health is so high on national political agendas that most governments do not want the EU interfering with it. The EU was given powers to spend money on European level health projects but to date has not passed laws harmonizing public health measures in member states.

The professional role and the scope of practice for all professions have evolved and developed in line with the individual health care policies of each country. A significant factor across countries is professional regulation through various forms of authority. In the majority of member states regulation is conducted through a statutory body in the form of a Nursing Board and in Eastern Europe there is an absence of statutory nursing bodies and such a function is most often undertaken within the Ministry of Health.

Given the diverse circumstances influencing care of the mentally ill, there is much variance in the education and training and role of the psychiatric nurse in Europe. Unlike general nursing there is a lack of specific European Directives governing the education and training of the psychiatric nurse. In the 1970s the introduction of Sectoral Directives for general nursing created a European identity for general nurses and facilitated freedom of movement for general nurses to practice in all European member states including reciprocal recognition of qualifications. The lack of such a system for psychiatric nurses has resulted in them not enjoying the same freedom of movement and right to practice across the health services of European countries. The enlargement in the number of countries in the European Union in recent years has further exacerbated the lack of commonality in the education and training and role of the psychiatric nurse across Europe.

*Seamus Cowman is Professor and Head of Nursing at the Royal College of Surgeons in Dublin, Ireland. As a registered Psychiatric and General Nurse and Nurse Tutor, Seamus has worked across the health services in Ireland and the UK. He was an undergraduate at London University and took his MSc at the University of Surrey before embarking on his PhD at Dublin City University, becoming the first nurse in Ireland to obtain a PhD from an Irish University in 1994.

This chapter will review the significant historical developments as they have influenced the evolution of psychiatric nursing in Europe. The different and changing perspectives on the role of the nurse in Europe will be examined. A prospective view on the role of the nurse in mental health care in the years ahead is presented and the case is made for European agreement on the education and training of the psychiatric nurse and the essential elements that constitute the essence of psychiatric nursing.

HISTORICAL REFLECTIONS

The literature on psychiatric nursing in Western Europe is rich in historical discourse and it provides a strong sense of the role of the nurse as it evolved in the traditional mental hospital setting. In those early days a major element of nursing role involved the enforcement of rules and psychiatric nursing was the cornerstone of service delivery.[2] During the later part of the 20th century there was a major shift in mental health care policy away from institutional care to a more community-based service. Taylor[3] contends that psychiatric nursing was a major health profession when most people with mental illness were cared for in large institutions, and the suggestion is made that the value of psychiatric nursing is now being questioned as the large mental hospitals are closing.

In the past little was known about the practice of psychiatric nursing in Central and Eastern Europe. In recent times there have been major changes and social upheaval in Central and Eastern Europe with social and political revolutions leading to radical changes in health care systems. The resulting greater transparency has focused attention on levels of abuse and misuse of the mental health care systems, including its use to discipline and punish social dissidents.[4] Such was the environment for the practice of psychiatric nursing, which was delivered by individuals, who were lacking specialist education and training, and with an impoverished ability to provide any meaningful therapeutic engagement with clients of the system. The recognition of the importance of mental health nursing as a force in enhancing service delivery led to the WHO Nursing in Action project.[5] Primarily due to the influence of the WHO initiatives a number of Eastern European countries are in the process of radically reforming their education programmes for the preparation of psychiatric nurses. Countries like Romania, Poland, are in various stages of policy development with phased implementation of new and reformed education programmes for psychiatric nursing.

A predominant feature of psychiatric nursing history in all of Europe is the extent to which the role was pre-scribed by medical staff and included participation in many questionable interventions with no scientific basis. Such roles included warm and cold baths, malaria treatment, insulin coma, lobectomy, lobotomy and more recently ECT. Domestic manual and farm work was undertaken by patients and supervised by nurses. In those early days, the nursing role, which was carried out with little autonomy, is eloquently captured in an Irish context by a resident physician:

> The idea of a keeper (psychiatric nurse) comprehends a person constantly supervising the madmen. In this institution therefore the apartments, where the patients are confined during the day should never be without keepers. They should be locked in with the patients and the porter should let them out only at times stated by the regulations. They should be considered as sentinels and be constant to their post and vigilant on duty.[6]

With the exception of the Eastern European bloc, in the early 1970s governments across Europe became increasingly concerned about the large mental institutions and the custodial nature of mental health services. In the Federal Republic of Germany there was concerted government effort to establish smaller psychiatric units and to introduce therapeutic and rehabilitative psychiatry as had occurred in the UK in the 1950s, the US 1960s, and Italy 1970s. Weurth[7] described it as being 'like a wave of liberation'. Following this the picture of psychiatry in Germany changed considerably. For example in 1961 a newly admitted patient expected to stay in a psychiatric hospital for 6–9 years, by 1985 half the patients left the facility after less than 4 weeks. Only one of 100 stays was longer than one year.[7]

The earliest days of mental health care and the evolutionary pathways of Eastern and Western Europe are not dissimilar, except that the early mental health history of Western Europe is reflective of a more recent history of Eastern Europe, which is now undergoing rapid change.

EUROPEAN STRUCTURES

The concept of a European Union commenced with the Treaty of Rome in 1957. It now applies to 15 member states of Europe and the three Economic Area States (EEA). The relationship between economic integration, migration and welfare were some of the basic ideas behind the European Community and such principles having been established in the Treaty of Rome was extended in the Treaty of Mastricht in 1992. Notably the original Treaty of Rome did not include health nor did it enhance greater movement of people in Europe through mutual recognition of qualifications.

It was only in the early 1970s that the necessary procedures and directives were first established which facilitated freedom of movement and reciprocal recognition of qualifications across the Europe Union. Today professional recognition within the EU occurs by means of two different regimes:

❑ Sectoral Directives.
❑ General Systems Directives.

Sectoral Directives bestow a rather privileged position on certain individual health professions including medical doctor, dental practitioner, pharmacist, general care nurse and midwife. The directives provide for minimum harmonization of training and automatic recognition of title throughout the European Union. Their operation is strongly supported by the intensive work of EU advisory committees for each individual profession. The advisory committees comprise representation of each member state, which exchange information, develop documentation and suggest change. The Sectoral Directives[8,9] for general nursing were introduced in 1977 and allowed general nurses to enjoy freedom of movement and automatic recognition of their nursing qualification across EU member states. Most significantly psychiatric nurses were not included in the Sectoral Directives.

The *General Systems Directives*[10] were introduced in 1994 in an attempt to harmonize a greater number of academic and professional qualifications. They apply across a wide range of professions, which follow varying levels, and duration of education and training. Unlike the Sectoral Directives they do not guarantee immediate and automatic recognition of different qualifications and the host country may require additional training and testing and supervised practice as part of the recognition process. Psychiatric nursing falls within the control of the General Systems Directive.

Primarily due to the application of a Sectoral Directives general nursing has a much stronger identity in Europe than does psychiatric nursing. General nurses enjoy greater privileges and rights to practice across EU member states than do psychiatric nurses. The lack of Sectoral Directive for psychiatric nursing means that there is no minimum stated education and training requirement for psychiatric nursing in Europe with resultant implications for psychiatric nursing practice.

There is an increasing need for mobility among health professions in Europe. Some countries such as Germany educate more professionals than they need while others are in need of certain professionals. It is also the case that an increasing need for health services along with service imbalances may lead to increased movement of nurses in years to come. This requires that the EU political, legal and administrative systems put in place to facilitate such movement are improved and perfected.[11] The right of every European citizen to live and work in other member states is fundamental and a basic assumption is that freedom of movement will give EU citizen's opportunities to develop their skills and experiences.

Recent efforts in Europe have been focused on simplifying EU rules in order to facilitate the free movement of qualified people between member states particularly in view of an enlarged European Union.[12] The proposed changes include greater liberalization of the provision of services and more automatic recognition of qualifications. It is important that psychiatric nursing qualifications are part of the changes to the recognition of evidence of training. In looking to the future and in a European context much work needs to be done to ensure that:

❑ Psychiatric nurses are better informed about EU documentation and its importance to psychiatric nurses.
❑ Psychiatric nurses across Europe are agreed in principle on the minimum acceptable education and training requirements for psychiatric nursing in Europe.
❑ Psychiatric nurses recognize the importance and potential influence of the EU agenda generally in strengthening the care of mentally ill and in particular the practice of psychiatric nursing in Europe.
❑ Psychiatric nurses create a forum and proactive agenda in pursuance of common goals in the best interest of psychiatric nursing in Europe.

NURSING EDUCATION IN EUROPE

There are many differences in psychiatric nursing education across Europe. In Eastern and Central Europe regulated education and training for psychiatric nursing is in its infancy, whereas in Western Europe regulation through a national nursing board is well established. Welch[13] as recently as 1995 described the limitations in Eastern and Central Europe, in particular a lack of regulatory structures and significantly the lack of clinical experiences in education programmes for psychiatric nursing.

Psychiatric nursing education commenced as a certificated training programme in a hospital based school of nursing in the early 1900s. Across most of Europe nursing education has now been integrated into or linked to the third level university based education system of member states, with nursing students receiving their education alongside other students. It should be noted that integration into the third level system exists in various forms from full integration into third level education to rather tenuous links. The removal of students from the nursing labour force of mental health services is a significant factor in the changes, which have taken place in nursing education.

MODELS OF NURSING EDUCATION

Across Europe three different models of psychiatric nursing registration education programme are discernible with different types and levels of professional regulation and academic awards. The three models are:

❑ Specialist Model.
❑ Generic Core and Specialist Pathway Model.
❑ Generic Programme.

Specialist Model

The specialist model represents the earliest formalized approach to psychiatric nursing education. Students had direct entry to a programme of training which was entirely focused on psychiatric nursing and when completed it entitled the nurse to work exclusively in the psychiatric setting. For the training programme psychiatric nursing students were recruited by hospitals and they formed an essential part of the nursing workforce. Students therefore had to fulfil the requirements of dual roles as employee and student. Such a model having commenced in the early 20th century was implemented widely across countries such as the Netherlands, the UK and Ireland. Today Ireland remains as the only EU country to have maintained a specialist entry programme for psychiatric nurses. This programme is now totally integrated into the third level education sector and in Ireland from September 2002 will be conducted as a four-year degree psychiatric nurse registration programme.

Generic Core and Specialist Pathway Model

The recognition and acceptance that there are central tenets of a clinical and theoretical nature underpinning nursing education irrespective of clinical setting led to the establishment of a core programme for nursing education. Such a programme was introduced into the UK in the later part of the 1980s and remains as the predominant model of nursing education in the UK. The UK model involves a Common Foundation Programme of 18 months' duration, followed by a second 18 months, which is focused on psychiatric nursing and is much more practice-based.

Generic Model

The generic model is the most common educational model for the preparation of psychiatric nurses across Europe. In this model, which is promoted through the WHO, all nursing students including psychiatric nursing students enter a similar programme of registration usually of three years' duration. The generic model is well established in EU member states such as Italy, Norway, Sweden and Spain. Internationally there is a move towards the generic model, for example Australia in the late 1980s replaced the specialist model with a generic model. In more recent years the Netherlands changed from a traditional specialist programme to a generic model. In the Netherlands all students obtain psychiatric nursing experience but there is no specialist qualification. Students in the final six months may if they wish, choose a psychiatric specialist element. During the programme students gain experience in many clinical settings.

There are many criticisms of the core and generic models as the most appropriate approach to the educational preparation of psychiatric nurses. Bowers et al.[14] point to the implications for the skill and expertise of graduating nurses and point out the need for specific action to safeguard psychiatric nursing skills within the generic curriculum. In an Australian context a similar concern was expressed[15] about the movement of psychiatric nursing education to a generic model in Victoria, Australia and in particular a devaluing of the skills and practice of psychiatric nursing to the extent that the very survival of the specialist branch of nursing is in serious jeopardy. A position paper from the Australian and New Zealand Mental Health Nurses[16] highlighted the constraining effects on practice of Generic Nurse training. The paper suggested that the Generic programme resulted in minimal clinical experiences for psychiatric nurses, and the regulation of mental health nursing is seriously undermined.

In looking towards a future agenda it is important that the concerns of some psychiatric nurse leaders about the suitability of the generic model of psychiatric nursing education be taken seriously. Therefore a European study to examine and evaluate the impact of the different models of psychiatric nursing education in Europe must be commissioned with an aim of ensuring best educational approaches in the preparation of psychiatric nurses.

Ideological positions

There is a strong tradition of institutional care in Europe and primarily because of this it may be argued that nurses are trapped within a medical and institutional model, which adversely affects the type and level of service that they provide. In particular psychiatric nursing has been dominated by therapeutic shifts within the discipline of psychiatry and an expanded scope of practice. It has been identified[17] that primarily due to the wide-ranging role, psychiatric nurses now occupy a pivotal and central role in services for mentally ill people in many care and treatment locations.

Given the strong historical association between psychiatric medicine and psychiatric nursing, the challenging question is, to what extent can the psychiatric nursing role develop outside of medicine. In Europe psychiatric nursing remains strongly institutionally based and medically dominated. Psychiatric nurses in Western Europe, much more so than in Eastern or Central Europe, have achieved a level of autonomous practice and have in a significant way diversified their practice into settings outside of the institution including the community and the home.

The reduced reliance on custodial care, changing mental health care legislation, and the requirement for multidisciplinary patterns in the care of the mentally ill have profound implications for the role of the nurse. Psychiatric nurses will be expected to provide care to different groups, with whom they have had minimal contact in the past. There is a new emphasis on health promotion, early intervention, community development and on nursing being provided closer to where people live and work, as well as making access to services easier for vulnerable groups of the population.

The search for a universal ideology to guide nursing practice has been raised, and in terms of practice, psychiatric nurses are involved in all forms of treatment from merely monitoring medication to introducing psychotherapeutic modalities. There is clearly a lack of a single unifying ideological approach to psychiatric nursing in Europe; indeed ideological eclecticism may represent a core foundation for the practice of nursing. However the lack of an agreed understanding and a single ideology for psychiatric nursing in Europe introduces serious limitations, and it is suggested that psychiatric nurses are hard pressed to define or predict outcomes of nursing.[18]

Across Europe there is a lack of authoritative information on psychiatric nursing roles. However there is general agreement that mental health problems require patterns of care which draws on psychological, spiritual, and social well-being as well as the physical aspects of the person. The juxtaposition between traditional custodial roles and the evolving therapeutic role of the nurse is eloquently summed up by Pepleau,[19] when she suggests that there is a significant difference between taking responsibility for the care of people and being therapeutically responsive to each person.

A number of studies have been undertaken to describe the role of the psychiatric nurse in different Europe countries. In one of the earliest UK studies, Altschul[20] concluded that it had proved impossible to obtain any picture of the treatment ideologies that prevailed among nurses. Cormack[21] found little evidence of therapeutic activity. In a more recent study[17] nine categories of the psychiatric nursing role were identified. These included assessing patients' needs and evaluating care, planning care, nurse–patient interactions, pharmaceutical interventions, education, documenting information, co-ordinating the services of nurses and other professionals for patients, communicating with other professionals and grades of staff, and the administration and organization of clinical work. Importantly psychiatric nurses performed independent functions as well as collaborating with other professional groups to provide patient/client care. The study identified that psychiatric nurses considered the central tenet of psychiatric nursing to be that of the caring relationship between patient and nurse. It was reported[17] that psychiatric nurses cared for patients at different levels; for example, for patients with greater dependency levels nursing meant 'doing for' patients those activities that they could not do for themselves. In other cases the nurse's role involved care at a level of 'doing with' individuals, which meant supporting, supervising and working alongside patients in a way that recognized their strengths. At another level nurses at times provided a presence 'being with' patients where other more active interventions were not possible, not required or inappropriate.

Clearly the psychiatric nursing role is evolving and it is important that the future role of the psychiatric nurse develops in a centrally co-ordinated way across Europe.

THE PRACTICE OF PSYCHIATRIC NURSING

As previously indicated, across the EU region there is much variance in the level of investment in the environment for care and this impacts directly on psychiatric nursing. Across the EU psychiatric nursing environments range from outdated overcrowded Dickensian institutions to purpose built modern units. High staff turnover, problems with recruitment and retention are a salient feature of psychiatric nursing in Europe. It is therefore important that there be concerted EU efforts to make psychiatric nursing more attractive so as to stabilize the psychiatric nursing workforce across Europe.

There have been no dramatic scientific discoveries, which provide an understanding of the nature and aetiology of mental illness. The lack of discoveries in cures for the major illnesses of schizophrenia and depression at this point in history distinguishes the mental health

3 **Assessing patient's ability to perform ADL**. It was also noted that nurses were able to observe changes in patients' activities of daily living (ADL). When patients became unable to carry out their ADL – for example, when they could no longer cope with daily activities, ate almost nothing or did not take medication at all – the nurse's visiting care could no longer meet the patient's needs.

4 **Disposition of patients**. On perceiving a patient's failure regarding their ADL, visiting nurses reported directly to the patient's doctor, and then decided how to support the patient as a team from then on. The decision involved making a choice between supporting patients continuously on an outpatient basis, or admitting patients to hospital so that they could reorganize their living.

5 **Suggesting hospital visits or admission**. Visiting nurses tried to help patients become aware of their own symptoms, so that they could recognize the development of breakdown in their daily living activities. In such circumstances, the nurses suggested that a visit or admission to a hospital might be necessary for them. When the nurses thought it would be difficult for the patient to transfer from home to hospital, they would consider accompanying the patient.

THE JAPANESE SYSTEM OF NURSING LICENSE: RN AND PHN

Under the Japanese system of nursing license, there are two kinds of certification for making home visits. These are RN (Registered Nurse) and PHN (Public Health Nursing). All PHN have an RN license and take the national PHN examination after receiving a further 6–12 months of special education. The roles of the two licenses are different. Most PHNs work at public health centres as civil servants. In contrast, Many RNs work at private hospitals. PHNs are expected to be co-ordinators or supporters of RNs, but today, the rapid increase in aging populations has led to a change of roles RN and PHN in home visiting.

In 1992 a revised health and medical insurance system launched the system of a visiting nurses service station (VNSS).[2] The VNSS is sponsored by a psychiatric hospital, a physician's association, the Japanese Nursing Association, or established by the private capital of a nurse manager. VNSS chiefly provide home visits to the elderly but also provide care for mentally disabled people. VNSS also employ *home-helps*. The Home-help's licenses are of various kinds. Many of these are based on a 6-month period of communication education. The home-helps do not have an educational background in medicine.

In general most staffs of VNSS do not have experience of psychiatric nursing. They are often fearful about caring for people with mental illness and seek special skills to enhance their home visiting work. As mentioned before, many of them were trained as care providers for elderly people and often ask psychiatric nurses to lecture on psychiatric care.

CURRENT EXPECTATIONS OF PSYCHIATRIC NURSING

As mentioned above, expectations for psychiatric nursing are changing. Nurses have the responsibility of building trust between not only themselves and their patients but also with other staff who may need consultation support or supervision. If they are all nurses, they can use their common knowledge to teach skills of trust-building with patients. However, in many cases people who need help do not have nursing backgrounds, so psychiatric nurses need to develop a description of the essential issues of their practice.

This situation requires Japanese psychiatric nurses to employ more suitable research methods to define psychiatric nursing practice. Nojima[3] pointed out that the theme of nursing science for next quarter century is to construct serviceable middle-range theories of Japanese nursing. The development of such a theoretical description of nursing is important for nurses and the other specialists nurses work with.

In addition to research, nurses can provide a direct service to staff dealing with mentally disordered people. Clinical supervision or clinical consultations are specific ways of accomplishing this. As specialists in human services, nurses should expand their service to other care staff, applying our knowledge of empowerment and caring. Barker has described the process of clinical supervision as 'an effective communication mechanism'.[4] Nurses are aware of the expectations of both clients and staff. Responding to such expectations will be a great challenge for all of us in the next ten years.

FORENSIC PSYCHIATRY AND PSYCHIATRIC NURSING

The years 2000 and 2001 were notable in Japan because of media publicity concerning offenders who had a history of inpatient psychiatric care.

In May 2001 a juvenile delinquent hijacked a highway bus. He had been on overnight leave from a psychiatric unit. The young man had a DSM diagnosis of conduct disorder. He killed a person with a sword and held 16 passengers captive inside the bus for 17 hours. Many members of the public were critical of the care this young man received.

The next year witnessed an extremely brutal event. A 30-year-old male killed eight pupils in a primary school with a knife. All of the victims were 7 or 8 years old. The offender had been admitted to psychiatric inpatient units many times. Citizens felt strong fear of psychiatric patients after this crime and many primary schools built strict security systems. Today people regard the killer as a malingerer, not a psychiatric patient, but many neighbours of mentally ill people fear that they also will commit violent crimes.

Fear that mentally disordered people will commit crimes has been very common for a long time, not only in Japan, but also throughout the world. Barker[4] has pointed out that 'many of us come to believe that our prejudices are no less than a recognition of a social reality – a reality which we have helped construct, through our expressions of prejudice'.

One lesson we have learned from these crimes is not to return to using asylum as the main form of treatment. We have to recognize that everyone has the possibility of becoming mentally ill. On such occasions without appropriate care, people can experience severe difficulties. The problem does not so much involve mentally ill people, but the shortage of primary or secondary care to support them. We need many specialists who can deal with them.

Secondly, we must alter our policies to create more constructive ways to provide care for mentally disordered people in the community, changing the attitudes of citizens, teaching skills to understand clients and how to deal with them, and how to prevent more serious problems. This represents a big challenge for psychiatric nurses in Japan.

THE EXPANDING ROLE OF HUMAN COMMUNICATION

All the issues mentioned here point to the need to expand and develop our capacity for human communication. Nurses cannot remain inside the psychiatric hospital or health centre, encircled only by medical staff. We must go out to meet with citizens, write papers and promote understanding of mental illness and psychiatric nursing.

If citizens feel psychiatric nurses are accessible, we will become practical specialists for them. However, this will be a big challenge. Japanese psychiatric nurses used to be like the gatekeepers of psychiatric hospitals, but in the future their role will be to use psychiatric nursing as a means of expanding human communication.

REFERENCES

1. Kayama M, Zerwech J, Thornton K, Murashima S. Japanese expert public health nurses empower Clients with schizophrenia living in the community. *Journal of Psycho-social Nursing and Mental Health Services*, 2001; **39**: 40–45.
2. Murashima S, Nagata S, Magilvy J, Fukui S, Kayama M. Home care nursing in Japan: a challenge for providing good care at home. *Public Health Nursing* 2002; **19**(2): 94–103.
3. Nojima Y, Sawai N. The way for mature nursing science. *Quality Nursing* 2002; **8**(1): 4–8.
4. Barker P. *The philosophy and practice of psychiatric and mental health nursing*. Edinburgh: Churchill Livingstone, 1999.

Chapter 70

THE UNITED STATES CONTEXT

Shirley A Smoyak*

INTRODUCTION

Change is rarely embraced with open arms, even when there is acknowledgement that something needs fixing. Although the clinical practice of psychiatric nursing is based solidly on communication skills, reframing difficult situations, systems thinking and being articulate, nurses can be as resistant to change as any other group. In my near half-century as a professional nurse, I never cease to be amazed by how we manage to ignore or resist good ideas, common sense and golden opportunities. For this chapter, I have selected three changes which I believe are not only inevitable, but will dramatically affect, in a positive way, the practice of psychiatric nurses and the care received by our consumers. These are:

1 The professional practices of nurses and physicians will be re-examined, and what they do will be organized by the skills and knowledge needed, not by turf issues. Payment mechanisms will drive these changes.

2 Consumers will become more knowledgeable about their health needs and demand a collaborative working model with their health care providers.

They will select their providers more easily when professional barriers are altered.

3 Public health and mental health will again be partners, thus providing the bedrock needed for working in communities. With this realignment, prevention and population based strategies will be possible.

REALIGNED ROLES

In the United States, in the late 1950s and early 1960s, physicians, nurses and patients or clients were distressed with the dysfunctional health care system. Several nationally funded studies documented the animosity between the professions and the reasons for nurses leaving the field. In the 1970s, the *National Joint Practice Commission* (NJPC), comprised of eight physicians appointed by the *American Medical Association* (AMA) and eight nurses, appointed by the *American Nurses Association* (ANA) worked to repair the discord and attempted to institute collaboration and colleagueship in primary care settings. Problems in educational systems and service delivery settings were addressed. Advanced practice nurses were at the centre of the debates. New

---

*Shirley A Smoyak was a psychiatric nurse before Thorazine (chlorpromazine). This says it all – that she had only her wits to deal with the people on the wards of the state mental hospitals where she worked. She currently is Professor II (Distinguished Professor) at the Rutgers University Edward J. Bloustein School of Planning and Public Policy. She has been Editor of the *Journal of Psychosocial Nursing and Mental Health Services* since 1981.

strategies were developed and promulgated by conferences and publications. Many lessons were learned in that decade and the following years. Ironically, there was never a psychiatrist on the NJPC, so I had no partner to dialogue and plan with during this decade.

New ways of relating to each other can be realized when basic questions about assumptions and beliefs are placed squarely on the table. 'Who owns what?' and 'Who has the knowledge and/or skills to do what?' are basic questions to begin the dialogue. The fact that no-one can 'own' knowledge, in the sense that this is licensed or controlled is critical. The needed negotiations are then more clearly seen as dialogues about time, place, populations and politics. As psychiatric nurses expand their practices to include prescriptive authority, such dialogue will be very important.

The legacy of Hildegard E. Peplau

How and why advanced practice nurses developed as they did in the United States is a story, which takes more space than allotted here. It is a fascinating tale, and one which could offer some direction to countries just setting out to incorporate this level of nursing into the health care arena.

Hildegard E. Peplau is the acknowledged leader of the movement to prepare psychiatric nurses with Master's degrees. In the late 1950s at Rutgers, the State University of New Jersey, College of Nursing, Newark, NJ, she developed a Master of Science programme, which prepared clinical specialists in psychiatric nursing. The two-year academic programme required 16–20 hours of work with severely ill patients with mental illness in state hospitals. Her seminars about the interpersonal relationships were conducted at the hospitals. Before this, Master's degrees had an administrative or education focus, not clinical. This change to a clinical focus was met with great scepticism by many.

Dr Peplau managed to secure the clinical settings for these Master's students by explaining to the physician superintendents that what they were doing was 'group work'. If the word 'therapy' had been used, the programme would not have had a clinical site. Fifty years later, the words 'therapy' and 'psychotherapy' are used easily and forthrightly to describe what these nurses do.

After I graduated from this programme and joined the faculty, my assignment was to develop collaborative relationships with the Department of Psychiatry in the Rutgers Medical School. This was a relatively easy assignment, since the academic milieu was one where collaboration and colleagueship were voiced expectations. In other settings, however, nurses found barriers to any joint practice arrangements in psychiatric settings.

Through the years, it became clear that joint practice arrangements needed to be guided by mutually agreed upon principles. MDs and RNs work as colleagues, collaboratively, when there is:

1 mutual agreement on a goal;

2 equality in status and personal interactions;

3 a shared base of scientific and professional knowledge with complementary diversity in skills, expertise and practices;

4 mutual trust and respect for each other's competence;

Professional practice choices and decisions will continue to change as patients and consumers enter as full partners.

CONSUMERS AS PARTNERS

Even in mid-century, as Dr Peplau was teaching graduate students and the continuing education workshops across the United States, the notion that psychiatric patients needed to be considered as people with full citizenship rights was emphasized. This was a time before patient advocates, usually lawyers, became a part of the government system at the federal and state levels. Ward staff were not pleased when they were reminded that patients had rights and that their wishes needed to be appreciated and implemented wherever possible.

In the United States, consumers began to make it clear that they expected to be treated as partners, and not just recipients of care when the psycho-social rehabilitation movement began in the late 1970s. The *National Alliance for the Mentally Ill* (NAMI), was founded in 1980 by groups of parents championing the cause for their mentally ill sons and daughters. Today this group is a significant factor in Congressional decisions about funding for mental illness, including insurance requirements. Many nurses are members of and partners with NAMI.

Consumers share strategies with each other about identifying and accessing professional providers who are resonant with their needs. They know, for instance, that although they may find many psychiatrists in the yellow pages of the phone book, that only a small minority of these actually practice in ways that the consumers find useful. Consumers may also find it difficult to locate a psychiatric nurse, who may be their preferred provider. Advanced practice nurses are fewer in number than psychiatrists.

As a psychiatric nurse, I had never thought of myself as a minority. However, having perused the new *Mental Health, United States, 2000*, just released by the U.S. Department of Health and Human Services (USDHSS), I realize that I am. All 15,330 Master's-prepared psychiatric nurses are a minority in the mental health field. We are a tiny group, compared with 40,731 psychiatrists, 77,456 psychologists, 31,278 school psychologists, 96,407 social workers and 44,225 marriage and family therapists. Perhaps the most startling statistic is that there are now 100,000 professionals with Master's degrees in psycho-social rehabilitation. This group is the newest addition to the ranks of mental health professionals and is graduating a significant number of people. Counsellors – also a relatively new field, but also licensed – number 108,104.

Ronald Manderscheid and Marilyn Henderson served as editors for this new volume.[1] Dr Manderscheid has been involved with the production of this statistical reporting document for nearly 20 years, from the time when the National Institute for Mental Health was organized with services, education and research under one administration. The document is now under the administrative authority of the *Substance Abuse and Mental Health Services Administration* (SAMHSA), Center for Mental Health Services.

INTERDISCIPLINARY COLLABORATION

Professionals from all disciplines will need to learn how to collaborate fully with people for whom they are offering care. Frances Hughes, a Commonwealth Fellow (2002), has also forecast this projected change.[2] She adds a Type III to the practice models identified by the National Joint Practice Commission in the 1970s.[3] Type I describes work that is highly specific, with practitioners undergoing rigorous training for the specialty. Type II work can be accomplished by generalist practitioners from different backgrounds. Type III work is accomplished in a collaborative mode, with patients and practitioners sharing in the assessment and decision-making about treatment strategies (see Table 70.1).

Data presented in the USDHSS document reflect information only on nurses with graduate degrees in psychiatric/mental health nursing. The obvious reason that I did not feel like a minority, before looking at the reported statistics, is that I see many psychiatric nurses in the hospital and community settings where my teaching, monitoring and research activities take me. As I serve as a court-appointed monitor at Greystone Park Psychiatric Hospital in northern New Jersey, visiting wards in all areas, I see many nurses, but only an occasional psychiatrist or psychologist. Some of these nurses are Master's-prepared, but the majority are not. Such is the case in clinical settings across the country. It is impossible to produce an accurate accounting of the educational background and post-graduation training for the nurses in psychiatric settings who had their basic preparation in diploma, associate degree or baccalaure-

TABLE 70.1 Types of work

Type I Work (highly specific)
Workers are highly specialized and have considerable technical training.
Few clashes or conflicts among workers.
Workers know their places and what they have to do

Examples:
Baseball – pitchers and catchers
Health care – operating suites or emergency centres

Type II Work (general)
Workers from different backgrounds can do the work equally well.
Many conflicts over jurisdictions and relationships.
Competition, rivalry, blaming.

Examples:
Baseball – the outfield (left, centre, right)
Health care – primary care settings

ate degree programmes. The good news is that in the actual clinical settings, a spirit of collegiality and team building is the case in most instances. Clinical specialists and the newer psychiatric nurse practitioners serve as mentors and guides for the other nurses. My guess would be that in settings where there are no Master's-prepared nurses, the nurses there rise to the challenge of care delivery for their patients. The bad news is that we do not have the data to address the question of how academic preparation affects care delivery. In this age of outcome measures, we are handicapped by not having basic statistics on our entire workforce.

There are some interesting comparative statistics in the area of gender and race. Nurses are still overwhelmingly women (6% men). Even social workers, also a predominantly female occupation historically, now have proportionately more men (about 23%). Women members of the American Psychiatric Association in 1999 totalled 29%, while nearly half (48%) of psychologists were women. Nurses have the highest proportion reporting their race as white (94.6%), with psychologists next at 91.7% and social workers at 89%. Psychiatrists, on the other hand, report 73.8% as white, with 13.3% as Asian/Pacific Islander. There is more diversity in their ranks, than in the other three.

Less than 5% of female graduate-prepared nurses are younger than 35 years today. In 1988, 18% were under 35. The aging trend continues, with the current average age at 48 years. Regionally, the greatest percentage of advance practice nurses reside in the South Atlantic, East North Central and Middle Atlantic. More than 50% of the nurses received their highest degree more than 10 years ago. Employment practices indicate that 65% of the nurses hold just one position, while the others report two or more practice positions.

For those nurses with graduate degrees, 94% were prepared as clinical nurse specialists (CNS) and 13% as psychiatric nurse practitioners. However, Merwin, Lyon and Fox suggest a more accurate count as: 86% CNS, 6% NPs and 8% dually CNS and NP (p. 300). State licensure or regulation recognizes 32% as advanced practice nurses.

While the nurse practitioner movement is more than 30 years old, psychiatric nursing has just recently moved in this direction. In 1991, few nurse practitioner students (89 or 2%) specialized in psychiatric nursing. In 1994, there were 364 enrollees with 70 graduates. In 1996 there were 483 enrollees with 100 graduates (p. 301).

Issues and debates about certification mechanisms and boards continue. The current three types of preparation, CNS, NP, and combined, present dilemmas for those who write the certification examinations. Further, while other disciplines/professions reserve certification processes for those with advanced preparation, nursing has muddied the waters considerably by certifying generalists.

As consumers become stronger advocates for themselves, and are joined by family members and professionals who value accountability, the outcome will surely be closer scrutiny about how practices are conducted. The bottom line will be: are things better for the client? Ways to measure outcomes in psychiatric practice, when the consumer-professional relationship is the focus, need to be developed. When consumers and nurses are equally knowledgeable about medications, side-effects, alternative approaches to therapy, the value of dialogue, and action-oriented treatment, mental illness will surely lose considerable stigma. Nurses and consumers will enjoy new respect at work and in communities.

INTEGRATING PUBLIC HEALTH AND MENTAL HEALTH

Americans like convenience, and they like to have what they need or want instantly. In the USA, we have grouped materials and services in interesting ways. For instance, we can fill our car with gasoline and fill ourselves with coffee and a donut at the same time. We can shop for almost anything in grander and grander malls, and eat at the same time (sitting down or walking around). Some new malls even have exercise spas. Banks used to have one focus per institution; now we have one-stop banking in most urban settings where we can do checking, saving, mortgaging and getting a loan all in one visit. Grocery stores have become mini-malls and

include pharmacies (with blood-pressure checking devices), flower shops and photography centres.

And we apparently believe that providing good health care requires that it also be integrated. The advent of primary care a quarter century ago was heralded as the way to assure accessible, affordable, appropriate services. Fragmentation was supposed to end when practitioners adopted the new ways of organizing care. The associated frustrations with various barriers to care were supposed to become history. Ironically, parallel to this new interest in providing one-stop shopping for patients, the old fragmentation and animosity between nurses and physicians continued. As noted above, the NJPC attempted to address these problems, and turned their attention to primary care settings and how the practitioners arranged their work.[3]

When I tried to engage nurses in a discussion then about why 'primary nursing' was used in a different way from 'primary care', the positions taken were very clear. Nurses believed that they had to strengthen their own profession and image first, before engaging in any new collaboration with physicians. They saw MDs as the enemy, and they were acting on a need to draw the wagons around and keep their territory safe from invasion. Of course, MDs were also feeling attacked by the articulate, uppity, new breed of nurse practitioner who 'didn't know her place'.

Now, 25 years later, we are supposed to be working on integrating mental health in primary health. Surgeon General David Satcher convened a meeting in late 2000 'to advance the integration of mental health services and primary health care'.[4] This meeting was an outgrowth of the 1999 Surgeon General's Report on Mental Health.[5] A nurse, Brenda Reiss-Brennan, MS, APRN, CS, President of Primary Care Family Therapy Clinics, served as the consultant and meeting organizer, conducting over 90 interviews in preparation for the deliberations among the participants representing health care professionals, consumers, families, foundations and government agencies. Included among the interviewees were experts representing businesses, researchers, employers, economists, epidemiologists, providers, health care consultants and payors, as well as the participants listed above.

Among the group's recommendations were the following:

1   Convene a group under the auspices of the DHHS to develop a framework for the integration of mental health care and primary care, including a focus on comorbidities, diverse modalities, and diverse populations. (Note: This is very similar to the mission of the NJPC, but including mental health.)

2   Incorporate a list of skills, knowledges, attitudes, and

simple tools that reflects evidence-based 'best practices' and treatment management, leading to improved outcomes. (Note: The providers of such services are not named. The NJPC's idea of 'those who learn together earn together'[6] might yet be a reality.)

3 Design education and training standards for the integration of mental health care and primary care with all stakeholders, including accreditation bodies and promote implementation of those standards by schools of health and behavioural health. (Note: Stay tuned to see how these new schools evolve. Will we be talking about a 'fifth profession' again? With a primary care twist or spin?)

Those among us who have vested interests in keeping identities intact, and are resistant to change will not have an easy time of what is to come. On the other hand, we could adopt John Gardner's position, 'Life is full of golden opportunities carefully disguised as irresolvable problems'.[7]

REFERENCES

1. Center for Mental Health Services. Manderscheid RW, Henderson MJ (eds). (2001) *Mental Health, United States, 2000.* DHHS Publication No. (SMA) 01-3537. Washington, D.C.: Supt. of Docs, U.S. Government Printing Office. (This publication can be accessed electronically – http://www.samhsa.gov. Free single copies may be requested from the National Mental Health Services Knowledge Exchange Network – 1-800-789-2647.)

2. Hughes F. *Healthcare delivery issues: key lessons from the United States.* Paper prepared for the Commonwealth Fund, Harkness Fellowship, April, 2002 at the University of Pennsylvania, Philadelphia, PA, 2002.

3. Smoyak S. Problems in interprofessional relationships. *Bulletin of the New York Academy of Medicine* 1977; **53**: 51–9.

4. U.S. Department of Health and Human Services (DHHS). *Report of a Surgeon General's working meeting on the integration of mental health services and primary health care.* November 30–December 1, 2000, Atlanta, Georgia (Carter Center) Rockville, MD: USDHHS, Public Health Service, Office of the Surgeon General, 2001.

5. U.S. Department of Health and Human Services (DHHS). *Mental Health: A Report of the Surgeon General.* Rockville, MD: Substance Abuse and Mental Health Services Administration, Center for Mental Health Services, National Institute for Mental Health Substance Abuse and Mental Health Services Administration, Center for Mental Health Services, National Institute for Mental Health, 1999.

6. Hoekelman R. *Nurse–physician relationships: problems and solutions.* Commencement address to graduates of the Pediatric and Medical Nurse Associate Training Programmes, Rush-Presbyterian, St. Luke's Medical Center, Chicago, Illinois, June 26, 1974.

7. Quoted by Dr Satcher, in his opening remarks on November 30, 2000, who noted that John Gardner was Secretary of Health, Education and Welfare in the 1960s.

Chapter 71

THE AUSTRALIAN AND NEW ZEALAND CONTEXT: PROSPECTS FOR MENTAL HEALTH NURSING 'DOWN UNDER'

Jon Chesterson* and Michael Hazelton**

> May your joys be as deep as the ocean
> And your sorrows be as light as its foam[a]

INTRODUCTION

This chapter considers the current situation and future prospects for mental health nursing 'down under'. Discussion centres mainly on the situation in Australia, with reference to developments in New Zealand, noting the close cooperation between the two countries, the very significant historical and cultural differences, and origin and influence of *Te Tiriti o Waitangi* (The Treaty of Waitangi) in New Zealand. The chapter begins with an overview of the mental health policy context in Australia. This is followed by a discussion of the current situation faced by mental health nursing, focusing especially on questions of professional governance, practice development, and strategic partnerships involving service users and service providers. The final section presents a longer-term vision for the development of mental health nursing in the region, addressing questions of therapeutic attitude, ethics, social justice and public image. The main thrust of the chapter is to suggest that while mental health nursing faces many challenges in Australia and New Zealand, the current policy directions present many opportunities for advancement. How current challenges are resolved will heavily influence what mental health nursing can become by the year 2020.

THE POLICY CONTEXT

Australia's federal system of government involves power-sharing between the Commonwealth Government and the various State and Territory governments. The implementation of national policies thus requires close cooperation between these two tiers of government. While the role of the Commonwealth in mental health policy is mainly to co-ordinate the response to major issues nationally and to facilitate reform, responsibility for the funding and delivery of mental health services largely rests with the State and Territory governments.

*Jon Chesterson is the promotion and prevention officer, Hunter Mental Health, New South Wales, Australia and conjoint Lecturer, University of Newcastle. His interests include psychiatric rehabilitation recovery, practice development, conference management and group facilitation. President of the Australian and New Zealand College of Mental Health Nurses 1997–1999, Jon is currently an advisor to the ICN on mental health nursing in Australia.

*Mike Hazelton is Professor of Mental Health Nursing at the University of Newcastle and Hunter Mental Health, New South Wales, Australia. His interests include mental health services research, rural mental health, international health and health sociology. Mike is the current editor of the *International Journal of Mental Health Nursing*.

[a] From a poem by an unknown patient, in: *A private World on a Nameless Bay*, Morriset Hospital Historical Society 2001, Cooranbong, NSW, Australia. As much a reflection of hope for the future of someone with a mental illness, this was in fact written as a tribute to a psychiatric nurse sometime around the late 1930s.

Australia's first National Mental Health Policy and Plan[1] was implemented over a five-year period commencing in 1992 under the National Mental Health Strategy (NMHS). The Second National Mental Health Plan[2] covers the five-year period from 1998 to 2003. The Strategy and plan have emphasized the importance of mental health as a public issue and differentiated the old institutional approach to service provision from the new community-based approach (see Fig. 71.1). The key policy aims are to:

❏ Promote the mental health of the Australian community and where possible, prevent the development of mental health problems and disorders.
❏ Reduce the impact of mental disorders on individuals, families and the community.
❏ Assure the rights of people with mental illness.

During the first five years (1992–1997), significant improvements were reported in the range, quality, responsiveness and community orientation of mental health services. In addition, mental health services were more closely integrated with mainstream health services. However, improvements were less than expected in a number of areas. Service users continued to report difficulties in accessing services; the quality of services remained uneven within and across jurisdictions; many primary care providers pointed to the continuing insularity of mental health services; and stigma and discrimination remained major problems for those using mental health services.[3]

NATIONAL MENTAL HEALTH STRATEGY

Achievements of First National Mental Health Plan

■ Structural reform of mental health services
■ Improved consumer/carer participation in decision making and advocacy
■ Collection/analysis of mental health information, development of data systems, accountability and monitoring
■ Improved service quality
■ Improved linkages between sectors, governments, external stakeholders
■ Improved understanding of mental illness, prevention and promotion
■ Identification, development, trialing of innovative service/funding models

Priorities for Second National Mental Health Plan

■ Promotion, prevention and early intervention
■ Development of partnerships in service reform
■ Quality and effectiveness of service delivery

FIGURE 71.1 National Mental Health Strategy. Adapted from 2nd National Mental Health Plan, Australian Health Ministers, 1998

During the second five years (1998–2003), priority has been given to reforms in mental health promotion and prevention; building partnerships in service reform; and further enhancing service quality and effectiveness. Moreover, surveys commissioned in the first stage of the Strategy indicated a high level of unmet need for mental health care.[4] Accordingly, an initial policy focus on the long-term mentally ill was now expanded to give greater emphasis to population health issues.[3]

The Strategy is often seen as a policy success story,[5] but doubts remain as to whether the reforms will resolve 'the historical problem of the marginalized and excluded mental patient'.[6] Recent studies have shown that many people with long-term mental disorders live marginal lives, characterized by severe disability, stigma and discrimination, social isolation, unemployment, homelessness, and poverty. Moreover, there remains a serious lack of community-based rehabilitation services, and of behavioural and psycho-social treatments such as cognitive-behavioural therapy, social skills training, psycho-education and supportive therapies.[4] For many service users the reforms have fallen well short of the desired 'democratization of human services provision'.[7]

THE IMMEDIATE YEARS AHEAD

There is no doubt that the Strategy has brought both opportunities and challenges for mental health nursing in Australia, and that similar developments have also occurred in New Zealand. The further development of mental health nursing in the region will be heavily influenced by responses to emerging issues and the drivers that shape the social infrastructure and context in which mental health nursing services are provided. The context and some of the challenges for the discipline have been discussed in greater detail elsewhere.[8–12] The following section discusses prospects for the immediate future to 2010, focusing on key initiatives and trends at regional and international levels with reference to the concept of clinical governance.

Clinical (professional) governance

The International Council of Nurses (ICN) has defined 'governance' as 'the process of controlling or guiding the profession'. Used interchangeably with the term 'regulation', this refers to governmental, professional, private, and individual means whereby order, identity, consistency, and control are brought to the profession. The concept also pertains to how the profession and its members are defined; how its scope and standards of practice, education, and ethics are determined; and how systems of accountability are established.[13]

<table>
<tr><td colspan="2">

STANDARDS OF PRACTICE

Mental health nurses

- Ensure their practice is culturally safe and sensitive
- Establish partnership as a basis for therapeutic relationships
- Provide systematic care that reflects contemporary nursing practice and client's health care/treatment plan
- Promote health and wellness of individuals, families and communities
- Commit to ongoing education, professional growth, and practice development based on appropriate research
- Practice ethically with respect to professional identity, independence, inter-dependence, authority, and partnership

</td></tr>
</table>

FIGURE 71.2 Standards of Practice. Adapted from Australian & New Zealand College of Mental Health Nurses, 1995

CODE OF ETHICS

Nurses

- Respect persons' individual needs, values and culture
- Respect the rights of persons to make informed choices
- Promote and uphold the provision of quality nursing care for all people
- Hold in confidence any information obtained in a professional capacity, and use professional judgment in sharing such information
- Accept accountability and responsibility in their roles
- Promote an ecological, social and economic environment which supports and sustains health and well being

FIGURE 71.3 Code of Ethics. Adapted from Australian Nursing Council, 1993

Similarly to other professions, mental health nursing is regulated. However, it is important to find an appropriate balance between over-regulation and under-regulation.[14] In Australia and New Zealand the external regulatory mechanisms affecting mental health nursing include nursing legislation, the Trans Tasman Mutual Recognition Act and mental health legislation. At a broader level, sociopolitical and economic forces also exert a regulatory effect, through national mental health policy, planning, and standards,[1,2,15-18] funding for education and health,[19] and workforce planning and industrial relations.

Although mental health nursing is subject to numerous external regulatory mechanisms, the profession has so far failed to develop a framework for self-regulation, a point of differentiation from other health professions such as psychiatry and psychology. Nevertheless, standards of practice have been developed,[20,21] and codes of conduct[22] and ethics[23] are in widespread use[24] (see Figs. 71.2 and 71.3). Since the 1970s the Australian and New Zealand College of Mental Health Nurses (ANZCMHN) has evolved as the professional body representing mental health nurses in Australia and New Zealand with a membership of approximately 12% of the mental health nursing workforce in both countries.[25] These factors touch on some aspects of clinical governance, but they do not provide a robust basis for the delivery of consistent, reliable standards of mental health care from all members of the profession within the region. The key to gaining greater public recognition and confidence is to demonstrate professional accountability and improved performance through clinical governance. Figure 71.4 represents a proposed clinical governance framework for mental health nursing within the context of current national policies, education, regulation, and mental health service provision.

Credentialing and accreditation

Credentialing may be defined as, 'the evaluation of an individual nurse's performance against relevant practice standards'.[26] Accreditation is a process by which educational programmes and/or educational and health care providers are evaluated for quality, relevance and performance. In a recent report to the Commonwealth Government, the Royal College of Nursing Australia[27] outlined the feasibility of a national approach in relation to advanced and specialist nursing practice. In an earlier report to the Nursing Board of Tasmania, the ANZCMHN[28] outlined credentialing and accreditation options specific to mental health nursing, and recommended that a collaborative approach, involving the College and the Nursing Board, be piloted in Tasmania (forerunner to a national framework). At present only a small number of specialist professional nursing organizations in Australia have moved to develop credentialing programmes.

Further consultation between the Nursing Board of Tasmania and the ANZCMHN has resulted in a proposal to establish a Credential for Practice Program (CPP) for mental health nurses (MHN) in that State. The CPP would be based on a formal application and review process involving periodic renewal. Applicants would be evaluated using set criteria, including the accrual of continuing education and practice development points, the provision of supporting evidence, and the support of professional referees.[29] The evaluation criteria would include:

- Specialist/postgraduate mental health nursing qualifications.
- Licensure as a Registered Nurse within Australia or New Zealand.

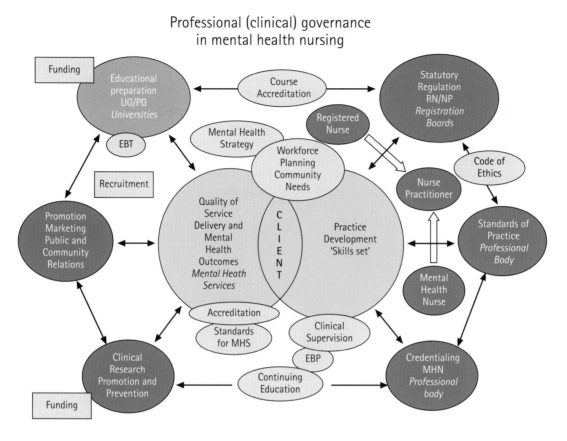

FIGURE 71.4 Professional (clinical) governance in mental health nursing.

❏ Practice experience including minimum duration and recency.
❏ Continuing professional education with points system over set period.
❏ Continuing practice development with points system over set period.
❏ Maintenance of an evidence-based record subject to random periodic audit.
❏ Referees and professional declarations.

Some State Nursing Boards within Australia currently review and endorse postgraduate courses in mental health nursing. It is anticipated that these arrangements will be replaced during the next decade by collaborative accreditation programmes involving the nursing boards, employers and the ANZCMHN.

Workforce planning, education and practice development

Serious gaps have been identified in mental health workforce planning at all levels in Australia. Mental health services face serious problems in recruiting and retaining staff, and too few registered nurses (RN) currently progress beyond the initial nursing qualification to complete postgraduate studies in mental health nursing. It has recently been reported that workforce morale is low and that the skill base and professional aspirations of mental health nurses have declined.[10] A number of solutions have been proposed to improve workforce planning for mental health nursing and to bring the development of the discipline into closer alignment with current mental health policy aims:[30-34]

1 Establishment of a comprehensive and reliable data set on the national mental health workforce. Existing data collection arrangements are ad hoc and poorly co-ordinated across jurisdictions, and thus provide a poor basis for workforce planning.

2 Workforce planning for the mental health nursing workforce by Commonwealth and State and Territory health planners needs to be more closely aligned with the needs of the community, employers and course planning arrangements in universities.

3 Greater emphasis should be placed on evidence-based practice (EBP) and evidence-based training (EBT) in mental health services, and undergraduate and postgraduate courses in the university schools of nursing.[35,36]

MENTAL HEALTH SERVICE STANDARDS	
Australia	**New Zealand**
Rights	Tangata Whenua (People of the land)
Safety	Pacific people
Consumer/carer participation	Cultural awareness
Promotes community acceptance	Children and young people
Privacy and confidentiality	Rights
Prevention and promotion	Safety
Cultural awareness	Consumer record and documentation
Integration	Privacy and confidentiality
Service development	Consumer participation
Documentation	Family and carer participation
Delivery of care	Prevention and early intervention
Access and entry	Leadership and management
Assessment and review	Access
Treatment and support	Entry
Community living	Consumer assessment
Supported accommodation	Quality care and treatment
Medical and other technologies	Community support options
Therapies	Discharge planning
Inpatient care	Follow-up and re-entry
Exit planning	Promotes mental health/community acceptance
Exit and re-entry	

FIGURE 71.5 National standards for mental health services. Adapted from Commonwealth of Australia, 1996 and Ministry of Health New Zealand, 1997.

4 Clinical supervision and mentorship programmes[37] should be established for mental health nurses and other health professionals in all mental health services.

5 Mental health nurses should be prepared for practice at both sub-specialist and advanced levels.[38,39]

6 The clinical effectiveness of nursing and multidisciplinary treatment and care practices should become a priority for mental health research.

Development of the nurse practitioner in mental health

The coming decade will also see the widespread introduction of the nurse practitioner (NP), and this will include mental health services. This important development has already necessitated the development of postgraduate nurse practitioner programmes at Master level in New South Wales, with similar initiatives at both Postgraduate Diploma and Master level also taking place elsewhere in Australia and New Zealand. The advent of the mental health nurse practitioner will augment developments in at least four aspects of a population health approach:

❑ Stronger alliances between primary health and mental health services including shared care services with general practitioners.[40]

❑ Improved services in rural and remote regions.

❑ Building prevention and mental health promotion programmes.

❑ Improving the capacity of mental health services to deal with unmet need for mental health care.

Mental health outcomes

Between 2001 and 2003 the New South Wales mental health workforce was given standardized mental health outcomes and assessment training (MHOAT).[41] While this innovative framework, or similar, is likely to be adopted in other parts of the country, it should be acknowledged that successful outcomes for people with mental illness depend on many other factors, besides comprehensive assessment, documentation and outcomes protocols. More needs to be done to lift the skill base and overall performance of the mental health workforce, including mental health nursing. Mental health outcomes foreshadowed by accreditation procedures and national standards for mental health services (see Fig. 71.5)[17,18] depend on a number of factors, including:

raised throughout the chapter. Developments in the first decade of the 21st century are already shaping the future identity and scope of mental health nursing 'down under'. The prospects outlined in this chapter are also, in part, a reflection of hope by the authors as much as attempting to envision the future. The capacity of the discipline to determine it's own place in society rests with its members, its practices, the partnerships forged, and the degree to which mental health nursing is able to assertively reach out into the community it serves.

USEFUL WEBSITES

ANZ College of Mental Health Nurses:
www.anzcmhn.org
ANZCMHN Email Discussion List:
ANZCMHN-subscribe@yahoogroups.com
International. Journal of Mental Health Nursing:
www.blackwellpublishing.com/journals/inm
Centre Psychiatric Nursing Research, Australia:
www.nursing.unimelb.edu.au/cpnrp
Joanna Briggs Institute, Australia:
www.joanna briggs.edu.au
Australian Nursing Council:
www.anci.org.au
Nursing Council of New Zealand:
www.nursingcouncil.org.nz
Royal College of Nursing, Australia: www.rcna.org.au
College of Nurses, NZ: www.nurse.org.nz
Commonwealth Health & Aged Care, Australia:
www.mentalhealth.gov.au
Ministry of Health, NZ: www.moh.govt.nz
Mental Health Council of Australia: www.mhca.com.au
Mental Health Commission, NZ: www.mhc.govt.nz
Nat Health Medical Research Council, Australia:
www.health.gov.au/nhmrc
Health Research Council, NZ: www.hrc.govt.nz
Nursing Review, Australia: www.nursing.camrev.com.au
New Zealand Nursing Review:
www.nursingreview.co.nz
Nursing Careers: www.ncah.com

REFERENCES

1. Australian Health Ministers. *National Mental Health Policy*: 4th reprint, first published 1992. Canberra: Commonwealth Department of Human Services and Health, Australian Government Publishing Service, 1995.
2. Australian Health Ministers. *Second National Mental Health Plan*. Canberra: Mental Health Branch, Commonwealth Department of Health and Family Services, Australian Government Publishing Service, 1998.
3. Mental Health and Special Programs Branch of the Commonwealth Department of Health and Aged Care. *National Mental Health Report 2000: 6th Annual Report*. Changes in Australia's Mental Health Services under the First National Mental Health Plan of the National Mental Health Strategy 1993–98. Canberra: Australian Government Publishing Service, 2000.
4. Jablensky A, McGrath J, Herrman H, *et al*. Psychotic disorders in urban areas: an overview of the study on low prevalence. *Australian and New Zealand Journal of Psychiatry* 2000; **34**: 221–36.
5. Whiteford H, Thompson I, Casey D. The Australian mental health system. *International Journal of Law and Psychiatry* 2000; **23**(3–4): 403–17.
6. Barham P. *Closing the asylum: the mental health patient in modern society*. London: Penguin Books, 1992.
7. Epstein M, Rechter D. Service users as educators, consultants and trainers. In: Deakin Human Services Australia (ed.) *Learning together: education and training partnerships in mental health services*. Final Report. Canberra: Commonwealth Department of Health and Aged Care, Australian Government Publishing Service, 1999: 21–7.
8. Clinton M, Hazelton M. Towards a Foucauldian reading of the Australian mental health nursing workforce. *International Journal of Mental Health Nursing* 2002; **11**(1): 18–23.
9. Clinton M. Why revised standards of practice will not be enough: Guest Editorial. *Australian and New Zealand Journal of Mental Health Nursing* 2001; **10**(1): 1–2.
10. Chesterson J, Clinton M. Scoping the present and planning the future: mental health nursing in Australia and New Zealand. *Journal of the American Psychiatric Nurses Association* 2000; **6**(5):165–9.
11. Chesterson J. Guest Editorial. *Australian and New Zealand Journal of Mental Health Nursing* 1999; **8**(4):121–2.
12. Chesterson J, Clinton M, Muir-Cochrane E. Cutting into the challenges of mental health nursing in the new millennium: mental health special report. *Nursing Review* October 1999; Sect. 15–16.
13. International Council of Nurses. *ICN on regulation: towards 21st century models, 3rd in a series on regulation*. Geneva: ICN, 1998.
14. Durkheim E. *Suicide*. New York: Free Press, 1951.
15. Mental Health and Special Programs Branch of the Commonwealth Department of Health and Aged Care. *Promotion, prevention and early intervention for mental health – a monograph*. Canberra: Australian Government Publishing Service, 2000.
16. Mental Health Commission. *Blueprint for Mental Health Services in New Zealand: how things need to be*. Wellington, NZ: Mental Health Commission, December 1998.
17. Ministry of Health Project Team. *The national

mental health standards. Wellington, NZ: Ministry of Health, Manatu Hauora, June 1997.

18. Project Consortium for the Mental Health Branch of the Commonwealth Department of Health and Family Services. *National standards for mental health services.* Canberra: Commonwealth Department of Health and Family Services, January 1997.

19. Mental Health Commission. *The funding needed for mental health services in New Zealand.* Wellington, NZ: Mental Health Commission, December 1998.

20. Australian and New Zealand College of Mental Health Nurses. *Standards of practice for mental health nursing in Australia.* PO Box 126, Greenacres, SA 5086: ANZCMHN, 1995.

21. Australian and New Zealand College of Mental Health Nurses. *Standards of practice for mental health nursing in New Zealand.* PO Box 83–111 Edmonton Road, Auckland, NZ: ANZCMHN, 1995.

22. Australian Nursing Council. *Code of professional conduct for nurses in Australia.* Canberra: ANCI, 1995.

23. Australian Nursing Council. *Code of ethics for nurses in Australia.* Canberra: ANCI, 1993.

24. Horsfall J, Cleary M, Jordan R. *Towards ethical mental health nursing practice: monograph.* PO Box 126, Greenacres, SA 5086: Australian and New Zealand College of Mental Health Nurses, 1999.

25. Australian and New Zealand College of Mental Health Nurses. *Setting the standard: a history of the Australian and New Zealand College of Mental Health Nurses.* PO Box 126, Greenacres, SA 5086: ANZCMHN, 1999.

26. Royal College of Nursing Australia. *Credentialing advanced nursing practice and accreditation of continuing education programs: an exploration of issues and perspectives,* Discussion Paper No. 4. Canberra: RCNA, September 1996.

27. Royal College of Nursing Australia. *The feasibility of a national approach for the credentialing of advanced practice nurses and the accreditation of related educational programs;* Final Report. Canberra: RCNA, July 2001.

28. Hazelton M, Farrell G, Biro P. *Self-regulation and credentialing in mental health nursing: a report to the Nursing Board of Tasmania.* PO Box 126, Greenacres, SA: Steering Committee, for the Australian and New Zealand College of Mental Health Nurses, October 1998.

29. Chesterson J. *Credential for practice program (CPP): Report to Council* – Unpublished. PO Box 126, Greenacres, SA 5086: Australian and New Zealand College of Mental Health Nurses, April 2002.

30. Clinton M. *Scoping study of the Australian mental health nursing workforce 1999.* Report from the Australian and New Zealand College of Mental Health Nurses to the Mental Health and Specials Programs Branch of the Commonwealth Department of Health and Aged Care. Canberra: Commonwealth Department of Health and Aged Care, Australian Government Publishing Service, May 2001.

31. Clinton M, Hazelton M. Scoping the prospects of Australian mental health nursing. *Australian and New Zealand College of Mental Health Nurses* 2000; 9(4):159–65.

32. Clinton M, Hazelton M. Scoping practice issues on the Australian mental health nursing workforce. *Australian and New Zealand Journal of Mental Health Nursing* 2000; 9(3):100–109.

33. Clinton M, Hazelton M. Scoping the Australian mental health nursing workforce. *Australian and New Zealand Journal of Mental Health Nursing* 2000; 9(2): 50–64.

34. Clinton M, Hazelton M. Scoping mental health nursing education. *Australian and New Zealand Journal of Mental Health Nursing* 2000; 9(1): 2–10.

35. Newell R, Gournay K (eds). *Mental health nursing: an evidence-based approach.* Edinburgh: Churchill Livingstone, 2000.

36. Farrell G. *Getting up to speed with evidence-based practice: monograph.* PO Box 126, Greenacres, SA 5086: Australian and New Zealand College of Mental Health Nurses, 1997.

37. Butterworth T, Faugier J (eds). *Clinical supervision and mentorship in nursing.* London: Chapman and Hall, 1992.

38. Clinton M, Nelson S (eds). *Advanced practice in mental health nursing.* Oxford: Blackwell Science, 1999.

39. Shea CA, Pelletier LR, Poster EC, Stuart GW, Verhey MP (eds). *Advanced practice nursing in psychiatric and mental health care.* St Louis: Mosby, 1999.

40. Davies J. *A manual of mental health care in general practice.* Canberra: Mental Health and Special Programs Branch, of the Commonwealth Department of Health and Aged Care, Australian Government Publishing Service, 2000.

41. Centre for Mental Health. *Mental health outcomes and assessment training (MH-OAT).* [online] 2001 [cited 2002 May 18]: NSW Health. Available from: URL: www.health.nsw.gov.au/policy/cmh/mhoat.

42. Hazelton M, Farrell G. *Evaluating the outcomes of mental health care: an introduction, monograph.* PO Box 126, Greenacres, SA 5086: Australian and New Zealand College of Mental Health Nurses, 1998.

43. Andrews G, Peters L, Teesson M. *The measurement of consumer outcome in mental health.* Canberra: AHMAC, National Mental Health Working Group, Mental Health Branch, Commonwealth Department of Human Services and Health, October 1994.

44. Mental Health and Special Programs Branch of the Commonwealth Department of Health and Aged Care.

National Action Plan for Promotion, Prevention and Early Intervention for Mental Health. Canberra: Australian Government Publishing Service, 2000.

45. Barker P. *The philosophy and practice of psychiatric nursing.* Edinburgh: Churchill Livingston, 1999.

46. Peplau H. *Interpersonal relations in nursing.* New York: G.P. Putnam, 1952.

47. Barker P. The Tidal Model: developing an empowering, person-centred approach to recovery within psychiatric and mental health nursing. *Journal of Psychiatric and Mental Health Nursing* 2001; 8(3): 233–40.

48. Barker P. *The Tidal Model: international mental health recovery model.* [online] 1999 [cited 2002 May 18]: Clan Unity PLC. Available from: URL: www.tidal–model.co.uk.

49. Barker P, Campbell P, Davidson B (eds). *From the ashes of experience.* London: Whurr, 1999.

50. Barker P, Chesterson J. The logic of experience: developing appropriate care through effective collaboration. In: Barker P (ed.) *The philosophy and practice of psychiatric nursing.* Edinburgh: Churchill Livingstone, 1999: 117–32.

51. Commonwealth Department of Human Services and Health. Mental Health Statement of Rights and Responsibilities: 2nd reprint, first published 1991. Canberra: Commonwealth of Australia, AGPS, 1995.

52. Human Rights and Equal Opportunity Commission. Human Rights and Mental Illness: Report of the National Inquiry into the Human Rights of People with Mental Illness. Canberra: Australian Government Publishing Service, 1993.

53. Department of Foreign Affairs and Trade. *Human rights manual.* Canberra: Australian Government Publishing Service, 1993.

54. Commonwealth Department of Health Housing and Community Services. *Social justice for people with disabilities.* Canberra: Commonwealth of Australia, AGPS, 1991.

55. Barker P, Davidson B (eds). *Ethical strife.* London: Arnold, 1998.

56. Barker P, Baldwin S (eds). *Ethical issues in mental health.* London: Chapman and Hall, 1991.

57. Bloch S, Choldoff P, Green A (eds). *Psychiatric ethics*, 3rd edn. Oxford: Oxford University Press, 1999.

Chapter 72

THE PRIMACY OF CARING

Phil Barker

INTRODUCTION

One hopes that the future of mental health nursing will be defined by an inquisitive approach to what constitutes mental health *care* and mental health *promotion*. One would hope, also, that nurses will consider to what extent *health* care actually exists within, if not beyond, the complex facades of the mental *illness*-focused systems, which dominate the field of mental health.

Increasingly, I have come to doubt that any such ethos of inquiry holds much currency in the disputes over 'knowledge' and 'evidence' in health care. Although the *science*, which is increasingly touted as the Royal Road to Mental Health, may have originated in the armchair reflections of Enlightenment philosophers, philosophical reflection about the nature of science and scientific inquiry, and the validity of research findings has become, almost, a red card offence in the halls of psychiatric academe.

Almost since its inception, psychiatry was a divided realm; split between those who sought to explain 'mentally aberrant' phenomena, by reference to some putative underlying, physical cause; and those who appeared to be in search of understanding of the many different ways of being human, that disturb society, the person, or both. If a blunt distinction between the two camps is necessary, the former are represented by a medical (or medicalized) practice, which locates itself, firmly – if not always appropriately – within the realm of science. The latter is a ragbag non-medical grouping, more concerned with addressing the immediate needs of dispossessed and disadvantaged people, than with winning Nobel prizes. Clarke saw this distinction personified in the classic confrontation between the assertively biological approach that begat the physical treatments of ECT and psychosurgery, and the libertarian approaches that spawned therapeutic communities, if not the whole 'anti-psychiatry' movement.[1] The former was enacted best, in his view, by the English psychiatrist William Sargant, who saw himself as 'a physician in the practice of psychological medicine'.[2] The latter was best illustrated by the hero with feet of clay – R.D. Laing[3] – who postulated the possibilities of a 'philosophical psychiatry', in which the madman might be co-opted as brother-philosopher.[4]

Even a casual study of the archives of the Psychiatric Nursing Internet List,[5] referred to by several authors in this book, reveals that the practising nurses and academics who represent its international membership, belong to similarly divided realms; albeit influenced by differing, and changeable, economic and political forces. However, if the Internet nursing list is in any way a representative sample of the constituency of mental health nursing, then beyond the banal assumptions of the need for 'holistic care' or the curse of 'illness' and the ambition of 'wellness', little consensus exists as to the virtue, far less the value, of *care* as a core construct for practice.

This book has covered a broad, though by no means comprehensive, canvas of psychiatric/mental health nursing practice. Although the majority of the authors have emphasized the creative nature of 'caring' for people in mental distress, others have addressed the role of various theoretical positions in shaping 'protocols' of treatment for 'patients' or 'clients. Given the shifting nature of mental health services and the policies that underpin them, it has been possible in this book only to address some of the more important elements of nursing, illustrated by some examples of the clinical population that nurses serve, and some of the theories and models that frame contemporary practice. It seems fitting, in this conclusion, to return to the seedbed of nursing practice, to consider the nature of caring, which – at least traditionally – has been the key feature of the discipline.

RECOVERING NURSING CARE

Recovery and reclamation

Given that the subtext of this book, if not its overarching ambition, has been the development of mental health and the minimization of mental distress, it seems obvious that we should consider what these phenomena represent and how they relate to being human. At the beginning of the 21st century, curiosity about what it means to be human appears to be waning. A century ago modern psychiatry chased the vain ambition of curing all the ills that might, literally or metaphorically, afflict the human soul. Today, it is largely focused on the genetic and biochemical underbelly of human experience. The soul or the *psyche* has been lost from the field of psychiatric vision. Interest in the nature of what it means to be human – well or ill – has become the province of the human development or 'personal growth' movement which, it has to be said, is largely disinterested in anyone who might be classed as 'mentally ill'. Personal growth is a euphemism for capitalistic iconography. In Brandon's view,[6] this was an exercise in self-diminishment. People who are attracted to the notion of 'improving' or 'growing' themselves, must first begin by buying the notion that they are faulty or stunted. Jerome Frank saw the folly of this, arguably, more clearly than most:

> Ironically, mental health education, which aims to teach people how to cope more effectively with life, has instead increased the demand for psychotherapeutic help. By calling attention to symptoms they might otherwise ignore and by labelling those symptoms as signs of neurosis, mental health education can create unwarranted anxieties, leading those to seek psychotherapy who do not need it. The demand for psychotherapy keeps pace with the supply, and at times one has the uneasy feeling that the supply may be creating the demand.[7]

This view makes a lot of sense to me, a 'baby-boomer' from working-class stock. In Scotland we used to say, 'the working class man doesn't suffer from stress. He has to get up for work in the morning'. Certainly that was true of my father, and in an egalitarian sense, of my mother, who rose before him, to pave the way for his 5 a.m. start. Neither would have understood the question, far less had an answer, if we had asked about the state of their self-*esteem* or self-*concept*. Brandon, who emerged from a similar background, noted wryly that today people are rapidly becoming like characters in a Woody Allen film, living 'intentionally' and, in trying:

> to increase our options and estimate every conceivable consequence; fun and spontaneity are reserved for the annual fortnight holiday in Benidorm, Ibiza or river rafting along the Amazon.[8]

This culture shift[9] has rippled out to the shores of mental health where:

> Consumers demand services that are easier to access. Everything from education upwards and downwards must be glycerined. (But) As Kenyon (1997) wrote: 'The fact is that Brahms needs effort, not just on the part of the performer but from the listener. And we underestimate that at our peril. The big classical works – not just the huge symphonies of Bruckner and Mahler and the operas of Wagner, but also Handel operas, Bach cantatas – make demands on the listener just as do a great book or a great picture'.[10]

Recovery in mental health – or the engagement process that might be part of its genesis – must be hard work and must occupy a very different territory from the sunny horizons of much personal growth psychology. I have met few, if any, 'survivors' who said that they had no difficulty in buying their ticket to 'recovery-land' or that they dithered idly over which of the many therapeutic options might be *easiest* for them. Yet, the ravenous, 'I-want-it-yesterday', attitude, which is part of the fallout from the follies of the Me-generation, looks set to consume the narrative about recovery, and human possibility, in the way that only the best (or worst) consumerist models can.

Already we have imported the American obsession with litigation, not just to recover appropriate compensation for malpractice, but also to use as another way to vent our anger at the vagaries of fate. We need, however, to ask what is the value of such compensation. Can any such loss ever be fully compensated and, more importantly, is this a distraction from the necessary work of *reclamation*? I cannot prove it, but the evidence of the need to embrace the pain and suffering of madness, as part of the recovery process, rather than to rail against it, litters my everyday experience.[11] Recovery involves a strenuous journey, taken over very rocky ground. The engagement process, that seeks to aid and abet recovery, is an equally daunting task, that can take the helper close to the edge of their own core humanity, and can – on occasions – tip them over, into the abyss of their own human incompetence. Those who seek to help people make these journeys – through the desert of their distress, hopefully to quench their thirst for wholeness at the well of genuine well-ness, may need to accept that their role is more that of support, confidante and witness, rather than active healer. Perhaps the healing lies not in the destination but in the taking of the recovery journey itself; in the whole process of trying to re-claim one's self, one's life, and one's place in the wider community of souls.

The nonsense of 'effective' nursing

I remind myself, at least of some of these human facts, before proceeding. The twin pursuits of happiness and human excellence, which have become the mainstays of the humanistic, personal growth camps, have bred, albeit inadvertently, the contemporary obsession with celebrity, the beauty myth and the vicarious pleasures that are the virtual fuel of the mass media. If my parents' generation spent most of their waking hours engaged with the everyday business of working, laughing, weeping and loving, today people spend a fair proportion of their time watching the carefully rehearsed, or disingenuously candid lifestyles of people behind the Big Brother camera, facilitated through a Jerry Springer-type panel, or enacted in one soap opera or another. These distractions – for they take us away from our 'lived experience' of being here and now – gloss over the true complexity of life, as it is lived, as surely as our eyes glaze over before the one-eyed god in the corner of our living room. Orwell would, doubtless, be distressed that not only has his National Lottery become fact but also that his nightmarish Big Brother has become a post-modern icon. These concerns have generalized to mental health where, as Clarke noted, nursing has become self-satisfied with its:

> pursuit of 'professionalism', accompanied by the easy acceptance of forensic incarceration, the happy embrace of the techniques of 'control and restraint', the abysmal absence of irony at the sinister language of 'assertive outreach'. The benightedness that refuses to accept the complexities, conscious or otherwise, that lead some patients to decline treatments; the accompanying denial

that civil liberties may be violated when compulsorily 'treating' patients 'in the community' are all typical of such modern discourse.[12]

In his essay on 'The Nonsense of Effectiveness', Don Bannister[13] famously said that, were he to ask how *effective* a conversation was, he would need to begin by questioning the question. Given the many possible meanings of 'effective' it would be nonsense simply to ask it. Mental health professionals have largely 'bought' the nonsense of 'effectiveness' and abandoned the inquisitiveness that Bannister thought *de rigeur.* In Clarke's view there is no greater offender than nursing, which appears most comfortable in offering grossly institutionalized responses to people in mental distress. This is not a problem, since we cannot see the people diminished by such institutionalized responses, hidden as they are, by the multiple barriers to human engagement that bolster the bureaucracy of mental health services.

What has any of this to do with mental health care and, specifically, the discipline of nursing? Given that nursing has, traditionally, been caught in the long shadow cast by psychiatric medicine, and has frequently been coloured by changing sociopolitical mores, it is not surprising that, today, mental health nursing (as it euphemistically describes itself) is undergoing radical changes. Ironically, few of these changes (in these self-directed times) are of nursing's own making. In this concluding reflection on the state of the craft of nursing, I beg some simple questions about the basis of the discipline of caring for people in mental distress[a] and consider what a radical[b] model of caring in mental health might involve.

If nursing, as a discipline, were based on the reflective practitioner models in common academic currency, nurses might ask, routinely, the following question:

> Would I be happy (or content, or satisfied) to be committed for care and/or treatment within the service in which I presently am working?

More importantly, they might reflect on the most vulnerable member of their family or social circle: someone whom they love – a parent, or a child or a friend. In reflecting on that person's essential vulnerability, they might become aware of how they are touched, invisibly, in the way that the power of emotions touches everyone. For every patient[c] is someone's parent, or child, or sibling, or lover or friend. They might well ask:

> Would I be happy to commit this person to the care of the services of which I am a part?

---

[a] I assume that the contractual relationship between nurses and the people in their care involves addressing the human distress that people, or others, believe exists in the abstract space called the mind. In that sense, the person is distressed by, or distressing to, others.

[b] In the sense of addressing the *root*, or fundamentals, of the process of caring.

[c] Although the term *patient* increasingly has been replaced by the euphemisms, client, user or consumer, the term patient remains true, at least in the sense that it denotes the potential for suffering. It also can be used, ironically, to suggest the patience required of people awaiting mental health workers to do something to help them with their distress.

Few nurses ask this question, framed as it is within this highly personal context. Moreover, when I have asked nurses to offer a heartfelt response to this question, some find the interrogation painful, others view it as a manipulative assignment. Although statistics always flatter to deceive, less than 5% of any audience has ever answered 'yes'. The catch – for indeed the question is manipulative – lies in the context of commitment.

Conversational realities

The answer to these questions says something about our attitude to commitment, in its dual senses, since it means both to pledge oneself – involving the act of charitable giving – but also means (or used to mean) the act of consigning someone to the care of another. Today, the caring destination to which society consigns people in mental distress is more likely to be characterized by little more than confinement. Indeed the commitment embraced by many care agencies is framed in the manner of Pilate, who through his literal act of washing his hands of Jesus, provided us with the apt metaphor for consigning (or committing) people to the hands of others. Although it may be unfashionable, there may be a virtue in recalling what words, at least, used to mean.

Commitment reminds us that we have the power to pledge ourselves and, at the same time, the power to abdicate – leaving people and their problems to be addressed by others or, as can be the case, leaving people to be exposed to the vagaries of fortune. Commitment might, therefore, mean opting in but it can also mean opting out. For a discipline that emerged from a one-thousand-year-old vocational history[14,15] nursing in the 21st century might care to ask itself, to what extent it is still involved in providing the conditions under which the person might be healed, by Nature or by God. Or, in its pursuit of institutionalized power[16] has it surrendered its lofty if diffuse ideals in favour of a more pragmatic social-policing role?[17]

Power comes in a variety of forms and few of these are not disguises. The everyday business of engaging with others involves a careful balancing act – ensuring that we display just enough vulnerability to complement the power of the other, while at the same time hoping that they will reciprocate in much the same way. Such engagement is always risky since, by exposing our vulnerability, however fleetingly, we risk losing the chance to influence the proceedings. We risk losing the advantage, which often we feign not to possess. At times, the boundaries of our selves can become blurred within such exchanges as we dance a verbal tango, weaving our

words – and the selves for which they advocate – seamlessly, yet provocatively, with the words of the other. The interpersonal paradigm, framed famously by Hildegard Peplau in the 1950s, is viewed by some as outmoded, in this era of 'case management' and 'brief intervention'.[18] However, when invited to explore the possible basis of their unique role, most nurses quickly identify the abstract, but all too real, interpersonal exchange – whether verbal or non-verbal – that takes place when nurse meets patient.[19] The comparison of a conversation with a dance may be apposite, since – at least from the observer's standpoint – it is not entirely clear who is leading, and who is following. In functional terms, we could say that all true human relationships involve a temporary sacrifice of the self. As the Irish poet W.B. Yeats wisely remarked, 'how can we know the dancer from the dance?' This begs the question, of course: 'how true are our therapeutic relations?' Are we pledging ourselves as helping (i.e. potentially helpful) agent? Or are our relations with people in care no more than political in character, paying only lip-service to the notion of human engagement?

METAPHORS AND MADNESS

We began this century with lofty ideals about furthering the medical notion of finding various cures for *mental illness*. Increasingly, however, we have come to doubt the validity of that core construct. Despite the fashionable assumption, predicated on a largely North American infatuation with genetics and biomedicine, that the riddle of madness[d] will, ultimately, be found in the gene pool, or in the size of one's ventricles, madness, in its various guises, is enjoying a renaissance. Perhaps we only have more ways of classifying and categorizing it, but the mad world recognized by Laing in the mid 1960s, where one in four would be manifestly distressed, if not disabled, by some form of madness, has come to pass. Indeed, Laing's figures seem a little conservative, for such a supposedly radical voice. To some extent the contemporary classification of any or all human foibles as one form of mental disorder or dysfunction or another provides an echo of Freud's once provocative thesis concerning the predatory way that our deepest pathology insinuates its way into our everyday lives.

History may well conclude that Thomas Szasz's assertion that mental illness was a myth was finally found to be right, although many would say, for all the wrong reasons.[20] The human phenomenon called 'mental illness' or 'mental disorder' has many correlates – biological, chemical, psychological and social. However, as Szasz has

---

[d] I have been encouraged by several friends in the survivor/user movement to prefer this expression, which conveys something of the majesty and horror of mental distress. It is, at the very least, preferable to the ludicrous euphemisms – such as 'mental health problems' – which increasingly hold sway.

recently noted, in physics, we use the same laws to explain why planes fly, and why they crash. However, psychiatry uses one set of laws to explain so-called *sane* behaviour, attributable to choices (reason) and another set to explain *insane* behaviour, attributed to causes (disease). For Szasz this was akin to the theory of phlogiston, once presumed to be a part of the nature of combustion.[21] What is actually *going on* within and around people when they are described as in states of 'mental illness' is, to say the least, highly complex, but is predicated on the same laws of choosing and reasoning as other aspects of the person's life. These ways of being human[22] involve a different set of behaviours, but stem from the same root of reason and choice. A frivolous, but meaningful example might be the all too common experience of encountering someone, described as in a 'florid psychosis' (and, according to traditional psychiatric wisdom, completely out of touch with reality) who manages to suspend the psychotic state long enough to beg, light and subsequently smoke a cigarette. Coleman offered similar examples, from his own experience, of how the apparently irrational behaviour of the person in psychosis, is a mask for the highly intentional choices of the person.[23] The reality of madness is that others – family, friends, neighbours, professionals – do not appreciate the choices of the 'mad' person. Indeed, on reflection, some people regret the choices they made when in a state of mental distress. However, this does not diminish their status as choices.

Despite all the presumed advances made in the recognition of different forms of mental illness or disorder, no clinical tests have been developed to establish, scientifically, whether or not a person *has* schizophrenia, bipolar disorder or any one of the forms of personality disorder that currently abound. Instead, practitioners continue to reply on diagnostic tests, which differ only in structure, from the social or personal constructs that frame our ideas of beauty or ugliness. This is hardly surprising since, mental distress/illness/disorder is a metaphor and, as such, is beyond clinical measurement. Any 'mental' disorders for which formal diagnostic test exist, become 'physical' disorders – like Huntington's chorea or cerebrovascular dementia. These are physical disorders with mental symptoms, no more and no less.

The metaphor of problems

In a remarkable body-swerve, some sections of the contemporary mental health community have abandoned the debate about the phlogiston status of mental illness, in favour of talking about 'mental health problems'. Ironically, they are echoing Szasz's original advocacy of Harry Stack Sullivan's use of the term 'problems of living', which he coined to describe the ways of being human shown by people in psychotic states.[24] 'Problems'

connote the kind of things that disturb people in the social world, rather than in the abstract world occupied by concepts such as health and illness. However, this also implies that such problems will be amenable to solutions. The English poet and critic, Al Alvarez, writing of his own suicide attempt, observed how, initially, as in a dream, he believed that his death would solve the problem of his life.

> I thought death would be like that: a synoptic vision of life, crisis by crisis, all suddenly explained, justified, redeemed, a Last Judgement in the coils and circuits of the brain. Instead, all I got was a hole in the head, a round zero, nothing. I'd been swindled.[25]

With remarkable foresight, Alvarez anticipated the emergence of the 'problem-solving' ethos that underpins many of today's services.

> The despair that had led me to try to kill myself had been pure and unadulterated, like the final, unanswerable despair a child feels, with no before or after. And childishly, I had expected death not merely to end it but also to explain it. Then, when death let me down, I gradually saw that I had been using the wrong language: I had translated the thing into Americanese. Too many movies, too many novels, too many trips to the States had switched my understanding into a hopeful, alien tongue. I no longer thought of myself as unhappy; instead I had 'problems'. Which is an optimistic way of putting it, since problems imply solutions, whereas unhappiness is merely a condition of life, which you must live with, like the weather. Once I had accepted that there weren't ever going to be any answers, even in death, I found to my surprise that I didn't much care whether I was happy or unhappy: 'problems' and 'the problem of problems', no longer existed. And that in itself is already the beginning of happiness.[26]

In some respects, Alvarez remains *avant-garde*. Today, even the mental health user/consumer movement has embraced the notion of 'problems' without appreciating how they have surrendered to the American obsession with solving (often aggressively), every difficulty that life throws up. Alvarez's gentle alternative is more provocative and draws from an Oriental tradition concerning acceptance, which is only slowly gaining ground in the West. In re-defining as problems, the wildest vagaries of heart and mind, we suggest that all such disruptions are amenable to solutions. Of course, in so doing we aid and abet, perhaps unwittingly, the generation of more and more 'prescribed solutions' for our various human ills. If Jenner *et al.* are right, and 'serious' forms of madness, like schizophrenia, are more a 'way of being human' than an 'illness' or 'disorder', then the challenge is to work out how to help people live with, accept, or make human sense of such experiences, rather than to 'fix' them.[27]

The metaphor of nursing

While political correctness clearly has changed the surface texture of madness, the phenomena that our linguistic contortions signify remain much the same. Some mental health 'problems' are malign forces, disabling and ultimately destroying personhood, if we fail to address them. Others are little more than signs that we are alive and smarting from the teachings of the resident philosopher within us all, called experience. However, in both cases, we need to consider how we respond to such human distress – whether it is called a serious mental illness, or some presumably trivial form of human upset.[28] These are not lofty philosophical issues. This is the very stuff of everyday life. What, exactly, are we dealing with when we talk about *nursing* people with mental health problems? Nurses, perhaps more than any other discipline, appear content to talk about applying *mental health nursing* to various forms of mental *illness*, when clearly health and illness lie at opposite ends of some hypothetical spectrum. Sadly, this is all too typical of the monocular vision bred of political correctness. More important, stands the question – how do we go about dealing with such phenomena?

Today, more than at any time in psychiatric history, we have become obsessed with certain kinds of evidence, and questions about the efficacy and efficiency of interventions. An all too common question, increasingly asked by nurses, keen not to be viewed as *passé*, is – does this or that intervention 'work'? An intriguing if naïve question, since everything 'works' in some way, even when it seems to be doing nothing – which is an outcome in itself. Alvarez's 'solution' *worked*, although he did nothing, other than to accept his state of mind. Perhaps the question we need to be asking is:

❏ in *what way* does any intervention work;
❏ to *whose specific end*; and
❏ to *what particular purpose* (or outcome)?'[e]

When people called nurses are involved in a process that they, or others, call human *engagement* we need to ask: 'what (exactly) is going on?' Rather than focus blindly on what might happen, as a (presumed) consequence of this process, we might try to understand the shifting patterns that characterize the quality of this engagement.

Of course, all of this is metaphorical. Things don't *work* in the way people called 'workers' work. We simply can't find any other way to describe such happenings, without comparing it to something else. Metaphor is vital to the world of mental illness since, as Tom Szasz[29] has repeatedly pointed out, whatever it is that we are dealing with – and he was in no doubt that people were in distress – such distress was not an illness, as such.[30]

Today we talk about buildings being *sick* and the economy being *sick*, reminding us, perhaps, that the sickness that overtakes these inanimate things might be close to the sickness of the soul or the spirit that we call mental illness. Given the context of nursing, where many of the functions involved in caring, involve the manipulation (metaphorically) of abstract elements – support, platonic love, respect, dignity, power – it is important that nursing, as a discipline, recognizes that its vocation belongs to a quite different territory of evidence: the world of human experience and, arguably, aesthetics.

The Tidal Metaphor

The *Tidal Model* [31] is predicated on the assumption that human experience is fluid. Experience ebbs and flows, like the tides of our seas and river estuaries. The Tidal Model also acknowledges that the life force – or *prajna* as it is called in the East – flows in and out of us, with each inhalation and exhalation. As we breathe in and out, we balance – literally – on the cusp of life and death.[32–34] The power of water is not something that can be controlled. However, if we learn to acknowledge how it *works*, it may be understood. Such understanding can illuminate us. We know that we can drown in a few inches of water, but the same amount of water can cleanse our system. It is a strange force that can kill or cure. The Tidal Model, which began as a *professional* nursing model of care[35] has been extended to embrace the nursing relationship that might be engaged in by any helping agent.[36] Wilkin wisely noted in Chapter 64 that in all human relationships, there is no exact science to help us to navigate our relations with others, far less ourselves.

> The light which experience gives is a lantern on the stern, which shines only on the waves behind us!

One person's experience (the nurse) of another (the patient) flows in and through the other, in a constantly changing narrative.[37] It is true that if a nurse gives a person a drug, the drug will have an effect on the bodily chemistry of the person who is the patient. However, if we recognize that nursing is fundamentally about relating to people through the exchange and development of narratives – as opposed to giving drugs for example – it becomes clear that it is folly to ask if such relating 'works'. The question that needs to be asked is 'how' does it work? In what way does it work? What 'happens' when the nurse encounters the person who is patient?

The power of water, as used within the Tidal Model, is a metaphor for the killing or curing of the spirit that we used to call madness. That at least a few people have

---

[e] I am indebted to my friend Thomas Szasz for helping me appreciate the simple, yet challenging, logic of 'efficacy'.

described the process of emergence from madness in positive terms, illustrates the *spiritual* nature of the experience itself.[38,39] Although it is hardly popular, I no longer apologize for talking about psychiatric care in *spiritual* terms, for madness does appear to be the place where the spirit of women and men risks extinction.[40] When we stop to consider the importance of even the simplest of interactions with this valuable, vulnerable person who – temporarily – is the patient, we realize that this is a sacred space, and we need to tread carefully and sensitively. We need to consider to what extent we might have the wisdom, rather than the technical know-how, to help facilitate this process of recovery, re-emergence and reclamation.

RECOVERY PARADIGMS

What are nurses talking about when they talk of *engaging* people in mental distress? We engage with nothing more than their stories – the representations of themselves and their experiences, which have come to represent their understanding of who they are what they mean as *persons*. It seems axiomatic that people can – at one moment – appear to be in great distress, and – at another moment – can appear to be *relieved* of their suffering, discomfort or pain. Nurses working within the assumptions of the Tidal Model are interested to know how such change occurs. In particular, they are interested to know what part the person played in this change and what part the nurse can play in fostering this positive change. The Model assumes that nurses learn from people about the nature of their distress, here and now and, in so doing, learn what, if anything, might 'need to be done'[f] to help alleviate it.

However we should urge caution against rushing in to alleviate distress, or at least we should avoid forcing the re-shaping of the narrative that is a person's life. Too many of our contemporary models emphasize what Szasz[41] has called a 'cruel compassion'. *Psychoeducation* may be one such example of cruel compassion. In their *Cochrane Centre* review, Pekkala and Merinder[42] noted that:

> schizophrenia can be a severe and chronic illness characterized by lack of insight and poor compliance with treatment. Psychoeducational approaches have been developed to increase patients' awareness of their illness and its treatment.

I defy Pekkala and Merinder to tell me, unequivocally, what is the nature of this *illness* called schizophrenia. What do they know of the illness that is not visible to my eyes and audible to my ears? They talk 'as if' schizophrenia is like diabetes, or some form of cancer, or HIV – and can be confirmed by some laboratory test, or refined medical examination. In truth, it can only be *judged* to be present (or absent) by the subjective impressions of the diagnostician. This is not to deny the emotional severity and, often, the social disability that can accompany a person who is *in* the human state, which we call schizophrenia (or any other psychiatric *condition*). I do not doubt their sincerity, but Pekkala and Merinder shine little light on the phenomena of madness (like schizophrenia) but merely ask us to try harder in accepting the darkness.

Similarly '*compliance* therapy' (sic) may also be a cruel euphemism for obliging people to see the world from our perspective and ours alone.[43] Given the contemporary ambition of nursing to 'empower' itself, it is unsurprising that many nurses are keen to adopt such approaches, which blatantly dis-empower the person further. Sadly, the fact that they can only gain such power, at the expense of the person in their care, escapes most nurses. Having cast ourselves in the role of psychiatric experts, it is rarely easy to acknowledge that really we know nothing of any consequence about the experience of mental distress. Humility and professionalism appear to live at opposite ends of the psychiatric street.

The story of recovery

We need to remember that the current page of the storybook of a person's life – how anyone is *here and now* – is only the latest entry in a story that has a meaningful beginning. For many people, their understanding of where they are, *now*, and what they need to do, *now*, to move forward, lies in an appreciation of where they first began to experience their distress.

For Pat Deegan[44] the first real signs of that distress originated in what she has called the desolation of winter – the season of anguish. For anguish involves living in terrible pain, which seems endless and futile, and leads to nothing more than more pain. When people begin to take a stand against that anguish they transform it into suffering. In Pat Deegan's own experience of madness, this stand was 'redemptive'. Ron Coleman[45] took a stand against his own anguish, as well as against the psychiatric system that heaped grief on top of anguish. Ron learned how to suffer for others as well as himself. Therein lay the seeds of his recovery. Suffering breaks the cycle of anguish when pain becomes something that will never be forgotten, but can be used to help people to move forward. We need to ask:

---

[f] This idea is borrowed from Japanese Morita Therapy, which in turn is heavily influenced by Zen thought about the need to learn from the 'reality of experience.

- ❑ How do nurses help people transform their anguish into suffering?
- ❑ How do they help them to use their spiritual pain to step from the darkness of alienation into the light?

There are no easy answers to these questions. What seems clear is that much of what passes as standard 'mental health nursing' practice is far removed from such facilitation. Many people who have been forcibly drugged, injected, restrained, placed under 'observation', or otherwise 'treated', describe such experiences as rape. A loaded word if ever there was one, but the cowering Self, who has witnessed the savage power of madness might be forgiven for expecting mental health nurses to represent *psychiatric rescue*, rather than what someone in one of my studies called 'adding insult to injury'. How can we assure the people committed to our care that they will not be subjected to the rape of the Self?

The enigma of empowerment

Addressing disempowerment is rarely easy, especially in traditional custodial institutions – and I use the term advisedly – like acute psychiatric wards and more secure settings. We talk about participating and collaborating with people in our care. But how do we do this? Cahill identified five attributes, which were necessary for participation to occur.[46]

- ❑ A relationship needs to exist. We are not talking here about simply interacting – but of relating. I interact with a computer but I do not have a relationship with it.
- ❑ The knowledge and information gap between the nurse and the person needs to be narrowed – the person needs to know what is going on and why.
- ❑ Power needs to be surrendered to a degree. It is folly to talk of giving this up entirely. Even if you wished to do so, you cannot shake off the invisible power of psychiatric authority.
- ❑ Selective intellectual and/or physical activities need to occur, which will lead to
- ❑ Some positive benefit for the person who is the patient.

In essence, the nurse needs to 'do' something '*with*' the person, which might be construed as empowering. This kind of relatedness is what Irene Whitehill – the user-advocate – and I have called 'caring with' the person.[47] We need to care *about* the person – which is the basis of our compassion. Sometimes we may show that by caring *for* the person, when they are vulnerable. But the empowering basis of participatory care involves *caring with*. If we do this, at the very least, we avoid contributing further to their disempowerment.

When the spirit of the person begins to break, the loss of hope and, ultimately, the will to live isn't far behind. The loss of hope inspires the need to develop what I have called 'hopelines'. The instillation of hope, even if only the hope for a peaceful death, lies at the heart of care. We cannot afford to ignore the power of hopelessness and its partner helplessness. Some of the finest accounts of how people submit to hopelessness and how they also kept the flame of the spirit alive, are to be found in the accounts of Holocaust survivors. Viktor Frankl touched his own spirit when he experienced torture and medical experimentation at the hands of Nazi doctors.[48] Frankl experienced his epiphany when one day he realized that no matter what they did to him, they could never touch his human essence. In that moment he made contact with the invisible spirit within him and he grasped his own power. Holding, metaphorically, on to the invisible power of Viktor Frankl he knew that he could never be defeated. Killed perhaps, in body, but never destroyed in spirit.

It was perhaps no accident that Frankl went on to establish a psychotherapy that helped develop a focus on the spirit. Logotherapy[49] focused on helping people to find the personal meaning of their distress and from this meaning to build hope for change and the future.

Only a few of us have had the kind of human schooling, that sensitized Frankl to 'what needs to be done' to help people in distress. However, we all have the same potential to *care with* people, to empower them. However, we must take some risks with our own selfhood to make such an engagement.

I–Thou and I–It

We might consider the possibility that some of the 'problems' shown by the people in our care might be examples of their taking a stand against the rape of the Self. Nurses often talk glibly of people being *non-compliant, treatment resistive, lacking insight* or *passive–aggressive*. These are not simply highly judgemental terms, for which we need to find a politically correct euphemism. These are simply the wrong way to 'read' people, at least if we care to understand them. People Like Pat Deegan, Sally Clay, Irene Whitehill and Ron Coleman have taught us how such kinds of active resistance can be life-enhancing. These may be signs of the person's strength and refusal to succumb to hopelessness. This 'resistance' is something we need to build on, through mutual understanding, not crush through further manipulation. As Anne Helm illustrated in Chapter 7, such resistances are the building blocks of the process of recovery and reclamation.

I am aware that such a view will not satisfy our political masters, at least some of whom see some mentally ill people as a nuisance. Why can't people just fit in? why can't they just take their medication? why can't they just do, exactly, as the care programme approach says they should? Why can't they just accept the tough hand that life has dealt them? Working with people in great mental distress brings us into close contact with our own vulnerabilities if not also our own spiritual wounds. The theologian Martin Buber provided us with an elegant means of appreciating the cycle of dehumanization in care when he distinguished the I–Thou and the I–It relationships.[50] The I–Thou relationship is marked by compassion, love and recognition of the sanctity of life. When we are sufficiently open to encounter the 'thou', we embrace, revere and honour the sanctity of the person's humanity. We encounter the 'Thou' each time we see a reflection of our own most valued – most vulnerable – family member or friend, in the eyes of the person who is the patient or client.

For many of us such true compassion is difficult and, instead, we settle for I–It relationships, where we objectify the person. Of course, when we treat others as objects – requiring 'observation', for example, rather than human engagement – we strip ourselves of our own humanity, as well. When we enter into the compassionate caring of the I–Thou relationship, we deepen our own humanity. Compassionate care (*com* = with, *passio* = to suffer) requires as, literally, to *suffer with* someone.

Emotional rescue

Within the Tidal Model I have talked about the need to get into the water with people. A lifesaver cannot rescue without getting wet. Similarly, we cannot do the necessary business of compassionate caring, without encountering at least something of what it is like to be in at the deep end. Frieda Fromm Reichman, who developed a psychoanalytic framework for working with people in psychosis, famously sat on the floor with a man who was playing with his own shit and began to handle it herself.[51] The bravery of such an encounter – which illustrated the starting point for a true *engagement* with the person in the sacred space of his distress – is largely denied us now. Most of us cannot even contemplate the possibilities of such a close encounter. Instead we try to develop ways of manipulating people from a distance: hence the re-emergence of the panopticon of observation. Few would stand, idly by, watching someone in great physical distress, but this is often what passes for 'care' in acute psychiatric settings. Increasingly, all our efforts at psychiatric rescue are like deep-sea fishing from the relative comfort of the shore.

When I entered the psychiatric field Neil Armstrong had just taken his famous one small step for man on the moon that was heralded as a huge leap for humankind.

Thirty years later the ambitions of the psychiatric system – at least at the political level – is to ensure that our services are 'safe, secure and supportive'.[52] Strategy is important but is worthless, if we do not have the level of commitment and capacity at the care face to ensure that people in deep human, if not spiritual crisis, are engaged in a manner that befitting the nature of their plight.

Fitness to practice

A sports team can have the best coach, equipped with the best strategy that can be mustered. However, if the team does not possess the highest level of fitness, supporting the highest level of commitment to winning, then they are beaten before the game begins. Sport provides a crude, but useful analogy for what is expected of people who are asked to nurse people in great mental distress. In the USA some hospitals hire university students to take over the menial task of observing suicidal patients, asserting that such surveillance is not appropriate for professional nurses. In the UK some Trusts have even employed security firms to do a similar surveillance work on acute wards. These post-psychiatric developments are either a clarion call to re-engage with caring for people in great distress, or a signal that nursing, and those who manage them, have abandoned care in favour of physical containment. Arguably, anyone with even a modicum of medical preparation could monitor and advise the psychiatric team of the 'presentation' of the patient – which is often all some psychiatrists ask for in a 'good nurse'. However, the only people who can provide the necessary conditions for the promotion of human growth and development – acknowledging the root definition of nursing – to *nourish* – will be those with a heart big enough for the task.

It is over one hundred years since Freud founded psychoanalysis, which, at least for a time, promised to solve the riddle of madness. When someone asked him why he always sat behind the patient during the analysis, Freud answered honestly that he wasn't the kind of person who could sit looking people full in the face for 8 hours a day. What Freud needed, and what his clientele needed were, clearly, two quite different things. Things haven't changed much. Today, we still find it difficult to confront madness. For many professionals, and many patients, their family members and friends, gain reassurance if not succour, from the idea that some abstract 'other' is responsible (at least temporarily) for directing the human tragedy of their lives. It seems to escape us that our 'scientific' conceptualizations of schizophrenia, bipolar disorder or borderline personality, differ little – at least in their function – from the abstract, highly malicious demons, which once were thought to have taken charge of our psyches. We still find it difficult to look at people simply, yet profoundly, as people at the centre of a metaphorical maelstrom, which threatens to engulf, and ultimately, drown them. We find it hard to face the kid who had dreams of being an astronaut or maybe just a father or lover, but who ended up as just another 'service user' with a 'serious and enduring mental illness'. We find it hard to face the dreamer who won't take his medication, won't fit in to this grossly misshapen society, and who has ended up as either a nuisance to his family or to the politicians who ultimately direct the mental health care traffic[g].

THE BASE LANGUAGE OF CARING

I can understand why nurses might find it difficult to engage patients as *people*. We haven't spend all this time trying to figure out what to call the people in our care – patients, clients, users or consumers – when the simple fact that we could just call them *people* was staring us in the face. Maybe – like Freud – all this language is a clever way of avoiding eye contact. Certainly, it reflects the political nature of our relations with those whom we are charged to care for. By redefining their basic humanity as some other – most often now in the language of capitalist consumerism – we avoid confronting the fact that, their pain is as much ours, as it is theirs.

These language games remind us how far we have travelled away from the root language of Greek, where the notion of *pity* for others reflected a common understanding that the 'other' was in a very real sense part of us, by dint of its otherness. The Greeks had no need for self-pity, for it was understood that others would fulfil this function on behalf of the pitiable person. In another, and more specific sense, the emotion of pity could not be self-administered since, one could no more feel pity for oneself than one could envy oneself: all such emotions served social functions.

Pity may no longer be part of the therapeutic canon, but this might simply illustrate how far we have descended, rather than progressed, since Hellenic times. William Blake's famous image of Pity illustrates Macbeth's soliloquy on the contemplation of Duncan's murder. Blake unites Shakespeare's two images of pity – the babe 'striding the blast' and heaven's cherubim on horseback. His image shows an angel, flying across the night sky, on a brilliant white charger, dropping the tiny, naked child into the sleeping figure of the mother below.

> And pity, like a naked new-born babe
> Striding the blast, or heaven's cherubim horsed
> Upon the sightless couriers of the air,

> Shall blow the horrid deed in every eye
> That tears shall drown the wind.

Blake clearly draws a connection between the *sacred*, which is weighed out carefully, and the profane, characterized perhaps by everything that is terrestrially bound.

In most mental health services – hospital or community – nurses greatly outnumber other disciplines. Nurses may have little overt power but, as the psychiatrist Len Stein long ago acknowledged, they have great covert power, which they can – and often do – use to influence the care (and indeed treatment) that people in distress receive. The general public may believe that the psychiatrist is the all-knowing, psychiatric professional but, in many settings, psychiatrists are rendered impotent by the subtle machinations of nurses' underground power base. Whoever replaces nurses as the 'foot soldiers' of mental health care, will likely possess the same power albeit with the same perceived lack of authority.[53]

The real challenge to developing a genuinely engaging relationship with people in mental distress, involves not so much the putative 'illness' from which they 'suffer', but the person on whose shoulders we erect these absurd concepts. The next person to whom we pay a 'domiciliary visit', or whom we interview in a 'consulting room', or whom we wrestle to the floor, in a 'de-escalation manoeuvre', is someone's mother, or someone's son. This is a *person* who may well have once dreamed of being somebody, rather than just another mental health statistic. When (s)he welcomes us in, or bars the door – literally or metaphorically – we shall begin to know what the politics of engagement is really all about.

This is the challenge that faces all those who would use the everyday discourse of human contact and conversation as the primary medium for the delivery of 'help'. For the present, such people are called nurses. However, in the post-psychiatric future, all manner of professionals, para-professionals or genuine *amateurs*, might replace professional nurses as the genuine 'nurses of the mind'. Whatever the name or the distinguishing features of the agent, the challenge will likely be the same: to establish how to use ordinary human-to-human interaction in an extraordinary way.

Even if nursing – as a distinct discipline – were to disappear in the years ahead, to be replaced by some ubiquitous 'mental health worker', people would still *need*, and likely ask for, 'nursing'. People would still need to be supported in the nurturing manner long associated with genuine nursing. Patients would still need to believed in, *as persons*, so that they might take the necessary steps that would prove sufficient for their own idea of recovery and reclamation, if not personal

---

[g] In his foreword to the National Service Framework for Mental health, published by the British government, the Health Minister, Frank Dobson, referred to some people with mental illness as 'a nuisance'.

redemption. Such a belief in the need for nursing is fundamental to the craft of caring. This is not so much something that can be proven or demonstrated but is taken as read: it is part of the faith system of all those who would seek to nurture the healing of the troubled mind, and its associated soul, through the virtue of caring.

REFERENCES

1. Clarke L. *Contemporary nursing: culture, education and practice*. Academic Publishing Services: Salisbury, 2001.

2. Sargant W. *The unquiet mind*. London: Heinemann, 1967.

3. Laing RD. *The divided self*. Harmondsworth: Penguin Books, 1961.

4. Burston D. *The crucible of experience: RD Laing and the crisis of psychotherapy*. Cambridge, MA: Harvard University Press, 2001.

5. http://www.jiscmail.ac.uk/lists/psychiatric-nursing.html

6. Brandon D. *The Tao of survival: spirituality in social care and counselling*. Birmingham: Venture Press, 2001.

7. Cited in Dineen T. *Manufacturing victims – what the psychology industry is doing to people*. Quebec: Robert Davies, 1996.

8. Brandon p. 3, *op. cit.*

9. Toffler A. *The third wave*. London: Pan Books, 1980.

10. Brandon p. 57, *op. cit.*

11. Barker P, Campbell P, Davidson B. *From the ashes of experience: reflections on madness, recovery and growth*. London: Whurr, 1999.

12. Clarke p. 97, *op. cit.*

13. Bannister D. The nonsense of effectiveness. *Changes* 1998; **16**(3): 218–20.

14. Barker P. *The philosophy and practice of psychiatric nursing*. Edinburgh: Churchill Livingstone, 1999.

15. Clarke, *op. cit.*

16. Barker P. Working with the metaphor of life and death. *Journal of Medical Ethics: Medical Humanities* 2000; **26**: 97–102.

17. Morall P. *Mental health nursing and social control*. London: Whurr, 1998.

18. Gournay K. Commentaries and reflections on mental health nursing in the UK at the dawn of the new millennium: Commentary 2. *Journal of Mental Health* 2000; **9**(6): 621–3.

19. If the reader cares to browse through the archives of the past five years of 'conversations' on the psychiatric nursing list, (s)he will find that nurse–patient interaction, and all that it entails, remains the major focus of interest of most practising nurses.

20. Szasz TS. *The myth of mental illness*. New York: Hoeber-Harper, 1961.

21. Szasz TS. Mental illness; psychiatry's phlogiston. *Journal of Medical Ethics* 2001; **27**(5): 297–301.

22. Jenner FA, Monteiro ACD, Zagalo-Cardosa JA, Cunha-Oliveira JA. *Schizophrenia: a disease or some ways of being human?* Sheffield: Sheffield Academic Press, 1993.

23. Coleman R. The politics of the illness. In: Barker P and Stevenson C (eds). The *construction of power and authority in psychiatry*. London: Butterworth Heinemann, 2000.

24. Evans FB. *Harry Stack Sullivan: interpersonal theory and psychotherapy*. London: Routledge, 1996.

25. Alvarez A. *The Savage God: a study of suicide*. New York: Random House, 1971: 282.

26. Alvarez, ibid.

27. Jenner *et al.*, *op. cit.*

28. Barker P, Keady J, Croom S, Stevenson C, Adams T, Reynolds W. The concept of serious mental illness: modern myths and grim realities. *Journal of Psychiatric and Mental Health Nursing* 1998; **5**(4): 247–54.

29. Szasz TS. *Insanity: The idea and its consequences*. New York: Wiley, 1987.

30. Barker, 2000, *op. cit.*

31. http://www.tidal-model.co.uk

32. Barker P. The Tidal Model: developing an empowering, person-centred approach to recovery within psychiatric and mental health nursing. *Journal of Psychiatric and Mental Health Nursing* 2001; **8**(3): 233–40.

33. Barker P. The Tidal Model: the lived experience in person-centred mental health care. *Nursing Philosophy* 2000; **2**(3): 213–23.

34. Barker P. The Tidal Model of mental health care: personal caring within the chaos paradigm. *Mental Health Care* 2000; **4**(2): 59–63.

35. Barker P. It's time to turn the tide. *Nursing Times* 1998; **94**(46): 70–2.

36. Barker P. The Tidal Model: a radical approach to person-centred care. *Perspectives in Psychiatric Care* 2001; **37**(2). 42–50.

37. Barker PJ. Chaos and the way of Zen: psychiatric nursing and the 'uncertainty principle'. *Journal of Psychiatric and Mental Health Nursing* 1996; **3**(4): 235–43.

38. Clay S. Madness and reality. In: Barker P, Campbell P, Davidson B (eds). *From the ashes of experience: reflections on madness, survival and growth*. London: Whurr, 1993.

39. Deegan PE. Recovering our sense of value after being labelled mentally ill. *Journal of Psycho-social Nursing and Mental Health Services* 1993; **4**: 7–11.

40. Clay, *op. cit.*

41. Szasz TS. *Cruel compassion: psychiatric control of society's unwanted*. New York: Wiley, 1994.

42. Pekkala E, Merinder L. *Psychoeducation for schizophrenia* (Cochrane Review). Oxford: The Cochrane Library, 1: 2002.

43. Perkins R, Repper J. Compliance or informed choice. *Journal of Mental Health* 1999; 8(2): 117–29.

44. Barker P. *Interview with Dr Patricia Deegan, 1999.* CD recording available from the author.

45. Coleman, *op. cit.*

46. Cahill J. Patient participation – a review of the literature. *Journal of Clinical Nursing* 1998; 7: 119–28.

47. Barker P, Whitehill I. The craft of care: towards collaborative caring in psychiatric nursing. In: Tilley S (ed.) *The mental health nurse: Views of practice and education.* Oxford: Blackwell Science, 1997.

48. Frankl V. *Man's search for meaning.* London: Hodder and Stoughton, 1964.

49. Frankl, ibid.

50. Buber M. *I and Thou.* T. Edinburgh: Clark, 1970.

51. Fromm Reichman F. *Principles of intensive psychotherapy.* Chicago: Chicago University Press, 1950.

52. Department of Health. *The National Service Framework for Mental Health.* London: DoH, 1999.

53. Barker P, Stevenson C. *The construction of power and authority in psychiatry.* Oxford: Butterworth Heinemann, 2000.

Index

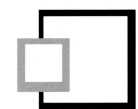